Minimal Access Cardiothoracic Surgery

Minimal Access Cardiothoracic Surgery

Anthony P. C. Yim, MD
Chief, Division of Cardiothoracic Surgery
The Chinese University of Hong Kong
Prince of Wales Hospital
Hong Kong, China

Stephen R. Hazelrigg, MD
Professor and Chairman
Division of Cardiothoracic Surgery
Southern Illinois University School of Medicine
Springfield, Illinois

Mohammad Bashar Izzat, MD
Consultant Cardiothoracic Surgeon
Damascus University Cardiovascular Surgical Center
Damascus University Hospitals
Damascus, Syria
Formerly:
Associate Professor of Surgery
Head, Section of Cardiac Surgery
The Chinese University of Hong Kong
Prince of Wales Hospital
Hong Kong, China

Rodney J. Landreneau, MD
Professor of Surgery and Human Oncology
Division Director, General Thoracic Surgery
Director, Allegheny Center of Lung and Thoracic Disease
Allegheny University of the Health Sciences
Pittsburgh, Pennsylvania

Michael J. Mack, MD
Assistant Professor of Thoracic Surgery
University of Texas Southwest Medical Center
Dallas, Texas

Keith S. Naunheim, MD
Professor and Acting Chief, Cardiothoracic Surgery
St. Louis University Medical School
Chief, Cardiothoracic Surgery
John Cochran Veterans Hospital
St. Louis, Missouri

With Foreword by:
Thomas B. Ferguson, MD
Professor Emeritus
Division of Cardiothoracic Surgery
Department of Surgery
Washington University School of Medicine
St. Louis, Missouri

W.B. Saunders Company
A Division of Harcourt Brace and Company
Philadelphia London Sydney Toronto

W.B. SAUNDERS COMPANY
A Harcourt Health Sciences Company

The Curtis Center
Independence Square West
Philadelphia, Pennsylvania 19106

Library of Congress Cataloging-in-Publication Data

Minimal access cardiothoracic surgery / editors, Anthony P.C. Yim . . . [et al.].

p. cm.

ISBN 0-7216-7723-1

1. Heart—Surgery. 2. Chest—Surgery. 3. Heart—Endoscopic surgery. 4. Chest—Endoscopic surgery. I. Yim, Anthony P.C.

[DNLM: 1. Thoracic Surgical Procedures—methods. 2. Surgical Procedures, Minimally Invasive—methods. WF 980 M6645 2000]

RD597.M55 2000 617.4′12—dc21

DNLM/DLC 99-36532

MINIMAL ACCESS CARDIOTHORACIC SURGERY ISBN 0-7216-7723-1

Printed in the United States of America

Last digit is the print number: 9 8 7 6 5 4 3 2 1

To Esther, for her love, understanding, and support.

APCY

To my loving and supportive wife, Shari, and our wonderful children, Andy, Lindsey, and Matthew.

SRH

To Hanna, Walid, and Mustafa.

MBI

To my parents, Rodney E. Landreneau, Jr., MD, and Colleen Fraser Landreneau, and to my four sons—Jerome, John, Joshua, and James.

RJL

To Barb, Annie, Andrew, Kate, Molly, and Ryan. Y'all make it all worthwhile.

MJM

To my wife, Rosanne, and to my children, Kate, Ted, Matt, and Molly. Their patience, understanding, and support foster my career and make me whole.

KSN

CONTRIBUTORS

Firass Abiad, MD
Chief Resident, Division of General Surgery, American University of Beirut, Beirut, Lebanon
Thoracoscopic Treatment of Hydatid Cysts of the Lung

Takashi Akaishi, MD, PhD
Associate Professor, Second Department of Surgery, Tohoku University School of Medicine, Sendai; Chief of Surgery, Akaishi Hospital, Shiogama, Japan
Thoracoscopic Esophagectomy With Extended Mediastinal Lymphadenectomy for Cancer

Zohair Al Halees, MD
Chief, Department of Cardiovascular Surgery, King Faisal Specialist Hospital, Riyadh, Saudi Arabia
Commentary 54B

Mark S. Allen, MD
Associate Professor of Surgery, Mayo Medical School; Consultant in General Thoracic Surgery, Mayo Clinic, Rochester, Minnesota
Interstitial Lung Diseases

Scott K. Alpard, MD
Surgical Research Fellow, Division of Cardiothoracic Surgery, University of Texas Medical Branch, Galveston, Texas
Resection for Pulmonary Metastases; Interventional Radiology in the Chest

Tomás Angelillo-Mackinlay, MD
Director, Postgraduate Program for Thoracic Surgery, University of Buenos Aires Medical School; Chief of Thoracic Surgery, British Hospital of Buenos Aires, Buenos Aires, Argentina
Empyema and Hemothorax

Gianni D. Angelini, MCh, FRCS
Professor of Cardiac Surgery, Bristol Heart Institute, University of Bristol, Bristol, United Kingdom
Echocardiography in Minimally Invasive Cardiac Surgery; Combined Minimally Invasive Coronary Artery Bypass and Angioplasty: An Integrated Approach; Myocardial Function and Metabolism During Beating Heart Coronary Revascularization; Commentary 77B

Kit V. Arom, MD, PhD
Staff Surgeon, Minneapolis Heart Institute, Minneapolis; St. Paul Heart & Lung Institute, St. Paul, Minnesota
Alternative Incisions for Cardiac Surgery; Mini-Sternotomy for Coronary Artery Bypass Surgery; Commentary 51A

Wassim Atassi, MD
Cardiovascular Research Fellow, The Chinese University of Hong Kong; Prince of Wales Hospital, Hong Kong, China
Graft Assessment in Off-Pump Coronary Artery Bypass Surgery

John R. Benfield, MD
Chief and Emeritus Professor of Thoracic Surgery, Department of Surgery, University of California–Davis, Davis, California
Commentary 6A; Commentary 20A

Theresa M. Boley, RN, MSN
Assistant Professor of Clinical Surgery, Division of Cardiothoracic Surgery, Southern Illinois University School of Medicine, Springfield, Illinois
Spontaneous Pneumothorax; Mediastinal Cysts

Piet W. Boonstra, MD
Thorax Center, University Hospital Gröningen, Gröningen, The Netherlands
Commentary 55A

Cornelius Borst, MD, PhD
Professor of Experimental Cardiology, Director, Experimental Cardiology Laboratory, Department of Cardiology, Heart Lung Institute, Utrecht University Hospital, Utrecht, The Netherlands
Facilitated Approaches to Vascular End-to-Side Anastomoses

Mark V. Braimbridge, MA, FRCS
Consultant Cardiothoracic Surgeon, St. Thomas' Medical School; Consultant Cardiothoracic Surgeon, St. Thomas' Hospital, London, United Kingdom
Thoracoscopy—A Historical Perspective

Johan J. Bredée, MD
Professor of Cardiothoracic Surgery, Utrecht University; Cardiothoracic Surgeon, Heart Lung Institute, Utrecht University Hospital, Utrecht, The Netherlands
Off-Pump Coronary Artery Bypass Grafting Using the "Octopus" Device

Alan J. Bryan, FRCS
Consultant Cardiac Surgeon, Bristol Royal Infirmary, Bristol, United Kingdom
Combined Minimally Invasive Coronary Artery Bypass and Angioplasty: An Integrated Approach; Commentary 64A; Commentary 66C; Commentary 71A

Raphael Bueno, MD
Instructor of Surgery, Harvard Medical School; Associate Surgeon, Thoracic Surgery, Brigham and Women's Hospital, Boston, Massachusetts
Posterior Mediastinal Masses

Enio Buffolo, MD
Professor of Cardiovascular Surgery, Head of Cardiac Surgery, Paulista School of Medicine, Federal University of São Paulo, São Paulo, SP Brazil
Off-Pump Coronary Artery Surgery; Commentary 63A

Thomas A. Burdon, MD
Clinical Assistant Professor, Department of Cardiothoracic Surgery, Standford University, Stanford, California
Port Access Coronary Artery Bypass Grafting; Port Access Heart Valve Surgery

Redmond P. Burke, MD
Chief, Division of Cardiovascular Surgery, Miami Children's Hospital, Miami, Florida
Commentary 74A

Robert J. Caccavale, MD
Associate Clinical Professor of Surgery, University of Medicine and Dentistry of New Jersey, Robert Wood Johnson Medical School, Piscataway; Chief of Thoracic Surgery, St. Peter's Medical Center, New Brunswick, New Jersey
Video-Assisted Thoracic Surgical Non–Rib-Spreading Simultaneously Stapled Lobectomy

Antonio M. Calafiore, MD
Professor, School of Specialization in Cardiac Surgery; Chief of the Department of Cardiac Surgery, University of Chieti, San Camillo de Lellis Hospital, Chieti, Italy
Minimally Invasive Direct Coronary Artery Bypass (MIDCAB); Combined Minimally Invasive Coronary Artery Bypass with Angioplasty: An Integrated Approach; Commentary 65A; Commentary 67A

Fabio Capasso, MD
Consultant in Cardiology, Casa di Cura San Michele, Caserta, Italy
Echocardiography in Minimally Invasive Cardiac Surgery; Myocardial Function and Metabolism During Beating Heart Coronary Revascularization

Henrik Casimir-Ahn, MD, PhD
Linköping Heart Center, University Hospital, Department of Cardiothoracic Surgery, Linköping, Sweden
Axial Blood Flow Pumps: An Alternative to Cardiopulmonary Bypass for Coronary Surgery

Filip P. Casselman, MD
Fellow, Department of Thoracic and Cardiovascular Surgery, The Cleveland Clinic Foundation, Cleveland, Ohio
Minimally Invasive Heart Valve Surgery: Operative Technique and Results

Angus C. W. Chan, FRCS(Edin)
Associate Professor, Department of Surgery, The Chinese University of Hong Kong, Prince of Wales Hospital, Hong Kong, China
Interventional Esophagoscopy

Chau-Hsiung Chang, MD
Professor, President, Chang Gung University, Taoyuan, Taiwan
Limited Incision Coronary Surgery With Cardiopulmonary Bypass Support; Minimally Invasive Surgery for Congenital Heart Defects

W. Randolph Chitwood, Jr., MD
Professor, East Carolina University School of Medicine; Chairman, Department of Surgery, Chief, Division of Cardiothoracic Surgery, Pitt County Memorial Hospital, Greenville, North Carolina
Video Assisted Minimally Invasive Mitral Valve Surgery; Commentary 73A; Commentary 79A

Jaw-Ji Chu, MD
Lecturer, Chang Gung University, Taoyuan; Attending Staff, Division of Thoracic and Cardiovascular Surgery, Chang Gung Memorial Hospital, Taipei, Taiwan
Limited Incision Coronary Surgery With Cardiopulmonary Bypass Support; Minimally Invasive Surgery for Congenital Heart Defects

S. C. Sydney Chung, MD, FRCS
Professor, Department of Surgery, The Chinese University of Hong Kong, Prince of Wales Hospital, Hong Kong, China
Interventional Esophagoscopy

C. Peter Clarke, MBBS, FRACS, FACS, FCCP
Professorial Associate, Senior Thoracic Surgeon, Department of Surgery, Austin and Repatriation Medical Centre, University of Melbourne, Melbourne, Australia
The Diaphragm

William E. Cohn, MD
Instructor in Surgery, Harvard Medical School; Cardiothoracic Surgeon, Beth Israel Deaconess Medical Center, Boston, Massachusetts
The H-Graft MIDCAB

Giorgio Furio Coloni, MD
Professor of Thoracic Surgery, Section Head, General Thoracic Surgery, University of Rome (La Sapienza), Rome, Italy
Diagnostic Thoracoscopy for Mediastinal Masses

Denton A. Cooley, MD
Clinical Professor of Surgery, University of Texas Medical School; President and Surgeon-in-Chief, Chief, Cardiovascular Surgery, Texas Heart Institute; Chief, Cardiovascular Surgery, St. Luke's Episcopal Hospital, Houston, Texas
Commentary 54A; Commentary 66B

Joel D. Cooper, MD
Evarts A. Graham Professor of Surgery, Washington University School of Medicine; Chief of Cardiothoracic Surgery, Barnes-Jewish Hospital, St. Louis, Missouri
Transcervical Approach to the Thymus

Delos M. Cosgrove, MD
Chairman; Department of Thoracic and Cardiovascular Surgery, The Cleveland Clinic Foundation, Cleveland, Ohio
Minimally Invasive Heart Valve Surgery: Operative Technique and Results

Stewart R. Craig, FRCS
Specialist Registrar in Cardiothoracic Surgery, Royal Infirmary of Edinburgh, Edinburgh, Scotland
The Immune Response to Surgery: Conventional and VATS Lobectomy

Alvin H. Crawford, MD
Professor of Pediatrics, University of Cincinnati; Director, Pediatric Orthopaedics, Children's Hospital Medical Center, Cincinnati, Ohio
Spinal Deformities; Thoracoscopic First Rib Resection for Thoracic Outlet Syndrome

Ralph J. Damiano, MD
Professor and Chief, Cardiothoracic Surgery, Co-director Cardiovascular Center, The Milton S. Hershey Medical Center, The Pennsylvania State University, Hershey, Pennsylvania
Commentary 83A

Tiziano DeGiacomo, MD
Assistant Professor of Thoracic Surgery, Department of Thoracic Surgery, University of Rome (La Sapienza), Rome, Italy
Diagnostic Thoracoscopy for Mediastinal Masses

Paul De Leyn, MD
Professor, University of Leuven, Consultant, Department of Thoracic Surgery, University Hospitals Leuven, Leuven, Belgium
Videomediastinoscopy

Jan A. Deprest, MD
Research Director, Centre for Surgical Technologies; Consultant, Obstetrics and Gynecology, University Hospital Gasthuisberg, Leuven, Belgium
Endoscopic Fetal Surgery

Patrick A. Dillon, MD
Assistant Professor of Surgery, St. Louis University School of Medicine; Attending Surgeon, Cardinal Glennon Children's Hospital, St. Louis, Missouri
Pediatric Minimal Access Cardiothoracic Surgery

Carolyn M. Dresler, MD
Director, Medical Affairs for Smoking Control, SmithKline Beecham Consumer Healthcare, Parsippany, New Jersey
Malignant Pleural Effusion

Robert W. Emery, MD
Director of Transplantation, Minneapolis Heart Institute, Minneapolis; St. Paul Heart and Lung Institute, St. Paul, Minnesota
Alternative Incisions for Cardiac Surgery; Ministernotomy for Coronary Artery Bypass Surgery; Commentary 62A

Volkmar Falk, MD
Heartcenter, University of Leipzig, Leipzig, Germany
Robotic Surgery

James I. Fann, MD
Clinical Assistant Professor, Department of Cardiothoracic Surgery, Stanford University, Stanford, California
Port Access Coronary Artery Bypass Grafting; Port Access Heart Valve Surgery

Mark K. Ferguson, MD
Professor of Surgery, Pritzker School of Medicine, The University of Chicago, Chicago, Illinois
Chylothorax

Thomas B. Ferguson, MD
Professor Emeritus, Division of Cardiothoracic Surgery, Department of Surgery, Washington University School of Medicine, St. Louis, Missouri
Foreword

Peter F. Ferson, MD
Professor of Surgery, University of Pittsburgh Medical Center; Chief of Thoracic Surgery, Veterans Administration Medical Center, Pittsburgh, Pennsylvania
Interventional Bronchoscopy

Luiz Tarcisio B. Filomeno, MD
Assistant Professor, Division of Thoracic Surgery, University of São Paulo Medical School, São Paulo, Brazil
Partial Sternotomy Approach to the Thymus

Manson Fok, FRCS
Honorary Associate Professor, Department of Surgery, The University of Hong Kong; Queen Mary Hospital, Hong Kong, China
Commentary 24A; Commentary 34C

Thierry A. Folliguet, MD, FACS
Cardiothoracic Surgeon, Institut Mutualiste Montsouris, Paris, France
Minimal Access Surgery for Patent Ductus Arteriosus; Commentary 77A

James D. Fonger, MD
Director of Cardiac Surgery, Washington Adventist Hospital, Takoma Park, Maryland
Reoperative Minimally Invasive Direct Coronary Artery Bypass (MIDCAB) Coronary Grafting

W. D. Andrew Ford, MD
Director, Department of Pediatric Surgery, Women's and Children's Hospital, North Adelaide, Australia
Commentary 45A

Erik Fosse, MD, PhD
Professor of Minimally Invasive and Image Guided Therapy, University of Oslo; Head of Department of Surgery, The Interventional Centre, Rikshospitalet, Oslo, Norway
Commentary 56C

Mohammad Fouda, MD
Head, Cardiac Surgery, College of Medicine, King Khalid University Hospital, Riyadh, Saudi Arabia
Commentary 66A

Inderjit S. Gill, MD
Department of Thoracic and Cardiovascular Surgery, Metrohealth Hospital, Cleveland Clinic Foundation, Cleveland, Ohio
Quality of Life Assessment in Minimally Invasive Coronary Surgery

A. Marc Gillinov, MD
Staff Surgeon, Department of Thoracic and Cardiovascular Surgery, The Cleveland Clinic Foundation, Cleveland, Ohio
Minimally Invasive Heart Valve Surgery: Operative Technique and Results

Brian W. Goodacre, MD
Associate Professor of Radiology, Director, Residency Program, University of Texas Medical Branch, Galveston, Texas
Interventional Radiology in the Chest

Dominique Gossot, MD
Department of Surgery, Saint-Louis Hospital, Paris, France
Commentary 30A; Commentary 34B

Geoffrey M. Graeber, MD
Professor of Surgery, Director of Surgical Research, West Virginia University School of Medicine; Staff Cardiothoracic Surgeon, Ruby Memorial Hospital; Staff Cardiothoracic Surgeon, Monongalia General Hospital, Morgantown, West Virginia
Chest Trauma

Edward Gratacos, MD, PhD
Research Fellow, Centre for Surgical Technologies, Leuven, Belgium
Endoscopic Fetal Surgery

Paul F. Gründeman, MD, PhD
Assistant Professor of Experimental Cardiac Surgery, Experimental Cardiology Laboratory, Department of Cardiology, Heart Lung Institute, Utrecht University Hospital, Utrecht, The Netherlands
Facilitated Approaches to Vascular End-to-Side Anastomoses

Y. John Gu, MD
Blood Interaction Research, Department of Cardiothoracic Surgery, University of Gröningen, The Netherlands
Commentary 61B

Beverly Hahn, RN, BES
Special Project Assistant, Cardiovascular and Thoracic Surgeons, Inc., Cincinnati, Ohio
Thoracoscopic First Rib Resection for Thoracic Outlet Syndrome

Stephen R. Hazelrigg, MD
Professor and Chairman, Division of Cardiothoracic Surgery, Southern Illinois University School of Medicine; Memorial Medical Center; St. John's Hospital, Springfield, Illinois
Spontaneous Pneumothorax; Mediastinal Cysts; Commentary 2A; Commentary 7A; Commentary 13A; Commentary 21A; Commentary 29A; Commentary 38A; Commentary 39A; Commentary 41A; Commentary 48A; Commentary 78A

Robin H. Heijmen, MD, PhD
Resident in Cardiothoracic Surgery, Utrecht University Hospital, Utrecht, The Netherlands
Facilitated Approaches to Vascular End-to-Side Anastomoses

Norio Higuchi, MD
Staff Surgeon, Ishinomaki Red Cross Hospital, Ishinomaki, Japan
Thoracoscopic Esophagectomy with Extended Mediastinal Lymphadenectomy for Cancer

Santiago Horgan, MD
Assistant Professor, Attending Surgeon, Director, Minimally Invasive Surgery, College of Medicine, University of Illinois, Chicago
Achalasia

John S. Ikonomidis, MD, PhD
Resident, Cardiothoracic Surgery, Stanford University Medical Center, Stanford, California
Port Access Coronary Artery Bypass Grafting; Port Access Heart Valve Surgery

Mohammad Bashar Izzat, MCh, FRCS(CTh)
Consultant Cardiothoracic Surgeon, Damascus University Cardiovascular Surgical Center, Damascus University Hospitals, Damascus, Syria; formerly Associate Professor of Surgery, Head, Section of Cardiac Surgery, Prince of Wales Hospital, The Chinese University of Hong Kong, Hong Kong, China
Pleuropulmonary Tuberculosis; VATS Approach to the Thymus; Echocardiography in Minimally Invasive Cardiac Surgery; Role of Cytokines in Coronary Artery Bypass Grafting With or Without Cardiopulmonary Bypass; Graft Assessment in Off-Pump Coronary Artery Bypass Surgery; Commentary 56B

Salik Jahania, MD
Research Fellow, Division of Cardiovascular Surgery, University of Kentucky College of Medicine; A. B. Chandler Medical Center, Lexington, Kentucky
Pharmacologic and Mechanical Stabilization During Minimally Invasive Coronary Artery Surgery

Erik W. L. Jansen, MD
Cardiothoracic Surgeon, Heart Lung Institute, Utrecht University Hospital, Utrecht, Netherlands
Off-Pump Coronary Artery Bypass Grafting Using the "Octopus" Device

Alfred Jaretzki III, MD
Associate Clinical Professor of Surgery, College of Physicians and Surgeons, Columbia University; Attending Surgeon, Presbyterian Hospital, New York, New York
Commentary 28A (Dr. Jaretzki's commentary applies to Chapters 26, 27, and 28.)

Fabio Biscegli Jatene, MD, PhD
Associate Professor, Director of Thoracic Surgery, University of São Paulo Medical School, São Paulo, Brazil
Partial Sternotomy Approach to the Thymus

David W. Johnstone, MD
Assistant Professor of Surgery, University of Rochester, Rochester, New York
Malignant Pleural Effusion

Shaun B. Jones, MD
Assistant Professor of Surgery, Uniformed Services University of Health Sciences (USUHS), Bethesda, Maryland
Future Technologies for Surgical Applications

Sami Kabbani, MD
Director, Cardiovascular Surgical Center, Professor of Surgery, Damascus University, Damascus, Syria
Commentary 59A

Iwao Kaneda, MD, PhD
Vice President and Chief of Surgery, Ishinomaki Red Cross Hospital, Ishinomaki, Japan
Thoracoscopic Esophagectomy With Extended Mediastinal Lymphadenectomy for Cancer

Robert J. Keenan, MD
Associate Professor of Surgery, Vice Chief, Cardiothoracic Surgery, Director, Cardiopulmonary Transplantation, Principal Investigator for National Emphysema Treatment Trial, University of Pittsburgh Medical Center, Pittsburgh, Pennsylvania
Interventional Bronchoscopy

Cesar A. Keller, MD
Division of Pulmonology and Occupational Pulmonary Medicine, Department of Internal Medicine, St. Louis University Health Sciences Center, St. Louis, Missouri
Thoracoscopic Lung Volume Reduction for End-Stage Emphysema

Simon R. Knight, FRACS
Lecturer in Surgery, Thoracic Surgeon, Department of Surgery, Austin and Repatriation Medical Centre, University of Melbourne, Melbourne, Australia
The Diaphragm

Tadasu Kohno, MD
Chief, Department of Thoracic Surgery, Toranomon Hospital, Tokyo, Japan
Thoracoscopic Thoracic Sympathectomy

Evan R. Kokoska, MD
Surgery Resident, St. Louis University Health Sciences Center, St. Louis, Missouri
Pediatric Minimal Access Cardiothoracic Surgery

Evgenii V. Kolesov, MD
Professor of Cardiac Surgery, The State University, Dnepropetrovsk, Ukraine
Pioneering Minimally Invasive Coronary Surgery: A Historical Perspective

Mark J. Krasna, MD
Associate Professor of Surgery, Head, Division of Thoracic Surgery, University of Maryland Medical School, Baltimore, Maryland
Thoracoscopic Staging for Intrathoracic Malignancy

Catherine P. Krucylak, MD
Assistant Professor, Department of Anesthesiology, Washington University School of Medicine; Staff Anesthesiologist, St. Louis Children's Hospital, St. Louis, Missouri
Anesthetic Considerations for Pediatric Thoracoscopic Procedures

Peter E. Krucylak, MD
Assistant Professor, Department of Anesthesiology, Washington University School of Medicine; Barnes-Jewish Hospital, Saint Louis, Missouri
Anesthetic Considerations for Minimally Invasive Cardiac Surgery

François Laborde, MD
Chief, Department of Surgery, Institut Mutualiste Montsouris, Paris, France
Minimal Access Surgery for Patent Ductus Arteriosus

Jaap R. Lahpor, MD
Cardiothoracic Surgeon, Heart Lung Institute, Utrecht University Hospital, Utrecht, The Netherlands
Off-Pump Coronary Artery Bypass Grafting Using the "Octopus" Device

Buu-Khanh Lam, MD
Senior Cardiac Surgery Resident, University of Ottawa Heart Institute, University of Ottawa, Ottawa, Ontario, Canada
Quality of Life Assessment in Minimally Invasive Coronary Surgery

Rodney J. Landreneau, MD
Professor of Surgery and Human Oncology, Division Director, General Thoracic Surgery; Director, Allegheny Center of Lung and Thoracic Disease, Allegheny University of the Health Sciences, Pittsburgh, Pennsylvania
Strategic Planning for Video-Assisted Thoracic Surgery; Interventional Bronchoscopy

H. Ann Leaver, PhD
Senior Scientist, Department of Pharmacology, University of Edinburgh, Edinburgh, Scotland
The Immune Response to Surgery: Conventional and VATS Lobectomy

Toni Lerut, MD, PhD
Professor of Surgery, Director, Centre for Surgical Technologies; Professor and Head, Department of Thoracic Surgery, Catholic University Hospital Gasthuisberg, Leuven, Belgium
Videomediastinoscopy; Endoscopic Fetal Surgery; Commentary 28C; Commentary 34A

Ralph J. Lewis, MD
Clinical Professor of Surgery, University of Medicine & Dentistry of New Jersey; Chief of Thoracic Surgery, University of Thoracic Surgery, Surgical Service, Robert Wood Johnson University Hospital; St. Peter's University Hospital, New Brunswick, New Jersey
Video-Assisted Thoracic Surgical Non–Rib-Spreading Simultaneously Stapled Lobectomy; Commentary 18A

Leonardo Esteves Lima, MD
Associate Surgeon, La Pite Hospital, Paris, France
Minimally Invasive Vein Harvesting for Coronary Artery Bypass

Jeffrey C. Lin, MD
Chief Resident, Thoracic Surgery, Allegheny General Hospital, Pittsburgh, Pennsylvania
Strategic Planning for Video-Assisted Thoracic Surgery

Pyng Jing Lin, MD
Professor, Chang Gung University, Taoyuan; Chief, Division of Thoracic and Cardiovascular Surgery, Chang Gung Memorial Hospital, Taipei, Taiwan
Limited Incision Coronary Surgery with Cardiopulmonary Bypass Support; Minimally Invasive Surgery for Congenital Heart Defects

Alex G. Little, MD
Professor and Chairman, Department of Surgery, University of Nevada School of Medicine; Chief of Surgery, University Medical Center, Las Vegas, Nevada
Esophageal Leiomyoma, Diverticulum, and Duplication Cyst

Hui-Ping Liu, MD
Lecturer, Chang Gung University; Associate Professor, Head, Section of Thoracic Surgery, Division of Thoracic and Cardiovascular Surgery, Chang Gung Memorial Hospital, Taipei, Taiwan
Cost-Containing Strategies; Minimally Invasive Surgery for Pericardial Diseases

Clinton T. Lloyd, FRCS
Registrar in Cardiac Surgery; Bristol Mears Institute, Bristol, United Kingdom
Combined Minimally Invasive Artery Bypass and Angioplasty—An Integrated Approach; Commentary 77B

Joseph LoCicero, III, MD
Associate Professor, Harvard University; Chief General Thoracic Surgery, Cardiothoracic Surgery, Beth Israel Deaconess Medical Center, Boston, Massachusetts
Diagnostic Thoracoscopy for Pleural Disease

Urban Lönn, MD, PhD
Linköping Heart Center, University Hospital, Department of Cardiothoracic Surgery, Linköping, Sweden
Axial Blood Flow Pumps: An Alternative to Cardiopulmonary Bypass for Coronary Surgery

John M. Low, FRCA
Associate Professor, Chinese University of Hong Kong; Honorary Consultant, Department of Anesthesia and Intensive Care, Prince of Wales Hospital; Honorary Consultant, Tai Po Nethersole Hospital, Hong Kong, China
Anesthesia for Video-Assisted Thoracoscopic Surgery (VATS)

Vincenzo Lucchetti, MD
Director of Cardiac Surgery, Consultant Cardiac Surgeon, Casa di Cura San Michele, Caserta, Italy
Echocardiography in Minimally Invasive Cardiac Surgery; Myocardial Function and Metabolism During Beating Heart Coronary Revascularization

Jeanne M. Lukanich, MD
Instructor in Surgery, Harvard Medical School; Staff Surgeon, Division of Thoracic Surgery, Brigham and Women's Hospital; Dana Farber Cancer Institute, Boston; Faulkner Hospital, Jamaica Plain, Massachusetts
Posterior Mediastinal Masses

James D. Luketich, MD
Assistant Professor of Surgery, Section Head Thoracic Surgery, Co-Director of Minimally Invasive Surgery, Co-Director, Lung Cancer Center, University of Pittsburgh Medical Center, Pittsburgh, Pennsylvania
Minimal Access Approach to Esophagectomy; Interventional Bronchoscopy

Marco Maciocco, MD
Assistant Professor, Department of General Surgery; San Giuseppe Hospital, Department of Surgery, University of Milan, Milan, Italy
Anatomic Lung Resection

Michael J. Mack, MD
Assistant Professor of Surgery, University of Texas Southwest Medical Center, Dallas, Texas
Localization of Pulmonary Nodules; Future of Minimally Invasive Cardiac Surgery; Commentary 1A; Commentary 28B

Mitchell J. Magee, MD
Cardiothoracic Surgeon, Cardiothoracic Surgeon's Association of North Texas; Dallas City Hospital; Presbyterian Hospital, Dallas; Plano Hospital, Plano, Texas
Spontaneous Pneumothorax; Mediastinal Cysts

Robert J. March, MD
Assistant Professor of Surgery, Department of Cardiovascular and Thoracic Surgery, Rush Medical College; Director, Cardiovascular Research, Department of Cardiovascular and Thoracic Surgery, Rush–Presbyterian–St. Luke's Medical Center, Chicago, Illinois
Laser Revascularization of Ischemic Myocardium

Paulo E. Marchiori, MD
Assistant Professor, Division of Neurology, University of São Paulo Medical School, São Paulo, Brazil
Partial Sternotomy Approach to the Thymus

William R. Mayfield, MD
Cardiovascular Surgeon, Piedmont Hospital; Saint Joseph's Hospital, Atlanta, Georgia
Commentary 56A; Commentary 68A

Robert J. McKenna, Jr., MD
Director, Lung Center, Cedars-Sinai Medical Center, Los Angeles, California
Commentary 17A

Martin F. McKneally, MD, PhD
Professor of Surgery, Department of Surgery and Joint Centre for Bioethics, University of Toronto; Professor of Surgery, The Toronto Hospital, Toronto, Canada
Ethical Aspects of Introducing New Surgical Technology

Dan M. Meyer, MD
The Sarah M. and Charles E. Seay Distinguished Chair in Thoracic Surgery, Director, Mechanical Assist Program, Associate Director, Pulmonary Transplantation, University of Texas Southwestern Medical Center; Director, Mechanical Assist Program, Baylor University, Dallas, Texas
Preoperative Assessment for Video-Assisted Thoracic Surgery (VATS); Preoperative Assessment for Minimally Invasive Cardiac Surgery

José Ribas Milanez de Campos, MD
Assistant Professor, Division of Thoracic Surgery, University of São Paulo Medical School, São Paulo, Brazil
Partial Sternotomy Approach to the Thymus

Chris Monk, FRCA
Consultant Anesthetist, Bristol Royal Infirmary, Bristol, United Kingdom
Combined Minimally Invasive Coronary Artery Bypass and Angioplasty—An Integrated Approach

Kenric M. Murayama, MD
Director, Minimally Invasive Surgery, Saint Louis University Health Sciences Center, Department of Surgery, Saint Louis, Missouri
Laparoscopic Antireflux Surgery

Tsuguo Naruke, MD, PhD
Professor of Surgery, Keio University School of Medicine; Deputy Director, Chairman, Department of Surgery, Chief, Division of Thoracic Surgery, National Cancer Center Hospital, Tokyo, Japan
Thoracoscopic Lobectomy With Mediastinal Lymph Node Dissection or Sampling

Keith S. Naunheim, MD
Professor and Acting Chief, Cardiothoracic Surgery, St. Louis University Medical School; Chief, Cardiothoracic Surgery, John Cochran Veterans Hospital, St. Louis, Missouri
Thoracoscopic Lung Volume Reduction for End-Stage Emphysema; Laparoscopic Antireflux Surgery; Commentary 9A; Commentary 32A; Commentary 33A

Ninh T. Nguyen, MD
Assistant Professor, University of California-Davis; Director, Center for Minimally Invasive Surgery, University of California-Davis Medical Center, Sacramento, California
Minimal Access Approach to Esophagectomy

Arno P. Nierich, MD
Cardiac Anesthesiologist and Intensivist; Institute of Anesthesiology; Utrecht University Hospital, Utrecht, The Netherlands
Off-Pump Coronary Artery Bypass Grafting Using the "Octopus" Device

Jemi Olak, MD
Attending Surgeon, Lutheran General Hospital, Park Ridge, Illinois
Wedge Resection

Kelly C. O'Neal, MD
Staff General Surgeon, Kaiser Oakland Hospital, Oakland, California
Commentary 40A

Mehmet C. Oz, MD
Associate Professor in Cardiac Surgery, Columbia University School of Medicine; Department of Surgery, Columbia Presbyterian Medical Center, New York, New York
Commentary 67B

Leonardo Paloscia, MD
Cardiologist, Ospedale San Carillo de Lellis, Chieti, Italy
Combined Minimally Invasive Coronary Artery Bypass and Angioplasty: An Integrated Approach

Ugo Pastorino, MD
Director, Division of Thoracic Surgery, European Institute of Oncology, Milan, Italy
Commentary 21B

F. Griffith Pearson, MD
Professor Emeritus, University of Toronto, Toronto, Ontario, Canada
Commentary 20B

Carlos A. Pellegrini, MD
Professor and Chairman, Department of Surgery, University of Washington School of Medicine; Attending Surgeon, University of Washington Medical Center, Seattle, Washington
Achalasia

William S. Peters, MD
Department of Cardiothoracic Surgery, Alfred Hospital, Prahran, Australia
Commentary 73B

George D. Picetti III, MD
Director, Orthopedic Spine Clinic, Sacramento Region, Kaiser-Permanente, Roseville, California
Commentary 40A

Mario F. Pompili, MD
Clinical Assistant Professor, Department of Cardiothoracic Surgery, Stanford University, Stanford, California
Port Access Coronary Artery Bypass Grafting; Port Access Heart Valve Surgery

Ganga Prabhakar, MD, FRCS
Fellow, Cardiothoracic Surgery, Department of Surgery, West Virginia University Hospital, Morgantown, West Virginia
Chest Trauma

W. Gerald Rainer, MD, MS
Distinguished Clinical Professor of Surgery, University of Colorado Health Sciences Center, Denver, Colorado
Commentary 49A; Commentary 69A

Erino Angelo Rendina, MD
Assistant Professor of Thoracic Surgery, University of Rome (La Sapienza), Department of Thoracic Surgery, Rome, Italy
Diagnostic Thoracoscopy for Mediastinal Masses

M. Clive Robinson, MD
Associate Professor, Division of Cardiothoracic Surgery, University of Kentucky College of Medicine, A. B. Chandler Medical Center, Lexington, Kentucky
Pharmacologic and Mechanical Stabilization During Minimally Invasive Coronary Artery Surgery

Giancarlo Roviaro, MD
Professor of General Surgery, Department of General Surgery, University of Milan; Head, Department of General Surgery, San Giuseppe Hospital, Milan, Italy
Anatomic Lung Resection

Valerie W. Rusch, MD
Professor of Surgery, Cornell University Medical College; Attending Surgeon and Alfred P. Sloan Chair, Division of Thoracic Surgery, Department of Surgery, Memorial Sloan-Kettering Cancer Center, New York, New York
Commentary 8A

John E. Sanderson, MD, FRCP
Professor, Department of Medicine and Therapeutics, The Chinese University of Hong Kong; Honorary Consultant Cardiologist, Head, Division of Cardiology, Prince of Wales Hospital, Hong Kong, China
Commentary 68A; Commentary 76A

Richard M. Satava, MD
Professor of Surgery, Yale University School of Medicine, New Haven, Connecticut
Future Technologies for Surgical Applications

Basem R. Shabb, MD
Associate Professor, Division of Cardiothoracic Surgery, American University of Beirut, Beirut, Lebanon
Thoracoscopic Treatment of Hydatid Cysts of the Lung

Hani Shennib, MD
Associate Professor of Surgery, Division of Cardiothoracic Surgery, McGill University, Montreal, Canada, Quebec
Instrumentation for Minimally Invasive Cardiac Surgery

Mark L. Silen, MD
Associate Professor of Surgery and Pediatrics, St. Louis University Health Sciences Center, St. Louis, Missouri
Pediatric Minimal Access Cardiothoracic Surgery

Eugene K. W. Sim, MD
Associate Professor of Surgery, Head, Cardiothoracic Surgery, National University of Singapore, Singapore
Commentary 50A

Joshua R. Sonett, MD
Assistant Professor, Division of Thoracic Surgery, Director of Lung Transplantation, University of Maryland Medical School, Baltimore, Maryland
Thoracoscopic Staging for Intrathoracic Malignancy

Pieter R. Stella, MD
Interventional Cardiologist, Heart Lung Institute, Utrecht University Hospital, Utrecht, The Netherlands
Off-Pump Coronary Artery Bypass Crafting Using the "Octopus" Device

Valavanur A. Subramanian, MD
Director, Department of Surgery, Lenox Hill Hospital, New York, New York
Patient Selection for Minimally Invasive Coronary Artery Bypass

Hon Chi Suen, FRCS
Chief Resident, Division of Cardiothoracic Surgery, Washington University School of Medicine; Chief Resident in Cardiothoracic Surgery, Barnes-Jewish Hospital, St. Louis, Missouri
Transcervical Approach to the Thymus

David J. Sugarbaker, MD
Associate Professor of Surgery, Harvard Medical School; Vice Chair, Department of Surgery, Chief, Division of Thoracic Surgery, Brigham and Women's Hospital; Philip L. Lowe Senior Surgeon, Chief, Department of Surgical Services, Dana Farber Cancer Institute, Boston, Massachusetts
Posterior Mediastinal Masses

Mohammed-Saadeh Suleiman, PhD
Senior Lecturer in Physiology, Bristol Heart Institute, University of Bristol, Bristol, United Kingdom
Myocardial Function and Metabolism During Beating Heart Coronary Revascularization

James F. Symes, MD, MSC, FRCS(C), FACS
Professor of Surgery, Tufts University School of Medicine; Chief, Cardiothoracic Surgery, St. Elizabeth's Medical Center, Boston, Massachusetts
Therapeutic Angiogenesis

Shinichi Takamoto, MD
Professor and Chairman, Department of Cardiothoracic Surgery, Graduate School of Medicine, University of Tokyo, Tokyo, Japan
Thoracoscopic Thoracic Sympathectomy

Hock Lim Tan, MD
Staff Surgeon, Department of Paediatric Surgery, Gleneagles Hospital, Singapore
Commentary 37A

Malcolm J. Underwood, MD, FRCS(CTh)
Senior Registrar, Bristol Heart Institute, Bristol Royal Infirmary, Bristol, United Kingdom
Myocardial Function and Metabolism During Beating Heart Coronary Revascularization

Egidius van Aarnhem, MD
Resident, Heart Lung Institute, Utrecht University Hospital, Utrecht, The Netherlands
Off-Pump Coronary Artery Bypass Grafting Using the "Octopus" Device

Willem van Oeveren, MD
Blood Interaction Research, Department of Cardiothoracic Surgery, University of Gröningen, Gröningen, The Netherlands
Commentary 61B

Eric vanSonnenberg, MD
Professor of Radiology and Medicine, University of Texas Medical Branch, Galveston, Texas
Interventional Radiology in the Chest

Federico Varoli, MD
Associate Professor, Department of General Surgery, University of Milan, Milan, Italy
Anatomic Lung Resection

Federico Venuta, MD
Assistant Professor of Thoracic Surgery, University of Rome (La Sapienza), Department of Thoracic Surgery, Rome, Italy
Diagnostic Thoracoscopy for Mediastinal Masses

Contardo Vergani, MD
Assistant Professor, Department of General Surgery; S. Giuseppe Hospital, Department of Surgery, University of Milan, Milan, Italy
Anatomic Lung Resection

Giuseppe Vitolla, MD
Resident in Cardiac Surgery, University of Chieti, Chieti, Italy
Minimally Invasive Direct Coronary Artery Bypass

William S. Walker, FRCS
Consultant Cardiothoracic Surgeon, Clinical Director, Cardiothoracic Surgery, Royal Infirmary of Edinburgh, Edinburgh, Scotland
The Immune Response to Surgery: Conventional and VATS Lobectomy; Complications and Pitfalls in Video-Assisted Thoracic Surgery

Song Wan, MD, PhD
Division of Cardiothoracic Surgery, Department of Surgery, Prince of Wales Hospital, The Chinese University of Hong Kong, Hong Kong, China
Role of Cytokines in Coronary Artery Bypass Grafting With or Without Cardiopulmonary Bypass

Andrew S. Wechsler, MD
Professor and Chairman, Department of Cardiothoracic Surgery, Medical College of Physicians—Hahnemann University Hospital, Philadelphia, Pennsylvania
Commentary 60A; Commentary 61A

Tracey L. Weigel, MD
Assistant Professor of Surgery, University of Pittsburgh Medical Center, Pittsburgh, Pennsylvania
Interventional Bronchoscopy

Peter Wilde, FRCR
Consultant Radiologist, Bristol Royal Infirmary, Bristol, United Kingdom
Combined Minimally Invasive Coronary Artery Bypass with Angioplasty—An Integrated Approach; Commentary 53A

Randall K. Wolf, MD
Associate Professor of Surgery, Director of Minimally Invasive Cardiac Surgery and Robotics, The Ohio State University Medical Center, Columbus, Ohio
Room Setup and Instrumentation; Spinal Deformities; Thoracoscopic First Rib Resection for Thoracic Outlet Syndrome; Quality Assessment in Off-Pump Coronary Artery Bypass Surgery

Jun Wu, MD, PhD
Research Fellow, Centre for Surgical Technologies, Leuven, Belgium
Endoscopic Fetal Surgery

Hirotoshi Yamamoto, MD, PhD
Research Fellow, Centre for Surgical Technologies, Leuven, Belgium
Endoscopic Fetal Surgery

Peng Lee Yap, PhD, FRCPath
Consultant Immunologist, Southeast Scotland Blood Transfusion Service, Edinburgh, Scotland
The Immune Response to Surgery: Conventional and VATS Lobectomy

Anthony P. C. Yim, MD, FRCS
Chief, Division of Cardiothoracic Surgery, The Chinese University of Hong Kong, Honorary Consultant Cardiothoracic Surgeon, Prince of Wales Hospital, Tai Po Nethersole Hospital, Hong Kong, China
Pleuropulmonary Tuberculosis; VATS Approach to the Thymus; Role of Cytokines in Coronary Artery Bypass Grafting With or Without Cardiopulmonary Bypass; Graft Assessment in Off-Pump Coronary Artery Bypass Surgery; Commentary 3A; Commentary 5A; Commentary 10A; Commentary 11A; Commentary 19A; Commentary 22A; Commentary 25A; Commentary 36A; Commentary 42A; Commentary 44A

Joseph B. Zwischenberger, MD
Professor of Surgery, Medicine, and Radiology, Director, General Thoracic Surgery and ECMO Programs, University of Texas Medical Branch, Galveston, Texas
Resection for Pulmonary Metastases; Interventional Radiology in the Chest

FOREWORD

This book is about a revolution in evolution. When surgeons of my generation were in training, we were taught that adequate exposure was *the* essential element of any surgical procedure. I can still remember as a general surgical house officer trying to learn from Glover Copher the complex method he used for packing the right upper quadrant of the abdomen with Mikulicz pads so that the gallbladder seemed to "fall out" of the wound. On operations for cancer, exposure was considered even more vital. I can still hear the dictum ringing in my ears: "To cure cancer, do the largest possible operation for the smallest possible lesion." This thought was so ingrained in many of us that for much too long we continued to consider pneumonectomy the gold standard for lung cancer and were blind to the accumulating mountain of data favoring lobectomy as the operation of choice whenever possible.

We must heed these lessons from the past. Whenever new ideas and techniques arrive on the scene, our responsibility is to evaluate them critically, compare and contrast them with current practices, and if they are found to be more worthy, embrace them. The easy path in medicine, and especially in surgery, is to build walls and roadblocks around change, with such rubrics as "Is it as safe?" or "Is it as effective?"

This is one of the many reasons I am so attracted to this book. It is edited by a group of six young surgeons, each of whom has been on the forefront in the development of a totally new concept in surgery, namely, testing the lower limits of access for a given operative procedure while maintaining previously defined objectives and standards of safety. "Minimal access" is the name they give to this revolution, which effectively began in 1974 with fallopian tube ligation and 25 years later has changed the way procedures are performed in every surgical discipline. I fully agree with the authors in their choice of "minimal access" over "minimally invasive," a term that somehow has crept into use in the cardiothoracic literature, and one that I personally find repugnant. It should be reserved for use by troops of infantry on the battlefield.

Everything about this volume speaks with vigor and the excitement of change. The Contents Table is carefully thought out so as to be comprehensive and yet provide a template that can be easily expanded, both for the sections presently covered as well as for subjects and techniques not yet on the scene. The 173 contributors are all recognized for their seminal contributions in this new field and have written authoritatively in their special areas of expertise.

Clearly, however, the editors have emphasized to each the ephemeral nature of their subject matter, so while the chapters are state of the art as of 1999, they essentially are a look at one frame of a rapidly moving film.

The above point is stressed by one of the features of this book I find most valuable, namely, the use of commentaries. Almost every chapter (subject) has at least one commentary, and several of them have two or three. These comments are all written by experts, although not necessarily those who embrace this new technology. The sum effect is to provide not only balanced, honest differences of opinion, but again to emphasize that, because of the nature of this field, much of which is captured in print in this edition may be modified or even rejected in the next edition. What a healthy attitude!

As the editors say in their preface, the book is divided into two parts: endoscopy and general thoracic procedures and cardiac surgery and evolving technology. I would comment on the last section, because I believe it points clearly to a direction for the future. Minimal access procedures have one overriding downside, and that is, in order to use them, surgeons have had to abandon techniques they spent the better part of a decade learning, and become proficient in a whole new set of complex skills. Detractors of minimal access surgery say that we are now approaching a limit to the number of manipulations that can be performed with instruments designed to work through ports of the minimal access type. The use of robotic engineering to perform the same procedures we now do with video-assisted thoracic surgery (VATS) technology may at this juncture sound expensive and "Buck Rogers-ish," but the greatest plus for these devices is not that they minimize tremor but that they restore for surgeons some of the traditional "feel" we were taught when dissecting with scissors or placing a stitch. When the expense and availability of these complex systems have been resolved, surely the restoration of what we semireverently call "surgical skills" will propel minimal access surgery to new heights we cannot yet even envision.

This volume is totally in tune with the rapidly changing field it covers, and I predict that the second and following editions will be also, because the editors want this to be the case. But in the meantime, this is the first edition, Enjoy!

THOMAS B. FERGUSON, MD

"To exist is to change, to change is to mature, to mature is to go on creating oneself endlessly."

Henri Louis Bergson
(1859–1941)
translated from *L'évolution créatrice*
Paris: Alcan, 1907

PREFACE

In 1869, Benjamin Disraeli noted, "Change is inevitable. In a progressive country, change is constant." Although this remark pertained to the political climate in Victorian England, it seems equally applicable to medicine at the close of the 20th century. As the new millennium approaches, cardiothoracic surgery is experiencing a paradigm shift with regard to the conduct of operative procedures. Many surgeons have come to recognize that the process of obtaining intrathoracic access is sometimes more traumatic than the procedure to be performed. We are entering a very exciting era as we continue to develop innovative approaches to established cardiac and thoracic procedures. This volume includes 83 chapters that describe just such innovative approaches, many of which were devised by the authors themselves, all of whom represent recognized authorities in their fields. Many issues regarding operative technique, indications, and patient selection remain controversial; therefore, we have also invited other experts to lend their opinions. Although their beliefs may not necessarily be consonant with those of the editors, it is important to present both supportive and critical views because these will yield a more balanced perspective. We believe this approach will also assist the reader to determine the proper place for these techniques in his or her own practice.

We chose to name this book *minimal access* rather than *minimally invasive* cardiothoracic surgery because the former term is less ambiguous and more easily understood. On the other hand, *minimal invasiveness,* although a commonly used term, can connote different meanings to different readers. The true value of these new approaches could only be defined by carefully planned studies designed to document clear and significant advantages over conventional techniques.

This book is divided into 10 sections in 2 parts. The first part, consisting of 6 sections, deals with video-assisted thoracic surgery and interventional endoscopy. The second part, consisting of the remaining 4 sections, deals with minimal access cardiac surgery and *off-pump* coronary artery bypass grafting. The editors are grateful to the 173 authors who kindly contributed to this work. Because this is a rapidly evolving field, it is probable that some of the information herein may be outdated soon after publication. Nonetheless, we believe this book will serve its purpose as a point of reference for the current application and development of minimal access cardiothoracic surgery.

In addition to the contributors, the editors are grateful to many individuals. We are indebted to Richard Lampert, senior medical editor at W.B. Saunders Company, and his capable assistant, Beth LoGiudice. Both alternated in their roles as guiding lights and relentless taskmasters. Natalie Ware and Mary Reinwald proved to be the most efficient production manager and copy editor, respectively. Connie Yeung, Pat Schafer, Cheryl Candler, and Laura Bianchi provided invaluable help to the editors on a day-to-day basis. Without the expertise, diligence, and dedication of these individuals, this textbook would not have seen daylight.

We realize that there will be omissions and oversights in this book. Therefore, we would personally like to invite the readers to communicate their comments and suggestions so that we may improve the content when a second edition is warranted.

APCY
SRH
MBI
RJL
MJM
KSN

NOTICE

Medicine is an ever-changing field. Standard safety precautions must be followed, but as new research and clinical experience broaden our knowledge, changes in treatment and drug therapy become necessary or appropriate. Readers are advised to check the product information currently provided by the manufacturer of each drug to be administered to verify the recommended dose, the method and duration of administration, and the contraindications. It is the responsibility of the treating physician, relying on experience and knowledge of the patient, to determine dosages and the best treatment for the patient. Neither the Publisher nor the editor assumes any responsibility for any injury and/or damage to persons or property.

THE PUBLISHER

CONTENTS

* Dr. Jaretzki's commentary applies to Chapters 26, 27, and 28.

Section I

General Aspects

Chapter 1

Thoracoscopy—A Historical Perspective

Mark V. Braimbridge

The Three Decades

Thoracoscopy was invented in the first decade of the 20th century. It was a Swedish internist's response to the pressing thoracic medical problem of pleural adhesions complicating artificial pneumothorax. Subsequently, thoracoscopy was taken over by surgeons and became widely used throughout the world. In the 1940s, the advent of streptomycin caused this procedure to be virtually abandoned with the exception of some European centers. During the century's last decade, the advance of technology with the development of the video monitor led to an explosion of renewed interest in thoracoscopy.

Artificial Pneumothorax

In 1882, Koch discovered the tubercle bacillus. By coincidence, in the same year, Forlanini noticed that tuberculous cavities collapsed and healed when the patient developed a spontaneous pneumothorax or a massive effusion. He performed the first *pneumotorace artificiale,* news of which was published that year in a series of chatty articles in the *Gazzetta degli Ospitali.*[19] The article occupied the top half of the opening page (Fig 1–1), extended to the top of the next page, and was continued as the lead page in 10 subsequent issues. Forlanini's technique required inserting a needle obliquely into the anterior axillary line and injecting air or nitrogen under water pressure, inserting 200 ml initially. This technique became widely adopted.

Closed Intrapleural Pneumonolysis

It soon became clear that many artificial pneumothoraces could not be completed because of adhesions between the lung and the chest wall. In response to this limitation of the technique, Hans Christian Jacobaeus of the Serafimerlasarettet Hospital in Stockholm—or Serafen, as it was familiarly known (Fig 1–2)—performed the first therapeutic thoracoscopy to divide these adhesions.[31] It is ironic, in view of the often quoted anxiety that pulmonologists might expropriate thoracoscopy as they did bronchoscopy, that Jacobaeus, a professor of internal medicine and head of the Medical Department II at the hospital, was himself not a surgeon.

Jacobaeus 1910

The first article by Jacobaeus was written in German and appeared in the Munich medical journal of 1910 (Fig 1–3). The article dealt with the possibility of using the cystoscope in investigating serous cavities.[31] Jacobaeus described his two-cannula technique (Fig 1–4) first as it was used in the peritoneum (laparoskopie) and then, only at the end of his article, as it was used in the pleura (thorakoskopie). His simple equipment was illustrated by a line diagram.

Jacobaeus 1922 to 1923

Jacobaeus published twice in *Surgery, Gynecology and Obstetrics*, in 1921[29] and 1922,[30] but his definitive article appeared in *Proceedings of the Royal Society of Medicine* of London in 1922–1923.[27] The Royal Society of Medicine has separate Sections that meet regularly and publish their proceedings: His presentation, surprisingly, was not delivered to thoracic internists or surgeons, but to the Section of Electro-Therapeutics (Fig 1–5). A composite photograph of his equipment was featured (Fig 1–6). This publication was reprinted word for word in the United States in 1923 in two sections of *Archives of Radiology and Electrotherapy*[28]—again, not where it would be published today.

Technique. Jacobaeus' technique was to sedate his patients with bromide or phenobarbital (Luminal). Using fluoroscopy, he would mark the exact position of the adhesion on the chest wall and insert the thoracoscope nearby. He would then insert the galvanocautery into the anterior axillary line (see Fig 1–4) and heat it to a red glow.

Classification of Adhesions. Jacobaeus classified adhesions by their position, shape, and surgical difficulty. Lateral adhesions tended to be long and thin; apical adhesions were likely to be short and painful to cauterize; and diaphragmatic adhesions presented a moving target or necessitated the patient's holding his or her breath. He noted that cauterization was usually more difficult than would be expected from the radiograph. Adhesions were cord-like, membranous, or surface. Cord-like adhesions were the simplest to cauterize, and surface adhesions

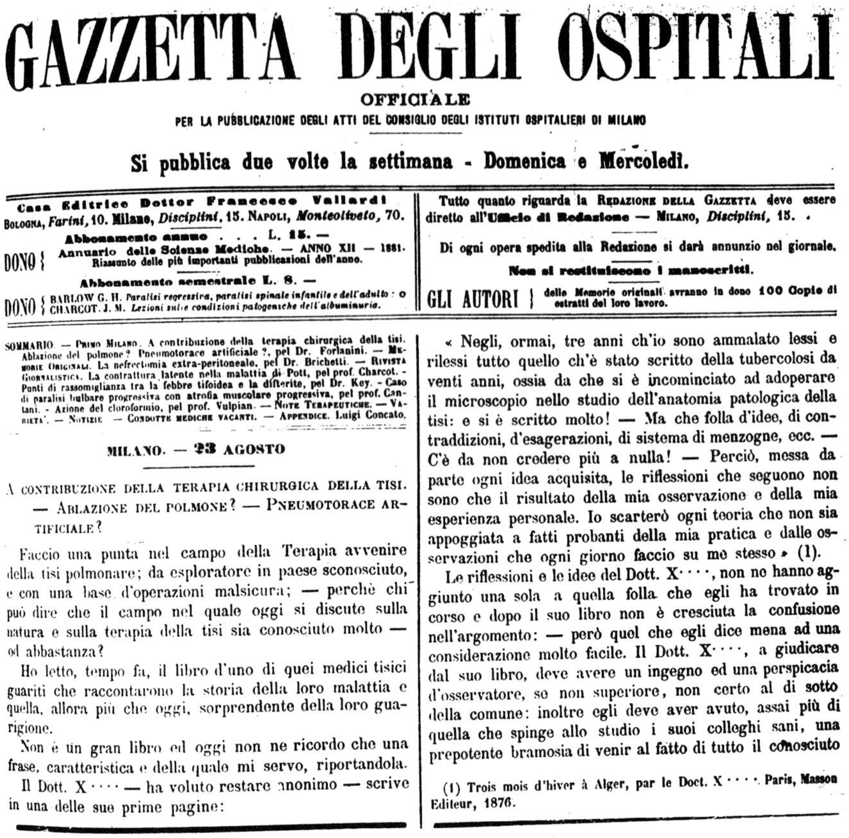

GAZZETTA DEGLI OSPITALI

OFFICIALE

PER LA PUBBLICAZIONE DEGLI ATTI DEL CONSIGLIO DEGLI ISTITUTI OSPITALIERI DI MILANO

Si pubblica due volte la settimana - Domenica e Mercoledì.

Casa Editrice Dottor Francesco Vallardi
BOLOGNA, *Farini*, 10. Milano, *Disciplini*, 15. NAPOLI, *Monteoliveto*, 70.

Abbonamento annuo . . . L. 15. —

DONO { Annuario delle Scienze Mediche. — ANNO XII — 1881. Riassunto delle più importanti pubblicazioni dell'anno.

Abbonamento semestrale L. 8. —

DONO { BARLOW G. H. *Paralisi regressiva, paralisi spinale infantile e dell'adulto*: o CHARCOT. J. M. *Lezioni sulle condizioni patogeniche dell'albuminuria.*

Tutto quanto riguarda la REDAZIONE DELLA GAZZETTA deve essere diretto all'Ufficio di Redazione — MILANO, *Disciplini*, 15.

Di ogni opera spedita alla Redazione si darà annunzio nel giornale.

Non si restituiscono i manoscritti.

GLI AUTORI { delle Memorie originali avranno in dono 100 Copie di estratti del loro lavoro.

SOMMARIO. — PRIMO MILANO. A contribuzione della terapia chirurgica della tisi. Ablazione del polmone? Pneumotorace artificiale?, pel Dr. Forlanini. — MEMORIE ORIGINALI. La nefrectomia extra-peritoneale, pel Dr. Brichetti. — RIVISTA GIORNALISTICA. La contrattura latente nella malattia di Pott, pel prof. Charcot. - Punti di rassomiglianza tra la febbre tifoidea e la difterite, pel Dr. Key. - Caso di paralisi bulbare progressiva con atrofia muscolare progressiva, pel prof. Cantani. - Azione del cloroformio, pel prof. Vulpian. — NOTE TERAPEUTICHE. — VARIETÀ. — NOTIZIE — CONDOTTE MEDICHE VACANTI. — APPENDICE. Luigi Concato.

MILANO. — 23 AGOSTO

A CONTRIBUZIONE DELLA TERAPIA CHIRURGICA DELLA TISI. — ABLAZIONE DEL POLMONE? — PNEUMOTORACE ARTIFICIALE?

Faccio una punta nel campo della Terapia avvenire della tisi polmonare; da esploratore in paese sconosciuto, e con una base d'operazioni malsicura; — perchè chi può dire che il campo nel quale oggi si discute sulla natura e sulla terapia della tisi sia conosciuto molto — od abbastanza?

Ho letto, tempo fa, il libro d'uno di quei medici tisici guariti che raccontarono la storia della loro malattia e quella, allora più che oggi, sorprendente della loro guarigione.

Non è un gran libro ed oggi non ne ricordo che una frase, caratteristica e della quale mi servo, riportandola.

Il Dott. X···· — ha voluto restare anonimo — scrive in una delle sue prime pagine:

« Negli, ormai, tre anni ch'io sono ammalato lessi e rilessi tutto quello ch'è stato scritto della tubercolosi da venti anni, ossia da che si è incominciato ad adoperare il microscopio nello studio dell'anatomia patologica della tisi: e si è scritto molto! — Ma che folla d'idee, di contraddizioni, d'esagerazioni, di sistema di menzogne, ecc. — C'è da non credere più a nulla! — Perciò, messa da parte ogni idea acquisita, le riflessioni che seguono non sono che il risultato della mia osservazione e della mia esperienza personale. Io scarterò ogni teoria che non sia appoggiata a fatti probanti della mia pratica e dalle osservazioni che ogni giorno faccio su me stesso » (1).

Le riflessioni e le idee del Dott. X····, non ne hanno aggiunto una sola a quella folla che egli ha trovato in corso e dopo il suo libro non è cresciuta la confusione nell'argomento: — però quel che egli dice mena ad una considerazione molto facile. Il Dott. X····, a giudicare dal suo libro, deve avere un ingegno ed una perspicacia d'osservatore, se non superiore, non certo al di sotto della comune: inoltre egli deve aver avuto, assai più di quella che spinge allo studio i suoi colleghi sani, una prepotente bramosia di venir al fatto di tutto il conosciuto

(1) Trois mois d'hiver à Alger, par le Doct. X····. Paris, Masson Editeur, 1876.

Figure 1–1. The upper half of the first page of the Gazetta degli Ospitali with Forlanini's report. (Reprinted with permission from the Society of Thoracic Surgeons [The Annals of Thoracic Surgery 56:611, 1993].)

were short and had to be treated with great caution for fear of air leak.

Material. Jacobaeus reported 121 cases: seventy-five of his own, together with 46 from the series of Holmboe, Gravesen, and Saugman, and Somme and Unverricht.

Results. Eighty-three percent of cases involved the relatively easy, lateral adhesions. Seventy percent of the total series had complete collapse of the cavities; 62% had a good clinical result, but 29% were classified as "incomplete cauterization."

Complications. Jacobaeus reported complications only in his own series of 75 cases. Seventy-three percent showed

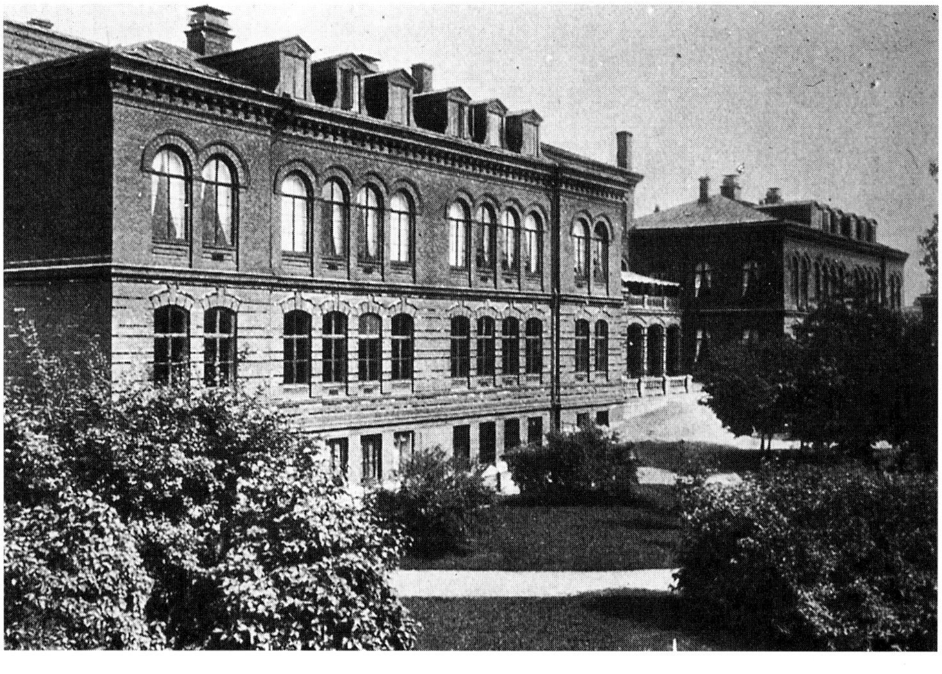

Figure 1–2. The Serafimerlasarettet Hospital in 1910. (Reprinted with permission from the Society of Thoracic Surgeons [The Annals of Thoracic Surgery 56:611, 1993].)

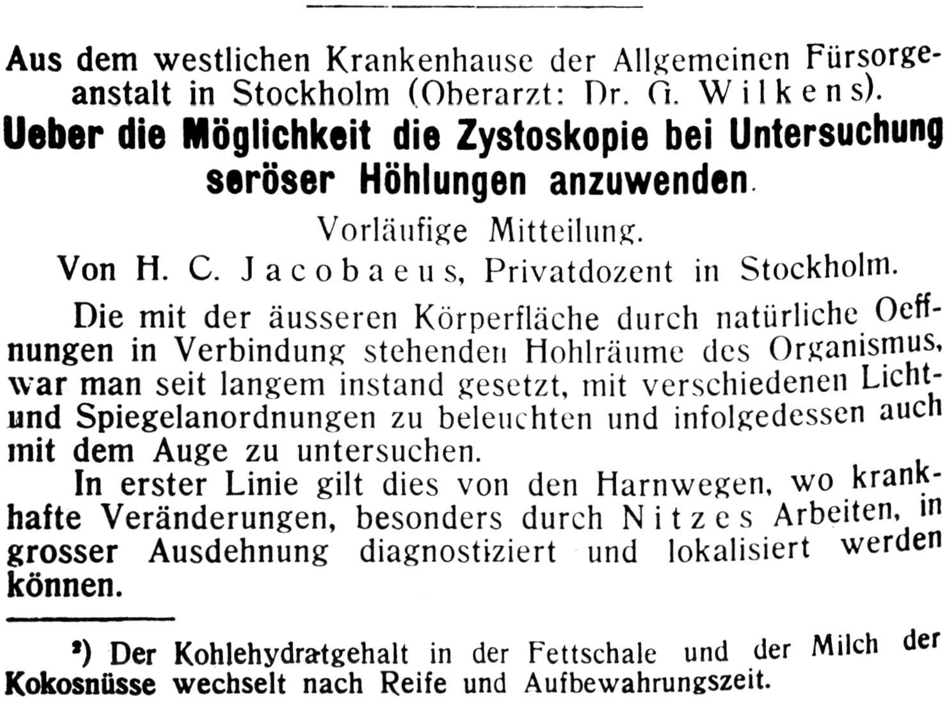

Aus dem westlichen Krankenhause der Allgemeinen Fürsorge-anstalt in Stockholm (Oberarzt: Dr. G. Wilkens).

Ueber die Möglichkeit die Zystoskopie bei Untersuchung seröser Höhlungen anzuwenden.

Vorläufige Mitteilung.

Von H. C. Jacobaeus, Privatdozent in Stockholm.

Die mit der äusseren Körperfläche durch natürliche Oeffnungen in Verbindung stehenden Hohlräume des Organismus, war man seit langem instand gesetzt, mit verschiedenen Licht- und Spiegelanordnungen zu beleuchten und infolgedessen auch mit dem Auge zu untersuchen.

In erster Linie gilt dies von den Harnwegen, wo krankhafte Veränderungen, besonders durch Nitzes Arbeiten, in grosser Ausdehnung diagnostiziert und lokalisiert werden können.

*) Der Kohlehydratgehalt in der Fettschale und der Milch der Kokosnüsse wechselt nach Reife und Aufbewahrungszeit.

Figure 1–3. The title page of Jacobaeus' first article. (Reprinted with permission from the Society of Thoracic Surgeons [The Annals of Thoracic Surgery 56: 611, 1993].)

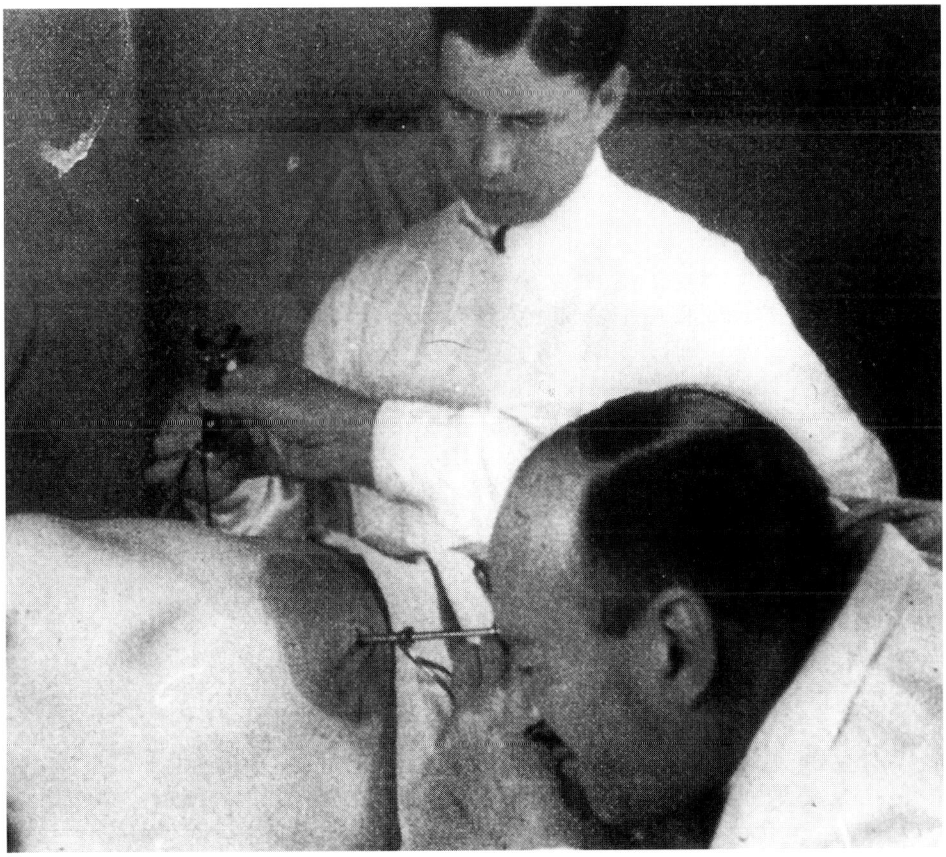

Figure 1–4. Jacobaeus and his assistant with his two-cannula technique. (Reprinted with permission from the Society of Thoracic Surgeons [The Annals of Thoracic Surgery 56:611, 1993].)

Section of Electro-Therapeutics.

President—Dr. Robert Knox.

The Cauterization of Adhesions in Artificial Pneumothorax Treatment of Pulmonary Tuberculosis under Thoracoscopic Control.

By H. C. Jacobaeus, M.D.[1]

(From the Medical Service II of the Serafimerlasarett, Stockholm, Sweden, Professor H. C. Jacobaeus, Director.)

For about ten years I have been occupied with endoscopy of the serous cavities, peritoneum and pleura. At first, I was interested only in the diagnostic advantages which could be gained by such a method. In a case of ascites, after tapping and replacing the fluid by air, I could by endoscopy get a clear view of the abdominal organs. There was thus no difficulty in diagnosing liver cirrhosis, malignant tumour, Pick's disease, syphilis, &c. Further, in carcinoma and tuberculosis of the peritoneum, I could see changes characteristic of these diseases. After first performing endoscopy, or laparoscopy, only

Figure 1–5. The title page of Jacobaeus' 1922/1923 publication in the Section of Electro-Therapeutics of the Royal Society of Medicine. (Reprinted with permission from the Society of Thoracic Surgeons [The Annals of Thoracic Surgery 56:612, 1993].)

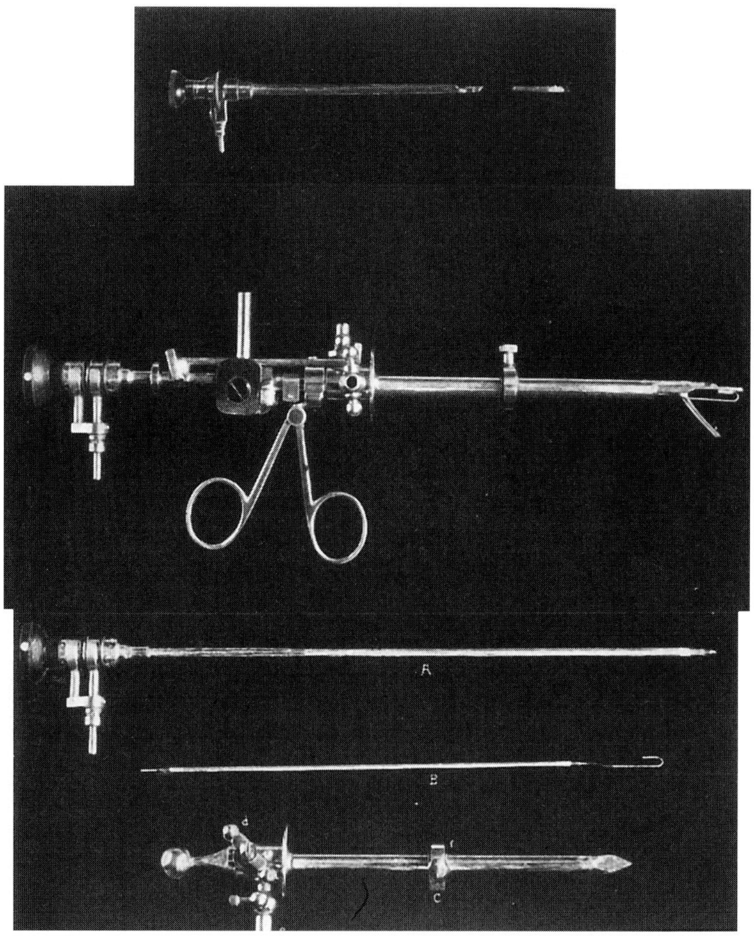

Figure 1–6. Jacobaeus' 1922 equipment. (Reprinted with permission from the Society of Thoracic Surgeons [The Annals of Thoracic Surgery 56:612, 1993].)

either no or slight pleural exudate; 15% had an exudate accompanied by fever; 9% developed an empyema; and a late exudate occurred in 3%.

Case Reports. Jacobaeus added two illustrative case reports with accompanying chest radiographs.

Operative (Therapeutic) Thoracoscopy: The Era of Enthusiasm

Jacobaeus' technique was adopted with enthusiasm throughout Europe and the United States.

Development of Equipment. The modified cystoscope and the two-cannula approach of Jacobaeus were inevitably improved by the development of better instruments. Cutler[13] used a single instrument in 1933, but found it was more expensive and had poorer visibility than the two-cannula method. He suggested that "the necessary experience is best gained by repeated experimentation on raw meat well moistened"! A more acceptable practice milieu was the cardboard box which was used in Britain to develop the spatial skills of two-cannula thoracoscopy (Fig 1–7). In 1929, Davidson[14] also used a single instrument, because the concern at that time was to minimize the number of ports.

A retrograde step was made by Friedel[20] in 1970, who used a bronchoscope in the pleura with an inevitable incidence of severe surgical emphysema, hemorrhage, and death.

Clinical Series. In 1938, Drash[16] reported 231 cases of thoracoscopy, with sputum conversion in 93.5% and cavity closure in 74.8%. There were no deaths, but there were six cases of tuberculous empyemata. Moore[56] reported 1830 cases in 1934.

There were numerous other reports, but perhaps the most careful review at the end of the era of enthusiasm was that of Day, Chapman, and O'Brien[15] in 1948. They reported on an analysis of 1000 consecutive closed intrapleural pneumonolyses, as they were termed in the United States (though more often appearing as "thoracoscopy and division of adhesions" and "thorakokaustik" on British and German operating lists, respectively). Day, using Davidson's single instrument, reported only two deaths in 923 patients, but there were 50 cases of empyemata, mostly tuberculous. At follow-up 6 months to 7 years later, tuberculosis was arrested in 52% but was still active in 20%, and 28% of the patients had died.

The age of enthusiasm for operative—later termed therapeutic—thoracoscopy ended in 1945 with the introduction of streptomycin, and the era of neglect began, with thoracoscopy confined mainly to diagnostic measures.

Therapeutic Thoracoscopy—The Era of Neglect

After 1945, biopsy—diagnostic thoracoscopy—became virtually the only operative procedure within the pleura, and interest in thoracoscopy waned. There was a symposium on thoracoscopy in 1980 in Marseilles, where Le Tacon gave a brief historical review,[41] mainly of the French literature. In 1978, Kock[35] looked at the early history of both laparoscopy and thoracoscopy in the German literature. In spite of the diminished role of thoracoscopy, Viskum and Enk[67] in 1981 listed a formidable number of complications from their Copenhagen experience, including hemorrhage, air embolism, and surgical emphysema; wound infection and malignant spread; empyema, cardiac arrhythmias, and hypotension; and respiratory insufficiency and persistent pneumothorax.

But it was Bloomberg[5] from the Bronx who in 1978 best summarized the history of thoracoscopy and its position in surgical management. He stated, "While some older surgical techniques are still being used, there are some that have been put aside and all but forgotten. One of these . . . is thoracoscopy." In 1978, his remaining indi-

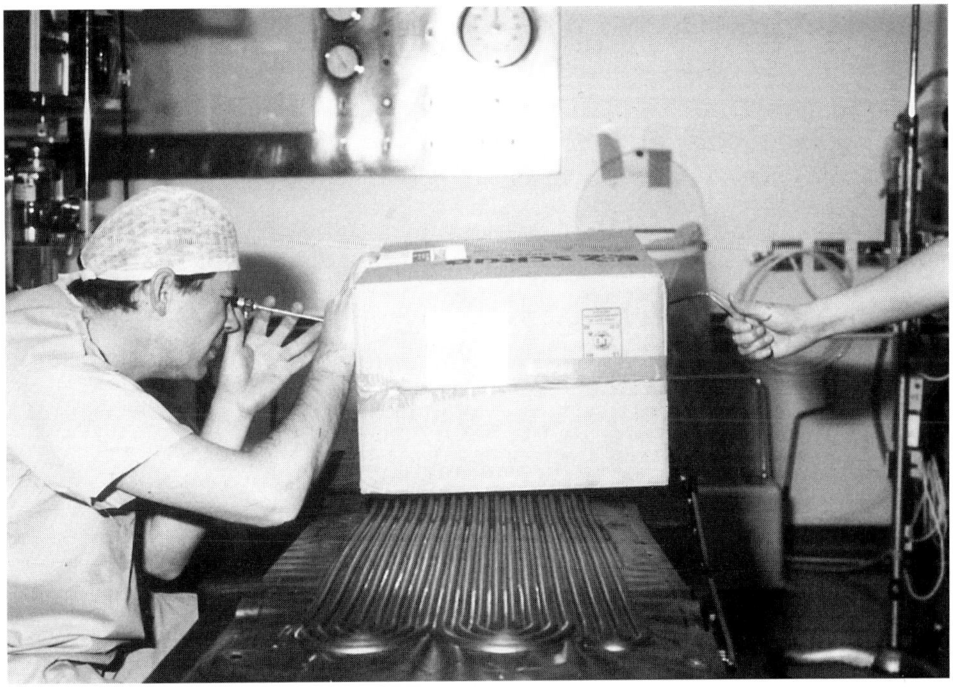

Figure 1–7. The cardboard box used as a thoracoscopy simulator. (Reprinted with permission from the Society of Thoracic Surgeons [The Annals of Thoracic Surgery 56:612, 1993].)

cations for thoracoscopy were undiagnosed pleural, pulmonary, and mediastinal disease requiring biopsy; preoperative screening for spontaneous pneumothorax and malignant disease surgery; trauma; "and, of course, . . . intrapleural pneumonolysis," a strange inclusion, as he concluded, "even after artificial pneumothorax and intrapleural pneumonolysis had been abandoned in many countries, European surgeons continued to use thoracoscopy for diagnosis and, in some areas, for therapy."

One of these areas was empyema, for which a technique was developed at St. Thomas' Hospital in London[26] in an attempt to avoid the usual long attendance of those outpatients who had an indwelling tube after rib resection and drainage. The technique was modified from that of Rosenfeldt and colleagues[63] and consisted of inserting a Jacobs-Palmer laparoscope[65] (long, and with an offset eyepiece unlike other thoracoscopes of the time) to break down loculi and debride fibrin. A tight-fitting Argyle drain was placed in the thoracoscope port, with a smaller one above, and the space was irrigated twice a day with alternating doses of 1% noxythiolin—an antiseptic—and saline. Tubes were removed after three successive sterile cultures.

The results of the first 12 cases, referred initially by pulmonologists for rib resection and drainage, showed that in all cases, including two of tuberculous origin, patients left hospital cured with no in-dwelling tube, but this was accomplished at the cost of a 4.8-week average stay—arguably acceptable in Great Britain, where health-care costs are regulated by the National Health Service, but not, as Ferguson[18] pointed out, in cost-conscious America. Also, extending the technique to chronic and malignant empyemata was less successful.[62] Even in Europe, therefore, therapeutic thoracoscopy rarely surfaced during the era of neglect.

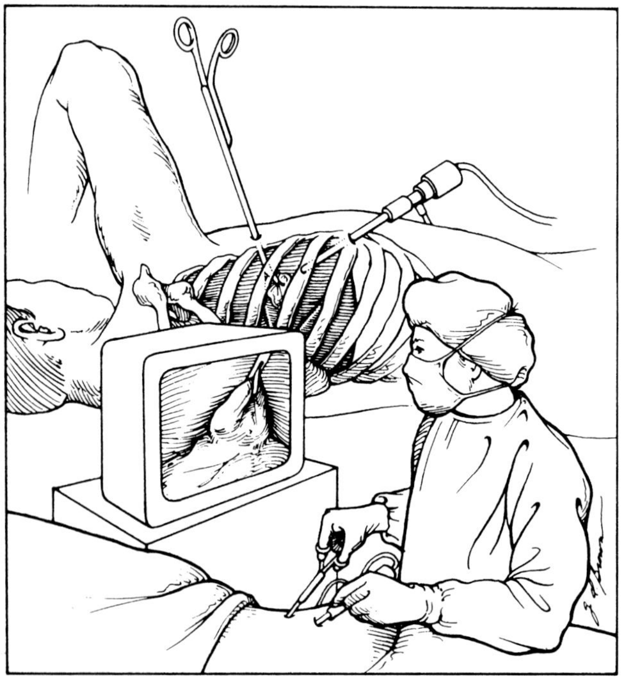

Figure 1–8. The advent of the video monitor. (Reprinted with permission from the Society of Thoracic Surgeons [The Annals of Thoracic Surgery 54:404, 1991].)

The Last Decade—Video-Assisted Thoracic Surgery

Technological advances in the 1990s, with the development of the video monitor, the instrument-tip camera, and percutaneous endoscopic instruments (Fig 1–8), caused the same level of magnitude of change in cardiothoracic surgery as the advent of cardiopulmonary bypass had in the 1950s. By 1992, Mack was able to report a series with no mortality, morbidity, or emergency thoracotomy,[50] as did Lewis.[42] The video monitor removed the awkward and potentially unsterile necessity for the surgeon's head to be at the end of a telescope close to the chest wall and also allowed the use of assistants.[55] Diagnostic thoracoscopy developed once again into therapeutic thoracoscopy, which then progressed to minimally invasive, direct-vision surgery. By this time, all three were, by definition, video-assisted thoracic surgery (VATS).

Nomenclature

Thoracoscopy was the title for this surgery at the beginning of the decade,[50,54] but it was soon changed to video-assisted thorascopic surgery (VATS).[44] The boundary be-

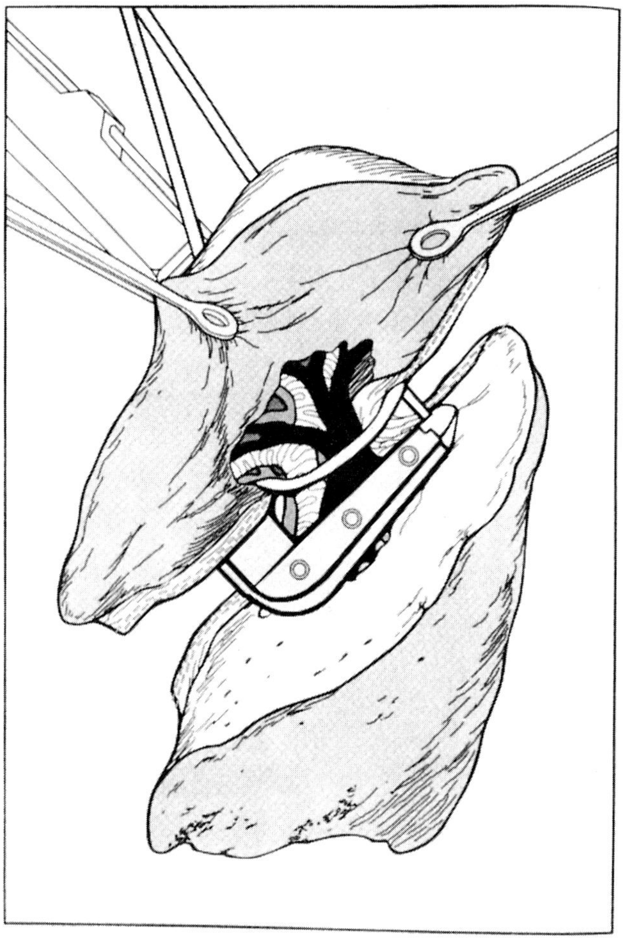

Figure 1–9. Thoracoscopic lobectomy. (Reprinted with permission from the Society of Thoracic Surgeons [The Annals of Thoracic Surgery 56:766, 1993].)

tween diagnostic and therapeutic thoracoscopy was clear, although sometimes it was confused by classifying some diagnostic techniques as therapeutic procedures.[55] Diagnostic thoracoscopy had biopsy as its sole instrumental procedure, whereas therapeutic thoracoscopy extended its techniques into operations on the *lung:* wedge,[38,55] lobe[43,45] (Fig 1–9), lung,[64] and excision of bullae[38,69,70]; the *pleura:* empyema,[18] effusion,[48] and pneumothorax,[23,69]; the *diaphragm:* eventration[57]; the *mediastinum:* thymectomy,[51] tumor excision,[22,37,60] and chylothorax management[18]; the *esophagus:* myotomy[39,61] and excision[21]; the *pericardium:* excision[50]; *extracardiac congenital anomalies:* patent ductus arteriosus[1,11,36] and vascular rings[10]; the *autonomic system:* thoracic sympathectomy[50]; and *orthopedics:* intervertebral discs.[52,53] The historian notes that in the early 1990s, one surgeon, Michael Mack, was a protagonist in virtually every one of these fields. He was an enthusiastic promoter of the new science, and was, to a large extent, responsible for its wide dissemination.

The boundary was not so clear between therapeutic thoracoscopy and direct-vision VATS. "VATS is not thoracoscopy," Lewis stated in 1996,[46] citing 11 points of difference. He had a simplistic view of thoracoscopy, and his distinction between *direct* and *indirect* vision was equivocal, but he was right—it was not thoracoscopy.

The critical difference between thoracoscopy and VATS is vision. Thoracoscopy implies telescopic vision only, precluding thoracotomy, though the necessity for a small, non–rib-spreading incision to remove larger resected specimens blurs this distinction. Rib-spreading thoracotomy was necessarily a part of direct, that is, non-telescopic vision VATS, but, as all surgeons know, the word "thoracotomy," or even "mini-thoracotomy," disturbs pulmonologists—it became the T-word of the 1990s. *Minimally invasive*[7] and *port access*[17,49] were the referral-friendly substitutes, reflecting the general trend of surgery toward smaller incisions. Minimally invasive, direct access coronary artery bypass grafts (MIDCAB grafts),[2,4,17] mitral[47] and aortic valve surgery,[3] and atrial septal defect closure,[12,66] with or without peripheral access cardiopulmonary bypass,[12] and cardioplegia[17] (Fig 1–10), entered surgical practice, though usually assisted by indirect vision thoracoscopic techniques—for instance, in mobilization of the internal mammary artery[6] and caval cannulation. A far cry from the Serafimerlasarettet in Stockholm!

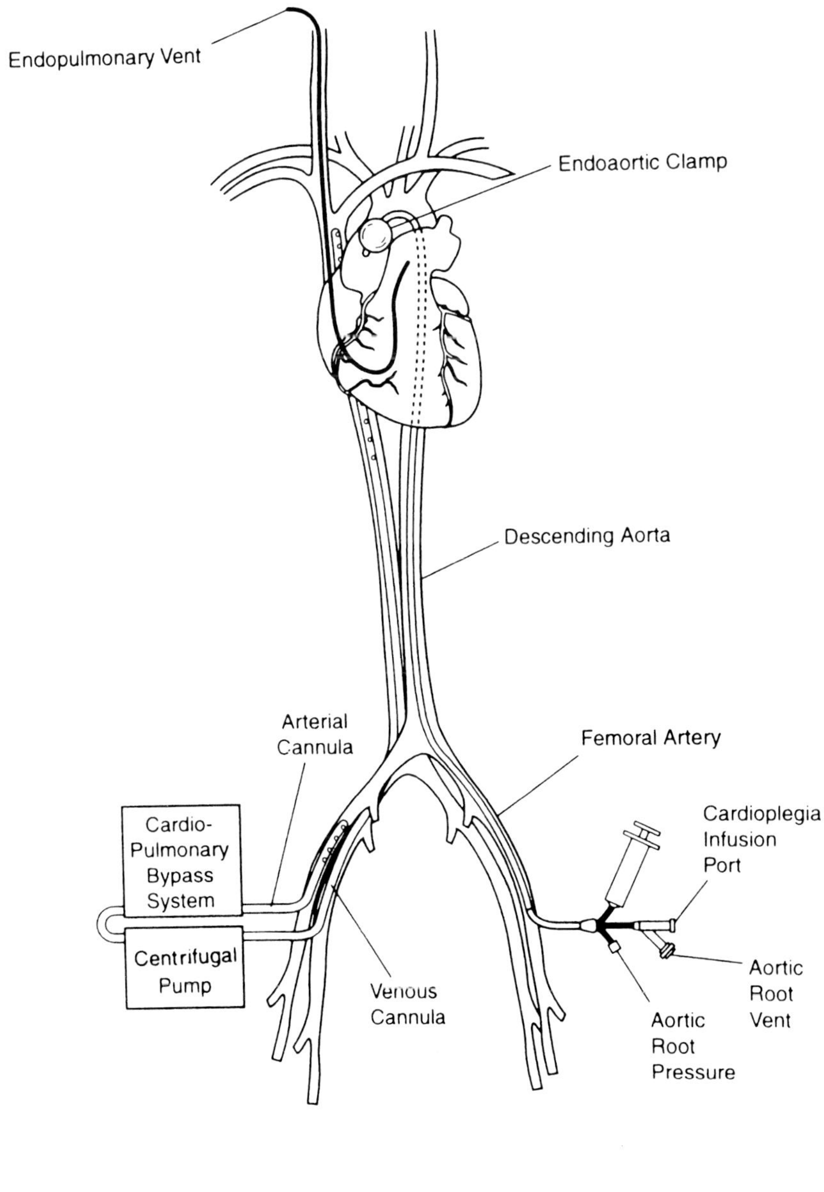

Figure 1–10. VATS with cardiopulmonary bypass and cardioplegia. (Reprinted with permission from the Society of Thoracic Surgeons [The Annals of Thoracic Surgery 63:536, 1997].)

The Two Revolutions

The VATS revolution of the 1990s, as dramatic in its impact on cardiothoracic surgery as the cardiopulmonary bypass in the 1950s, was similar in two respects to its predecessor. First, it was spearheaded in America. Apart from an early thoracoscopic technique for bullous ligation, notable for its complicated knot, which was reported from Scotland[59] (Fig 1–11), the early technological advances and the surgical enterprise all came from North America—indeed, at the 1993 San Antonio Thoracoscopy Symposium, the paper on "Thoracoscopy in Europe" was presented by a Canadian![58] Second, the bulk of early publications came mainly from North American centers—Minneapolis, Rochester, and Houston in the 1950s and Dallas, Pittsburgh, and Milwaukee in the 1990s.

The two revolutions differed, however, in several respects. The three centers that published in the 1950s did so separately, using different cardiopulmonary bypass techniques, whereas the centers that published in the 1990s produced joint papers, using essentially the same technique, thus emphasizing general applicability and also multiplying statistical experience.[39,40] This characteristic feature of joint publication soon became intercontinental—North America with Asia[51] and Europe,[49] and Europe with South America.[4]

This multiplication of surgical experiences allowed emphasis to be placed on the importance of cost-effectiveness, balancing equipment cost with decreased hospital stay[24,34,40]; of surgical training in indirect techniques[39,40,68]; and of safety monitoring[25] and complication rates.[9,32,33,71] All these considerations were critical in the financial and litigious environment of the 1990s, which was so different from that of the 1950s when, basically, money was no object and the surgeon's word was law.

The 1990s revolution, moreover, was led from the operating room rather than the dog laboratory, as had been the revolution of the 1950s. This difference was emphasized by the fact that virtually all early references to VATS appeared in *Annals of Thoracic Surgery*.

Finally, the 1990s revolution affected every aspect of intrathoracic surgery—cardiac, pulmonary, and esophageal—rather than cardiac alone, and brought pulmonary surgery back into the mainstream of thoracic progress and research.[8]

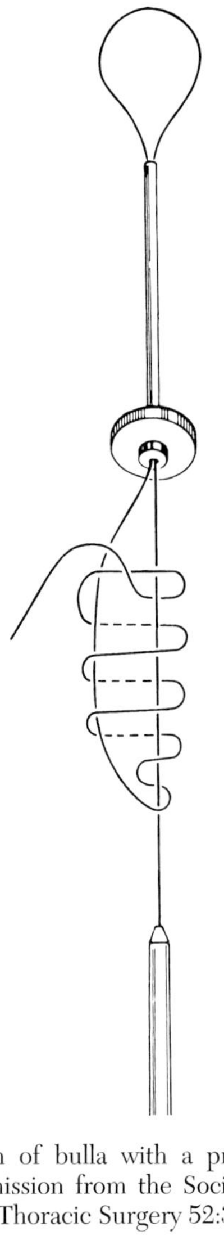

Figure 1–11. Ligation of bulla with a pre-tied Roeder knot. (Reprinted with permission from the Society of Thoracic Surgeons [The Annals of Thoracic Surgery 52:318, 1991].)

Conclusion

Eight decades later, Jacobaeus, that professor of medicine in Stockholm, would be proud of the way his simple adaptation of a cystoscope to treat pleural adhesions has been developed by surgeons into a treatment for diseases of every intrathoracic organ. His minimalist approach of 1910 has become the wide-ranging, innovative theme of cardiothoracic surgery in the 1990s.

ACKNOWLEDGEMENT

My grateful thanks are due to Prof. Stig Ekestrom of the Karolinska Hospital, Stockholm, for the early photographs of Jacobaeus and his hospital.

References

1. Alvarez-Tostado RA, Millan MA, Tovar LA, et al: Thoracoscopic clipping and ligation of a patent ductus arteriosus. Ann Thorac Surg 57:755–757, 1994.
2. Benetti FJ, Ballester C: Use of thoracoscopy and a minimal thoracotomy in mammary-coronary bypass to left anterior descending artery without extracorporeal circulation. J Card Surg (Torino) 36:159–161, 1995.
3. Benetti FJ, Mariani MA, Rizzardi JL, et al: Minimally invasive aortic valve surgery. J Thorac Cardiovasc Surg 113:806–807, 1997.
4. Benetti FJ, Mariani MA, Sani G, et al: Video-assisted minimally invasive coronary operations without cardiopulmonary bypass: A multicenter study. J Thorac Cardiovasc Surg 112:1478–1484, 1996.
5. Bloomberg AE: Thoracoscopy in perspective. Surg Gynecol Obstet 147:433–443, 1978.
6. Boonstra PW, Grandjean JG, Mariani MA: Local immobilization of the left anterior descending artery for minimally invasive coronary bypass grafting. Ann Thorac Surg 63(6 Suppl): S76–S78, 1997.
7. Borst C, Santamore WP, Smedira NG, et al: Minimally invasive coronary artery bypass grafting: On the beating heart and via limited access. Ann Thorac Surg 63(6 Suppl):S1–S5, 1997.

8. Braimbridge MV: The history of thoracoscopic surgery. Ann Thorac Surg 56:610–614, 1993.
9. Buhr J, Hürtgen M, Kelm C, et al: Tumor dissemination after thoracoscopic resection for lung cancer. J Thorac Cardiovasc Surg 110:855–856, 1995.
10. Burke RP, Chang AC: Video-assisted thoracoscopic division of a vascular ring in an infant: A new operative technique. J Card Surg 8:537–540, 1993.
11. Burke RP, Wernovsky G, van der Velde M, et al: Video-assisted thoracoscopic surgery for congenital heart disease. J Thorac Cardiovasc Surg 109:499–507, 1995.
12. Chang CH, Lin PJ, Chu JJ, et al: Video-assisted cardiac surgery in closure of atrial septal defect. Ann Thorac Surg 62:697–701, 1996.
13. Cutler JW: A technique and apparatus for intrapleural pneumonolysis. Am Rev Tuberc 28:528–536, 1933.
14. Davidson LR: A simplified operating thoracoscope. Am Rev Tuberc 19:306–309, 1929.
15. Day JC, Chapman PT, O'Brien EJ: Closed intrapleural pneumonolysis: An analysis of 1000 consecutive operations. J Thorac Surg 17:537–554, 1948.
16. Drash EC: An appraisal of closed internal pneumonolysis in pulmonary tuberculosis. Relation of tuberculous empyema to the operation. J Thorac Surg 7:411–419, 1938.
17. Fann JI, Pompili MF, Stevens JH, et al: Port-access cardiac operations with cardioplegic arrest. Ann Thorac Surg 63(6 Suppl): S35–S39, 1997.
18. Ferguson MK: Thoracoscopy for empyema, bronchopleural fistula, and chylothorax. Ann Thorac Surg 56:644–645, 1993.
19. Forlanini C: A contribuzioni della terapia chirurgica della tisi—Ablazione del polmone? Pneumotorace artificiale? Gazzetta degli Ospitali 3:537–539; 585–587; 601, 602; 609, 610; 617–619; 625–627; 641–643; 657–660; 665–667; 689–691; 705–707, 1882.
20. Friedel H: Importance of bronchological examination in case of pleural disease. Bronches 20:77–82, 1970.
21. Gossot D, Fourquier P, Celerier M: Thoracoscopic esophagectomy: Technique and initial results. Ann Thorac Surg 56:667–670, 1993.
22. Hazelrigg SR, Landreneau RJ, Mack MJ, et al: Thoracoscopic resection of mediastinal cysts. Ann Thorac Surg 56:659–660, 1993.
23. Hazelrigg SR, Landreneau RJ, Mack MJ, et al: Thoracoscopic stapled resection for spontaneous pneumothorax. J Thorac Cardiovasc Surg 105:389–393, 1993.
24. Hazelrigg SR, Nunchuck SK, Landreneau RJ, et al: Cost analysis for thoracoscopy: Thoracoscopic wedge resection. Ann Thorac Surg 56:633–635, 1993.
25. Horswell MS: Anesthetic techniques for thoracoscopy. Ann Thorac Surg 56:624–629, 1993.
26. Hutter JA, Harari D, Braimbridge MV: The management of empyema thoracis by thoracoscopy and irrigation. Ann Thorac Surg 39:517–520, 1985.
27. Jacobaeus HC: The cauterization of adhesions in artificial pneumothorax treatment of pulmonary tuberculosis under thoracoscopic control. Proc Roy Soc Med 16(Jul)(Parts 1&2, Section of Electrotherapeutics):45–60, 1922, 1923.
28. Jacobaeus HC: The cauterization of adhesions in artificial pneumothorax treatment of pulmonary tuberculosis under thoracoscopic control. Arch Radiol Electrotherapy 28:97–105; 136–146, 1923.
29. Jacobaeus HC: The cauterization of adhesions in pneumothorax treatment of tuberculosis. Surg Gynecol Obstet 32:493–500, 1921.
30. Jacobaeus HC. The practical importance of thoracoscopy in surgery of the chest. Surg Gynecol Obstet 34:289–296, 1922.
31. Jacobaeus HC: Ueber die Möglichkeit die Zystoskopie bei Untersuchung seröser Höhlungen anzuwenden. München Med Wchenschr 57:2090–2092, 1910.
32. Jancovici R, Lang-Lazdunski L, Pons F, et al: Complications of video-assisted thoracic surgery: A five year experience. Ann Thorac Surg 61:533–537, 1996.
33. Kaiser LR, Bavaria JE: Complications of thoracoscopy. Ann Thorac Surg 56:796–798, 1993.
34. Kirby TJ, Mack MJ, Landreneau RJ, et al: Lobectomy—video-assisted thoracic surgery versus muscle-sparing thoracotomy—a randomized trial. J Thorac Cardiovasc Surg 109: 997–1002, 1995.
35. Kock W: Frühgeschichte der Laparoskopie, der Thorakoskopie und der Thorakokaustik. Neue Munch Beitr Gesch Med Naturwiss Medizinhist Reihe 7, 8:517–527, 1978.
36. Laborde F, Noirhomme P, Karan J, et al: A new video-assisted thoracoscopic surgical technique for interruption of patent ductus arteriosus in infants and children. J Thorac Cardiovasc Surg 105:278–280, 1993.
37. Landreneau RJ, Hazelrigg SR, Ferson PF, et al: Thoracoscopic resection of 85 pulmonary lesions. Ann Thorac Surg 54: 142–144, 1992.
38. Landreneau RJ, Herlan DB, Johnson JA: Thoracoscopic neodymium:yttrium-aluminum garnet laser-assisted pulmonary resection. Ann Thorac Surg 52:1176–1178, 1991.
39. Landreneau RJ, Mack MJ, Hazelrigg SR, et al: Video-assisted thoracic surgery: Basic technical concepts and intercostal approach strategies. Ann Thorac Surg 54:800–807, 1992.
40. Landreneau RJ, Mack MJ, Keenan RJ, et al: Strategic planning for video-assisted thoracic surgery. Ann Thorac Surg 56:624–629, 1993.
41. Le Tacon J: La pleuroscopie. Rappel historique. Poumon-Coeur 37:5,6, 1981.
42. Lewis RJ, Caccavale RJ, Sisler GE, et al: One hundred consecutive patients undergoing video-assisted thoracic operations. Ann Thorac Surg 54:421–426, 1992.
43. Lewis RJ, Caccavale RJ, Sisler GE, et al: One hundred video-assisted thoracic surgical simultaneously stapled lobectomies without rib spreading. Ann Thorac Surg 63:1415–1422, 1997.
44. Lewis RJ, Caccavale RJ, Sisler GE: Special report: Videoendoscopic thoracic surgery. N J Med 88:473–475, 1991.
45. Lewis RJ: Simultaneously stapled lobectomy: A safe technique for video-assisted thoracic surgery. J Thorac Cardiovasc Surg 109:619–625, 1995.
46. Lewis RJ: VATS is not thoracoscopy. Ann Thorac Surg 62: 631–632, 1996.
47. Lin PJ, Chang CH, Chu JJ, et al: Video-assisted mitral valve operations. Ann Thorac Surg 61:1781–1787, 1996.
48. Lo Cicero J: Thoracoscopic management of malignant pleural effusion. Ann Thorac Surg 56:641–643, 1993.
49. Mack MJ, Acuff TE, Casimir-Ahn H, et al: Videoassisted coronary bypass grafting on the beating heart. Ann Thorac Surg 63(6 Suppl):S100–S103, 1997.
50. Mack MJ, Aronoff RJ, Acuff TE, et al: Present role of thoracoscopy in the diagnosis and treatment of diseases of the chest. Ann Thorac Surg 54:403–409, 1992.
51. Mack MJ, Landreneau RJ, Yim AP, et al: Results of video-assisted thymectomy in patients with myasthenia gravis. J Thorac Cardiovasc Surg 112:1352–1360, 1996.
52. Mack MJ, Regan JJ, Bobechko WP, et al: Application of thoracoscopy for diseases of the spine. Ann Thorac Surg 56: 736–738, 1993.
53. Mack MJ, Regan JJ, McAfee PC, et al: Video-assisted thoracic surgery for the anterior approach to the thoracic spine. Ann Thorac Surg 59:1100–1106, 1995.
54. Miller DL, Allen MS, Trastek VF, et al: Videothorascopic wedge excision of the lung. Ann Thorac Surg 54:410–414, 1992.
55. Miller JI, Jr: Therapeutic thoracoscopy: New horizons for an established procedure (Editorial). Ann Thorac Surg 52:1036–1037, 1991.
56. Moore JA: Intrapleural pneumonolysis. A critical review. J Thorac Surg 3:276–299, 1934.

57. Mouroux J, Padovani B, Poirier NC, et al: Technique for the repair of diaphragmatic eventration. Ann Thorac Surg 62: 905–907, 1996.
58. Mulder DS: Thoracoscopy in Europe: Views from North America. Ann Thorac Surg 56:731–733, 1993.
59. Nathanson LK, Shimi SM, Wood RA, et al: Videothoracoscopic ligation of bulla and pleurectomy for spontaneous pneumothorax. Ann Thorac Surg 52:316–319, 1991.
60. Naunheim KS: Video thoracoscopy for masses of the posterior mediastinum. Ann Thorac Surg 56:653–656, 1993.
61. Pellegrini CA, Leichter R, Patti M, et al: Thoracoscopic esophageal myotomy in the treatment of achalasia. Ann Thorac Surg 56:680–682, 1993.
62. Ridley PD, Braimbridge MV: Thoracoscopic debridement and pleural irrigation of empyema thoracis. Ann Thorac Surg 51: 461–464, 1991.
63. Rosenfeldt FL, McGibney D, Braimbridge MV, et al: Comparison between irrigation and conventional treatment for empyema and pneumonectomy space infection. Thorax 36:272–277, 1981.
64. Roviaro G, Varoli F, Rebuffat C, et al: Major pulmonary resections: Pneumonectomies and lobectomies. Ann Thorac Surg 56:779–783, 1993.
65. Sang CTM, Braimbridge MV: Thoracoscopy simplified using the laparoscope. Thorac Cardiovasc Surg 29:129–130, 1981.
66. Shetty DF, Dixit MD, Gan MD, et al: Video-assisted closure of atrial septal defect (Letter). Ann Thorac Surg 62:940, 1996.
67. Viskum K, Enk B: Complications of thoracoscopy. Poumon-Coeur 37:25–28, 1981.
68. Wain JC: Thoracoscopy training in a residency program. Ann Thorac Surg 56:799–800, 1993.
69. Wakabayashi A, Brenner M, Wilson AF, et al: Thoracoscopic treatment of spontaneous pneumothorax using carbon dioxide laser. Ann Thorac Surg 50:786–790, 1990.
70. Wakabayashi A: Thoracoscopic technique for management of giant bullous lung disease. Ann Thorac Surg 56:708–712, 1993.
71. Yim AP, Liu HP: Complications and failures of video-assisted thoracic surgery: Experience from two centers in Asia. Ann Thorac Surg 61:538–541, 1996.

COMMENTARY

Michael J. Mack

It is only appropriate to begin this book with a historical perspective from a true giant of thoracic surgery. Upon acceptance of the task of compiling a complete history, and again upon submission of his completed chapter, Mr. Braimbridge apologized profusely regarding his perspective on video-assisted thoracic surgery (VATS), because he had no hands-on experience. Rather than viewing this as a shortcoming, I myself believe, and I think the reader will agree, that this distance actually lends credibility to his perspective. Sometimes, when we are too close to an event, it is impossible to place it in its proper historical context. I was somewhat surprised—and indeed humbled—to read this chapter and learn Mr. Braimbridge's opinions about VATS. We have the added advantage of being able to enjoy this historical narrative in the King's English.

Whether the impact of VATS in minimal access surgery is truly a revolution, as Mr. Braimbridge indicates, remains to be seen. It has been only a few years since the introduction of VATS into thoracic surgery in 1990, and an even shorter time since minimal access cardiac surgery was first described. Even today, only a minority of procedures in each specialty are performed using minimally invasive techniques. Although controversy has been generated, it remains to be seen whether it constitutes a true revolution or merely an interesting sidelight. The real contribution, however, may be in the paradigm shift of the way surgery is viewed by its practitioners, and the stimulation and rejuvenation that has occurred in mature surgical specialties. Innovative thinking is alive and well in thoracic and cardiac surgery.

Chapter 2

Preoperative Assessment for Video-Assisted Thoracic Surgery

Dan M. Meyer

The recent emergence of minimally invasive techniques in cardiothoracic surgery has led to a modification of many of the indications for surgery that had been standard for many years. This has resulted in the option of surgical therapy for patients who before the introduction of video-assisted thoracic surgery (VATS) may not have been considered surgical candidates. As a result, the preoperative assessment of the patient has been altered to focus on issues specifically related to minimally invasive surgical procedures. However, while the assessment of patients may be modified, key standard guidelines for evaluating thoracic surgical patients are maintained.

Assessment

Preoperative assessment of patients considered for minimally invasive thoracic surgery must include the same attention to detail and scrutiny that would typically be directed toward patients undergoing surgery using a conventional incision. Only the means to access the thoracic cavity is changed. Current candidates for minimally invasive thoracic procedures include patients requiring diagnosis and treatment of selected neoplasms, and those who have infections, trauma, persistent or recurrent pneumothoraces, pericardial processes, and selected congenital abnormalities. Moreover, in patients with emphysema, lung volume reduction surgery (LVRS) may be performed through this route.[5,6] Thymectomy has been reported to be safely performed via thoracoscopy.[8] A survey of 200 North American thoracic surgeons[4] detailed some of the more common applications of VATS (Table 2–1). While this list does comprise the classic indications for thoracoscopic procedure, the surgeons who were questioned expressed concern over the appropriate use of VATS, with 38% still feeling that this technology has been significantly overused. This is in contrast to a survey of thoracic surgeons outside of North America, which found a much higher proportion of surgeons favoring VATS (APC Yim, personal communication).

Interestingly, there are no specific groups of patients who would not be considered for minimally invasive surgery. Early in the thoracoscopic experience, the profile of patients who were denied candidacy for these procedures included a prior thoracotomy, although this is no longer thought to be an absolute contraindication. A study by Yim and associates[10] reviewed their experience with 40 patients who underwent VATS procedures after a prior thoracic procedure on that side. They found that although adhesions, ranging from minimal to strong fibrous adhesions, were present in all cases, in only two cases (5%) was the procedure aborted because of the adhesions requiring conversion to an open procedure. Those patients who have had a prior pleurodesis, however, with no evidence of a free pleural space, may be less attractive candidates for minimally invasive techniques. Means to assess for pleural symphysis have included the creation of a pneumothorax followed by a chest radiograph (CXR) to help plan the positioning of the thoracoscopic ports. Carbon dioxide insufflation is another option that may facilitate adhesiolysis by collapsing the lung. Overall, the investigators quoted no mortality or intraoperative complications, concluding that VATS is safe and technically feasible in the reoperated chest. Moreover, they stated that the experience of the surgeon and the nature of the surgical procedure are the important factors in deciding whether VATS should be attempted in this patient population.

Patients at relatively high risk, such as the elderly, who in the past would not have been offered surgical therapy requiring a thoracotomy, may actually be candidates for VATS. A study by DeCamp and associates[1] reviewed their experience with 895 consecutive VATS cases. In a prospective manner, they evaluated outcome in three high-risk groups: Age over 70 years, forced expiratory volume in the first second (FEV_1) of <1.0 L, and Karnofsky performance index of less than 8. The overall mortality rate in the series was 1.0%, with a morbidity rate of 14%. In the elderly, low FEV_1, and depressed performance status cohorts, the mortality rates were 1.5%, 2.1%, and 9.8%, respectively. Correspondingly, the morbidity rates in these high-risk patients were 19%, 30%, and 18%, respectively. The authors concluded that VATS offered a surgical option to patients who up until this point would not have been candidates for standard surgical therapy. A review by Yim reported fully acceptable results of VATS in patients who were older than 75 years.[7] There was no mortality, and morbidity was isolated to prolonged thoracostomy tube drainage in two patients (9.1%). The findings of such low postoperative complications allowed the author to conclude that VATS is safe in the elderly population. Age alone should not be a deterrent when deciding upon offering major lung or mediastinal surgery to the elderly patient, a finding confirmed by other smaller studies.[2] Nevertheless, both the surgeon and the patient should realize that for any major VATS procedure, the possibility exists for conversion to formal thoracotomy. Therefore, the patient and the operating suite should be prepared accordingly.

Overall, contraindications to thoracoscopy are quite limited. Patients who cannot tolerate single-lung ventilation, such as those who are dependent on a ventilator or who have pulmonary hypertension, would not be ideal candidates for thoracoscopic procedures, nor would patients who have selected metastatic pulmonary lesions, al-

Table 2–1. Indications for Use of Video-Assisted Thoracoscopy

Diagnostics
- Pleural effusions
- Pleural-based masses
- Indeterminate pulmonary nodule
- Diffuse parenchymal lung disease (nonintubated patient)
- Anterior and posterior mediastinal masses
- Staging for esophageal and pulmonary malignancies

Therapeutics
- Neoplasms
  - Wedge resection (patients with limited pulmonary function)
  - VATS Lobectomy
- Trauma
  - Retained hemothorax
- Resection of mediastinal masses
- Infections
  - Early empyema
- Persistent or recurrent pneumothoraces
- Pericardial processes
- Selected congenital abnormalities
- Sympathectomy
- Transthoracic vagotomy
- Benign esophageal disorders
- Lung volume reduction surgery (LVRS)
- Thymectomy

though minimally invasive procedures would be technically feasible (see Chapter 21). These patients may be better served by an open thoracotomy, allowing the surgeon to palpate the smaller lesions that may not be visible on CT scan.

History

Even in this new age of minimal access surgery, the history of the present illness remains the initial phase of the preoperative assessment. The goal of the assessment, as in any patient evaluation, is the determination of the nature of the problem and the assignment of an appropriate management algorithm. For minimally invasive thoracic surgery, much of the specific information in the history is similar to that obtained when conventional procedures are performed. To exclude neoplastic processes in a patient with a solitary pulmonary nodule, history of a prior normal chest radiograph is likely the most important standard information, along with an inventory of associated risk factors. For acquired conditions, such as chronic obstructive pulmonary disease (COPD), a history of oxygen dependency, incapacitating shortness of breath, and significant impairment of daily activities is elicited. For infectious etiologies, such as the common empyema, the duration of symptoms may allow the physician to predict the feasibility of attempting a minimally invasive approach. Typically, a process of less than 2 weeks' duration is manageable thoracoscopically.

In the acute trauma setting, the history is of somewhat less importance, with the stability of the patient being central. Patients who have spontaneous pneumothoraces may give a history of acute pleuritic chest pain after a cough or minimal exertion. The number of previous episodes, as well as the occupational history, influences the timing of the operative intervention.

Finally, for congenital lesions, such as mediastinal cysts, symptomatic complaints, such as pain, or, more importantly, fever, are the critical factors, because in these situations operative indications are not clear cut. Aspects of the history that may influence recovery from surgical procedures should be identified preoperatively and include comorbid conditions, such as cardiac disease, hypertension, underlying pulmonary disease, diabetes mellitus, recent weight loss of greater than 10% of ideal body weight, and age greater than 70 years.

Physical Examination

Preoperative assessment of candidates for minimally invasive procedures demands the same careful inspection on physical examination as would be performed on any individual, regardless of the type of incision planned. For patients who have neoplastic or potentially neoplastic conditions, a full examination focusing on evidence of metastatic disease would be of importance. Cervical, axillary, or supraclavicular adenopathy would not only change the operative plan, but could also give a simpler means of obtaining a diagnosis. Assessing a patient with an infectious process would necessitate a survey to ensure that no other ongoing source of infection is present. Moreover, examination should detect if there is a safer or more rapid method to access the problem.

The trauma patient would undergo full evaluation to guard against the presence of serious injuries that would necessitate more rapid management. Minimally invasive techniques are typically applied to nonemergency processes, because the hemodynamically unstable patient may not tolerate the positioning needed for thoracoscopic procedures, or the time required to place the double-lumen endotracheal tube adequately.

Patients who have spontaneous pneumothoraces are usually stable, with tube thoracostomy in place before consideration for thoracoscopic exploration. These patients are typically young males with a tall, thin physique. Patients who have pericardial effusions referred for drainage are assessed for hemodynamic stability and their ability to tolerate anesthetic induction. Individuals who have posterior mediastinal masses, such as neurogenic tumors, should undergo a full neurologic examination to prevent involvement of the spinal cord, because this could change the planned minimally invasive operative approach.

Radiographic Evaluation

Standard CXR and chest computed tomography (CT) are typically obtained on patients undergoing thoracoscopic procedures. While a simple CXR may suffice in many cases, the additional information obtained from a CT is often a useful adjunct, because the ability to palpate within the chest cavity is largely lost in thoracoscopic surgery. The CXR gives enough initial information to indicate whether a pulmonary lesion is accessible by minimally invasive techniques. Most nodules must have a peripheral location to be considered for thoracoscopic removal. More central lesions may require a video-assisted approach, involving a small utility incision for palpation along with thoracoscopic visualization.

Computed tomography may also be helpful in localizing lesions in subpleural locations. In some cases, CT-directed needle localization may be of use. A guide wire placed into the lesion before surgery may help localize a lesion situated deep within the lung parenchyma (see Chapter 15).[3] These wires are of small caliber and have a tendency to become dislodged with undue movement of the patient. An additional maneuver to help localize small lesions preoperatively is by instillation of methylene blue to the site localized by chest CT. This does not offer as accurate a localization as obtained with the guide-wire technique, but it may be of some assistance in finding subpleural nodules. An adjunctive or perhaps alternative maneuver to help localize subpleural peripheral nodules includes digital localization. Additional small, nonspreading intercostal incisions have been reported to yield excellent results in identifying these nodules.[9] CT is also useful in identifying enlarged lymph nodes, which can be biopsied if indicated.

In cases of infected pleural collections, CT helps to detail the areas in the pleural space where the predominant collections are present and identifies any fluid sequestered within the fissures or subdiaphragmatic regions. In the trauma setting, CXR may be a useful tool in determining the path of the missile and the extent of nonpenetrating injury. Importantly, CXR also serves to detect any pneumo- or hemothoraces. Subsequent films are used to monitor any changes on the CXR consistent with retained or recurrent hemothoraces or pneumothoraces. Computed tomography is of use in the preoperative assessment of patients who have retained hemothoraces, again detecting areas of loculated fluid collections. In patients who have spontaneous pneumothoraces, CXR alone is a sufficient assessment to direct surgical therapy. Frequently, no abnormality can be seen on CXR, but thickening of the apex of the lung may be identified. Occasionally, blebs can be detected in the remaining lung. CT adds little to the assessment of these patients, because exploration at the time of surgery is necessary regardless of the results of the study.

Candidates for LVRS require at least radiographic assessments as part of their evaluation. A chest radiograph shows findings of end-stage chronic obstructive pulmonary disease, and the chest CT demonstrates diffuse emphysematous changes. Finally, in congenital conditions, CXR and CT are important in first identifying the abnormality and characterizing the lesion. Dense adhesions to the mediastinum may be important when considering minimal access surgery. Furthermore, possible involvement of the spinal canal can be a concern in patients who have a posterior mediastinal mass.

Pulmonary Function

As stressed in the preceding sections, patients who are candidates for minimally invasive thoracic procedures require the same comprehensive evaluation typically as patients who are undergoing formal open procedures. While these less invasive thoracoscopic techniques may enable the borderline surgical candidate to be considered for surgical therapy, the standard minimal pulmonary assessment guidelines should still be satisfied. If the patient is a current smoker, elective surgery could be made less eventful if cessation of tobacco use could be achieved for 1 to 2 weeks preoperatively. Patients who do not have the motivation or physical ability to generate an adequate cough pose problems in the postoperative period. The importance of an effective cough should not be overlooked, even after minimal access thoracic procedures.

For most thoracoscopic procedures in which significant resection is not planned, formal pulmonary function testing is not necessary. The majority of patients tolerate the recommended single-lung ventilation during the operation. Exceptions to this include the groups of patients described earlier who would not be good candidates for thoracoscopic procedures, such as the elderly and those with chronic obstructive pulmonary disease. However, in situations where clinical suspicion of poor pulmonary function exists, spirometry studies, or graded exercise testing, such as stair climbing, is an accurate method of determining pulmonary reserve (Table 2–2). If a major pulmonary resection is planned, testing is necessary, as it would be if a conventional incision were to be used. This would include use of technetium 99m quantitative perfusion lung scans in some situations.

Assessment of arterial blood gas may be of importance in patients undergoing formal pulmonary resection. A low preoperative oxygen pressure may trigger further cardiopulmonary testing prior to surgery. Similarly, desaturation of oxygen with exertion should also encourage additional assessment. Patients with hypercapnia must be closely evaluated, as they may have cor pulmonale and therefore not tolerate a major resection. Despite all attempts to stratify patients according to their risk for tho-

Table 2–2. Pulmonary Function Criteria for Lung Resection

PFT	Normal	Pneumonectomy	Lobectomy	Wedge
FEV_1	>2L	>2L	>1L	>0.8L
$FEF_{25\%-75\%}$	>2L	>1.6L	>0.6L	>0.6L
MVV	>80%	>55%	>40%	>35%
Stair-climbing	>2 flights	2 flights	1 flight	<1 flight

FEV_1 = forced expiratory volume in 1 second; $FEF_{25\%-75\%}$ = forced expiratory flow, midexpiratory phase; MVV = maximal ventilatory volume.

Modified from Miller JI: Thallium imaging in perioperative evaluation of the pulmonary resection candidate. Ann Thorac Surg 54:249, 1992, with permission from the Society of Thoracic Surgeons.

racoscopic surgery, an experienced clinician must make the final decision. The VATS technique has enabled poor operative candidates to be considered for surgical therapy, but the preoperative assessment must be conducted systematically, and the basic guidelines for surgical resection essentially remain the same.

Cardiovascular Assessment

Information obtained from the history helps tailor the preoperative cardiovascular assessment. The critical information revolves around the presence or absence of cardiac symptoms, previous history or evidence of myocardial infarction, congestive heart failure, dysrhythmias, or unstable angina. Moreover, an inclusive list of the patient's cardiac medications is of importance. Based upon the response from the history, standard exercise stress testing and exercise thallium testing could be performed. This information may help identify patients who have ischemia, and, more specifically, reversible ischemia. In most situations, this latter scenario may require myocardial revascularization before the elective thoracic procedure.

Conclusion

Preoperative assessment of patients undergoing minimally invasive thoracic surgery requires a focused history and physical examination as well as CXR and chest CT to obtain a visual image of the pleural space. The information gathered from these studies must give the surgeon full coordinates for which to care for the problem. Additional studies to assist in risk assessment may also have utility in the overall evaluation. At no time should the length of planned incision jeopardize the patient's immediate course or long-term outcome.

References

1. DeCamp MM, Jaklitsch MT, Mentzer SJ, et al: The safety and versatility of video-thoracoscopy: A prospective analysis of 895 consecutive cases. J Am Coll Surg 181:113–120, 1995.
2. Ishida T, Ishii T, Yamazaki K, et al: Thoracoscopic limited resection of bronchogenic carcinoma in patients over the age of 80. Int Surg 81:237–240, 1996.
3. Mack MJ, Gordon MJ, Postma TW, et al: Percutaneous localization of pulmonary nodules for thoracoscopic lung resection. Ann Thorac Surg 53:1123–1124, 1992.
4. Mack MJ, Scruggs GR, Kelly KM, et al: Video-assisted thoracic surgery: Has technology found its place? Ann Thorac Surg 64:211–215, 1997.
5. McKenna RJ Jr, Brenner M, Fischel RJ, et al: Should lung volume reduction for emphysema be unilateral or bilateral? J Thorac Cardiovasc Surg 112:1331–1338, 1996.
6. Weder W, Schmid RA, Russi EW: Thoracoscopic lung volume reduction surgery for emphysema. Int Surg 81:229–234, 1996.
7. Yim AP: Thoracoscopic surgery in the elderly population. Surg Endosc 10:880–882, 1996.
8. Yim AP: Video-assisted thoracoscopic resection of anterior mediastinal masses. Int Surg 81:350–353, 1996.
9. Yim AP, Ho JK: Digital localization of peripheral lung nodules with video-assisted thoracic surgery [letter] Chest 107:886, 1995.
10. Yim APC, Liu HP, Hazelrigg SR, et al: Thoracoscopic surgery on reoperated chests. Ann Thorac Surg 65:328–330, 1998.

COMMENTARY

Stephen R. Hazelrigg

Although video-assisted thoracic surgery has been demonstrated to reduce early perioperative pain over open thoracotomy, it still requires general anesthesia in most cases, and patients need to be evaluated critically for the procedure. There has been a tendency to offer surgical intervention to patients who may have been denied surgery before VATS techniques were available. Recognizing their increased comorbidity before surgery can help to anticipate and treat potential postoperative problems. It may be difficult to list absolute contraindications to VATS procedures, but good judgment is invaluable in weighing risk-benefit ratios.

Attempting to predict pleural adhesions is difficult. Pleural thickening on computed tomography (CT) scans is helpful but not absolute. As noted, the presence of adhesions does not prevent performance of the procedure in most settings. However, adhesions may significantly increase the difficulty and time required. Preoperative risk factors are the same for VATS as for open procedures. The only advantage offered by VATS is decreased early postoperative pain, which may allow fewer pulmonary complications (e.g., atelectasis or pneumonia) and the ability to mobilize the patient more quickly.

Chapter 3

Room Setup and Instrumentation

Randall K. Wolf

With the advent of minimal access procedures, a revolution in cardiothoracic surgery was set in motion. This revolution is now in a state of evolution, and with it there have been many major changes in operating room setup and instrumentation. The use of video cameras alone has changed the thoracic operating setup dramatically. The technology in the operating room has increased exponentially and, therefore, unfortunately, so has the surgeon's dependence on this new technology. However, this technology now allows the surgeon to perform procedures that were not technically possible 10 years ago, and patients ultimately benefit. The new technology can sometimes frustrate everyone in the operating room, which usually manifests itself when insufficient understanding of the technology impedes proper troubleshooting of the new equipment. Frustration can lead to a jaded view of this new paradigm, and this must be avoided. The revolution in minimal access cardiothoracic surgery is allowing the surgeon to evolve his or her right hemispheric visual-spatial intuition to heights never before imagined.

We are entering an exciting phase of new technology, which must be carefully incorporated into the room setup and instrumentation to achieve maximum benefit for all. Our operating rooms had changed little over the last 40 years. We are all capable of making the changes necessary so that we may embrace and benefit from this new technology.

Setup

Most minimal access cardiothoracic surgery requires a scope, a light source, and a camera. Cameras have evolved to standard, three-chip, high-definition color models that are readily available because they are used routinely in laparoscopic and orthopedic procedures. The light source and scope attach to the camera to form a practical unit. This unit is ubiquitous in operating rooms now, because it is the mainstay for performing laparoscopic cholecystectomy procedures.

The most practical setup of video equipment for the cardiothoracic surgeon is to mount a monitor near each side of the head of the operating table (Fig 3–1). This allows viewing from either side of the table for most thoracic work. The monitor, camera, light source, recorder, and scope should be checked by the surgeon before the incision is made. To help manage the many wires and cords leaving the field in the minimally invasive setup, a standard placement is recommended. The camera, light cord, and insufflation tubing are passed toward the head of the table, and the cords are placed on the sterile field in a trough alongside the patient. The trough is fashioned from the drapes and provides a repository for instruments as well as keeping the cords comfortably away from the field. This setup also allows the surgeon to switch from one side of the patient to the other without disturbing the lines exiting the field. Advanced computer technology now allows integrated voice control of most of the devices in the operating room. This involves voice-activated control of electrocautery, insufflation, and other units into one thought processor that responds to the surgeon's voice commands (Fig 3–2). As the commands are executed (such as changing the setting of the cautery), the settings are displayed on the monitors. Clinical trials of this system are taking place at selected centers. Another integrated control system for the equipment in the operating room involves a command station that allows a nurse to operate all the endoscopic equipment from a simple touch screen central panel on the side of the tower. A sterile control panel could also be made available for the surgeon.

Tower

The cabinet that contains many of the video components is known as the tower or cabinet. The camera is connected to a video monitor, which is mounted on the tower (Fig 3–3). The monitor can be slaved to a second video monitor on the opposite side of the operating room table. These should be situated at eye level on portable cabinets. The cabinet usually contains, from top to bottom (see Fig 3–3), a monitor, a camera processing unit, an insufflator, an additional camera source (optional), a light source, a Super VHS recorder, and a color printer.

Cameras

The imaging system that revolutionized surgical endoscopy is the miniaturized television camera, which consists of a light-sensitive silicone chip. The chips typically measure about 1 cm^2 in size. One silicone chip is called a charged coupling device (CCD). Color pictures require special techniques; for example, the CCD can be divided into red, green, and blue areas. Proper processing of the electrical impulses from the CCD forms a color image. The resolution is only fair with this method because only one third of the CCD detects each color. Alternatively, three CCDs may be placed in one camera with a prism splitting the light into red, green, and blue wavelengths. Each group of wavelengths is detected by a separate CCD. This method improves resolution.[3,4] These three-chip cameras are often used in today's operating suite. CCD chips can be mounted at the distal end of the thoracoscope. With this type of mounting, the thoracoscope does not require a rigid design to house mirrors (Hopkins lens design). Instead, the thoracoscope contains the wires that lead to the processor, and the

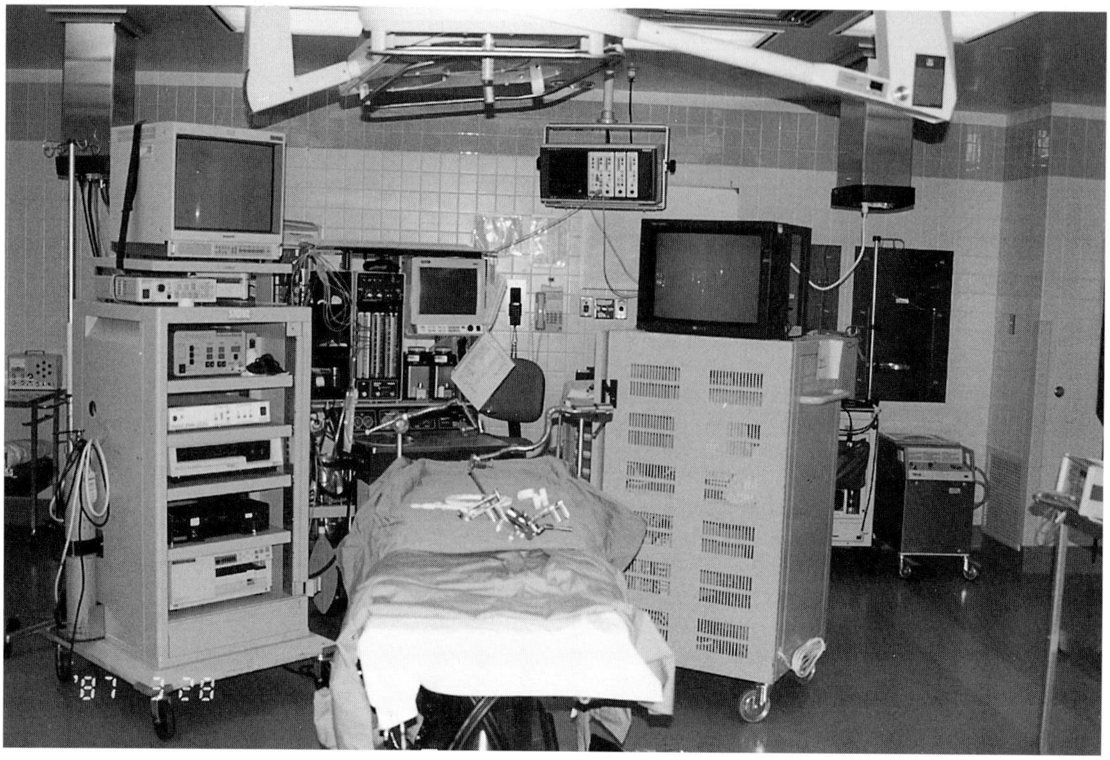

Figure 3–1. Typical operating room setup for minimally invasive procedures.

scope is flexible. Until recently, the flexible thoracoscope lacked the resolution of a rigid scope with a Hopkins lens system. The newest generation of flexible thoracoscopes has resolution that rivals that of rigid scopes, which are more expensive. Four hundred eighty lines of horizontal resolution are available with the flexible scope (Olympus Corp, Tokyo, Japan).

At least four manufacturers produce three-dimensional (3-D) cameras for thoracoscopic procedures. Generally, they are superior to the three-chip two-dimensional (2-D) cameras, but the use of special glasses is required to produce the 3-D image. One particular system requires the operator to wear a headset that contains two light-emitting

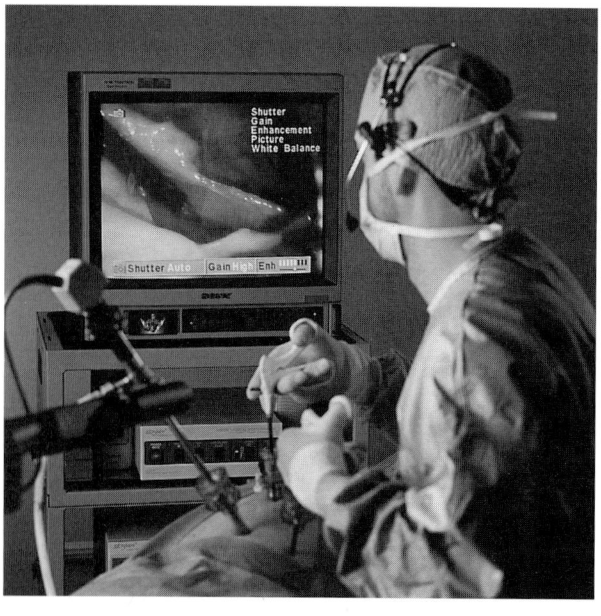

Figure 3–2. Robotic device with voice-activated, integrated controls with monitor display (Courtesy of Stryker Corporation, Kalamazoo, MI.)

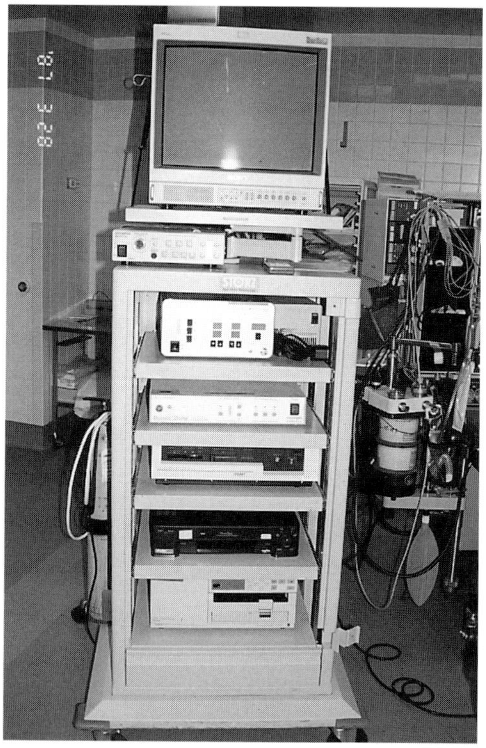

Figure 3–3. Video component tower. (Courtesy of Karl Storz Endoscopy America, Inc., Culver City, CA.)

diode (LED) screens (Vista, Inc., Westborough, MA). The visualization system incorporates a head-mounted display (Fig 3–4) based on a design that was originally developed for critical applications in military aerospace. The head-mounted display provides 3-D visualization of an endoscopic or microscopic image, and presents the images to the surgeon in an optically correct, intuitive, and ergonomic mode. Future plans for this platform include the ability to project additional inputs, such as angiograms or echocardiograms, directly onto the viewer's screen. The Vista system, as well as the other 3-D systems, is evolving rapidly and promises to be increasingly user friendly. However, these systems are presently very expensive and may not add much to routine surgery, such as video-assisted thoracic surgery (VATS), for pleural or lung procedures. For procedures requiring magnification, such as endoscopic coronary suturing, these 3-D camera systems may prove valuable.

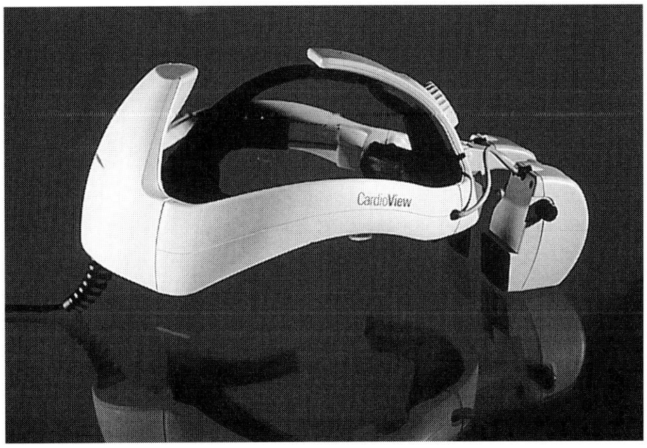

Figure 3–4. Visualization system incorporating a head-mounted display. (Courtesy of Vista, Inc., Westborough, MA)

Scopes

Generally, rigid zero-degree or 30-degree scopes are used. A 30- or 45-degree scope allows better visualization of the thorax. Angled scopes require more training than the zero-degree scope, but the operator will be rewarded by their advantages. Flexible scopes (Olympus Corp) are also available and are described in the earlier section on cameras (Fig 3–5). Flexible thoracoscopes require less light than rigid scopes because the CCD chip is on the distal end of the scope and light is not reflected through any mirrors to the proximal end of the scope. On the horizon are smaller, brighter 2-D scopes. Several manufacturers have developed 2- to 2.7-mm endoscopes for pediatric thoracoscopic procedures to accommodate smaller intercostal spaces. Five-mm thoracoscopes are also available in adult lengths to decrease intercostal trauma and improve mobility of the scope in the intercostal space.

Recording Devices

Pictured in Figure 3–3 are two recording devices: a Sony printer and a VHS video recorder. The printer can document operative findings that can be used as part of the patient's permanent record. The videocassette recorder (VCR) is indispensable for the surgeon to review his or her operative technique critically and is an important tool in teaching residents, fellows, and colleagues. Although a standard home VCR is often used in the operating suite, a higher quality VCR is recommended if editing is anticipated, such as the Super VHS video recorder shown in Figure 3–3. With a Super VHS recorder, the image quality is well maintained if copies are made. All VHS recorders convert the digital signal from the camera to an analog signal. However, it is possible to record the digital signal directly onto a computer in the operating room. This technique has been developed by Wolf and Scott. Currently used is a six-gigabyte, hard-drive, desktop computer with hardware and software that allows video capture, editing, compression, and writing onto a cassette disk (CD). This system is recommended for surgeons who wish to edit and present their video material as the recording is made directly onto the computer and the digital image is superior. Editing can be performed precisely and in a fraction of the time it takes to edit a standard VCR tape. The edited, compressed video can then be written onto a CD that can be played later on a laptop computer. With this system, the surgeon no longer needs to depend on a specific VCR (such as NTSC, SECAM, or PAL). The CD player can

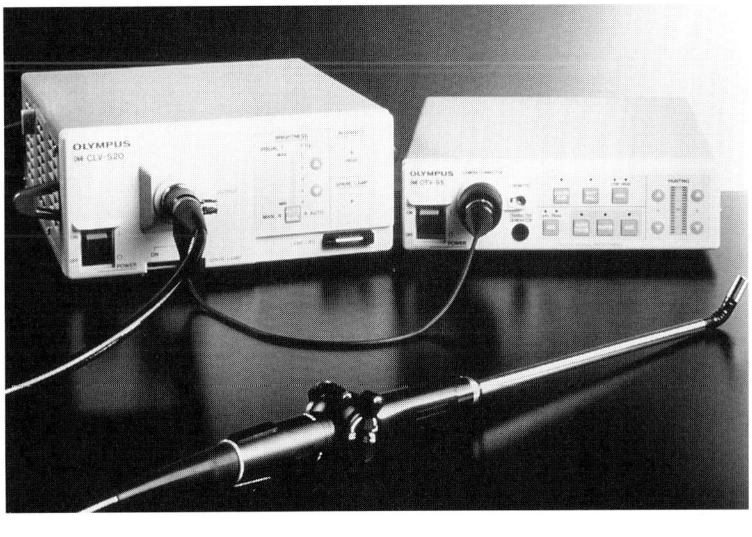

Figure 3–5. Flexible thoracoscopes. (Courtesy of Olympus Corp., America, Inc.; Melville, NY.)

produce a superior image. With a jazz drive, two gigabytes of data can be archived onto one disk.

Enabling Technologies

Besides the basic operating room setup, there are many enabling technologies that will soon be available to the practicing minimal access cardiothoracic surgeon. Readers are referred to Chapters 55 and 83 on future technologies. The Aesop 3000 device (available from Computer Motion, Inc., Goleta, CA) is a voice-controlled thoracoscopic camera holder that allows the operator hands-free control of scope movements (Fig 3–6). This device responds quickly to the surgeon's voice commands. The technology is expensive, but it does decrease scope maneuvering, increases efficiency, and allows a very steady view. This may prove helpful as we move toward endoscopic vessel anastomoses. The voice-activated device is particularly valuable in video-assisted mammary artery mobilization for minimally invasive coronary artery bypass grafting and mitral valve procedures.[3]

Additional technology includes transesophageal echocardiography, which cardiac surgeons already use for standard procedures, angiography equipment, open magnetic resonance imaging (MRI), and navigational devices. The latter use preoperative or intraoperative imaging to pinpoint actual endoscopic positions in real time in the operating suite. Several of these systems are now in prototype form.

Instrumentation

For noncardiac minimal access thoracic procedures, little in the way of disposable thoracoscopic instrumentation is necessary, and many experienced minimal access thoracic surgeons use conventional thoracic instrumentation.[1,4–7] Nonetheless, there are a few sets of reusable thoracoscopic instruments that can be helpful. Kaiser produces one such set of thoracoscopic instruments (available from the Pilling Weck Company, Research Triangle Park, NC). Kaiser-Pilling large modified sponge sticks and Yankour sucker can be particularly helpful. Landreneau has also developed a set of reusable thoracoscopic instruments that include a long, straight endoscopic clamp that can be applied to the lung to compress the tissue and assists in placement of an endoscopic stapler.

An innovative set of reusable thoracoscopic instruments with detachable, interchangeable tips has been developed by Linder (manufactured by the Aesculap Company, Tuttlingen, Germany). All the instruments can be completely dismantled for cleaning and can be assembled in any combination of handle and tip. Angled and straight shafts are available as well as angled tips. The axial handle has the most ergonomic design. Rotation of the instruments around the longitudinal axis is much easier than with pistol-shaped handles. The instrument set also includes a reusable and in situ reloadable clip applier with cartridges containing eight clips. These instruments have been available since 1966 and have proven their worth in terms of precision, stability, and durability.

Burke at Miami Children's Hospital has released a complete set of minimal access thoracoscopic instruments for pediatric cardiothoracic VATS procedures, including repair of congenital heart defects. These instruments accommodate the small size of the pediatric mediastinum and the relative vulnerability of neonatal tissues to mechanical stress. The pediatric intercostal space varies from 2 mm in the premature newborn to 6 mm in the adolescent child, limiting instrumentation to this diameter range to avoid intercostal trauma.

Mechanical stabilization of the imaging system is critical in a confined operative space and can be facilitated by such a device as the mechanical Leonard arm (Leonard Medical, Huntingdon Valley, PA), which has double universal joints operated by a suction system. Instrumentation in this area is evolving rapidly, and many of our current tools are in prototype form. These instruments are particularly suited not only to pediatric work but also to adult work in which 2- to 4-mm instruments and scopes are used [Burke R., personal communication].

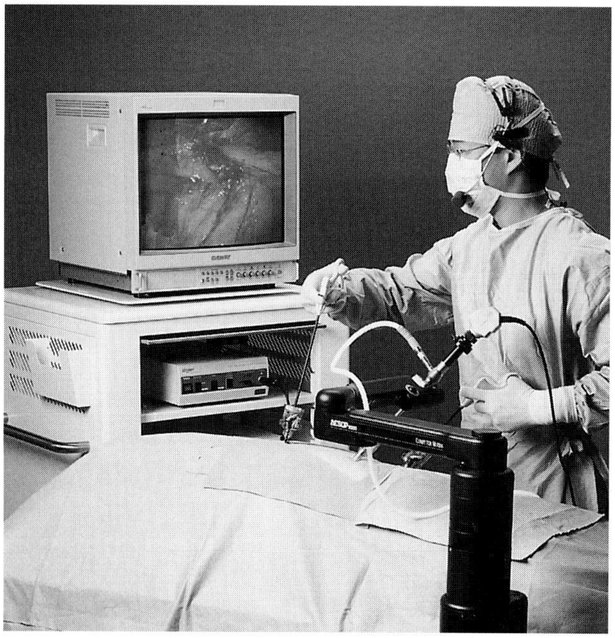

Figure 3–6. Voice-controlled robot AESOP 3000. (Courtesy of Computer Motion, Inc., Goleta, CA.)

Trocars

Trocars are not always necessary, but are usually used for the scope port. Disposable or reusable trocars are available. In minimal access thoracoscopic spine procedures, disposable flexible trocars (Ethicon Endo-Surgery, Cincinnati, OH) allow the use of standard orthopedic spine instruments. Usually 12- to 15-mm ports suffice for most instrumentation. Ports of 2 to 5 mm are available when smaller instruments are used. An instrument between the ribs works best with no port and operates with less trauma to the neurovascular bundle as long as access can be maintained. To increase the mobility of a particular instrument in a rigid port, it is recommended that the rigid port be simply pulled back from the chest wall. The port remains on the instrument outside the chest wall and can be replaced when the instrument is removed. The increased mobility obtained by retracting the trocar may also decrease trauma to the neurovascular bundle.

Retractors

Two reusable mini-thoracotomy retractors (Genzyme Surgical or Naruke) are very easily placed through a 5-cm intercostal incision without distracting the ribs. They are low-profile retractors and provide excellent tactile feedback on rib tension.

Mayo Stand

The Mayo stand contains the instruments needed to begin a minimally invasive thoracic procedure. A scope, a camera, a light cord, one disposable port, graspers, monopolar and bipolar electrocautery, and standard instruments are included. The instrument tray contents are decreased to a minimum. This decreases setup and count time.

Insufflators

Insufflators are not usually helpful in noncardiac minimally access thoracic procedures, but are readily available on laparoscopic carts. For the occasional situation in which it is advantageous to use insufflation (e.g., to hasten lung atelectasis), sealed ports are necessary. In thoracoscopic mammary artery immobilization, insufflation is extremely helpful. A heated CO_2 insufflator is recommended. The pressure limit should be set to 6 to 8 mm Hg. Blood pressure must be continually monitored by arterial line. If hypotension occurs, the insufflation should be stopped immediately.

Instrumentation for Specific Procedures

In general, most noncardiac minimal access thoracic surgery can be performed with a few 12- to 15-mm ports, straight sponge sticks, reusable endoscopic graspers, endoscopic scissors, and disposable endoscopic staplers. In some cases, disposable endoscopic kittners (Ethicon Endo-Surgery, Cincinnati, OH, or U.S. Surgical Corporation, Norwalk, CT) are handy. Instrumentation is discussed in more detail in the appropriate chapters. The brief descriptions here reflect the author's preference.

Wedge Resections

For wedge resections, disposable atraumatic stapling devices are preferred. These are available in 30- to 60-mm lengths and are easy-to-use, reliable devices. For vascular stapling of the hilar vessels, special disposable staplers are also available. For bronchial stapling, endoscopic or open staplers are employed. A knot pusher, tissue bag, disposable bipolar cautery, and endoscopic clip applier are kept available in the operating suite. When dealing with known or possible neoplastic disease, all tissue must be removed after it is placed in a protective tissue bag in the thorax. This should theoretically reduce the potential for port site recurrences of cancer.

VATS Lobectomy

Instruments used for hilar dissection include the Semb clamp and Shallcross clamp. These conventional surgical instruments have very gently curved blunt tips and are generally safer than the standard right-angle clamp. For lung grasping and manipulation, reusable endoscopic graspers and standard or long sponge sticks are ideal.[8] In training programs and with assistants, it is recommended that clamps with ratchets be avoided. If an assistant is distracted from the monitor and his or her position changes, the grip of the nonratcheted device is usually released, avoiding undue inadvertent traction on important structures. The mini-thoracotomy retractors, mentioned previously, can be used for the accessory thoracotomy.

Mediastinal Procedures

Posterior neurogenic tumors, as well as anterior benign tumors and the thymus, can be biopsied and resected utilizing well-discussed thoracoscopic techniques. For hemostastis, disposable endoscopic scissors and bipolar endoscopic cautery are commonly used as well as endoscopic clips. The stone-crushing clamp is an excellent biopsy tool for mediastinal masses. The ports and other instruments are the same as mentioned under Wedge Resections.

Pleural and Pericardial Procedures

For pleural and pericardial procedures, the Harmonic scalpel (Ethicon Endo-Surgery, Cincinnati, OH) can be used in place of electrocautery.[9] This scalpel can coagulate and divide blood vessels. In pericardial procedures, the Harmonic Scalpel can be used near the heart without fear of electrical stimulation because it employs only ultrasound energy. Disposable endoscopic tips for the Harmonic Scalpel are commercially available.

Esophageal Procedures

For esophageal procedures near the diaphragm, it is recommended that the monitors be placed toward the foot of the bed, so the operators can view the screen comfortably while manipulating the instruments. A gastroscope should be available and can be invaluable in delineating areas of interest in the esophagus. The gastroscope transilluminates the esophageal wall and can thus guide the surgeon. Additional thoracoscopic instruments that are commonly used for esophageal procedures can be found in the standard tray outlined earlier.

Operating Room of the Future

Operating suites of the future are being built now. Two of these are in Oslo, Norway. Fosse has outfitted one operating room with monoplane angiography and another with an open MRI system. As use of enabling technology increases, operating rooms will increasingly resemble a hybrid of a sterile operating suite and an interventional suite. These advanced suites will make possible high-risk interventional procedures with increased patient safety. Also, hybrid interventional and operative techniques will be possible in one safe setting. A future goal is to eliminate the necessity of transporting a patient who has failed an interventional procedure to another area of the hospital that is equipped to handle a critically ill patient.

The Zeus project (Computer Motion) incorporates remotely controlled robots that not only control the thoracoscope but also control all instruments placed in the chest. The surgeon can manipulate precise robotic movements using advanced hand controls.

In the future, a surgeon may one day perform a procedure while seated comfortably outside the sterile operating room environment by manipulating robots and utilizing interventional imaging techniques. These scenarios are being developed.

The da Vinci system of advanced robotic controls (Intuitive Surgical, Inc., Mountainview, CA) allows the surgeon to manipulate instruments and successfully suture coronary anastomoses thoracoscopically. This system is currently available in Europe and will soon be available in the United States.[2]

Conclusion

With trained personnel, including a minimally invasive scrub nurse, a circulating nurse, an attentive anesthesiologist, and an assistant who is comfortable with endoscopic procedures, the setup and initiation of a VATS procedure can be routine and enjoyable. There is little question that the patient benefits from a properly outfitted and manned minimally invasive thoracic surgery suite. This type of suite is increasingly technology dependent and will continue to evolve rapidly over the next few years. Ultimately, robots and interventional setups may be commonplace in the operating room as we pass into the next millennium.

References

1. Boutin C, Viallat JR, Aelony Y: Practical Thoracoscopy. Berlin, Springer-Verlag, 1991.
2. Falk V, Walther T, Autschbach R, et al: Robot-assisted minimally invasive solo mitral valve operation. Thorac Cardiovasc Surg 115:470–471, 1998.
3. Harshbarger JH: Standardization of the television raster for non-broadcast applications. SMPTE J 804, 1982.
4. Kaiser CR, Daniel TM: Thoracoscopic Surgery. Boston, Little, Brown, 1993.
5. Krasna MJ, Mack MJ: Atlas of Thoracoscopic Surgery. St. Louis, Quality Medical Publishing, 1994.
6. Landreneau RJ, Dowling RD, Castillo W, et al: Thoracoscopic resection of an anterior mediastinal mass. Ann Thorac Surg 54:142, 1992.
7. Mack MJ, Aronoff RJ, Acuff TE, et al: Present role of thoracoscopy in the diagnosis and treatment of diseases of the chest. Ann Thorac Surg 54:403, 1992.
8. McKenna RJ: VATS lobectomy with mediastinal lymph node sampling or dissection. Chest Surg Clin North Am 5:2, 223–232, 1995.
9. Ohtsuka T, Wolf RK, Dunsker SB: Port-access first rib resection with new instruments: A report of two cases. J Surg Endosc (in press).

COMMENTARY

Anthony P. C. Yim

This chapter by Wolf gives a detailed description of his personal choice of equipment as well as what is available. One important difference between laparoscopy and video-assisted thoracic surgery (VATS) is that in the latter, the chest is bound by a rigid rib cage. As the lung is collapsed with selective one-lung vertilation, there is ample room for instrument maneuvering. Carbon dioxide insufflation (and hence valved ports) is usually unnecessary. Conventional thoracic instruments can be used, and these can be placed directly through stab incisions without trocars as mentioned by the author. The whole setup requires a low level of technology, yet is effective and safe, without having dazzling technology that could potentially distract the surgeon from focusing on the patient.

Chapter 4

Anesthesia for Video-Assisted Thoracic Surgery

John M. Low

Minimally invasive, or limited access, surgery has provided an enormous stimulus to the development of new techniques and ingenious equipment. Over the past two decades, nearly every procedure has been attempted with varying degrees of success. The first thoracoscopy has generally been attributed to Jacobaeus in 1910, in which he performed intrapleural pneumolysis for tuberculosis under local analgesia. However, it has really been since the early 1990s that developments in the technology have allowed widespread, and relatively safe, clinical applications of thoracoscopic techniques.[24] By its very nature, thoracoscopy is more demanding on the ability of the anesthetist to provide the satisfactory conditions for surgical access, usually achieved by one-lung ventilation.[1,15,20,24,27,33,39]

Risks, Benefits, and Complications

As the technology continues to evolve, so does the level of expertise achieved by the operator. The balance between the risk of the procedure and the benefits of minimal access techniques[1,14,20,24,32,39] is continually changing. It is, therefore, prudent to adopt a flexible attitude toward recommending such procedures to high-risk patients. Although an uncomplicated video-assisted thoracic surgery (VATS) procedure can be very well tolerated by many patients, representing a wide range of preoperative conditions, one significant consideration is the possibility of conversion to open thoracotomy and its implicit risks. The risks and benefits of VATS, and the possibility of open thoracotomy, must therefore be fully explained to the patient.

Anesthesia for VATS should be undertaken by specialists who have interest and experience in thoracic or cardiothoracic surgery. The proximity of the lungs to the major cardiac structures has an important impact on the nature of anesthesia for thoracic surgery. The anesthesiologist and the thoracic surgeon need to collaborate in choosing the correct anesthetic technique for the individual patient. One-lung ventilation (OLV) has always represented a challenge for the anesthesiologist.[1,4,15,20,25,27,29,33,39] However, because of the limited access available to the surgeon performing VATS, it is not possible to compensate for a partially deflated lung by the use of a lung retractor. Failure to isolate the ipsilateral lung completely renders the procedure unnecessarily difficult. Some movement of the lung and the mediastinum can be tolerated in all but the most demanding surgery. Anesthetic techniques for VATS in the pediatric population are covered in a chapter 36.

Preoperative Assessment

As with all contemporary anesthetic practice, the prelude to smooth anesthetic management is a thorough preoperative assessment of the patient, with both clinical and objective tests of cardiac and pulmonary function. During this visit, the anesthesiologist discusses with the patient not only the risk factors associated with the surgical procedure, but also the options for perioperative care and pain relief. The objective is to allay the patient's fear and anxiety by communicating information to the patient, as well as providing premedication drugs.[1,14,15,27,32,33,39]

All thoracic and thoracoscopic surgeries should be treated as major procedures, from the consideration of pathophysiologic changes to the body as well as the potential for major morbidity and mortality.[1,4,14,32,33] Ambulatory surgery in the strict sense is, therefore, not appropriate, except for the simplest procedures. Patients should be fully assessed and screened, as is usual in the preparation for major surgery.[1,14,15,20,27]

In addition, emphasis should be placed on the preoperative assessment of the cardiovascular and pulmonary systems, because these systems bear the major consequences of major surgery, lateral positioning, and OLV. By optimizing the patient's condition before administration of general anesthesia, there is a reduction in perioperative morbidity and mortality. This is particularly beneficial in regard to anesthesia for thoracic surgery, in which the process of surgery may compromise respiratory function sufficiently to cause early postoperative morbidity, resulting in a prolonged hospital stay. The known stress factors of thoracoscopy include hypoxemia, hypercapnia, and sympathetic nervous system activation, resulting in hypertension and tachycardia. Therefore, it is imperative to assess not only the risk of ischemic heart disease but also pulmonary function and respiratory reserve.[1,14,20,24,32,34,39]

During history taking, specific, unbiased questions should be asked, relating to risk factors associated with thoracic surgery, such as age (exceeding 60 years), and exercise tolerance. A history of smoking and symptoms related to bronchospasm and increased bronchial secretions are especially important, because preoperative physiotherapy and antibiotic prophylaxis may reduce the risk of complications. Lung function tests are simple and economical and should be undertaken routinely.

During preoperative respiratory care, the following should be considered [1,15,28]:

1. Discontinuation of smoking is mandatory. Apart from its major contribution to ischemic heart disease, chronic particulate irritation to the airways increases

the likelihood of bronchospasm and increased bronchial secretions.

2. If reversible airway obstruction is detected clinically or following pulmonary function tests, measures should be taken to dilate the airways. These include administration of β_2-adrenergic antagonists; phosphodiesterase inhibitors (aminophylline, theophylline); nebulized steroids; and, if time allows, sodium dichromoglycate.
3. Reduced secretions should be achieved by a combination of mucolytic agents (i.e., humidification, rehydration, acetylcysteine, expectorant drugs) and physical drainage (i.e., coughing, postural drainage, chest physiotherapy by percussion and vibration).
4. Medical therapy, in relation to possible anemia, sepsis, cor pulmonale, and cardiac dysrhythmias should be optimized. Digitalization, even in the absence of atrial fibrillation, should be considered.
5. A positive psychological state in a patient expedites recovery, and he or she can be motivated with this objective. The patient who is aware that medical therapy has been carefully optimized also benefits subjectively from attention to his or her nutritional state and motivation, such as the use of incentive spirometry.
6. The use of anticholinergic drugs may be of benefit only in those patients who have copious secretions. Their routine use is unnecessary because current inhalation anesthetic agents are far less prone to stimulate bronchial secretions than the classic agents, such as ether and trichloroethylene.

Technique of General Anesthesia

An anesthesiologist who has a thorough understanding of the nature and duration of the VATS procedure is able to draw upon a wide range of available anesthetic drugs and inhalation agents. A wide choice of drugs is available for inducing balanced anesthesia for VATS. Our common practice is to use either diazepam (0.2–0.3 mg/kg) or midazolam (0.1 mg/kg) as an anxiolytic before transferring the patient to the operating suite. As our operating room schedule accommodates 16,800 cases per annum, it is not possible to estimate the timing of the premedication with a high degree of precision, and diazepam has greater flexibility than midazolam in this respect. General anesthesia is frequently induced with fentanyl (1–2 μg/kg),[1] propofol (1–2 mg/kg), and vecuronium (0.1 mg/kg) with morphine (0.1 mg/kg) supplementation for longer procedures and for postoperative analgesia. Maintenance of anesthesia is provided by ventilation with 0.5% to 1.5% isoflurane in nitrous oxide and oxygen. Postoperative analgesia (see Postoperative Management) is implemented in the postanesthesia care unit (PACU).

Anesthesia Workstation

Our institution has installed the North American Drager (NAD) Narkomed 4 as the standard anesthesia workstation. The major advantages include an excellent ventilator (AV2) offering ventilation rates of 1 to 99 breaths/min^{-1}, pressure limitation to reduce pulmonary barotrauma, and the facility of positive end expiratory pressure (PEEP) (Fig 4–1) as standard at every workstation. In particular, the inclusion of an auxiliary oxygen flowmeter (Fig 4–2) allows the connection of a simple and inexpensive device for maintaining a continuous positive airway pressure (CPAP) circuit to the collapsed lung (Fig 4–3).

Monitoring

In accordance with the monitoring requirements of the Hong Kong College of Anaesthesiologists (http://www.hkca.edu.hk), our institution uses the standard mandatory monitoring for anesthesia during VATS. The physiologic variables monitored include noninvasive blood pressure (NIBP), a 3- or 5-lead electrocardiograph (ECG), pulse oximetry (SpO_2), airway pressure (Paw), and spirometry (tidal and minute volume) of the expired breathing circuit. The objective of close monitoring is to maintain the range of the patient's vital signs within 15% of preoperative readings. Inspired and expired gas analyses allow the continuous measurement of oxygen, nitrous oxide, carbon dioxide, and volatile anesthetic concentration from the patient's breathing circuit.

Future Monitoring Options

Pressure-volume (P-V) loop monitoring is not a standard feature on many anesthetic machines, with the exception of the Datex AS/3 ADU (Datex-Engstrom Division, Instrumentation Corp., Helsinki, Finland). The considerable information provided by P-V loops can be of enormous

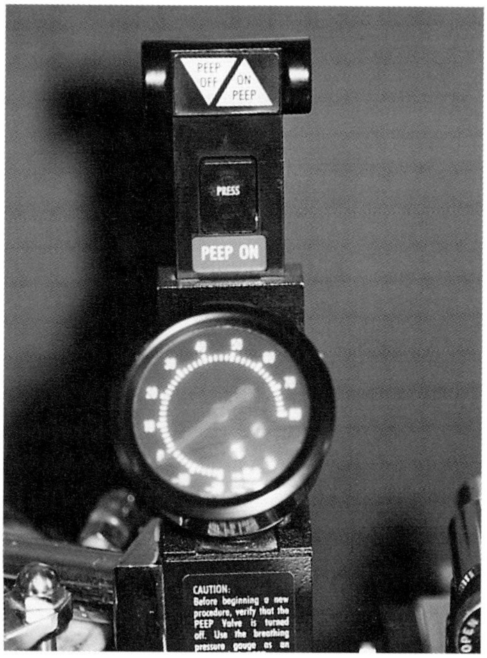

Figure 4–1. Adjustable positive end expiratory pressure (PEEP) valve available as a standard feature of the anesthesia workstation. Activation of the PEEP valve automatically displays a warning red flag. The amount of PEEP is displayed on an analog gauge as well as on the airway pressure monitor.

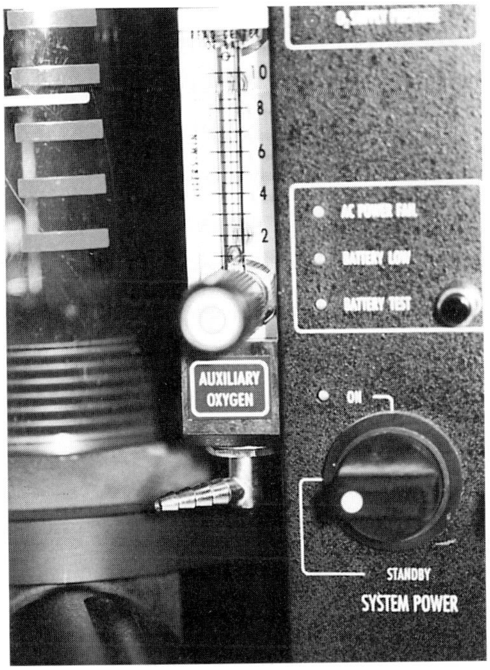

Figure 4–2. Auxiliary oxygen flowmeter allows the control of supplementary oxygen independently of the fresh gas supply to the patient circuit.

benefit to the thoracic anesthesiologist because these data make possible very early detection of leaks in the circuit as well as decreased lung compliance and changes in lung elastance.

One-Lung Ventilation

The best surgical field is achieved by the use of endobronchial intubation and single-lung ventilation.[1,4,17,20,34,39] However, in trying to provide the best surgical conditions, the technique of one-lung ventilation (OLV) compromises ventilation-perfusion balance in the lungs and increases venous admixture, leading to reduced arterial oxygenation. A full description of the normal anatomy and physiology of the lung, as well as the pathophysiologic changes during single-lung ventilation, is to be found in the definitive text on the subject by Dr. Jonathan Benumof.[1] In practice, it is impossible to undertake adequate thoracoscopy without isolation and collapse of the lung. Although thoracoscopy can be performed under local analgesia,[15,35] the mainstay technique is the use of a double-lumen tube (DLT) for endobronchial intubation, with intentional collapse of the lung ipsilateral to the pathology. Another means of isolating the lung is by the use of bronchial blockers (Univent™).[23] Some centers favor the use of carbon dioxide insufflation using a Veres needle, for improved surgical access and vision.[20] Recently, the use of oxygen insufflation through a single-lumen endotracheal tube for short VATS procedures has been described.[44]

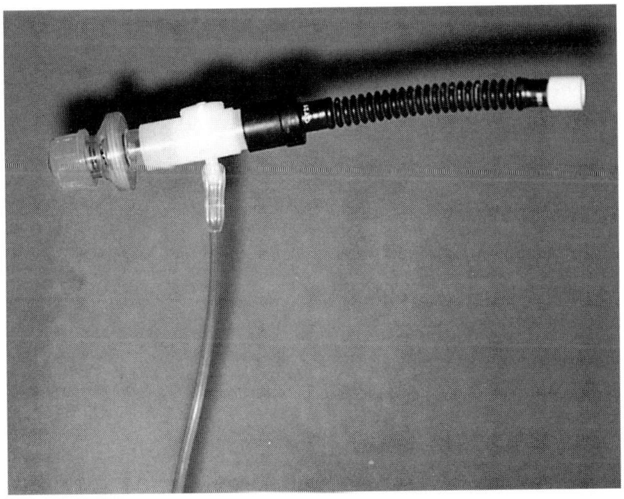

Figure 4–3. A simple and economical apparatus assembled from commonly available anesthetic items, capable of delivering adjustable continuous positive airway pressure (CPAP) to the collapsed lung during one-lung ventilation.

Placement of Endobronchial Tube

There are many methods for the "blind" placement of the endobronchial tube. The classic endobronchial tube still in use is the Robertshaw DLT, which is anatomically shaped for right or left endobronchial use and available in small, medium, and large sizes. The pronounced curvature of the left Robertshaw pattern makes it suitable for easy intubation by direct laryngoscopy. More often than not, a malleable stylet is needed for passing the right Robertshaw tube through the vocal cords. However, the advantage of the Robertshaw pattern is that the anatomic shape lends itself to easy placement once it has been passed through the vocal cords.

Right Side or Left?

The classic dilemma over which side of the lung to isolate prompted the choice of an endobronchial tube, which isolates the bronchus contralateral to the lung containing the pathology. However, current teaching about the choice of endobronchial intubation favors left-sided intubation in the majority of cases, whichever lung contains the pathology, unless there is a chance of surgery on the left main bronchial stem. In that case, right-sided endobronchial intubation is recommended. Because of anatomic considerations, there is a high risk of occluding the right upper lobe if right endobronchial intubation is performed, and, therefore, current practice favors left-sided intubation, unless otherwise specifically indicated.

Choice of Endobronchial Tube Size

The size of the endobronchial tube can be assessed by clincial experience in the majority of cases, but a more accurate prediction of endobronchial tube size can be made from the computed tomography (CT) scan,[22] and the tracheal size seen on chest radiograph (CXR).[10] Correct sizing is important because the complications of misplacement and obstruction to the bronchi often occur when the endobronchial tube size is inappropriately small for the patient and the tube is unintentionally advanced beyond the optimal position.

Fiberoptic Bronchoscopy

That fiberoptic bronchoscopy (FOB) should be the standard of care in the placement of endobronchial tubes is still controversial. Some protagonists,[2,19,43] would like bronchoscopy to become an established practice in every endobronchial intubation. Others[7,9] consider the use of FOB extremely important, but in selective situations. There are some institutions where FOB is performed routinely both in the supine position and also in the lateral decubitus position. Ideally, this procedure should be performed. However, it is costly and time consuming to enforce this as a rigid protocol. Fiberoptic scopes require capital expenditure as well as maintenance and labor costs in terms of preparation and sterilization for the next patient.

The practice in our institution is to insert a Robertshaw endobronchial tube by direct laryngoscopy, and if the placement is clinically unquestionably correct, including the presence of breath sounds in the right apex, the tube is secured and the patient is placed in the decubitus position. If there is some distortion of the patient's bronchial anatomy, or if auscultation or a poor end tidal carbon dioxide trace casts any doubt about the placement of the tube, the threshold for using FOB is very low. In actual practice, we often share the FOB equipment with the surgical team, and thus the scope, the light source, and the video camera are always at hand. If FOB is required, the use of a video camera and monitor provides an educational exercise for all the staff members in attendance.

We emphasize the need to inspect the endobronchial tube (passing the fiberoptic scope through the tracheal lumen) and then confirm placement of the endobronchial portion of the tube (via endobronchial lumen), checking for the right upper lobe orifice, which requires a 70-degree flexion of the scope. Herniation of either cuff leading to airway obstruction can also be excluded by FOB. This procedure is repeated with the patient in the lateral decubitus position in preparation for surgery. The FOB and light source are then kept on standby, and FOB is repeated during periods of unexplained desaturation. Our experience is that FOB is nearly always required for bronchial blockers (Univent) and the PVC-type, double-lumen tubes (Portex, Mallinckrodt). Finally, we believe that FOB is of enormous value in aiding the removal of secretions that occur at the end of any major VATS procedure. Our practice is to keep the FOB equipment available until the end of the VATS procedure for the purpose of performing bronchial toilet.

Problems with Placement

Unintentional placement of the endobronchial tube in the contralateral bronchus is common, but, fortunately, it is an easy problem to recognize and to rectify. Even when the correct side is intubated, the optimal position must be obtained by adjusting how far the tube is inserted. Careful auscultation and confirmation by FOB helps the operator to achieve correct tube placement. It is important to check the placement of the tube once again after the patient has been placed in the lateral decubitus position, and the operating table has been articulated,[45] because during this part of the procedure the tube can easily be displaced. Herniation of the endobronchial and endotracheal cuff is a possibility that should always be borne in mind, so that obstruction of one or the other lumens can be corrected promptly. If there is failure to isolate the lung, FOB should be performed. In addition, high-frequency ventilation may need to be implemented or conventional ventilation may need to be applied to the operated lung. In some centers, the use of a Veres needle to insufflate the pleural cavity with carbon dioxide is helpful.

Management of Arterial Hypoxemia

An inescapable consequence of OLV is that the majority of cardiac output entering the immobile and collapsed lung is unoxygenated. This imbalance between ventilation (V) and perfusion (Q) leads to arterial hypoxemia. Increasing the fraction of inspired oxygen (FiO_2) and adding positive end expiratory pressure (PEEP) to the ventilated lung improve oxygenation immediately. Other approaches are usually followed to reduce the effect of this shunting. In the first place, residual blood flow in the collapsed lung can be oxygenated by using apneic insufflation with oxygen (sometimes labeled "continuous positive airway pressure" [CPAP]) by means of an auxiliary oxygen source. Intermittent reinflation of the lung also achieves this, although surgical access is compromised or interrupted. The other approach is to limit the blood flowing through the nonventilated lung. In this respect, gravity is helpful in favoring blood flow to the ventilated lung. Low concentrations of oxygen in residual alveoli of the collapsed lung would normally stimulate the hypoxic vasoconstrictor response in the pulmonary arteries. Furthermore, the increased vascular resistance in a collapsed lung tends to result in reduced flow.[1,3,4,33,41]

There has been an interest in the pharmacologic control of pulmonary blood flow. Canine studies have demonstrated the ability to achieve selective pulmonary artery vasoconstriction by the infusion of prostaglandin $F_{2\alpha}$.[12] Another approach has been the selective ventilation of one lung with nitric oxide, which obviates the systemic effects of using nitric oxide donor drugs (e.g., sodium nitroprusside, nitroglycerin).[21,40]

A novel approach described by Rozenberg uses single-lumen ventilation, postural changes (the patient is raised 60 to 70 degrees from the horizontal position), and carbon dioxide insufflation via a Veres needle to help induce an artificial pneumothorax and collapse of the operated lung.[41] However, there would be a major problem should the patient develop hypotension, and reinflation of a collapsed lung is less easily achieved with a single-lumen tube, as predicted by the Laplace principle (Table 4–1).

Positioning

After ensuring satisfactory induction of anesthesia and correct placement of the double-lumen endotracheal tube,

Table 4–1. Complications of One-Lung Ventilation (OLV)

1. Failure to isolate one lung
2. Obstruction by cuff herniation
3. Cardiovascular instability
4. Hypoxemia
5. Bronchopleural fistula
6. Pleural effusion
7. Persistent pneumothorax
8. Hypercapnia and air embolism (from CO_2 insufflation)

the next priority is to prepare the patient for surgery by safe and suitable positioning. Most VATS requires a patient to be placed in a lateral decubitus position with arching of the operating table to widen the intercostal spaces on the operated side.[45] Care should be taken during the change to the lateral position, and attention should be given to potential pressure areas in the lateral position. Deliberate disconnection of the ventilator circuit just before turning the patient reduces the chance of accidental extubation or displacement of the endobronchial tube. A soft axillary support is placed. The eyelids are carefully taped to avoid the risk of corneal abrasion during the procedure. After placing the arms in a comfortable position, care is taken to ensure that both ulnar nerves are protected from pressure damage. A waterproof sheet is placed under the patient's head to collect potential oral secretions, which may be spilled in the lateral position. Depending on the anticipated duration of the procedure, measures to maintain body temperature should be used, including a heated water blanket or air blanket, a warm covering, and humidification of anesthetic gases. Finally, the anesthesiologist should ensure adequate access to monitoring leads, arterial and venous lines, and easy access to the patient's airway and ventilator connections. It should be possible to perform bronchoscopy readily in the lateral position should there be an episode of hypoxemia or incomplete lung isolation.

Transport of the Patient

Safety and care of the patient in the postoperative period should be commensurate with a meticulous intraoperative technique. Extreme care should be taken during transfer of the patient from the operating table to the bed or transport trolley. The anesthesiologist should be dedicated to care for the patient's head, neck, and airway, and all movement should be directed by the anesthesiologist. Intravascular catheters should be secured, and care should be taken that monitoring and intravenous lines do not become entangled during transfer. Before transfer is attempted, all chest drains should be clamped securely to prevent siphoning of fluid into the pleural cavity, and the clamps should be released as soon as the underwater seals are secured below the level of the patient. Allowing the patient to sit upright at a 45-degree angle improves ventilatory function. Finally, the patient's transport trolley or bed should allow easy positioning for a portable CXR to assess re-expansion of the collapsed lung postoperatively. Patients at risk should be monitored fully, and many self-powered portable monitors allow a comprehensive range of physiologic variables to be recorded during transport. Following extubation, all patients who have had VATS should be given supplemental oxygen by mask, nasal cannula, or nebulizer. A comfortable bed not only allows adequate support for monitors when necessary, but also provides space for underwater seals and a portable oxygen source. Furthermore, mechanical adjustment of the bed may allow an upright posture for the patient to improve functional residual capacity by 0.5 to 1.0 L.[16,28,34]

Postoperative Management

The vast majority of patients undergoing VATS follow an uneventful perioperative course, and few difficulties should be encountered during extubation in the operating room. The effect of postoperative pain and residual muscle paralysis is to impair ventilatory function and the ability to cough and clear mucous secretions. There is a significant reduction in vital capacity and functional residual capacity. In addition, patients undergoing pulmonary surgery may have pre-existing chronic obstructive airway disease. In such cases, the already diminished pulmonary function is further compromised by surgery, especially resection of pulmonary tissue. Careful and thorough bronchial toilet, using flexible-suction catheters through each lumen of the endobronchial tube, can overcome the problem of bronchial secretions. However, more complete bronchial toilet may be achieved by the routine use of FOB at the end of the procedure, just before extubation. Changing to a single-lumen endotracheal tube facilitates bronchial toilet by allowing a larger size FOB.

Patients who have severely diminished pulmonary function can benefit from a comprehensive perioperative management plan aimed at maximizing pulmonary function, before administration of general anesthesia and ventilation.[1,14,15,27] Postoperative elective ventilation may, however, be anticipated for some patients who will be weaned off the ventilation gradually over a period of time ranging from several hours to several days. Single-lumen endotracheal tubes are suitable for postoperative ventilation and should preferably be exchanged before transfer to an intensive care unit (ICU). Following a period of rewarming, fluid balance, adequate analgesia, lung re-expansion, and optimization of physiologic variables, the patient with severely compromised pulmonary function has every chance of successful extubation.

Postoperative CXR is mandatory, and this excludes residual pneumothorax and rarely, hemothorax. The position of the chest drain is confirmed and similarly, the central venous pressure line, if present. Mediastinal shift should be minimal following VATS. Atelectasis is best avoided by applying controlled positive pressure to each lung to re-expand the lung following surgery, and before extubation. Sustained positive pressure to both lungs simultaneously is not as effective as that applied to a single lung, because greater pressure is required to re-expand a collapsed lung. Following extubation, continuous gentle suction (10 to 20 cm H_2O) should ensure that any residual pneumothorax, if present, remains minimal.

Postoperative Analgesia

Adequate analgesia without excessive sedation also facilitates the process of extubation by allowing deeper inspiratory efforts and the ability to cough without pain. There are many fuller texts that deal with this topic at length, and the reader is referred to these. The method of postoperative analgesia may take various forms. Immediate postoperative analgesia may also be provided by intercostal nerve blocks. Performed under direct vison of the nerve during VATS, such blocks are particularly effective, and if bupivacaine is combined with adrenaline, pain relief may last for several hours. Intravenous opioid analgesia is commonly used intraoperatively, and this may be continued postoperatively in the postanesthetic care unit (PACU). When resources are limited, a simple protocol to administer 1 to 3 mg of intravenous (IV) morphine (appropriately diluted), at 5-minute intervals, helps to ensure a comfortable patient by titrating the analgesia without producing excessive sedation. This may be followed by patient-administered analgesia (PCA), using simple disposable or electronic PCA devices available. Thoracic epidural analgesia is rarely required in VATS. Some centers, however, have developed the routine use of patient-controlled epidural analgesia (PCEA), using bupivacaine 0.1%, and ropivacaine 0.25%, with or without fentanyl 10 μg/ml added to the infusion. Under supervision of a well-established acute pain service, this can be very beneficial. Nonsteroidal anti-inflammatory drugs (NSAIDs) may also be used as an adjunct to opioid analgesia, and ketorolac is the most suitable, as it may be administered by IV and intramuscular (IM) routes. However, caution should always be used, because these drugs can aggravate conditions such as peptic ulcer, asthma, or coagulation disorders. Renal impairment is a contraindication to the use of this drug. Recent interest has been shown in the use of continuous extrapleural intercostal analgesia[18,37] and continuous paravertebral infusion.[30,38]

Summary

VATS presents a challenge to the surgeon and the anesthesiologist alike, with the introduction of new techniques and equipment. There are extra demands for the anesthesiologist to provide excellent surgical conditions for the procedure, not only to make it possible, but also to ensure a high level of patient safety. Practical anesthetic techniques to achieve these objectives have been described.

References

1. Benumof JL (ed): Anesthesia for Thoracic Surgery, 2nd ed. Philadelphia, WB Saunders, 1995.
2. Benumof JL, Partiridge BL, Salvatierra C, et al: Margin of safety in positioning modern double-lumen endotracheal tubes. Anesthesiology 67:729–738, 1987.
3. Benumof J: Mechanisms of decreased blood flow to atelectatic lung. J Appl Physiol 46:1047–1048, 1978.
4. Benumof J: One-lung ventilation and hypoxic pulmonary vasoconstriction: Implications for anesthetic management. Anesth Analg 64:821–833, 1985.
5. Body SC: Thoracic epidural analgesia. *In* Ferrante FM, Vadeboncouer TR (eds): Postoperative Pain Management. New York, Churchill Livingstone, 1993, pp 417–440.
6. Brodner G: Pain management in patients undergoing thoracic surgery. Curr Opin Anaesthesiol (serial online) 10:54–59, 1997. Available at: http://anaesthesiology.currentopinion.com
7. Brodsky JB, Macario A, Cannon WB, et al: 'Blind' placement of plastic left double lumen tubes. Anaesth Intensive Care 23: 583–586, 1995.
8. Brodsky JB, Mark JBD: A simple technique for accurate placement of double-lumen endotrachael tubes. Anesthesiol Rev 10: 26–30, 1983.
9. Brodsky JB: Proper positioning of a double-lumen endobronchial tube can only be accomplished with endoscopy. J Cardiothorac Vasc Anesth 2:105–109, 1988.
10. Brodsky JB, Mackey S, Cannon WB: Selecting the correct size left double lumen tube (Letter). J Cardiothorac Vasc Anesth 11:924–925, 1997.
11. Brodsky JB, Macario A, Mark JBD: Tracheal diameter predicts double lumen tube size: A method for selecting left double lumen tubes. Anaesth Analg 82:861–864, 1996.
12. Chen T-L, Ueng T-H, Huang C-H, et al: Improvement of arterial oxygenation by selective infusion of prostaglandin E_1 to ventilated lung during one-lung ventilation. Acta Anaesthesiol Scand 40:7–13, 1996.
13. Chui PT, Gin T, Oh TE: Anaesthesia for laparoscopic general surgery. Anaesth Intensive Care 21:163–171, 1993.
14. Coosemans W, Lerut T: Risks and benefits of thoracoscopic surgery. Curr Opin Anaesthesiol 10:48–53, 1997.
15. Craigo P: Anaesthesia for thoracoscopic procedures. Department of Anesthesia and Critical Care, The University of Chicago. Vascular Thoracic Manual. Available at: http://dacc.bsd.uchicago.edu/library/manuals/vtmanual/thoracoscopy.html.
16. Craig DB, Wahba WM, Don HF, et al: "Closing volume" and its relationship to gas exchange in seated and supine positions. J Appl Physiol 31:717, 1971.
17. Desiderio DP, Burt M, Kolker AC, et al: The effects of endobronchial cuff inflation on double-lumen endobronchial tube movement after lateral decubitus positioning. J Cardiothorac Vasc Anesth 11:595–598, 1997.
18. Downs CS, Cooper MG: Continuous extrapleural intercostal nerve block for post thoracotomy analgesia in children. Anaesth Intensive Care 25:390–397, 1997.
19. Ehrenwerth J: Proper positioning of a double-lumen endobronchial tube can only be accomplished with endoscopy. J Cardiothorac Vasc Anesth 2:101–104, 1988.
20. Fredman B, Olsfanger D, Jedeikin R: Thoracoscopic sympathectomy in the treatment of palmar hyperhidrosis: Anaesthetic implications. Br J Anaesth 79:113–119, 1997.
21. Hambraeus-Jonzon K, Bindslev L, Frostell C, et al: Effect of unilaterally inhaled NO during selective lung ventilation in anesthetized humans. Anesthesiology 81:A1457, 1994.
22. Hannallah M, Benumof JL, Silverman PM, et al: Evaluation of an approach to choosing a left double lumen tube size based on chest computed tomographic scan measurement of left mainstem bronchial diameter. J Cardiothorac Vasc Anaesth 11:168–171, 1997.
23. Hannallah M: The Univent tube: Bronchial cuff inflation. Anesthesiology 75:165–166, 1991.
24. Harris RJ, Kavuru MS, Rice TW, et al: The diagnostic and therapeutic utility of thoracoscopy. Chest 108:828–841, 1995.
25. Hedenstierna G: Gas exchange during anaesthesia. Br J Anaesth 64:507–514, 1990.
26. Hill RC, Jones DR, Vance RA, et al: Selective lung ventilation during thoracoscopy: Effects of insufflation on haemodynamics. Ann Thorac Surg 61:945–948, 1996.
27. Horswell JL: Anesthetic techniques for thoracoscopy. Ann Thorac Surg 56:624, 1993.
28. Jacobsohn E: The management of the patient after thoracic surgery. Department of Anesthesia and Critical Care, The Uni-

versity of Chicago. Vascular Thoracic Manual. Available at: Webmaster@dacc.uchicago.edu.

29. Katz Y, Zisman E, Isserles SA, et al: Left but not right, one-lung ventilation causes hypoxaemia during endoscopic transthoracic sympathectomy. J Cardiothorac Vasc Anesth 10:207–209, 1996.
30. Karmakar MK, Booker PD, Franks R, et al: Continuous extrapleural paravertebral infusion of bupivacaine for post-thoracotomy analgesia in young infants. Br J Anaesth 76:811–815, 1996.
31. Kavanagh BP: Pain control after thoracic surgery. A review of current techniques. Anesthesiology 81:737–759, 1994.
32. Krasna MJ, Deshmuhk S, McLaughlin JS: Complications of thoracoscopy. Ann Thorac Surg 61:1066–1069, 1996.
33. Larbuisson R, Lamy M: Anaesthesia for thoracoscopic surgery. Curr Opin Anaesthesiol 10:44–47, 1997.
34. Lumb AB, Nunn JF: Respiratory function and ribcage contribution to ventilation in body positions commonly used during anaesthesia. Anaesth Analg 73:422–426, 1991.
35. Morton JR, Guinn GA: Thoracoscopy using local anaesthesia. Am J Surg 122:696–698, 1971.
36. Mulder DS: Pain management principles and anesthesia techniques for thoracoscopy. Ann Thorac Surg 56:630, 1993.
37. Murphy DF: Interpleural analgesia. Br J Anaesth 71:426–434, 1993.
38. Perttunen K, Nilsson E, Heinonen J, et al: Extradural, paravertebral and intercostal nerve blocks for post-thoracotomy pain. Br J Anaesth 75:541–547, 1995.
39. Plummer S, Hartley M, Vaughan RS: Anaesthesia for telescopic procedures in the thorax. Br J Anaesth 80:223–234, 1998.
40. Rich GF, Lowson SM, Johns RA, et al: Inhaled nitric oxide selectively decreases pulmonary vascular resistance without impairing oxygenation during one-lung ventilation in patients undergoing cardiac surgery. Anesthesiology 8:57–62, 1994.
41. Rozenberg B, Katz Y, Isserles SA, et al: Near-sitting position and two-lung ventilation for endoscopic transthoracic sympathectomy. J Cardiothorac Vasc Anesth 10:210–212, 1996.
42. Schultz A-M, Werba A, Ulbing S, et al: Peri-operative thoracic epidural analgesia for thoracotomy. Eur J Anaesthesiol 14:600–603, 1997.
43. Smith GB, Hirsh NP, Ehrenwerth J: Placement of double-lumen endobronchial tubes. Br J Anaesth 58:1317–1320, 1986.
44. Tseng C-C, Wu M-H, Day Y-B, et al: Clinical application of transorotracheal tube tracheal insufflation of oxygen in patients undergoing simple video-assisted thoracoscopic surgery. Anesth Analg 84:20–25, 1997.
45. Yim APC: Minimizing chest wall trauma in video assisted thoracic surgery. J. Thorac Cardiovasc Surg 109:1255–1256, 1995.

Chapter 5

Strategic Planning for Video-Assisted Thoracic Surgery

Jeffrey C. Lin and Rodney J. Landreneau

Advances in video and endoscopic instrumentation, endoscopic surgical instruments, and the evolution of proper endosurgical techniques[1, 2] have allowed rapid expansion in video-assisted operative approaches in nearly every surgical discipline. Thoracic surgery is no exception. The development of endoscopic surgical instruments and techniques has facilitated the evolution of thoracoscopy from a diagnostic to a therapeutic modality. In less than 10 years, minimally invasive video-assisted thoracic surgery (VATS) has evolved from a concept to the preferred approach for many common thoracic surgery problems. There has been an exponential increase in the number and variety of operations now performed with VATS techniques. The VATS approach has pervaded the practice of general thoracic surgery today, just as laparoscopic approaches now dominate many aspects of general surgery.

The central goal of VATS approaches is to reduce postoperative pain and other post–thoracotomy-related morbidity that follows thoracic surgery without compromising the therapeutic principles of open thoracic surgery.[1, 3, 4] Successful implementation of these goals has made VATS the preferred approach for diagnostic and therapeutic interventions in many intrathoracic disease processes.

Because of the vital role of appropriate instrumentation and associated equipment in the performance of VATS, a brief outline of the necessary video and operative instruments is covered in this chapter. The basic VATS approach strategies that are important in accomplishing safe and efficacious VATS procedures are then detailed.

Instrumentation for Imaging

The 10-mm, zero-degree, rigid "operating" thoracoscope (Karl Storz Endoscopy-America, Inc., Culver City, CA) is preferred in our practice for the vast majority of VATS procedures. In contrast to the instrumentation used in standard thoracolaparoscopies, this thoracoscope has a 5-mm biopsy channel that can accommodate most 5-mm endoscopic instruments. This feature allows added flexibility, and thus, this type of instrument is preferable to the view-only thoracoscopes and laparoscopes that are used in most VATS procedures (Figs. 5–1 and 5–2). When used with 5-mm biopsy forceps, this operative thoracoscope offers single intercostal access for the management and biopsy of many pleural-related problems. Similarly, the performance of more complex VATS interventions with one less intercostal access site may be possible with 5-mm grasping forceps through the scope.[1, 2] Furthermore, when use of the Nd:YAG laser is considered, the biopsy channel of the operating thoracoscope allows for direct end-on viewing of the laser's effect on the target pathology. The need for the angled thoracoscope is rare with proper planning of the trocar sites, but it may be helpful in selected instances.

A modern high-resolution "three-chip" charged coupling device (CCD) video camera and high-resolution video monitors are paramount for accurately depicting the operative field. Our institution currently uses the Karl Storz Endovision system, consisting of the Tricam SL camera (see Fig. 5–2) and image processing module (Fig. 5–3). Similar high-quality three-chip CCD cameras are available (e.g., Stryker Endoscopy, San Jose, CA; Olympus, New Hyde Park, NY), but the Storz system offers a built-in zoom capability and digital image enhancement features. A photographic printer, video tape recorder, and dual high-resolution video monitors (Sony Electronics, Toyko, Japan) complete the videoscopic equipment setup used by our thoracic surgical team (see Fig. 5–3).

Given the technological limitations of presently available three-dimensional (3-D) systems, we have found little need for this technology. Headsets, visors, and other devices typically employed by these systems are unwieldly and uncomfortable. Furthermore, the focal distance and depth of field at which most systems provide "3-D" or binocular vision are rather narrow, making thoracoscope manipulation difficult. Attempts at a closer view by advancing the thoracoscope result in a loss of accommodation, which causes a blurred image. The limitations of monocular vision can usually be accommodated as experience with VATS increases. A 3-D stereotactic sense is generally acquired with increasing operative experience. Appropriate placement of the instrument ports and the thoracoscope in relation to the target also aids in maintaining the proper spatial orientation. The technique of intermittently "zooming" the thoracoscope back to garner a broad view of the operative field and then readvancing the thoracoscope for detailed magnification of the operative field is very useful in maintaining perspective of the various instruments to the field.

Stapling Devices

The development of effective and reliable endoscopic staple-and-divide instruments significantly broadened the appeal of VATS for pulmonary diseases for most thoracic surgeons.[5] The endoscopic stapling devices are quick and convenient, and they reliably divide pulmonary parenchyma and vessels while maintaining excellent hemostasis and pneumostasis. Commonly available models include the EVC/ELC staplers from Ethicon (Cincinnati, OH) and EndoGIA from U.S. Surgical (Norwalk, CT). A variety of staple sizes and stapler lengths is now available. The "one grip" type, such as the Ethicon EZ-45, has opposing sta-

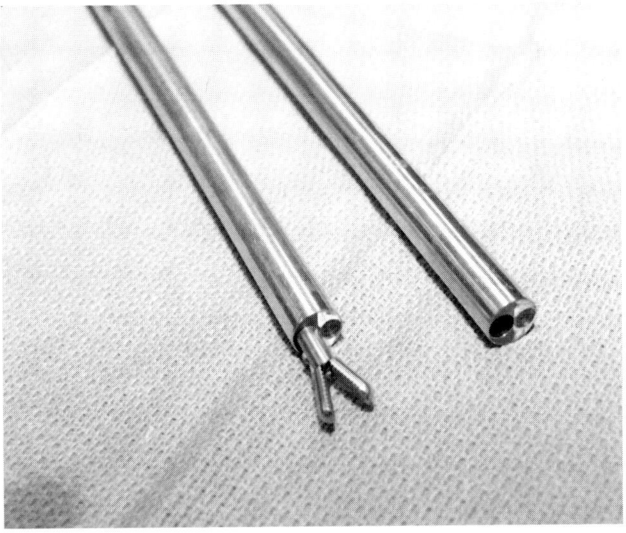

Figure 5–1. Storz operating thoracoscope. Note the 5-mm grasper in the biopsy channel of the thoracoscope, left. (Courtesy of Karl Storz Endoscopy-America, Inc., Culver City, CA.)

pler jaws, thus allowing for the application of the staples without the surgeon having to change the grip. Roticulating stapler designs also are now available from U.S. Surgical, Ethicon, and Richard Allen and are of benefit in certain instances, such as VATS lobectomy.

Hand-Held Instruments and Instrument Design

A problem facing the surgeon performing VATS relates to the "pistol grip" design that has been incorporated into many endosurgical instruments. Although the "pistol-grip" design works well for some applications, such as endostaplers, it is awkward to use for detailed manipulation and dissection of tissues (Fig. 5–4). As a result, some surgeons have adapated the use of standard thoracic surgery instruments via a "utility" or "limited" thoracotomy access incision. The best alternative is the use of "coaxial" endosurgical instruments that allow for unimpeded access through the intercostal port (Fig. 5–5) (Starr Medical Instruments, Inc., New York, NY) for true port-access VATS. These coaxial instruments retain the tactile feel of "standard" open surgical instruments by replicating the grasping end, the handles, and the ratchet-and-hinge mechanism of conventional surgical forceps and clamps while requiring a minimal intercostal access incision (Fig. 5–6A–D).

Basic VATS Operative Strategies

The first maneuver for VATS is proper patient selection. Although the range of indications for VATS thoracic surgery has widened dramatically with increasing experience, the proper patient candidate is still vital for successful surgical results. Suggested guidelines of indications and contraindications for VATS are listed (Table 5–1). As with any major operative procedure, a careful assessment of the patient's physiological reserve is mandatory.[6] Another major preoperative concern facing the thoracic surgeon beginning VATS is determining the adequacy of anesthesia team support available in his or her hospital. It is vital that anesthesia personnel be experienced in open thoracic procedures and additionally be well versed in the principles and applications of selective "one-lung" ventilation during the operation.[7] VATS procedures cannot be accomplished without suffcient unilateral pulmonary atelectasis. Thus, it is critically important that the anesthesia team is well acquainted with the techniques of double-lumen endotracheal intubation, bronchial blockers, and other means to achieve single-lung ventilation. Invasive intravascular monitoring is used as determined by the patient's cardiovascular status and comorbidities.

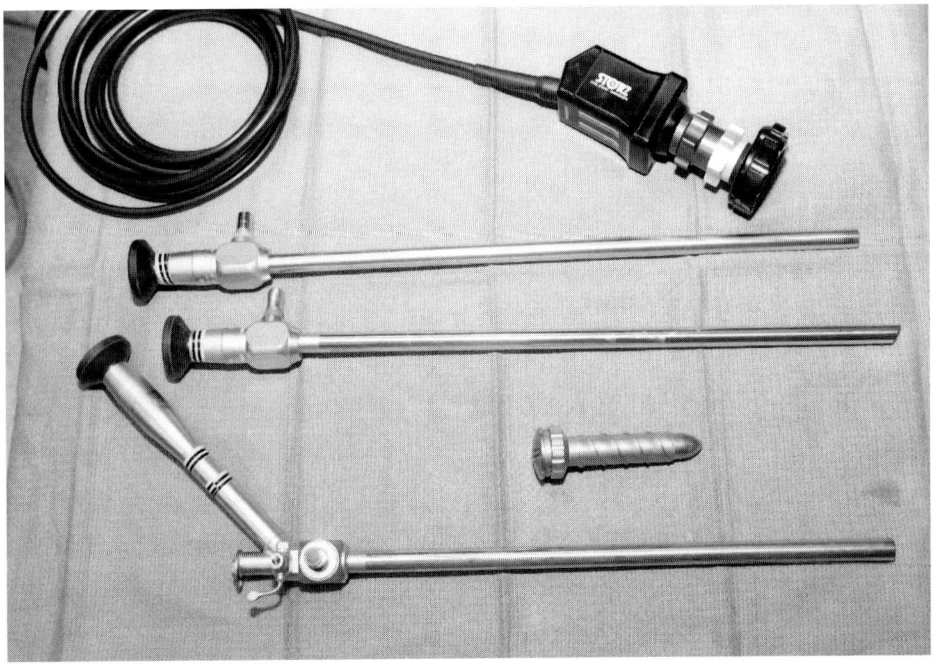

Figure 5–2. From top to bottom: Storz Endovision Camera, 0-degree standard laparoscope, 30-degree laparoscope, reusable blunt-tip thoracoscopic port, Storz thoracoscope with biopsy channel. (Courtesy of Karl Storz Endoscopy-America, Inc., Culver City, CA.)

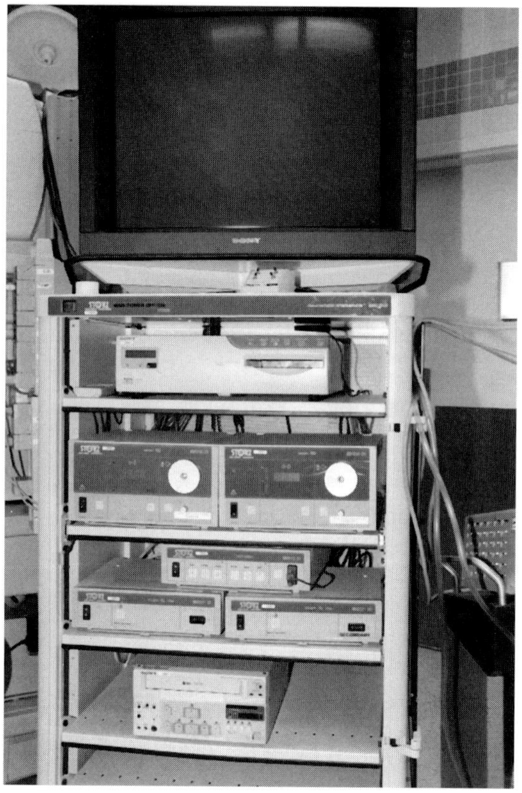

Figure 5–3. Video endoscopic equipment, top to bottom: High-resolution video monitor, video image printer, xenon light sources (×2), video processing units (×3), videotape recorder. (Courtesy of Karl Storz Endoscopy-America, Inc., Culver City, CA.)

A careful preoperative review of the chest roentgenogram and the CT scan is vital to formulate the plan for the initial and subsequent intercostal access for the thoracoscopic and surgical instruments,[2] because often, the initial trocar locations determine the subsequent ease or difficulty of the operation. In comparison, a large open thoracotomy is more flexible because of the larger space in which the instruments and view of the field can be manipulated. Anatomic considerations of both the patho-logic lesion and of the patient are important in preoperative assessment. For instance, in VATS lung biopsy of diffuse bilateral interstitial pulmonary disease, a right-sided approach is favored. Because of the trilobar anatomy of the right lung, there are simply more lung "edges" available for obtaining a stapled wedge biopsy. On the other hand, for a bilateral discrete nodular pulmonary process that requires biopsy, a left-sided approach has been more successful because more reliable complete atelectasis is required to discretely identify the nodules for biopsy. In addition, a left-sided approach is helpful for VATS biopsy for diffuse processes in smaller patients, in whom the employment of a double-lumen endotracheal tube is more difficult, but where bronchial blockers are generally easier to deploy in the left main bronchus.[2, 8–10]

Similarly, because of anatomic considerations, we have altered our approach to VATS thymectomies. From our accumulated experience in VATS thymectomy, a right-sided approach is now advocated instead of the left, as was previously described.[11] The left-sided approach was initially chosen for more reliable ipsilateral lung collapse and to visualize the aortopulmonary window lymph nodes. However, because of potential troublesome bleeding from the caval-innominate vein junction that can occur during the dissection, a right-sided approach, which allows for direct visualization of the caval-innominate vein region, is now preferred.

Intraoperative bronchoscopic examination is likewise important to rule out the presence of endobronchial pathology. After placement of the double-lumen endotracheal tube is confirmed, the patient is positioned in a full lateral decubitus position with appropriate padding and with the operating table extended to maximize the intercostal distances on the operative side (Fig. 5–7). The patient should be safely secured to the table to allow for any table position changes needed. The thorax is prepared and draped for open thoracotomy, should this necessity arise. it is vital that the surgical team preparing to perform VATS interventions be personally familiar with standard thoracic surgical procedures. VATS procedures share the

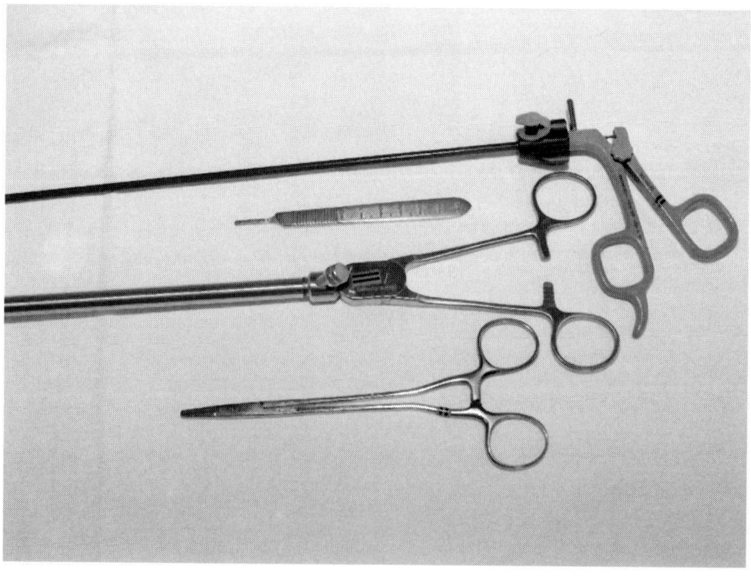

Figure 5–4. Thoracoscopic instrument design: Pistol versus coaxial grip. Top to bottom: pistol and coaxial grips, with standard open instrument for comparison.

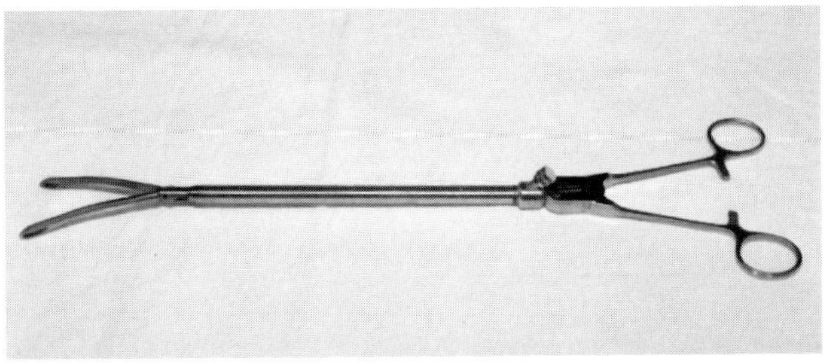

Figure 5–5. Example of coaxially designed thoracoscopic grasper. (Courtesy of Starr Medical Instruments, Inc., New York, NY.)

same potential intraoperative complications as their thoracotomy counterpart; accordingly, VATS procedures should be performed in an operating room where facilities for immediate conversion to thoracotomy are available if necessary.

The operation is begun by choosing an appropriate intercostal site of access for exploratory thoracoscopy.[1] The skin incision is made directly over the intercostal space to be entered, as opposed to the traditional subcutaneous "tunnel" made for simple chest tubes. This allows for a full 360-degree arc of mobility of the port and reduces the incidence of postoperative neuritis secondary to excessive pressure due to improper port placement.[2] Careful introduction of a small, curved pointed clamp (e.g., Kelly or Crile) through the intercostal muscles and pleura is made, avoiding the intercostal vessels and nerve along the inferior edge of the more cephalad rib. The clamp is opened to widen the intercostal space. *Direct digital exploration* of the intercostal access site, rather than blind trocar placement into the chest, is used to identify the presence of local pleural adhesions and to confirm actelectesis of the lung (see Fig. 5–7). Pleural adhesions to the lung can impede the introduction of instruments and potentially result in pulmonary parenchymal injury. Flimsy local adhesions

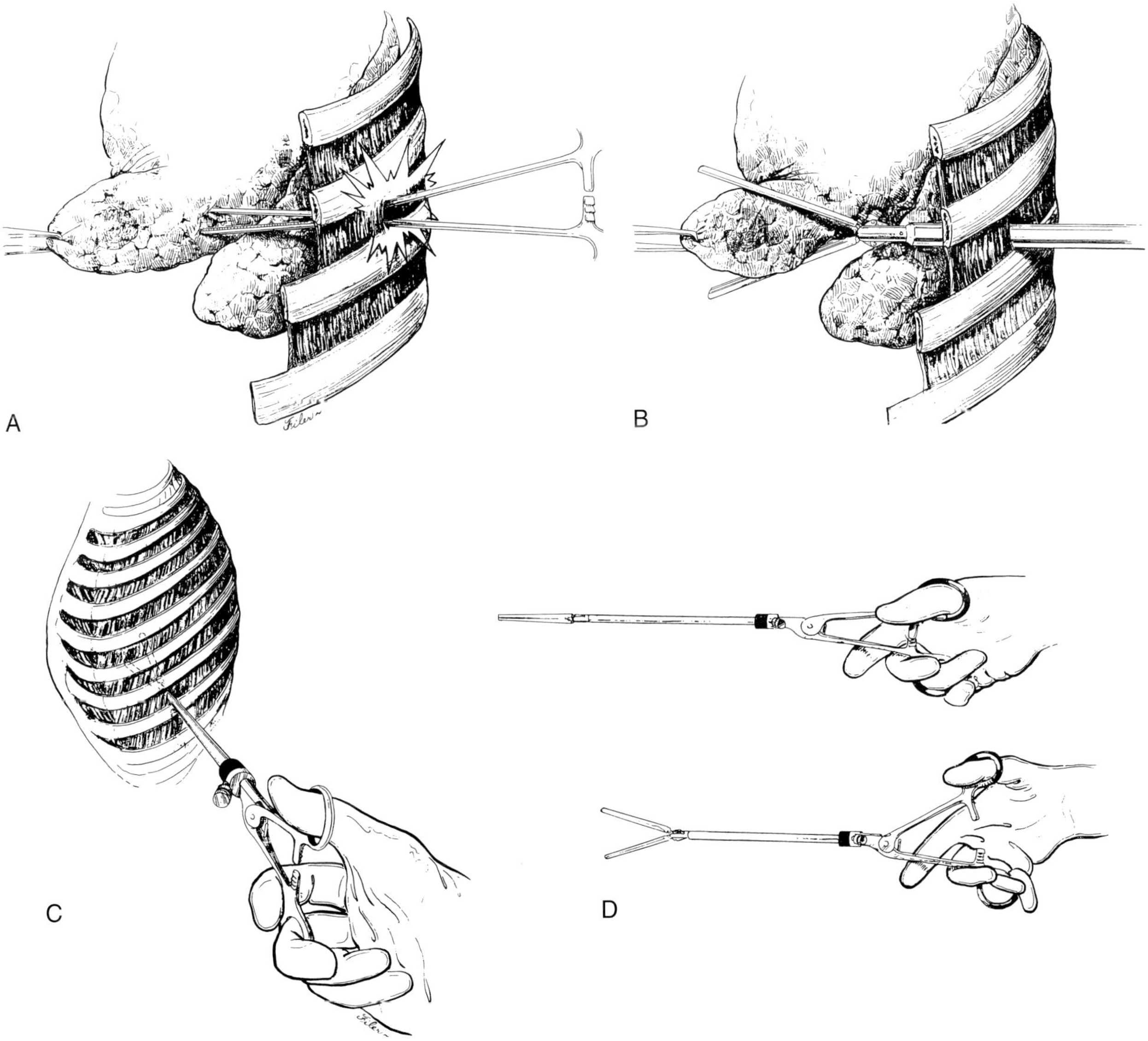

Figure 5–6. *A,* Narrow intercostal space prevents use of standard open instruments. *B–D,* Coaxial thoracoscopic instruments allow use of small port incisions but retain instrument feel of standard open instruments.

Table 5–1. Potential Indications and Contraindications for VATS

Indications

Diagnostic

Indeterminate pleural effusion (benign vs. malignant)
Tissue diagnosis
  Pleural-based masses (metastatic adenocarcinoma vs. mesothelioma)
  Wedge resection lung biopsy (for diffuse disease or for indeterminate nodule smaller than 3 cm in diameter)
  Mediastinal lymph node biopsy
  Mediastinal mass biopsy

Therapeutic

Pleuropulmonary
  Pleural effusion/empyema
  Pleurodesis (thermal/mechanical/chemical)
  Bullous disease ablation/resection
  Resect "early stage" lung cancer
Esophageal
  Resection of leiomyomata
  Resection of enteric cysts
  Esophagomyotomy
  Antireflex surgery
  Video-assisted esophagectomy
Mediastinal
  Thymectomy for myasthenia gravis
  Thymectomy for stage one thymoma
  Resection of posterior mediastinal (neurogenic) masses
  Excision of bronchogenic/enteric cysts
  Pericardiectomy

Miscellaneous

Dorsal sympathectomy/splanchnicectomy
Drainage of paravertebral abscess
Orthopedic discectomy
Internal mammary artery harvest for coronary artery bypass graft

Contraindications

Dense pleural symphysis
Ventilator dependency
Noncompliant lung
Severe emphysema
Pulmonary hilar lesions
Pulmonary lesions abutting the upper mediastinum or posterior paravertebral gutter
Small (< 1 cm), deeply located pulmonary nodules
Large pulmonary nodules (> 3 cm)
Chest wall involvement
"Small" thoracic cavity or significant anatomic restrictions (i.e., severe scoliosis)
Inability to achieve or tolerate single-lung ventilation
Inability to achieve ipsilateral pulmonary atelectasis
Inadequate visualization or instrumentation to perform procedure

can be divided with blunt finger dissection. More extensive pleural symphysis in the location of the proposed initial access site may require alternative intercostal access to conduct the VATS procedure. Hemostasis of the port site should be meticulous, as even small amounts of bleeding will dribble down the trocar and onto the endoscope, interfering with the view.

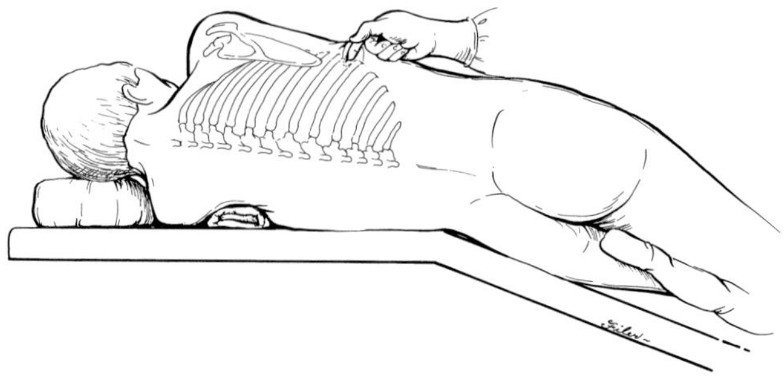

Figure 5–7. Patient in the left lateral decubitus position; digital exploration of the proposed initial trocar site is performed to confirm that a free pleural space is present. (Reprinted with permission from the Society of Thoracic Surgeons. From Landreneau RJ, Hazelrigg SR, Mack MJ, et al: Video-assisted surgery: Basic technical concepts and intercostal approach strategies. Ann Thorac Surg 54;800, 1992.)

In general, the sixth or seventh intercostal space in the midaxillary line is ideal for "trocar-protected" thoracoscope access to the pleural cavity. This initial thoracoscope location usually provides a clear view of the mediastinum, all pleural surfaces, and the pulmonary parenchyma. The intercostal port is important to prevent contamination of the thoracoscope lens surface, resulting in a "smudged" view. Agents such as FRED (Dexide, Inc., Fort Worth, TX) can be applied to the lens to reduce lens fogging. Prewarming of the thoracoscope in a warm water bath (Circon Co., Santa Barbara, CA) will further reduce lens fogging from condensation by reducing the temperature differential between the warm moist air within the pleural cavity and the cooler thoracoscope. Carbon dioxide insufflation is rarely needed to conduct VATS. Occasionally, this is used at the beginning of the procedure to facilitate a more complex and expeditious collapse of the lung. If carbon dioxide insufflation is used, the intrapleural pressure is kept below 10 mm Hg to avoid mediastinal tension and hemodynamic compromise. Exploratory thoracoscopy is then performed.

The visibility of the entire thoracic cavity obtained through the VATS approach contrasts favorably with the direct view obtained through a limited axillary, inframammary or lateral thoracotomy.[1, 2] After the initial thoracoscopic exploration of the pleural cavity is concluded, further intercostal access for VATS instrumentation is achieved under direct thoracoscopic vision (Fig. 5–8). The specific locations of the additional port sites are determined by the site of the primary pathology, but in general, the ports are placed across the (ipsilateral) pleural cavity to allow for some "working room" between the port site and the lesion. It is also very useful to conceptualize the 3-D location of the target lesion within the thorax, then place the port access sites to "triangulate" the lesion. With proper port placement and by keeping adequate distance between the ports, crossing over or "fencing" of the instruments can be avoided while enhancing the surgeon's spatial perception of the operative field. The VATS instruments and the thoracoscopic camera must be oriented so that they all are being utilized to face the target pathology from the same direction (Fig. 5–9); otherwise, difficulties in instrument manipulation will occur because of "mirror

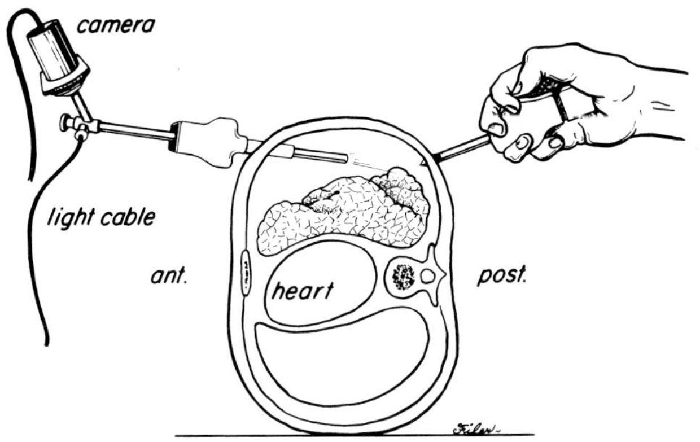

Figure 5–8. All subsequent instruments, including trocars, are introduced under direct thoracoscopic visualization to ensure proper location and to avoid trauma to the intercostal neurovascular bundle or intrathoracic structures. (Reprinted with permission from the Society of Thoracic Surgeons. From Landreneau RJ, Hazelrigg SR, Mack MJ, et al: Video-assisted thoracic surgery: Basic technical concepts and intercostal approach strategies. Ann Thorac Surg 54;800, 1992.)

imaging" when the instruments are directed toward the thoracoscopic camera. In addition to the thoracoscope, trocared ports are required to protect endostaplers during their insertion into the thorax. On the other hand, most other instruments do not require a trocar port, and increased instrument mobility can be gained by omitting the trocar once the intercostal incision has been made. Strategic positioning of the thoracoscopic camera and the endoscopic instruments is vital to the success and efficiency of the procedure (Table 5–2).

There are several procedures and techniques that greatly help facilitate VATS when employed for nodular processes of the lung. First, complete ipsilateral pulmonary atelectasis is critical, and both the surgeon and anesthesiologist should work to achieve this. With collapse of the pulmonary parenchyma, most pleural and subpleural based nodules of 1 cm or larger should be evident. Smaller nodules or nodules situated deeper in the lung parenchyma may reveal themselves as a subtle puckering of the visceral pleural surface. If not, then a sweeping motion over the lung parenchyma with a blunt instrument may allow the surgeon to locate the mass. Lastly, if these maneuvers are unsuccessful, then the lung can be elevated toward the chest wall with a lung clamp, and direct digital palpation of the suspected area of the lung can be performed through one of the other port sites.[12, 13] Preoperative computed tomography–guided needle localization may be a useful adjunct in selected patients with a small but deeply located pulmonary lesion.[14]

Compared with the general strategies in trocar placement for most VATS procedures, the approach to a localized or loculated pleural inflammatory process such as an empyema[15, 16] is reversed. Because of the inflammatory reaction that results in degrees of pleural symphysis, there is a greater risk of injury to normal lung tissue when the empyema pocket is approached from across the pleural cavity. Instead, the initial trocar should be inserted toward the central portion of the process from a dependant approach, and the empyema is drained first, thus lessening the risk of contaminating the rest of the pleural cavity. Following drainage and decompression of the empyema pocket, the other trocars can be placed to facilitate the decortication, if needed.

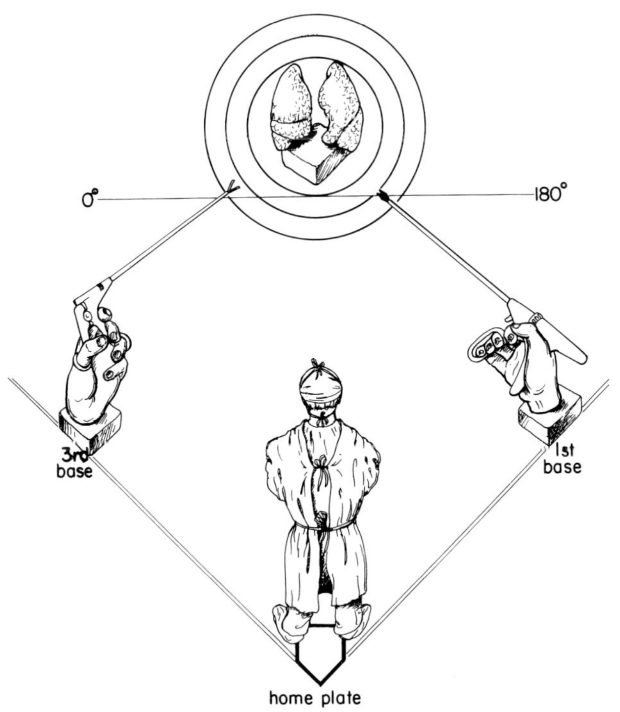

Figure 5–9. "Baseball diamond" concept for triangulation of the instruments and the thoracoscope for strategic visibility and manipulation of the target pathology. (Reprinted with permission from the Society of Thoracic Surgeons. From Landreneau RJ, Hazelrigg SR, Mack MJ, et al: Video-assisted surgery: Basic technical concepts and approach strategies. Ann Thorac Surg 54:800, 1992.)

Table 5–2. Basic VATS Operative Concepts

1. Place trocar sites and thoracoscope at a distance across the chest cavity from the lesion to achieve a panoramic view of the operative field and to provide room to manipulate the instruments.
2. Place the trocar sites appropriately apart to avoid instrument crowding and "fencing" during manipulation of the instruments.
3. Conceptualize the three dimensional location of the lesion from the computed tomography scans to "triangulate" the trocars.
4. Keep the operative instruments and the thoracoscope in the same 180-degree arc to maintain the same videoendoscopic perspective and avoiding "mirror imaging."
5. Utilize both hands to manipulate the instruments.
6. Conduct manipulation and movement of the instruments in an orderly fashion, preferably in a serial fashion instead of random movements of multiple instruments.
7. Become familiar with the required equipment (e.g., thoracoscope, video system, stapling devices) before operation.
8. Conversion to thoracotomy is an appropriate option when the performance of VATS is limited by availability of necessary equipment, technical assistance, or clinical condition of the patient.

Manipulation of the operative table is important in the course of a VATS procedure. Typically, the table is canted posteriorly to expose more of the anterior thorax. For cases involving an anterior lesion, a more posterior approach is achieved by canting the table anteriorly and placing the ports more posteriorly. The use of a Trendelenburg or a reverse Trendelenburg position is also helpful to allow gravity to keep the lung out of the operative field. Because of the nature of the endoscopic instruments protruding out of the thorax, the operative table should be kept low enough so that the surgeon can be comfortable. To minimize muscular tension and fatigue in the surgeon's arms and hands, the handles of the instruments should be at the level of his or her elbow or slightly lower, to keep the wrists in neutral position and the elbows in slight extension (elbows held slightly beyond 90 degrees).

Excessive torque should be avoided when manipulating the instruments in VATS to avoid damaging the instruments and to prevent the complications of postoperative neuritis. If the view is inadequate or if the angle of the instrument is inappropriate for the desired manipulation, then options include alternating the port sites or placing another port. Sometimes, by changing or alternating the location of the instruments and thoracoscope, a different perspective can be gained to achieve the task at hand (Fig. 5–10*A*,*B*). Lastly, if a diligent effort in performing the operation thoracoscopically is unsuccessful, performing a limited "utility" thoracotomy or converting to a standard open thoracotomy is wise and appropriate.

Extraction of Tissue Specimens

Removal of pathologic tissues from the thoracic cavity can be a problem encountered with VATS procedures. Extraction of a small specimen is facilitated by placing it within a sterile glove or a commercially available plastic sleeved device, such as the Pleatman sac (Cabot Medical, Langhorne, PA) or EndoCatch (U.S. Surgical, Norwalk, CT), for retrieval through one of the intercostal access sites. For larger specimens, a sterile plastic endoscopic video camera sleeve works well as a retrieval device. For retrieval of larger specimens, the intercostal access incision can be slightly lengthened without rib spreading to accommodate the size of the specimen.

Conclusions

The concepts of minimally invasive surgery and VATS have been readily incorporated into the practice of thoracic surgery over the past decade. Undoubtedly, the decreased postoperative pain and functional disability of the patient are advantageous compared with conventional thora-

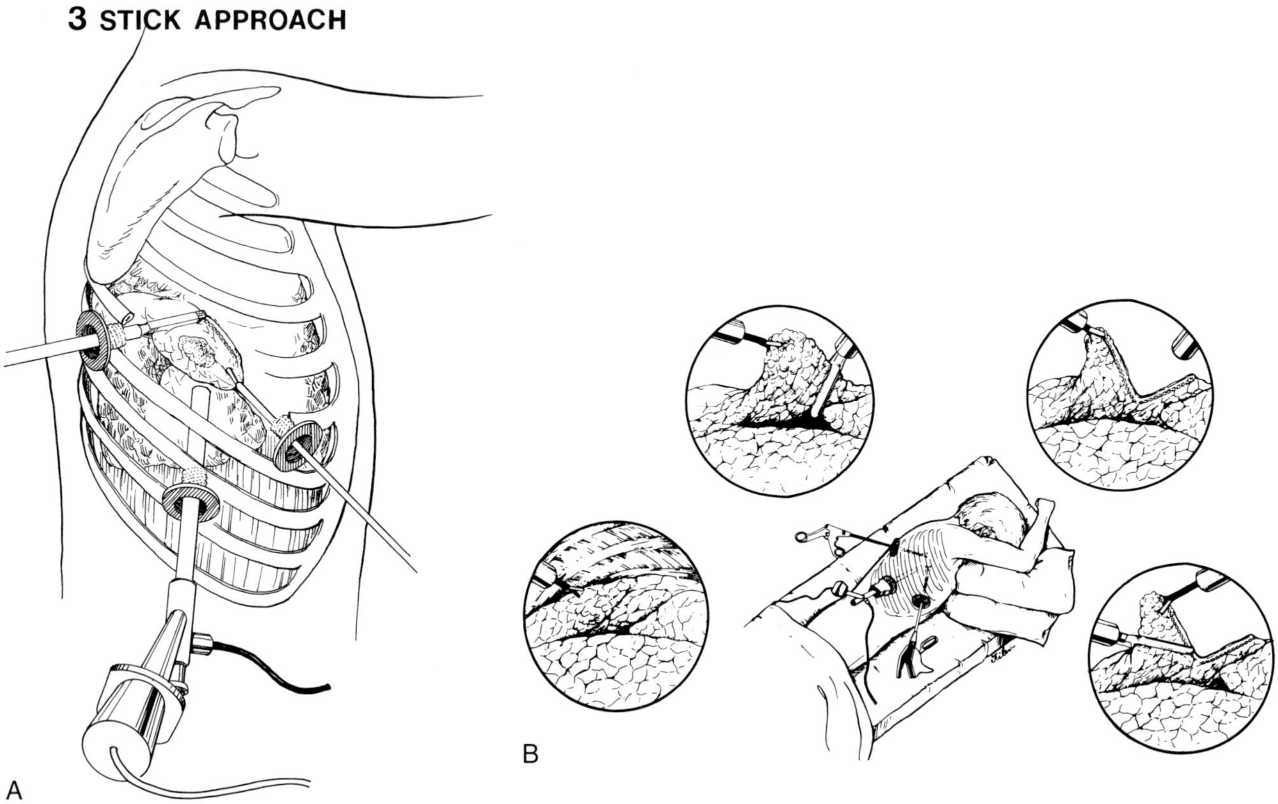

Figure 5–10. *A*, Drawing of a "three-stick" intercostal access approach typically used for a video-assisted thoracic surgical (VATS) wedge resection of the lung using the endoscopic stapling device. (From Ferson PF, Landreneau RJ, Dowling RD, et al: Comparison of open versus thoracoscopic lung biopsy for diffuse infiltrative pulmonary disease. J Thorac Cardiovasc Surg 106:194–199, 1993.) *B*, Serial application of the endostapling device to accomplish a standard "V" wedge resection of the lung with a three-stick technique. Note that the intercostal access position of the stapling device and the grasping instruments is reversed to complete the stapled wedge resection expeditiously. (From Dowling RD et al: Thoracoscopic wedge resection of the lung. Surgical Rounds 16;341, 1993.)

cotomy approaches. Most basic and many advanced thoracic surgery procedures can be performed by VATS, with good outcomes and without increased complications. As a result, the acceptance of VATS has imposed the need for many surgeons to acquire a new set of skills to perform these operations safely and expediently. It is our goal that the suggestions made in this chapter in regard to selection of equipment, as well as basic concepts and operative techniques employed in VATS, will allow for a smoother transition to VATS.

References

1. Landreneau RJ, Mack MJ, Hazelrigg SR, et al: Video-assisted thoracic surgery: Basic technical concepts and intercostal approach strategies. Ann Thorac Surg 54:800–807, 1992.
2. Landreneau RJ, Mack MJ, Keenan RJ, et al: Strategic planning for video-assisted thoracic surgery. Ann Thorac Surg 56:615–619, 1993.
3. Landreneau RJ, Hazelrigg SR, Mack MJ, et al: Postoperative pain-related morbidity: Video-assisted thoracic surgery versus muscle sparing "open" thoracotomies. Ann Thorac Surg 56:1285–1289, 1993.
4. Landreneau RJ, Mack MJ, Hazelrigg SR, et al: Prevalence of chronic postoperative pain following pulmonary resection by thoracotomy of video-assisted thoracic surgery. J Thorac Cardiovasc Surg 107:1079–1085, 1994.
5. Acuff TE, Mack MJ, Landreneau RJ, et al: Role of mechanical stapling devices in thoracoscopic pulmonary resection. Ann Thorac Surg 56:749–751, 1993.
6. Wernly JA, DeMeester TR: Preoperative assessment of patients undergoing lung resection for cancer. In Roth JA, Ruckedeschel JC, Weisenburger TH (eds): Thoracic Oncology. Philadelphia, WB Saunders, 1989, pp 156–176.
7. Benumof JL: Physiology of the open chest and one-lung ventilation. In Kaplan JA (ed): Thoracic Anesthesia. New York, Churchill Livingstone, 1983, pp 287–316.
8. Ferson PF, Landreneau RJ, Dowling RD, et al: Comparison of open versus thoracoscopic lung biopsy for diffuse infiltrative pulmonary disease. J Thorac Cardiovasc Surg 106:194–199, 1993.
9. Chechani V, Landreneau RJ, Schaikh S: Diffuse infiltrative lung disease: Where and how many open lung biopsies to perform. Ann Thorac Surg 54:296–300, 1992.
10. Gaensler EA, Carrington CB: Open biopsy for chronic diffuse infiltrative lung disease: Clinical, roentgenographic, and physiological correlations in 502 patients. Ann Thorac Surg 30:411–426, 1980.
11. Landreneau RJ, Dowling RD, Castillo W, et al: Thoracoscopic resection of an anterior mediastinal mass. Ann Thorac Surg 54:142–144, 1992.
12. Mack MJ, Shennib H, Landreneau RJ, et al: Techniques for localization of pulmonary nodules for thoracoscopic resection. J Thorac Cardiovasc Surg 106:550–553, 1993.
13. Nomori H, Hoirio H: Endofinger for tactile localization of pulmonary nodules during thoracoscopic resections. Thorac Cardiovasc Surgeon 44:50–53, 1996.
14. Mack MJ, Gordon MJ, Postma TW, et al: Percutaneous localization of pulmonary nodules for thoracoscopic lung resection. Ann Thorac Surg 53:1123–1124, 1992.
15. Landreneau RJ, et al: Thoracoscopy for empyema and hemothorax. Chest 109:18–24, 1996.
16. Ridley PD, Braimbridge MV: Thoracoscopic debridement and pleural irrigation in the management of empyema thoraces. Ann Thorac Surg 51:461–464, 1991.

COMMENTARY

Anthony P. C. Yim

The classic operative strategy in VATS is detailed in this chapter in which surgeon, camera, targeted pathology, and television monitor are kept along the same line to maintain the correct spatial relationship for instrument maneuvering. Paradoxical motion is generated when the camera and instruments are on opposite sides of the targeted pathology. This is difficult to avoid when there is a wide operating field. Experience has demonstrated that turning the camera 180 degrees restores a normal spatial relationship.[1] This simple maneuver allows the operator to use the existing camera and instrument ports to his or her best ergonomic advantage.

References

1. Yim APC, Izzat MB, Lee TW: Counteracting paradoxical motion in videoendoscopic operations. Ann Thorac Surg 66: 965, 1998.

Chapter 6

Ethical Aspects of Introducing New Surgical Technology

Martin F. McKneally

Innovations Should Be Valid

Innovation is a valued expression of problem-solving skills that are well developed in some members of society. In a progressive society, innovators are rewarded for providing useful solutions. Surgeons make innovative improvements in their handicraft as they seek to minimize discomfort, scarring, and other side effects of operations. These improvements earn the respect of the profession. Successful innovative procedures are sometimes named after the innovators, perpetuating their place of honor in surgical discourse through eponyms like Billroth's gastrectomy, Starr and Edwards' prosthetic valve, and Fontan's procedure to bypass the hypoplastic right ventricle.

There is an implicit expectation that surgeons faced with unanticipated findings in the operating room innovate to develop a solution that allows completion of the surgical mission: "We couldn't remove the obstruction, but we were able to bypass it"; "We couldn't fit the transplanted lung into the recipient, so we did a contralateral lung reduction."[37]

Surgery has strong traditions that protect patients and surgeons from less valid innovations that may be harmful. This conservative tendency is expressed almost ritually in the fixed routines of the operating room and the clinic. New procedures are carefully worked out in the animal laboratory and the dissecting room of the anatomy or pathology department. They are presented for approval to colleagues. New procedures may be disapproved by credentials committees, operating room committees, research ethics boards, or the surgeon-in-chief. Nurses, anesthesiologists, and other members of the operating room team—a moral community who have strongly felt, though generally implicit, standards—protect the patient and the surgeon from danger, including dangerous innovations. The discipline that provides this protection is under increased pressure as the more entrepreneurial and sometimes less patient-centered interests of equipment manufacturers, insurers, and others penetrate the sanctuary of the operating room.

I will use the term *nonvalidated* to describe the status of innovations such as minimally invasive coronary bypass or lung reduction surgery at the time this chapter is being written. Although many treatments that are accepted as standard therapy have not been formally validated, the term *nonvalidated,* introduced by Levine[14] to describe innovative therapies, is a well-chosen one that accurately captures the sense of moral hazard that should be attached to their use in vulnerable and trusting patients before they become widely accepted throughout the expert medical community. Acceptance does not ensure validity. Validation, the process by which a treatment receives authoritative confirmation that it is safe and effective in producing the desired result, is not well defined in surgery. Consensus within the expert medical community seems to confer implicit validation of surgical operations. In contrast, agencies such as the United States Food and Drug Administration (FDA) confer validation on pharmaceuticals by an explicit approval process. The lack of general agreement on validation has drawn a diverse group of stakeholders into the debate about innovative surgical procedures.[18]

There are many issues that can be teased out in an analysis of the introduction of innovative surgical technology. I will focus on the ethical questions of how new technology should be introduced to our patients and where we can turn for guidance about the ethical challenges inherent in surgical innovation. I will close with a suggestion for how the profession of surgery and our industrial partners might help us address these questions systematically.

Consent for Nonvalidated Treatments

Patients approach their surgeons in an unbalanced relationship. Patients are generally vulnerable, often suffering, and their knowledge of the disease and its treatment is incomplete. Novelty and media promotion of innovative treatments may increase their willingness to accept an unsound innovation. In contrast to their patients, surgeons have extensive knowledge, skill, and experience that can be intimidating, even when it is used to endorse a new technology that they may be minimally prepared to introduce. There are two general approaches to protect the patient's interest in this unbalanced relationship: The legal doctrine of informed consent and the ethical obligation of fidelity to trust in the fiduciary relationship.

The best known approach to protecting patients' interests in the unbalanced surgeon-patient relationship is the legal doctrine of informed consent. Informed consent is "the autonomous authorization of a medical intervention . . . by individual patients."[1] To be valid, consent must be (1) voluntary—free of constraint or pressure; (2) capable—the patient must be able to weigh the risks, benefits, and impact of the intervention in his or her own life situation; and (3) informed—the patient must be told and must comprehend all that a reasonable person would want to know about the risks, benefits, and impact of the proposed treatment.[8]

The doctrine of informed consent, extensively elaborated by Katz over the past several decades,[12] provides more theoretical than practical protection for the patient, because of the fundamental trust that dominates the relationship. It introduces a legalistic, contractual tone to the transaction that many patients and surgeons find awkward, because it implies distrust. Nevertheless, written documentation of informed consent has become a standard component of practice, because patients often fail to recall the information disclosed in the preoperative interval.[29] The written record of informed consent provides some legal protection for the surgeon against claims of *battery* (unconsented violation of personal integrity), or *negligence* (insufficient explanation of the intended intervention) when complications, mistakes, unsatisfactory outcomes, or other maloccurrences that arise during treatment lead to the consideration of legal action against the surgeon.

The standard of disclosure in informed consent that is accepted in most jurisdictions is "what the reasonable person in the same circumstances would want to be told."[7] A higher standard of disclosure for nonvalidated procedures has been required by research ethics boards* for many years.[16] This mechanism provided a relatively public review of new treatments before and after their introduction. However, the current tendency to bypass institutional review has allowed nonvalidated innovations to be smuggled into practice by declaring them to be "safe and effective" on marginal evidence. This particular phrase, quoted from the requirements of the FDA for the approval of new treatments, has been used inappropriately by some innovators to describe their preliminary results, accelerating but not validating adoption of the innovation.[30]

The consent process required by research ethics boards usually identifies the issue of novelty by requiring a statement in the consent form that the treatment is experimental. This may not be sufficient; novelty per se carries risks, including unfamiliarity on the part of the surgical team and other subsequent caregivers.

Introducing Nonvalidated Treatments in a Relationship of Vulnerability and Trust

Fiduciaries, such as physicians, lawyers, teachers, and clergy, have an ethical obligation to put the interests of their patients, clients, students, or congregation members above their own.[28] This obligation permits the patient to enter a relationship characterized by trust and confidence. Though ennobling and inspiring, the concept of fiduciary obligation is too vague to be helpful without further specification. Fiduciary duties require reflective analysis of the interests of the patient and the surgeon, and a specific and concrete plan for protecting them. Most surgeons work this problem out implicitly; most patients trust their surgeons implicitly. Here are some suggestions that can clarify the issue of introducing novel treatments in a fiduciary relationship, using explicit language and fair procedures for protecting the patients' interests.

- Recognize and discuss the magnitude of the imbalance of knowledge, skill, and power in the relationship, and its potential influence on the acceptance of the nonvalidated treatment you are proposing.
- Discuss your level of skill and experience, including the lack of skill and experience with the particular innovation. Specific discussion of analogous experience, for example, with open techniques, and its relationship to the innovative components is reassuring and appropriate, but smuggling innovations past the patient's critical faculties on the basis of competency in analogous but different procedures is an abuse of the fiduciary relationship.
- Discuss the general lack of certainty and the incomplete state of knowledge about the specific nonvalidated therapeutic procedure you are proposing.
- Tell the patient that he or she is participating in a validation process. Clarify the novelty and the risks inherent in the novel aspects of the procedure. This helps bring into focus the essential truth that the procedure is nonvalidated.
- Choose valid and relevant endpoints. The validation process should be designed to generate data and to allow analysis of well-chosen endpoints that will lead to adoption of the innovation as part of standard therapy, or to rejection. For example, an innovation such as minimally invasive coronary bypass, which potentially compromises the technique of constructing a coronary artery anastomosis, requires early imaging of the anastomosis as an endpoint to validate its continued use, guide improvement, or lead to rejection of the innovation. The length of hospital stay and the mortality rate are not sufficiently sensitive endpoints to establish validity, even if they are accepted as evidence by patients and by some members of the expert medical community.

Mack and associates[27] and Subramanian and associates[35] are conducting careful studies of minimally invasive coronary bypass surgery to document the endpoint of graft patency before discharge from the hospital. Izzat and Yim[11] and others[3,13] are studying anastomotic patency intraoperatively. This level of intellectual honesty and scientific scrutiny is commendable and necessary. Practitioners who are unable or unwilling to participate in such meticulous documentation of relevant endpoints in the early postoperative period may accept the apparent absence of mortality as a surrogate. Omission of evaluation of relevant endpoints is the greatest hazard during the early adoption phase, because expert management of complications and the strong placebo effect of surgery may lead patients and doctors to accept undetected suboptimal or harmful effects as apparent successes of the innovative technique. An innovation that is based on the hypothesis that there may be less disability because open thoracotomy, sternotomy, or the pump oxygenator is not employed should include endpoints specific to these components of the procedure, that is, assessment of chest wall pain and disability, and tests of the highest integrative functions of the brain. Addressing these issues is a responsibility of all who are introducing nonvalidated treatments, not just those who are conducting randomized trials.

Where Can We Turn for Guidance?

When the usual sources of scientific evidence in the literature and the traditions of surgery do not provide answers to the question "what should I do?," there are three "wells

* In the United States, research ethics boards are referred to as Institutional Review Boards (IRBs), an opaque term.

of wisdom" that physicians can turn to for guidance: Law, policy, and ethics.*

Law. The law provides guidance regarding the rights of patients and duties of practitioners in the conduct of customary accepted care and in the conduct of research trials. Epstein's articulate discussion of legal liability for medical innovation reduces the issues to the application of the standard legal frameworks of warning through disclosure of risks, assumption of risks by the patient once relevant information about them is received, and liability of manufacturers and practitioners for deviation from customary or applicable standards.[16] The problems introduced by the novelty of the treatment he leaves to independent review boards despite inconsistency between institutions. Because the law provides guidance from post hoc analysis of maloccurrences that develop in the course of treatment, it is less useful for making judgments about the introduction of novel treatments. The law tends to follow and to consolidate principles and procedures through judgments in case law about consent and liability.

An exception might be legislation or regulations prohibiting the use of government funds for certain innovations outside of designated centers or protocols, such as cardiac transplantation in the late 1960s in the United States, and lung reduction surgery today. It seems appropriate for legislators to make judgments on behalf of society about the allocation of public funds for expensive, nonvalidated surgical innovations. The responsibility for developing and validating them rests with the profession of surgery.

Policy. Ambiguous or troublesome problems that an individual surgeon faces can sometimes be resolved by the application of policies established at the institutional or organizational level for resolving similar cases using accepted values and principles. When a patient is desperately ill, it is tempting to offer innovative treatments that are unjustified by experience but carry an unrealistic hope that they could possibly help. Embedding values and principles in policy guidelines helps the patient, the family, the doctor, and the institution over difficult moral terrain.

Policies set or approved by research ethics boards as part of a research protocol regulate the conditions under which an innovation is appropriately offered to patients to ensure its validation or rejection. The entry criteria for a clinical trial are part of a policy protecting the integrity of the evaluation as well as the patients. It seems appropriate to use such policies more generally. I will suggest how we might do so shortly.

The fiduciary obligations of surgeons are described in a general way in the "Statements on Principles" of the American College of Surgeons. The Society of Thoracic Surgeons (STS) and American Association for Thoracic Surgery (AATS) refer to this statement and to the code of ethics of the American Medical Association for general guidance, and to their policy statements and guidelines. Each of the major organizations has an ethics committee that addresses ethical issues by formulating policy statements and guidelines, and by reviewing individual cases in which there are possible violations of the practice standards of the profession. The thoracic surgical organizations develop guidelines on issues such as training practitioners in emerging technology through ad hoc committees[22,23] and standing committees. Because the problem of emerging technology has proved to be a durable one, with new challenges developing so regularly, standing committees on emerging technology have been struck by both the American College of Surgeons and the AATS-STS as a joint activity. These committees attempt to detect important new technologies, set standards for education, provide courses of instruction, and provide guidance regarding the diffusion of new technology into practice.

Individual hospitals and clinics develop local policies reflecting the interests and values of the particular institution. These are generally focused on control of expenditures and safety issues rather than validation. Like policies on cardiopulmonary resuscitation, they often put a strong emphasis on procedural considerations and tend to avoid those that are value-laden. In contrast, the well-reasoned policy for deployment of the new technology of coronary stenting developed by Etchells and associates in 1996 uses evidence, cost benefit analysis, and ethics criteria.[9,32]

Ethics. Ethics is the study of what *should* be done, based on values and principles. Formally, ethics is a discipline within philosophy, emphasizing thorough knowledge of principles, values, classical writings on ethics, and moral codes. Clinical ethicists often have less knowledge of the philosophical foundations and more case-based knowledge of health-related moral quandaries; they are skilled at clarifying values, applying principles, and mediation. Despite extensive knowledge and skill, an ethicist may lack normative moral authority in a particular community because of lack of nuanced and expert knowledge of the values and beliefs of the community in which an ethical problem arises.[39] In contrast, respected members of a community may have moral authority (the authority to provide credible judgments about what should or should not be done) based on their fairness, wisdom, and knowledge of the values of the particular community, without formal education in ethics. Within the thoracic surgical community, Chairman Frank Spencer and the ethics committee of the AATS, or Chairman Nick Kouchoukas and the ethics committee of the STS provide case by case judgments and occasional policy positions on morally hazardous issues. Their moral authority is derived from the surgical community's recognition of their leadership in action, scholarly writing, and reflection in the field of surgery, not their formal study of ethics.

Surgeons can be considered to belong to a moral community locally if the department or operating room shares the same values and beliefs. A clear example is provided by Catholic hospitals with a univocal policy on abortion: "We don't do that here!" Individual members of the surgical team may hold different values and beliefs privately; the department chief, the operating room committee, the hospital trustees, and the hospital ethics committee help with the delineation of commonly held values and limits. These values form the basis for policies that guide judgments about issues that may be hazardous physically, financially, legally, or morally. For example, a hospital surgery depart-

* I learned this formulation from Peter A. Singer, MD, Director of the University of Toronto's Joint Centre for Bioethics, during many illuminating discussions.

ment might develop a priority scale for emergency operations, ranking life-threatening illnesses such as ruptured aneurysm ahead of less urgent ones such as appendicitis, and establish a fair procedure for priority ranking of elective cases when facilities, personnel, or other resources are limited. Such ethical guidelines or codes of conduct achieve binding authority by consensus when the community is small and all members accept their legitimacy. Whether the world community of surgeons can be considered to be a more general moral community, sharing common values is problematic because of the diversity of membership. There are reasonable arguments that can be forwarded to support such a claim that I will not develop here.[19]

Local clinical ethics committees and research ethics boards can provide helpful consultation and serve as a source of multidisciplinary and community advice, adding balance, breadth, and a measure of protection for all stakeholders in the important experiment that we are all engaged in when we introduce nonvalidated innovative therapy.

A Proposal for Introduction and Validation of New Surgical Technology

Given that there is an inherent drive among innovative surgeons to discover and promote new innovative treatments,* and given that there is a bias among members of program committees and editorial boards toward positive results even when they are preliminary,[21] we will always be confronted by noteworthy fragments of promising clinical experience in our meetings and journals. Qualifying statements that "these results require confirmation in large randomized clinical trials" are scientifically devout references to events that rarely occur because of their cost and complexity.

As research ethics has developed as a distinct domain of knowledge within bioethics over the past three decades, there has been a heavy emphasis in the literature on randomized trials because of their scientific strengths and the myriad ethical problems and enlightened solutions they have engendered.[15] The randomized controlled trial (RCT)[25,31] of innovative versus standard treatment has many safeguards. To counteract bias, sealed envelopes or a blinded central randomizing mechanism are used. To counteract misunderstanding or deception, extensive disclosure is distinctly emphasized in the process of informed consent. To protect the hospital and patients from the infectious enthusiasm of investigators,† a diverse group of reviewers, including lay members, are recruited to the research ethics board. To provide early detection of unacceptable effects, safety monitoring procedures are built into the protocol.

These safety features have strengthened the credibility of the clinical research process. The complexity and expense of setting up and maintaining an RCT[25] have led to less rigorous alternatives. It is here that we should focus our scrutiny, and help with the development of reasonable and credible alternatives to the RCT without losing the safeguards. The power of data to convince practitioners is not limited to RCTs; in fact, some (particularly small ones, such as my own testing the effect of bacillus Calmette Guérin (BCG) in lung cancer[24]) can be misleading, and a substantial number of RCTs have little impact on practice. In contrast, some observational studies are overwhelmingly persuasive, such as Morton and Warren's demonstration of the effect of ether anesthesia.

Debates on the merits of the innovation are reasonable and responsibled,[5,20] but our debates and pro and con panel discussions are often arranged by ardent technophiles with token "reasonable" opponents. The power of data, organized into information through thoughtful analysis, can be harnessed to provide the profession and society with useful solutions. The outcomes movement[4] and the "report card" approach to the analysis of the results of cardiac surgery[10,26] are strong indicators of society's need for this information. We could develop the data and analyses to meet this need using the resources of our surgical societies; our colleagues in industry, who have a strong interest in finding out what works best; and the technical and intellectual skills of surgeons, all of whom are scientists.[17,38] If large databases can be linked, we can sort out the questions about which treatments are appropriate.[4]

I would like to propose the conduct of a linked set of observational studies, reviewed by the research ethics board of each surgeon's institution and conforming to some general principles agreed upon by the participating surgeons and the major surgical societies. The use of a principle-based policy without a rigid protocol specifying and limiting the techniques would allow development of the adaptations and adjustments that are needed during the evolution of surgical innovation. This is what was done during the preapproved, precisely documented innovative phase of lung transplantation.[2] The protocol, selection criteria, and the particular patients to be transplanted were reviewed and approved by a panel of experts who were not involved in the transplant program. The protocol was approved by the research ethics board and presented to the administration of the Toronto General Hospital. After the first four transplants, a careful review of results led to approval for continuing the program. Singer and associates at the University of Chicago[33,34] clearly described a similar process for the introduction of liver transplantation from living related donors. They recommend a formal sequence of steps to ensure that new technology is evaluated in a timely way under defined conditions. First, the novel procedure is published in the medical literature; this public statement commits the workers to give a follow-up when their clinical observations on a defined number of patients become available. Second, a working paper is submitted to the hospital or clinic where the procedure will be conducted. This summarizes and explains the research plan. Third, after a defined number of patients have been

* Innovators gain notoriety within their community, attract patients, appear on panels, give invited lectures, and contribute papers and chapters to the surgical literature. These perquisites create a conflict of interest with their patients that is often unrecognized.[36]

† Francis D. Moore described "funkenluste," the enthusiasm for doing what you become proficient at doing, as a catalyst for promoting the use of novel treatments irrespective of their validity, in his discussion of M.R. Harrison's presentation on "Fetal Surgery" at the Colloquium on Ethics: An Ethics "M and M" during the American College of Surgeons Clinical Congress in Chicago on October 12, 1994.

exposed to the new treatment (e.g., after 20 living related donor liver transplants), a follow-up publication is submitted to share the experience, regardless of the success or failure of the program. Close attention to recording short- and intermediate-term endpoints might improve patient selection and early results. Exchange of information learned from experience also strengthens the program; this was a highly valued benefit of membership on the teaching team assembled by the AATS-STS Joint Committee on Video-Assisted Thoracic Surgery during the introduction of that new technology.

Socially responsible investment in research benefits our colleagues in industry who are producing a cornucopia of innovative products. By testing their products systematically, surgeons can help manufacturers secure the outcome data they need for marketing. The existence of a research structure to which the surgeon can refer facilitates discussion with patients about the novelty and nonvalidated status of the intervention without diminishing its worthiness. The status of national or international organizations sponsoring the trial assures patients that the treatment is on the leading edge of medical science without obscuring its experimental status. Limited experience of the surgeon with the intervention is an acceptable inherent element when the treatment is presented as part of a research program. It is not difficult to envision the structure and procedures of such a program. We have several excellent models, such as the Congenital Heart Surgery Group, the Lung Cancer Study Group, and the collaborating team comprising the editors of this book. The challenge for surgeons is to overcome the established entrepreneurial competition between institutions and practices, in order to develop a credible, cooperative team approach that will clarify and facilitate the introduction and validation of new technology.

References

1. Beauchamp TL, Faden RR: Informed consent: II. Meaning and elements of informed consent. *In* Reich WT (ed): Encyclopedia of Bioethics, rev ed, vol 3. New York, Simon & Schuster Macmillan, 1995, pp 1238–1241.
2. Cooper J: Personal communication, 1997.
3. Elbeery JR, Chitwood WR Jr: Intraoperative catheterization of the left internal mammary artery via the left radial artery. Ann Thorac Surg 64:1840–1842, 1997.
4. Ellwood PM: Shattuck lecture—outcomes management: A technology of patient experience. N Engl J Med 318:1549–1556, 1988.
5. Emery RW vs Ullyot DJ: Mini Debate, Minimally Invasive Coronary Bypass Surgery: Way of the Future vs Flash in the Pan. Society of Thoracic Surgeons. New Orleans, Jan 25, 1998.
6. Epstein RA: Legal liability for medical innovation. *In* Siegler M, Toulmin S, Zimring FE, et al (eds): Medical Innovation and Bad Outcomes. Ann Arbor, MI, Health Administration Press, 1987, pp 163–184.
7. Etchells E, Sharpe G, Burgess MM, et al: Bioethics for Clinicians: 2. Disclosure. Can Med Assoc J 155:387–391, 1996.
8. Etchells E, Sharpe G, Walsh P, et al: Bioethics for Clinicians: 1. Consent. Can Med Assoc J 155:177–180, 1996.
9. Etchells E, Singer P, Lazzam C, et al: Coronary artery stents: Report of the advisory group for coronary artery stenting at The Toronto Hospital. June 12, 1996.
10. Green J, Wintfeld N: Report cards on cardiac surgeons—assessing New York State's approach. N Engl J Med 332: 1229–1232, 1995.
11. Izzat MB, Yim APC: Letter: MIDCABG: Lessons learned from routine "on-table" angiography. Ann Thorac Surg 64:1872–1874, 1997.
12. Katz J: The Silent World of Doctor and Patient. New York, The Free Press, 1984.
13. Lazzara RR, McLellan BA, Kidwell FE, et al: Intraoperative angiography during minimally invasive direct coronary artery bypass operations. Ann Thorac Surg 64:1725–1727, 1997.
14. Levine RJ: Ethics and Regulation of Clinical Research, 2nd ed. New Haven, CT, Yale University Press, 1988, p 4.
15. Levine RJ: Randomized clinical trials. *In* Levine RJ: Ethics and Regulation of Clinical Research, 2nd ed. New Haven, CT, Yale University Press, 1988, pp 185–212.
16. Levine RJ: Standards for informed consent to research and practice. *In* Levine RJ: Ethics and Regulation of Clinical Research, 2nd ed. New Haven, CT, Yale University Press, 1988, pp 127–131.
17. McKenna RJ Jr: Developing new knowledge in community practice. *In* Troidl H, McKneally MF, Mulder DS, et al (eds): Surgical Research: Basic Principles and Clinical Practice, 3rd ed. New York, Springer Verlag, 1997, pp 15–22.
18. McKneally MF: Can surgical innovation survive? Bull Am Coll Surg 81:8–21, 1996.
19. McKneally MF: Ethical issues in surgical trials and practice. Lecture, University of Cologne, Germany, Symposium on Evolution, Cognition, and Surgical Research. July 5, 1996.
20. McKneally MF: It is appropriate for pulmonologists to perform thoracoscopy for pleural disease? Debate, Second International Symposium on Video Assisted Thoracic Surgery. New York, April 1994.
21. McKneally MF, Cassivi S, Troidl H: Publications do not always reflect the real world. *In* Troidl H, McKneally MF, Mulder DS, et al (eds): Surgical Research: Basic Principles and Clinical Practice, 3rd ed. New York, Springer Verlag, 1997, pp 75–82.
22. McKneally MF, Lewis R, Anderson RP, et al (Joint Committee for Video Assisted Thoracic Surgery): Guidelines for courses from the AATS/STS Joint Committee on Video Assisted Thoracic Surgery. Ann Thorac Surg 56:591–592, 1993.
23. McKneally MF, Lewis R, Anderson RP, et al (Joint Committee for Video Assisted Thoracic Surgery): Report: Guidelines for granting hospital privileges in video-assisted thoracic surgery. Ann Thorac Surg 60:1456, 1995; and J Thorac Cardiovasc Surg 110:1, 1995.
24. McKneally MF, Maver C, Kausel HW: Regional immunotherapy of lung cancer with intrapleural BCG. Lancet 1:377–379, 1976.
25. McKneally MF, McPeek B, Mosteller F, et al: Clinical trials. *In* Troidl H, McKneally MF, Mulder DS, et al (eds): Surgical Research: Basic Principles and Clinical Practice, 3rd ed. New York, Springer Verlag, 1997, pp 197–210.
26. New York State Department of Health: Coronary artery bypass surgery in New York State 1990–1992. *In* Vibbert S, Migdail KJ, Strickland D, et al (eds): The 1995 Medical Outcomes & Guidelines Sourcebook. Washington, DC, Faulkner & Gray, 1994, pp 466–480.
27. Osborne J: Personal communication, 1997.
28. Pellegrino ED, Thomasma DC: The Virtues in Medical Practice. New York, Oxford University Press, 1993, p 67.
29. Robinson G, Merav A: Informed consent: Recall by patients tested postoperatively. Ann Thorac Surg 22:209, 1976.
30. Rose E: Discussion of "Minimally Invasive CABG" panel discussion by DJ Ullyot, TA Burdon, NW Salomon, et al. Western Thoracic Surgical Association, Napa, CA, June 27, 1997.
31. Roy DJ, Black P, McPeek B, et al: Ethical principles in research. *In* Troidl H, McKneally MF, Mulder DS, et al (eds): Surgical Research: Basic Principles and Clinical Practice, 3rd ed. New York, Springer Verlag, 1997, pp 581–604.

32. Singer PA: Editorial: Resource allocation: Beyond evidence-based medicine and cost-effectiveness analysis. ACP Journal Club 127:A16–A18, 1997.
33. Singer PA, Siegler M, Lantos JD, et al: The ethical assessment of innovative therapies: Liver transplantation using living donors. Theor Med 11:87–94, 1990.
34. Singer PA, Siegler M, Whitington PF, et al: Ethics of liver transplantation with living donors. N Engl J Med 321:620–622, 1989.
35. Subramanian VA, McCabe CJ, Geller CM: Minimally invasive direct coronary artery bypass grafting: Two-year clinical experience. Ann Thorac Surg 64:1648–1655, 1997.
36. Thompson DF: Understanding financial conflicts of interest. N Engl J Med 329:573–576, 1993.
37. Todd TR, Perron J, Winton TL, et al: Simultaneous single lung transplant and lung volume reduction. Ann Thorac Surg 63:1468–1470, 1997.
38. Troidl H, McKneally MF: Toward a definition of surgical research. *In* Troidl H, McKneally MF, Mulder DS, et al (eds): Surgical Research: Basic Principles and Clinical Practice, 3rd ed. New York, Springer Verlag, 1997, pp 3–8.
39. Wildes KW: Healthy skepticism: The emperor has very few clothes. J Med Philos 22:365–371, 1997.

COMMENTARY

John R. Benfield

Martin McKneally's thoughtful discourse about ethical considerations associated with the introduction of new surgical technology includes key concepts, such as the vulnerability of patients when they are being asked to give informed consent for "nonvalidated procedures." He discusses the "moral authority" of the medical profession, the "unbalanced relationship" between patients and their surgeons, and the guidance that the profession receives from the law, public policy, and ethical axioms. His hope for better methods to "overcome the . . . entrepreneurial competition between institutions and practices" is laudable, but probably unrealistic. Competition for leadership in the implementation of new methods will persist. I believe such competition can be in the patient's best interest if it remains ethical. This means that patients who are the subjects of new methods are completely informed of the novelty, and that surgeons embark on the use of new methods after they have been as well prepared as possible, and not primarily to achieve economic advantage.

Consideration of ethics pertaining to new surgical technology should include a discussion of the role of public information media, such as newspapers and television. Journalists wish to report newsworthy information as promptly as possible, because rapidity in publication helps to sell their products. Thus, information regularly appears in the press after it has been presented at scientific meetings and before it has been published in professional journals. Such information can, and often does, mislead vulnerable patients into false hopes that they pursue at great emotional and monetary expense without realistic hope of true benefit. Is it ethical for journalists to insist upon distribution of information about new surgical technology before such technology has matured within the profession?

Freedom of the press, the right to information, and freedom of speech are sacrosanct to me and to the society in which I am privileged to live. Thus, I oppose censorship. I recognize that scientifically presented information about new technology is in the public domain, but I believe it is never crucial to distribute it via the media within hours after its initial presentation. It is imperative that the information given by the media be as accurate as possible, and that it be presented in ways that protect patients from unwarranted hopes and potential profiteering. Cohesion and cooperation among journalists and investigators are the ways to achieve this goal.

It is common for journalists to take notes and then to present their findings promptly in the media. With regard to new technology in health care, a different method should become routine. Journalists should provide investigators with drafts of what they wish to say and how they wish to say it to the public. Ethical journalists and ethical developers of new surgical technology should commit themselves to taking the time and making the effort to be accurate and not misleading. This may require several drafts of a proposed communication. The idea that today's events must be reported in tomorrow's press does not pertain to new surgical technology.

Patients, their families, and their referring physicians are the major decision-makers concerning how quickly, where, and by whom new surgical technology is used. An example of this was seen when laparoscopic cholecystectomy was first performed. Patients were demanding the method before it was as safe as the tried-and-true method of removing the gallbladder. Similarly, patients and incompletely informed referring physicians have sometimes insisted upon video-assisted thoracic surgery (VATS) when traditional methods are safer and better.

Balance, judgment, and honesty are key ingredients in implementing new technology. There is no clear-cut and uniform answer as to how much preparation a surgeon needs before he or she embarks on the independent learning curve of a new operation. It is clear, however, that each surgeon needs to communicate honestly with patients and to believe that he or she is as well prepared as possible to use any new method that promises to be advantageous to them. The use of new technology should not be seen as a badge of courage, and adherence or return to a proven older technology must not be perceived as defeat or inadequacy.

All the issues discussed by McKneally in this chapter are important, and many others remain to be considered. Ethics evolves as society matures. Some of the clear-cut ethical concepts of the past are no longer acceptable today, and, certainly, some of today's wisdom will be unacceptable in the future. The most ethical things we can do are to continue to be true to our patients and to ourselves, and to resist self-serving entrepreneurial behavior in the realm of new technology in health care.

Section II

Pleural Diseases

Chapter 7

Diagnostic Thoracoscopy for Pleural Disease

Joseph LoCicero III

Physicians use diagnostic procedures as the first test of new invasive technology. Thoracoscopy is no exception. Simple observation and selective small biopsies can show the value of the procedure without causing undue risk to the patient. Dr. Jacobaeus, the famous Swedish physician, performed and reported on the first thoracoscopy, which was performed for diagnosis.[1] He became an excellent diagnostician, writing about the phases of tuberculosis and describing how primary and secondary tumors cause malignant pleural effusions.[2]

Three decades later, vehement criticism in the United States over the use of the technique by less than qualified personnel led thoracoscopy to be relegated to the level of a museum piece on the western side of the Atlantic. However, since there was no such denunciation in Europe, practitioners have performed diagnostic thoracoscopy essentially using the original format up to today. Other than refined optics and a camera, little has changed over the decades.

Indications

The most common presentation of a patient for a diagnosis of pleural disease is a pleural effusion (Fig. 7–1). This seems to state the obvious, but there are actually many potential reasons to explore the pleura. Other indications may include chest trauma with hemothorax or hemopneumothorax, thickening of the pleura, persistent pleuritic pain without evidence of an effusion, or suspicion of mesothelioma in a patient who has had heavy asbestos exposure with or without an effusion. Also, in the case of trauma victims, Frame and associates suggest that patients who suffer blunt torso trauma requiring abdominal exploration should have a diagnostic thoracoscopy before the abdomen is opened to assess structures at or near the diaphragm as well as the diaphragm itself.[3]

Prethoracoscopy Testing

Thoracocentesis, not thoracoscopy, is the first diagnostic step in the nonemergent evaluation of a pleural effusion. When thoracocentesis is performed, as much fluid as possible should be removed. This not only ensures an adequate number of samples of fluid for performance of all possible studies, but also allows assessment of improvement in the patient's condition. Such information is invaluable in determining whether a therapeutic procedure, such as pleurodesis, might be beneficial.

Patients require little in the way of preparation for diagnostic thoracoscopy. Especially significant in this era of cost containment is the fact that almost no routine testing is necessary. Most patients who are evaluated for a pleural problem, including acute trauma, have usually already had a variety of laboratory and radiologic examinations performed.

Minimal required testing includes a radiogram of the chest, a complete blood count, and an electrocardiogram for those who are older than 45 years of age. However, most patients will have had computed tomography (CT) of the chest, a chemical profile, and coagulation studies. Acute trauma patients will have had a variety of tests, including a complete blood count, blood chemistries, and blood gases; a chest tube will frequently have been inserted and sometimes a CT of the chest and abdomen will have been performed.

The most direct way to assess the potential space is by thoracocentesis. This helps to determine the ability of the operator to access the pleural space in question. Sometimes, this assessment can be made by observing changes on the CT of the chest. Scalloping of the lung at the edge of the pleural process is a sign of a solid process that may not yield a space for the thoracoscope (Fig. 7–2). Another sign of potential difficulty is a zone of enhancement at the edge of the pleural fluid, suggesting an organized fibrinous mass or a fibrin peel on the lung that would prevent lung expansion (Fig. 7–3).

Preparation

Minimal preparation is required for pleural exploration. Most patients breathe better when the pleural fluid is removed during the procedure. However, preoperative pulmonary hygiene can be helpful for improving postoperative pulmonary toilet and maintaining lung expansion. Teaching the patient simple incentive spirometry and breathing exercises is very helpful.

Equipment

Basic equipment is all that is required for standard diagnostic thoracoscopy. Standard endoscopic equipment in-

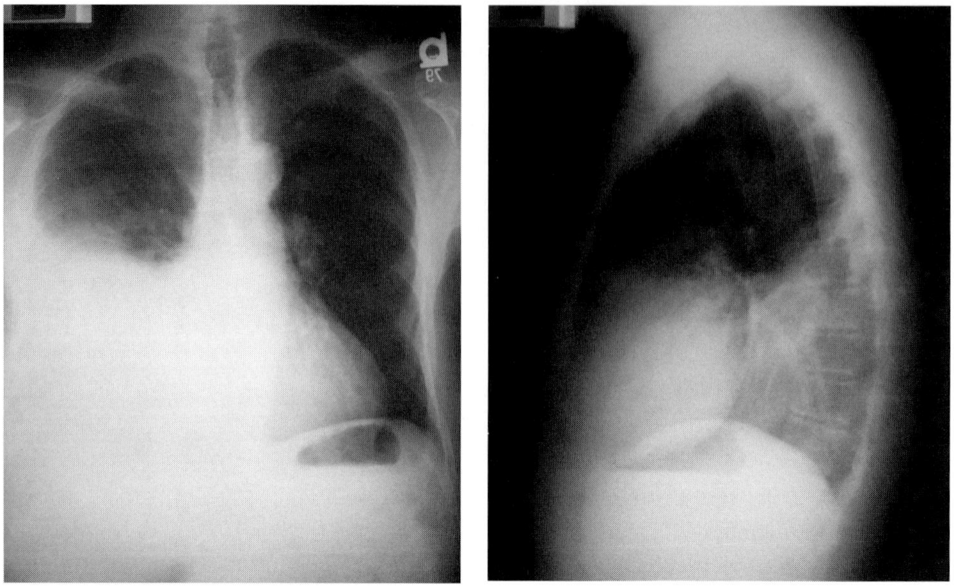

Figure 7–1. Anteroposterior and lateral views of a pleural effusion.

cludes a scope and a camera, three ports, two graspers, and a scissors. Additional equipment that may be helpful under special circumstances includes a cautery or spatula, a large grasping forceps, such as a gallbladder forceps, and a straight and curved ring forceps.

When less invasive or limited procedures are planned, miniaturized equipment is available. A 2-mm scope and biopsy forceps that fit through a Veres needle may be used with local anesthesia in an outpatient setting. However, these instruments give very limited visualization and maneuverability. In a small closed space, such as a joint, where the background color is white, the light from this small optic device is adequate for excellent viewing. However, in the capacious chest cavity, the light generated is weak and may be inadequate for evaluation of the large area. Therefore, the cases for which this instrumentation is considered must be carefully evaluated preoperatively. A small scope that has been used successfully is the cystoscope, which has better optics and lighting than the 2-mm size.[4]

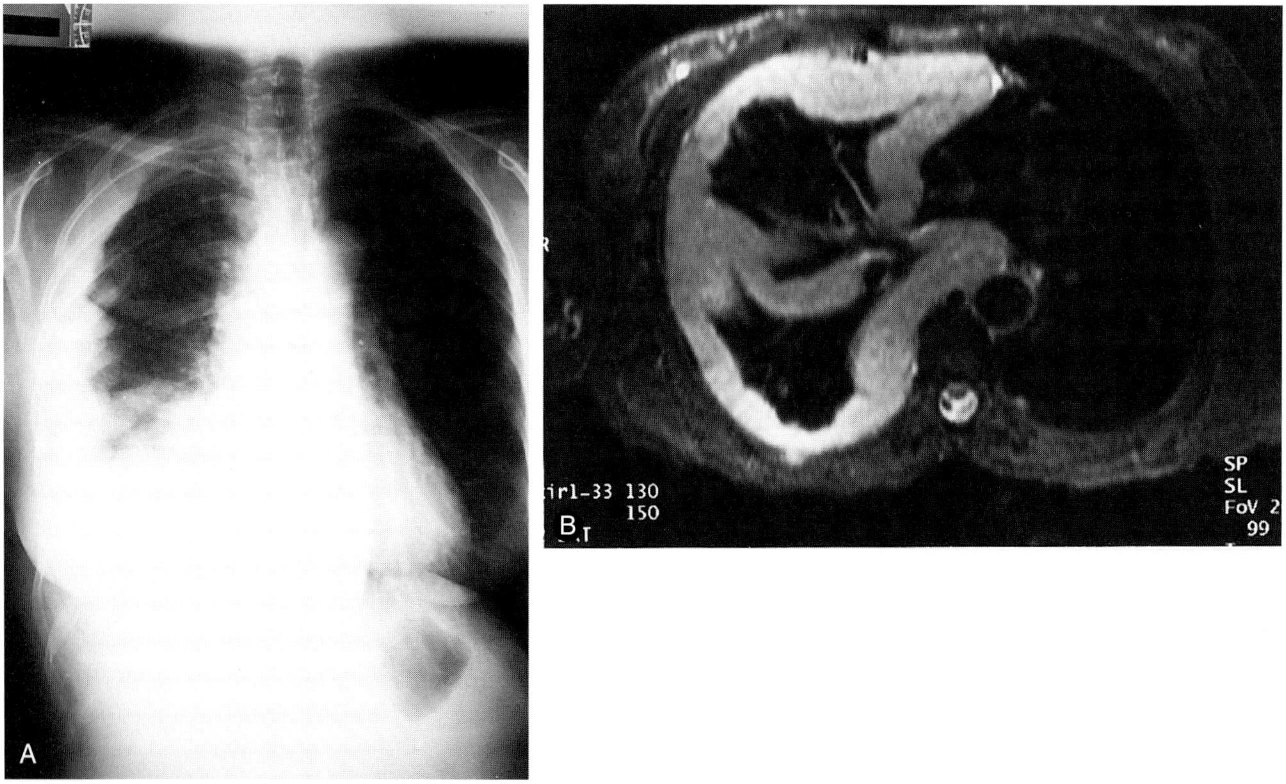

Figure 7–2. Scalloping of the lung. *A*, Plain film view. *B*, Computed tomography (CT).

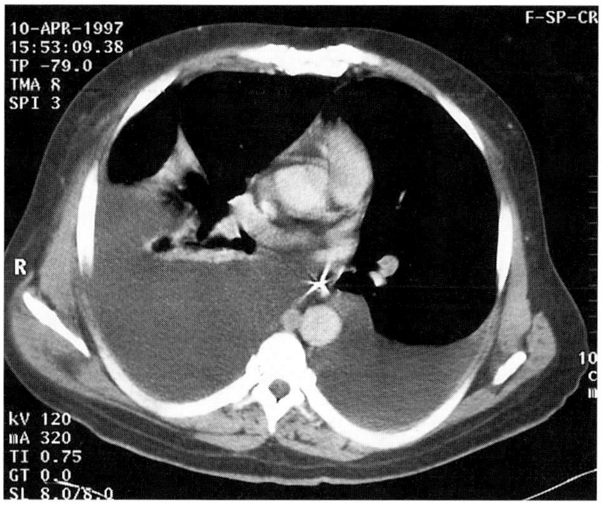

Figure 7–3. Computed tomography showing zone of enhancement at the edge of the pleural fluid.

Another scope that is helpful in minimally invasive procedures is the operating laparoscope. This 10-mm scope has a 5-mm channel that is parallel to the viewing optics and the light source, allowing easy access for grasping, suctioning, and biopsy. Instruments can be exchanged through the operating channel without another port having to be created. The channel can be fitted with an optional airtight cap. Disadvantages of this scope are that it allows only one operating function at a time, and it has a limited field of view for performing maneuvers. This latter problem limits the size of the biopsy because the view changes with the movement of the instrument. In my experience, the usual size of biopsy obtainable with one port and an operating scope is a pleural strip measuring 3 cm by 3 cm.

Procedure

Procedures may be conducted under local or general anesthesia. Techniques are similar, but there are a few subtle differences worth noting.

Local Anesthesia

For simple, straightforward cases of pleural disease, a thoracoscopy can be performed under local anesthesia with monitored conscious sedation. This procedure should be performed on carefully selected patients who have a good performance status. In addition, this procedure should be performed in an operating room because of the potential for conversion to an open procedure if complications develop.

Patients should be prepared as if for an open thoracotomy. At a minimum, they should have cardiac monitoring, noninvasive blood pressure monitoring, and pulse oximetry. After baseline readings have been obtained, the patient is placed in the thoracotomy position and prepared and draped as for a thoracotomy. During the preparation, conscious sedation is begun, usually with midazolam. Local anesthesia is important in helping to maintain a quiet field. The port sites are infiltrated with 3 to 5 ml of 0.5% lidocaine or bupivacaine with or without epinephrine.

General Anesthesia

Patients who require more than a small biopsy should be candidates for thoracoscopy under general anesthesia. Lysis of adhesions, biopsy of lymph nodes, large pleural or lung biopsies, or other advanced thoracoscopic procedures are best done under completely controlled conditions. General anesthesia requires positive pressure ventilation; therefore, a double-lumen tube is necessary for split-lung ventilation.

Once asleep and intubated, the patient is positioned as for a posterolateral thoracotomy. If the major pathology is in the apex of the chest, the patient is positioned as if for an axillary thoracotomy. The remainder of the procedure is performed in the same way as any other thoracoscopic operation. At the point the patient is prepared, the lung is isolated and allowed to collapse. This permits the air in the lung to begin to be absorbed, which speeds the collapse of the lung at the start of the procedure.

At the conclusion of the procedure, regardless of anesthetic technique, a chest tube is inserted and the lung is slowly expanded. To minimize the postoperative pain, bupivacaine is infiltrated around all the incisions, including the chest tube insertion site. Because of the systemic absorption of local anesthetics through the pleura, most surgeons do not instill bupivacaine into the chest cavity.

Conduct of the Operation

Positioning of the first port in the chest varies, depending upon the location of interest. The scope should be sufficiently far away (about 10 cm) from the pathology to allow easy viewing. In practical terms, this usually means at least two interspaces and 6 cm anterior or posterior to the pathology; anterior and inferior placement is usually best. Sometimes, owing to adhesions or loculation, such distances are not possible. In these cases, the scope is placed in the line of a potential thoracotomy.

In a case of local anesthesia, an artificial pneumothorax must be created. This is done using a Veres needle, which is inserted at the same site as the scope.[5] Atmospheric air or carbon dioxide can be insufflated through the needle to collapse the lung. Approximately 800 ml of gas at 8 mm Hg is necessary to collapse the lung. In the case of general anesthesia, insufflation is not necessary, because the lung can be collapsed by using the double-lumen tube. Thus, the first incision to insert the scope is the size of a chest tube insertion site.

Once the scope is in the chest, the entire hemithorax should be examined. This is a principle retained from exploratory thoracotomy. Lysis of adhesions may be required unless the operation is a limited examination in which the pathology is readily apparent. All structures should be examined, including the aorta and its branches or the vena cava and its tributaries, the lungs, the mediastinum, the esophagus, the pleura, and the sympathetic chain.

A unique feature of thoracoscopy is that it facilitates obtaining quality photographs of the intrathoracic pathology. No opportunity should be allowed to pass without obtaining photo documentation of all pathologies.

Biopsy of any of the chest structures is possible. Wedge resection of the lung is covered elsewhere. Biopsy of the pleura is begun by making an incision over a rib to avoid injury of the intercostal bundle. Once the pleural flap is begun, it is continued by undermining it with a blunt instrument until there is sufficient tissue for all the required studies. The specimen is removed by incising it with scissors or cautery. Sometimes, a hook with a cautery attached works just as well. Biopsies of the mediastinal structures require incision of the pleura over the pathology. Blunt dissection usually delivers the specimen of interest. The remaining connections contain the blood supply and can be cauterized or clipped.

When large masses or matted nodes are encountered, a core biopsy is indicated. The capsule can be very well vascularized, and bleeding can be significant. Needle aspiration is performed first to ensure that the structure is not highly vascularized on the inside beyond the capsule. A figure-of-eight stitch is placed in the mass as a biopsy traction anchor. Cautery is used to coagulate the capsule in the area of incision. Once this is accomplished, a long scalpel is inserted and a cone-shaped biopsy is taken. Any additional bleeding may be cauterized with a guarded suction cautery. Local pressure can be applied with an endoscopic Kitner or with a small gauze pad applied to the area with a sponge forceps.

All specimens are examined by frozen section for three reasons: first, to confirm that abnormal tissue has been obtained; second, to confirm that sufficient tissue has been obtained to perform all the tests necessary to arrive at a diagnosis; third, and much less important, to have a preliminary diagnosis to tell the patient and family after the procedure.

Postoperative Care

When a diagnostic thoracoscopy is the only procedure performed, a chest tube is not always required. A temporary catheter can be placed and the lung re-expanded. The catheter can be removed in the operating room or in the recovery room after radiologic confirmation of lung expansion. In the case of a chronic pleural effusion, the length of time the chest tube remains in place is dependent upon the amount of drainage.

Pain is not usually a major issue because of the limited nature of the procedure. Usually acetaminophen (Tylenol) is sufficient for pain relief. Local care of the incisions is standard. Most patients can return to normal activity within a few days.

Results

The yield of diagnostic thoracoscopy is dependent on the perseverance of the operator. If the pathology is not readily apparent, the surgeon must continue an exhaustive search for abnormal tissue. When this is done, a diagnosis can be made almost all the time. However, the etiology of some pleural effusions is never found. Light points out that there are myriad causes, including malignancy, congestive heart failure, renal failure, infection, pulmonary infarction, and collagen vascular diseases.[6] Maitre and associates followed a series of pleural effusions with unknown etiologies after thorough thoracoscopic evaluations.[7] He and his colleagues discovered that of the 10% without etiology, one third were eventually proven to be of malignant origin. Canto and associates studied 622 malignant pleural effusions to shed some light on this subject.[8] They noted that the likelihood of finding pleural metastasis in patients with an effusion and lung cancer was 77%. However, when there was an effusion of less than 500 ml, only 22% had cancer. When the metastasis was small and localized, only 19% had positive cytology. But in generalized cases, the yield was 73%.

Complications

Problems are uncommon when only diagnostic thoracoscopy is performed. However, all the usual problems do occur from time to time. These include bleeding, infection, nerve injury resulting from a biopsy or pressure on an intercostal nerve, postthoracotomy pain syndrome, pleural effusion, air leak, atelectasis, and pneumonia. Each problem is addressed in the same manner as any other thoracic procedure.

References

1. Jacobaeus HC: Über die Möglichkeit der Zystoskopischen unter suchung Serösser höhlunger enzuwenden. München Med Wochenschr 40:2090, 1910.
2. Jacobaeus HC: Die Thoraskopie und ihre Praktische Bedeutung. Dtsch Med Wochenschr 25:702–705, 1921.
3. Frame SB: Thoracoscopy for trauma. Int Surg 82:223–228, 1997.
4. Sakurai S, Ohura M, Ogawa J, et al: Video-assisted bedside pleuroscopy under local anesthesia: Use of a rigid cystouretero-scope in patients with undiagnosed pleural effusion. Nippon Kyobu Shikkan Gakkai Zasshi 34(Suppl):148–154, 1996.
5. Faurschou P, Viskum K: Artificial pneumothorax by the Veress cannula: Efficacy and safety. Respir Med 91:402–405, 1997.
6. Light RW: Pleural diseases. Dis Mon 38:261–331, 1992.
7. Maitre B, Atassi K, Housset B: Diagnosis of pleurisy. Rev Pract 47:1298–1303, 1997.
8. Canto A, Arnau A, Galbis J, et al: The so-called malignant pleural effusion: A new review of direct data obtained with diagnostic pleuroscopy. Arch Bronconeumol 32:453–458, 1996.

COMMENTARY

Stephen R. Hazelrigg

Diagnostic thoracoscopy is a simple procedure to obtain tissue from any intrathoracic location. This procedure is tolerated well, requires short-term anesthesia, and is not very controversial. Because of its simplicity and excellent visualization, it has made blind pleural biopsies almost obsolete.

There are advocates of performing more of these procedures under local anesthetic. The arguments for this are that it decreases costs and may be performed in the endoscopy suite instead of the more costly operating room. Our experience has been that local procedures require more experience and are tolerated less well by patients. The short-term general anesthesia is usually tolerated well, and performance in the operating room provides safe alternatives should intraoperative problems occur. Except in very carefully selected cases, we recommend general anesthesia even for simple diagnostic procedures.

Chapter 8

Empyema and Hemothorax

Tomás Angelillo-Mackinlay

Video-assisted thoracic surgery (VATS) is an approach that avoids the undesirable sequelae of thoracotomy without altering the nature of the proper surgical procedure. Complete resolution of the disease is mandatory and to advocate its use, results equal to those obtained by means of thoracotomy are essential. The aim of this chapter is to describe when and how VATS can replace thoracotomy in the treatment of empyema thoracis and hemothorax. Both of these conditions have similar operative indications as well as similar sequelae resulting from suboptimal treatment.

The application of VATS requires prior cessation or marked decrease of the offending causes, namely, control of hemorrhage in the hemothorax, and control of the source of infection in empyema. Therefore, VATS debridement replaces thoracotomy *only* in *residual* infections or *residual* hemorrhages, *not* in ongoing processes, such as open bronchopleural fistula, esophageal perforation, or major active bleeding. In these cases, thoracotomy is indicated, with a different degree of urgency, depending on the individual case. Early surgical intervention is the key for a successful outcome at a point when the collection can still be suctioned out through a few small incisions.

Finally, it must be noted that if treatment is lacking or delayed, empyema and hemothorax lead to fibroblastic invasion of the fibrinous collection, with resultant lung encasement. In this situation, minimally invasive surgery has no place, and full thoracotomy is indicated to restore lung expansion.

Empyema

During the 20th century, the impressive evolution of technology and the better understanding of the pathogenesis of the disease process dramatically changed the surgical management of empyema, particularly after the discovery and clinical application of antibiotics. At the beginning of World War I, empyema thoracis among US military forces was associated with a mortality rate greater than 30% in patients treated by open drainage. The ad hoc "Empyema Commission" created by Evarts Graham and associates[22] recommended closed-tube rather than open drainage in the early stages of empyema, thus lowering the lethal outcome to less than 10%. The basic principles of this new approach were the following:

1. Avoidance of pneumothorax caused by open drainage, which was responsible for most of the immediate postoperative mortality
2. Prevention of chronicity by early evacuation of septic material and obliteration of the infected cavity
3. Careful preservation of the nutritional state of the patient

Since then, tube drainage, with or without rib resection, has remained the mainstay of surgical therapy. Empyema thoracis is a septic complication secondary to many different causes, and it has a variable biological evolution. Therefore, different technical modalities have a role and an appropriate time and place in the treatment of acute and chronic thoracic empyema.

The procedures used are thoracotomy for early fibrinous debridement or late peel decortication; pleurocutaneous thoracostomy windows[12–17] for bronchopleural fistula; thoracoplasty[1] and space-filling techniques that use muscle transposition for residual pleural pockets associated with unexpandable lungs[45]; open-tube thoracoscopy,[59–64] with or without fibrinolytic irrigation,[8–48, 49] for loculated empyema; and, more recently, video-assisted thoracic surgery (VATS).[4, 20, 26–31, 38, 53, 58–66]

Empyema is a collection of pus or infected effusion within the pleural cavity. It can involve the entire cavity or it can be loculated. Most frequently, empyema is caused by underlying pneumonia (65%), although it can develop after surgery or trauma (25%), or as a result of mediastinal or subdiaphragmatic infections (Fig. 8–1). The causative agent may be anaerobic, aerobic, or mixed. In the preantibiotic era, empyemas were generally caused by pneumococci or streptococci. With better antibiotic control of these germs, a wide variety of gram-negative and gram-positive bacteria can be commonly found, such as *Escherichia coli, Klebsiella, Staphylococcus aureus, Bacteroides, Enterobacter aerogenes, Pseudomonas,* and *Proteus.*[10] These organisms usually reach the pleural cavity by extending directly from the lung, the mediastinum, the diaphragm, the chest wall, or the neck. Occasionally, there may be hematogenous or lymphatic spread, particularly in immunocompromised patients.

The American Thoracic Society describes three stages in the biologic evolution of an empyema.[3] Initially, the exudative effusion remains fluid and the pleural membrane becomes edematous (stage I, or the exudative phase). As the infected effusion progresses, fibrin is deposited over the visceral or parietal pleuras, or both (stage II, or the fibrinopurulent phase). Because of the specific gravity of the effusion, the deposition begins in the partially compressed lower lobe and follows an irregular distribution, which results in formation of septa. Up to this point, the pleura is still well preserved, so good re-expansion of the lung can occur after removal of the empyema. Within 3 to 4 weeks, the outer aspect of the peel becomes firm, fibrous tissue (stage III, or the organizational phase), with massive ingrowth of fibroblast and formation of collagen fibers over the pleural surface. The lung is trapped and can no longer re-expand except through decortication.

The evolution of an infected effusion from the exudative stage to fibrotic encasement represents a continuous process that has no sharply defined boundaries. Fibrin

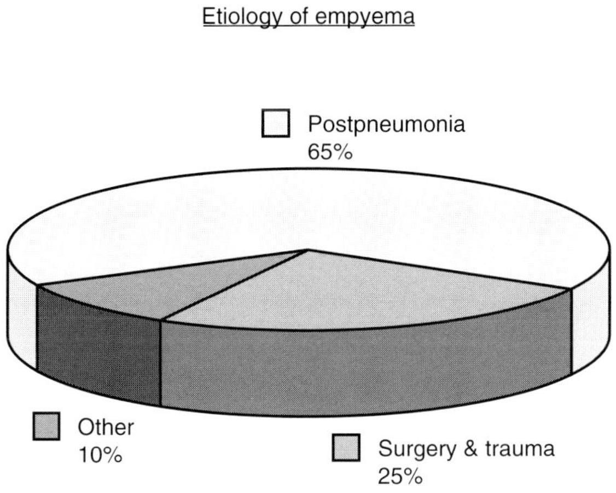

Figure 8–1. Etiology of empyema.

deposition within the pleural cavity is variable, depending on individual biologic reaction. It seems to occur earlier and be more pronounced when anaerobic bacteria, either alone or in combination with aerobic germs, are the causative agent. For this reason, empyemas resulting from surgery or trauma are usually associated with a worse clinical course and faster development of fibrotic lung encasement than those that are a complicating factor of underlying pneumonia. Sahn and associates[51] have proved in an elegant experimental study that both leukocyte phagocytosis and bacterial metabolism contribute to the presence of low pH empyema fluid, which indicates infection even when bacteria cannot be identified or cultured. Therefore, pH and glucose levels below 7 and 40 mg/100 ml, respectively, and lactate dehydrogenase (LDH) units above 1000 IU/1000 ml may predict the development of empyema.[34]

Diagnosis

Diagnosis is usually made on clinical grounds, according to the cause of origin, radiographic signs, and demonstration of infected fluid on thoracocentesis. The most common initial symptoms are dyspnea (82%), fever (81%), cough (70%), and chest pain (67%).[2–61]

Once the diagnosis of empyema thoracis has been firmly established, it is necessary to know whether the collection is *free* or *loculated.* Many loculated effusions or empyemas contain no frank pus, but rather a large number of fibrin clots and membranes, forming several compartments filled with seropurulent fluid. Ultrasonography and computed tomography (CT) scans are highly sensitive in detecting the presence of septa or loculation. We prefer CT scans because they render additional information about the lungs and the mediastinum. The most suggestive sign of empyema on chest radiograph is an encapsulated effusion in an atypical position. On CT scan, empyema are usually encapsulated and bioconvex, showing thickening of the parietal pleura and the endothoracic fascia, along with increased contrast uptake of the parietal pleura as shown by Kirsh and associates.[29] In their experience, CT scans were unable to differentiate between early and late phases of empyema.

Personal Experience

For years, surgeons have sought a less aggressive approach than posterolateral thoracotomy for the evacuation of loculated empyema. Open-tube thoracoscopy by mediastinoscope,[59] large-bore tube drainage in conjunction with fibrinolytic agents,[8, 28, 33, 49] and several types[4–60] of limited thoracotomies have been extensively used with different rates of success.

Long before the advent of VATS, we systematically used to debride an empyemic collection through a 10-cm lateral thoracotomy along the seventh or eighth intercostal space (Fig. 8–2). Palpation allowed complete evacuation of fibrin clots, disruption breakdown of septa, and destruction of septic pouches, especially in fissures and the subpneumonic area.

If fibrotic peel was found, the thoracotomy was extended as much as necessary to allow complete pulmonary decortication. In 1992, we realized that these same goals could be achieved by using VATS, with the advantages of more accurate and magnified direct visual inspection of the whole cavity, and visual command of surgical maneuvers and instrumentation.

Our first experience[4] with VATS in this setting showed encouraging results.

Surgical Technique

Patient Preparation

All patients were operated on under general anesthesia, and a double-lumen tube was used for selective ventilation. The usual vital parameters (e.g., median arterial pressure, arterial blood gases, electrocardiogram, hourly urinary output) were always registered. After induction of anesthesia, fiberoptic bronchoscopic examination was performed on all patients to rule out the presence of obstructive endobronchial lesions. Conversion to a double-lumen endotracheal tube was then accomplished to achieve selective lung ventilation.

Patients were placed in the usual full lateral thoracotomy position. The operating table was flexed downward to widen the intercostal spaces and to avoid bulking the shoulder and pelvis, thus allowing a 360 degree free rota-

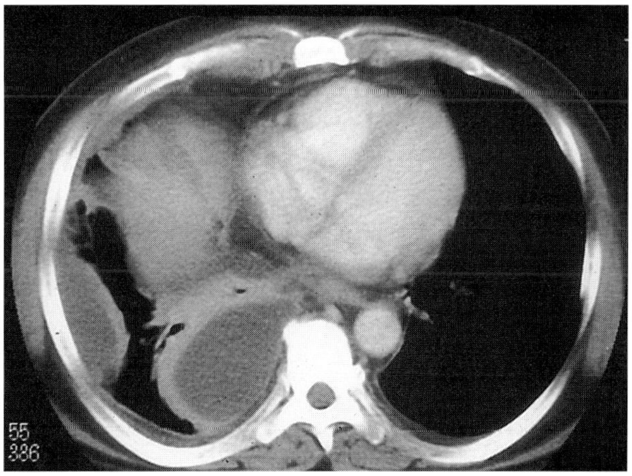

Figure 8–2. Computed tomographic scan showing loculated effusion.

tion of the scope and instruments. The hemithorax was prepared and draped for possible open thoracotomy.

Thoracotomy

When thoracotomy was performed, the thorax was approached through muscle-sparing lateral incisions (see Fig. 8–2), that were long enough to allow the introduction of one hand for manual exploration and blind debridement (Fig. 8–3). Rib spreaders were not used. Once complete digital debridement was accomplished, one or two large-bore chest tubes were placed in the lower part of the cavity through separate incisions. A sample of the pleural exudate was removed for culture, Gram's stain, and fungal stain.

Video-Assisted Thoracic Surgery (VATS)

When VATS is used, we divide the thorax into four areas by two lines: one is drawn longitudinally (cephalocaudal) along the midaxillary line, and the other is drawn transversely (ventrodorsal) along the nipple level (Fig. 8–4). This division results in four zones: ventrocephalic, dorsocephalic, ventrocaudal, and dorsocaudal. We have learned that, in most cases, the degree of difficulty in freeing the lung from the thoracic wall follows this order. Therefore, we designed a four-port approach that represents our present technique (Fig. 8–5).

The first incision is made in the fourth intercostal space outside the pectoral rim, usually the least involved area. First, a finger is introduced to perform careful lysis of any adhesions that might exist, thus creating a cavity. A 7.5-mm diameter working channel scope (Storz, Tuttlingen, Germany) is inserted through a 12-mm trocar, and, by means of a blunt-tipped suction cannula, the lung is mobilized in its upper and dorsal areas. Samples are taken for bacteriologic culture, physiochemical examination, and so forth.

The second incision is made in the subscapular zone under videoscopic control. Through this post, instruments, such as curved-ring forceps, curettes, and specially designed, high-pressure suction cannulae, are introduced directly through skin incisions. In this way, fibrin clots from both visceral and parietal pleural surfaces can be removed under direct visualization. The scope is then placed in the second port and the ventrocaudal region is freed, with special care given to separating the lung from the pericardial fat pad. The anterior end of the fifth intercostal space is individualized, and the third port is placed at that level.

Reintroducing the scope through the first port frees the ventrodorsal area—usually the area with the most tenacious adhesions. The insertion of instruments in different combinations through these ports makes debridement complete. This four-port approach can be reduced to

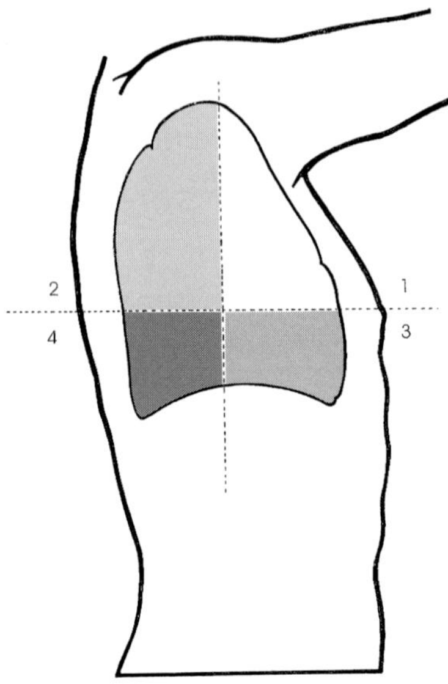

Figure 8–4. Schematic division of the pleural cavity. Ordinal numbers indicate increasing degree of difficulty in debridement: 1 = easiest, 4 = most difficult.

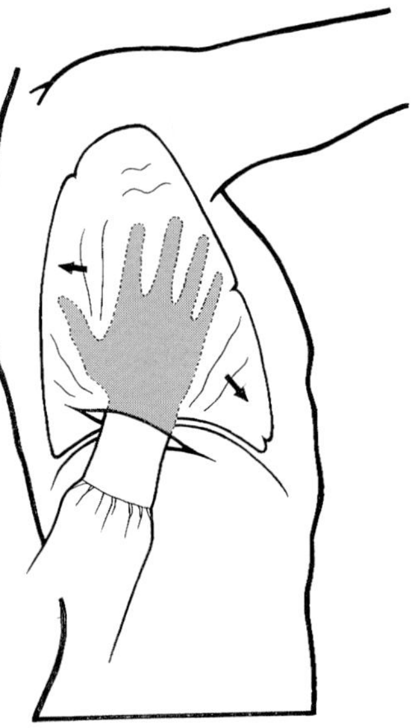

Figure 8–3. Blind loculated empyema debridement.

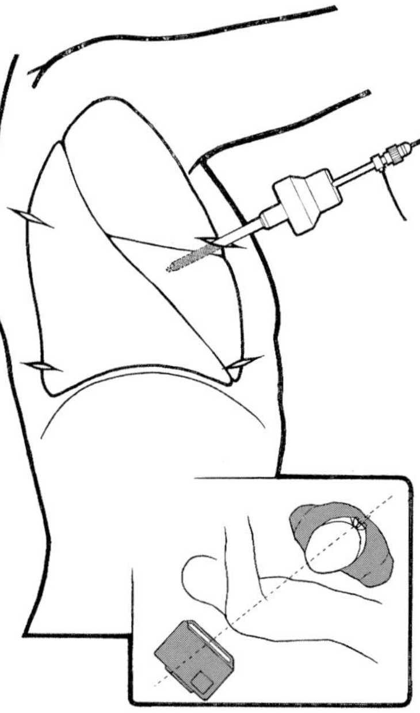

Figure 8–5. Four-port approach. Exploration starts through Port 1. Inset: Surgeon-monitor alignment.

three, or even two, incisions, when the effusion is tackled in its earliest stages, and fibrin adhesions can be removed easily by suction.

The alignment of the second and third ports closely follows the greater fissure orientation and allows for the drainage of encapsulated pus pockets that could have developed within the fissure, whereas the alignment of the first and second ports follows the lesser fissure orientation and proceeds similarly (Fig. 8–6). The alignment of the third and fourth ports frees the subpulmonary area, which is facilitated by grasping the lung upwards from the second and fourth ports. When necessary, the fourth port can be extended several centimeters to perform a partial fibrotic decortication, thus avoiding a full thoracotomy. Should conversion be needed, posterolateral thoracotomy can be done by joining the second and third incisions, and axillary thoracotomy can be achieved by joining the first and third incisions to form a curved longitudinal skin wound. In any circumstance, we keep the VATS equipment on the operative field so that continued video assistance can be used during the open intervention to facilitate the procedure in hard-to-visualize areas. The lung is then re-expanded and checked for air leakage. One or two drainage tubes are left in place under endoscopic vision.

The procedure is completed with standard closure of all other intercostal access sites and the establishment of 20 cm of negative pressure suction to the underwater seal chest-drainage system.

Postoperative Care

Patients from both series are alternatively sent to the intensive care unit or to a room on the floor, depending on the degree of illness. Antibiotics are administered for at least 3 weeks. The clinical course, body temperature, leukocyte count, and duration of chest tube insertion are always recorded. Chest radiographs are obtained at different intervals, beginning immediately postoperatively and continuing up to 6 months later, when patients are discharged.

Patients and Methods

The following data attest to our experience with all types of phase II empyemas, including postpneumonic and other related etiologies, such as postsurgical, posttramatic, and miscellaneous empyemas. Since 1985, 161 cases of acute empyema have been operated on at our institution.

To compare the relative values of VATS and thoracotomy in phase II empyemas, *all* other procedures, such

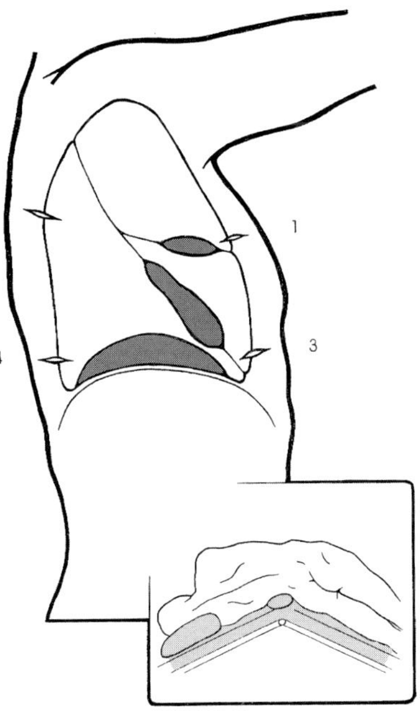

Figure 8–6. Encapsulated pus collections within fissures and subpulmonary area. Inset: Patient positioned on flexed operating table.

as Eloesser flaps, ab initio (or planned) thoracotomies, and drainage tubes were excluded from the analysis because they were usually associated with ongoing infection. Analysis, therefore, was made of only 125 cases treated either by VATS (80) or thoracotomy (45).

The 86 postpneumonic cases were divided into two groups, depending on whether they were treated by thoracotomy (Group I = 33 cases) or by VATS (Group II = 53 cases). Similarly, the 39 cases that had origins *other* than pneumonia were divided into Group III (12 cases) and Group IV (27 cases).

These data were analyzed prospectively in Groups II and IV and retrospectively in Groups I and III. All populations were essentially similar in terms of age and gender ratio (Table 8–1).

Statistical Analysis

Results are expressed as mean values plus or minus standard deviation. A student's t test for paired data was employed for quantitative variables, and either χ^2 or Fisher's test was used for qualitative variables. Statistical significance was determined at a P value of less than 0.05.

Table 8–1. Population Features (N = 125)

Variable	Group I	Group II	Group III	Group IV	*P*
Number	33	53	12	27	
Gender (M/F)	13/20	14/39	3/9	6/21	NS
Age (mean)	51	55	50	54	NS

NS = not significant

Results

In the postpneumonic group, the preoperative length of stay dropped significantly after the introduction of VATS, reflecting an earlier referral to surgery when this minimally invasive technique became available ($P < 0.05$) (Table 8–2).

The postpneumonic patients had lower mortality and relapse rates than others, but the rates did not have statistical significance. Mortality in all thoracotomy cases versus all VATS cases showed no statistical difference.

Mortality ranged from 1.8% in the postpneumonic VATS group to 8.3% in the other etiology thoracotomy subset. Global morbidity was 12%, and global mortality was 4%.

After VATS debridement, relapse was much higher in the other etiology groups than in postpneumonic cases, where it was zero. The conversion rate was lower in the postpneumonic groups than in the other group, but again there was no statistical difference.

In the last 22 cases of postpneumonic empyemas added to our original experience, VATS debridement resulted in 0% mortality and 0% conversion rate as well as 0% relapse.

Our entire experience in these 125 cases has shown that VATS debridement for fibrinopurulent empyema of *any* origin offers excellent results in terms of the following:

1. Resolution of the disease (92.5%)
2. Morbidity (12.5%)
3. Mortality (3.75%)
4. Conversion rate (8.75%)
5. Cost
6. Labor impediment

Discussion

The surgical treatment of empyema thoracis should accomplish three goals:

1. Evacuation of all infected material
2. Re-expansion of the lung
3. Correction of the etiologic factor.

It is estimated that in the United States, 90,000 cases of empyema thoracis are registered every year; two thirds (60,000) of them are postpneumonic and one third are due to other causes. Disregarding the cause of origin, 35%[25–42] of them are loculated at the time of the surgical consultation; hence, they do not respond to tube drainage.[13] Those patients need some other procedure that can achieve complete evacuation of the whole infected collection. Historically, such a procedure has been thoracotomy, which is currently being replaced by VATS. Delay in achieving this is currently associated with a high mortality rate, which averages about 20%.

Early surgical treatment has been urged by many authors[47–50, 52–57] before and after VATS became available. In spite of the relatively high incidence of loculated effusions and the widespread use of VATS worldwide, there is a relative paucity of literature assessing its value in treating this disease. Some reports[20–35] mention its use among other indications for VATS, whereas some others[27–37] refer to it in retrospective experiences. Few of these operations are prospectively undertaken,[4–31] and one[62] has been randomized versus pleural drainage plus fibrinolytic therapy. Nonetheless, most reports recommend early intervention and complete evacuation of all infected material. They also show uniformly good outcomes associated with low morbidity and mortality. In spite of these obvious advantages, some recent reports[49] still insist on the use of fibrinolytic agents in dealing with loculated effusions. These treatments demand long hospitalization, high cost, high morbidity stemming from drug toxicity, and poor results. A randomized prospective trial[62] comparing pleural drainage plus fibrinolytic therapy versus VATS in 20 cases of loculated postpneumonic empyema, showed higher primary treatment success (91%, or 10/11, vs. 44%, or 4/9; $P < 0.05$) lower chest tube duration, shorter hospital stays, and lower costs when VATS was used. There was one death in each group. Noticeably, VATS debridement resolved all cases that had failed fibrinolytic treatment.

A well-conducted experimental study[52] used a new rabbit animal model to demonstrate the impact of timing of pleural drainage on the outcome of treatment for

Table 8–2. Comparative Results (N = 125)

Variable	Group I	Group II	Group III	Group IV	P
Number	33	53	12	27	
Conversion rate		3/53 (5.6%)		4/27 (14.8%)	NS
Tube Duration					
Mean	6.1	5.37	7.95	7.94	NS
Range	2/13	2/15	2/14	2/25	NS
SD	2.3	2.9	2.9	6.1	NS
Relapse	4/33 (12.1%)	3/53 (5.6%)	0/12 (0%)	8/27 (29.6%)	NS
Mortality	1/33 (3%)	1/53 (1.8%)	1/12 (8.3%)	2/27 (7.4%)	NS
Preoperative length of stay	17.2*	3.5	3.2	4.8	<0.05
Postoperative length of stay	11.8	8.8*	12	11.7	<0.05

*Group with statistical difference; $P < .05$ compared with other groups.

empyema. This study supports previous expert opinions and conclusions from retrospective analyses by maintaining that early drainage is beneficial in the treatment of empyema.[11–42, 47–50]

As indicated previously, the evacuation of all infected material depends on whether the collection is free or loculated and whether the offending cause has ceased or whether it persists. Tube-drainage treatment is effective if the collection is free and if its origin has been controlled or is being corrected (e.g., postpneumonic empyema). If the source of infection persists, open procedures are usually required to deal with the underlying pathology (e.g., bronchopleural fistula, esophageal perforation, subphrenic abscess). In our experience, modified liposuction cannulae attached to a high-vacuum source are the most adequate instruments to break through the septa and aspirate all infected material. Ring forceps and conventional curettes are also useful tools to accomplish complete evacuation of all infected material in the general cavity, fissures, and recesses. Another clear indication for the use of VATS is an infection not associated with a bronchopleural fistula, which is located in the residual postpneumonectomy cavity. In this situation, VATS toilet can be achieved through local anesthesia.

The state of the underlying lung must be taken into account in choosing the proper technique and instrumentation during thoracoscopic exploration. The lung can be normal or lightly pneumonic, frankly pneumonic, necrotic, or entrapped by a fibrous peel. In the first two cases, VATS debridement can be performed with varying degrees of difficulty, whereas in the latter two instances, another technique must be selected. Peripheral lung abscess, which can pour necrotic material into the pleural cavity, is better dealt with by creating a pleurocutaneous window, whereas fibrotic lung encasement must be treated by open decortication.

Based on our experience, we proceed according to an established algorithm (Fig. 8–7). Whenever an empyema thoracis or infected effusion is clinically suspected, we recommend the following measures:

1. Prove (directly or indirectly) the presence of infection by performing thoracocentesis.
2. Assess whether the collection is free or loculated (by CT scan or ultrasonography).
3. Determine whether the origin of the infection has been corrected by antibiotics or whether it still persists (ongoing infection).
4. Perform VATS for exploration and evacuation of all residual collections, using conventional liposuction cannulae attached to a high-volume vacuum source.
5. Clean the entire cavity, especially fissures and subpulmonary areas.
6. Do not hesitate to convert the procedure to open thoracotomy if fibrotic peel is found or other causes indicate the advisability of open thoracotomy.

In summary, VATS has proved to be an effective method of dealing with loculated effusions in the fibrinopurulent phase (method of choice).

Care should be taken to remove *all* infected material, with special reference to missed pockets within the fissures or in the subpulmonary area. The patient and the surgical team should be prepared for the procedure to be converted to open decortication whenever videoscopic findings indicate the advisability of doing so. Lung encasement with fibrotic peel is the most frequent cause for conversion.

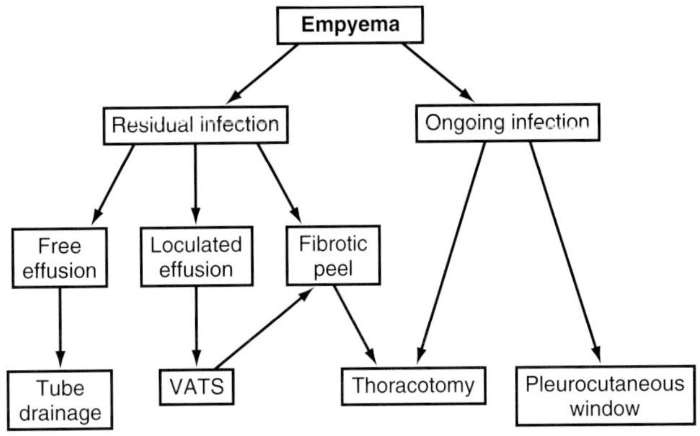

Figure 8–7. Strategic algorithm for empyema treatment.

According to the literature, VATS treatment of loculated empyema seems to be underutilized in relation to the estimated incidence of this disease.

Hemothorax

In major cities, the incidence of thoracic trauma is increasing. This trend is generally occurring because of penetrating trauma caused by stabbbing and gunshot wounds. In a 20-year review of penetrating injuries in the city of Montreal, there is striking notation made that 50% of the incidences occurred in the last 5 years of the review, with gunshot wounds accounting for 62% of the injuries.[5] The overall assessment and management of patients who survive the initial thoracic injury and arrive in an emergency room has been well established.[41] These patients can generally be classified into two groups: those requiring emergent thoracotomy for massive blood loss, and those who can be managed successfully with tube drainage.

Before videothoracoscopy became available, a clotted hemothorax or continued hemorrhage after chest-tube placement represented a clear indication for thoracotomy.

Diaphragmatic injuries are frequently undetectable at first, but they can lead to intestinal strangulation, which is a devastating, and frequently fatal, complication.[6–19, 24–39, 44]

Videothoracoscopy is a proven technique in the investigation, diagnosis, staging, and treatment of intrathoracic disease. It facilitates safe and effective removal of retained blood from the thoracic cavity, eliminating the need for a major thoracotomy incision.

Previous studies[17–30, 40, 41] indicate that early evacuation of blood collected in a hemothorax results in decreased operative blood loss, decreased morbidity and mortality, shortened hospital stay, limited thoracic incision, and avoidance of complications of empyema and fibrothorax.

Personal Experience

From February 1992 to February 1997, 27 patients who had hemothorax underwent VATS treatment at our institution, which is not a trauma center.

This figure represents only 3.6% of our whole VATS experience. There were 17 male and 10 female patients. Their ages ranged from 16 to 84 years (mean = 33 years). All patients were hemodynamically stable at surgery, and, except for postoperative cases, all were evaluated by CT scans. The interval between initial hemothorax production and VATS treatment ranged from 4 hours to 30 days (mean = 152 hr). There were 25 cases of chest trauma (18 blunt, 5 postoperative, 1 stab wound, 1 gunshot) and 2 were cases of spontaneous hemothorax. Only 1 case had to be converted to thoracotomy (3.7% conversion rate). This was an 80-year-old patient who had spontaneous hemothorax without pneumothorax. Active bleeding caused poor visibility and a limited thoracotomy was required. A broken vascularized pleural adhesion was found to be responsible for the hemorrhage, which was arrested by clipping the artery. A hemothorax that had not been promptly resolved proved to be infected, and fibrinopurulent debridement was accomplished by VATS. In 3 cases (1 right stab wound and 2 left blunt traumas), diaphragmatic lacerations were thoracoscopically sutured through a purposely placed, 3-cm long incision. Two ports were used in 15 patients, and three ports were used in the other 12 patients; length of hospital stay ranged between 3 and 15 days (mean = 7.2 days), and duration of drainage tube insertion was between 2 and 8 days (mean = 3.8 days). Two cases were complicated by pneumonia (morbidity = 7.4%), and the patients recovered after antibiotic treatment. There was no mortality. All patients recovered uneventfully and were followed up to 6 months postoperatively, after which they were definitively discharged.

Surgical Technique

Anesthesia, patient positioning, and general surgical setup were identical to those employed for empyema debridement. The main difference was in the placement of the ports, with the videothoracoscopic exploration commencing through a single 1-cm incision made in the sixth intercostal space at the level of the anterior axillary line (the third port of Fig. 8–6). Many times, the hemothorax can be resolved solely through this approach. Occasionally, in stab wound cases, the initial exploration can be done through the same wound, if it fits the purpose.

In some cases, another 3- to 4-cm incision is needed to liberate tenaciously adherent fibrin or to suture a torn diaphragm or disrupted lung tissue. The placement of this utility incision depends on the location of the internal lesion. Whenever a mild bleeding source is discovered, clipping or electrocoagulation is sufficient. Removal of foreign bodies, such as bullets or rib fragments, is generally carried out easily by this method. Disruption of clots or fibrin membranes is best handled by high-volume suction cannulae. Ring forceps, curettes, and grasping instruments complete the surgical armamentarium. Should any inconveniences arise—usually uncontrollable hemorrhage—the procedure must be converted to an open approach. Closure and drainage of the thoracic cavity is similar to cases of empyema. (Fig. 8–8).

Discussion

Surgical treatment of hemothorax aims at three objectives:

1. Arrest the bleeding source.
2. Evacuate the pleural cavity.
3. Re-expand the lung.

To fulfill these requirements and select the appropriate surgical procedure, the following conditions should be considered:

1. Type of blood collection: Define whether hemothorax is residual or actively bleeding.
2. Hemorrhage magnitude: In actively bleeding patients, assess whether the loss is massive or moderate (up to 1500 ml/24 hr).

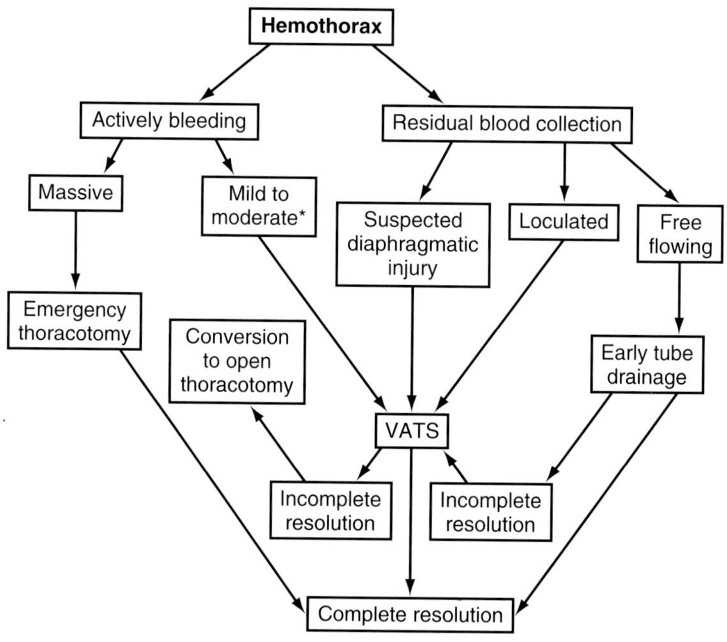

Figure 8–8. Strategic algorithm for treatment of hemothorax.

3. State of the collection: In residual hemothoraces, state whether the effusion is free flowing or clotted.
4. Laceration of the diaphragm: In low, penetrating wounds, this circumstance should always be suspected, especially on the left side.

In hemodynamically compromised patients, hemostasis should be promptly attained through an expeditious anterolateral thoracotomy. Mildly to moderately active bleeding can be resolved by VATS: should visualization reveal difficulties, or if the patient should decompensate, immediate conversion to thoracotomy is mandatory.

Evacuation of the pleural cavity should be performed completely and promptly; long-standing hemothoraces can result in empyema thoracis or fibrotic lung encasement.

Retained blood within the pleural cavity can evolve in any of the following ways:

1. Resorption
2. Progression to fibrothorax
3. Infection with empyema formation

In free-flowing residual collections, early tube drainage usually achieves complete resolution. Helling and associates[23] found that 18% of patients who had hemothorax initially treated with tube thoracostomy developed a clotted hemothorax, and that 39% of these patients eventually required decortication.

Early evacuation of hemothorax is also essential in the prevention of empyema, which occurs in 2 to 6% of cases.[43–46, 54]

Long before the introduction of videothoracoscopy, many investigators stressed the need for *early* and *complete* evacuation of residual hemothoraces, either by tube drainage or thoracotomy.[7–14, 15, 16, 30] Recent reports[10–21, 40–43] adhere to the same classic principles by advocating a minimally invasive technique, such as VATS, that attains the same outcomes with additional benefits.

Whenever CT scans demonstrate loculated or clotted hemothorax, early VATS debridement is the intervention of choice. Conventional instruments (e.g., ring forceps, high-volume suction cannulae) render excellent results. Moreover, VATS is also able to be performed under local anesthesia when postpneumonectomy collections become clotted, which often represents an early sign of infection.

In postsurgical bleeding, VATS exploration through one of the drainage tube incisions may resolve the complication, thus avoiding the need for reopening the thoracotomy incision.

In long-standing hemothoraces, VATS exploration may reveal fibrotic peel encasement. If the clinical condition of the patient is stable, the procedure should be converted and conventional decortication must be performed.

In crippled or unstable patients, this has to be judiciously evaluated and may need to be postponed until a more favorable opportunity arises.

Enzymatic dissolution has yielded poor outcomes and can produce fever and allergic reaction along with higher costs and longer hospital stays.[62]

Small diaphragmatic perforations usually present no symptoms, but they may cause very severe complications later. It is estimated that 20% of diaphragmatic lacerations eventually end up in strangulation, which is associated with a mortality rate as high as 36%.[39] For this reason, exploratory videothoracoscopy is advocated for penetrating injuries of the lower thorax and in cases of blunt trauma with inward protruding rib segments.[6–18, 63]

Laparoscopy should not be attempted as a first exploratory method because of the risk of tension pneumothorax resulting from carbon dioxide insufflation.[55] Should abdominal exploration be needed, laparoscopy can be performed after the diaphragmatic laceration has been closed by thoracoscopy and the pleural cavity has been properly drained.

According to recent literature, VATS treatment of hemothorax is gaining widespread application in a variety of clinical settings.[32–36, 56–65]

In summary, VATS treatment of hemothorax of any origin has proved to be a sound strategic approach. Comparing it with thoracotomy, the same results can be achieved with less trauma, lower cost, shorter hospital stay, better cosmesis, shorter overall recovery, and more prompt return to work.

ACKNOWLEDGMENTS

To my wife, Diana, my colleagues Domingo Chimondeguy, Gustavo Lyons, and Diego Angelillo-Mackinlay, for their invaluable assistance in the preparation of this chapter.

References

1. Alexander J: The collapse therapy of pulmonary tuberculosis. Springfield, IL, Charles C. Thomas, 1937.
2. Alfageme I, Munoz F, Pena N, et al: Empyema of the thorax in adults. Etiology, microbiologic findings, and management. Chest 103:839–843, 1993.
3. American Thoracic Association, Medical Section of the National Tuberculosis Association: Management of nontuberculous empyema. Am Rev Respir Dis 85:935, 1962.
4. Angelillo-Mackinlay TA, Lyons G, Chimondeguy DJ, et al: VATS debridement versus thoracotomy in the treatment of loculated postpneumonia empyema. Ann Thorac Surg 61:1626–1630, 1996.
5. Baillot R, Dontigny L, Verdant A, et al: Penetrating chest trauma: A 20-year experience. J Trauma 27:994, 1987.
6. Beal SL, McKennan M: Blunt diaphragmatic rupture: A morbid injury. Arch Surg 123:828–832, 1988.
7. Beall A, Crawford H, De Bakey M: Considerations in the management of acute traumatic hemothorax. Scand J Thorac Cardiovasc Surg 11:265–268, 1977.
8. Bergh NP, Ekroth R, Larsson S, et al: Intrapleural streptokinase in the treatment of the hemothorax and empyema. Scand J Thorac Cardiovasc Surg 11:265, 1977.
9. Bhattacharyva N, Umland ET, Kosloske AM: A bacteriologic basis for the evolution and severity of empyema. J Pediatr Surg 29:667–670, 1994.
10. Carrillo EH, Heniford BT, Etoch SW, et al: Video-assisted thoracic surgery in trauma patients. J Am Coll Surg 184:316–324, 1997.
11. Cham CW, Haq SM, Rahamin J: Empyema thoracis: A problem with late referral? Thorax 48:925–927, 1993.
12. Clagett OT, Geraci JE: A procedure for the management of post-pneumonectomy empyema. J Thorac Cardiovasc Surg 45: 141, 1963.
13. Coon J, Shuck J: Failure of tube thoracostomy for posttraumatic empyema: An indication for early decortication. J Trauma 15:588, 1975.
14. Cordice J, Cabezon J: Chest trauma with pneumothorax and hemothorax. Chest Trauma 50:316, 1965.

15. Coselli J, Mattox K, Beall A: Reevaluation of early evacuation of clotted hemothorax. Am Surg 50:21, 1984.
16. Culiner M, Roe B, Grimes O: The early elective surgical approach to the treatment of traumatic hemothorax. J Thorac Cardiovasc Surg 38:780, 1959.
17. Eloesser L: An operation for tuberculous empyema. Surg Gynecol Obstet 60:1096, 1935.
18. Fallazadeh H, Mays ET: Disruptions of the diaphragm by blunt trauma: New dimensions of diagnosis. Am Surg 41:337–341, 1975.
19. Feliciano DV, Cruse PA, Mattox KL, et al: Delayed diagnosis of injury to the diaphragm after penetrating wounds. J Trauma 28:1135–1143, 1989.
20. Ferguson MK: Thoracoscopy for empyema, bronchopleural fistula, and chylothorax. Ann Thorac Surg 56:644, 645, 1993.
21. Freixinet J, Rodriguez de Castro F, Quevedo S, et al: Traumatic hemothorax treated by video-assisted thoracoscopic surgery. Arch Bronconeumol 31:424–425, 1995.
22. Graham EA: Some fundamental considerations in the treatment of empyema thoracis. St. Louis, CV Mosby, 1925.
23. Helling TS, Gyles NR, Eisenstein CL, et al: Complications following blunt and penetrating injuries in 216 victims of chest trauma requiring tube thoracostomy. J Trauma 29:1367–1370, 1989.
24. Hood RM: Traumatic diaphragmatic hernia. Ann Thorac Surg 12:311–324, 1971.
25. Hoover EL, Hsu HK, Webb H, et al: The surgical management of empyema thoracis in substance abuse patients: A 5 year experience. Ann Thorac Surg 46:563–566, 1988.
26. Hornick P, Towsend ER, Clark D, et al: Videothoracoscopy in the treatment of early empyema: An initial experience. Ann R Coll Surg Engl 78:45–48, 1996.
27. Hurley JP, McCarthy J, Wood AE: Retrospective analysis of the utility of video-assisted thoracic surgery in 100 consecutive procedures. Eur J Cardiothorac Surg 8:589–592, 1994.
28. Hutter JA, Harari D, Braimbridge MV: The management of empyema thoracis by thoracoscopy and irrigation. Ann Thorac Surg 39:517–520, 1985.
29. Kirsh E, Guckel C, Kaim A, et al: The findings and value of computed tomography in pleural empyema. Rofo Forstchr Geb Rontsgenstr Neuen Bildgeb Verfahr 162:404–411, 1994.
30. Kish G, Kozoll L, Joseph WL, et al: Indications for early thoracotomy in the management of chest trauma. Ann Thorac Surg 22:23–30, 1976.
31. Landrenau RJ, Keenan RJ, Hazelrig SR, et al: Thoracoscopy for empyema and hemothorax. Chest 109:18–24,1995.
32. Lazdunski L, Mouroux J, Pons F, et al: Role of videothoracoscopy in chest trauma. Ann Thorac Surg 63:327–333, 1997.
33. Lema L, Hutter JA, Harari D, et al: The management of empyema thoracis by thoracoscopy and irrigation. Cent Afr J Med 36:20–22, 1990.
34. Light RW, Girard WM, Jenkinson SG, et al: Parapneumonic effusions. Am J Med 69:507, 1980.
35. Linder A, Friedel G, Toomes H: Prerequisites, indications, and techniques of video-assisted thoracoscopy surgery. Thorac Cardiovasc Surg 41:140–146, 1993.
36. Liu DW, Liu HP, Lin PJ, et al: Video-assisted thoracic surgery in treatment of chest trauma. J Trauma 42:670–674, 1997.
37. Liu HP, Chang CH, Lin PJ, et al: Video-assisted thoracic surgery. The Chang Gung experience. J Thorac Cardiovasc Surg 108:834–840, 1994.
38. Mackenzie JW: Video-assisted thoracoscopy. Treatment for empyema and hemothorax. Chest 109:18–24, 1996.
39. Madden MR, Paull DE, Finkelstein JL, et al: Occult diaphragmatic injury from stab wounds of the lower chest and abdomen. J Trauma 33:101–109, 1989.
40. Mancini M, Smith L, Nein A, et al: Early evacuation of clotted blood in hemothorax using thoracoscopy: Case reports. J Trauma 34:144–147, 1993.
41. Milfeld DJ, Mattox KL, Beall A: Early evacuation of clotted hemothorax. Am J Surg 136:686–692, 1978.
42. Miller JI: Empyema thoracis. Ann Thorac Surg 50:343–347, 1990.
43. O'Brien J, Cohen M, Solit R, et al: Thoracoscopic drainage and decortication as definitive treatment for empyema thoracis following penetrating chest injury. J Trauma 36:536–540, 1994.
44. Oparah SS, Mandal AK: Operative management of penetrating wounds of the chest in civilian practice. J Thorac Cardiovasc Surg 77:162–167, 1979.
45. Pairolero PC, Arnold PG, Phieler JM: Intrathoracic transposition of extrathoracic skeletal muscle. J Thorac Cardiovasc Surg 86: 809, 1983.
46. Patterson LT, Schmitt HJ, Armstrong RG: Intermediate care of war wounds of the chest. J Thorac Cardiovasc Surg 55:16–23, 1968.
47. Pothula V, Krellenstein DJ: Early aggressive surgical management of parapneumonic empyemas. Chest 105:832–836, 1994.
48. Ridley PD, Braimbridge MV: Thoracoscopic debridement and pleural irrigation in the management of empyema thoracis. Ann Thorac Surg 51:461–466, 1991.
49. Robinson LA, Moulton AL, Fleming WH, et al: Intrapleural fibrinolytic treatment of multiloculated empyemas. Ann Thorac Surg 57:803, 1994.
50. Sahn SA, Light RW: The sun should never set on a parapneumonic effusion. Chest 95:945, 1989.
51. Sahn SA, Reller LB, Taryle DA, et al: The contribution of leukocytes and bacteria to the low pH of empyema fluid. Am Rev Respir Dis 128:811–815, 1983.
52. Sasse S, Nguyen TK, Mulligan M, et al: The effects of early chest tube placement on empyema resolution. Chest 111: 1679–1683, 1997.
53. Silen ML, Naunheim KS: Thoracoscopic approach to the management of empyema thoracis. Indications and results. Chest Surg Clin North Am. 6:491–499, 1996.
54. Smith RS, Fry WR, Tsoi EK, et al: Preliminary report on videothoracoscopy in the evaluation and treatment of thoracis injury. Am J Surg 166:690–695, 1993.
55. Smith RS, Tsoi EK, Fry WR, et al: Laparoscopic evaluation of abdominal trauma: A preliminary report. Contemp Surg 42:13–18, 1993.
56. Sosa JL, Puente I, Lemasters L, et al: Videothoracoscopy in trauma: Early experience. J Laparoendosc Surg 4:295–300, 1994.
57. Strange C, Sahn SA: The clinician's perspective on parapneumonic effusions and empyema. Chest 103:259–261, 1993.
58. Striffeler H, Ris HB, Wursten HU, et al: Video-assisted thoracoscopy of pleural empyema. A new therapeutic approach. Eur J Cardiothorac Surg 1994;8:585–588.
59. Urschel JD, Pearson RJ, Fraser RE: Open tube thoracoscopy: Does it have a role in modern thoracic surgery? J Laparoendosc Surg 4:37–39, 1994.
60. Van Way III C, Narrot JK, Hopeman A: The role of early limited thoracotomy in the treatment of empyema. J Thorac Cardiovasc Surg 96:436, 1988.
61. Varkey B, Rose HD, Kesavan-Kutty CP, et al: Empyema thoracis during a ten-year period. Analysis of 72 cases and comparison to a previous study (1952 to 1967). Arch Intern Med 141:1771, 1981.
62. Wait MA, Sharma S, Hohn J, et al: A randomized trial of empyema therapy. Chest 111:1548–1551, 1997.
63. Ward RE, Flynn TC, Clark WP: Diaphragmatic disruption secondary to blunt abdominal trauma. J Trauma 21:35–38, 1981.
64. Weissberg D, Refaely Y: Pleuroscopy: Therapeutic applications. Scand J Thorac Cardiovasc Surg 30:1–10, 1996.
65. Wong MS, Tsoi EK, Henderson VJ, et al: Videothoracoscopy: An effective method for evaluating and managing thoracic trauma patients. Surg Endosc 10:118–121, 1996.
66. Yim AP, Ho JK, Lee TW, et al: Thoracoscopic management of pleural effusions revisited. Aust N Z J Surg 65:308–311, 1995.

COMMENTARY

Valerie W. Rusch

In this chapter, Dr. Angelillo-Mackinlay from the British Hospital of Buenos Aires discusses the use of video-assisted thoracic surgery (VATS) in the management of empyema and hemothorax, based on his personal experience with this approach. Since 1991, he has used VATS to drain fibrinopurulent empyemas in 80 patients. This was most successful in patients who had postpneumonic empyemas. Only 3 of 53 (5.6%) patients required conversion to a thoracotomy, operative mortality was low (1.8%), and the length of hospital stay was shorter compared with the historical experience with thoracotomy in similar patients. However, VATS performed for patients who had post-traumatic empyemas did not appear to shorten hospital stay, perhaps because these patients often have additional medical problems that prolong recovery. A smaller number of patients (27 cases) underwent VATS for subacute hemothorax. Only one patient required conversion to thoracotomy, there were no operative deaths, and all patients apparently had satisfactory long-term results.

This report places the role of VATS in perspective. Since the advent of videothoracoscopic technology, surgeons have often taken the position of favoring or opposing its use with vehemence, mainly on the basis of personal prejudice. VATS is frequently compared with thoracotomy, but assuming that the two techniques are competitive, or mutually exclusive, overlooks the possibility that VATS may simply be a more appropriate procedure for certain subsets of patients. After all, mediastinoscopy and parasternal mediastinotomy (Chamberlain procedure) are understood to play an important role in the diagnosis and staging of lung cancer and mediastinal masses. They are complementary to thoracotomy, not mutually exclusive. Why should VATS not be considered in a similar vein?

Dr. Angelillo-Mackinlay describes very nicely the precise technique for VATS in the management of empyema and hemothorax. He has obviously developed a specific approach to proper port placement and debridement of the pleural space in empyema, which has gradually led to very low rates of morbidity and conversion to thoracotomy. Likewise, he clearly articulates the important technical points about port placement and the addition of a utility incision for the treatment of hemothorax. Refinement of patient selection and surgical technique are pivotal to the appropriate and successful use of VATS, and this report illustrates how a systematic surgical approach leads to excellent results.

Finally, Dr. Angelillo-Mackinlay defines very carefully the circumstances under which VATS is not effective. Recognition of when a thoracotomy is a better procedure than VATS is critical to the success of surgical management and to patient safety. Too often, surgeons wish to be perceived as doing "minimally invasive surgery." Under that guise, VATS is sometimes considered to include a thoracotomy incision of varying dimensions (albeit perhaps non–rib-spreading) with various and sundry port sites. Dr. Angelillo-Mackinlay recognizes what he can accomplish via a small number of port incisions, and what he cannot. Such honesty is noticeably absent in some publications about VATS.

This report emphasizes that VATS is an integral part of our thoracic surgical armamentarium. It occasionally obviates the need for thoracotomy, but is not appropriate for the management of technically complex problems. As pointed out by the author, both empyema and hemothorax are easiest to manage when diagnosed early. We hope this experience will encourage primary care physicians to refer their patients to thoracic surgeons early in the disease process, when VATS is most likely to be successful.

Chapter 9

Chylothorax

Mark K. Ferguson

A chylothorax is an uncommon condition that arises from a broad range of etiologies, including cancer, trauma, and congenital abnormalities. Although the diagnosis of chylothorax rarely presents a clinical challenge, the treatment of this entity requires a detailed knowledge of anatomy, pathophysiology, and, in many cases, surgical technique, to effect a cure. The introduction of thoracoscopic techniques for the management of postoperative chylothorax has opened possibilities that may alter the current algorithm for the timing and approach to operative intervention.

History

The first description of lymph channels is attributed to Aselli, who made detailed observations in the early 17th century.[41] Within two decades, several authors, including Pecquet, Bartholen, and Rudbeck, described the thoracic duct.[2] Although the first detailed description of the thoracic duct was published by Mascagni in the late 18th century, pathology of the thoracic duct was not comprehensively reviewed until nearly 100 years later.[11] Chylothorax was first described by Longelot in 1663, 36 years after the first description of the lymphatic system, and only 12 years after the discovery of the thoracic duct.[11]

Until the middle of the 20th century, nearly 100% of patients who had nontraumatic chylothorax and 50% of patients who had traumatic chylothorax died.[2] Treatment before that time included multiple thoracocenteses (after which the aspirated chyle was often infused intravenously) and pleural sclerosis. Although thoracic duct ligation was thought to be possible, the procedure was generally considered too dangerous to attempt. However, in 1948, Lampson introduced thoracic duct ligation for the management of chylothorax, forever changing the approach to this problem.[30] The next summary of chylothorax management reported the mortality after thoracic duct ligation to be only 10%.[2] Since that time, progress has been made in both medical and surgical therapy for these patients, with a resultant improvement in overall survival.

Anatomy

The human lymphatic system consists of right and left divisions. Lymph from the lower half of the body (including most of the abdomen), as well as the left arm, the left side of the chest and head, and the left upper lobe of the lung, flows into the left lymphatic system, which culminates in the thoracic duct. Lymph from the right arm, all of the remaining lung lobes, the right side of the chest and head, the right diaphragm, and the liver flows into the right system, which culminates in the right lymphatic duct.[11,19]

The thoracic duct has an overall length of 36 to 45 cm and is 2 to 4 mm in diameter.[50] It arises from the cisterna chyli and ascends into the chest on the anterior surface of the vertebral column and to the right of the aorta through the aortic hiatus (Fig 9–1). It continues behind the esophagus and between the azygos vein and the aorta to the level of the fifth or sixth thoracic vertebra, where it crosses to the left and ascends behind the aortic arch. The duct continues along the left lateral wall of the esophagus and crosses the thoracic inlet behind the subclavian artery. The duct joins the venous system at or near the confluence of the subclavian and left internal jugular veins. The right lymphatic duct is the main drainage pathway of the tracheobronchial lymph nodes and of the heart. It ascends in the posterior mediastinum to the right of the esophagus and terminates near the junction of the right subclavian and internal jugular veins.

There is considerable variability in the anatomy of the thoracic duct. A persistent left lymphatic duct is present at the level of the diaphragm in 15% of people, and a bilateral duct system is present above the level of the fifth thoracic vertebra in 35% of people.[9,26,50] The thoracic and right lymphatic ducts have numerous communications between them and with the mediastinal venous system via lymphaticovenous communications. Valves present in lymph vessels provide unidirectional lymph flow cephalad and prevent retrograde flow of blood into the vessels through the venous communications.

Physiology of the Thoracic Duct

The thoracic duct fluid is alkaline, odorless, and sterile, and ranges in appearance from serous to milky white, depending on the postprandial state.[45] The contents of chyle include protein, fat, electrolytes, and cellular elements. The most striking chemical difference between chyle and serum is the triglyceride content, which is substantially higher in chyle, especially after ingestion of a fatty meal (Table 9–1). White blood cells found in chyle (400 to 6800/mm^3) are primarily T-lymphocytes, and there are only a few segmented white blood cells present, most of which are eosinophils. The erythrocyte count ranges from 50 to 600/mm^3 and increases after meals.[35]

The volume of flow through the thoracic duct varies from 14 to 110 ml/hr, or 500 to 2500 ml/day, and is dependent in part on the volume of food or fluid ingested and the fat content of the ingestant.[43,46] Flow is controlled by extrinsic factors, such as motion, transmitted pulsations from adjacent blood vessels, pressure differentials between the thoracic and abdominal cavities, and the respiratory cycle.[6,19,29,38] More importantly, a variety of intrinsic factors regulate flow through the thoracic duct, particularly intrinsic spontaneous contractions of the smooth muscle in the duct and the transmural pressure to which the duct is exposed.[14,18,28,32,34] Spontaneous smooth

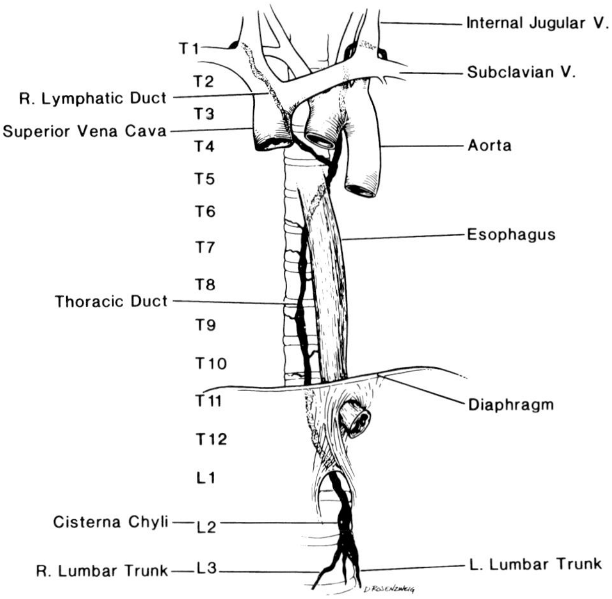

Figure 9–1. The anatomy of the thoracic duct. (From Ferguson M: The anatomy and physiology of the thoracic duct. *In* Deslauriers J, Lacquet LK [eds]: Thoracic Surgery: Surgical Management of Pleural Diseases. Thoracic Surgery: The Pleural Space, Vol 6. St. Louis, CV Mosby, 1990, p 353, with permission.)

muscle contractions are under both neural and pharmacologic control.[12,13,16,17,42,47]

Etiology

A wide variety of causes of chylothorax have been described (Table 9–2). Congenital chylothoraces are related to anatomic abnormalities of the thoracic duct or the entire lymphatic vascular system and will not be discussed. Traumatic chylothoraces are most often iatrogenic. They are usually associated with major thoracic or cardiac surgical procedures, and have an overall rate of occurrence of 0.2 to 0.4%.[3–5,15] The most common operative causes of thoracic duct injury are esophagectomy, which has an incidence of 3 to 4%,[10,36] and major lung resection, which has an incidence of 0.3 to 1.8%.[3,21]

Chylothoraces associated with obstruction are usually due to neoplasms, a condition that accounts for more than half of chylothoraces in adults. The most common underlying cancer is lymphoma, although Kaposi's sarcoma associated with the autoimmune deficiency syndrome has recently been reported to be associated with the development of chylothorax.[25,37] A large variety of infectious, obstructive, and miscellaneous etiologies account for the remaining small number of reported cases of chylothorax.

Table 9–2. Etiology of Chylothorax

Congenital
- Absence or atresia of thoracic duct
- Lymphangiectasia
- Tracheoesophageal fistula
- Noonan's syndrome
- Down's syndrome

Traumatic
- Postoperative
  - Esophagectomy
  - Lung resection
  - Other
- Other iatrogenic
- Blunt
- Penetrating

Obstructive
- Nonmalignant
  - Tuberculosis
  - Mediastinal fibrosis
  - Filariasis
- Malignant
  - Lymphoma
  - Kaposi's sarcoma
  - Other

Idiopathic

Miscellaneous
- Pulmonary lymphangiomyomatosis
- Lymph node hyperplasia
- Cirrhosis
- Heart failure
- Lymphangitis of the thoracic duct
- Aortic aneurysm
- Intestinal lymphangiectasia
- Reticular hyperplasia
- Nephrotic syndrome
- Hypothyroidism
- Pancreatitis
- Mediastinal irradiation

Table 9–1. Relative Composition of Chyle and Serum

Component	Chyle	Serum
Protein (g/dl)	2.2–6.0	6.5–7.9
Albumin	1.2–4.2	3.2–5.0
Globulin	1.1–3.1	2.2–3.1
Fibrinogen	0.16–0.24	0.26–0.33
Lipids (mg/dl)	800–4600	450–750
Cholesterol	60–220	140–220
Cholesterol esters	20–180	30–100
Triglycerides	100–2200	50–220
Urea nitrogen (mg/dl)	8–18	14–40
Nonprotein nitrogen (mg/dl)	6–14	15–31
Electrolytes (mEq/L)		
Sodium	104–148	134–149
Potassium	3.8–5.0	3.5–5.2
Chloride	85–130	95–108
Calcium	3.4–6.0	4.6–5.2
Specific gravity	1.012–1.025	1.024–1.028

From Ferguson M: The anatomy and physiology of the thoracic duct. *In* Deslauriers J, Lacquet LK (eds): Thoracic Surgery: Surgical Management of Pleural Diseases. Thoracic Surgery: The Pleural Space, Vol 6. St. Louis, CV Mosby, 1990, pp 353–356.

Pathophysiology

Any clinically apparent chylothorax entails a substantial loss of chyle into the pleural space. This fact has both nutritional and immunologic consequences. Unless the lost fluid is replaced, volume depletion can occur, which results in hypovolemia and hypotension. The loss of chyle also causes a measurable decrease in serum total protein and albumin and is accompanied by a continued loss in total body weight.[15] The use of enteral or parenteral nutrition to prevent or reverse these trends is rarely entirely successful.

The loss of chyle is also accompanied by lymphocyte depletion. This produces a measurable decrease in the peripheral lymphocyte count and results in depression of immunologic function.[15] Indeed, thoracic duct drainage was an early technique for immunosuppression in transplant patients. Interestingly, a high rate of infectious complications has not been reported routinely in patients who undergo prolonged drainage of a chylothorax. Most authors cite a low or absent incidence of empyema associated with chylothorax, which may be due to the bacteriostatic properties of chyle.[4,15,21] Nevertheless, infection has been reported as a complication in up to 40% of patients with chylothorax, suggesting that the immunologic consequences of prolonged drainage must be considered when planning therapy.[10,15]

Diagnosis

A diagnosis of chylothorax in the postoperative setting is usually suspected on the basis of an excess volume of thoracostomy tube drainage. Fluid may also accumulate in the pleural space if that space is loculated or undrained. If the patient is taking enteral nutrition, whether it consists of clear liquids or a general diet, the fluid is usually milky white in appearance and somewhat thick in consistency. In patients who are taking no enteral nutrition, the fluid may be serous or serosanguineous. In other clinical settings, most patients are on a regular diet at the time a pleural effusion is diagnosed. Diagnostic thoracocentesis usually demonstrates milky white fluid, leading to the diagnosis of chylothorax.

Under most circumstances, it is useful to confirm the clinical suspicion of chylothorax by performing pleural fluid analysis. This is also important if the pleural fluid lacks the characteristic milky appearance of chyle but the suspicion of chylothorax is entertained in the differential diagnosis. The main alternative diagnoses that are usually considered are empyema and, in some patients, pseudochylothorax. In empyema, the cloudy appearance of the fluid is caused by suspended white blood cells and cellular debris. Centrifugation leaves a clear supernatant in the empyema fluid, but in both chylothorax and pseudochylothorax the supernatant remains opaque. To differentiate between chylothorax and pseudochylothorax, microscopic examination of the pleural fluid sediment reveals cholesterol crystals in the latter condition but none in true chylothorax.

Chemical analysis of the pleural fluid is also useful in making a diagnosis of chylothorax. Measurement of triglycerides is the single most important test. If the triglyceride level exceeds 110 mg/dl, the chance of fluid's being chylous is nearly 100%, whereas, if the level is less than 50 mg/dl, there is almost no chance that the fluid is chylous.[45] If the triglyceride level falls between these values, lipoprotein electrophoresis is performed, and the demonstration of chylomicrons confirms the diagnosis of chylothorax. Lipoprotein electrophoresis is also useful in distinguishing between chylothorax and pseudochylothorax because, in the latter condition, the fluid may have elevated triglyceride levels but does not contain chylomicrons.

Management

Initial Management

The general principles followed in the initial management of chylothorax are complete drainage of the pleural space and re-expansion of the lung, fluid repletion, nutritional support, and reduction of lymph flow. Drainage of the pleural space may be accomplished initially by thoracocentesis, but a single episode of thoracocentesis is rarely sufficient to provide adequate long-term evacuation, and the risk of complications increases with repeated procedures. Thoracostomy tube drainage is more reliable in attaining complete initial drainage and in maintaining drainage of the pleural space. These factors help prevent the development of pleural loculations, which can affect the outcome of conservative therapy. Insufflation of talc through the thoracostomy tube to sclerose the pleural space and the addition of fibrin glue through the tube to seal the chyle leak have been reported as adjuncts to thoracostomy tube management of chylothorax.[1,51,52]

Fluid repletion is accomplished initially by means of standard electrolyte solutions. Some physicians recommend the use of albumin as a fluid replacement to help avoid hypoproteinemia. Reduction of lymph flow is accomplished by decreasing oral fluid intake and eliminating ingested fats. It is possible to provide a high-calorie, nonfat diet that is palatable for a short while. The substitution of medium-chain triglycerides for fats is also commonly recommended. Both of these measures can sustain a patient's nutritional status and promote the spontaneous closure of the lymphatic leak. However, the success of these measures has been variable, partly because triglycerides derive from both endogenous and exogenous sources, and because oral intake of any kind has been found to increase thoracic duct lymph flow.[23,24,40] A more common technique of nutritional management is total elimination of oral intake and administration of parenteral nutrition.

In postoperative or traumatic chylothoraces, in which there is usually no obstruction of the thoracic lymphatics, adherence to these general principles, including thoracostomy tube drainage, sometimes promotes spontaneous closure of the chyle leak within 5 days to 2 weeks. After the chest drainage has subsided, the patient is started on a general diet. The thoracostomy tube is removed subsequently if no increase in drainage occurs and if no pleural effusion develops after 1 or 2 days. The success rate of conservative management under these circumstances is about 25% in adult patients and 80% in pediatric patients.[3,4,10,15,31,33] Nontraumatic chylothoraces, which are usually associated with malignancy, are typically caused by lymphatic obstruction, and respond much more slowly to conservative management than postoperative or traumatic chylothoraces. Issues regarding fluid replenishment, nutritional support, and immunologic compromise take on long-term significance.

Surgical Management

For patients in whom conservative management fails, surgical intervention is considered. The timing and type of intervention depend on the underlying cause of the chylothorax and on the clinical condition of the patient. The smaller the daily volume of chyle loss is, the longer conservative management can be considered. However, losses in excess of 500 ml daily suggest that spontaneous cessation of chyle leak is unlikely in the short term, and that surgical intervention should be considered within a week or so after the diagnosis is established. Patients who suffer postoperative chylothorax are likely to have a single injury to a major lymphatic vessel, which is amenable to surgical intervention. This suggests that relatively early operative intervention is appropriate in postoperative patients as long as their overall condition permits it. Early intervention is particularly important in patients who are likely to have a major thoracic duct injury and who are already nutritionally depleted, such as patients who suffer a postoperative chylothorax after esophagectomy.[36] Early surgical management is avoided in patients who are in poor overall medical condition caused by other underlying medical causes; in very young patients who have a postoperative chylothorax, because this age group seems to respond well to conservative management; and in patients whose chylothorax is caused by a malignancy with a presumed obstructive etiology.

Options for surgical intervention include thoracic duct ligation, placement of a pleuroperitoneal shunt, or thoracoscopy and pleurodesis. The choice among these options is based on the condition of the patient, the cause of the chylothorax, and the surgeon's preference. There are no comparative studies that demonstrate the superiority of one method of management over another.

Thoracoscopy and Pleural Sclerosis. The use of thoracoscopy to drain the pleural space, identify the source of the chyle leak, and perform talc sclerosis has been reported by several authors.[8,52] The advantages include lysis of any adhesions to provide complete drainage and lung expansion, placement of drainage tubes in optimal locations, and optimal instillation and coating with talc. Thoracoscopy is associated with less morbidity than occurs after major thoracotomy, and may be more appropriate in debilitated patients.

The procedure is performed under general anesthesia with selective ventilation of the contralateral lung. It is feasible to perform this operation under sedation without positive pressure ventilation, although the successful use of such an approach has not yet been described. Two ports are usually required, one for the telescope and a separate working port for suction and administration of the talc. After complete evacuation of the pleural space and division of any adhesions, the lung is examined to ensure that there is no pleural peel or other pathology that would inhibit its complete expansion. Sterile, asbestos-free, iodized talc (2 to 4 g) is then insufflated into the pleural space, and one or two thoracostomy tubes are placed for postoperative drainage. The patient is maintained on nothing by mouth until drainage from the tubes subsides to a minimum. The patient is then given a regular diet and, if there is no additional drainage and the chest radiograph remains clear, the thoracostomy tubes are removed. The likelihood of success in highly selected patients is about 80%.[8,52]

Pleuroperitoneal Shunt. The pleuroperitoneal shunt was originally described in 1982 for the management of malignant pleural effusion and was adapted for the management of chylothorax shortly thereafter.[33] The advantages of shunting are reduced operative morbidity compared with open thoracotomy; retention of the volume, nutritional components, and immunologic components of chyle that leaks into the pleural space; and treatment of chylothorax primarily on an outpatient basis. Candidates for the shunt procedure are patients who are personally able to pump the shunt's compression chamber for 4 to 6 periods of time per day (or who have caregivers to perform this function), who are motivated, and who do not require hospitalization for other medical problems. Patients must have no evidence of pleural space infection or other ongoing infection; must not have an abdomen frozen by adhesions from previous surgery; and should not have ascites. In general, long-term thoracostomy tube drainage is not advisable if pleuroperitoneal shunting is to be used, because of the risk of contamination of the pleural space along the tract of the indwelling tube before the shunt placement.

Shunts are comprised of a pleural limb and a peritoneal limb joined by a pumping chamber, which is fitted with one-way valves at each end that provide unidirectional flow from the pleural cavity to the peritoneal cavities. The chamber capacity is about 2 ml, and each compression moves about 1.5 ml of fluid. Shunt placement is performed under either general anesthesia or sedation without positive pressure ventilation. After performing a thoracocentesis to ensure that access to free pleural fluid is possible, the pleural limb of the shunt is inserted using a Seldinger technique. A subcutaneous pocket is fashioned on the surface of the rib cage, and a 2-cm incision is made in the upper quadrant of the abdomen into the peritoneum to receive the peritoneal limb of the device. After evacuating any air from the pleural space and priming the shunt by pumping on the chamber, the shunt is tunneled through the pocket, where the pumping chamber is anchored, and the peritoneal limb is inserted into the abdomen (Fig 9–2). Purse-string sutures in the fascia are tied around the peritoneal limb to secure it and prevent leakage into the wound. The shunt is pumped to evacuate the pleural space, and pumping sessions are performed thereafter every 6 hours for 5 to 10 minutes or until the pleural space is evacuated (Fig 9–3). This schedule permits over 1500 ml of fluid to be shunted from the pleural space every 24 hours.

Patients in good general health are started on a regular diet and discharged once it is clear that the shunt is functioning satisfactorily, which usually is on the first or second postoperative day. Shunt malfunctions occur primarily because of clotting of fibrinous exudate in the shunt chamber, which is not a common problem in patients with chylothorax, but the frequency of this complication may be increased by the failure of patients to pump their shunts frequently enough or use appropriate techniques.[48] This underscores the importance of patient education when using this device. The shunt is left in place and is not pumped for several days after cessation of the chyle leak to ensure that no recurrence develops, after which the device

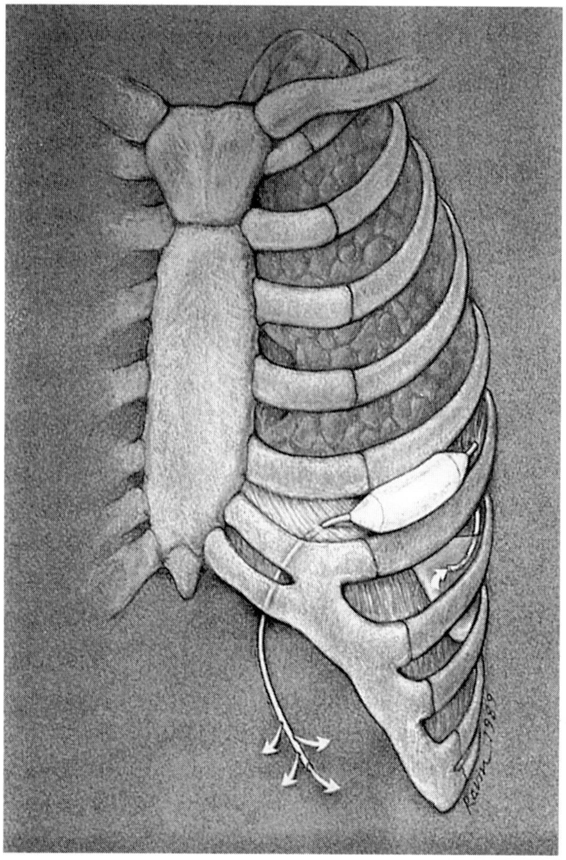

Figure 9–2. The position of a pleuroperitoneal shunt for draining a chylothorax. (From Thurer R, Cimochowski G, Feun LG, et al: Malignant pleural effusions. Contemp Surg 35:79–104, 1989, with permission.)

is removed under local anesthetic (Fig 9–4). The success rate in selected patients approaches 95%.[7,39,48]

Thoracic Duct Ligation. Since the landmark report by Lampson in 1948, thoracic duct ligation has been the mainstay of surgical therapy for chylothorax. However, reports of open ligation have been supplanted by descriptions of thoracoscopic techniques. There is no consensus as to which approach is optimal, and no comparative data exist.

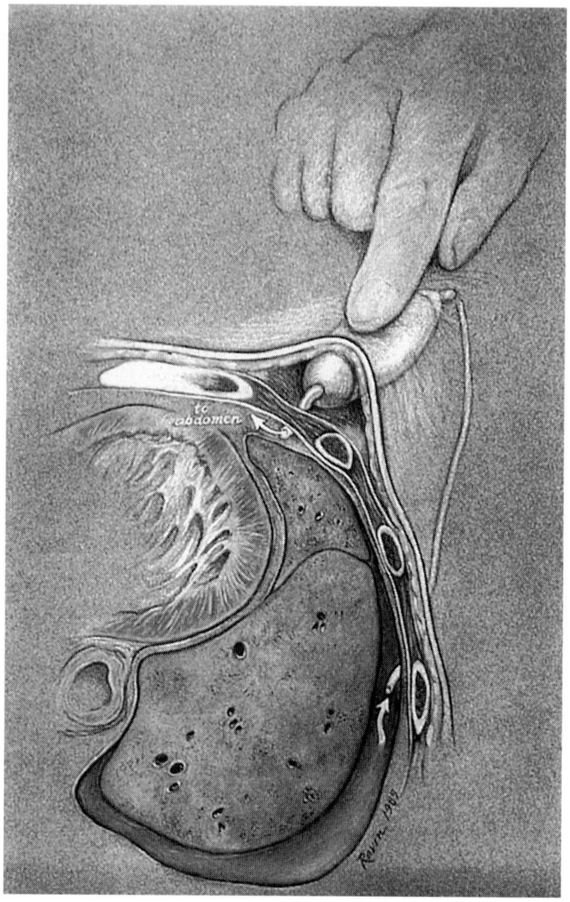

Figure 9–3. Technique for pumping on a pleuroperitoneal shunt to move fluid from the pleural to the peritoneal space. (From Thurer R, Cimochowski G, Feun LG, et al: Malignant pleural effusions. Contemp Surg 35:79–104, 1989, with permission.)

The open approach to thoracic duct ligation is performed either through a thoracotomy or, rarely, through an upper abdominal incision. If a thoracotomy is to be used, most surgeons recommend approaching the patient

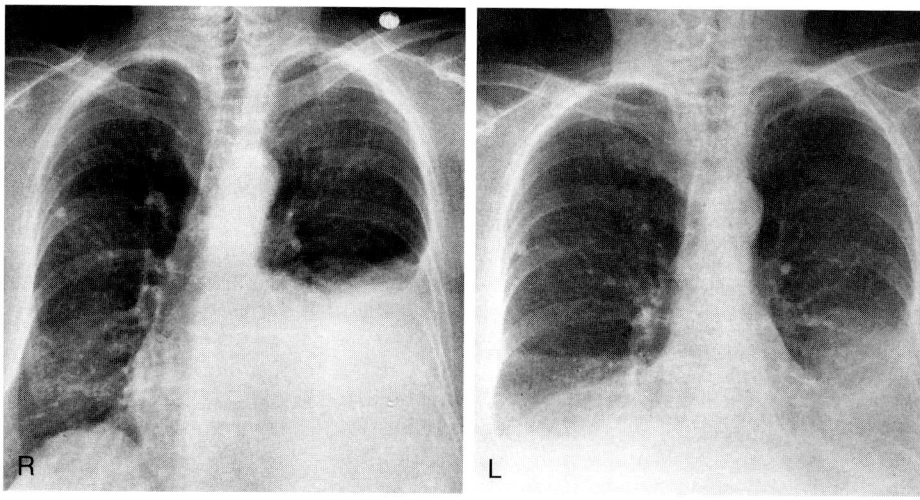

Figure 9–4. Chest radiographs demonstrating a chylothorax before treatment (*left*) and after insertion of a pleuroperitoneal shunt (*right*). (From Brofman JD, Hall JB, Scott W, et al: Yellow nails, lymphedema, and pleural effusion. Chest 97:743–745, 1990, with permission.)

through the affected side. This enables identification and closure of the site of the lymph leak, regardless of whether the leak is from the thoracic duct itself or another major lymphatic channel. However, it is also an option to proceed with the simple objective of ligating the thoracic duct, in which case the easiest approach is through the right chest.

Identification of the site of the chyle leak is usually straightforward if the volume of lymph loss is sufficient to warrant an operation. Aids to identification include the enteral administration of high-fat liquids, such as heavy cream or a lipophilic dye, shortly before the planned operation. Once the site of the lymph leak is identified, it is ligated or sutured. Given the location of the thoracic duct, which is found on the surface of the vertebral bodies between the azygos vein and the aorta, many surgeons recommend encompassing all tissues from the lateral aspect of the azygos vein to the aorta in a single large ligature to gain control of the thoracic duct (Fig 9–5). Heavy suture material is used to avoid cutting through the delicate tissues. Once the duct has been ligated, the site is observed for several minutes to ensure that no further leakage occurs. Some surgeons recommend performing mechanical or talc pleurodesis before closing the thoracotomy incision to increase the chances of successful control of the leak.

Thoracoscopic approaches to thoracic duct ligation have recently been described. The timing of thoracoscopic intervention is similar to that of open thoracotomy, usually within the first week after the diagnosis of chylothorax if conservative measures are unsuccessful. The operation is performed under general anesthesia through the right side of the chest with isolated left lung ventilation. The camera port is placed in the midaxillary line in the sixth interspace, and two or three additional ports are placed at or below this level, focusing activity in the supradiaphragmatic region of the posterior mediastinum (Fig 9–6). The pulmonary ligament is divided. The parietal pleura is incised adjacent to the azygos vein, and the site of leakage is identified. The duct is controlled with clips or suture ligature, or by sectioning of the vessel and ligature of the open, caudad cut end. The site is observed for several minutes to ensure that the lymph leak has been controlled. Mechanical or talc pleurodesis is recommended by some surgeons as an adjunct to thoracic duct ligation.

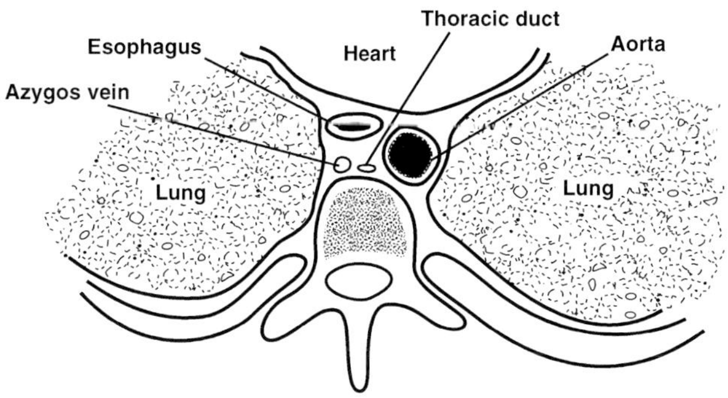

Figure 9–5. The cross-sectional anatomy of the thoracic duct and its relationships to surrounding structures.

Whether the operation is performed by open thoracotomy or by using thoracoscopic techniques, a thoracostomy drain is placed. The patient is placed on a general diet in the early postoperative period if the drainage is sufficiently low, which indicates a successful duct ligation. If there is no increase in the thoracostomy tube output and no fluid accumulates in the hemithorax, the drain is removed. Successful control of the chylothorax by oversewing of the site of the leak or by simple thoracic duct ligation, performed either patently or thoracoscopically, is reported in 90 to 95% of patients.[3,4,10,15,20–22,27,31,33,36,53]

A challenging, but, fortunately, rare, type of chylothorax is that which occurs after pneumonectomy. The diagnosis of this condition is straightforward once a thoracocentesis is performed. Prolonged thoracostomy tube drainage and dietary manipulation are of some benefit in these patients, particularly if the onset of the chylothorax is late, if the amount of ongoing drainage is relatively small, and if the drainage decreases in size after cessation of oral intake. Some authors also suggest that the finding on lymphangiography of a small accessory lymph vessel leak rather than a thoracic duct injury indicates the possibility of spontaneous closure of the leak. The success rate of conservative management approaches 90% in selected patients.[49] In other patients, early reoperation is indicated to permit ligation or suture closure of the site of the leak. This may be performed through the original incision or thoraco-

Figure 9–6. Thoracoscopic techniques for ligating the thoracic duct.

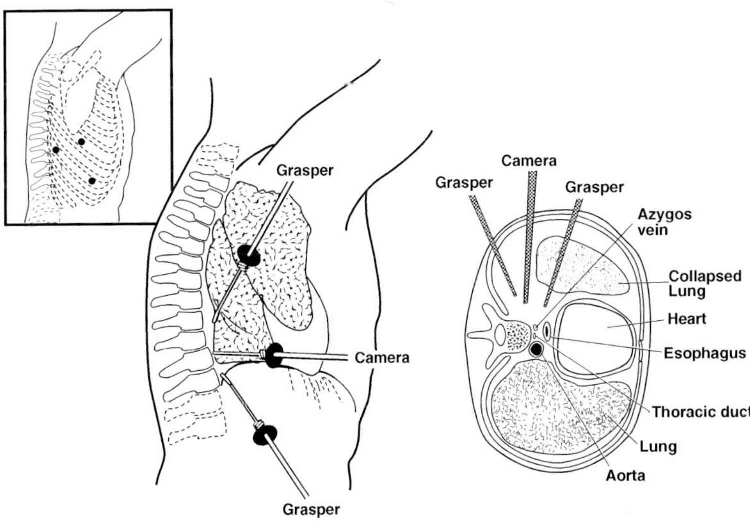

scopically. Management of the site of the leak is similar to that described for other postoperative chylothoraces.[44,49] The success of operative management of postpneumonectomy chylothorax is between 85 and 90% in selected patients.[49]

References

1. Akaogi E, Mitsui K, Sohara Y, et al: Treatment of postoperative chylothorax with intrapleural fibrin glue. Ann Thorac Surg 48: 116–118, 1989.
2. Bessone LN, Ferguson TB, Burford TH: Chylothorax. Ann Thorac Surg 12:527–550, 1971.
3. Brie M, Deslauriers J, Michaud P, et al: Chylothorax complicating pulmonary resection. *In* Deslauriers J, Lacquet LK (eds): Thoracic Surgery: Surgical Management of Pleural Diseases. International Trends in General Thoracic Surgery, Vol 6. St. Louis, CV Mosby, 1990, p 373.
4. Cerfolio RJ, Allen MS, Deschamps C, et al: Postoperative chylothorax. J Thorac Cardiovasc Surg 112:1361–1366, 1996.
5. Cevese PG, Vecchioni R, D'Amico DF, et al: Postoperative chylothorax. J Thorac Cardiovasc Surg 69:966–971, 1975.
6. Cressman RD, Blalock A: The effect of the pulse upon the flow of lymph. Proc Soc Exp Biol Med 41:140–144, 1939.
7. Cummings SP, Wyatt DA, Baker JW, et al: Successful treatment of postoperative chylothorax using an external pleuroperitoneal shunt. Ann Thorac Surg 54:276–278, 1992.
8. Daniel TM, Tribble CG, Rodgers BM: Thoracoscopy and talc poudrage for pneumothoraces and effusions. Ann Thorac Surg 50:186–189, 1990.
9. Davis HK: A statistical study of the thoracic duct in man. Am J Anat 17:211–244, 1914 and 1915.
10. Dougenis D, Walker WS, Cameron EWJ, et al: Management of chylothorax complicating extensive esophageal resection. Surg Gynecol Obstet 174:501–506, 1992.
11. Ferguson M: The anatomy and physiology of the thoracic duct. *In* Deslauriers J, Lacquet LK (eds): Thoracic Surgery: Surgical Management of Pleural Diseases. International Trends in General Thoracic Surgery, Vol 6. St. Louis, CV Mosby, 1990, p 353.
12. Ferguson MK: Modulation of lymphatic smooth muscle contractile responses by the endothelium. J Surg Res 52:359–363, 1992.
13. Ferguson MK, DeFilippi VJ: Nitric oxide and endothelium-dependent relaxation in tracheobronchial lymph vessels. Microvasc Res 47:308–317, 1994.
14. Ferguson MK, DeFilippi VJ, Reeder LB: Characterization of contractile properties of porcine mesenteric and tracheobronchial lymphatic smooth muscle. Lymphology 27:71–81, 1994.
15. Ferguson MK, Little AG, Skinner DB: Current concepts in the management of postoperative chylothorax. Ann Thorac Surg 40:542–545, 1985.
16. Ferguson MK, Tzeng E: Attenuation of histamine-induced lymphatic smooth muscle contractility by arachidonic acid. J Surg Res 51:500–505, 1991.
17. Ferguson MK, Williams U, Leff AR, et al: Heterogeneity of tracheobronchial lymphatic smooth muscle responses to histamine and 5-hydroxytryptamine. Lymphology 26:113–119, 1993.
18. Ferguson MK, Williams U, Leff AR, et al: Length-tension characteristics of bovine tracheobronchial lymphatic smooth muscle. Lymphology 26:19–24, 1993.
19. Gnepp DR: Lymphatics. *In* Staub NC, Taylor AE (eds): Edema. New York, Raven Press, 1984, pp 263–298.
20. Graham DD, McGahren ED, Tribble CG, et al: Use of video-assisted thoracic surgery in the treatment of chylothorax. Ann Thorac Surg 57:1507–1512, 1994.
21. Haniuda M, Nishimura H, Kobayashi O, et al: Management of chylothorax after pulmonary resection. J Am Coll Surg 180:537–540, 1995.
22. Jannssen JP, Joosten HJM, Postmus PE: Thoracoscopic treatment of postoperative chylothorax after coronary bypass surgery. Thorax 49:1273, 1994.
23. Jensen GL, Masciolo EA, Meyer LP, et al: Dietary modifications of chyle composition in chylothorax. Gastroenterology 97:761–765, 1989.
24. Johnstone DW, Feins RH: Chylothorax. Chest Surg Clin N Am 4:617–628, 1994.
25. Judson MA, Postic B: Chylothorax in a patient with AIDS and Kaposi's sarcoma. South Med J 83:322–324, 1990.
26. Kausel HW, Reeve TS, Stein AA, et al: Anatomic and pathologic studies of the thoracic duct. J Thorac Surg 34:631–642, 1957.
27. Kent RB III, Pinson TW: Thoracoscopic ligation of the thoracic duct. Surg Endosc 7:52–53, 1993.
28. Kinmouth JB, Sharpey-Schafer EP: Pressure waves in the human thoracic duct. J Physiol 145:3P, 1959.
29. Kinnaert P: Pressure measurements in the cervical portion of the thoracic duct in man. Br J Surg 60:558–561, 1973.
30. Lampson RS: Traumatic chylothorax. J Thorac Surg 17:778–791, 1948.
31. Marts BC, Naunheim KS, Fiore AC, et al: Conservative versus surgical management of chylothorax. Am J Surg 164:532–535, 1992.
32. McHale NG, Roddie IC: The effect of transmural pressure on pumping activity in isolated bovine lymphatic vessels. J Physiol 261:255–269, 1976.
33. Milsom JW, Kron IL, Rheuban KS, et al: Chylothorax: An assessment of current surgical management. J Thorac Cardiovasc Surg 89:221–227, 1985.
34. Mislin H: Active contractility of the lymphangion and coordination of lymphangion chains. Experientia 32:820–821, 1976.
35. Niblack GD, Richie RE: Thoracic duct drainage—an overview. Heart Transplant 2:197–203, 1983.
36. Orringer MB, Bluett M, Deeb GM: Aggressive treatment of chylothorax complicating transhiatal esophagectomy without thoracotomy. Surgery 104:720–726, 1988.
37. Pandya K, Lal C, Tuchschmidt J, et al: Bilateral chylothorax with pulmonary Kaposi's sarcoma. Chest 94:1316–1367, 1988.
38. Pflug J, Calnan J: The valves of the thoracic duct at the angulus venosus. Br J Surg 55:911–916, 1968.
39. Rheuban KS, Kron IL, Carpenter MA, et al: Pleuroperitoneal shunts for refractory chylothorax after operation for congenital heart disease. Ann Thorac Surg 53:85–87, 1992.
40. Robinson CL: The management of chylothorax. Ann Thorac Surg 39:90–95, 1985.
41. Ross JK: A review of the surgery of the thoracic duct. Thorax 16:12–21, 1961.
42. Russell JA, Zimmerman K, Middendorf WF: Evidence of alpha-adrenergic innervation of the isolated canine thoracic duct. J Appl Physiol 49:1010–1015, 1980.
43. Shafiroff GP, Kau QY: Cannulation of the human thoracic lymph duct. Surgery 45:814–819, 1959.
44. Shirai T, Amano J, Takabe K: Thoracoscopic diagnosis and treatment of chylothorax after pneumonectomy. Ann Thorac Surg 52:306–307, 1991.
45. Staats BA, Ellefson RD, Budahn LL, et al: The lipoprotein profile of chylous and nonchylous pleural effusions. Mayo Clinic Proc 55:700–704, 1980.
46. Tilney NL, Murray JE: Chronic thoracic duct fistula. Ann Surg 167:1–8, 1968.
47. Tirone P, Schiantarelli P, Rosati G: Pharmacological activity of

some neuro-transmitters in the isolated thoracic duct of dogs. Lymphology 6:65–68, 1973.
48. Tzeng E, Ferguson MK: Predicting failure following shunting of pleural effusions. Chest 98:890–893, 1990.
49. Vallieres E, Shamji FM, Todd TR: Postpneumonectomy chylothorax. Ann Thorac Surg 55:1006–1008, 1993.
50. Van Pernis PA: Variations of the thoracic duct. Surgery 26:806–809, 1949.
51. Vargas FS, Milanez JRC, Filomeno LTB, et al: Intrapleural talc for the prevention of recurrence in benign or undiagnosed pleural effusions. Chest 106:1771–1775, 1994.
52. Weissberg D, Ben-Zeev I: Talc pleurodesis. J Thorac Cardiovasc Surg 106:689–695, 1993.
53. Zoetmulder F, Rutgers E, Baas P: Thoracoscopic ligation of a thoracic duct leakage. Chest 106:1233–1234, 1994.

COMMENTARY

Keith S. Naunheim

This is a balanced and thorough review of the anatomy, physiology, diagnosis, and management of chylothorax. The only additional item I feel important to mention is the expertise required to manage chylothorax with video-assisted thoracic surgery (VATS) techniques. On the one hand, it is a relatively simple matter to visualize the pleural cavity, achieve complete drainage of the chylothorax, and instill talc for sclerosis. Although this is certainly an option, many of the patients seen with chylothorax are relatively young people in whom talc sclerosis produces a fused pleural space, which makes it quite difficult to perform thoracotomy if it should be required for a new disease in the future. Thus, the advisability of this particular option in young patients is, in my opinion, questionable. In such patients, I believe it far better to proceed with direct suture ligation of the leak itself, or en bloc ligation of the thoracic duct above the diaphragm. Using VATS to perform these procedures can be quite challenging technically. Very often, isolation of the thoracic duct above the diaphragm requires significant mobilization of the esophagus, and circumnavigation of the thoracic duct with thoracoscopic instruments can be difficult. Simple ligature with a 2-0 silk tie just above the hiatus is my management option of choice, and this can be done with intracorporeal or extracorporeal knot-tying techniques. Suture ligation of the thoracic duct deep into the mediastinum can be difficult to perform, especially given the fragility of the thoracic duct tissues. Thus, I am writing not so much a commentary as a caveat for those readers wishing to undertake thoracoscopic management of chylothorax. One should not be hesitant to convert the procedure to an open one if difficulty is encountered in achieving the goals of safe and reliable ligation of the duct.

Chapter 10

Malignant Pleural Effusion

David W. Johnstone and Carolyn M. Dresler

Diagnosis and management of malignant pleural effusion (MPE) have historically involved minimally invasive techniques compared with other malignant thoracic diagnoses. There are approximately 250,000 diagnoses of MPE per year in the United States, and these patients usually have a limited life expectancy. In most cases, the tumors are incurable and therapies should be tailored to minimize suffering while providing as much palliation of symptoms as possible. Technologies developed in the 1990s have improved diagnostic accuracy and may offer more effective palliation.

Definition

Pleural effusion, the collection of fluid within the pleural space, is a common complication of malignant disease, which, in many cases, results in disabling respiratory symptoms. The presence of malignant cells within the pleural fluid constitutes the diagnosis. Pleural effusion may be the initial presentation of a patient who has a malignancy, or it may herald recurrent or progressive disease. Though occasional patients who have malignancy develop a pleural effusion due to a benign disorder, the vast majority of effusions in this setting—even if initial thoracentesis yields no malignant cells—are a direct result of the malignancy. Prognosis in most patients with MPE is poor, with survival measured in months. Prompt evaluation and management of MPE result in considerable relief of symptoms and improved quality of life for many patients.

Pathophysiology

The pleural space is bounded by the parietal and visceral pleural surfaces, each consisting of a nearly confluent mesothelial layer. The visceral pleura is supplied by high-pressure systemic capillaries, and the parietal pleura by low-pressure pulmonary capillaries. This results in a hydrostatic gradient from the chest wall to the lung, which allows diffusion of up to 10 L of low-protein fluid per day.[10] The normal pleural space contains a scant (5 to 10 ml) volume of fluid.

Fluid accumulation in malignant pleural disease is a result of several possible etiologies or their interactions[6,9,29]:

1. Obstruction of subpleural lymphatics and visceral pleural capillaries by tumor cells
2. Obstruction of lymphatic outflow by nodal metastases
3. Release of vasoactive amines by tumor cells, resulting in changes in capillary permeability
4. Associated conditions, such as hypoalbuminemia, pericardial involvement, congestive heart failure, superior vena cava obstruction, malignant ascites, and lymphatic changes associated with radiation fibrosis and chemotherapy

Progressive entrapment of the lung, which can occur because of tumor implantation or fibrosis on the visceral pleura, results in an obligatory pleural effusion that fills the residual pleural space. Thus, the lung is restricted, or trapped, in a contracted state, and simple drainage of the pleural fluid does not result in reinflation of the lung. Such entrapment is a considerable obstacle to the permanent resolution of the malignant effusion. Therefore, care should be taken to address the diagnosis and treatment of MPE at an early phase to avoid lung entrapment.

Clinical Manifestations

Most patients who have MPEs are symptomatic. Local symptoms include nonproductive cough, dyspnea, pleuritic chest pain, and a sense of fullness or pressure in the chest. Constitutional symptoms, which include anorexia, weight loss, fatigue, and malaise, are usually related to the underlying malignant process. Physical examination reveals diminished breath sounds and dullness to percussion on the involved side. Upright chest x-ray (CXR) typically demonstrates opacification of a portion of the hemithorax with a lateral meniscus (Fig. 10–1). Lateral decubitus films help discriminate free-flowing effusion from loculated fluid, a distinction that influences drainage technique. Computed tomography and ultrasound are not necessary for most patients but may be helpful in defining loculations for percutaneous drainage. In patients without a previous diagnosis, computed tomography as a diagnostic tool is very informative after large effusions are drained, because the effusion often obscures the underlying lung pathology.

Cancers of the breast, lung, and ovary, as well as lymphoma, account for about 75% of MPEs. Malignancies of the gastrointestinal and genitourinary tracts, melanoma, and various solid tumors account for the bulk of the remainder. About 3% of patients have unknown primary malignancies.[15]

Thoracentesis

Thoracentesis is the primary method of diagnosis. The procedure is simple and safe in the presence of a large effusion, but may require image guidance when the volume is small or the fluid is loculated. Complications of thoracentesis are uncommon. An exaggerated vagal response to pleural puncture is easily managed with position, intravenous (IV) fluids, and, possibly, atropine. If a large volume (>1 L) is drained rapidly, re-expansion pulmonary edema may occur, with potentially dangerous results;

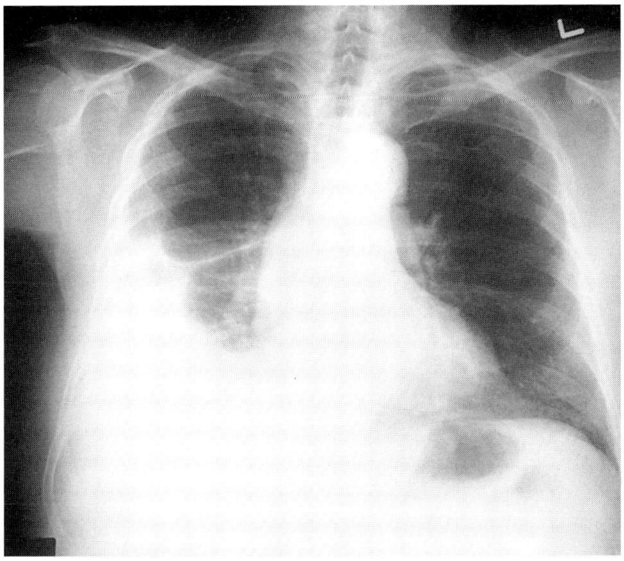

Figure 10–1. Chest radiograph demonstrating large right malignant pleural effusion with typical lateral meniscus. The scalloped appearance of the underlying lung surface may indicate entrapment, which was found in this case.

therefore, large effusions should be drained slowly. Pneumothorax and bleeding are other potential complications, but they are unusual if the draining needle or catheter is placed carefully.

The diagnostic yield of thoracentesis is about 50% after the first procedure, increasing to about 70% after the second and third attempts.[15] If closed pleural biopsy is added, the yield may increase to 80%.[28] The major disadvantage of closed pleural biopsy is the small random sample obtained, which may easily miss scattered pleural metastases. The diagnosis of mesothelioma by these methods maybe difficult because of the scant material obtained, relatively low sensitivity of positive fluid cytology (32%), and cytologic similarities to adenocarcinoma.[25] Lymphomas also have a low diagnostic yield because the predominant mechanism of effusion is central lymphatic obstruction rather than pleural implantation. Of all the lung cancers, adenocarcinoma has the greatest propensity for pleural metastases and associated effusions.

Therapeutic thoracentesis relieves symptoms quickly but transiently, because the pleural fluid reaccumulates rapidly. Simple drainage of MPE is associated with prompt relief of dyspnea. If there is no further intervention, this is followed by reaccumulation of the effusion, with a mean time to recurrence of 4.2 days; 97% recur within 1 month.[3] Repeated thoracenteses should be discouraged in favor of definitive drainage and pleurodesis. Therapeutic thoracentesis, in which the majority of the volume is removed, does permit an estimate of the degree of pulmonary entrapment and a sense of how much symptomatic improvement is likely with definitive relief of the effusion. This may be important in patients with other potential sources of dyspnea (e.g., pericardial effusion, cardiac failure, parenchymal disease) that are not addressed by drainage of the pleural space.

Thoracoscopy

Despite thoracentesis and pleural biopsy, approximately 15 to 20% of pleural effusions remain undiagnosed.[18] Thoracoscopy is a safe and effective method of diagnosis in these cases. The major advantages over previous methods are the acquisition of directed biopsies and the breakdown of adhesions. Despite the generally poor condition of many patients, current techniques carry minimal morbidity and low mortality. Mediastinoscopes and rigid thoracoscopes have been used for this purpose for many years, and these procedures are often performed with the patient under local anesthesia.[7] The major disadvantage of these instruments is the limited view of the pleural space, although they certainly afford better diagnostic accuracy than closed pleural biopsy. Hucker and associates[16] obtained a positive diagnosis in 80.3% of 102 patients who had rigid thoracoscopy performed for recurrent pleural effusions. These were patients in whom a diagnosis had not been achieved by conventional methods. Menzies and associates[21] reported a positive diagnosis in 96% of 86 patients who had undiagnosed pleural effusion, and found a negative predictive value of 93% for the diagnosis of pleural malignancy. Boutin and associates[5] showed a diagnostic accuracy of 96% in 215 patients undergoing thoracoscopy for effusion.

Video-Assisted Thoracoscopy (VATS)

Video-assisted thoracic surgery (VATS), now a well-refined technique, has probably been the most frequently used method of thoracoscopy in the 1990s. Single-lung ventilation under general anesthesia is necessary, and is tolerated by most patients who have MPE for the time necessary to drain, diagnose, and treat the effusion. Current optics and image reproduction afford unparalleled visual access to the entire pleural space and permit accurate biopsies (Fig. 10–2*A*). Morbidity related to the procedure is extremely low and most cases can be completed in less than 30 minutes.

Yim and associates[35] performed VATS for MPE in 69 patients, including 46 biopsies, 34 talc pleurodeses, and 16 limited decortications. No mortality or intraoperative complications occurred, though there were postoperative complications in 10% of cases. Diagnostic sensitivity was 87%. Talc pleurodesis was successful in 94% at the 6-month follow-up. This group of investigators also reported a case of re-expansion pulmonary edema immediately following thoracoscopic drainage and talc pleurodesis for MPE.[11] Kendall and associates[18] following standard methods performed VATS on 48 patients who had undiagnosed effusions, and found diagnostic sensitivity of 83%, specificity of 100%, and negative predictive value of 25%. Six of eight patients who did not have a diagnosis following VATS were subsequently found to have malignancy with further intervention.

Besides the great accuracy of VATS, other advantages include the ability to break down thin loculations, ensure complete evacuation of fluid, assess lung re-expansion directly, and achieve uniform distribution of sclerosant (see Fig. 10–2*B*). Additional procedures can be performed, such as lung biopsy and mediastinal node sampling,

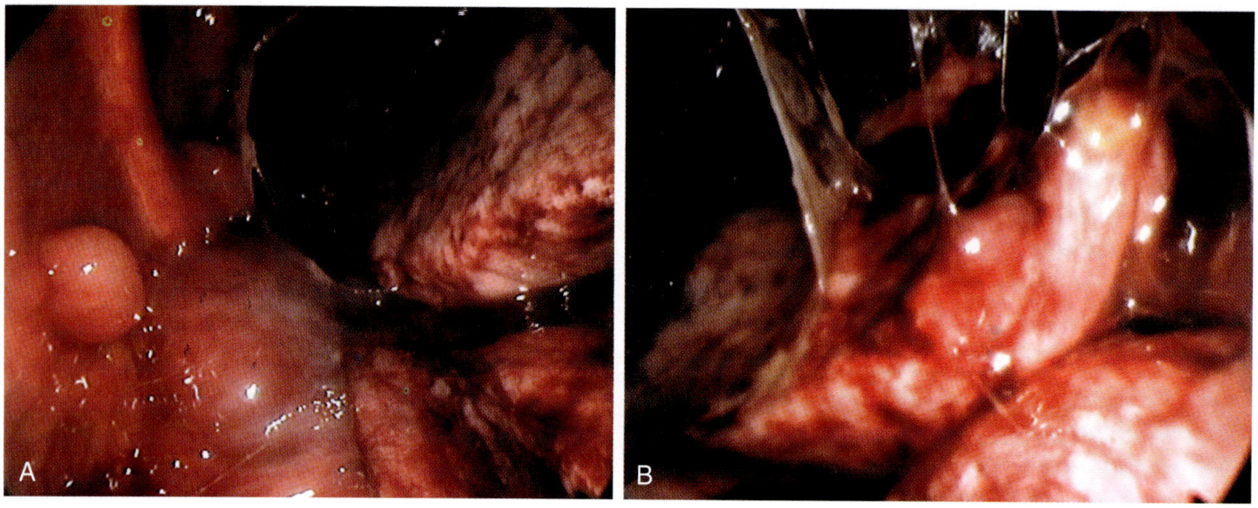

Figure 10–2. *A*, Video-thoracoscopic image of right pleural space involved with metastatic tumor to parietal and visceral pleura. Note rim of thin loculation apically. *B*, Intrapleural adhesions can easily be lysed thoracoscopically to permit complete drainage of pleural fluid and improve the distribution of sclerosant.

though these are not commonly required. Treatment of malignant pleural effusion is possible in some cases with mechanical pleurodesis or parietal pleurectomy. Visceral pleural decortication is usually impossible if tumor encasement is present, but if the lung expands well, obliteration of the pleural space is often achieved with parietal pleurectomy. Waller and associates[32] reported VATS pleurectomy in 19 patients who had MPE (13 who had a mesothelioma and six who had an adenocarcinoma). The median operating time was 35 minutes, the median hospital stay was 5 days, and there was no operative mortality. At the 12-month follow-up, 11 of 13 survivors remained free of effusion; six patients died of underlying disease during the follow-up.

Chemical Pleurodesis

Fluid drainage followed by chemical pleurodesis is effective and widely recognized as standard therapy for MPE. The majority of symptomatic MPEs require pleurodesis, but effusions caused by chemoresponsive tumors (e.g., lymphomas) should be treated with chemotherapy and radiation directed at the primary malignancy. Symptomatic effusions associated with tumor types that respond poorly to systemic treatment are appropriate for chemical pleurodesis.

Obliteration of the pleural space is necessary to prevent reaccumulation of fluid. The mean control rate for tube thoracostomy alone is only 22%.[15] Successful pleurodesis depends upon complete re-expansion of the lung and creation of an inflammatory pleural symphysis by chemical or mechanical means. It is unnecessary to postpone chemical pleurodesis until daily drainage has reached a certain threshold; once the lung is fully expanded, as demonstrated on CXR, pleurodesis should be performed. Placement of chest tubes for more than a few days may hinder the dispersion of the sclerosant within the pleural space because of the formation of loculations. After pleurodesis, the tube is left to drain until the daily output is about 150 ml or less.

Chemical sclerosants are given through the chest drain, whether done on an outpatient basis, or intraoperatively via the thoracoscope. The optimal agent continues to be a point of controversy, but it is agreed that the ideal agent should be effective, cause few side effects, be simple to deliver, and cost little. Many agents have been used, including radioactive phosphorus or gold, thiotepa, 5-fluorouracil (5FU), quinacrine, talc, nitrogen mustard, tetracycline (now unavailable), doxycycline, minocycline, bleomycin, doxorubicin, and *Corynebacterium parvum*. Clinical trials of these agents are hampered by patients' short life expectancy, lung entrapment, concurrent cancer therapy, and lack of standard criteria for successful pleurodesis. Clinical studies of sclerosing agents have generally been small, uncontrolled, retrospective trials. At present, the most commonly used agents are talc, doxycycline, and bleomycin.

Putnam and associates[24] reported the results of a phase III trial of treatment for MPE using the Pleurx (Denver Biomaterials, Golden, CO) pleural catheter versus conventional chest tube drainage plus doxycycline. The Pleurx catheter is a 15.5 French fenestrated silicone catheter that is placed into the pleural space under local anesthesia; tunneled subcutaneously to allow fixation of tissues to a polyester cuff; and accessed at the exposed end through a safety valve, which prevents inadvertent passage of fluid or air through the catheter. The patient can drain the fluid at home with a simple vacuum bottle kit to relieve dyspnea and achieve pleural apposition. One hundred forty-four patients who had MPE were randomized (99 catheter, 45 chest tube + sclerosis). Successful pleurodesis at 90 days was seen in 52% of the chest tube group versus 58% of the Pleurx catheter group (P = NS). It is worth noting that better results are historically obtained with talc pleurodesis, and talc could certainly be instilled through this catheter. Though this study was designed to measure the efficacy of pleurodesis, the device offers the best means available for outpatient external drainage of MPE. Since most patients have a life expectancy of only a few months, the likelihood of long-term complications seems low.

Pleurodesis Agents

Bleomycin, Tetracycline

Bleomycin and the tetracyclines are moderately effective sclerosing agents for MPE. In an extensive review of the pleurodesis literature, the success rates of bleomycin, the tetracyclines, and talc are 54%, 67%, and 93%, respectively; doxycycline appears to be an effective tetracycline replacement, with a success rate of 72%.[31] The main side effect reported with intrapleural bleomycin is fever. Although hematologic, pulmonary, and skin toxicity reactions have not been described, approximately 45% of an intracavitary dose is absorbed systemically.[2] High serum levels associated with one death, and three additional probable drug-related deaths, have been reported in the literature.[22,27,30]

Early randomized trials comparing intrapleural tetracycline with bleomycin for control of MPE have been inconclusive.[17,19] In at least one of these trials, bleomycin-treated patients had a higher incidence of nausea, vomiting, and rigors associated with therapy than did those treated with tetracycline.[19]

A large prospective, randomized trial in which 85 patients were evaluable after receiving either 60 units of bleomycin or 1 g of tetracycline intrapleurally found that bleomycin was superior to tetracycline in terms of median time to effusion recurrence (>46 days vs 32 days, P = .037), 30-day recurrence rate (36% vs 67%, P = .023), and 90-day recurrence rate (30% vs 53%, P = .047).[27] There were no significant differences in incidence of fever, pain, or other adverse reactions. This study failed to control for the use of intrapleural lidocaine, did not consider the need for retreatment after initial sclerotherapy, and did not address cost considerations. Bleomycin is expensive. In addition, it needs to be prepared by pharmacy personnel using chemotherapy precautions.

Talc

Intrapleurally administered talc has been shown to cause an intense chemical pleuritis with the formation of dense adhesions. Most published studies have examined thoracoscopic insufflation of talc under general anesthesia and report greater than 80% success rates (Fig. 10–3*A*, *B*). Bedside instillation of a talc slurry via thoracostomy tube is also reported to be effective in the management of MPE without the extreme pleural pain that may accompany talc poudrage application. Chambers[8] initially reported successful pleurodesis using a suspension of talc in 1% procaine in 17 of 20 patients who had MPE. More recently, Webb and associates[33] treated 34 patients with 5 g of iodized talc mixed with lidocaine. Of the 28 patients who had MPE, 100% achieved control of the effusion; two of the treated patients had previously failed tetracycline pleurodesis. Most patients were premedicated with a narcotic and a sedative and still reported mild to moderate discomfort.

Two small randomized studies have suggested that talc is more effective than bleomycin or tetracycline for control of MPE. Fentiman and associates[12] randomly assigned 33 evaluable breast cancer patients to receive talc (N = 12) via thoracoscopic insufflation, or tetracycline 500 mg via chest tube (N = 21). Successful sclerosis was achieved in 92% of the talc-treated patients versus 48% of those treated with tetracycline. In addition, 11 tetracycline failures were subsequently salvaged by talc. Hamed and associates[13] compared intracavitary bleomycin (N = 15) with talc insufflation (N = 10) in 25 evaluable breast cancer patients. With a mean follow-up of 9 months, they reported 100% control with talc versus 66% control after bleomycin. One half of bleomycin failures were successfully salvaged with talc. Of note, pleuritic pain was not observed in the talc group. In both studies, talc was adminis-

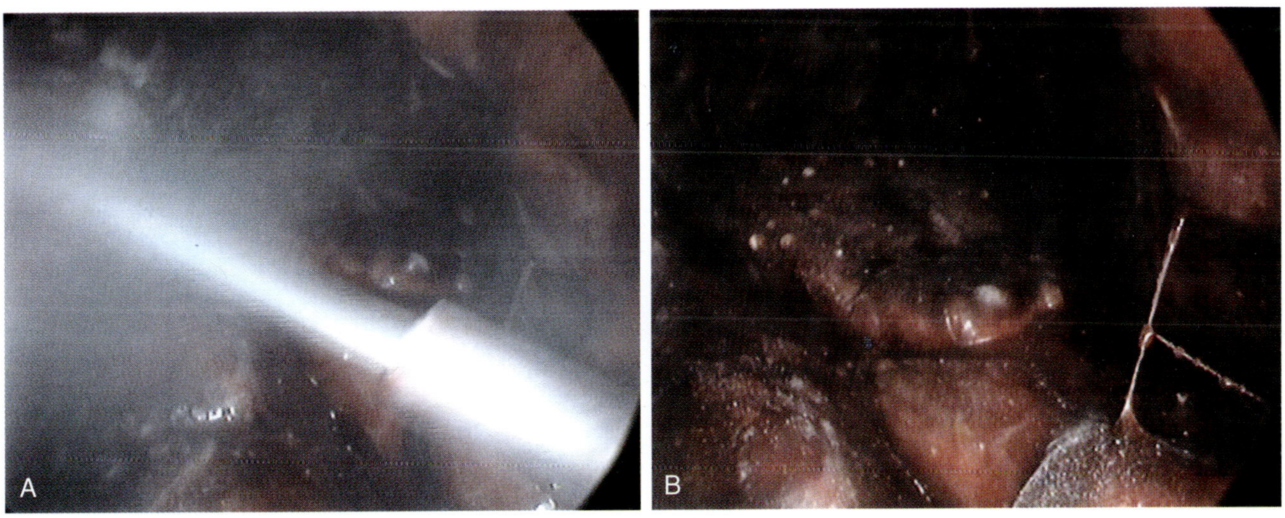

Figure 10–3. *A*, Talc insufflation during thoracoscopy should achieve as uniform a distribution as possible. *B*, A visual "snowstorm" results, which subsides to reveal scattered fine deposits of talc over all surfaces.

tered by insufflation under general anesthesia, any reaccumulation of effusion was called a treatment failure, and the patient population under study was only breast cancer patients.

A third study by Hartman and associates[14] compared insufflated talc under local anesthesia with 85 historical controls using tetracycline and bleomycin. Thirty-nine patients underwent talc pleurodesis with 3 to 6 g of talc, followed by chest tube drainage until output was less than 100 ml per day. Success rates at 90 days were 95% for talc compared with 70% for bleomycin and 47% for tetracycline.

The short-term morbidity with intrapleural talc appears to be minimal. Pain is thought to be less in patients with cancer compared with those being treated for recurrent pneumothorax. Most reports have advocated the use of general anesthesia for talc insufflation, but in all the above-referenced reports of bedside instillation of a talc suspension, only local anesthesia was given with no reports of severe or unmanageable pain. Thoracoscopic exploration and insufflation may similarly be carefully performed under local anesthesia with IV sedation.

Yim and associates performed a prospective, randomized study of VATS talc insufflation versus bedside talc slurry for MPE.[34] Fifty-seven patients were randomized to receive 5 g of talc by one of these methods. There was no statistically significant difference between the two groups with respect to complications, chest tube duration, or recurrence (3.5% VATS vs 10.3% talc slurry, P = NS).

Adverse reactions reported after the instillation of talc include a report of acute respiratory distress syndrome (ARDS) in three patients after intrapleural instillation of 10 g talc, and acute respiratory failure with diffuse bilateral pulmonary infiltrates a few hours after instillation of 2 g of talc in another report.[4,26] Adler and Sayek described 22 steroid-dependent patients who experienced transient hypotension following instillation of talc by poudrage; symptoms rapidly resolved with IV fluids and steroids.[1] In the study by Hamed and associates,[13] two patients in the talc group had an unexplained asystolic arrest under general anesthesia while being turned after the poudrage procedure. In the study by Hartman and associates,[14] one patient had severe chest pain; however, a myocardial infarction was ruled out. Fever occurred in seven patients, lasting 24 hours, and six patients had nonclinically significant subcutaneous emphysema.

The other issue associated with talc is concern about asbestos contamination. Currently, all talc used for medical purposes is labeled and available as "USP" (United States Pharmacopeia), and is asbestos free.

Two prospective, randomized, cooperative group trials are under way. The first is a three-arm comparison of talc, doxycycline, and bleomycin delivered via chest tube or small-bore catheter. This will provide a prospective comparison of the relative efficacy of these agents. The second trial compares talc slurry pleurodesis via chest tube versus talc insufflation pleurodesis via thoracoscopy. This trial will provide excellent data on the efficacy of talc overall, and indicate whether operative techniques have a therapeutic advantage over simple chest tube management in the setting of established MPE.

Management of the Entrapped Lung

Entrapment of the lung poses a significant problem in the setting of MPE because formal decortication is not possible. Pleural apposition and symphysis cannot take place and the effusion recurs rapidly (Fig. 10–4). Many of these patients are symptomatically improved despite incomplete re-expansion. Maintenance of a minimal volume of pleural fluid should be the goal in these patients. The available methods include repeated thoracentesis, pleuroperitoneal shunting, and, possibly, a permanent external catheter. Repeated thoracentesis entails frequent procedures, risk of bleeding, pneumothorax, and infection; moreover, it is often limited by gradual loculation of the pleural effusion. Pleuroperitoneal shunts may be appropriate as second-line treatment in young, motivated patients who do not have ascites, who are able to pump the chamber repeatedly (up to 1000 times per day), and who have a life expectancy that warrants implantation of a permanent device. Successful palliation is reported in 70 to 95% of patients who have occlusion or revision rates of 12 to 17%.[20,23] Finally, the Pleurx catheter, or devices of similar design, may offer a simple means of intermittent external drainage in patients with a short life expectancy.[24]

Summary

Malignant pleural effusion remains a common complication of malignant disease. Diagnostic and therapeutic approaches have always been minimally invasive, but the advent of video-assisted thoracoscopy offers improved visualization and instrumentation. Methods of pleurodesis are the subject of ongoing investigation, and the most effective and economical pleurodesis agent appears to be sterile talc. Better palliation for patients who have an entrapped lung remains an elusive goal.

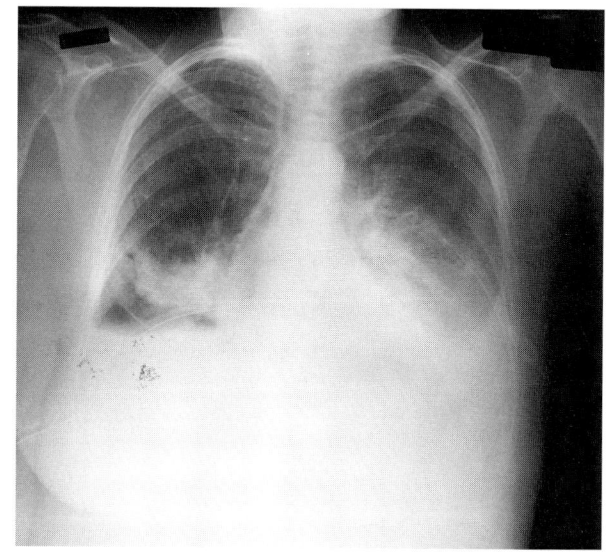

Figure 10–4. Chest radiograph demonstrating entrapment of the right lower lobe. The obligatory pleural space refills once the drain is removed. Pleuroperitoneal shunting and intermittent external drainage are potential palliative options in this case.

References

1. Adler RH, Sayek I: Treatment of malignant pleural effusion: A method using tube thoracoscopy and talc. Ann Thorac Surg 28:8–15, 1976.
2. Albert DS, Chen HSG, Mayersohn M, et al: Bleomycin pharmacokinetics in man: II. Intracavitary Admin Cancer Chemother Pharmacol 2:127–132, 1979.
3. Anderson CB, Philpott GW, Ferguson TB: The treatment of malignant pleural effusions. Cancer 33:916–922, 1974.
4. Bouchama A, Chastre J, Gaudichet A, et al: Acute pneumonitis with bilateral pleural effusion after talc pleurodesis. Chest 86:795–797, 1984.
5. Boutin C, Viallat JR, Gugnino P, et al: Thoracoscopy in malignant pleural effusion. Am Rev Respir Dis 124:558–592, 1981.
6. Black LF: The pleural space and pleural fluid. Mayo Clin Proc 47:493–506, 1972.
7. Brandt HJ, Mai J: Differential diagnosis of pleural effusions using thoracoscopy. Pneumonologie 145:192–203, 1971.
8. Chambers JS: Palliative treatment of neoplastic pleural effusion with intercostal intubation and talc instillation. West J Surg 66:26–28, 1958.
9. Chernow B, Shan SA: Carcinomatous involvement of the pleura. Am J Med 63:695–702, 1977.
10. Claus RH, Yacoubian NH, Barker HG: Dynamics of pleural effusion. Surg Forum 7:201–204, 1956.
11. Critchley LA, Au HK, Yim AP: Reexpansion pulmonary edema occurring after thoracoscopic drainage of a pleural effusion. J Clin Anesth 8:591–594, 1996.
12. Fentiman IS, Rubens RD, Hayward JL: A comparison of intracavitary talc and tetracycline for the control of pleural effusions secondary to breast cancer. Curr J Cancer Clin Oncol 9:1079–1081, 1986.
13. Hamed H, Fentiman IS, Chaudary MA, et al: Comparison of intracavitary bleomycin and talc for control of pleural effusions secondary to carcinoma of the breast. Br J Surg 76:1266–1267, 1989.
14. Hartman DL, Gaither JM, Kesler KA, et al: Comparison of insufflated talc under thoracoscopic guidance with standard tetracycline and bleomycin pleurodesis for control of malignant pleural effusions. J Thorac Cardiovasc Surg 105:743–748, 1993.
15. Hausheer FH, Yarbro JW: Diagnosis and treatment of malignant pleural effusion. Semin Oncol 12:54, 1985.
16. Hucker J, Bhatnagar NK, Al-Jilaihawi AN, et al: Thoracoscopy in the diagnosis and management of recurrent pleural effusions. Ann Thorac Surg 52:1145–1147, 1991.
17. Johnston CE, Curzon PGD: Comparison of intrapleural bleomycin and tetracycline in the treatment of malignant pleural effusion. Thorax 40:210, 1985.
18. Kendall SW, Bryan AJ, Large SR, Wells LC: Pleural effusions: Is thoracoscopy a reliable investigation? A retrospective review. Respir Med 86:437–440, 1992.
19. Kessinger A, Wigton RS: Intracavitary bleomycin and tetracycline in the management of malignant pleural effusions: A randomized study. J Surg Oncol 36:81–83, 1987.
20. Little AG, Kadowaki MH, Ferguson MK, et al: Pleuro-peritoneal shunting: Alternative therapy for pleural effusions. Ann Surg 208:443–450, 1988.
21. Menzies R, Charbonneau M: Thoracoscopy for the diagnosis of pleural disease. Ann Intern Med 114:271–276, 1991.
22. Ostrowski MJ: An assessment of the long term results of controlling the reaccumulation of malignant effusions using intracavitary bleomycin. Cancer 57:721–727, 1986.
23. Petrou M, Kaplan D, Goldstraw P: Management of recurrent malignant pleural effusions. The complementary role of talc pleurodesis and pleuroperitioneal shunting. Cancer 75: 801–805, 1995.
24. Putnam JB, Ponn R, Olak J, et al: A phase III trial of treatment for malignant pleural effusions: Pleurx pleural catheter versus chest tube + doxycycline sclerosis (abstract). Chest 112 (Suppl)–126S, 1997.
25. Renshaw AA, Dean BR, Antman KH, et al: The role of cytologic evaluation of pleural fluid in the diagnosis of malignant mesothelioma. Chest 111:106–109, 1997.
26. Rinaldo JE, Owens GR, Rogers RM: Adult respiratory distress syndrome following intrapleural instillation of talc. J Thorac Cardiovasc Surg 85:523–526, 1983.
27. Ruckdeschel JC, Moores D, Lee JY, et al: Intrapleural therapy for malignant pleural effusions: A randomized comparison of bleomycin and tetracycline. Chest 100:1528–1535, 1991.
28. Sahn SA: The pleura. Am Rev Respir Dis 138:184, 1988.
29. Sahn SA: Pleural effusion in lung cancer. Clin Chest Med 14:189–200, 1993.
30. Trotter JM, Stuart JFB, McBeth F, et al: The management of malignant effusions with bleomycin. Br J Cancer 40:310, 1979.
31. Walker-Renard PB, Vaughan LM, Shan SA: Chemical pleurodesis for malignant pleural effusions. Ann Intern Med 120:56–94, 1994.
32. Walker DA, Morritt GN, Forty J: Video-assisted thoracoscopic pleurectomy in the management of malignant pleural effusion. Chest 78:1454–1456, 1995.
33. Webb WR, Ozman V, Moulder PV, et al: Iodized talc pleurodesis for the treatment of pleural effusion. J Thorac Cardiovasc Surg 103:881–886, 1992.
34. Yim AP, Chan AT, Lee TW, et al: Thoracoscopic talc insufflation versus talc slurry for symptomatic malignant pleural effusion. Ann Thorac Surg 62:1655–1658, 1996.
35. Yim AP, Chung SS, Lee TW, et al: Thoracoscopic management of pleural effusions. Chest 109:1234–1238, 1996.

COMMENTARY

Anthony P. C. Yim

Malignant pleural effusion remains a common condition that could be difficult to treat. The authors cover the subject very nicely. As they point out, talc is probably the most effective sclerosant, although the optimal route of administration is yet to be determined. In a small randomized, prospective study, we have not found any statistical difference in results between giving the talc as a slurry versus thoracoscopic insufflation as long as the lung is not significantly trapped. The advantage of the former is that it can be administered at the bedside, whereas the latter necessitates general anesthesia. It will be interesting to see if our conclusion will be substantiated by a larger multicenter study. Nonetheless, it is important to realize that the treatment goal here is palliation and not extended survival. Simple treatment should probably be tried first, and the temptation to utilize VATS nonselectively in every patient must be resisted.

Section III

Parenchymal Lung Diseases

Chapter 11

Spontaneous Pneumothorax

Stephen R. Hazelrigg, Mitchell J. Magee, and Theresa M. Boley

Spontaneous pneumothorax is a disease with an estimated incidence of 4 to 9 out of 100,000 patients per year and a 5:1 male predominance.[17] Its management differs depending upon its etiology, duration, previous occurrence, patient occupation, and general health. The ability to treat this disease by video-assisted thoracic surgery (VATS) has raised several questions and caused us to re-evaluate the treatment of spontaneous pneumothorax.

Pathophysiology

Spontaneous pneumothorax tends to be distributed between two distinct age groups. The first group comprises young patients, 85% of whom are less than 40 years of age. The disease in these patients is called primary spontaneous pneumothorax (PSP). The typical patient in this group is a man between the ages of 25 and 30 years who is tall, thin, and who often has a history of smoking. Pain is the most frequent symptom, followed by mild dyspnea. Upon examination, these patients generally have ruptured blebs, which are small (<1 cm), blister-like areas (Fig 11–1) composed of parietal pleura and located on the surface of the lung. Because of their otherwise normal pulmonary function, patients in this group tolerate the pneumothorax well and have minimal symptoms. Rarely, a pneumothorax may lead to hemorrhage from a torn adhesion, or to a tension pneumothorax.

The precise etiology for the formation of blebs is not completely understood. There is increased incidence in asthmatic patients and smokers, and it is believed that any disorder that increases the pressure at the alveolar level may enhance the development of a bleb. As noted, blebs are made up of parietal pleura from a ruptured alveolus and they have no epithelial lining. Congenital cysts that are epithelially lined also occur rarely, but they tend to have bronchial connections. Rarely, PSP may occur without the presence of blebs from an adhesion that tears the surface of the lung at the time of a cough.

The second group of patients who develop spontaneous pneumothorax are older (60 to 65 years of age) and have more comorbid medical problems than patients who have PSP. The most common etiology of a pneumothorax in this group is the rupture of a bulla. Bullae are larger than blebs (usually >2.5 cm) and occur in patients with obstructive lung disease and emphysema (Fig 11–2). This type of pneumothorax is defined as a secondary spontaneous pneumothorax (SSP), because there is known pre-existing lung disease. Because of their underlying lung disease, these patients do not tolerate the pneumothorax nearly as well as those who have PSP and, commonly, SSP patients have significant levels of dyspnea and hypoxia on presentation. Mortality rates as high as 16% have been reported.[31]

There are several other causes of SSP that are less common than ruptured bullae. Included on this list are necrotic peripheral malignancies, trauma, infection, interstitial lung disease, congenital cysts, connective tissue diseases, lymphangioleiomyomatosis, endometriosis, and AIDS. In the immune-compromised patient, *Pneumocystis carinii* pneumonia (PCP) may produce pneumothorax as a result of peripheral tissue necrosis. This tends to occur as a late problem in the overall course of AIDS as demonstrated by a mean survival of about 5 months after development of a pneumothorax. Bilateral disease is the norm with PCP, and this should be appreciated in developing treatment strategies.[8,9]

Traumatic pneumothorax may occur from either blunt or penetrating trauma or iatrogenic injury (e.g., thoracentesis, barotrauma, central line placement). Catamenial pneumothorax occurs during menstruation as a result of endometrial implants, and occurs on the right side in 90% of cases. Oral contraceptives have been used to avoid future recurrences

Radiographic Evaluation

The typical radiologic evaluation of spontaneous pneumothorax has been simply performed using chest radiograph (CXR). The CXR is used to look for evidence of large cysts or bullae and to ensure complete re-expansion of the lung. There have been reports of the use of computed tomography (CT) scans in the evaluation of these patients. The support for CT scans has been suggested because the presence of cysts, blebs, and bullae visualized on CT scan predict frequent recurrence and prolonged air leaks and, hence, dictate aggressive treatment. Thus far, the use of CT scans in the decision tree for management is not clear, and these scans are not generally used because of their additional cost. Further evaluation of this modality is needed to see if it will indeed allow us to stratify patients and individualize their treatments.

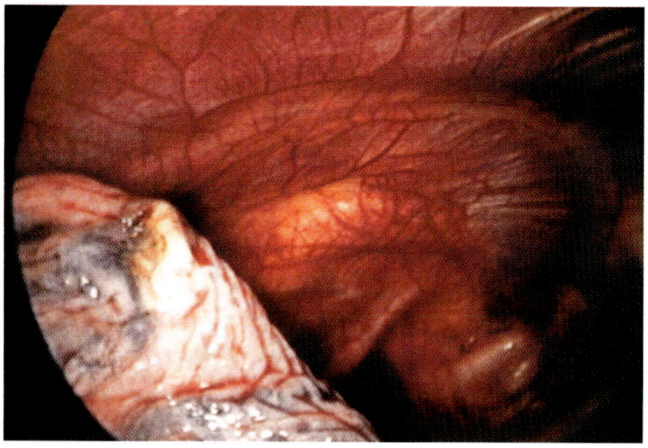

Figure 11–1. Thoracoscopic view of a ruptured bulla in the left upper lobe. (From Yim APC, Ho JKS, Chung SS, et al: Video-assisted thoracoscopic surgery for primary spontaneous pneumothorax. Aust NZ J Surg 64:667–670, 1994, with permission.)

Treatment

The etiologies of PSP and SSP are separate and distinct. For this reason, they also have separate and distinct treatment strategies. Whereas PSP occurs in an otherwise normal lung, SSP is related to emphysematous, and often diffusely diseased, underlying lung tissue. The general goals of treatment, however, are the same, regardless of the etiology, and include the elimination of the source of the leak, full lung re-expansion, and minimization of the risk of recurrence, all done at the lowest possible financial cost, and with the lowest possible incidence of morbidity and mortality.

The options for treatment of spontaneous pneumothorax remain many, and it has often been difficult to compare these varied forms of therapy. For asymptomatic patients with a small pneumothorax (<20%), conservative treatment with observation, and possibly oxygen therapy, is appropriate. For most patients, however, some intervention is required. Options for intervention include the following:

1. Aspiration
2. Chest tube placement
3. Pleurodesis (chemical)
4. Surgical intervention by open incision (i.e., thoracotomy) or video-assisted thoracic surgery (VATS).

Indications

Surgical indications generally include recurrent pneumothoraces, prolonged air leaks, associated complications (e.g., hemothorax), recognized large cysts, and unique employment or residence (e.g., pilots, scuba divers, patients living in remote areas). Timing of intervention for recurrences must be made based on understanding of the risk of future recurrent episodes.

Recurrent Pneumothorax. There have been estimates that the risk of a recurrence is between 20 and 40% after the first episode of spontaneous pneumothorax. This incidence generally rises to 50% or greater after a second

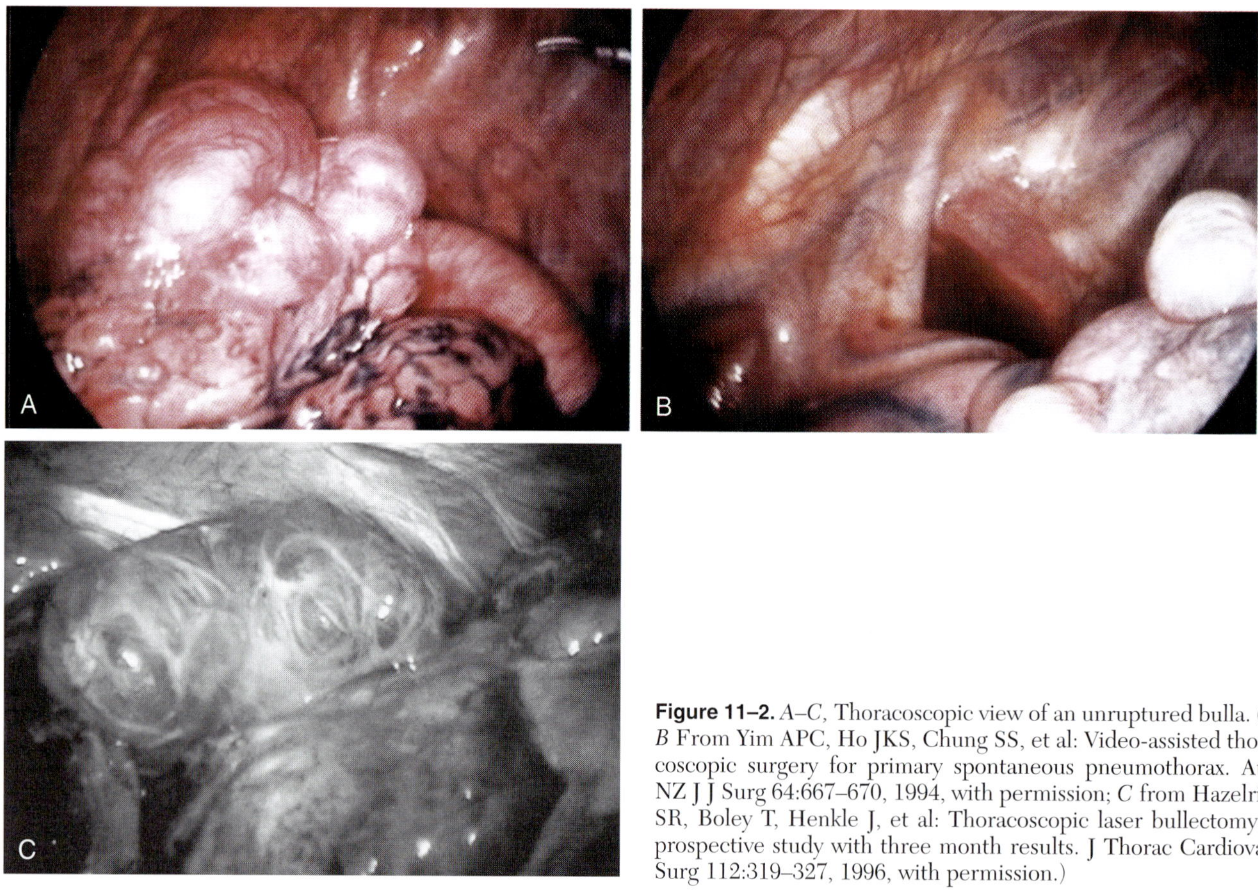

Figure 11–2. *A–C,* Thoracoscopic view of an unruptured bulla. (*A, B* From Yim APC, Ho JKS, Chung SS, et al: Video-assisted thoracoscopic surgery for primary spontaneous pneumothorax. Aust NZ J J Surg 64:667–670, 1994, with permission; *C* from Hazelrigg SR, Boley T, Henkle J, et al: Thoracoscopic laser bullectomy: A prospective study with three month results. J Thorac Cardiovasc Surg 112:319–327, 1996, with permission.)

episode, and the risk of recurrence continues to rise with each subsequent episode.[10–12,28,29] Boutin estimated the risk of recurrence at 21% after a first episode based on review of data collected from 4982 cases treated with chest tube alone.[4] Almind, in 1986, reported a recurrence rate of 36% in a prospective study of patients treated with chest tube alone.[1] There is a suggestion that the risk of recurrence may be higher for SSP than for PSP, but the exact difference is not clear. Traditionally, open surgery was recommended after the third episode. The emergence of VATS has altered this approach, so that many centers now recommend surgery after the second episode of PSP, but they remain more conservative in surgical treatment of SSP based on the overall health status of the patient.

Prolonged Air Leak. The optimal timing of surgical intervention for continued air leak is uncertain. Data suggest that the majority of air leaks seal within 72 hours. Leaks persisting after this time may lead to a very prolonged waiting period before there is complete sealing. As a general rule in cases of PSP, we have recommended intervention after 72 hours if the leak has not resolved or shown evidence of significant resolution. Full-lung expansion must be achieved and may require additional chest tubes. Failure to resolve the leak by manipulating the chest tubes leaves options for additional treatment that include chemical pleurodesis or surgical intervention. With the availability of VATS, it has become our preferred treatment for most prolonged air leaks. We prefer general anesthesia (and double-lumen endotrachael intubation); however, alternatives are pleuroscopy under local anesthesia, instillation of a chemical sclerosant, or both.

Treatment Options

Chemical Pleurodesis. Many different substances have been used for chemical sclerosis in the pleural space. All these agents have in common the side effects of pleural inflammation and adherence of the visceral and parietal pleura. The effectiveness of any sclerosant is dependent on complete expansion of the lung, apposition of the pleural surfaces, and development of adhesions.

There have been many comparisons of different sclerosing agents, but, at present, the most common choices are doxycycline, bleomycin, and talc. Both doxycycline and talc are inexpensive; however, bleomycin generally costs $1000 to $2000 per treatment dose.

Many of the sclerosant agents used alone have been associated with high rates of recurrent pneumothoraces. Silver nitrate was used for airmen in the Royal Air Force, but the recurrence rate of 28% was considered too high and led to the abandonment of this treatment.[18] A prospective study comparing treatment with chest tube alone, chest tube with tetracycline, and chest tube with talc instillation revealed recurrence rates for pneumothoraces of 36%, 13%, and 8%, respectively.[1] Most comparative studies have shown talc to be more effective than tetracycline (or doxycycline), and animal studies have demonstrated that tetracycline produces rather flimsy adhesions. Talc, on the other hand, tends to produce obliteration of the pleural space. Direct animal experiments comparing various methods of pleurodesis revealed mechanical abrasion and talc to be more effective than tetracycline, laser (Nd:YAG), or the argon beam coagulator.[5]

Talc instillation has raised concern about possible contamination with asbestos and the resultant risk of mesothelioma. At present, the preparation of talc is asbestos free and quite safe from this standpoint. The typical dose of talc ranges from 2 to 5 g, and the incidence of intense inflammation and focal granulomas seems to occur more frequently when doses greater than 10 g are used. Talc does seem to have some variation in its exact composition. Some reports have suggested a systemic identification of talc after intrapleural insufflation, but the clinical significance of this is unclear. Many patients develop pleuritic pain and fever in the first 24 to 48 hours after chemical pleurodesis; these symptoms are presumably related to the inflammation produced.

Another concern related to chemical pleurodesis is the long-term impact upon the pleural space and pulmonary function. One study that examined this issue did not yield any evidence of restrictive pulmonary changes in patients seen 20 years after undergoing pleurodesis.[22] Talc has, however, been reported to produce acute pneumonitis and, rarely, a respiratory distress syndrome.[3,27] The obliteration of the pleural space likely makes any future ipsilateral surgery difficult and should be avoided in patients who have a high likelihood of future operation or transplantation (e.g., patients who have cystic fibrosis).

Surgical Treatment. Operative intervention is generally weighed against the risk of future recurrence or a prolonged hospital stay occasioned by a persistent leak. Thoracotomy has been the traditional surgical approach and may be performed by several different types of incision. A formal lateral thoracotomy offers an excellent view of the lung and the thoracic cavity, but is the most invasive method from the perspective of pain and postoperative disability. Limited thoracotomy through the auscultatory triangle has been reported, but axillary thoracotomy has been the most frequently used open incision. Axillary thoracotomy entails a limited incision at the inferior axillary hair line and entrance into the chest at the third or fourth intercostal space.[17] This approach reportedly produces less pain than a lateral thoracotomy but offers a more limited view of the lung. Since the majority of blebs are located in the apex of the upper lobe, or the superior segment of the lower lobe, they can be seen satisfactorily. Several years ago, VATS began to be used for the treatment of spontaneous pneumothorax. This allows smaller incisions with better visualization, and with the availability of endoscopic staples, the operation could be performed endoscopically in the same way as the open procedure.

VATS Techniques

Thoracoscopic evaluation of the pleural space may be performed using local or general anesthesia.[20] The majority of procedures, however, have been performed using general anesthesia and double-lumen endotracheal intubation, because this allows one-lung ventilation and maximizes the working space and visualization of the pleural cavity.

Typically, we have used three access ports for the performance of bleb or bulla resection (Fig 11–3).[13] The ini-

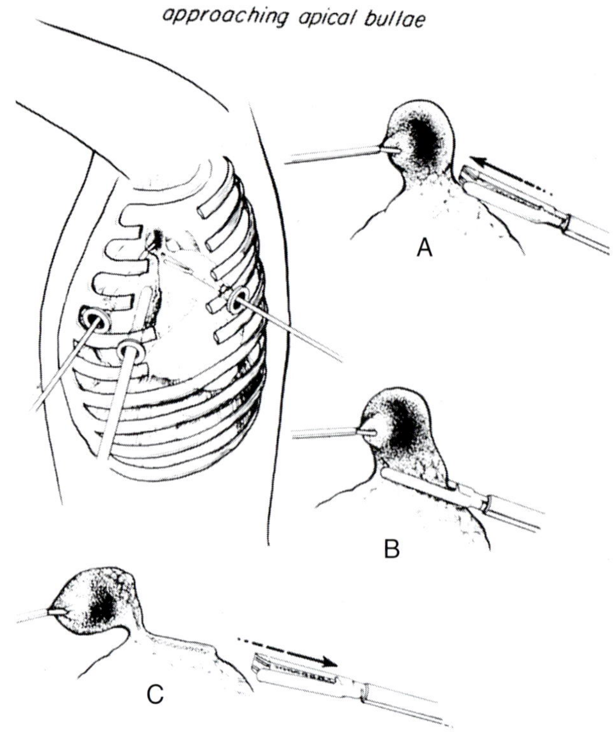

Figure 11–3. Approximate sites of routine trocar placement for spontaneous pneumothorax and demonstration of stapled resection of bleb or bulla. The bleb is initiallly grasped. *A,* The endoscopic stapler is applied with a rim of normal lung tissue; *B, C,* each staple application cuts between multiple rows of staples. (From Hazelrigg SR, Landreneau RJ, Mack M, et al: Thoracoscopic stapled resection for spontaneous pneumothorax. J Thorac Cardiovasc Surg 105:389–393, 1993, with permission.)

tial port is placed in the midaxillary line of the seventh intercostal space (ICS). The incision is probed initially to ensure the absence of significant adhesions and a port is placed. The size of the trocar used depends upon the size of the thoracoscope. Scopes are available in sizes ranging from 2 to 10 mm. The larger scopes provide more light and a wider operative field; however, for simple bleb resection, a small scope can offer satisfactory visualization. The 2-mm scope can be placed through small introducers and theoretically reduces the risk of postoperative intercostal pain.

After the scope is introduced, two other incisions are made at higher interspaces for introduction of instruments. Our preference for management is resection of the blebs or bullae using the endoscopic stapler, which requires an incision large enough for introduction (>10 mm). We attempt to place all access ports anterior to the posterior axillary line, recognizing that the ICSs become progressively narrower posteriorly with increased risk of intercostal nerve injury.

The typical trocar placement results in the three sites being triangulated, with the upper two sites in the fifth ICS at the anterior and posterior axillary lines. We do not use trocars unless the amount of subcutaneous tissue prevents easy introduction of instruments. A ring forceps or 5-mm grasper is used to move the lung and inspect the entire surface. Attention is directed particularly to the apical region of the lung; however, it must be recognized that multiple blebs are common, and the entire lung surface should be inspected.

After identification, the blebs or bullae are resected with the stapler, which is applied at the base to a rim of normal lung tissue (Fig 11–4). Other methods of treatment are available, including cauterization, laser, ablation[36] or endoloop ligation.[23] We prefer stapled excision, but endoloop ligation has been reported with success in large numbers of patients.[37]

A pleural procedure is typically performed in addition to the elimination of the air leak source. This is usually done by apical mechanical pleural abrasion. We introduce an unraveled gauze sponge and use it to abrade the apical pleura, but many other, more costly, substances, including rolled-up Marlex mesh, have been used (Fig 11–5). Apical abrasion is thought to decrease the risk of recurrence in open and VATS procedures.

Another option is partial or complete pleurectomy. The more extensive the pleurectomy, the lower the risk of recurrent pneumothoraces, but the higher the morbidity caused by hemothorax and fibrothorax. When pleurectomy

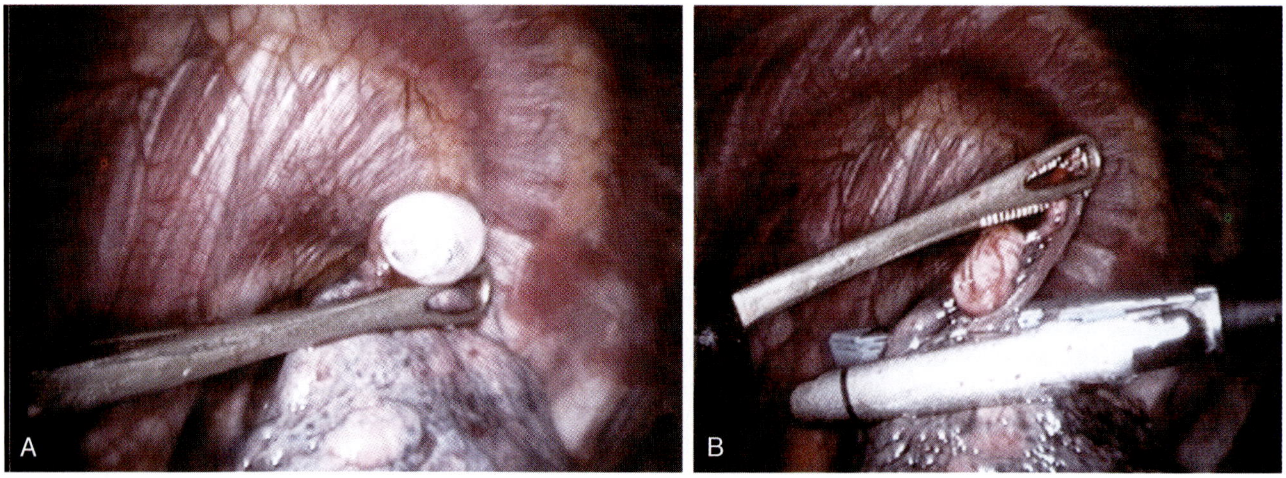

Figure 11–4. Stapled resection of a bulla. (From Yim APC, Ho JKS, Lai CKW, et al: Primary spontaneous pneumothorax treated by video assisted thoracoscopic surgery—results of intermediate follow up. Aust N Z J Med 25:146–150, 1995, with permission.)

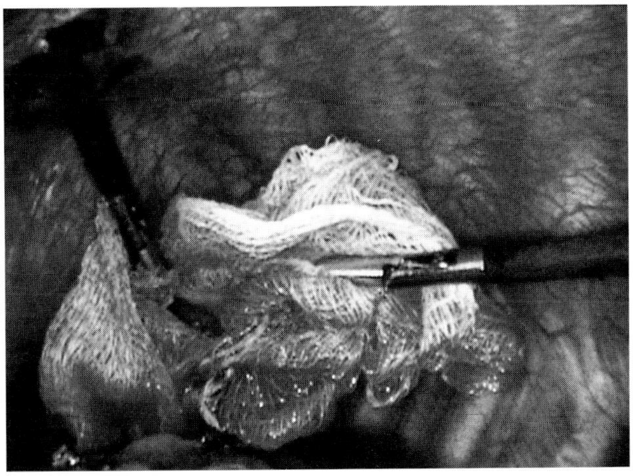

Figure 11–5. Sponge gauze used to create a mechanical abrasion of the apex of the parietal pleura. (From Yim APC, Ho JKS, Lai CWK, et al: Primary spontaneous pneumothorax treated by video assisted thoracoscopic surgery—results of intermediate follow up. Aust N Z J Med 25:146–150, 1995, with permission.)

is performed, it is generally limited to the apex of the chest, although there are a few instances, such as with PCP, in which a more extensive pleurectomy may be warranted.

Apical parietal pleurectomy can be performed satisfactorily under thoracoscopic guidance. We generally use the cautery on the fourth or fifth rib to start the pleurectomy and continue with traction and cautery to develop the plane. In most cases, the pleura comes down easily and takes no more than 15 to 20 minutes of additional operative time. We have not routinely attempted to remove the mediastinal pleura.

Results

Several facts have been noted in the literature on spontaneous pneumothorax. For SSP, the rate of recurrence after open stapled resection and pleural abrasion is 1 to 5%.[30,33,38] The addition of pleurectomy seems to decrease recurrence, which is related to the extent of the pleurectomy. Thoracoscopic and open surgical procedures are identical in virtually all cases. As with all new techniques, there is a learning curve, and there are reports of elevated recurrence rates in early experience with VATS, probably related to missed pathology and other technical issues.

Comparison of VATS with open thoracotomy has consistently demonstrated less pain with VATS, and the degree of difference probably depends upon the type of thoracotomy, the location of trocar sites, and the amount of crushing-type manipulation done to the intercostal nerves.[21] Long-term intercostal pain occurs with VATS at rates similar to thoracotomy because of inadvertent nerve injury. We recommend the use of anterior ports, especially for the stapling device, and avoidance of excessive crushing of the ICS to try to decrease the incidence of long-term pain.

We reported our early results of VATS resection of apical blebs in 26 patients and compared them with results in 20 patients who had axillary thoracotomy.[15] Our findings included a shorter hospital stay (2.9 days vs 4.5 days) and reduced need for intravenous IV narcotics in the VATS group. At 48 hours postoperatively, only 7.7% of VATS patients required (IV) narcotics, whereas 70% of the axillary thoracotomy patients were using IV analgesia. Many subsequent reports confirmed the early efficacy of VATS, with shortened hospital stays and less pain.[2,6,23,26,32,34] Inderbitzi reported on VATS partial pleurectomy in 12 patients, with no recurrences and a mean hospital stay of 3.3 days.[19]

As more patients have undergone VATS and as follow-up has become more extended, a slightly increased incidence of recurrence has been seen.[32] Naunheim reviewed more than 100 patients who were followed for more than a year and noted that when blebs were identified, the risk of recurrence was very low (1 to 2%), but when no blebs were seen, the recurrence risk was elevated. This led to a recommendation of apical pleurectomy or open thoracotomy for the group of patients in whom no blebs or bullae were found.[32]

It is likely that the increased recurrences reported in some series using VATS were due to missed blebs or bullae or to the incorrect application or malfunction of the endoscopic stapler. Most series continue to see progressively lower recurrence rates over time, approaching a 1 to 2% recurrence rate.

Cost-analysis interpretation depends upon the method used to manage blebs. The quantity of expensive disposable equipment used, as well as the length of the hospital stay, largely determines the overall cost.[16] At present, we do not use any disposable equipment with the exception of the endoscopic stapling device, and our average hospital stay is 2.4 days.

Some surgeons have advocated the use of the endoloop ligation technique to avoid the cost of using the stapler.[23,24,35] Although there are several reports of a large number of patients treated satisfactorily with endoloops, there are also reports of these loops slipping off. In addition, the endoloops may be difficult to use for large bullae that do not have a discrete "neck."

Surgical techniques may be more difficult in the setting of SSP. When the bullae are large and diffuse (without a discrete neck), their excision may be technically difficult. The more emphysematous the lung is, the higher the risk of prolonged leaks and recurrence. The use of bovine pericardial sleeves to buttress the staple lines has been proven to reduce the length of postoperative leaks in emphysema patients.[14] Surgical judgment based upon anatomic findings and the surgeon's own experience should dictate whether to perform the surgical resection by open techniques or VATS.

Conclusion

Spontaneous pneumothorax is a common problem that may have many different etiologies. The most common cause, however, is rupture of blebs or bullae, which tends to occur in different patient groups, but there are common themes in strategies for management of either blebs or bullae. Because spontaneous pneumothorax is a benign disorder that generally is not life threatening, it lends itself well to a low level of invasive treatment. Gradually, VATS is becoming the norm for the management of spontaneous pneumothorax; and in centers where large numbers of VATS are performed, recurrence rates are similar to the results obtained by traditional open surgery. Excellent visualization and improved instrumentation allow precise and complete surgical resection of the offending pathology, and the patient is returned rapidly to normal activity. As is true in all surgical procedures, sound judgment is required for complex cases in which a more extensive procedure or open approach may be advisable.

References

1. Almind M, Lange P, Viskum K: Spontaneous pneumothorax: Comparison of simple drainage, talc pleurodesis, and tetracycline pleurodesis. Thorax 44:627–630, 1989.
2. Bertrand PC, Regnard JF, Spaggiari L, et al: Immediate and long-term results after surgical treatment of primary spontaneous pneumothorax by VATS. Ann Thorac Surg 61:1641–1645, 1996.
3. Bouchama A, Chastre J, Gaudichel A, et al: Acute pneumonitis with bilateral pleural effusion after talc pleurodesis. Chest 86:795–797, 1984.
4. Boutin C: Thoracoscopy in the diagnosis and treatment of spontaneous pneumothorax. *In* Boutin C, Viallat JR, Aelony Y (eds): Practical Thoracoscopy, 1st ed. Berlin, Springer, 1990, pp 73–81.
5. Bresticker MA, Oba J, LoCicero J III, et al: Optimal pleurodesis: A comparison study. Ann Thorac Surg 55:364–367, 1993.
6. Cole FH, Khandekar A, Maxwell JM: Video-assisted thoracic surgery: Primary therapy for spontaneous pneumothorax? Ann Thorac Surg 60:931–935, 1995.
7. Deslauriers J, Beanlieu M, Despres JP, et al: Transaxillary pleurectomy for treatment of spontaneous pneumothorax. Ann Thorac Surg 30:569–574, 1980.
8. Fleisher AG, McElvaney G, Lawson L, et al: Surgical management of spontaneous pneumothorax in patients with acquired immunodeficiency syndrome. Ann Thorac Surg 45:21–23, 1988.
9. Gerein AN, Brumwell ML, Lawson LM, et al: Surgical management of pneumothorax in patients with acquired immunodeficiency syndrome. Arch Surg 126:1272–1277, 1991.
10. Getz SB Jr, Beasley WE III: Spontaneous pneumothorax. Am J Surg 145:823–827, 1983.
11. Gobbel WG Jr, Rhea WG Jr, Nelson IA, et al: Spontaneous pneumothorax. J Thorac Cardiovasc Surg 46:331–345, 1963.
12. Granke K, Fischer CR, Gago O, et al: The efficiency and timing of operative intervention for spontaneous pneumothorax. Ann Thorac Surg 42:540–542, 1986.
13. Hazelrigg SR: Thoracoscopic management of pulmonary blebs and bullae. Semin Thorac Cardiovasc Surg 5:327–331, 1993.
14. Hazelrigg SR, Boley TM, Naunheim KS, et al: Effect of bovine pericardial strips on air leak after stapled pulmonary resection. Ann Thorac Surg 63:1573–1575, 1997.
15. Hazelrigg SR, Landreneau RJ, Mack M, et al: Thoracoscopic stapled resection for spontaneous pneumothorax. J Thorac Cardiovasc Surg 105:389–393, 1993.
16. Hazelrigg SR, Nunchuck SK, Landreneau RJ, et al: Cost analysis for thoracoscopy: Thoracoscopic wedge resection. Ann Thorac Surg 56:633–635, 1993.
17. Hepper NGG, Melton LJ, Okford K: Incidence of spontaneous pneumothorax in Olmsted County, Minnesota, 1950–75. Am Rev Respir Dis 120:1379–1382, 1979.
18. Hopkirk JAC, Pullen MJ, Fraser JR: Pleurodesis: The results of treatment for spontaneous pneumothorax in the Royal Air Force. Aviat Space Environ Med 54:158–160, 1983.
19. Inderbitzi RGC, Furrer M, Striffeler H: Thoracoscopic pleurectomy for treatment of complicated spontaneous pneumothorax. J Thorac Cardiovasc Surg 105:84–88, 1993.
20. Landreneau RJ, Mack MJ, Hazelrigg SR, et al: Video-assisted thoracic surgery: Basic technical concepts and intercostal approach strategies. Ann Thorac Surg 54:800–807, 1992.
21. Landreneau RJ, Mack MJ, Hazelrigg SR, et al: Prevalence of chronic pain after pulmonary resection by thoracotomy or video-assisted thoracic surgery. J Thorac Cardiovasc Surg 107:1079–1086, 1994.
22. Lange P, Mortensen J, Groth S: Lung function 22–35 years after treatment of idiopathic spontaneous pneumothorax with talc poudrage or simple drainage. Thorax 43:559–561, 1988.
23. Liu HP, Lin PJ, Hsieh MJ, et al: Thoracoscopic surgery as a routine procedure for spontaneous pneumothorax. Results from 82 patients. Chest 107:559–562, 1995.
24. Nathanson LK, Shimi SM, Wood RAB, et al: Videothoracoscopic ligation of bulla and pleurectomy for spontaneous pneumothorax. Ann Thorac Surg 52:316–319, 1991.
25. Naunheim KS, Mack MJ, Hazelrigg SR, et al: Safety and efficacy of video-assisted thoracic surgical techniques for the treatment of spontaneous pneumothorax. J Thorac Cardiovasc Surg 109:1198–1203, 1995.
26. Passlick B, Born C, Häussinger K, et al: Efficiency of video-assisted thoracic surgery for primary and secondary spontaneous pneumothorax. Ann Thorac Surg 65:324–327, 1998.
27. Rinaldo JE, Owens GR, Rogers RM: Adult respiratory distress syndrome following intrapleural instillation of talc. J Thorac Cardiovasc Surg 85:523–526, 1983.
28. Saha SP, Arrants JE, Kosa A, et al: Management of spontaneous pneumothorax. Ann Thorac Surg 19:561–564, 1975.
29. Seremetis MG: The management of spontaneous pneumothorax. Chest 57:65–68, 1970.
30. Singh SV: The surgical treatment of spontaneous pneumothorax by parietal pleurectomy. Scand J Thorac Cardiovasc Surg 16:75–80, 1982.
31. Tanaka F, Itoh M, Esaki H, et al: Secondary spontaneous pneumothorax. Ann Thorac Surg 55:372–376, 1993.
32. Waller DA, Forty J, Morritt GN: Video-assisted thoracoscopic surgery versus thoracotomy for spontaneous pneumothorax. Ann Thorac Surg 58:372–376, 1994.
33. Weeden D, Smith GH: Surgical experience in the management of spontaneous pneumothorax 1972–82. Thorax 38:737–743, 1983.
34. Yim APC, Ho JK, Chung SS, et al: Video-assisted thoracoscopic surgery for primary spontaneous pneumothorax. Aust NZ J Surg 64:667–670, 1994.
35. Yim APC, Ho JKS, Lai CKW, et al: Primary spontaneous pneumothorax treated by video assisted thoracoscopic surgery—results of intermediate follow up. Aust NZ J Med 25:146–150, 1995.
36. Yim APC: Video assisted thoracoscopic suturing of apical bullae—an alternative to staple resection in the management of primary spontaneous pneumothorax. Surg Endosc 9:1013–1016, 1995.
37. Yim APC, Lin HP: Video-assisted thoracoscopic management of primary spontaneous pneumothorax. Surg Laparosc Endosc 7:236–240, 1997.
38. Youmans CR Jr, Williams RD, McMinn MR, et al: Surgical management of spontaneous pneumothorax by bleb ligation and pleural dry sponge abrasion. Am J Surg 120:644–648, 1970.

COMMENTARY

Anthony P. C. Yim

Video-assisted thoracic surgery (VATS) is quickly becoming the approach of choice for the surgical treatment of primary spontaneous pneumothorax (PSP) even though the timing of surgery and the optimal technique remain areas of contention. It is important to note that previous surgical algorithms were developed based on the morbidity of the thoracotomy. With the greatly reduced morbidity of VATS, such older protocols need to be re-evaluated. As a result of reduced morbidity, we have seen that many surgeons who are practicing VATS are willing to recommend earlier surgical intervention than in the past. Many centers now recommend VATS to patients with a first-time recurrence or an air leak that persists for more than 3 days. Cost of the consumables continues to be an important issue, especially for developing countries. We encourage surgeons to use conventional surgical instruments whenever possible. Alternative techniques to staple-resection the apical bullae (e.g., endoloop and endoscopic suturing) were developed.

Although VATS is applicable to almost all cases of PSP, careful clinical judgment is required to select patients for surgery who have secondary spontaneous pneumothorax, as pointed out by the authors. Nonoperative approaches (e.g., talc pleurodesis given as a slurry) should be considered for elderly patients who have comorbidities when full lung re-expansion could be achieved by tube thoracostomy with or without suction.

Chapter 12

Interstitial Lung Diseases

Mark S. Allen

Diffuse interstitial diseases of the lung comprise a diverse group of diseases (Table 12–1).[1] The thoracic surgeon's role is to obtain a sample of lung tissue from the patient so that an exact diagnosis can be achieved. Before the advent of thoracoscopic biopsy, tissue was obtained by a small anterior or axillary thoracotomy. Although these incisions are less morbid than a standard posterior lateral thoracotomy, they still cause a fair amount of disability and discomfort. Since the early 1990s, video-assisted thoracic surgical techniques (VATS) have allowed the thoracic surgeon to obtain a significant sample of lung parenchyma for analysis through small incisions in the chest wall. This has reduced the morbidity of an open lung biopsy. This technical improvement has increased the willingness of referring physicians to send patients with interstitial lung disease for lung biopsy.

Patient Selection

As with any operative procedure, patient selection is important. VATS is ideal for the ambulatory patient who has diffuse lung disease. The procedure can be done quickly, safely, and with minimal morbidity. The hospitalization is usually no more than 2 or 3 days. Normal activity or work can be resumed about 1 week after surgery, and appropriate therapy to correct the underlying disease can be started immediately after the diagnosis is reached. VATS is useful for obtaining tissue from any area of the lung; thus, the location of the lesions is not critical. However, the size of the lesions is sometimes an important factor when deciding whether or not to use VATS. If the lesions are nodular they can be too large to remove through the relatively small incisions used for VATS; moreover, it is sometimes difficult to remove a portion of a large nodular infiltrate using current VATS techniques. Another class of patients who may be problematic VATS candidates are those who have a dense infiltrate.

Complications and Contraindications

In these patients, the lung is sometimes hepatized, and application of the stapling devices may tear the lung with resultant bleeding or a large air leak. This is difficult to predict preoperatively; therefore, the procedure can begin with the intention of obtaining the biopsy using VATS, but if problems arise, the chest can be opened wider, the tear or air leak repaired, and the biopsy obtained via an open technique.

Patients who are intubated are questionable candidates for VATS biopsy, because they need reintubation with a double-lumen tube or placement of a bronchial blocker. Excessive manipulations by anesthesia may unnecessarily complicate an otherwise relatively simple open lung biopsy. In addition, intubated patients cannot leave the hospital shortly after an open lung biopsy, because, if their lung disease is serious enough to require intubation, they will likely need in-hospital care for an extended period. Thus, the benefits of early discharge after a VATS biopsy could not be realized for intubated patients. Therefore, for a number of reasons, VATS biopsy of the intubated patient is usually not indicated. However, it could be argued that the reduced morbidity of a VATS biopsy may help with the weaning process postoperatively and may reduce the fluid shifts that occur with a larger incision, but this hypothesis has never been tested, let alone proven.

Patients who need a lung biopsy are often immunosuppressed, but this is not a contraindication for VATS. However, patients with a coagulopathy are at higher risk with VATS. This is not an absolute contraindication, but liberal use of electrocautery should be employed in these patients. VATS is not useful for the patient with a fused pleural space. However, this cannot usually be determined preoperatively, so VATS can be started, and, if an obliterated pleural space is encountered, the procedure can be converted and the biopsy obtained through a small muscle-sparing incision.

Preoperative Testing

Preoperatively, the patient should have a lesion to biopsy that has been located by radiograph. Computed tomography (CT) of the chest is preferable but not absolutely necessary.[2] It can be omitted to reduce costs. The CT is useful to plan a specific area of biopsy and to choose a side on which to operate. If both lungs are equally involved, the right side has a theoretical advantage, because it has an additional fissure, so there are more edges to grasp and biopsy. The area to be biopsied should ideally contain normal and abnormal tissue. Sampling an area of the lung that is severely diseased may yield only fibrotic tissue and not a true representation of the pathologic process. At least two biopsies should be taken, ideally from separate areas to reduce the risk of sampling error.

After a specimen is obtained, it should be divided sterilely, a portion sent for culture, and the remainder reserved for pathologic examination. The tissue should be cultured for plausible pathogens but not for "everything," because this is expensive and unnecessary. If possible, the pathologist should be told the history and shown the radiologic examinations to help narrow the diagnostic possibilities. This also allows the pathologist to save some tissue for special handling, such as freezing or special stains.

Table 12–1. Etiology of Diffuse Lung Diseases

Adult respiratory distress syndrome
Connective tissue diseases
Eosinophilia
Hemorrhage
Histiocytosis X
Idiopathic (e.g., interstitial pulmonary fibrosis)
Infection
Neoplasm
Occupational/hypersensitivity
Protein
Pulmonary edema
Pulmonary embolism
Sarcoid

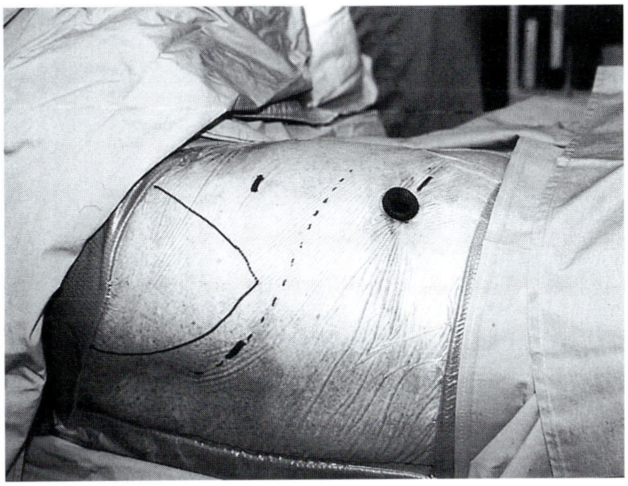

Figure 12–2. The lung has been deflated, and a metal trocar is placed into the chest wall. A black cylinder is slid over the trocar and left in place to allow the camera to go into the chest cavity without smearing the lens.

VATS in Interstitial Lung Disease

The technique of VATS for diffuse interstitial lung disease is similar to VATS for other pathologies in the lung.[3–5] Single-lung ventilation is usually necessary to collapse the lung and secure enough room to work in the pleural space. A double-lumen tube or a bronchial blocker can be used to isolate one lung. Rarely, both lungs can be ventilated with reduced tidal volume and enough space is available for a simple biopsy, but this is usually less than optimal. The patient is monitored with an arterial line, O_2 saturation probe, electrocardiograph (ECG), and CO_2 mass spectrometry. After general anesthesia is induced, the patient is placed in the lateral decubitus position. Biopsies can be performed under local anesthesia, but general anesthesia is more comfortable for the surgeon and the patient; furthermore, if local anesthesia is used, it is awkward to convert to an open procedure if necessary.

An initial incision is made in the midaxillary line to enter the chest just above the diaphragm. This is usually at the eighth interspace but can be higher if the diaphragm is elevated (Fig. 12–1). The pleural space is entered with a cautery, and a metal trocar is placed in the incision so the thoracoscope can be introduced without smearing the lens (Fig. 12–2). One lung is deflated; CO_2 is not required to deflate the lung. The pleural space is examined, and preliminary suitable sites for biopsies are determined. Two additional incisions, each about 1 cm long, are made. These incisions are superior to the initial incision; one is placed in the anterior and the other in the posterior axillary lines. The anterior incision can be made slightly larger, because the intercostal space is wider anteriorly than posteriorly, and the anterior incision is used to remove the specimens. By inserting lung clamps through the anterior

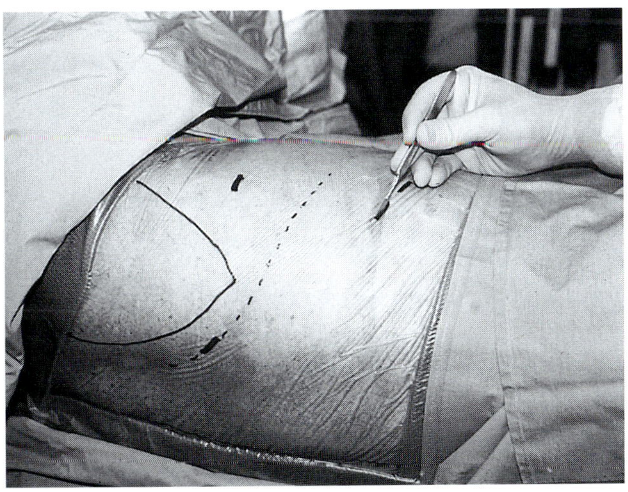

Figure 12–1. The patient is under general anesthesia, in the left lateral decubitus position, and an incision is made in the mid axillary line over the eighth rib.

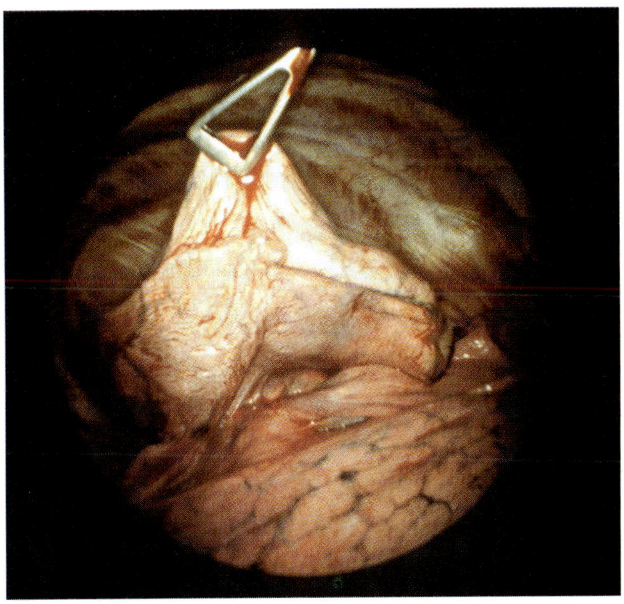

Figure 12–3. A lung clamp grasps the lung and positions it for examination to determine the ideal spot for a biopsy. No special tools are required for a VATS lung biopsy.

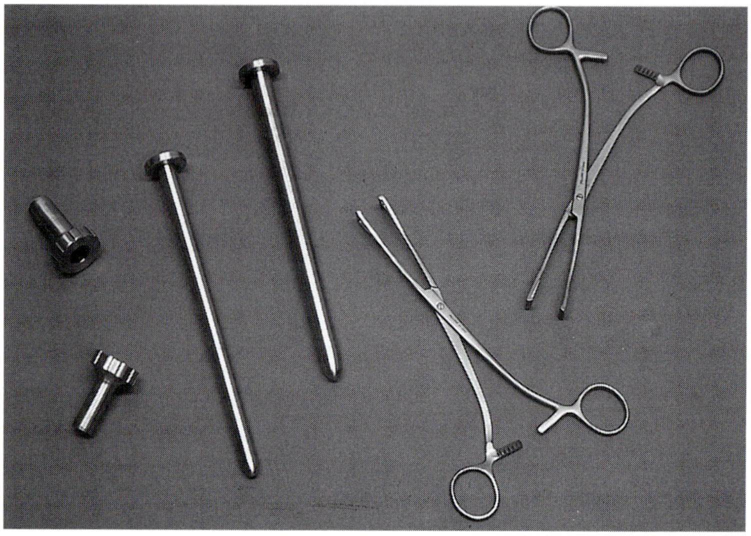

Figure 12–4. Photo of the reusable metal trocar, sleeves, and lung clamps used for VATS lung biopsy.

and posterior incisions, the lung can be manipulated and carefully examined to determine the best area for a biopsy (Figs. 12–3 and 12–4). As mentioned previously, the ideal area is one that has both normal and abnormal tissue present.

Once the site has been determined, one lung clamp is used to grasp the tissue and the stapler is introduced to cut the lung (Figs. 12–5 to 12–7). Usually the stapler has to be applied from each side to form a V-wedge excision. If the stapler is applied repeatedly from one incision, the edge of the lung is shaved off, and a long narrow sample is removed. This is referred to as the "banana peel effect," because the resection is like peeling a banana. By applying the stapler from two different incisions (i.e., different angles), less of the lung has to be resected and fewer staple cartridges are used (Fig. 12–8). After the specimen is resected, it is brought out through the anterior incision and sent for culture and pathologic examination as previously described.

When all the biopsies have been performed, each staple line is examined for hemostasis and dryness, and a chest tube is inserted through the inferior incision and passed to the apex of the chest. A tract separate from that of the thoracoscope is made for the chest tube, so when the tube is removed, air is not sucked into the chest. The thoracoscope is used to visualize the tube position and to ensure the lung is properly reinflated. The deep strata of the incisions are closed in layers, and the skin is approximated with a subcuticular stitch (Figs. 12–9 and 12–10). The chest tube is placed to 20-cm suction overnight and the waterseal is placed the next day. If there is no air leak and the drainage is less than 300 ml per 24 hours, the tube is removed and the patient is discharged from the hospital, usually on the second postoperative day.

VATS Patient Data

In the 2-year period from July 1994 to July 1996, we performed open lung biopsy on 121 patients at the Mayo Clinic using VATS.[4] The median age was 62 years (with a

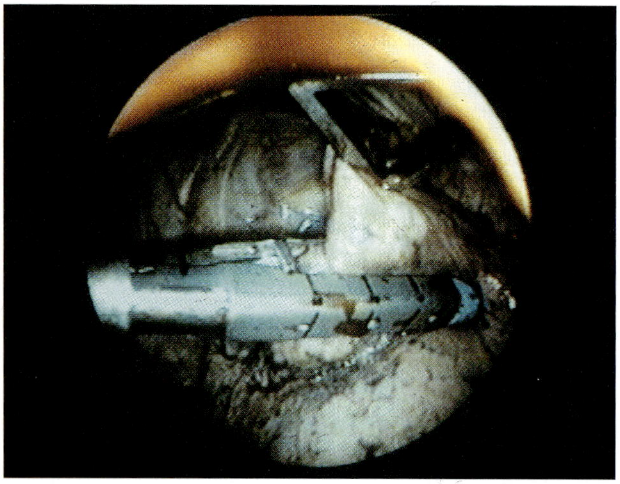

Figure 12–5. The stapler is applied from the posterior incision to begin the biopsy.

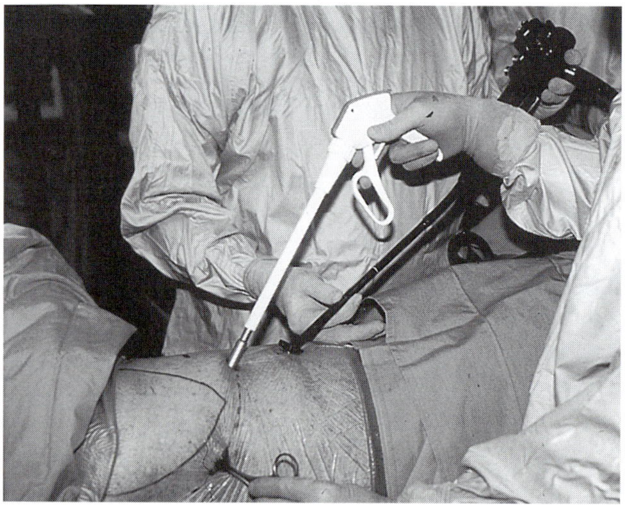

Figure 12–6. The second firing of the stapler is from the anterior incision to complete the "V" wedge excision.

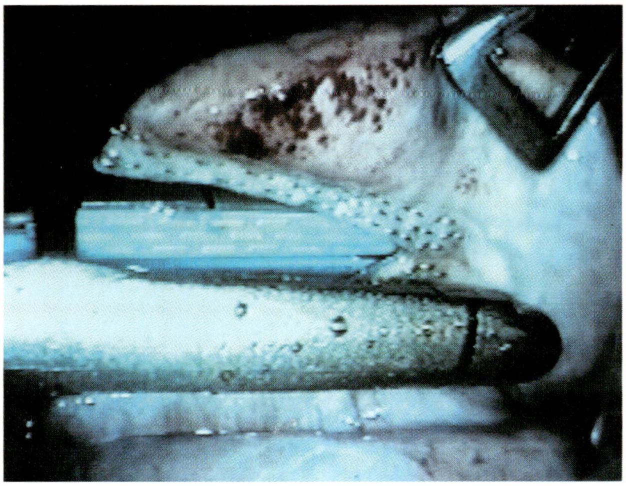

Figure 12–7. Close-up view of application of the stapler on the lung.

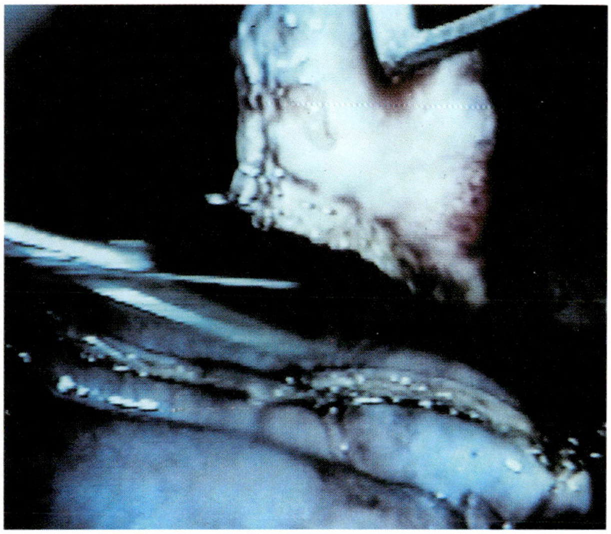

Figure 12–8. The biopsy has been completed and will be brought out through the anterior incision and sent for culture and pathologic examination.

range of 22 to 80 years), and the gender distribution was 72 men and 49 women. The reasons these patients underwent VATS approach as opposed to small thoracotomy varied among surgeons, but, in general, ambulatory patients, patients who had disease on the surface of the lung, and those who had normal coagulation underwent VATS. The technique used was as described previously: general anesthesia, double-lumen tube, no CO_2 insufflation, several biopsies, and a single chest tube.

Conversion to an open procedure was required in 14 (11.6%) patients. The reasons for conversion were an obliterated pleural space, bleeding, unconfirmed pathology, stapler malfunction, and the necessity of performing a complete resection of a diseased lung. Operative mortality was 6%, which is common in a group of patients who have severe lung disease. Complications occurred in 12% of patients and included prolonged air leak, respiratory failure requiring prolonged intubation, bleeding, and pneumothorax. Pathology included interstitial fibrosis or pneumonia in 82, sarcoidosis in 17, histiocytosis X in 6, tuberculosis in 6, vasculitis in 3, Wegener's granulomatosis in 2, and other causes in 5.

In summary, VATS for diffuse lung disease is a new technique that has the potential to provide an accurate diagnosis with reduced morbidity.[6] It should be done with careful attention to detail and cannot be used in all patients. The procedure should have similar morbidity and mortality to its open counterpart, and the diagnostic accuracy should be the same. As technology advances, morbidity and the cost of the procedure should fall, allowing an easier method for obtaining a diagnosis in this group of patients.

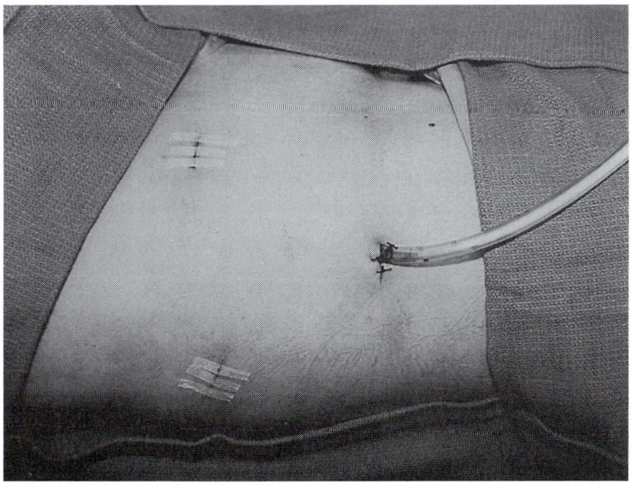

Figure 12–9. A single chest tube is in place, and the remaining incisions have been closed.

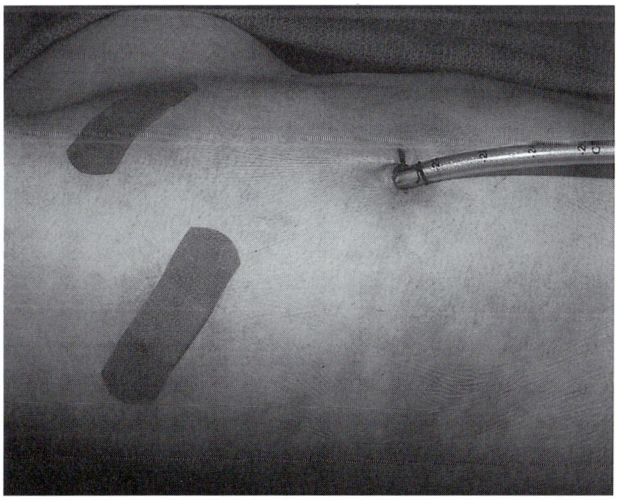

Figure 12–10. "Bandaids" are placed on the superior incision, and an occlusive dressing will be placed on the chest tube site.

References

1. Thurlbeck WM, Miller RR, Möller NL, et al (eds): Diffuse Disease of the Lung. A Team Approach, Philadelphia, BC Decker, 1991, p 19.
2. Krasna MJ, White CS, Aisner SC, et al: The role of thoracoscopy in the diagnosis of interstitial lung disease. Ann Thorac Surg 59:348–351, 1995.
3. Liu HP, Chang CH, Lin PJ, et al: Video-assisted thoracic surgery. The Chang Gung experience. J Thorac Cardiovasc Surg 108: 834–840, 1994.
4. Allen MS, Deschamps C, Jones DM, et al: Video-assisted thoracic surgical procedures: The Mayo experience. Mayo Clin Proc 71:351–359, 1996.
5. Allen MS, Deschamps C, Lee RE, et al: Video-assisted thoracoscopic stapled wedge excision for indeterminate pulmonary nodules. J Thorac Cardiovasc Surg 106:1048–1052, 1993.
6. Ferson PF, Landreneau RJ, Dowling RD, et al: Comparison of open versus thoracoscopic lung biopsy for diffuse infiltrative pulmonary disease. J Thorac Cardiovasc Surg 106:194–199, 1993.

Chapter 13

Lung Volume Reduction for End-Stage Emphysema

Keith S. Naunheim and Cesar A. Keller

Emphysema is a progressive disabling disease that affects almost 2 million people in the United States. Because of increasing tobacco use throughout the world, emphysema is likely to continue to be a major health problem in the coming millennium. Standard therapy for emphysema can help eliminate symptoms, but, unfortunately, it has a limited impact on the quality of life and survival of the patient. The concept of surgical treatment for emphysema is not new. Throughout the early and mid-1900s, multiple procedures were proposed to alleviate the symptoms of this chronic obstructive disease, including costochondrectomy, thoracoplasty with phrenic nerve paralysis, parietal pleurectomy, and tracheal stenting with bone grafts. Unfortunately, the results of these procedures were dismal, and they were rapidly abandoned.

In 1959, Brantigan and colleagues reported yet another surgical approach for emphysema.[1] This entailed multiple small resections that reduced the overall size of the lung. They believed that the remaining lung would re-expand to fill the enlarged chest cavity and in so doing help prevent early collapse of the terminal airways, a physiologic result of chronic obstructive disease. This operation was reintroduced by Cooper and colleagues in 1995 via a median sternotomy approach.[2] Shortly thereafter, proponents of minimally invasive thoracic surgery used a thoracoscopic approach to perform lung volume reduction in selected patients.[3–5] This chapter reviews the operative rationale, the indications for surgery, the preoperative workup and preparation, the surgical techniques, and the results of lung volume reduction surgery.

Operative Rationale

Emphysema is caused by a chronic inflammatory process within the lung parenchyma, which results in destruction of the alveolar walls and abnormal permanent enlargement of the air spaces distal to the terminal bronchioles. The parenchymal destruction leads to a decrease in the circumferential "tethering" effect by the normal lung parenchyma on the terminal bronchioles. It is this radial tethering that tends to hold small airways open throughout the expiratory cycle until a balance is achieved between the chest wall and lung elastic recoil forces at end expiration. The combination of a lessened alveolar driving force (secondary to alveolar destruction) and lessened tethering leads to early closure of small airways during expiration. This results in poor expiratory flow and hyperinflated lungs. Gas is trapped within the lung, which limits inspiratory capacity and impairs maximal breathing capacity, as evidenced by very low maximal voluntary ventilation indices. The rationale behind lung volume reduction (LVR) is that decreasing the amount of lung within the fixed chest cavity results in improved cardiopulmonary physiology. Ablation or resection of the most diseased portion of emphysematous lung limits the detrimental effect of resection and, in theory, maximizes the beneficial effects. The ideal patient is believed to be one in whom clear target zones appear on the ventilation and perfusion scans. Such zones are characterized by markedly decreased perfusion limited to a single region in both lungs (Fig. 13–1). Ideally, this regional hypoperfusion correlates with the site of gas retention on the ventilation scan. It is important to note that the remainder of the lungs should demonstrate relatively good perfusion if the patient is to be considered an optimal candidate. Hypoperfusion not limited to a single region of the lung (i.e., homogeneous or diffuse changes) was once thought to be a contraindication to LVR. However, investigators have performed operations on such patients and found that beneficial effects still occur from a volume reduction procedure, although they appear to be less than those found in the optimal patient with heterogeneous disease.[6]

The purpose of LVR is to resect the dysfunctional target zones and thus reduce the amount of trapped gas within the lungs. There are at least four mechanisms reported to be responsible for the respiratory improvement that occurs following LVR. It is important to remember that all these physiologic mechanisms are interrelated and may affect one another.

1. *Elastic recoil.* It was Brantigan's original theory that partial lung resection would result in expansion of the residual lung tissue to fill the thoracic cage, thus reinstituting the radial or circumferential tethering on the small airways. This would secondarily decrease airway resistance and cause some resolution of lung hyperinflation. Reports by Sciurba, Barnas, and Gelb and their associates documented improvements in elastic recoil and expiratory airway resistance.[7–9]
2. *Ventilation/perfusion mismatch.* The retention of expired gas in areas of decreased perfusion (characterized as the so-called target zone) may lead to elevated systemic levels of carbon dioxide. Such dilated, hyperinflated regions may lead to atelectasis of adjacent areas of less diseased lung, resulting in perfused but hypoventilated lung. This condition results in shunting and systemic hypoxia. Resection of this sort of dysfunctional lung could lead to improvements in hypoxia and hypercarbia by removing areas with the worst ventilation/perfusion mismatch.
3. *Respiratory musculature.* The hyperinflation that results from emphysema leads to severe distention of

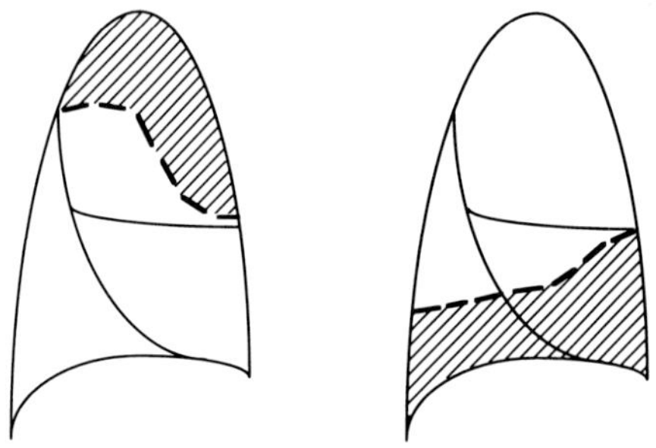

Figure 13–1. Extent and site of resection for patients with emphysema located predominantly in the apex (left) or basilar (right) areas of the lung.

the chest cage with marked diaphragmatic flattening and stretching. Both the intercostal musculature and the diaphragm have an optimal length at which maximal tension is developed. Distention of the chest and flattening of the diaphragm result in decreased efficiency and strength in the respiratory musculature in patients with emphysema. Resection of dysfunctional lung leads to reduced volume of the lung and allows the distended chest cage to return to a more normal diameter. The diaphragm also returns to its usual dome shape, thus improving the efficiency of the respiratory pump. Recent studies documented improved ventilatory mechanics and diaphragmatic function following LVR.[10, 11]

4. *Cardiovascular hemodynamics.* It has been suggested that LVR may have some beneficial effects on the right heart volume by virtue of the recruitment of hypoperfused pulmonary artery capillaries after expansion of atelectatic lung. In addition, it is recognized that patients with end-stage emphysema who suffer "auto PEEP" (positive end expiratory pressure) may deteriorate acutely when placed on mechanical ventilatory support owing to the phenomenon of air trapping that results in a form of pulmonary tamponade. Markedly elevated intrathoracic pressures can decrease systemic venous return, with disastrous consequences. This concept of impaired hemodynamics due to variations in intrathoracic pressure has been championed by Dahan and colleagues.[12]

Indications

Those patients believed to benefit most from LVR are those with "pure" emphysema unadulterated by other forms of chronic lung disease. Such patients are characterized by severe respiratory functional impairment, which usually corresponds to grade 3 or 4 (out of 4) on the modified Medical Research Council Dyspnea Scale. Clinical or radiographic signs of chronic bronchitis, bronchiectasis, and a significant component of reversible airway disease are felt to be relative contraindications to surgical intervention for emphysema. Processes that are likely to result in significant pleural adhesions greatly complicate the performance of LVR surgery. Taking down extensive adhesions can lead to multiple visceral pleural defects with large air leaks that may be uncontrollable by any means other than resection. Thus a history of extensive empyema, decortication, pleurodesis, or previous major thoracotomy is considered a contraindication to LVR surgery.

Preoperative Workup

The initial portion of the investigation is, of course, the initial history and physical examination. A clinical history that might contraindicate an LVR operation (see earlier) should be sought, along with physical findings confirmatory of end-stage emphysema (barrel chest, hyperinflated lungs, intercostal muscle retraction, use of accessory musculature). The remaining workup is generally divided into cardiopulmonary imaging studies and tests to measure functional status.

The pulmonary imaging studies consist of high-resolution computed tomography (CT) of the chest to define the structural changes associated with emphysema. This has also been helpful to rule out the presence of occult pulmonary nodules, which appear in as many as 11% of patients presenting for assessment.[13, 14] Most institutions include a quantitative ventilation/perfusion scan to assess regional differences in perfusion and ventilation within the lung fields. The ideal target area is one that shows a heterogeneous pattern with decreased or absent blood perfusion associated with decreased early ventilation and evidence of delayed air trapping. Ideally, the remainder of the lung away from this target area should demonstrate relatively good perfusion (see Fig. 13–1). This underventilated and hypoperfused target area is usually located in the area of most severe parenchymal destruction demonstrated in the CT scan. Although patients with more homogeneous or diffuse disease have been demonstrated to attain some benefit from LVR, most investigators believe that the patients with heterogeneous disease are better candidates.[2, 6, 15]

The patient's cardiac status is evaluated with Doppler echocardiography to assess both left- and right-sided cardiac function. Assessment of regional wall motion and valvular function helps rule out a cardiac cause for dyspnea. Examination of the right side of the heart is undertaken to identify changes that might indicate significant elevation of pulmonary artery pressures (valvular regurgitation, ventricular hypertrophy, or dilatation). If pulmonary hypertension is suspected, catheterization of the right side of the heart is performed to confirm or refute this suspicion. Evidence of segmental wall motion abnormalities suggestive of ischemia warrant further workup with a nuclear imaged stress test or catheterization, because 15% of this population demonstrates occult coronary artery disease.[16]

The physiologic parameters measured include spirometry, measurement of lung volume with plethysmography, and measurement of diffusion capacity. A 6-minute walking test has been used for many years in the assessment of functional status after lung transplantation and is commonly used in lung reduction candidates before and after surgery to assess functional improvement. Formal cardiopulmonary exercise evaluation may be performed, using a bicycle ergometer with measurement of exhaled ventilatory variables and arterial blood gases.[17]

Once formal testing has been completed, the decision whether to proceed with LVR is made using the following inclusion and exclusion criteria. Inclusion criteria include:

1. Diagnosis of end-stage emphysema
2. Disabling dyspnea (Modified Medical Research Council dyspnea grade 3 or 4)
3. Postbronchodilator forced expired volume in 1 second (FEV_1) less 35% predicted
4. Residual volume (plethysmography) greater than 200% predicted
5. Total lung capacity (plethysmography) greater than 120% predicted
6. Hyperinflated lungs on chest radiography
7. Regional heterogeneity perfusion on radionuclide lung scan
8. Ability to participate in a course of preoperative pulmonary rehabilitation

Exclusions criteria include:

1. Age older than 80 years
2. Any tobacco use (inhaled or oral) within 6 months
3. Pulmonary artery hypertension (systolic >45 mm Hg, mean >35 mm Hg)
4. Resting carbon dioxide tension greater than 55 mm Hg
5. Irreversible obesity (>1.25 ideal body weight) or cachexia (<0.75 ideal body weight)
6. Unstable coronary artery disease
7. Other life-limiting medical disease (e.g., uncontrollable malignancy, severe congestive heart failure, cirrhosis)
8. Ventilator dependence
9. Chronic bronchitis, bronchiectasis, asthma
10. History of pleurodesis, empyema, prior thoracotomy

Preoperative Preparation

Once a patient is accepted as a candidate, optimization of medical management is undertaken. Maximal medical therapy includes smoking abstinence, bronchodilators, antibiotics when indicated, and oxygen therapy for those with significant hypoxemia. Many patients are receiving significant steroid dosages, and the goal is to wean them off oral steroids before surgery if at all possible. Inhaled steroids can be helpful in this maneuver. All patients participate in a monitored pulmonary rehabilitation program, which includes attention to proper breathing exercises, pulmonary toilet, upper body strengthening, nutritional repletion, and overall conditioning using a treadmill or stationary bike. The eventual goal of conditioning is 30 minutes of uninterrupted exercise on the treadmill or bicycle. During exercise, supplemental oxygen is administered at whatever level necessary to maintain an arterial oxygen saturation of 90% or greater. A detailed description of optimal preoperative preparation is available elsewhere.[18]

Operative Procedure

The procedure begins with placement of an arterial line, peripheral intravenous line, central venous access, and urinary catheter. Pulmonary artery catheters with oximetric capability are not used routinely but are used selectively in those patients in whom borderline pulmonary hypertension is diagnosed or suspected. Exhaled gas capnography and pulse oximetry are constantly monitored. A left-sided double-lumen tube is placed, and its position is confirmed bronchoscopically. A thorough discussion of the anesthetic management is beyond the scope of this chapter but has been covered in detail elsewhere.[19]

The operation is performed either unilaterally or bilaterally. Initially, thoracoscopic lung reduction was performed only as a unilateral procedure owing to the uncertainty regarding its efficacy. However, within 2 years of its inception, reports had appeared demonstrating significant improvement in spirometric, functional, and oxygenation indices,[3–5] and practitioners progressed toward the simultaneous bilateral thoracoscopic procedure.[20–22]

There are two different thoracoscopic approaches being used for bilateral LVR. In one of these, a supine position is assumed by the patient, and the arms are extended at the shoulders upward toward the head. The elbows are crooked at 90 degrees, and the arms are supported in this position, thus exposing the upper chest and axillary areas bilaterally. Incisions for trocar sites are made in the fifth intercostal space in the submammary position, in the sixth intercostal space in the anterior axillary line, and in the third intercostal space in the midaxillary line. The chest is entered bluntly, and adhesions are carefully felt for. The lung is collapsed, and carbon dioxide insufflation can be used to help speed collapse of the lung. The zero-degree thoracoscope is placed through the anterior axillary trocar site, and instruments are placed at the midaxillary and submammary sites. Any adhesions are taken down by sharp or cautery dissection, and the lobe to be resected is identified. This is an excellent approach for upper lobe disease, and the goal is to resect approximately half the upper lobe so that 20 to 30% of the lung volume is resected on a given side. A grasper or ring forceps is placed through the axillary site to lift the lung, and an endoscopic stapling device is placed through the submammary incision. The staples are routinely buttressed with either expanded polytetrafluoroethylene (PTFE) or gluteraldehyde-fixed bovine pericardium. Sequential firings are made beginning anteriorly on the upper lobe and extending in a "hockey stick" or "horseshoe" fashion through the apical segment of the upper lobe. A specimen is then withdrawn through the submammary incision where the intercostal space is largest. One or two chest tubes are left positioned in the apex of the chest and exiting through a trocar site. The other trocar site is closed, and the lung is re-expanded. The chest drainage unit is left on underwater seal without suction after the lung is completely re-expanded. Our practice is also to perform an intercostal block throughout the affected ribs using 0.5% bupivacaine with epinephrine. On the contralateral side, the mirror image procedure is performed. Generally, somewhere between 60 and 80 g of lung are resected from either side in a normal-size (70-kg) adult. The chest tubes are left on underwater seal, and a chest radiograph is obtained in the recovery room. Only if there is a significant (greater than 25%) pneumothorax associated with hypoxia are the chest tubes placed to suction.

The second approach is a sequential thoracoscopic LVR performed first on one side and then on the other with the patient in the lateral thoracotomy position. This requires reprepping and redraping in between procedures. For this, we commonly use a fifth intercostal space submammary trocar site, a sixth intercostal space anterior axillary site, and a sixth intercostal space posterior axillary incision. With the patient in the lateral position, this same procedure is performed using a buttressed endoscopic stapler with sequential firings.

For patients in whom the upper lobes are the target areas (Fig. 13–2), either the supine or the lateral thoracotomy position is appropriate. For those in whom the lower lobe is the desired target, a sequential lateral thoracotomy approach appears to be the easiest.

Patients are then extubated either in the operating room or soon thereafter in the recovery room. Immediate postoperative maneuvers to facilitate extubation are covered at length elsewhere.[18, 19]

Postoperative Care and Morbidity

A great effort is made to provide superlative postoperative analgesia so that there is minimal respiratory impairment secondary to pain. In our institution, we use multiple-level intercostal blocks with 0.5% bupivacaine with epinephrine, but many other programs routinely use a thoracic epidural catheter with narcotic infusions. With good analgesia, it is possible and desirable to extubate all patients either in the operating room or shortly thereafter in the recovery room. Just before extubation, we perform a bronchoscopy both to achieve optimal pulmonary toilet and to obtain a microbiologic specimen to allow for accurate selection of antibiotics if an early respiratory infection occurs. Following extubation, the patient spends the first night in the intensive care unit, and respiratory therapy (including nebulization with bronchodilators and percussion with postural drainage) is instituted immediately. The patient is on a broad-spectrum antibiotic for 3 days until the results of the pre-extubation bronchoscopic culture are known. Patients begin physical therapy with ambulation on the first postoperative day, and cathartics are begun early because the vast majority of these patients tend to have intestinal ileus. Chest tubes are left to water seal as long as the lung remains expanded, and the tubes are switched from a chest drainage unit to a Heimlich valve at 3 days if a minor leak is present.

Although the vast majority of published reports suggest that the operative mortality of LVR is between 4 and 10%, it has been suggested that many institutions were performing this operation with markedly higher operative mortality rates, upward of 50%. These are fragile, high-risk patients who require meticulous care postoperatively. The most common complication is a prolonged air leak, which has been described in approximately one third to one half of patients. Although the majority of these leaks prove to be nothing more than a nuisance, a certain percentage of patients will have significant leaks that make it difficult to keep their lungs expanded. Such patients often require some level of suction on their chest tube drainage device, and occasionally the leak is so great that it impairs their ventilatory status. Reoperation for control of prolonged or vigorous air leaks has been required in less than 5% of our patients.

Respiratory infections, including purulent bronchitis and pneumonia, are also very real risks for these patients with significant pulmonary compromise. Virulent pneumonia, though infrequent, may require reintubation and mechanical ventilation, a series of events that may result in the need for tracheostomy and prolonged ventilatory support. It is imperative that optimal respiratory care be maintained throughout the postoperative period, including vigorous bronchodilator therapy, percussion with postural

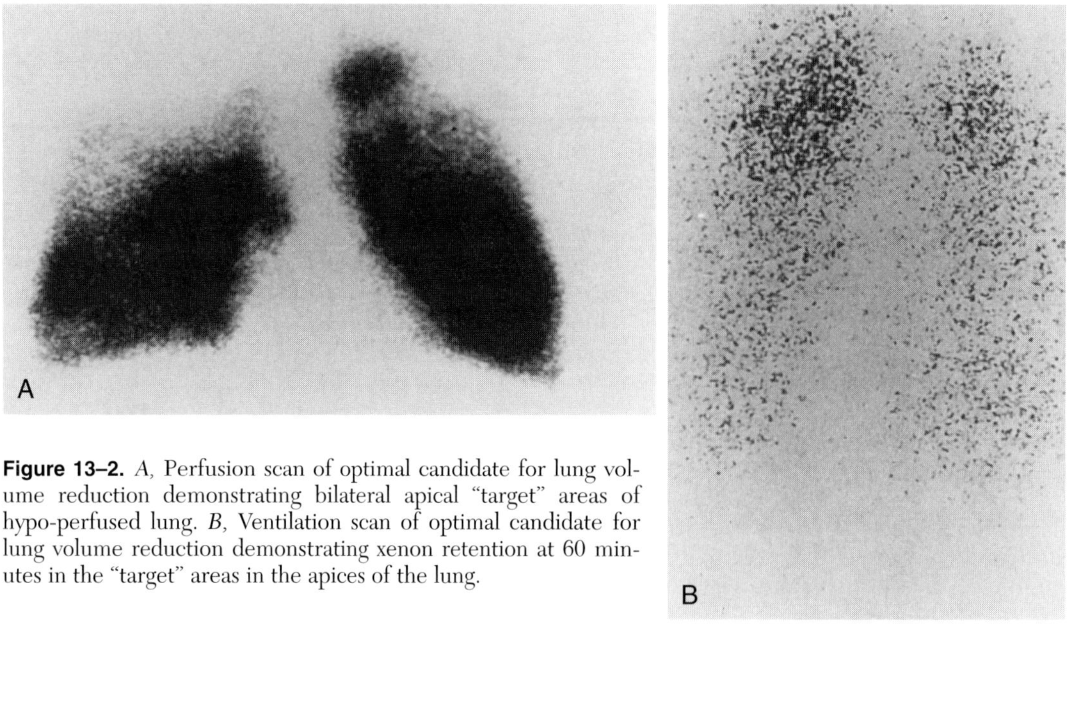

Figure 13–2. *A,* Perfusion scan of optimal candidate for lung volume reduction demonstrating bilateral apical "target" areas of hypo-perfused lung. *B,* Ventilation scan of optimal candidate for lung volume reduction demonstrating xenon retention at 60 minutes in the "target" areas in the apices of the lung.

drainage, and, when necessary, bronchoscopic clearance of the tracheobronchial tree.

Gastrointestinal complications are also a frequent occurrence in this patient subset and have been noted to occur in up to 15% of patients.[17] Gastric ulceration with bleeding, colonic perforation, pancreatitis, prolonged ileus, and ischemic bowel disease requiring surgical intervention have been reported in this patient subset.

Operative Results

Most larger series reporting LVR have suggested that up to 80% of patients have significant improvement with regard to their pulmonary status. These improvements occur in both subjective indices and objective measurements of pulmonary and functional parameters.

Subjective Indices

Many different dyspnea scoring systems have been used to evaluate the effects of LVR on patient dyspnea. Significant improvements in the dyspnea index have been noted by Keller,[17] Stammberger,[23] and Cooper[2] and their coworkers. Similarly, measurements of quality of life pre- and postoperatively also suggest a significant benefit from the LVR procedure.[2, 24] Cordova and colleagues followed the quality-of-life parameters over a 12- to 18-month period and found that the quality of life (as measured by a sickness impact profile) remained improved over that period.[24]

Objective Measurements

Many parameters have been followed in patients undergoing LVR in an attempt to evaluate the efficacy of this procedure. Spirometric indices, particularly FEV_1 and functional vital capacity (FVC), have consistently been demonstrated to improve following LVR, whether performed via median sternotomy or thoracoscopy.[2–5, 25] Although unilateral LVR has been demonstrated to significantly improve these spirometric indices, bilateral LVR has been demonstrated to yield even greater results (Table 13–1) and is currently felt to be indicated in those patients with bilateral disease and no contraindication to operation on either side. Lung volumes as determined by plethysmography have also consistently been shown to improve,[2, 4, 6, 8, 24] suggesting that there is indeed a decrease in the overall intrathoracic volume of trapped gas following the procedure. Postoperative radiographs demonstrating a decrease in the size of the chest cavity with reversal of the radiologic signs of hyperinflation corroborate this finding.

Improved gas exchange has been demonstrated by formal cardiopulmonary exercise testing[17, 23] and by a reduction in oxygen dependence.[4, 20] Finally, functional improvement has consistently been demonstrated whether assessed by 6-minute walk distance[4, 5, 23, 25] or by the more formal cardiopulmonary exercise testing assessing maximal exercise capacity or oxygen consumption.[17, 23, 24]

Controversies

The available literature suggests that LVR provides significant short-term improvement in the respiratory status of carefully selected patients. Although pulmonary rehabilitation alone has been demonstrated to improve dyspnea and functional status to some extent, LVR has been reported to provide a benefit in these areas far out of proportion to that provided by rehabilitation programs. In addition, it significantly improves spirometric indices and gas exchange, two benefits never reported for rehabilitation. However, in the pulmonology community at large, there remain significant doubts regarding the advisability of this procedure for patients with end-stage emphysema. Skeptics point to recognized but unreported examples of excessive operative mortality at some institutions, which caused many hospitals and physicians to back out of this high-risk surgery. The following questions and controversies persist, and it is hoped that the prospective randomized studies ongoing in the United States and Canada will help provide answers:

1. Is there a survival benefit from LVR? It is obvious that there is an initial "penalty" for operative intervention in terms of a 5 to 10% operative mortality that otherwise might not be incurred by this population. Will LVR provide for improved long-term survival at 2, 3, or 5 years?
2. What is the duration of symptomatic improvement? Although several studies have suggested that improvements in dyspnea, quality of life, and spirometric indices last for 1 to 2 years,[9, 25] it is not known whether these improvements will persist long term.

Table 13–1. Results of Unilateral and Bilateral VATS LVR Surgery

Investigator	Approach	FEV_1 Increase (%)	RV Decrease (%)	6-Minute Walk Increase (%)	Preoperative to Postoperative Oxygen Usage (%)
McKenna	Unilateral VATS	33	16	—	69–13
Keenan	Unilateral VATS	27	—	14	80–63
Naunheim	Unilateral VATS	35	33	20	74–40
McKenna	Bilateral VATS	52	—	—	56–18
Bingisser	Bilateral VATS	42	24	39	35–30
Kotloff	Bilateral VATS	34	28	17	—

LVR = lung volume reduction; RV = residual volume; VATS = video-assisted thoracic surgery.

Will this operation be justified if all patients return to their baseline levels within 2 to 3 years?

3. Does LVR reduce medication and hospital use? If so, how is the overall cost affected? Although LVR may decrease medication use and/or hospitalization in the short run, it is highly probable that the remaining emphysematous lung will worsen, and eventually the costs of progressive pulmonary deterioration will be incurred by the LVR patient. Thus, overall costs are merely delayed. However, if LVR provides a significant increase in quality-adjusted life-years of survival at a reasonable cost, this could still be a worthwhile procedure.
4. Who is the optimal candidate? Is there an upper age limit? Are active bronchitis, bronchiectasis, and pulmonary hypertension absolute contraindications? Are some patients too compromised to undergo LVR? Is a heterogeneous pattern absolutely necessary, or will patients with homogeneous perfusion benefit enough to warrant undergoing this procedure?
5. Is the median sternotomy approach better than a thoracoscopic one? Is a video-assisted thoracic surgical (VATS) approach truly minimally invasive, and will it have less morbidity than the open approach? The literature to date is sparse, and the results inconsistent. Whereas the report of Kotloff and associates suggested that the thoracoscopic approach has a significantly lower risk of morbidity and mortality than the sternotomy approach,[26] the paper by Wisser and colleagues reported similar risks and outcomes.[22] Both groups demonstrated that equivalent improvement in respiratory capacity and function occurs following the open and the minimally invasive approach.

LVR is an evolving discipline that provides a potentially beneficial treatment for patients with end-stage emphysema. The answers to the preceding questions will evolve as our understanding of the physiology of this disease progresses, and as the surgical procedure becomes further refined.

References

1. Brantigan OC, Mueller E, Kress MB: A surgical approach to pulmonary emphysema. Am Rev Respir Dis 80:194–206, 1959.
2. Cooper JD, Trulock EP, Triantafillou AN, et al: Bilateral pneumectomy (volume reduction) for chronic obstructive pulmonary disease. J Thorac Cardiovasc Surg 109:106–116, 1995.
3. McKenna RJ Jr, Brenner M, Gelb AF, et al: A randomized, prospective trial of stapled lung reduction versus laser bullectomy for diffuse emphysema. J Thorac Cardiovasc Surg 111:317–321, 1996.
4. Naunheim KS, Keller CA, Krucylak PE, et al: Unilateral video-assisted thoracic surgical lung reduction. Ann Thorac Surg 61:1092–1098, 1996.
5. Keenan RJ, Landreneau RJ, Sciurba FC, et al: Unilateral thoracoscopic surgical approach for diffuse emphysema. J Thorac Cardiovasc Surg 111:308–315, 1996.
6. Weder W, Thurnheer R, Stammberger U, et al: Radiologic emphysema morphology is associated with outcome after surgical lung volume reduction. Ann Thorac Surg 64:313–319, 1997.
7. Sciurba FC, Rogers RM, Keenan RJ, et al: Improvement in pulmonary function and elastic recoil after lung-reduction surgery for diffuse emphysema. N Engl J Med 334:1095–1099, 1996.
8. Barnas GM, Gilbert TB, Krasna MJ, et al: Acute effects of bilateral lung volume reduction surgery on lung and chest wall mechanical properties. Chest 114:61–68, 1998.
9. Gelb AF, Brenner M, McKenna RJ Jr, et al: Serial lung function and elastic recoil 2 years after lung volume reduction surgery for emphysema. Chest 113:1497–1506, 1998.
10. Criner G, Cordova FC, Leyenson V, et al: Effect of lung reduction surgery on diaphragm strength. Am J Respir Crit Care Med 157:1578–1585, 1998.
11. Russi EW, Stammberger U, Weder W: Lung volume reduction surgery for emphysema. Eur Respir J 10:208–218, 1997.
12. Dahan M, Salerin F, Berjaud J, et al: Interet de l'exploration hemodynamique dans les indications chirurgicales des emphysemes. Ann Chir 43:669–672, 1989.
13. Rozenshtein A, White CS, Austin JH, et al: Incidental lung carcinoma detected at CT in patients selected for lung volume reduction surgery to treat severe pulmonary emphysema. Radiology 207:487–490, 1998.
14. Hazelrigg SR, Boley TM, Weber D, et al: Incidence of lung nodules found in patients undergoing lung volume reduction. Ann Thorac Surg 64:303–306, 1997.
15. McKenna RJ Jr, Brenner M, Fischel RJ, et al: Patient selection criteria for lung volume reduction surgery. J Thorac Cardiovasc Surg 114:957–964, 1997.
16. Thurnheer R, Muntwyler J, Stammberger U, et al: Coronary artery disease in patients undergoing lung volume reduction surgery for emphysema. Chest 112:122–128, 1997.
17. Keller CA, Ruppel G, Hibbett A, et al: Thoracoscopic lung volume reduction surgery reduces dyspnea and improves exercise capacity in patients with emphysema. Am J Respir Crit Care Med 156:60–67, 1997.
18. Keller CA, Naunheim KS: Perioperative management of lung volume reduction patients. Clin Chest Med 18:285–300, 1997.
19. Krucylak PE, Naunheim KS, Keller CA, Baudendistel LJ: Anesthetic management of patients undergoing unilateral video-assisted lung reduction for treatment of end-stage emphysema. J Cardiothorac Vasc Anesth 10:850–853, 1996.
20. McKenna RJ Jr, Brenner M, Fischel RJ, Gelb AF: Should lung volume reduction for emphysema be unilateral or bilateral? J Thorac Cardiovasc Surg 112:1331–1338, 1996.
21. Kotloff RM, Tino G, Palevsky HI, et al: Comparison of short-term functional outcomes following unilateral and bilateral lung volume reduction surgery. Chest 113:890–895, 1998.
22. Wisser W, Tschernko E, Senbaklavaci O, et al: Functional improvement after volume reduction: Sternotomy vs. video endoscopic approach. Ann Thorac Surg 63:822–827, 1997.
23. Stammberger U, Thurnheer R, Bloch KE, et al: Thoracoscopic bilateral lung volume reduction for diffuse pulmonary emphysema. Eur J Cardiothorac Surg 11:1005–1010, 1997.
24. Cordova F, O'Brien G, Furukawa S, et al: Stability of improvements in exercise performance and quality of life following bilateral lung volume reduction surgery in severe COPD. Chest 112:907–915, 1997.
25. Cooper JD, Patterson GA, Sunderesan RS, et al: Results of 150 consecutive bilateral lung volume reduction procedures in patients with severe emphysema. J Thorac Cardiovasc Surg 112:1319–1330, 1996.
26. Kotloff RM, Tino G, Bavaria JE, et al: Bilateral lung volume reduction surgery for advanced emphysema. A comparison of median sternotomy and thoracoscopic approaches. Chest 110:1399–1406, 1996.

COMMENTARY

Stephen R. Hazelrigg

This chapter provides a broad overview of the current state of lung volume reduction surgery (LVRS). As noted, there still remain several unanswered questions about this procedure. There seems to be a consensus that hyperinflated emphysematous patients who have heterogeneous disease and who are still in relatively good physiologic shape are the ideal candidates. In this select group, which probably represents less than 25% of all emphysematous patients, the results have been uniformly excellent. A recent report from Washington University in St. Louis followed 22 patients who had been approved for LVRS but who were unable to undergo the procedure because of the decision of the Health Care Financing Administration (HCFA) to discontinue funding for the procedure.[1] These patients were compared with 65 matched patients who had LVRS just before this time. In spite of maximal medical therapy, the 22 patients demonstrated 16% *decline* in their forced expired volume in 1 second (FEV_1) at 1 year. Oxygen requirements rose from 32% to 88% at 2 years. The 1 year survival rate was 89% and the absolute survival rate was 64%. This was compared with the LVRS group, who had a 1 year *improvement* of 50% in FEV_1, a 49% decrease in O_2 use at rest, a 100% 1-year survival rate, and an 82% absolute survival rate. The difference in survival rates did not reach statistical significance.

These data lend support to the already existing literature and demonstrate significant improvements in breathing and exercise ability that are unobtainable without this operative procedure.

At present, there is weak support for the thoracoscopic approach to LVRS in preference to sternotomy. However, sternotomy remains a viable alternative, with identical long-term results. Video-assisted thoracic surgery (VATS) may be particularly advantageous for patients who take steroids (to avoid sternal healing problems) and those who have inferior or posterior lung nodules. Some data have demonstrated a lower occurrence of respiratory complications in the VATS group.

This procedure remains technically straightforward but requires strong hospital support for postoperative management of these demanding patients.

Reference

1. Meyers BF, Yusen RD, Lefrak SS, et al: Outcome of Medicare patients with emphysema selected for, but denied, a lung volume reduction operation. Ann Thorac Surg 66:331–366; 1998.

Chapter 14

Pleuropulmonary Tuberculosis

Anthony P. C. Yim and Mohammad Bashar Izzat

Pulmonary infection caused by *Mycobacterium tuberculosis* (TB) historically was a major impetus for the development of thoracic surgery.[4] As collapse therapy was the mainstay of operative management[1] before the advent of streptomycin, the earliest indication of thoracoscopy was, in fact, to lyse pleural adhesions under local anesthesia to allow the lungs to fully collapse in patients who had pulmonary tuberculosis (see Chapter 1).[9]

Today, TB continues to be a major health hazard and affects one third of the world's population, with nearly half of all new cases occurring in Southeast Asia.[17] Despite the effectiveness of short-course chemotherapy for sensitive disease,[8] the incidence of tuberculosis has been going up since 1985 because of a combination of factors: worsening social conditions, intravenous drug abuse, lack of access to health care, noncompliance with medication,[16] emergence of drug-resistant strains,[6] immigration,[11] immunosuppression resulting from disease (e.g., the human immunodeficiency virus [HIV] epidemic),[10,15] or the result of chemotherapy.

Pulmonary TB can present clinically in a variety of ways, and, in part, reflects the variable host response to *M. tuberculosis*.[5] The lesions may be localized to one part of one lung or involve both lungs diffusely (e.g., miliary TB); they may be liquefied caseous masses with cavity formation or progressive, locally destructive lesions. Complications include bronchopleural fistulae, aspergilloma formation, bronchiectasis with or without hemoptysis, empyemas, and trapped lungs. The role of surgery in the management of pulmonary TB appears to be threefold:

1. Establish the correct diagnosis after failed attempts with noninvasive or less invasive approaches
2. Treat multidrug-resistant TB
3. Treat TB complications[16,20]

Role of VATS in Pleuropulmonary TB

Video-assisted thoracic surgery (VATS) provides a new approach to the management of this condition. It has both a diagnostic and therapeutic role (Table 14–1). We have reported our experience with VATS in the management of pleuropulmonary TB.[20] We concluded first that VATS is safe and effective in achieving the diagnosis of TB through pleural biopsies or wedge lung resection of indeterminate pulmonary nodules. It is particularly useful for patients who are debilitated, thus making them poor candidates for conventional open surgery. Second, in patients with trapped lung or tuberculous empyema, VATS could achieve full lung re-expansion with minimal morbidity.

Diagnostic Modality

Pleural effusion is a common clinical condition. Approximately one quarter of all effusions remain undiagnosed despite conventional evaluation with multiple thoracocentesis and blind percutaneous biopsy of the pleura.[2,19] A transudate (specific gravity <1.018) usually reflects an alteration in the body's hydrostatic or colloid osmotic pressure. Primary pleural pathology is unlikely in this setting. On the other hand, an exudate (pleural fluid to serum protein ratio >0.5; pleural fluid to serum lactic dehydrogenase [LDH] ratio >0.6; pleural fluid LDH >200 IU) requires further investigation to exclude TB or pleural metastasis.[7] In our experience, about one third of indeterminate effusions turned out to be tuberculous in origin.[19] Early treatment is essential in minimizing progression of disease and development of complications. Likewise, TB remains the most common benign diagnosis of solitary lung nodules, accounting for just under one third of all the wedge resections in our experience. We have found the VATS approach particularly useful in patients who have a history of malignancy treated by chemotherapy and who develop new pulmonary nodules. Differentiation between infection (e.g., TB) and tumor recurrence is essential. Wedge resection provides a definitive diagnosis for further management.[22]

Therapeutic Modality

We have found VATS a useful approach in draining empyema and performing decortication. In the former, the goal is to break down loculations and allow the unified pleural space to be drained adequately. Every attempt is made to eradicate a residual space in the face of tuberculous pleurisy (see Chapter 8).

Timing of the operation is essential for therapeutic surgical procedures. Unless there is a medical emergency, such as massive hemoptysis or a large bronchopleural fistula, surgery should be delayed until the patient is covered adequately with antituberculous medication and the sputum smear is negative.[14] On the other hand, persistent sputum-positivity or pleuropulmonary pathology after a 6-month trial of multiple antituberculous medication is an indication for surgery.[14]

Operative Technique

Under general anesthesia in selective one-lung ventilation, the patient is placed in the full lateral decubitus position with the table flexed at 30 degrees to open up the intercostal spaces on the side of the surgery.[18] In young children, we use main stem intubation with a single-

Table 14–1. Applications of Video-Assisted Thoracic Surgery (VATS) in the Management of Tuberculosis (TB)

Diagnostic	Pleural biopsy
	Indeterminate pulmonary nodule
Therapeutic	Empyema drainage
	Decortication for trapped lung
	Resection for TB abscess, drug-resistant disease

lumen tube guided by a 3.5-mm outer diameter, fine, flexible bronchoscope (F1 10P Pentax, Tokyo, Japan) for selective ventilation[24] (Fig 14–1). Selective ventilation in this age group is not possible, but by reducing the tidal volume (together with intermittent apnea), we were able to achieve our goals of obtaining a diagnosis of TB and breaking down loculations to allow full lung re-expansion.[24]

For exploratory thoracoscopy, a zero-degree telescope (10 mm for adults and 5 mm for children) was placed through a reusable trocar (Thora-port, Snowden & Pencer, Tucker, GA) at the sixth or seventh intercostal space, midaxillary line, for exploration. For diagnostic purposes alone, we routinely use in adults an operating telescope (K. Storz, Germany) that carries a 5-mm instrument channel (for the biopsy forceps); thus, the number of ports used is minimized.

VATS decortication for mild and moderately trapped lungs is not only feasible, but often is not as difficult as it may sound initially (Fig 14–2). Using gentle blunt dissection, after the correct plane is reached, subtotal decortication can be performed using the standard three-port technique.[20] The surgical goal is full lung re-expansion, and this is achieved by a combination of mechanical removal of the encasing peel, positive pressure ventilation, and postoperative negative pressure chest drainage. Some postoperative air leak may be inevitable after decortication, but it is usually not a problem as long as the lung can be fully re-expanded.

For mass lesions, resections were indicated for diagnosis in cases of indeterminate nodules and for treatment in cases of failed antituberculous therapy for disease control. Thoracoscopic wedge lung resections (Fig 14–3) can be performed using an endoscopic stapler-cutter (Endo-GIA30, Autosuture, United States Surgical, Norwalk, CT; or EZ45, Ethicon EndoSurgery, Johnson and Johnson, Cincinnati, OH). Selection criteria include the following:

1. Nodules should be less than 3 cm in maximal diameter.
2. Nodules should be located over the peripheral one third of the lung, or close to a major fissure.

For small lesions lying deep against a flat surface of the lung, wedge resection using staplers may be technically difficult. In this situation, we have found it useful to place

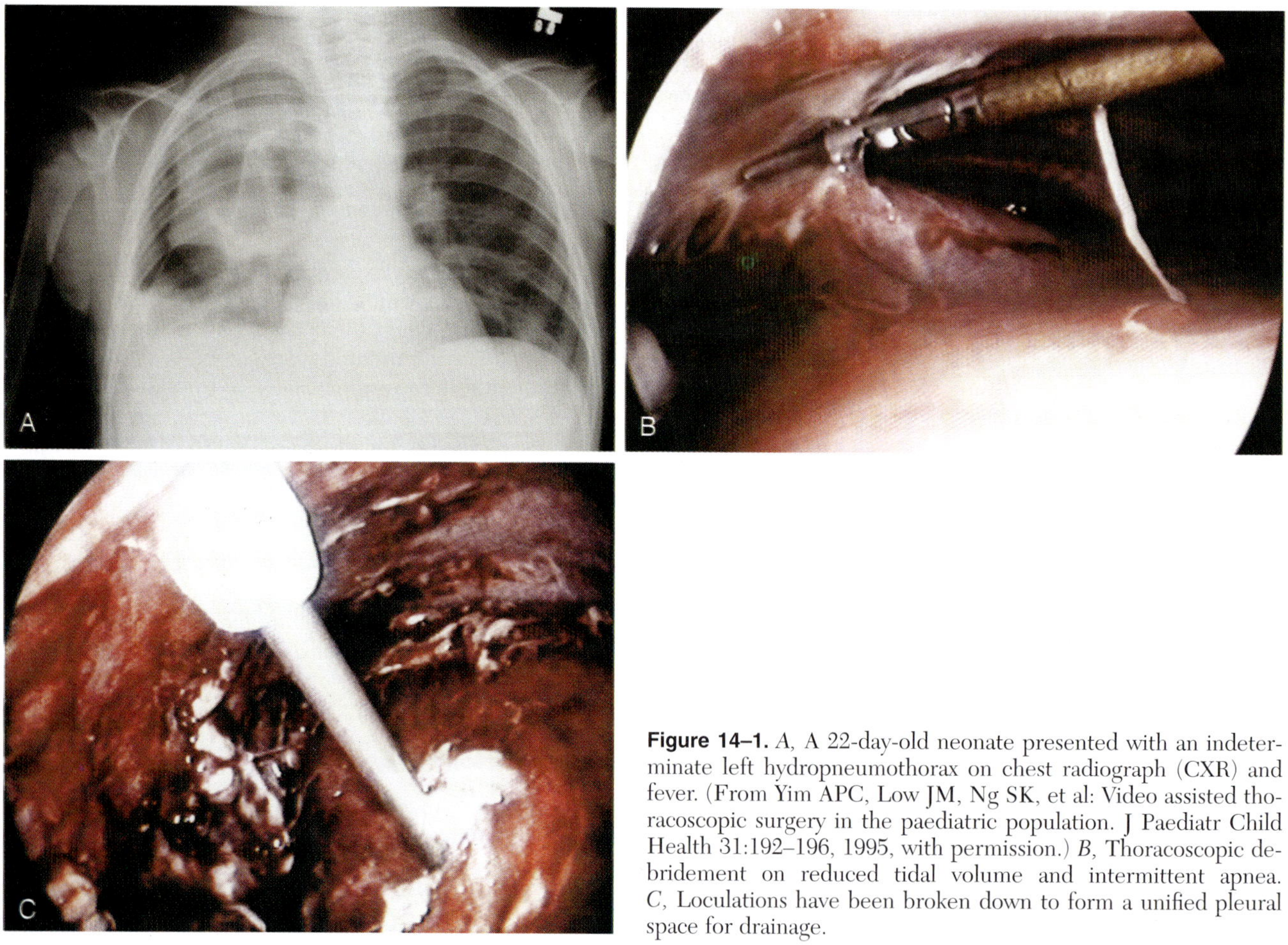

Figure 14–1. *A*, A 22-day-old neonate presented with an indeterminate left hydropneumothorax on chest radiograph (CXR) and fever. (From Yim APC, Low JM, Ng SK, et al: Video assisted thoracoscopic surgery in the paediatric population. J Paediatr Child Health 31:192–196, 1995, with permission.) *B*, Thoracoscopic debridement on reduced tidal volume and intermittent apnea. *C*, Loculations have been broken down to form a unified pleural space for drainage.

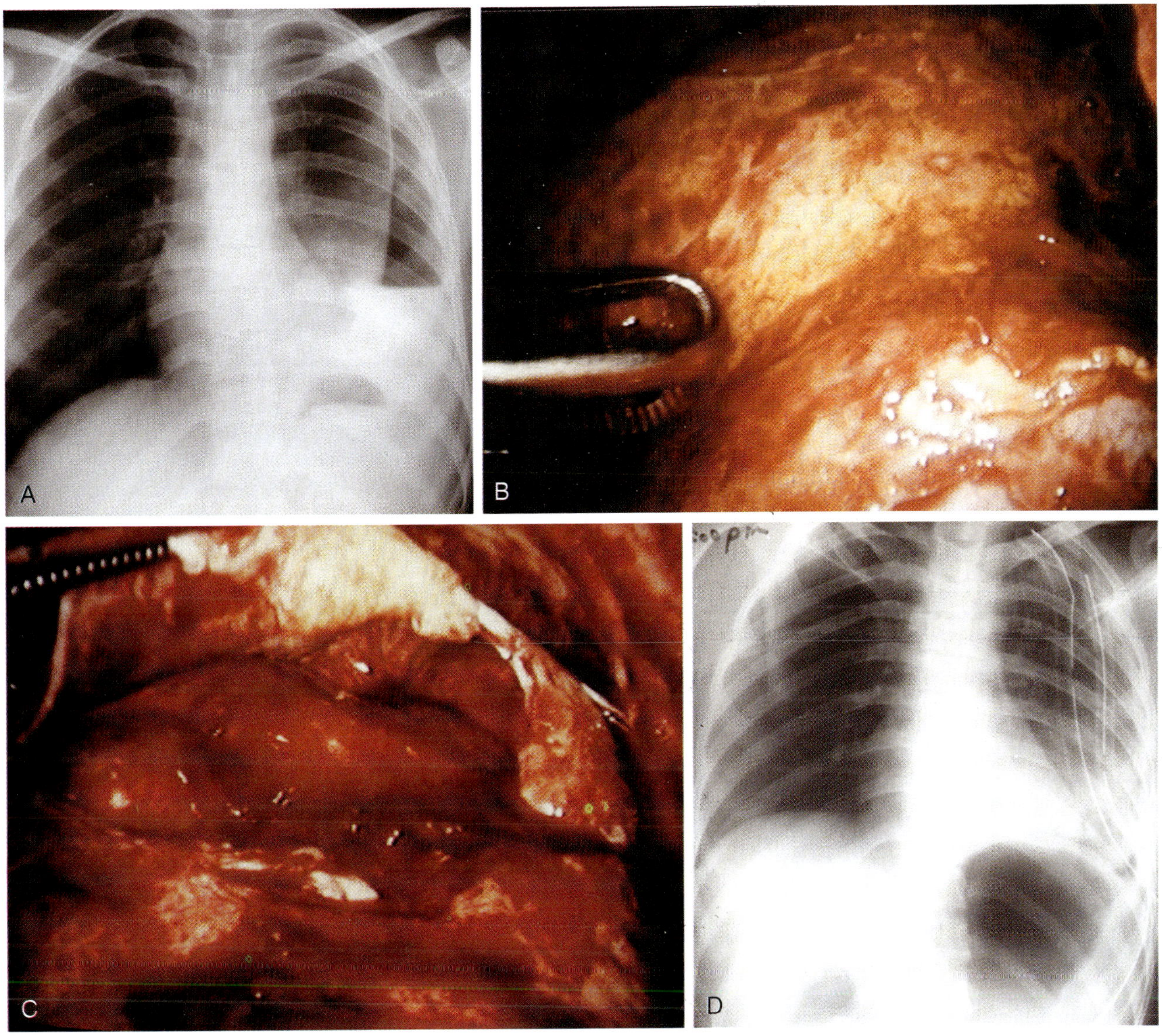

Figure 14–2. *A*, A 35-year-old female who has a right hydropneumothorax and a severely trapped lung caused by tuberculosis. (From Yim APC: The role of video-assisted thoracoscopic surgery in the management of pulmonary tuberculosis. Chest 110:829–832, 1996, with permission.) *B*, Thoracoscopic view of the encasing visceral pleural peel. *C*, Decortication of the peel to "liberate" the lung. *D*, Postoperative chest radiograph (CXR) in the recovery room shows full lung re-expansion.

a mini-thoracotomy over the lesion (for accurate localization and resection). The nodule can then be resected with a rim of normal lung using electrocautery under a combination of video assistance and direct vision. The lung can then be repaired with monofilament sutures. For large (>3 cm) or deep lesions, vascular control is often necessary, and, therefore, anatomic resection is required.[21]

Complications and Pitfalls

When patients are properly selected, surgical complications are few and relatively minor. In our experience on over 60 patients who had TB,[22] there was no incidence of surgical mortality or intraoperative complications. Persistent air leak remains the most common complication, and it occurred in 8% of patients.[22,23] As mentioned previously, timing of the surgical intervention is important, and unless there is a surgical emergency, the operation should be delayed until the patient is protected by anti-TB medication. Joint management of the perioperative care by surgeons and pulmonologists cannot be overemphasized, particularly with respect to nutrition and medical therapy.[13] For a more detailed discussion of complications and technical pitfalls, readers should refer to Chapter 43.

Major Lung Resection for TB

Although VATS major resection for TB is technically feasible,[20,21] it is generally not recommended because the anatomy is often distorted: The fibrotic hilum, which makes VATS dissection hazardous, and various degrees of lung destruction are often present. Localized multidrug-resistant TB remains the most common indication for ma-

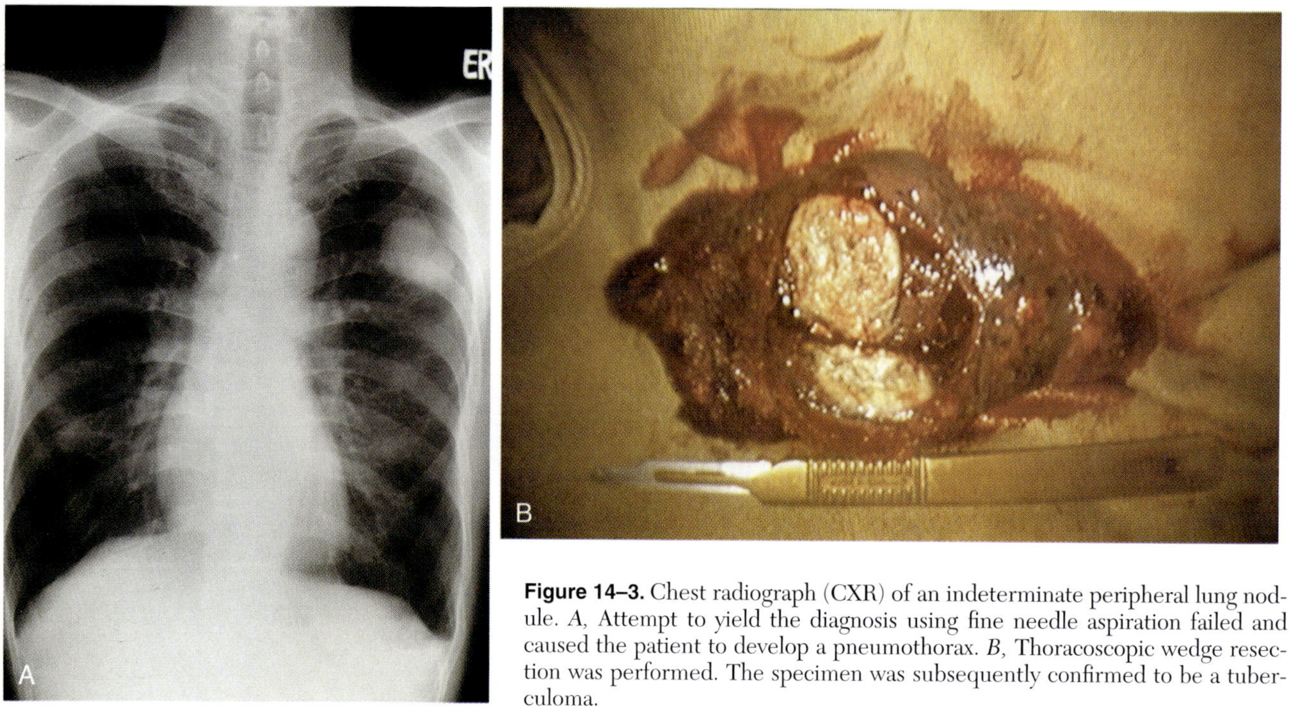

Figure 14–3. Chest radiograph (CXR) of an indeterminate peripheral lung nodule. *A*, Attempt to yield the diagnosis using fine needle aspiration failed and caused the patient to develop a pneumothorax. *B*, Thoracoscopic wedge resection was performed. The specimen was subsequently confirmed to be a tuberculoma.

jor lung resection.[12,13] Attention to details during intraoperative management is also crucial for success. An extrapleural approach may be required in cases of pleural symphysis, and muscle flaps or the omentum may be required to reinforce the bronchial stump closure.[3] Thoracoplasty is still occasionally necessary if residual space is an anticipated problem.

The complexity of the operative procedure renders the use of VATS inappropriate for most major lung resections in this group of patients. Nonetheless, the thoracoscope, which carries its own light source, could be a useful adjunct to open surgery by providing illumination and a magnified operative view during a difficult dissection (e.g., of the apex).

Conclusion

VATS has an established diagnostic role in the management of TB through pleural biopsy or wedge lung resection of indeterminate pulmonary nodules. It is particularly useful for patients who are elderly, debilitated, or who have multiple comorbidities, thus making them poor candidates for open surgery. We have also found it a very useful approach for patients who have a history of malignancy treated by chemotherapy and who have developed new pulmonary nodules. On the other hand, VATS also has a therapeutic role for some patients who have a moderately trapped lung or tuberculous empyema, for which decortication and guided drainage could be achieved, leading to full lung re-expansion with minimal perioperative morbidity. The role of VATS in major resection is limited because of the complex nature of the procedure. However, the thoracoscope, by providing illumination and a magnified view, could be a useful adjunct to open surgery.

References

1. Alexander J: The Collapse Therapy of Pulmonary Tuberculosis. Springfield, IL, Charles C. Thomas, 1937.
2. Boutin C, Astroul P, Seitz B: The role of thoracoscopy in the evaluation and management of pleural effusions. Lung 168: 1113–1121, 1990.
3. Brown J, Pomerantz M: Extrapleural pneumonectomy for tuberculosis. Chest Surg Clin North Am 5:289–296, 1995.
4. Churchill ED, Dlopstock R: Lobectomy for pulmonary tuberculosis. J Thorac Surg 20:843–853, 1950.
5. Edwards D, Kirkpatrick CH: The immunology of myocobacterial diseases. Am Rev Respir Dis 134:1062–1071, 1986.
6. Frieden TR, Sterling T, Pablos-Mendez A, et al: The emergence of drug-resistance in New York City. N Engl J Med 328:521–526, 1993.
7. Harris RJ, Kavura MS, Mehta AC, et al: The impact of thoracoscopy on the management of pleural disease. Chest 107:845–852, 1995.
8. Hong Kong Chest Service/British Research Council: Controlled trial of 2, 4 and 6 months of pyrazinamide in 6-month, three-times-weekly regimens for smear-positive pulmonary tuberculosis, including an assessment of a combined preparation isoniazid, rifampin and pyrazinamide: Results at 30 months. Am Rev Respir Dis 143:700–706, 1991.
9. Jacobaeus HC: Ueber die Möglichkeit die Zystoskopie bei untersuchung seröser Löhlungen anzuwenden. München Med Wochenschr 57:2090–2092, 1910.
10. McKenna MT, McCray E, Onorato I: The epidemiology of tuberculosis among foreign-born persons in the United States 1986 to 1993. N Engl J Med 332:1071–1076, 1995.
11. Narain JP, Raviglone MC, Kochi A: HIV-associated tuberculosis in developing countries: Epidemiology and strategies for prevention. World Health Organization WHO/TB 92.164, 1992.
12. Pomerantz M, Brown J: The surgical management of tuberculosis. Semin Thorac Cardiovasc Surg 7:108–111, 1995.
13. Pomerantz M, Brown JM: Surgery in the treatment of multidrug-resistant tuberculosis. Clin Chest Med 18:123–130, 1997.
14. Rizzi A, Rocco G, Bobustellini M, et al: Results of surgical man-

agement of tuberculosis: Experience in 206 patients undergoing operation. Ann Thorac Surg 59:896–900, 1995.

15. Selwyn PA, Sckell BM, Alcabes P, et al: High risk of active tuberculosis in HIV-infected drug users with cutaneous energy. JAMA 268:504–509, 1992.
16. Treasure RL, Seaworth BJ: Current role of surgery in *Mycobacterium tuberculosis.* Ann Thorac Surg 59:1405–1409, 1995.
17. Tuberculoses Programme, Division of Communicable Diseases, World Health Organization: Tuberculosis Notifications Update July 1992. World Health Organization. WHO/TB92.169, 1992.
18. Yim APC: Minimising chest wall trauma in video assisted thoracic surgery. J Thorac Cardiovasc Surg 109:1255–1256, 1995.
19. Yim APC, Ho JKS, Lee TW, et al: Thoracoscopic management of pleural effusion revisited. Aust NZ J Surg 65:308–311, 1995.
20. Yim APC: The role of video assisted thoracoscopic surgery in the management of pulmonary tuberculosis. Chest 110:829–832, 1996.
21. Yim APC, Ko KM, Ma CC, et al: Thoracoscopic lobectomy for benign diseases. Chest 109:554–556, 1996.
22. Yim APC, Izzat MB, Lee TW: Thoracoscopic surgery and pleuropulmonary tuberculosis. World J Surg (in press).
23. Yim APC, Liu HP: Complications and failures from video-assisted thoracic surgery: Experience from two centers in Asia. Ann Thorac Surg 61:538–541, 1996.
24. Yim APC, Low JM, Ng SK, et al: Video assisted thoracoscopic surgery in the paediatric population. J Paediatr Child Health 31:192–196, 1995.

Chapter 15

Localization of Pulmonary Nodules

Michael J. Mack

Although there are clear advantages to minimally invasive surgery, including less access trauma, there are significant disadvantages, such as the loss of the ability to manually palpate target organs and tissue. The ability to "operate by feel" and determine not only the location of target pathology but also vital structures by the proprioception gained by being able to place one's fingers in contact with tissue is an integral part of the traditional surgical armamentarium. When this valuable tool is lost because access is too small to introduce the hand into a body cavity, one must employ compensatory aids to be able to accomplish the desired result. These new learned skills and technical innovations that can be used to help locate target pulmonary pathology are listed in Table 15–1.

Preoperative Techniques to Localize Pulmonary Nodules

Successful localization of target pulmonary nodules begins with a preoperative selection of nodules that have a high likelihood of being located and resected. A surgeon with sufficient experience with thoracoscopic pulmonary resection should have no trouble detecting a lung nodule after proper preoperative assessment.

A successful VATS procedure begins with selection of appropriate nodules that are able to be located and resected by VATS techniques. For the most part, those nodules are smaller than 3 cm and located in the periphery of the lung (i.e., the outer third of the lung parenchyma) (Fig. 15–1). Nodules that are deep within the substance of the lung, on the medial aspect of the lung, or adjacent to the pulmonary hilum present difficult problems, in terms not only of location but also resection, and therefore are better approached by an open technique (Fig. 15–2). Nodules that are too small also present problems of localization. With the advent of spiral and high-resolution computed tomography (CT) scanning, many nodules smaller than 1 cm have been detected. VATS localization of nodules 3 mm and 4 mm in size may be somewhat difficult, even when they are in a subpleural location (Figure 15–3). Nodules that on initial cursory examination of the CT scan appear to be deep within the pulmonary parenchyma may in fact be adjacent to a fissure (Fig. 15–4). Note should be taken of the the location of fissures when determining the selection of appropriate nodules for VATS resection.

Assessment of Computed Tomography Scan for Location

The surgeon contemplating a VATS procedure should, of course, be cognizant of the lobe on which the nodule is located. Although this is also important for conventional lung surgery, in those cases, if the surgeon is in error about location of the nodule, the nodule can be easily palpated in an adjacent lobe. This is more difficult to do with VATS; therefore, the surgeon should be absolutely certain ahead of time of the location (i.e., on which lobe and where within that lobe the target nodule is located).

Notice should also be taken of adjacent landmarks. For instance, proximity to fissures is important in terms of determining resectability. Another important feature is the level in the chest of the nodule. By using the pulmonary hilum as a base point, the correct level usually can be ascertained. Determining location of the nodule in relation to the chest wall is also important, even though the relationship to the chest wall changes as the lung is collapsed. Knowing that the nodule is beneath the tip of the scapula, for example, certainly helps to delineate the location of the nodule within the lung (Fig. 15–5). By careful assessment of the CT scan and attention to adjacent landmarks, the surgeon should be able to narrow the area of lung to be examined by VATS to a target of 2 cm by 2 cm. It should also be noted that subtle pleural changes frequently are present adjacent to a lung nodule. Although these changes may go unrecognized in conventional surgery, they become crucial for adequate detection by VATS. Such an example is shown in Figure 15–6. Often, slight pleural puckering or retraction around a nodule, either inflammatory or malignant, gives a clue to the fact that the nodule lies in the immediate subjacent area of the visceral pleura.

If it is deemed that a nodule is going to be difficult to localize by VATS, either because of size or location, then a number of radiographic localization techniques can be used. The necessity for radiographic localization of nodules should be infrequent. At the present time, we use a localization technique in less than 5% of our VATS nodule resections. Nodules that are deep within the lobe and are difficult to detect are also difficult to resect. We approach these nodules by limited thoracotomy, so that a stapling device can be placed more easily adjacent to the nodule or so that a direct electrocautery technique can be employed to reach the nodule.

Nodules for which we employ a localization technique are those smaller than 7 mm or 8 mm in a subpleural location. This has been an increasing problem due to the frequency of detection of tiny nodules by high-resolution spiral CT scans. Frequently, these nodules are subpleural lymph nodes, but because the immediate subpleural area is a fertile area for metastatic disease, diagnosis of these nodules is crucial. Because these nodules are difficult to locate even by digital palpation in open thoracotomy, localization preoperatively is important to ascertain a correct location of the nodule (Fig. 15–7).

Table 15–1. Techniques to Locate Pulmonary Nodules by VATS

Preoperative

Selection of appropriate nodules
- Size ≥ 1 cm, ≤ 3 cm
- Location—periphery

Assessment of computed tomography scan for location
- Lobe
- Proximity to adjacent structures, fissures
- Pleural changes adjacent to nodule

Radiographic localization technique
- Hook-wire placement
- Methylene blue injection
- Polymer-coil injection
- Ultrasound

Intraoperative

Trocar placement over nodule
Visual inspection of suspected target area
Instrument palpation
Digital palpation

Intraoperative Techniques to Localize Pulmonary Nodules

Strategic planning for localization and subsequent resection of pulmonary nodules is based most importantly on strategic placement of trocars. Basic VATS principles of trocar placement as described by Landreneau (i.e., an inverted triangle with the scope at the bottom and working ports placed at the inverted base of the triangle; see Chapter 5) should be adhered to. Modification of this trocar placement should be based on location of the nodule within the lung. Specifically, one of the trocar sites should be placed as closely as possible to the adjacent chest wall over the target pulmonary nodule. Strategic placement of a trocar site over a nodule is important to allow digital palpation of the nodule. Introduction of the surgeon's index finger through an adjacent trocar site provides tactile confirmation of the positive location of a nodule in the subjacent lung tissue. Obviously, introduction of an examining digit is easier through an anterior trocar site over the lower lung field and more problematic for nodules underneath the scapula. Suffice it to say that placement of one trocar site in close proximity to the nodule optimizes the chance of being able to digitally palpate it.

Once the trocars have been placed, the first maneuver to locate a suspected nodule is visual inspection of the lung. As resorptive atelectasis occurs, a mounding of lung tissue over a subpleural nodule is likely to occur. If resorp-

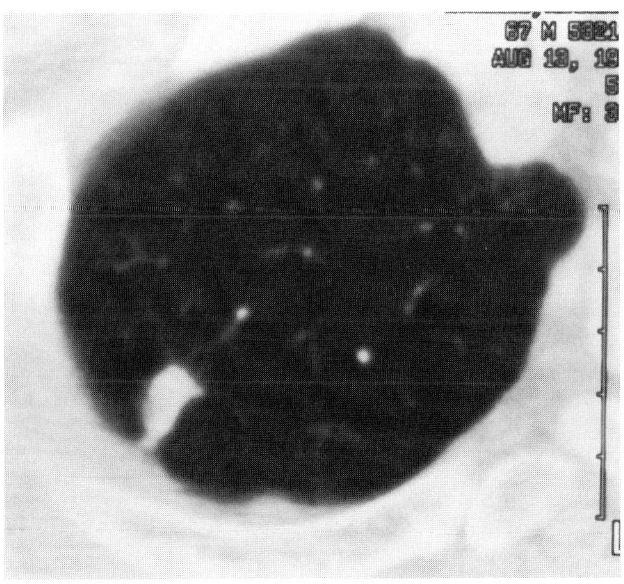

Figure 15–1. Nodule ideal in size and location for video-assisted thoracic surgery (VATS) resection.

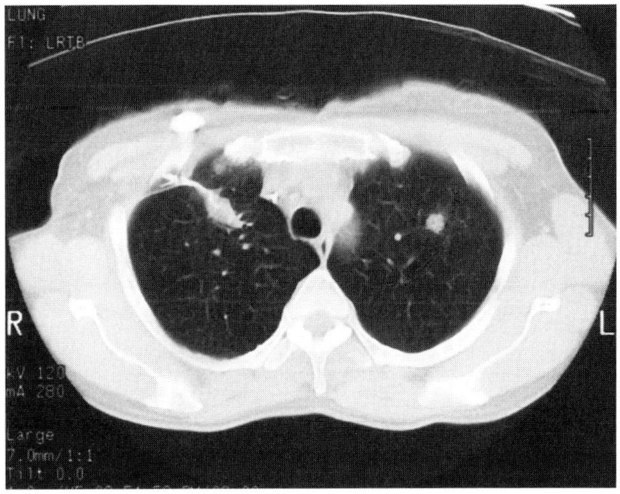

Figure 15–2. Nodule (left side) located too deep within the upper lobe for easy identification or resection.

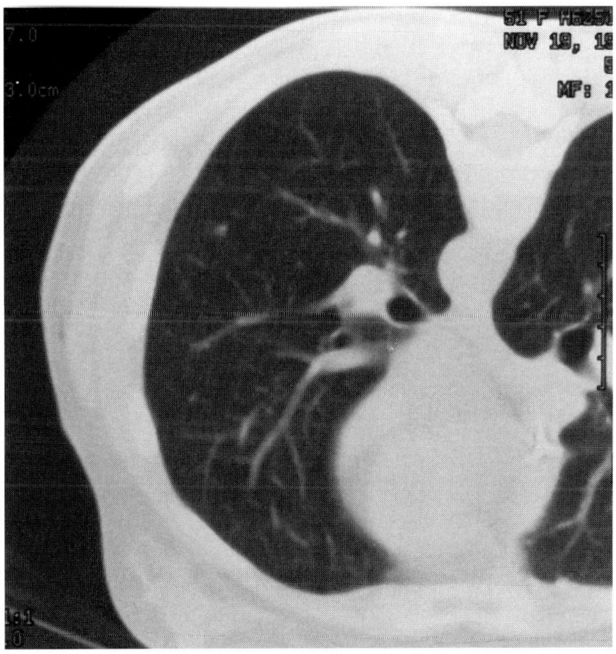

Figure 15–3. Four-mm nodule that is difficult to locate; even though it is in a subpleural location, it is too small to palpate easily.

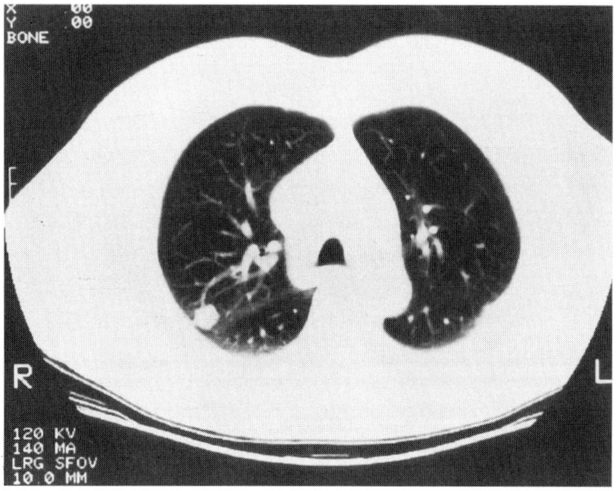

Figure 15–4. This pulmonary mass can be found adjacent to the interlobar fissure by VATS.

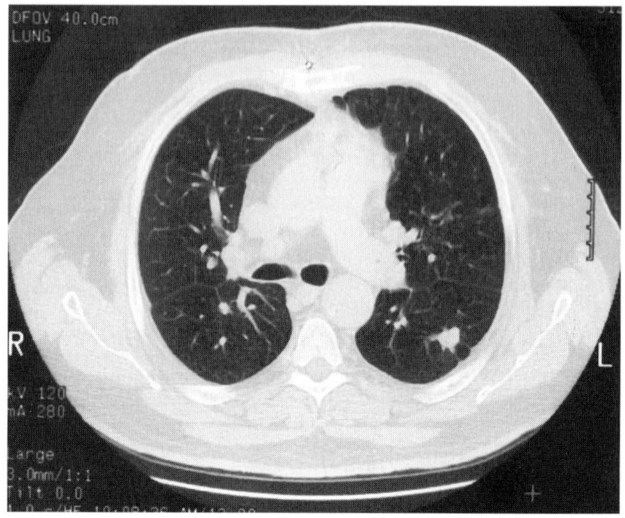

Figure 15–6. This subpleural nodule can be identified by VATS because of the adjacent pleural changes.

tive atelectasis is not prompt, suctioning of the collapsed lung by the anesthesiologist hastens the resorptive atelectasis and increases the contour of nodules located in the subpleural area. Of course, if pleural involvement with a nodule is present, then puckering of the pleural surface can be easily identified by visual inspection (Fig. 15–8). As mentioned previously, careful preoperative assessment with CT should be able to localize the area of lung surface to be examined to 2 cm by 2 cm.

If the suspected area of lung tissue containing the nodule has been ascertained, confirmation by palpation is often helpful. Palpation can be either with a surgical instrument or with the surgeon's index finger. If the nodule is not immediately adjacent to a trocar site, then introducing a curved ring forceps and "instrument palpating" the surface of the lung often confirm the presence of a nodule. The change in texture of the examined surface can be appreciated either through tactile feedback through the instrument or by visual confirmation by watching the instrument tip on the video screen.

The most confirmatory maneuver, however, is digital palpation. The trocar site should be large enough to allow a probing index finger to be placed through the trocar site. Placement of the finger through anterior and lower trocar sites where interspaces are wider is much easier. In addition, in thin, nonmuscular patients—specifically, patients with chronic obstructive pulmonary disease—palpation of the lung by the probing digit is easier. If the nodule is too remote in location from the nearest trocar site to allow direct digital palpation, a surgical grasping instrument, such as ring forceps, can often be placed through another trocar site, and the target lung tissue brought into apposition with

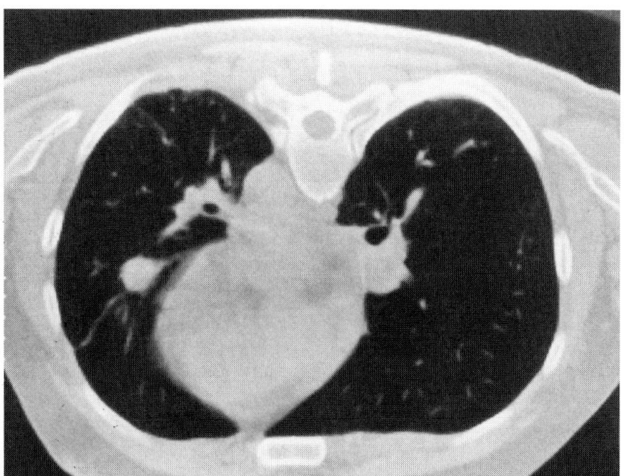

Figure 15–5. This nodule is located in the lung just subjacent to the tip of the scapula.

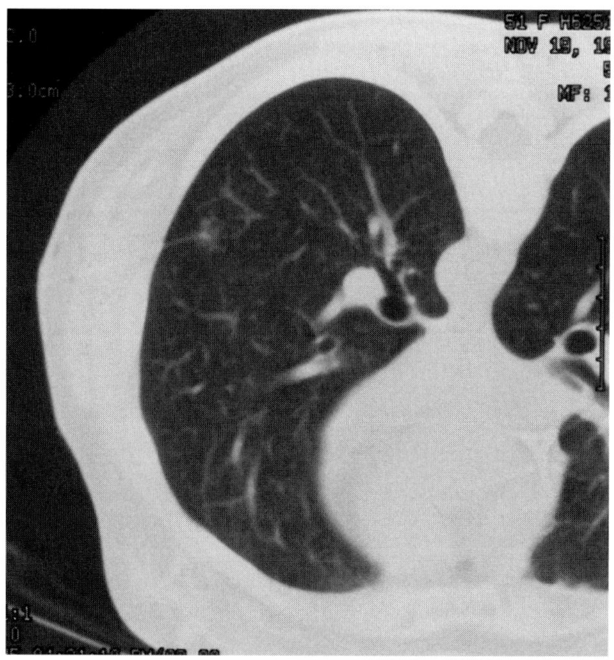

Figure 15–7. Preoperative hook-wire localization of a subpleural metastasis from a soft tissue sarcoma.

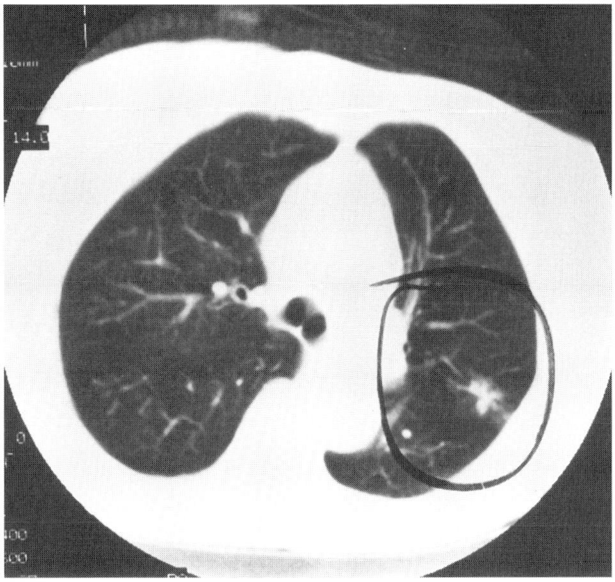

Figure 15–8. Pleural puckering is present over a subjacent lung cancer.

the probing finger (Fig. 15–9). Hard-to-discern nodules often can be located by using instrumentation to place the lung in approximation to the probing digital finger. We have found it helpful, once a difficult-to-ascertain nodule has been successfully localized, to score the surface of the lung over the nodule with electrocautery. This prevents confusion over the target lung to be resected once stapling has commenced. Confusion as to the portion of lung containing the target nodule is possible once distortion of the normal lung contour has occurred as the stapled resection continues.

If it has been determined by the criteria listed previously that a nodule is going to be difficult to locate at the time of thoracoscopy and preoperative localization has occurred, the localization target area is confirmed by visual inspection. A number of radiographic localization techniques can be used, including hook wire placement,[1] methylene blue injection,[2] or a combination of both. In addition, others have described injections of polymers or coils adjacent to a difficult-to-define target nodule. Ultrasound has been used in experimental studies in an attempt to define nodules, but because of the poor transmission of ultrasound frequencies through aerated lung tissue, this technique has not proved useful even when lung tissue is immersed in water. On the rare occasions when we have found localization to be necessary, we have used a hook wire placement. Under CT scan guidance, a breast localization hook wire is placed into the lung where the target nodule is located (see Fig. 15–7). The patient is then taken directly to the operating room, if possible, after the wire is taped to the chest wall. Once the patient is prepped and draped, we cut the wire flush with the chest wall before lung collapse occurs. We have found this to be helpful in preventing dislodgement of the nodule as the lung retracts away from the chest wall. Once the lung collapses, the wire can then be seen emanating from the surface of the lung (Fig. 15–10). On the rare occasion when the nodule does dislodge from the surface of the lung, entry point through the pleura can still be determined, and some subpleural hemorrhage occurring from the localization technique can be used as confirmatory evidence that the nodule is located in the subjacent tissue.

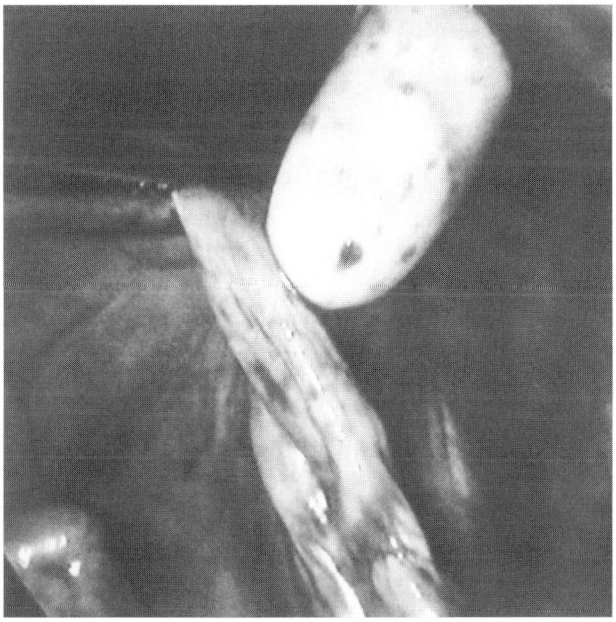

Figure 15–9. An instrument introduced through a second trocar site can bring distant part of the lung in opposition to a probing digit.

Conclusions

We have found thoracoscopy to be an extremely advantageous diagnostic and therapeutic modality for the management of pulmonary nodules. Success is based most importantly on selection of appropriate nodules for detection and resection. Once proper selection has occurred, adherence to the principles outlined in this chapter should yield a high degree of success in terms of identifying nodules for VATS resection. It should be emphasized,

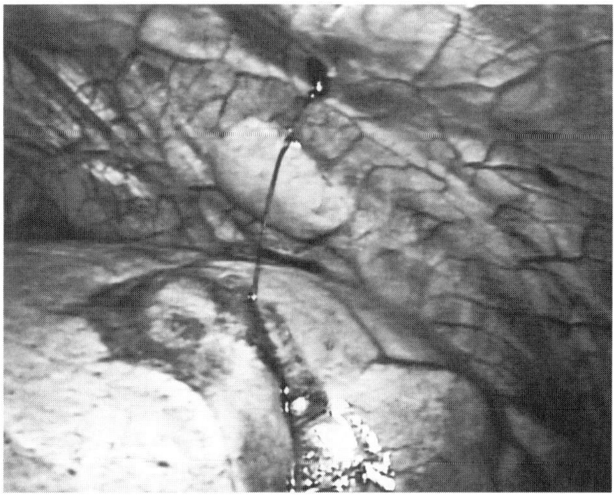

Figure 15–10. Hook wire localizing a lung nodule; the lung is stained with methylene blue.

however, that the goal of the surgical procedure is successful identification and removal of a suspicious pulmonary nodule. If the nodule cannot be successfully located despite adherence to the principles described here and the surgeon's skills, conversion to a thoracotomy should occur so that the lung nodule can be successfully resected. Conversion should not be viewed as a failure, but rather the exercise of mature surgical judgment. On occasions in which a suspected nodule cannot be located for resection by VATS technique, usually a mini-thoracotomy with minimal rib spreading to allow placement of a few fingers into the chest cavity will allow identification of the occult nodule.

References

1. Mack MJ, Gordon MJ, Postma TW, et al: Percutaneous localization of pulmonary nodules for thoracoscopic lung resection. Ann Thorac Surg 53:1123–1124, 1992.
2. Kerrigan DC, Spence PA, Crittenden MD, Tripp MD: Methylene blue guidance for simplified resection of a lung lesion. Ann Thorac Surg 53:163–164, 1992.

Chapter 16

Wedge Resection

Jemi Olak

Pulmonary wedge resection is indicated for both the diagnosis and treatment of indeterminate pulmonary nodules, for the treatment of benign lung tumors, and for the treatment of selected small (T1N0) lung cancers in patients who have medical contraindications to thoracotomy. Video-assisted thoracic surgery (VATS) is an acceptable approach to employ when the conditions outlined in this chapter apply.

Pulmonary nodules that are considered for stapled thoracoscopic resection generally fulfill all the following criteria:

1. Diameter between 5 mm and 3 cm
2. Peripheral location (outer one third of the lung)
3. Patient able to tolerate general anesthesia with one-lung ventilation

The chest radiograph (CXR) seen in Figure 16–1 demonstrates a solitary pulmonary nodule in the left upper lobe that might be suitable for wedge resection. The chest computed tomography (CT) scan seen in Figure 16–2 illustrates the same nodule and confirms that it is pleurally based and would indeed be amenable to a thoracoscopic wedge resection. The nodule illustrated in Figure 16–3 is also amenable to a thoracoscopic wedge resection, because it comes within 1 cm of the visceral pleural surface and is approximately 1.5 cm in diameter.

Deeper nodules, if they can be localized, may also be removed thoracoscopically using an Nd-YAG laser in addition to the endoscopic stapler. Clamps and suture are used infrequently to oversew the base of a nodule when a VATS approach is used.

Nodules that are either smaller or larger than those indicated have been successfully excised using thoracoscopic techniques; however, smaller nodules are more difficult to visualize and larger nodules are more difficult to circumscribe within the requisite 1-cm margin because of the thickness of the lung parenchyma at the inner limit of resection.

Technique

Preoperative Localization Technique

Preoperative examination of the relationship of the nodule to the chest wall and mediastinal structures on CT scan allows the surgeon to plan the placement of the camera port so visualization of the nodule is optimized.

Several investigators have described the preoperative needle localization of a pulmonary nodule using the long hook wire originally developed for the localization of breast nodules. Nodules are typically localized under guidance by either fluoroscopy or CT, after which the patient is taken to the operating room for excisional biopsy (see Chapter 15).[1–4]

The injection of methylene blue dye onto the visceral pleural surface overlying a nodule has also been advocated at the time of hook-wire placement because the hook wire can become dislodged either when the patient is moved or when the lung collapses.[2] Some surgeons have found that the methylene blue dye diffuses quickly from the point of injection, limiting its usefulness with regard to facilitating nodule localization. Nomori and associates have described the injection of colored collagen, noting that it stays at the injected site for a longer period of time than methylene blue dye.[5] In a series of 200 thoracoscopic wedge resections by Mack and associates, needle localization was used 51 times. The hook wire dislodged in four patients, but either the methylene blue dye or a visceral pleural hematoma allowed all four nodules to be located and successfully removed. The hook wire failed to aid the surgeon in two cases, and two patients developed pneumothoraces that required preoperative chest tube placement. Based upon this series, Mack and associates recommend the use of needle localization for nodules more than 2 cm below the visceral pleural surface.[2] Schwarz and associates reported a series of 30 patients who underwent a total of 33 needle localizations of nodules whose mean size was 7.9 ± 4.9 mm. Four complications occurred: a chylothorax, a persistent air leak, an arrhythmia, and a urinary tract infection. Forty-seven percent of the patients developed a 10 to 25% pneumothorax during the procedure; however, all were asymptomatic. The hook wire was successfully placed in 29 patients; one patient withdrew because of pain. All patients had a diagnosis established, and the authors concluded that needle localization was appropriate for 15 to 20% of nodules.[3]

Intraoperative Localization Technique

Successful localization of a pulmonary nodule depends upon complete collapse of the lobe in which it is located. This can be achieved by placing a double-lumen endotracheal tube with subsequent isolation of the lung undergoing the procedure, or by placing a bronchial blocker (e.g., No. 8–10 French venous Fogarty embolectomy catheter) in the main stem bronchus of the lung. Suctioning the main bronchus on the side to be operated upon also hastens lung collapse. For a lung that does not deflate readily because of underlying emphysema or a malpositioned double-lumen endotracheal tube, the use of CO_2 insufflation as a single bolus of 2 to 3 L, or at a continuous flow rate (with a maximal intrathoracic pressure of 10 mmHg), enhances resorptive atelectasis and improves the chance of visualizing the nodule. Once the lung collapses, the nodule is effaced.

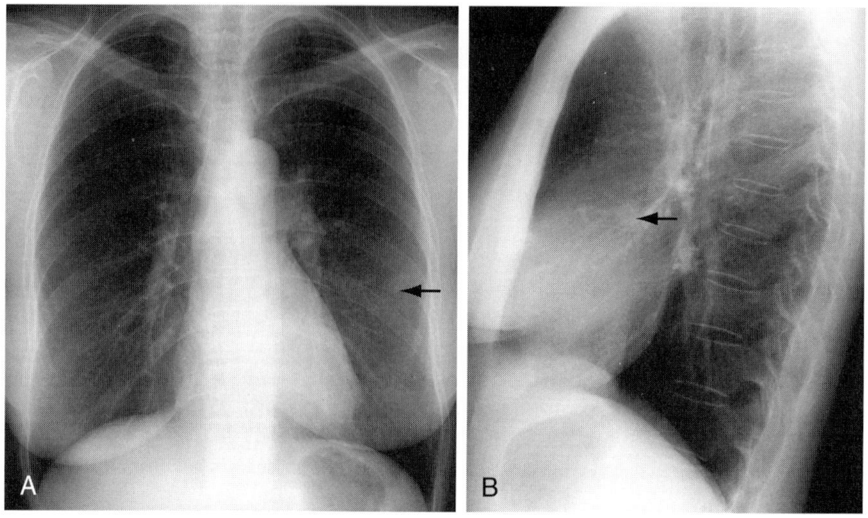

Figure 16–1. *A*, PA chest radiograph demonstrating a solitary pulmonary nodule (SPN) in the left mid-lung zone. *B*, Lateral chest radiograph localizing the solitary pulmonary nodule (SPN) to the lingular segment of the left upper lobe.

If the camera port has been positioned optimally, a pleural-based nodule larger than 8 to 10 mm (see Fig. 16–2) can almost always be seen. Occasionally, an instrument with a blunt tip can be used to palpate the nodule. For nodules positioned close to the apex of the lung or against the mediastinal or diaphragmatic surfaces, a 30-degree telescope can be used to enhance visibility.

Digital palpation is particularly useful for small nodules (<8 mm). It usually requires enlarging the incision closest to the nodule to approximately 2 in., through which a grasper and a finger or a thumb and index finger can be advanced to palpate the lung.

Intraoperative ultrasonography has also been reported to be helpful in the localization of small pulmonary nodules.[6] It requires that the lung be airless, and, as mentioned previously, this may be aided by CO_2 insufflation. Submerging the lung in fluid also improves visibility when using ultrasound. A 12-mm endovaginal or endorectal probe that has either an end or side transducer and that operates at 5 MHz is used.

Operative Technique

The patient is usually placed in the full lateral decubitus position, and the chest is prepared and draped in the same way as it would for a thoracotomy.

The skin, subcutaneous tissues, and parietal pleura at each port site may be infiltrated with .25% bupivacaine with epinephrine to decrease perioperative narcotic requirements.

The camera port (10- to 12-mm diameter) is usually placed in the fifth intercostal space in the midaxillary line, and the chest is explored to be certain that no unanticipated abnormalities (e.g., adhesions, pleural nodules) are found. The nodule is localized and placement of one or two additional ports is planned to facilitate a stapled resection of the nodule. Typically, one port (5 mm) is placed immediately above the nodule. A grasping instrument is advanced through this port to stabilize the lung in the region adjacent to the nodule. To minimize the risk of fracturing either the nodule or the visceral pleural sur-

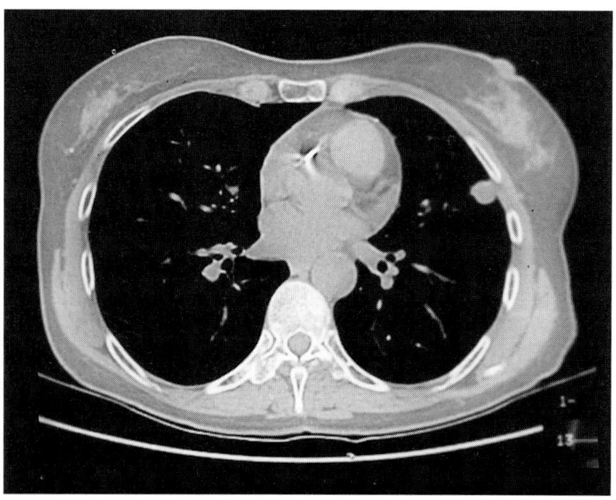

Figure 16–2. Computed tomographic scan demonstrating that the nodule seen in Figure 16–1 is pleurally based and suitable for VATS wedge resection.

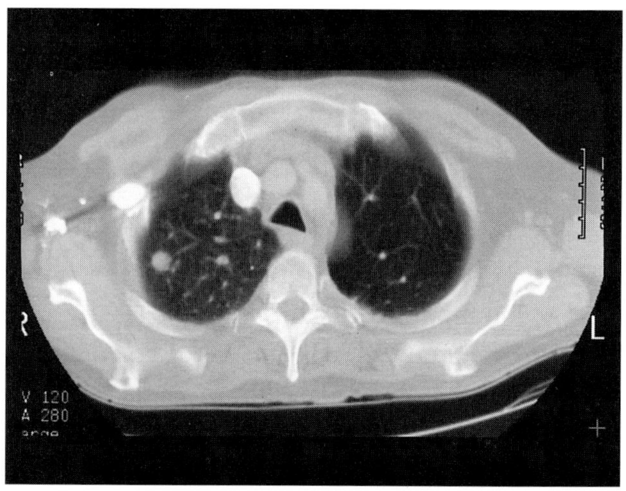

Figure 16–3. Computed tomographic scan demonstrating a nodule in the apical segment of the right upper lobe that is 8 mm beneath the pleural surface and suitable for video-assisted thoracic surgery (VATS) wedge resection.

face over it, care should be taken to avoid grasping the nodule directly.

The third port (12 mm) is placed at a distance from both the nodule and the camera port, forming a triangle to enable the wedge resection to be performed using an endoscopic stapling device. It is reasonable to place the camera though a 12-mm port, because this provides the option of applying the stapler from either one of the two working ports (see Chapter 5).

Specimens are placed in a plastic bag (or surgical glove) so they do not come into contract with the port site tissues when they are removed.

Results

Several retrospective series have been published documenting the spectrum of indications and results of VATS. A summary of the larger series of VATS resection of pulmonary nodules is presented in Table 16–1.

Indeterminate Pulmonary Nodule

VATS wedge resection of indeterminate solitary pulmonary nodules is therapeutic when the nodule is benign. When the nodule is malignant, wedge resection is diagnostic and occasionally therapeutic. The mortality and morbidity of VATS wedge resection of indeterminate pulmonary nodules are sufficiently low that its use can be recommended.[7–10]

Primary Lung Cancer

At present, VATS resection of primary lung cancer can only be recommended for diagnostic purposes. In the Mayo Clinic series, 64 of 333 patients who underwent excision of indeterminate pulmonary nodules by VATS proved to have primary lung cancers. These patients underwent conversion to an open thoracotomy for additional pulmonary resection and sampling or dissection of mediastinal and hilar lymph nodes.[7]

Therapeutic VATS wedge resection of primary lung cancer (T1N0) followed by postoperative radiation therapy is currently being evaluated in a phase II study conducted by the Cancer and Leukemia Group B (CALGB). Eligible patients must have cardiopulmonary dysfunction sufficient to preclude anatomic lobectomy. As of March 1998, 43 of 65 patients had been selected to participate in this study. The results of this study will help determine the merit of this approach.

Cancer Metastatic to the Lung

Cancers that are metastatic to the lung are discussed in Chapter 21.

Complications

General

A retrospective review of the complications of thoracoscopy by Krasna and associates forms the basis of this section. Three hundred forty-eight thoracoscopic procedures were performed on 321 patients between November 1991 and March 1995. The conversion rate to thoracotomy was 8% (27 of 321) for the following reasons:

1. Need for further resection (N = 12)
2. Adhesions (N = 6)
3. Lesion too large (N = 3)
4. Inability to find the lesion (N = 2)
5. Inability to achieve one-lung ventilation (N = 2)
6. Lost needle localization wire (N = 1)
7. Bleeding (N = 1).

In this series, there were 2 early postoperative explorations for bleeding, a total of 14 complications (4%), and no deaths.[11]

Specific

Port Site Seeding. The seeding of port sites or access incisions by tumor has been the subject of several case reports[12–15] and one survey of 50 surgeons participating in the VATSSG (Video-Assisted Thoracic Surgery Study Group).[16] For the most part, the complication occurred when specimens were removed without first being placed in a plastic bag or surgical glove. This was thought to have resulted in the tumor cells' seeding the port site through which they were withdrawn. In a few instances, however, a chest wall recurrence occurred at a port site other than the one through which the specimen had been removed. This

Table 16–1. VATS Resection of Pulmonary Nodules

Series	No. Wedge Resections (%)	No. Benign (%)	No. Malignant (%)	Mean Length of Stay (d)	Morbidity (%)	Mortality (%)
Allen MS et al (1996)[7]	333 (43.2)	158 (47)	175 (53)	5 (median)	17	8
DeCamp MM et al (1995)[8]	360 (40.2)	147 (40)	213 (60)	3	14	1
Liu HP et al (1994)[9]	76 (25.3)	29 (38)	47 (62)	4.5	2	0
Mack MJ et al (1993)[10]	242 (NA)	127 (52)	115 (48)	2.4	4	0

NA = not available.

was attributed to the reluctance of surgeons to maintain access to the pleural space by using ports that could allow instruments that might have become contaminated by tumor cells to come into direct contact with the chest wall tissues. There was at least one report of chest wall implantation by tumor in an area remote from any incisions. The authors postulated that this may have occurred secondary to spilling of tumor cells during performance of the resection. Further refinements in thoracoscopic techniques, development of instrumentation that will permit stabilization of lung tissue adjacent to a nodule without resultant damage to the nodule itself, and placement of all potentially malignant specimens in protective bags will likely minimize the occurrence of this complication in the future.

Air Leak. Prolonged air leaks are less common after VATS resection than after standard open resections in which standard gastrointestinal anastomosis (GIA) staplers are used. This is secondary to the use of endoscopic staplers that not only fire three rows of staggered staples on each side of the specimen, but also have smaller closing volumes that render them more pneumostatic. In two large series, prolonged air leaks occurred following 42 of 569 and 3 of 348 pulmonary procedures, respectively.[8,11]

Bleeding. Bleeding necessitated conversion to thoracotomy in 1 of 348 cases reported by Krasna and associates, and in 5 of 895 cases reported by DeCamp and associates.[8,11] In 2 of 348 other cases reported by Krasna and associates, reoperation for postoperative hemorrhage was required.

Pain. Landreneau and associates have published the results of a retrospective chronic pain survey of 343 patients, 178 of whom had undergone VATS and 165 of whom had undergone lateral thoracotomy. The authors found that the incidence of residual pain (assessed by a five-point Likert scale, need for specific treatment for pain, and arm and shoulder function) in patients who underwent VATS less than 1 year previously was reduced compared with patients who had had a lateral thoracotomy within the last year. These differences were not evident in patients who were more than 1 year postsurgery.[17]

Conversion to Thoracotomy Rate. Two large series have reported conversion rates from VATS to thoracotomy of 13 of 895 (1.5%) and 27 of 348 cases (7.8%), respectively.[8,11] The most common reason for conversion to thoracotomy in the former series was bleeding (5 patients), whereas in the latter series, it was the need to perform further resection (12 patients) and adhesions (6 patients). A third series reported a conversion rate of 78 of 352 (22.1%) among patients undergoing wedge resections, predominantly because of the need for further resection (46 patients).[7]

Conclusions

VATS wedge resection can be recommended for the diagnosis and treatment of benign lung tumors and the diagnosis of indeterminate pulmonary nodules. Its role in the treatment of both primary and metastatic malignant lung tumors awaits the results of the current and future clinical trials.

References

1. Mack MJ, Gordon MJ, Postma TW, et al: Percutaneous localization of pulmonary nodules for thoracoscopic lung resection. Ann Thorac Surg 53:1123–1124, 1992.
2. Mack MJ, Shennib H, Landreneau RJ, et al: Techniques for localization of pulmonary nodules for thoracoscopic resection. J Thorac Cardiovasc Surg 106:550–553, 1993.
3. Schwarz RE, Posner MC, Plunkett MB, et al: Needle-localized thoracoscopic resection of indeterminate pulmonary nodules: Impact on management of patients with malignant disease. Ann Surg Oncol 2:49–55, 1995.
4. Gossot D, Miauz Y, Guermazi A, et al: The hook-wire technique for localization of pulmonary nodules during the thoracoscopic resection. Chest 105:1467–1469, 1994.
5. Nomori H, Horio H: Colored collagen is a long-lasting point marker for small pulmonary nodules in thoracoscopic operations. Ann Thorac Surg 61:1070–1073, 1996.
6. Shennib H, Bret P: Intraoperative transthoracic ultrasonographic localization of occult lung lesions. Ann Thorac Surg 55:767–769, 1993.
7. Allen MS, Deschamps C, Jones DM, et al: Video-assisted thoracic surgical procedures: The Mayo Experience. Mayo Clin Proc 71:351–359, 1996.
8. DeCamp MM, Jaklitsch MT, Mentzer SJ, et al: The safety and versatility of video-thoracoscopy: A prospective analysis of 895 consecutive cases. J Am Coll Surg 181:113–120, 1995.
9. Liu HP, Chang CH, Lin PJ, et al: Video-assisted thoracic surgery: The Chang Gung Experience. J Thorac Cardiovasc Surg 108:834–840, 1994.
10. Mack MJ, Hazelrigg SR, Landreneau RJ, et al: Thoracoscopy for the diagnosis of the indeterminate solitary pulmonary nodule. Ann Thorac Surg 56:825–832, 1993.
11. Krasna MJ, Deshmukh S, McLaughlin JS: Complication of thoracoscopy. Ann Thorac Surg 61:1066–1069, 1996.
12. Walsh GL, Nesbitt JC: Tumor implants after thoracoscopic resection of a metastatic sarcoma. Ann Thorac Surg 59:215–216, 1995.
13. Fry WA, Siddiqui A, Pensler JM, et al: Thoracoscopic implantation of cancer with a fatal outcome. Ann Thorac Surg 59:42–45, 1995.
14. Wille GA, Gregory R, Guernsey JM: Tumor implantation at port site of video-assisted thoracoscopic resection of pulmonary metastasis. West J Med 166:65–66,1997.
15. Yim APC, Lin J, Chan ATC, et al: Video-assisted thoracoscopic wedge resection of pulmonary metastatic osteosarcoma: Should it be performed? Aust NZ J Surg 65:737–739, 1995.
16. Downey RJ, McCormack P, LoCicero J, et al: Dissemination of malignant tumors after video-assisted thoracic surgery: A report of twenty-one cases. J Thorac Cardiovasc Surg 111: 954–960, 1996.
17. Landreneau RJ, Mack MJ, Hazelrigg SR, et al: Prevalence of chronic pain after pulmonary resection by thoracotomy or video-assisted thoracic surgery. J Thorac Cardiovasc Surg 107:1079–1086, 1994.

Chapter 17

Anatomic Lung Resection

Giancarlo Roviaro, Federico Varoli, Contardo Vergani, and Marco Maciocco

Anatomic pulmonary resections, lobectomies, and pneumonectomies are the most difficult operations that can be attempted thoracoscopically, and a long training in conventional thoracic surgery is required to carry them out successfully.

The principles of videothoracoscopic resections do not differ from open surgery, because hilar elements, such as arteries, veins, and bronchi, must be separately isolated and transected.[1–5] The developments of mechanical endoscopic devices, such as clip appliers and automatic staplers, have allowed surgeons to perform all these maneuvers safely. Nevertheless, an endoscopic approach presents some special difficulties, such as the lack of manual palpation, three-dimensional vision, and the absence of a comprehensive view of the entire field. These factors significantly complicate the execution of this kind of surgery in comparison with traditional open surgery and, therefore, accurate and meticulous training in endoscopic surgery is mandatory.

For these reasons, anatomic pulmonary resections have not experienced the acceptance and success of other simpler procedures, such as wedge resections, bullectomies, or pleurectomies, and they are carried out in few centers, often using widely different techniques.[2–11]

Indications

As these techniques are still relatively new, indications are not yet defined owing to lack of sufficiently wide clinical experience. We regard the following main groups of diseases as indications:

1. Primary lung neoplasms at tumor-node-metastasis (TNM) stage 1, less than 4 cm in diameter, without intrabronchial growth and without atelectasis
2. Benign inflammatory disease or malformation, such as bronchiectasis, arteriovenous fistula, pulmonary sequestration, tuberculoma
3. Metastatic lesions that are located too deep within the parenchyma or too near the hilum to be amenable to wedge resection

Preoperative Evaluation

The patient is evaluated as for any major open pulmonary procedure. An accurate assessment of respiratory function and staging of the tumor are mandatory. In case of malignancy, bronchoscopy must be performed to rule out the presence of intrabronchial lesions or invasion of the bronchus, both of which would go undetected during an operation, and both of which represent absolute contraindications to carrying out the procedure. High-resolution computed tomography (CT) is helpful in defining the morphology of the mass and its relationship to neighboring pulmonary fissures. The patient must be prepared as for open surgery, because conversion to open surgery might be necessary.

Anesthesia, Position of the Patient, and Positions of the Operating Team

The patient is intubated with a double-lumen tube, which allows selective ventilation of each lung, and then placed in the lateral decubitus position as for a classic posterolateral thoracotomy. A pillow is placed under the chest, level with the inferior scapular angle, and the operating table is slanted downward on both sides from the center to ensure maximal stretching of the intercostal spaces and lowering of the patient's pelvis. This avoids hindrance to free movements of the camera (Fig 17–1). While inserting the trocars for initial exploration of the pleural cavity, the surgeon stands behind the patient; the first assistant stands in front of the surgeon; and the second assistant, who operates the camera, stands beside the latter. Two monitors are usually positioned on each side of the patient's head, because this offers the best view to all members of the team (Fig 17–2).

Port Insertion and Utility Thoracotomy

To carry out a thoracoscopic pulmonary resection, three trocars are usually required. A small incision is made that we have named the "utility thoracotomy." This is the incision through which the specimen is extracted at the end of the operation. The first trocar for the optics is inserted in the seventh or eighth intercostal space on the midaxillary line. Two other trocars are positioned under direct endoscopic vision on the anterior and posterior axillary lines between the fourth and sixth intercostal spaces, depending on the lobectomy to be carried out. Thus placed, each insertion site constitutes the vertex of a triangle, which offers optimal convergence of the instruments on the line of vision, prevents any interference between the instruments, and also prevents a mirror-imaging effect (Fig 17–3).

The first step to be carried out in every case of major pulmonary resection is a meticulous exploration of the entire pleural cavity, after first having dealt with adhesions, if present. Diffuse adhesions may take so much time and patience to overcome that conversion to open surgery would be an easier option.

Complete mobilization of the lung is essential for assessing the feasibility of the operation and ensuring the possibility of carrying out complex procedures. In a case of malignancy, this involves a veritable surgical staging procedure, which allows evaluation of the lesion, the fissures, the hilum, and the mediastinum. Thus, a decision on surgical intervention can be made and an alternative proce-

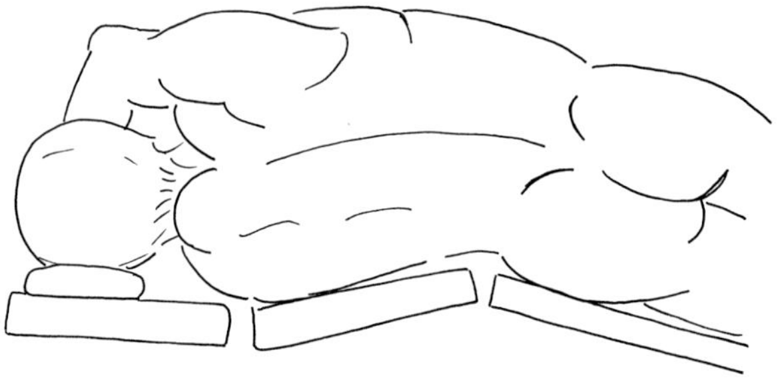

Figure 17–1. The patient lies on the table in the lateral decubitus position as for a classic posterolateral thoracotomy. The table is slanted downward from the center on both sides so that the iliac crest is lowered and does not interfere with the movements of the camera.

dure selected, if necessary. Furthermore, all thoracoscopic maneuvers are rather awkward when malignant lesions are larger than 4 cm, because weight and bulk hamper mobilization of the lung and potentiate injuries to the mass or to the parenchyma by the instruments. Such lesions, even though at TNM stage I, must be removed by video-assisted thoracotomy or conventional surgery.

Unlike other videothoracoscopic procedures, major pulmonary resections entail carrying out an additional incision—the utility thoracotomy—to withdraw the specimen. It is surprising to observe how easily a collapsed lobe or lung may be removed through a breach just a few centimeters wide (Fig 17–4). The utility thoracotomy is placed between the anterior axillary line and the sternum. In this region, the intercostal spaces are wider and there are no large muscles to incise other than the intercostal muscles and a few fibers of the serratus anterior muscle. Moreover, it is known in thoracic surgery that adhesions tend to be fewer here (Fig 17–5*A*).

For a cosmetic purpose in women, the site is marked preoperatively along the inframammary sulcus while the patient is upright; the breast then hides the incision nicely (see Fig 17–5*B*). The utility thoracotomy can be carried out at the beginning or the end of the operation. If carried out at the beginning, just after the resectability of the lesion is confirmed, it is extremely useful as a supplementary access for conventional instruments. It is also a useful emergency approach for applying a clamp on a vascular lesion and can be widened rapidly into an emergency thoracotomy. The utility thoracotomy is too small to provide direct vision of the field and, therefore, cannot be used as a "small" thoracotomy.

A rib spreader is not used unless there are difficulties in extracting the mass at the end of the procedure, and, even then, it is used as briefly and gently as possible, to avoid applying protracted pressure on the intercostal nerve and vessels, which could lead to severe postoperative pain. Retrieving the specimen requires particular precautions (see Fig 17–4). The specimen should not be extracted by grasping it at the hilum, because the bronchial branching, with its dependent increase in size, would wedge the specimen firmly within the breach. It is much better to grasp the edge closest to the tumor with a Duval forceps and extract the tumor first, so that greater traction may be applied safely to the remaining parenchyma.

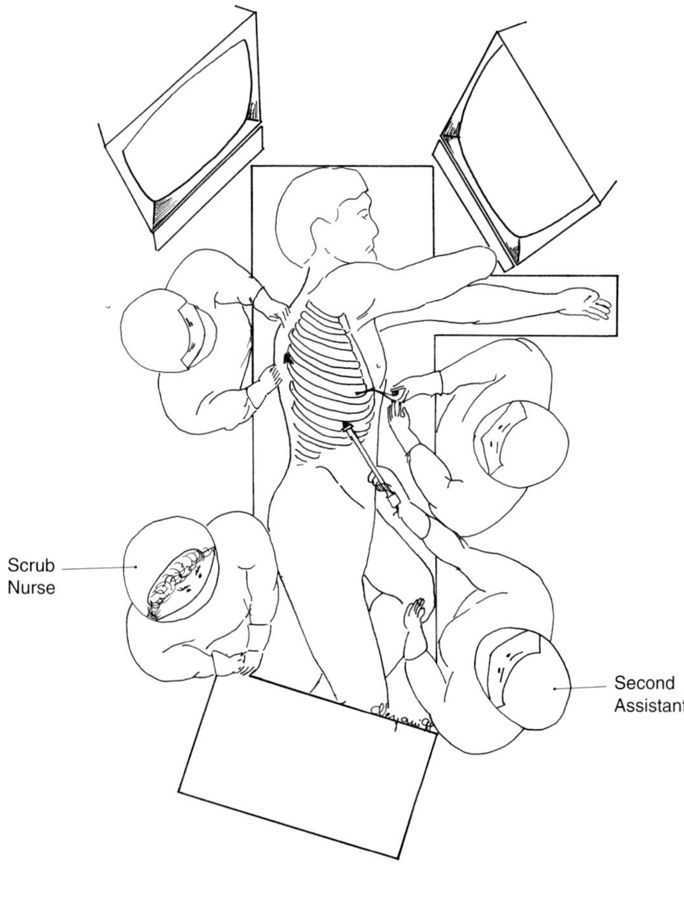

Figure 17–2. Positions of the operating team. The second assistant wields the camera. The surgeon and first assistant change position during the operation according to the different steps. At the beginning, the surgeon usually stands behind the patient while inserting the ports and for the general inspection. The surgeon then moves to the front of the patient to operate through the ports and the utility thoracotomy. Two monitors are essential to provide all members of the team with an optimal view.

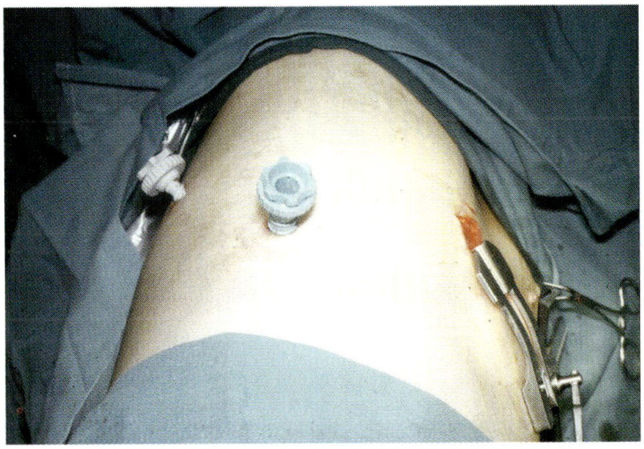

Figure 17–3. The intraoperative photo shows the sites of insertion of the trocars and of the utility thoracotomy. The utility thoracotomy has been carried out anteriorly along the inframammary sulcus. The camera is inserted through the most inferior central port positioned in the seventh or eighth intercostal space. The rib spreader is positioned at the end of the operation to withdraw the specimen, or, exceptionally, during the operation for particularly difficult steps.

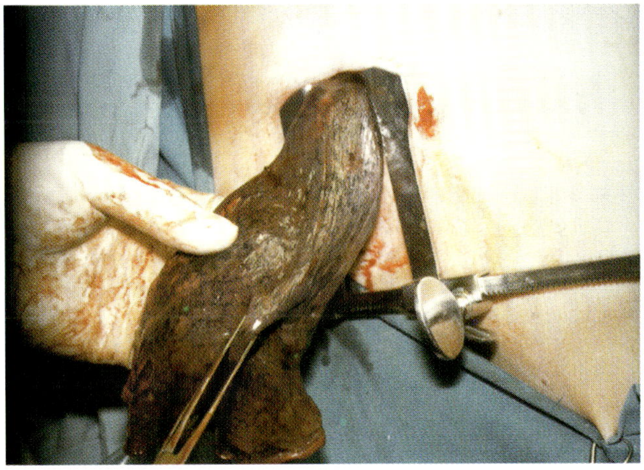

Figure 17–4. The resected specimen is easily extracted through the small utility thoracotomy incision. The rib spreader is positioned and widened for the final step to prevent postoperative pain from intercostal nerve trauma.

Following extraction of the tumor, the lung is engaged and extracted with gentle swinging movements. Neoplasms located deep within the parenchyma theoretically present no risk of seeding. Vice versa, when the tumor is superficial, protecting the edges of the wound is mandatory. We usually insert the specimen in a large plastic bag, the margins of which are drawn out and spread over the wound to protect the incision. The resected parenchyma is grasped within the bag and slipped simultaneously out of both bag and thorax.

The role of the utility thoracotomy may appear to be solely the extraction of the specimen; however, it is important in defining what exactly is meant by thoracoscopic, video-assisted, combined procedure, or conventional surgery.

Procedures that are strictly thoracoscopic are those in which all members of the operating team carry out the entire procedure by viewing a monitor exclusively; they, therefore, all have exactly the same view of the operative field, and all actions are synchronous because of the same view. In the case of video-assisted procedures, the first surgeon often looks through the thoracotomy, using the optics in this case merely to illuminate the limited operative field. The first surgeon's view differs from that of the other surgeons, who are, therefore, constrained to a rather passive function. Moreover, in this kind of surgery, as well as in all other middle or posterior thoracotomies, a rib spreader is used throughout the procedure; thus, the main advantage of thoracoscopy, namely, the diminution of postoperative pain, is thwarted.

General Principles

As previously described, exploration of the pleural cavity must be carried out after adequate mobilization of the lung

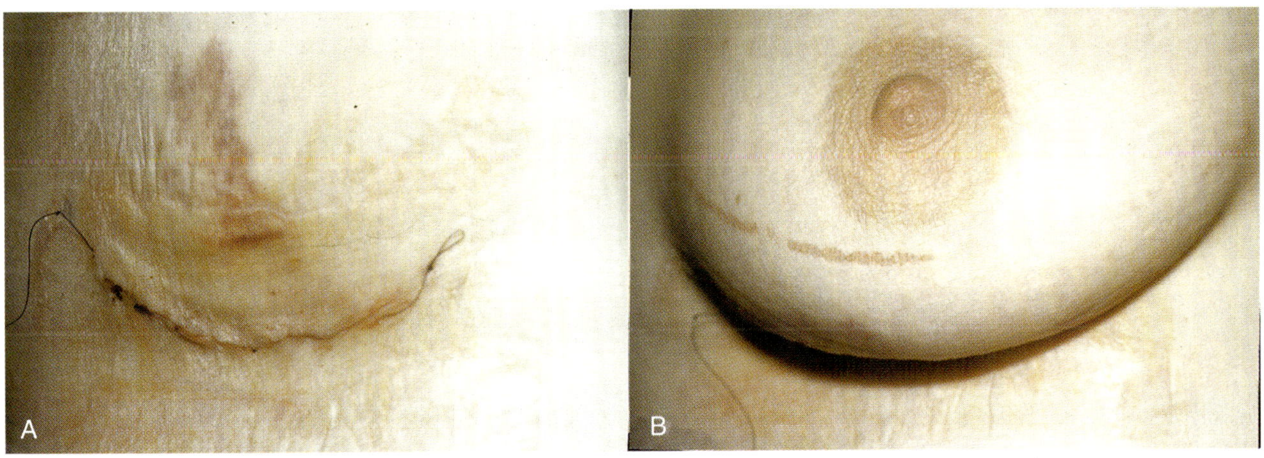

Figure 17–5. The utility thoracotomy incision is carried out along the inframammary sulcus. At this site there are no large muscles, the intercostal spaces are wider, and intracavitary adhesions generally tend to be fewer. *A*, The utility thoracotomy on the first postoperative day. The breast has been displaced upward. *B*, When the breast is back in its anatomic location, the incision is nicely hidden.

to stage the lesion, assess the resectability, and choose the approach for resection. A thorough evaluation of the fissure is of paramount importance, because, occasionally, the fissure is poorly developed and cannot be completed with endostaplers; in such circumstances, the procedure must be converted. In our experience, this was the most frequent cause for conversion. After the fissure and mediastinum are evaluated and the resectability of the lesion is confirmed, the true anatomic major thoracoscopic resection can be started. It must be borne in mind, however, that precautionary conversion for technical or oncologic reasons is by far preferable to an unjustified adventure and such a decision would speak for the maturity of the operator rather than representing a technical failure.

Assessment of thoracoscopic resectability proceeds along with the dissecting maneuvers, and the surgeon must always be prepared to change strategy and tactics of approach. The operative procedures follow the main principles of conventional open lobectomies. Schematically, three main phases can be described:

1. Mediastinal
2. Fissural
3. Bronchial

Mediastinal Phase

The mediastinum must be inspected accurately in close-up vision and explored by means of palpation with rigid endoscopic instruments.

Isolation and transection of the mediastinal vessels usually follow the same procedure in all types of major pulmonary resections. A solid knowledge of the anatomy of the main hilum is necessary, because difficulties are greater than in open surgery owing to the limited access and the relative inadequacy of the rigid endoscopic instruments. In this kind of surgery, all vessels must be isolated extensively to allow positioning of mechanical endostaplers, because these instruments are thicker than conventional ligature carriers. As a rule, the artery is divided before the vein, and the bronchus is sectioned last.

This should not be a rigid approach. Sometimes, it is more convenient to isolate and separate the vein before the artery. In much the same way, all other steps can follow a different sequence to facilitate the operation. When the loose outer coating of tissue (over the adventitia of vessels) that extends from the pericardium is thin, the vessels can be seen through it, and gentle swabbing toward the lung (never in the opposite direction) usually achieves isolation of the anterior and lateral surface of the vessels. If the tissue is thicker, it can be grasped and incised with scissors to obtain a cleavage plane between it and the vascular wall. The vessel is mobilized circumferentially, encircled with a ligature carrier or a Roticulator grasper, and encircled by a thread (Fig 17–6). Traction on this sling facilitates dissection of the deep aspect and, finally, positioning the endostapler.

Positioning the stapler is often a difficult and critical step. The rigidity of the ribs and the narrowness of the intercostal spaces limit the maneuverability of the instruments, which are too long and too rigidly rectilinear to allow much freedom of movement.

Several attempts may be required before the stapler is inserted at the correct angle. The jaws of the instrument should grip well beyond the vessel to staple and transect safely. The surgeons may have to change their positions repeatedly and insert the stapler through the trocars or even through the utility thoracotomy. Great care must be taken to avoid any dangerous traction on the instruments. It is difficult to evaluate intensity because leverage is determined by the length of the instruments from the fulcrum (the parietal insertion site). Furthermore, the lack of angulation of the staplers increases the difficulty of positioning.

Arteries and veins are transected in a similar fashion, with the realization that the arterial wall is less elastic and much more fragile than the venous one. If the stapler is correctly positioned, the two stumps immediately fall apart after firing. Some residual uncut adventitial fibers can be severed cautiously with scissors between the two triple-staggered rows of staples.

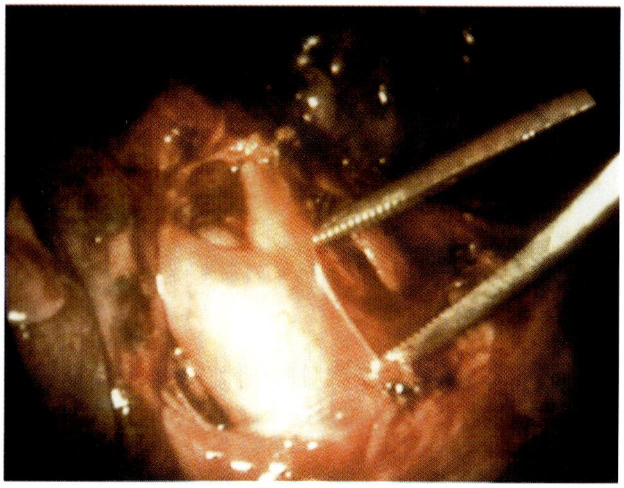

Figure 17–6. The vessel is isolated and encircled with thread by means of a conventional ligature carrier or with a Roticulator grasper. Gentle traction on the thread facilitates positioning the stapler. Here the superior right pulmonary vein has been isolated and encircled during a right upper lobectomy.

Fissural Phase

Isolating the artery within the fissure is a crucial step when performing a lobectomy. The lobar hilum is much more complex than the main hilum. Located deep in the parenchyma, it has adhering lymph nodes and more branchings. In young patients, the fissure is usually well defined and the artery can be seen clearly beating deep within the fissure. In these cases, isolating the vessel is a delicate but not difficult task if the general principles are respected. Once the vessel has been isolated, the artery or the arterial branches can be stapled or clipped according to their size (Fig 17–7). Smaller vessels, such as veins and arteries for the middle lobe, the lingula, the left upper lobe, or the posterior ascending artery, can usually be sectioned between clips. The parenchyma can usually be stapled to complete a partially fused fissure. In this case, it is sometimes necessary to compress the thick parenchyma with a clamp before positioning the stapler to avoid suboptimal closure of the device, which would lead to the

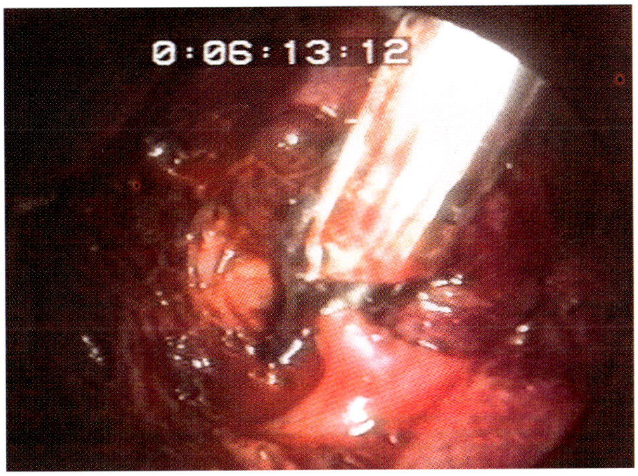

Figure 17–7. In this case of a right upper lobectomy, the lobar artery within the fissure is dissected. The posterior ascending artery has been isolated and can be clipped.

development of air leaks or bleeding when the lung is re-expanded.

When the fissure is markedly thickened because of emphysema or inflammatory reactions, or when the lymph nodes are enlarged and calcified, isolating the artery can be very difficult, and conversion to an open procedure is often recommended or even required.

Bronchial Phase

The bronchus is usually the last element to be divided, but tactics can be altered as required.

Many different techniques can be employed, and endostaplers have greatly simplified the procedure. Principles that must be followed to avoid fistulization of the bronchial stump are the same as for conventional surgery. The bronchial stump must be left with adequate vascularization, and to avoid stagnation of bronchial secretions, it must not be excessively long. Careful dissection of the bronchus can be accomplished using a mounted swab combined with electrocoagulation and sharp dissection. Peribronchial lymph nodes can be difficult to separate from the bronchus without causing excessive devascularization. Small bronchial vessels may be clipped easily.

When the bronchus has been isolated, it is stapled with an endostapler and divided. A lobar bronchus is usually resected using an endostapler that has 3.5-mm staples, whereas the main stem bronchus, or an abnormally thickened lobar bronchus, must be secured with 4.8-mm staples. Sometimes, an apical lower bronchus originates at the same level of the middle bronchus. In this case separate stapling of the common basal bronchus and the lower apical is required.

Dealing With Lymph Nodes

If enlarged mediastinal, fissural, and peribronchial lymph nodes are present, they generally complicate all dissecting maneuvers.

In the case of a benign disease, such as bronchiectasis or tuberculosis, the dissection of calcified lymph nodes from vascular structures to proceed with section suture can cause an accidental injury to adjacent vascular elements, and the ensuing bleeding can be difficult to control thoracoscopically. In such technically difficult circumstances, it is extremely dangerous to continue and much safer to proceed with conversion.

If there is a malignancy, the difficulties are increased by the oncologic radicality of the procedure. As mentioned, the indication for major lung resection in a case of malignancy is restricted to patients at TNM stage I. The presence of enlarged mediastinal or fissural lymph nodes detected during the procedure represents, therefore, understaging during the preoperative diagnosis, or merely reactive hyperplasia, such as is frequently encountered in smokers or patients who have chronic bronchitis. Such lymph nodes must be removed and sent for frozen section examination. In our opinion, if N1 or N2 disease is established, conversion to thoracotomy is mandatory, irrespective of whatever phase of the procedure has been reached. Lymphadenectomy is technically feasible thoracoscopically[2, 3, 8] and may be carried out in a fashion similar to conventional open procedures; however, available follow-up at present is insufficient, and the series are too small to confirm comparable results for conventional and thoracoscopic procedures. For these reasons, we prefer to limit indications to patients who are intraoperatively staged N0.

Of 152 patients who had major thoracoscopic lung resections for malignant disease, 17 were found to have N1 disease and 6 were found to have N2 disease at postoperative staging, even though the lymph nodes had seemed normal during the operation.

There are different opinions about what constitutes the best approach to dealing with lymph nodes in lung cancer, and different techniques when resection is considered. Many surgeons carry out radical lymphadenectomy routinely, but others perform lymph-node sampling to determine the stage of the disease before deciding how best to proceed. The correct answer will probably derive from a better understanding of tumor biology, which remains the decisive factor in determining the outcome, rather than from the exact surgical technique.

We usually carry out thoracoscopic lymphadenectomy similar to the way it is performed in any conventional open procedure. The mean number of lymph nodes removed by our team during thoracoscopic and thoracotomic resections for cancers at the same stage is similar. The steps followed during a thoracoscopic lymphadenectomy are the same as in conventional surgery, even though lymph nodes are not removed "en bloc," but rather one by one as they are encountered. Lymph nodes that are free from disease are usually removed rather easily. Whenever difficulties are encountered, frozen section examination must be performed to rule out any pathologic process. Small vessels sometimes bleed annoyingly, and great care must be taken when coagulating them. The removal of anterior mediastinal and paraesophageal lymph nodes does not usually present particular difficulties. Right paratracheal lymph nodes are usually easier to remove after the azygos vein is sectioned with an endostapler. On the left side, particular care must be taken to identify the left vagus and recurrent nerves before removing the left paratracheal nodes.

Greater technical difficulties may be encountered when

an attempt is made to remove the carinal lymph nodes, particularly from the left side, but patience and accurate dissection can usually accomplish the task.

Specific Aspects

Right Upper Lobectomy (RUL)

Right upper lobectomy (RUL) is one of the most difficult lobectomies that can be undertaken, because the artery must be isolated both in the mediastinum and within the fissure.

After the trocars have been positioned and the utility thoracotomy has been carried out opposite the mediastinal hilum, the upper lobe is gently drawn posteriorly by the assistant. The vena cava and the underlying vascular elements for the right lung dominate the field. The superior pulmonary vein is isolated first, and must be dissected until the venous branches from the upper and middle lobe are freed (see Fig 17–6). The upper branch is encircled with a Roticulator Endograsp (Autosuture, United States Surgical Corporation, Norwalk, CT) or a conventional dissector, and a sling is placed to facilitate positioning of the stapler without damaging the intermediate artery, which lies just behind the vein.

The artery is isolated with a mounted swab until the anterior (Boyden's) trunk and the intermediate artery for the fissure are visible. The latter is then approached through the fissure, which can be completed with the stapler, if necessary. Arterial dissection in the fissure is a delicate task, because the posterior ascending artery must also be exposed adequately. The anterior trunk is stapled, and the posterior ascending artery is usually severed between clips. The lung is displaced anteriorly to expose the upper bronchus, which is also surrounded with a sling and stapled.

If isolation of the posterior ascending artery is particularly difficult, it is sometimes better to divide the vein and the anterior trunk, and then section the bronchus. This sequence makes it easier to complete the fissure with an endoscopic stapler and include the posterior ascending artery within the stapled line.

Middle Lobectomy (ML)

Middle lobectomy (ML) is usually a simple procedure. The first step is the isolation of the superior pulmonary vein as for RUL. The branch for the middle lobe is isolated, encircled with a thread, and usually divided between clips. The fissure between the middle and lower lobe is incised, the artery is isolated, and the branch for the middle lobe is identified (see Fig 17–7). The dissection must be extended distally to rule out the presence of a possible second branch for the middle lobe. The middle bronchus can then be identified and stapled. The main fissure can be completed when necessary.

Right Lower Lobectomy (RLL) and Left Lower Lobectomy (LLL)

Right lower lobectomy (RLL) and left lower lobectomy (LLL) have many aspects in common. The first steps are dissection of the pulmonary ligament and isolation of the inferior pulmonary vein. The lung is grasped and drawn upward to achieve a mild tension of the ligament, which is then dissected up to the vein. The vein is encircled with a sling and stapled.

The artery must then be isolated within the fissure. On the right side, the isolation must also expose the branches for the middle lobe and for the apical lower segment (see Fig 17–7). During a left lobectomy, the artery must be isolated for a longer period of time to expose all the branches for the lingula. The branches for the basal segments and for the apical lower segment are then clipped and severed. The lung can then be displaced anteriorly to expose the bronchus, which is isolated with scissors and swab, encircled, and stapled. When required, the fissures can be completed with an endoscopic stapler. A poorly developed fissure can be identified more easily by partially inflating the lung after the bronchus has been stapled.

Left Upper Lobectomy (LUL)

A left upper lobectomy (LUL) is certainly the most difficult operation that can be carried out thoracoscopically, mostly because of the presence of arterial branches that originate from the fissure and those that originate from the arc of the pulmonary artery. We waited almost 2 years from the start of our experience before attempting such a procedure for fear of injuring the vascular elements, which are very easily damaged even in conventional open procedures. However, as our experience in major thoracoscopic surgery increased, we gradually devised some clever technical maneuvers. We now carry out LULs routinely. After the lung has been displaced posteriorly with an endograsp, the branches of the vein for the upper lobe and the lingula must be identified, and the vein to the upper lobe must be isolated. After anterior and lateral aspects of the vein have been isolated, a thread is passed around the vein. It is very important at this point to bear in mind that the bronchus for the upper lobe lies close to the vein's posterior aspect. When the vein is sectioned with an endostapler, the bronchi for the upper and lower lobes are exposed. Isolating the lobe for the upper bronchus is relatively easy. However, care must be taken because of the close proximity of the pulmonary artery to the posterior aspect of the vein. Keeping close to the bronchial wall, a thread can be passed using gentle and cautious widening movements of the ligature carrier. Once the sling is ready, the bronchus can be sectioned, exposing the spectacular sight of the pulsating pulmonary artery with its branches for the upper lobe. These branches must be isolated gently and very cautiously. Most of them can be sectioned between clips. Larger branches, particularly the first mediastinal branch, may require an endostapler.

Mastering the technique of thoracoscopic lobectomy was such a pleasant and fascinating discovery process, that we now carry out most of our LULs using this approach. With the surgeon standing in front of the patient, the operation proceeds as already described (see Figure 17–2).

Right and Left Pneumonectomy (RP, LP)

Pneumonectomies are technically simpler to carry through than lobectomies, because the main hilum is anatomically much simpler. Arteries and veins do not present abnormalities and anatomic variants, and, even more important, there is no fissural phase for isolating the artery throughout the procedure. The indications for carrying out a thoracoscopic pneumonectomy are rare, and include the following:

1. Two parenchymal tumors
2. A small tumor, located at the secondary carina, which cannot be removed by bronchoplasty techniques
3. Parenchymal tumors, smaller than 4 cm, which appear to infiltrate the fissure on high-definition CT

When the intended operation is a lobectomy, but thoracoscopic dissection proves extremely difficult or technically impossible, we believe the operation should not be changed to a thoracoscopic pneumonectomy, which is not an alternative to a difficult thoracoscopic lobectomy.

The operating time for a thoracoscopic pneumonectomy is much the same as for a conventional pneumonectomy. The first surgeon almost always takes a position in front of the patient, facing the mediastinal vascular hilum. The utility thoracotomy is usually carried out in the third or fourth space, at a slightly higher level than for a lobectomy. It must be carried out under direct thoracoscopic vision to face the mediastinal vascular hilum and to allow rapid insertion of conventional vascular clamps in case vascular lesions should occur.

The upper pulmonary vein is always isolated first, using the same maneuvers as described in cases of RUL or LUL. When the vein has been sectioned, the arteries are exposed: The common trunk on the left, the intermediate artery, and the anterior (Boyden's) trunk on the right. On the left side, the artery is usually larger, and isolation may require changing the position of the optics to improve the view, especially in its upper and lower aspects. When the artery is free, a sling should be passed to reduce the caliber of the vessel and facilitate placing the endostapler. On the left side, the artery can obviously be sectioned only on the common trunk, whereas, on the right side, when isolating the pulmonary artery on the common trunk proves difficult, the Boyden trunk and the intermediate artery can be sectioned separately.

The pulmonary ligament is sectioned, and the lower pulmonary vein is then isolated and sectioned with a stapler.

After all the other vascular elements have been sectioned, a sling is passed around the bronchus, which is then sectioned, taking care to draw the lung slightly upward so that the stapler can be positioned ideally, as closely or inferiorly as possible. The thickness of the bronchial wall requires 4.8-mm staples; either endoscopic or conventional staplers inserted through the utility thoracotomy can be employed.

Intraoperative Complications

Complications that can occur during the course of videothoracoscopic operations are the same as for conventional procedures and are mainly occasioned by the surgeon's limited experience, technical difficulties, or inadequate or improper use of instrumentation.

When a complication occurs, the surgeon is faced with the choice between attempting to solve the problem thoracoscopically or converting to an open procedure. The most frightening and dreaded complication that can occur during a thoracoscopic procedure is bleeding from a great vessel. Indeed, many thoracic surgeons avoid this technique because they fear this very complication. We believe the surgeon confronted with this complication should carry out temporary thoracoscopic control of the bleeding rapidly, and then convert to thoracotomy.

Vascular lesions can occur during fissural or hilar dissection of the artery, or while the attempt is being made to encircle the vessel with ligature carriers or staplers. Theoretically, stapler malfunction and failure to secure the margins of the vessel can also occur. For these reasons, many surgeons prefer to remove the blade before firing the stapler, and divide the vessel only after having applied the staples.

The utility thoracotomy is of the utmost importance in the case of vascular lesions, because a conventional vascular clamp can be inserted promptly. Sometimes, the bleeding can be controlled thoracoscopically by clipping or stapling the vessel with an endoscopic stapler. When this cannot be done, the utility thoracotomy must be rapidly extended while the bleeding is controlled by temporarily using a mounted swab inserted through the utility thoracotomy.

Postoperative Course and Complications

The advantage of not having a wide thoracotomic incision is the great reduction of postoperative pain. For the patient, this affords a quicker recovery of normal ventilation and cough reflex, as well as a more rapid return to normal life and activities than after an open procedure.

Postoperative hospital stay is usually shorter and the patient can be mobilized within a few hours after the operation. However, in the case of elderly patients, or when the fissure was not well defined and required much dissection, persistent air leaks can prevent removing the underwater seal drain. When the bubbling begins to decrease, a Heimlich valve can be adopted, which enables the patient to be discharged from the hospital.

Postoperative complications are usually the same as those that occur after conventional surgery and are, therefore, not peculiar to thoracoscopic surgery. The most frequent postoperative complications are bleeding, bronchial fistulae, and empyema. Whenever these occur, the surgeon must decide whether a conservative treatment will be adequate, or whether rethoracoscopy, or even thoracotomy, will serve best.

In case of hemothorax or empyema, both hemostasis and drainage can be carried out thoracoscopically.

Tumor seeding at the insertion site of the trocars, or on the utility thoracotomy incision, has been reported.[15, 16] In this case, insertion of the specimen into a plastic bag before extracting it from the chest can reduce the frequency of this complication.

Conclusions

Even though at present thoracoscopic anatomic lung resections are accepted as a feasible procedure, their routine application is still rare in thoracic surgery practice. The main reasons are that precise indications have not yet been stated definitively, particularly regarding resection for malignancy. Isolation of hilar vessels remains a technical challenge for surgeons, and major bleeding remains a dreaded potential complication. Moreover, these techniques still need to be standardized, and endoscopic instruments still need to be improved.

These procedures certainly offer greatly reduced trauma and marked decrease of postoperative pain. Consequently, postoperative hospital stay is shortened and patients can look forward to earlier resumption of usual daily activities. All these factors contribute to reduced costs. It is, therefore, reasonable to expect an increase in application, even though these techniques require solid conventional thoracic experience as well as specific endoscopic training. Wider acceptance, larger series, and longer follow-ups will provide data for assessment of the role of thoracoscopic anatomic lung resections in modern thoracic surgery practice.

References

1. Roviaro CG, Rebuffat C, Varoli F, et al: Videoendoscopic pulmonary lobectomy for cancer. Surg Laparosc Endosc 2:244–247, 1992.
2. Roviaro CG, Rebuffat C, Varoli F, et al: Major videothoracoscopic pulmonary resections. Endosc Surg 1:288–293, 1993.
3. Roviaro CG, Varoli F, Rebuffat C, et al: Videothoracoscopic major pulmonary resections. Ann Thorac Surg 56:779–783, 1993.
4. Kirby TJ, Mack MJ, Landreneau RJ, et al: Initial experience with video-assisted thoracoscopic lobectomy. Ann Thorac Surg 56: 1248–1253, 1993.
5. Yim APC, Kai-ming Ko, Wing-shun Chau, et al: Video-assisted thoracoscopic anatomic lung resections: The initial Hong Kong experience. Chest 109:13–17, 1996.
6. Lewis RJ, Caccavale RJ, Sisler GE, et al: One hundred consecutive patients undergoing video-assisted thoracic operations. Ann Thorac Surg 54:421–426, 1992.
7. Lewis RJ: The role of video-assisted thoracic surgery for carcinoma of the lung: Wedge resection to lobectomy by simultaneous individual stapling. Ann Thorac Surg 56:762–768, 1993.
8. McKenna RJ: Lobectomy by video-assisted thoracic surgery with mediastinal node sampling for lung cancer. J Thorac Cardiovasc Surg 107:879–882, 1994.
9. Lewis RJ: Simultaneous stapled lobectomy: A safe technique for video-assisted thoracic surgery. J Thorac Cardiovasc Surg 109:619–625, 1995.
10. Walker WS, Carnochan FM, et al: Thoracoscopic pulmonary lobectomy. Early operative experience and preliminary clinical results. J Thorac Cardiovasc Surg 106:1111–1117, 1993.
11. Walker WS, Carnochan FM, Matter S: Video-assisted thoracoscopic pneumonectomy. Br J Surg 81:81,82,1994.
12. Giudicelli R, Thomas P, Lonjon T, et al: Comparative study of lobectomy through thoracotomy and video-assisted thoracoscopy. Ann Thorac Surg 58:712–718, 1994.
13. Kirby TJ, Mack MJ, Landreneau RJ, et al: Lobectomy: VATS vs thoracotomy. A randomized study. Presented at the 74th Annual Meeting of the American Association for Thoracic Surgery, New York, April 24–27, 1994.
14. Kirby TJ, Mack MJ, Landreneau RJ, et al: Lobectomy: VATS vs thoracotomy: A randomized study. J Thorac Cardiovasc Surg 109:997–1002, 1995.
15. Yim APC: Port site recurrence following videoassisted thoracoscopic surgery. Surg Endosc 9:1133–1135, 1995.
16. Fry WA, Siddiqui A, Pensler JM, et al: Thoracoscopic implantation of cancer with a fatal outcome. Ann Thorac Surg 59:42–45, 1995.

COMMENTARY

Robert J. McKenna, Jr.

Many patients believe that a video-assisted thoracic surgical (VATS) approach for a lobectomy is preferable to a thoracotomy because it is less invasive. Although the worldwide experience with VATS lobectomy demonstrates that it can be performed with reasonable safety,[1–7] the medical community has questioned the adequacy of the cancer operation and whether there is any advantage to VATS lobectomy.

There are at present substantial data about the procedure from around the world, which facilitate assessment of the safety of VATS lobectomy. The results of the larger published series of VATS lobectomies and pneumonectomies (Table 17A–1) compare favorably with the results expected of a thoracotomy.[1–7] Complications occurred in 10 to 21.9% of patients after they underwent VATS lobectomy. These included prolonged air leak (5 to 10%), arrhythmias, pneumonia, and respiratory failure. Transfusions were necessary in 0 to 3% of patients. Bronchial stump leak required surgical repair in 4 (0.36%) cases. Seven (0.6%) deaths in 1120 patients were caused by venous mesenteric infarct, myocardial infarction, respiratory failure, or unknown reasons. The risk of massive intraoperative bleeding appeared to be

Table 17A–1. Mortality and Length of Stay for VATS Lobectomy

Reference	N	Cancer	Mortality (%)	LOS
Lewis	200	171	0	3.07
Yim	214	168	1 (0.4)	6.8
Kasada	145	103	1 (0.8)	NA
Hermansson	30	15	0	4.4
Walker	150	123	3 (2)	7.2
Roviaro	169	142	1 (0.5)	NA
McKenna	212	212	1 (0.5)	4.6
Total	1120	934	7 (0.6)	5.28

LOS = length of stay

quite small. A 1997 survey of 23 surgeons who performed 1560 VATS lobectomies found only one intraoperative death, which was related not to bleeding[8] but to an intraoperative myocardial infarction.

Although two prospective studies have shown that patients received some benefits from lobectomy by VATS compared with those received from lobectomy by thoracotomy,[9–10] these studies failed to prove conclusively any superiority for the VATS approach. Compared with lobectomy via thoracotomy, the VATS approach appeared to offer a shorter hospital stay and either comparable or reduced morbidity and mortality.

Patients generally appeared to have less pain after VATS lobectomy compared with that experienced by patients after lobectomy by thoracotomy. Walker[11] compared the requirement for narcotic pain medication in his 83 VATS resections with that of 110 patients who underwent thoracotomy during the same time period. On average, the VATS group used less morphine than did the thoracotomy group (57 vs 83 mg morphine, $P < 0.001$). The incidence of post-thoracotomy pain syndrome after VATS lobectomy (2.2%) was lower than that expected after thoracotomy.

A VATS lobectomy should be an adequate cancer operation because, as Roviaro describes, it is a standard anatomic resection. A 1997 international survey[8] of 1560 VATS lobectomies by 23 surgeons who had performed at least 20 of these procedures showed that during these operations mediastinal nodes were biopsied by mediastinoscopy alone (22.7%), mediastinoscopy, and lymph node sampling (32%), or lymph node dissection (45.5%). Kaseda[2] reported that lymph node dissection combined with VATS lobectomy yielded an average of 23 lymph nodes (range 10 to 51). Long-term, disease-free survival is the ultimate measure for the adequacy of any cancer operation.[12] Kaseda[2] reported a 94% 4-year survival rate for stage I lung cancer resected by VATS lobectomy. In another assessment of lung cancer resections, Lewis[3] found a 3-year survival rate of 94% for stage I, 57% for stage II, and 25% for stage III. This suggests that lung cancer surgery can be performed by VATS without compromising the survival rate achieved with a thoracotomy. Although seeding of VATS incisions has occurred,[13] the incidence of this appeared to be less than 0.5%.[1–7]

There will be further refinement of the VATS lobectomy technique in the future. This will come in part from the sharing of experiences in chapters such as this. For example, Roviaro[3] states that a right upper lobectomy, which is the most common lobectomy that we perform at present, is difficult to accomplish with VATS. Our approach is to operate from an anterior location.[14]

A cautious approach is recommended toward performance of lobectomy by VATS. The VATS procedure is not appropriate for all lobectomies or for all surgeons. It requires that the surgeon have excellent video skills and comprehensive knowledge of thoracic anatomy. The procedure should be performed only in appropriately selected patients by surgeons who have skills in VATS techniques that allow them to perform a complete cancer operation, rather than a compromise operation, with minimal morbidity and mortality. Care should be taken to minimize the risk of local recurrence by placing the specimen in a bag. Because there is a risk of bleeding, the surgeon must be prepared for this possibility.

References

1. Hermansson U, Konstantinov IE, Aren C: VATS lobectomy: The initial Swedish experience. Semin Thorac Cardiovasc Surg 10:285–290, 1998.
2. Kaseda S, Aoki T, Hangai N: VATS lobectomy: The Japanese experience. Semin Thorac Cardiovasc Surg 10:300–304, 1998.
3. Lewis RJ, Caccavale RJ: VATS lobectomy. Semin Thorac Cardiovasc Surg 332–339, 1998.
4. McKenna RJ Jr, Fischel RJ, Wurnig P, et al: VATS lobectomy: The Los Angeles experience, Semin Thorac Cardiovasc Surg 10:321–325, 1998.
5. Roviaro G, Varoli F, Vergani C, et al: VATS major pulmonary resections: The Italian experience. Semin Thorac Cardiovasc Surg 10:313–320, 1998.
6. Walker WS: VATS lobectomy: The Edinburgh experience. Semin Thorac Cardiovasc Surg 10:291–299, 1998.
7. Yim APC, Liu H, Izzat MB, et al: Thoracoscopic major lung resections—An Asian perspective. Semin Thorac Cardiovasc 10:326–331, 1998.
8. Mackinlay TA: VATS lobectomy: An international survey. Presented at the IVth International Symposium on Thoracoscopy and Video-Assisted Thoracic Surgery, Sao Paulo, Brazil, May 1997.
9. Giudicelli R, Thomas P, Lonjon T, et al: Video-assisted minithoracotomy versus muscle-sparing thoracotomy for performing lobectomy. Ann Thorac Surg 58:712–718, 1994.
10. Kirby TJ, Mack MJ, Landreneau RJ, et al: Lobectomy video assisted surgery versus muscle sparing thoracotomy. A randomized trial. J Thorac Cardiovasc Surg 109:997–1002, 1995.
11. Walker WS, Pugh GC, Craig SR, et al: Continued experience with thoracoscopic major pulmonary resection. Int Surg 81:255–258, 1996.
12. McKenna RJ Jr, Wolf RK, Brenner M, et al: Is VATS lobectomy an adequate cancer operation? Ann Thorac Surg 66:1903–1908, 1998.
13. Downey RJ, McCormick P, LoCicero J, et al: Dissemination of malignant tumors after video-assisted thoracic surgery: A report of twenty-one cases. J Thorac Cardiovasc Surg 111:954–960, 1996.
14. McKenna RJ Jr: VATS lobectomy with mediastinal lymph node sampling or dissection. Chest Surg Clin North Am 4:223–232, 1995.

Chapter 18

Thoracoscopic Lobectomy With Mediastinal Lymph Node Dissection or Sampling

Tsuguo Naruke

Video-assisted thoracoscopic surgery (VATS) should be recognized as a remarkable development in the history of medical science. The rapid evolution of VATS derives mostly from the emphasis put on the minimally invasive character of the technique itself. However, other factors have also played a role in the development of this technique. These include the enthusiasm of surgeons, demands of patients, and promotion by the media.

In addition, there have been rapid technical developments, including miniaturization of video components and innovation and invention of surgical instruments, especially the endoscopic stapling device.

The enthusiasm of surgeons for the VATS approach to thoracic disease has been spurred by its minimally invasive nature, because this approach results in reduced morbidity and rapid recuperation. Many surgeons believe these advantages make VATS the ideal approach for fragile, high-risk patients, such as the elderly or those who have significant underlying chronic lung disease.

One of the most controversial but most attractive indications for VATS is the performance of lobectomy for lung cancer. The critical determinant of success with the VATS procedure is not the feasibility of the technique but the assessment of morbidity and survival results compared with standard open lobectomy accompanied by lymph node dissection.

This chapter discusses VATS lobectomy for lung cancer with reference to the issues of patient selection, endoscopic instrumentation, lymph node dissection or sampling, and operative techniques.

Indication

Standard operative therapy for lung cancer is either lobectomy or pneumonectomy combined with systematic lymph node dissection. It is difficult to perform these tasks with the thoracoscope in the same way the standard open procedure is performed; nevertheless, by applying slight technical modifications, lobectomy or pneumonectomy, as well as lymph node sampling, can be accomplished with a VATS approach. Lymph node dissection has also become possible to a certain extent; however, at present it is practiced by only a small number of well-trained surgeons. When considering a VATS approach for lung cancer, certain criteria must be met:

- A peripheral tumor less than 2 cm at its greatest diameter, or an appropriate history (e.g. non–small-cell lung cancer) for which systematic lymph node dissection is not required.
- Elderly or high-risk patients who have stage IA (T1N0M0) or IB (T2N0M0) cancers for whom systematic lymph node dissection would not be performed in a standard open procedure
- Patients who have stage IA (T1N0M0) or IB (T2N0M0) tumors, which are found following complete lymph node sampling, and which do not have any sign of mediastinal lymph node involvement

Furthermore, in cases in which lymph node dissection similar to standard thoracotomy is possible, or, for those surgeons who are able to perform such surgery, the indications include non–high-risk patients who have stage IA (T1N0M0) or IB (T2N0M0) tumors, or who have tumors small enough to be removed through the intercostal space.

Contraindication

Lobectomy performed using VATS should not be attempted in patients who have clinical stage II or a more advanced stage of lung cancer; nor should it be performed after chemotherapy or radiation therapy because of fibrosis around blood vessels and lymph nodes. Mild pleural adhesions are not a contraindication, and, even for those patients who have pleural effusions, surgery can be performed if the fluid cytology shows no sign of tumor.

General Setup

After induction of general anesthesia, the patient is intubated with a double-lumen Carlens tube, and flexible bronchoscopy is performed to confirm proper placement. Precise positioning of the tube allows separate ventilation of the lungs and total collapse of the operative lung. The patient is placed in the lateral decubitus position as would be done for a standard posterolateral thoracotomy. A pillow or towel should be placed underneath the patient at the level of the scapular angle to widen the intercostal spaces maximally. This can also be aided by "breaking" the table and lowering the patient's pelvis. Lowering the iliac crest also avoids limitation of movement of the thoracoscope. After the positions of the trocars are marked and the accessory incision is made, the patient should be covered by a surgical drape. In case of an emergency, the instruments for standard thoracotomy should always be kept immediately available. In normal practice, two television monitors should be in position, one behind the operator and one behind the assistant. An alternative arrangement is placing both television sets at the head of the operating table on either side of the anesthesiologist.

The lung must be fully collapsed for this procedure. If

the lung does not collapse sufficiently, intrabronchial suctioning in the main bronchus may be helpful. Carbon dioxide insufflation into the pleural space is not necessary to collapse the lung. An arterial line and pulse oximeter are used to monitor the patient. If the oxygen saturation drops during single-lung ventilation, it is necessary to check the position of the tip of the endotracheal tube by using the bronchoscope, because improper positioning can cause a drop in oxygen saturation. Mucous plugs can also worsen oxygen saturation and should be suctioned out if identified. If improvement is not achieved with these maneuvers, intermittent bilateral lung ventilation may be necessary (see Chapter 4). If single-lung ventilation cannot be accomplished safely and reliably, VATS lobectomy should not be attempted, and immediate conversion to standard thoracotomy is advised.

Instruments for VATS Lobectomy

During the development of thoracoscopic surgery, numerous kinds of thoracoscopic instruments and equipment, which aided in the evolution of this discipline, have been introduced. To perform a VATS operation accurately and efficiently, the surgeon should have the kind of equipment best suited to his or her style and technique. The equipment can be chosen from many manufacturers worldwide. However, if the kind of equipment required has not yet been introduced, the surgeon should work with the manufacturer to devise what is needed. Several tools developed in this manner that greatly facilitate certain VATS procedures are the Cotton Finger, the Mini-Thoraco Retractor, specialized forceps, and others.

Cotton Finger

The Cotton Finger (KENTZMEDICO Co. Ltd., Saitama, Japan) was developed for multiple purposes, including localization of lesions, palpation of the lung, retraction, dissection and exposure of the pulmonary vein and artery, and hemostasis. This device is useful for both endoscopic and standard surgical procedures. Two sizes, 5 mm and 10 mm in diameter, are available.

Mini-Thoraco Retractor

The Mini-Thoraco Retractor (KENTZMEDICO Co. Ltd.) is a miniature rib spreader used for the small utility thoracotomies that are performed in thoracoscopic procedures. The retractor has a blade that retracts the intercostal muscle and is designed to allow the easy passage of long instruments into the chest.

Forceps

Forceps are used to grasp and manipulate organs for exposure, dissection, or both. The tip is designed in such a way as to permit easy and reliable grasping without damaging the tissue.

Ligation of blood vessels can be performed by using either an endoscopic stapler or a hemostatic clip. However, there are some disadvantages associated with each of these techniques. The stapler is an expensive tool and may have limited application. The clip can fall off or be dislodged during an operation, or it can obstruct the operative site and impair further dissection of structures.

The safest, and, in my opinion, the ideal, procedure for ligating blood vessels is conventional knotting with thread. The Naruke dissecting and knotting (D.K.) forceps (KENTZMEDICO Co. Ltd., Saitama, Japan) can be used not only for exposure and dissection but also for sliding down and tightening extracorporeally tied ligatures. This forceps is available in three different styles (Fig. 18–1). It has angled, notched limbs that allow the operator to slide the knot down to the structure being ligated. Once this technique is mastered, it allows the creation of knots as safe and smooth as manually tied ligatures (Fig. 18–2).

Lung Grasping Forceps and Lymph Node Forceps

Lung grasping forceps and lymph node forceps (KENTZMEDICO Co. Ltd.) are ring-shaped devices that are available with either angled or straight arms. The lymph node forceps can also be used for grasping the lung and other organs.

Intraoperative Techniques

With the patient in the complete lateral position, the first trocar is placed in the seventh intercostal space in the anterior axillary line. After the parietal pleura is opened through the intercostal space, a finger is inserted to make sure there are no adhesions, and then the thoracoscope is inserted.

The fissure is checked and the lung is retracted posteriorly to expose the superior pulmonary vein and to determine the proper placement of the utility thoracotomy incision. For an upper lobectomy, the incision is made in the fourth intercostal space, and the fifth space is used for the utility thoracotomy in middle and lower lobec-

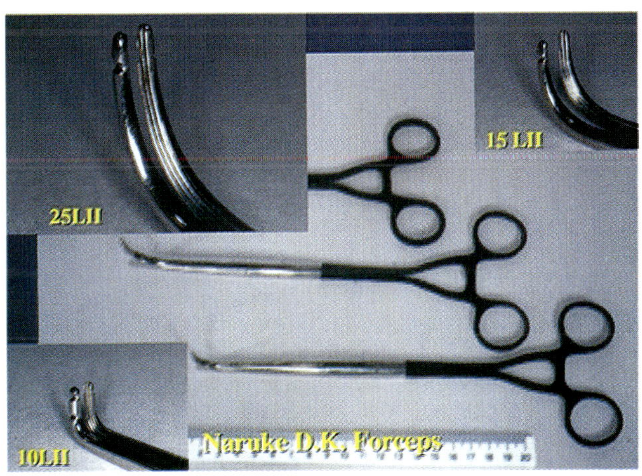

Figure 18–1. The Naruke D.K. forceps is an angled forceps designed with lateral notches used for sliding the suture to tighten knots safely within the thorax with ease and safety. This forceps is also suitable for dissecting.

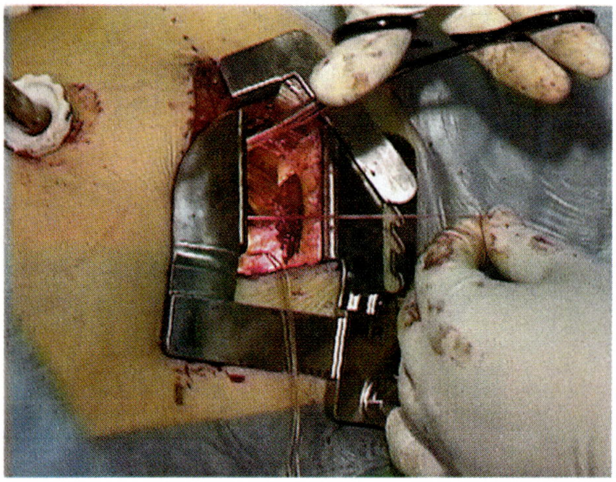

Figure 18–2. By slightly opening the forceps and sliding the suture along the notch of the forceps, the knot may be advanced or pushed down and tightened to occlude the vessel. One limb of the suture is grasped by the Naruke D.K. forceps and pulled deeper into the wound away from the other limb of suture, which is held by the hand outside the thorax. The knot is thus tightened to the appropriate tension.

tomies (Fig. 18–3). A 6- to 7-cm utility thoracotomy is made from the midaxillary line and carried anteriorly. A 1.5-cm incision is made in either the auscultatory triangle or the fifth intercostal space in the posterior axillary line. An additional trocar, placed through the seventh intercostal space in the posterior axillary line, is also used for insertion of the chest tube after the operation. Using these trocars and the utility thoracotomy, the thoracic cavity is examined for the presence of pleural dissemination, lymph node metastasis, or pulmonary nodules.

For the utility thoracotomy, the Mini-Thoraco Retractor is used. Trocars should be inserted along the line of the skin incision that may be required if it is necessary to convert to standard thoracotomy. It should be noted that the trocars are inserted with at least 5 to 7 cm of space between them. During mediastinal lymph node dissection, additional trocars may be placed along the anterior axillary line of the second or third intercostal space. In the case of an upper or middle lobectomy, the pulmonary vein is ligated and dissected, followed by ligation and dissection of the pulmonary artery, the bronchus, and the interlobar fissure, in that order. For a lower lobectomy, the pulmonary artery should first be ligated and divided, followed by ligation and dissection of the pulmonary vein and the bronchus. Lymph node dissection or lymph node sampling should be performed after completion of the lung resection.

VATS Lobectomy for Lung Cancer

Right Upper Lobectomy

The lung is retracted posteriorly, and the phrenic nerve is dissected and gently retracted. The superior pulmonary vein is doubly ligated, and ligatures are also tied around each of the segmental veins prior to their division (Fig. 18–4).

The segmental branches of the truncus anteriosus and the ascending posterior segment branch are then ligated and divided in similar fashion (Fig. 18–5). After ligation and division of the bronchial artery, a tape is passed around the upper lobe bronchus and a stapler is used to divide the bronchus (Fig. 18–6). A tape is placed through the interlobar fissure, which is divided by an endoscopic stapler.

It should be noted that the exposure of the bronchus is done at the same time as dissection of the lymphatic sump and lobar lymph nodes. Nodes are sent for frozen section. The specimen is placed in a retrieval bag and removed through the utility incision (Fig. 18–7).

Middle Lobectomy

This procedure, as with right upper lobectomy, is begun with ligation and dissection of the middle lobe vein, followed by dissection and ligation of the lobar pulmonary artery branches and the middle lobe bronchus. The hilar lymph nodes around the middle lobe bronchus are dissected en bloc with the specimen.

Left Upper Lobectomy

After the phrenic nerve is taped and retracted, the left superior pulmonary vein is dissected and ligated as discussed previously. In the case of a short pulmonary vein, the two sets of branches, V4 and V5, as well as V1, V2, and V3, are ligated and divided separately. A vascular endoscopic stapler may be useful for division if it can be placed around the blood vessel, but if it cannot, individual ligation is per-

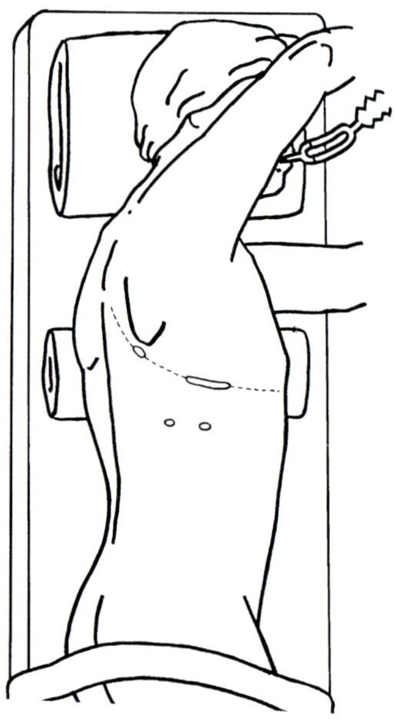

Figure 18–3. Incision for right VATS lobectomy. The utility thoracotomy incision is located in the fourth or fifth intercostal space at the anterior to the midaxillary line. Thoracoscopic port placement is also shown.

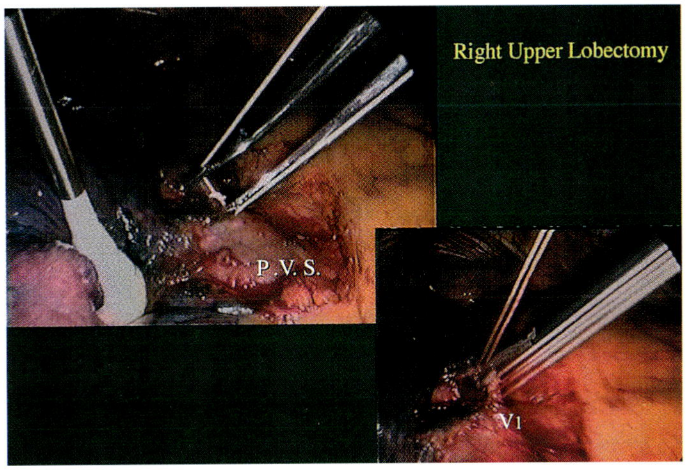

Figure 18–4. Left, Ligation of a segmental branch of the right superior pulmonary vein (PVS). The cotton finger is used for exposure of the vessels and bronchus and for retraction. **Right,** V1 is exposed and doubly ligated by the Naruke D.K. forceps and divided.

formed. For the pulmonary artery branches, great care is taken not to damage or avulse the segmental branches, which tend to be short and fragile.

Lower Lobectomy

On both right and left sides, the usual procedure involves dissection and double ligation of the pulmonary artery (Fig. 18–8) through the interlobar fissure. The pulmonary vein should be dissected and divided with an endoscopic stapler.

Lymph Node Dissection

Lymph node dissection or sampling should be performed systematically, using the standard lymph node map as a guide (see Chapter 24).[1]

The mediastinal lymph node stations and their designations are as follows.

#1. The superior mediastinal lymph nodes are located along the upper third of the trachea within the thorax. Included in this group are nodes around the trachea. Their location is defined by the horizontal line at the upper edge of the subclavian artery and the horizontal line at the center point of the trachea, where the upper edge of the brachiocephalic vein crosses the front of the trachea as the vein ascends to the left.

#2. The paratracheal lymph nodes are situated between stations #1 and #4 and are found on both sides of the trachea.

#3. These nodes are classified as pretracheal, #3; retrotracheal, #3p; and anterior mediastinal, #3a. The nodes located posterior to the trachea are called retrotracheal lymph nodes, #3p; and those in the prevascular compartment on the anterior aspect of the brachiocephalic vein and the upper portion of the superior vena cava are called #3a lymph nodes.

#4. The tracheobronchial lymph nodes are located at, or close to, the obtuse angle between the trachea and at either side of each main bronchus. The nodes on the right side are at an obtuse angle, level with the azygos vein. Those on the left side are found on the mediastinal aspect of the subaortic lymph nodes.

#5. The subaortic lymph nodes are those adjacent to the ligamentum arteriosum.

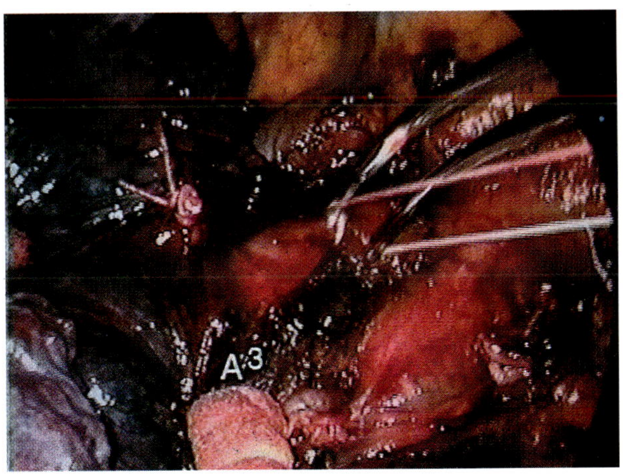

Figure 18–5. Pulmonary artery A3 is ligated by the Naruke D.K. forceps.

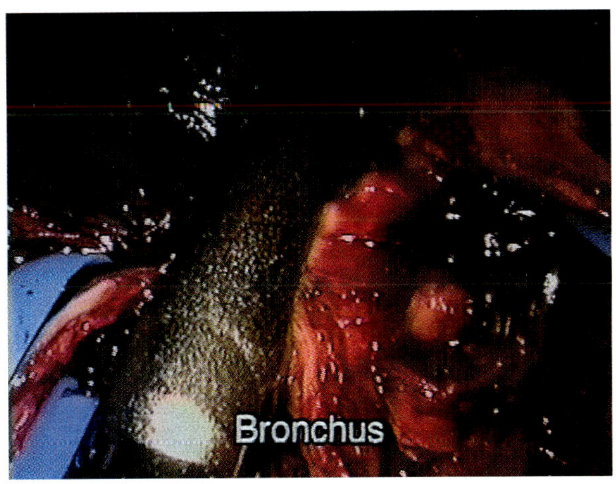

Figure 18–6. A lobar bronchus has been divided with an Endo-GIA30 (USSC, Norwalk, CT).

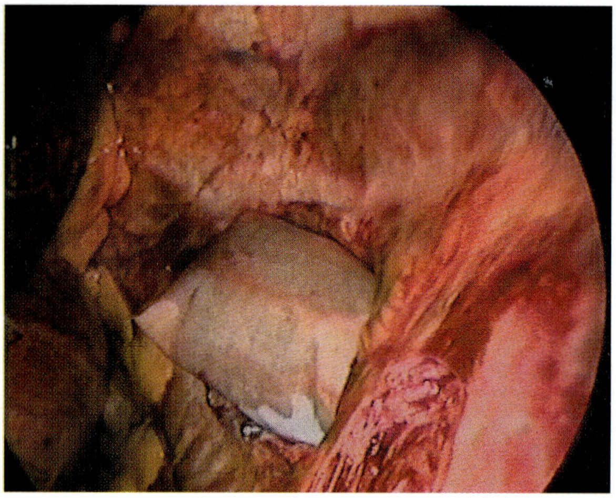

Figure 18–7. When the specimen is completely resected, it is put into the LAPSAC (Cook Urological Inc., Spencer, IN) and removed through the accessory thoracic incision.

#6. The para-aortic lymph nodes are located on the anterolateral walls of the ascending aorta and the aortic arch and anterior to the vagus nerve.
#7. The subcarinal lymph nodes are located just beneath the point where the trachea is divided into the two main bronchi.
#8. The paraesophageal lymph nodes are caudal to the level of the bifurcation of the trachea and adjacent to the esophagus.
#9. The pulmonary ligament lymph nodes are found within the ligament. The lymph nodes on the posterior wall and the lower edge of the inferior pulmonary vein are included in this designation.
#10. The lymph nodes just distal to the trachea and extending along the length of the main bronchi are also called hilar lymph nodes.
#11. The interlobar lymph nodes are located between the lobar bronchi. On the right side, these nodes are specifically classified as those between the upper and middle lobes, #11s; and as those between the middle and lower lobes, #11i.
#12. These nodes are found around the lobar bronchus.
#13. These nodes are located along the segmental bronchus.
#14. The lymph nodes are present around the subsegmental bronchus or distal to this site.

According to the Union Internationale Contre Cancer (UICC) Tumor, Nodes, and Metastasis (TNM) Classification of Malignant Tumors,[2] the relationships between the N classification and the sites of lymph nodes in the classification of stages can be defined as follows:

N0: No regional lymph node metastasis
N1: Metastasis in the hilar lymph nodes (#11) around the lobar bronchus (#12), the interpulmonary nodes (#13, #14), or both
N2: Metastasis in the ipsilateral mediastinal lymph nodes, (#1–#9), the subcarinal lymph node or nodes (#7), or both
N3: Metastasis in the contralateral mediastinal, contralateral hilar, ipsilateral or contralateral scalene, or supraclavicular lymph node or nodes

The dissection of N1 level lymph nodes, that is, those at stations #10, #11, #12, around the hilar area, involves en bloc removal of the fatty tissue containing the lymph nodes, and the pulmonary vein, the pulmonary artery, and the bronchus are also dissected and exposed. A pathologic diagnosis is required for the #11 sump node (Fig. 18–9).

The dissection of N2 level mediastinal lymph nodes, that is, those at stations #1 to #9, should be preceded by lobectomy. However, carinal lymph node dissection is done together with exposure of the main bronchus.

Dissection of the mediastinal lymph nodes is carried out by using electrocautery, scissors, or the Ultra Cision (by Ethicon Endo-Surgery, Cincinnati, OH).

For dissecting the right superior mediastinum, the azygos vein, which has already been taped, is pulled down and the mediastinal pleura is incised vertically through the upper edge of the azygos vein to the apex of the thorax, and the mediastinal structures are then opened

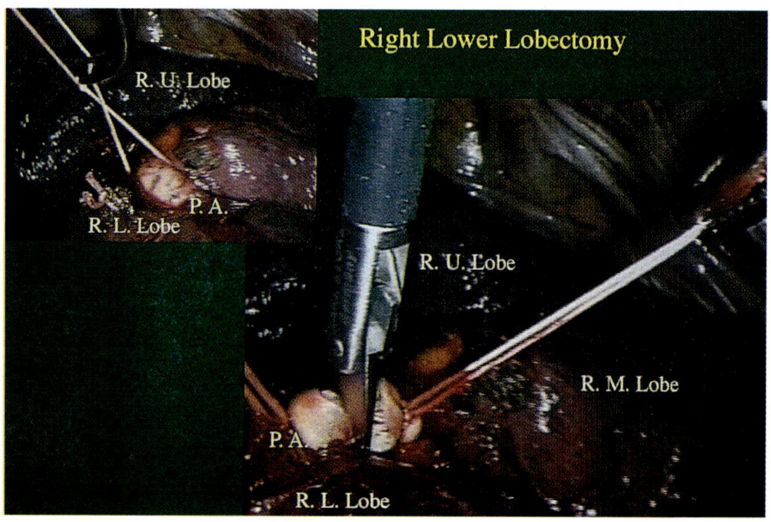

Figure 18–8. The main trunk of the pulmonary artery (PA) and the segmental branches to the lower lobe are exposed, and the trunk is ligated with suture tied through the accessory incision. The PA branch is being divided. RU = right upper; RL = right lower; RM = right middle.

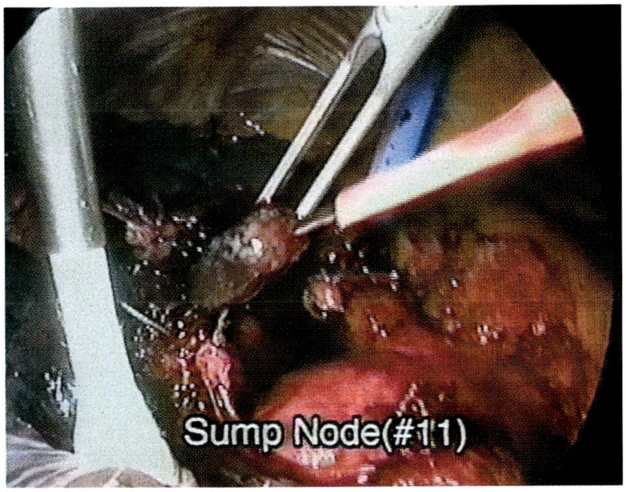

Figure 18–9. Level #11 lymphatic sump node is removed for pathologic examination

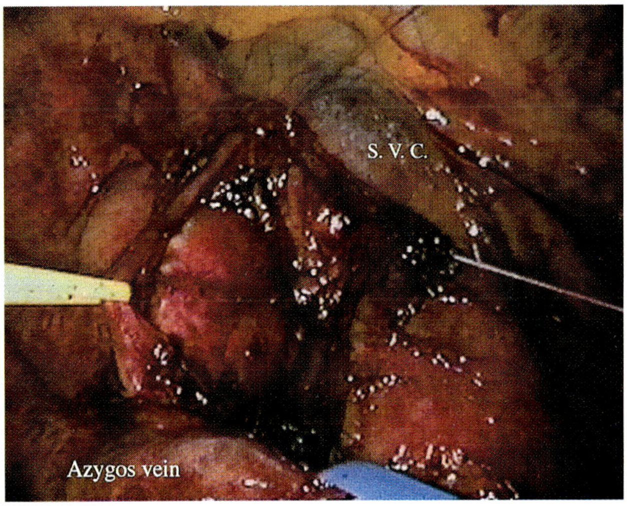

Figure 18–11. Posterior mediastinal lymph node dissection. The vagus nerve is retracted. SVC = superior vena cava.

up by using a retraction stay suture at the incised edge of the mediastinal pleura, as in the standard thoracotomy procedure. After the vagus nerve is taped, the highest #1 lymph node should be grasped by the lymph node forceps. When it has been ascertained that no damage has been done to the recurrent nerve, the right brachiocephalic artery and the superior pulmonary vein are exposed, as well as the #1 vagus nerve and the #3 trachea, while the #2 and #4 lymph nodes are undergoing dissection (Figs. 18–10 and 18–11). The fragile vein could show up when the superior pulmonary vein is exposed; therefore, it should be cauterized by an electroknife or controlled with a clip applier, or the Ultra Cision to prevent bleeding.

In the case of the #7 carinal lymph node dissection or sampling (Fig. 18–12), the patient's lung can be retracted by turning the operating table forward, thus enabling the exposure of the carina. Carinal node dissection becomes possible when the pericardium is exposed from the contralateral side to the median of the main bronchus, and from underneath (Fig. 18–13).

In the case of lower lobectomy, the dissection of the lower lobe bronchus is preceded by carinal lymph node dissection, and then both should be dissected together.

Regarding dissection of the left mediastinal node, it should be done mainly for #6, #5, and #4 nodes. As for the lower lobectomy, #8 paraesophageal and #9 ligamentum pulmonale lymph node dissections are required.

The important point in lymph node sampling is to be fully aware of the lymphatic route, that is, the tumor location and lymph nodes that are bound to metastasize. Lymph node sampling should take place at #3 and #4 in right upper lesions, #3 and #7 in middle lobe lesions, #7 in right lower lobe lesions, #5 and #6 in left upper lobe lesions, and #7 in left lower lobe lesions (Fig. 18–14).

In a case in which the pathologic diagnosis proves positive on lymph node sampling at the N1 level, the N2 level, or both, a systematic nodal dissection becomes necessary. However, lymph node dissection is not required for high-risk patients who, in the first place, would not undergo lymph node dissection in a standard operation.

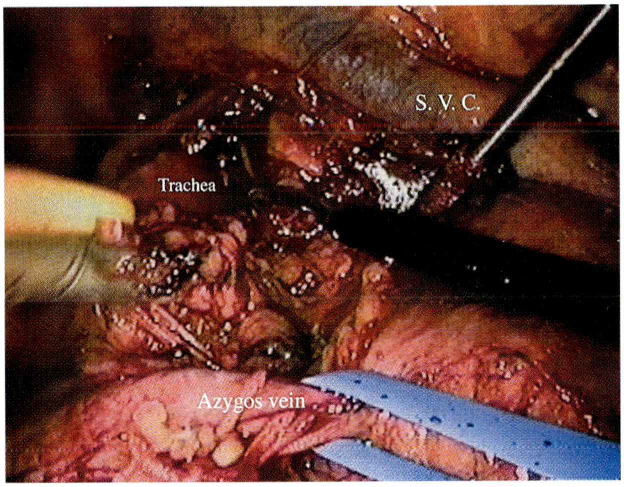

Figure 18–10. Upper mediastinal lymph node dissection. SVC = superior vena cava.

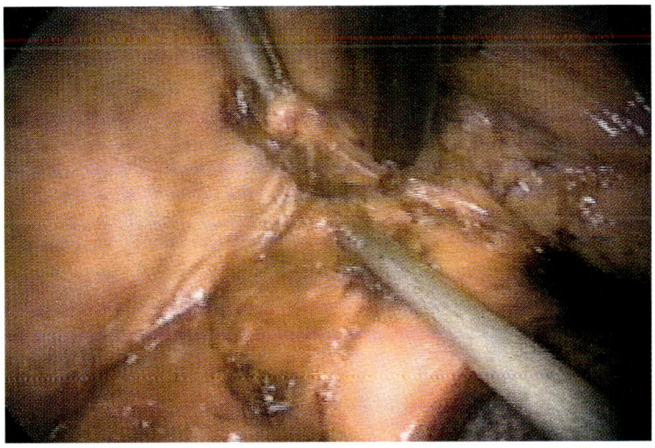

Figure 18–12. Carinal lymph node sampling.

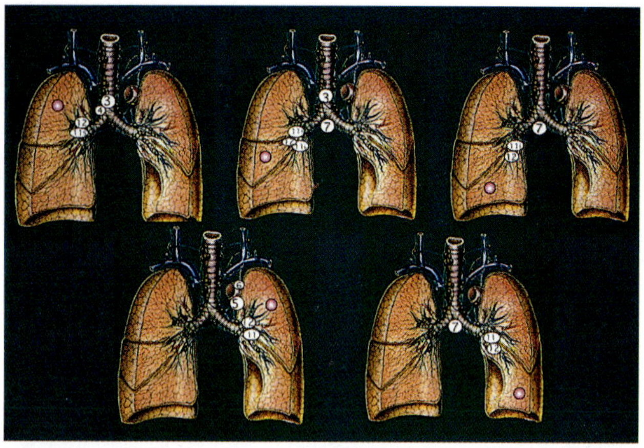

Figure 18–13. Primary lesion and sites of lymph node sampling. Lymph node station numbering is explained in the text.

Results

At the National Cancer Center Hospital, 315 thoracoscopic surgical procedures have been performed during the last 5 years, 79 of which were VATS lobectomies. Among these 79 cases, there were 17 conversions to thoracotomy for the following reasons: 4 for lymph node metastasis, 3 for pleural adhesion, 3 for bleeding, 2 for low oxygen saturation, 2 for technical trouble with staplers, 2 for inability to achieve adequate lymph node dissection, and 1 for inability to achieve lung ventilation.

In the remaining 62 VATS cases, the resections included 26 right upper lobectomies, 4 right middle lobectomies, 15 right lower lobectomies, 10 left upper lobectomies, 6 left lower lobectomies, and 1 middle and lower lobectomy. The pathologic stages in these 62 VATS lobectomies were T1N0M0 in 45, T2N0M0 in 15, T4N0M0 in 1, and T2N0M1 in 1. In the 17 converted cases, the pathologic stages were T1N0M0 in 9, T2N0M0 in 5, T3N0M0 in 1, T1N2M0 in 1, and T1N0M1 in 1. Long-term follow-up evaluation has revealed that 2 of the 62 VATS lobectomy patients and 2 of the 17 converted patients died within 3 years, yielding survival rates of 94.1% and 75.8%, respectively (Fig. 18–15). Forty-five of the 62 VATS lobectomy patients with pathological T1N0M0 were found on follow-up evaluation to be alive with no evidence of disease (Fig. 18–16).

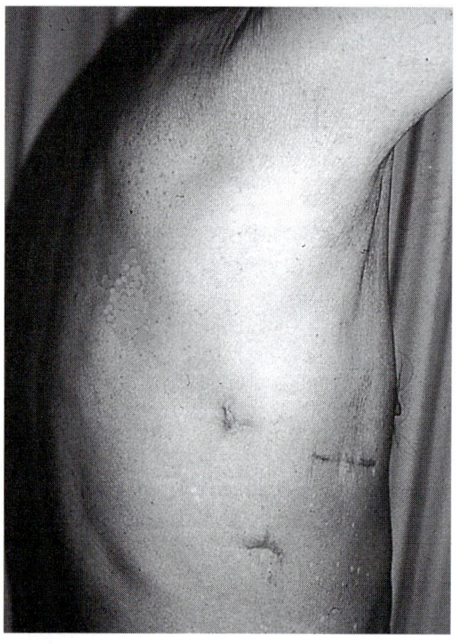

Figure 18–14. Incisions following a right upper lobectomy with mediastinal lymph node dissection by VATS approach.

Discussion

Major lung resection by VATS is a new approach to the treatment of lung cancer. The recent developments in thoracoscopic instruments, together with the innovative efforts of surgeons, have served to bring about improvements in VATS lobectomy. These advances have resulted in a procedure that many authorities believe can be performed as safely as a conventional lobectomy when undertaken in properly selected patients.[3–12]

The standard curative operation involves pneumonectomy or lobectomy combined with hilar and mediastinal lymph node dissection. The question as to what amount of lung should be resected for lung cancer has been answered by the Lung Cancer Study Group. Their randomized controlled study of wedge or segmental resection versus lobectomy reveals that limited resection resulted in a higher local recurrence rate; therefore, the acceptable procedure is lobectomy.[13]

There has been much argument and controversy over the issue of the necessity of lymph node dissection. What is generally agreed is that lymph node dissection yields accurate staging, and, even with N2 disease, selected patients undergoing complete resection have a reasonable chance for survival. Moreover, it is generally recognized that lymph node dissection does not increase the incidence of complications, and, thus, mediastinal lymph node dissection should be a standard maneuver during lung resection in low-risk patients.[14] However, certain questions remain: Is lymph node dissection mandatory in all patients? Is sampling adequate, or must a radical dissection be performed? One significant concern is that only a limited number of surgeons are able to perform mediastinal lymph node dissection with VATS lobectomy. Also, lymph node dissection is more easily and thoroughly performed in an open procedure than with VATS.

We believe there are patients in whom lymph node dissection is not indicated; for example, those who have in

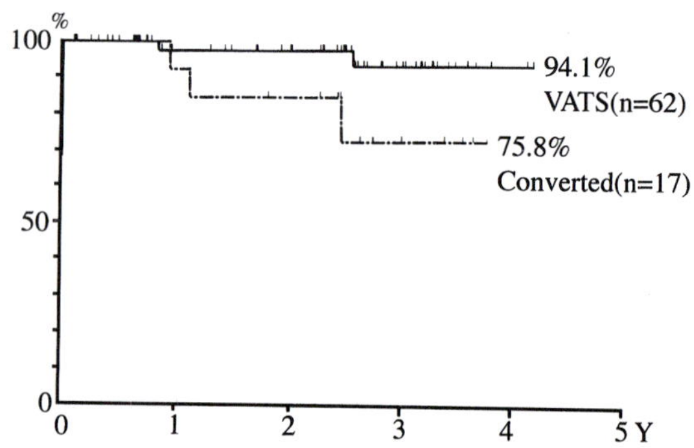

Figure 18–15. Survival rates for patients undergoing VATS lobectomy and for patients in whom the procedure was converted to thoracotomy.

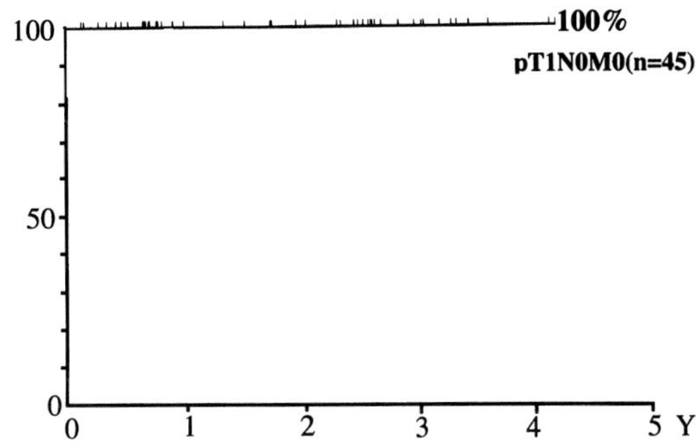

Figure 18–16. Survival rates for patients undergoing VATS lobectomy for pT1N0M0.

situ bronchioalveolar cell carcinoma or squamous cell cancer less than or equal to 2 cm in diameter,[16] in whom nodal metastases rarely occur. However, many authors believe that lymph node dissection is routinely indicated for T1N0M0 and T2N0M0 lung cancer.[4–6, 10–12] Currently, VATS lobectomy is performed in patients in whom we would not perform mediastinal lymph node dissection, including those who have T1N0M0 lung cancers, elderly patients, and those who are at high risk because of cardiopulmonary dysfunction, diabetes, or hepatic diseases. A conversion to thoracotomy with complete mediastinal lymph node dissection is indicated for low-risk patients who have clinical stage T1N0M0 disease and in whom a positive node is found following lymph node sampling.

Those few skillful and experienced thoracoscopic surgeons who are able to perform a complete VATS mediastinal lymph node dissection should not worry about the need for conversion to thoracotomy.

In conclusion, our experience at the National Cancer Center Hospital reinforces the notion that VATS lobectomy can be a standard option for the treatment of lung cancer in appropriately selected patients. We believe that there is less intraoperative blood loss than with standard thoracotomy, that complications are rare, and that the procedure is cost-effective given the early recovery and reduced postoperative stay. In comparison with conventional lobectomy, the amount of postoperative pain is reduced, especially within the first 6 months. Finally, in terms of prognosis, VATS lobectomy appears as promising as open lobectomy for the surgical treatment of T1N0M0 non–small-cell lung cancer.[17]

References

1. Naruke T, Suemasu K, Ishikawa S: Lymph node mapping and curability at various levels of metastasis in resected lung cancer. J Thorac Cardiovasc Surg 76:832–839, 1978.
2. Sobin LH, Wittekind CH (eds): UICC TNM Classification of Malignant Tumours, 5th ed. New York, Wiley-Liss, 1993–1997.
3. Landreneau RJ, Mack MJ, Hazelrigg SR, et al: Video-assisted thoracic surgery: Basic technical concepts and intercostal approach strategies. Ann Thorac Surg 54:800–807, 1992.
4. Kirby TJ, Rice TW: Thoracoscopic lobectomy. Ann Thorac Surg 56:784–786, 1993.
5. Roviaro G, Varoli F, Rebuffat C, et al: Major pulmonary resections: Pneumonectomies and lobectomies. Ann Thorac Surg 56:779, 1993.
6. Walker WS, Carnochan FM, Pugh GC: Thoracoscopic pulmonary lobectomy. Early operative experience and preliminary clinical results. J Thorac Cardiovasc Surg 106:1111–1117, 1993.
7. Kirby TJ, Mack MJ, Landreneau RJ, et al: Initial experience with video-assisted thoracoscopic lobectomy. Ann Thorac Surg 56: 1248–1253, 1993.
8. De Letter J, Proot L: Thoracoscopic assisted lobectomy. Surg Laparosc Endosc 5:12–16, 1993.
9. Roviaro GC, Rebuffat C, Varoli F, et al: Videothoracoscopic major pulmonary resections. Ann Thorac Surg 56:779–783, 1993.
10. Lewis RJ: Simultaneously stapled lobectomy: A safe technique for video-assisted thoracic surgery. J Thorac Cardiovasc Surg 109:619–625, 1995.
11. McKenna R: VATS lobectomy with mediastinal lymph node sampling or dissection. Chest Surg Clin North Am 2:223–232, 1995.
12. Yim AP, Ho JK: Video-assisted thoracoscopic lobectomy: A word of caution. Aust N Z J Surg 65:438–441, 1995.
13. Ginsberg RJ, Rubinstein LV: Randomized trial of lobectomy versus limited resection for T1N0 non–small-cell lung cancer. Ann Thorac Surg 60:615–623, 1995.
14. Naruke T: Significance of lymph node metastases in lung cancer. Semin Thorac Cardiovasc Surg 5:210–218, 1993.
15. Noguchi M, Morikawa A, Kawasaki M, et al: Small adenocarcinoma of the lung: Histologic characteristics and prognosis. Cancer 75:2844–2852, 1995.
16. Asamura H, Nakayama H, Kondo H, et al: Lymph node metastases, recurrence, and prognosis in resected small, peripheral, non–small-lung cell lung carcinomas: Are these carcinomas candidates for video-assisted lobectomy? J Thoracosc Cardiovasc Surg 110:1125–1134, 1996.
17. Naruke T, Tschiya R, Kondo H: The video-assisted thorascopic surgery for lung cancer: Indication and results. J Jpn Soc Endosc Surg 1:110–115, 1996.

COMMENTARY

Ralph J. Lewis

Once again, I must compliment Dr. Tsuguo Naruke—a renowned and internationally respected specialist in the surgical treatment of carcinoma of the lung—for another major contribution to the field. His pioneering efforts and extraordinary results with video-assisted thoracic surgery (VATS) lobectomy for malignancy will impact significantly on the approach to this disease in the future. It was not too long ago that Dr. Naruke provoked discussion and debate among thoracic surgeons by his landmark publication on the role of lymph nodes in cancer surgery.[1] His convictions, in combination with the vast and significant information that has emanated from numerous important studies conducted by the Lung Cancer Study Group, have helped to outline and determine the oncology for carcinoma of the lung that has been advocated, followed, and applied by all thoracic surgeons since the 1980s. Staging systems were devised to allow comparisons of various surgical resections performed by different surgeons for purportedly similar neoplasms. Because those staging systems were totally dependent upon the anatomic characteristics of the tumor, they proved to be poor barometers for biologic activity.[2] They were unreliable, inconsistent, and inaccurate for predicting survival. Although these were exciting times, unfortunately, the application and use of all these new concepts did not improve overall survival for patients with resected primary pulmonary neoplasms. Sadly, long-term survival for patients with resected carcinoma of the lung has not improved in over 50 years.

However, the excellent reports of long-term survival with VATS lobectomy are beginning to rekindle a small hope that real, valid progress is occurring. In the past, we were never able to alter the natural, intrinsic behavior of carcinoma of the lung. In fact, our current staging systems are more predictive for resection of the neoplasm than for survival of the patient. Interestingly, we thoracic surgeons have even formulated an oncology that would conform to our techniques and technologies rather than pursuing techniques that would more validly address the true, perplexing, and complex oncology of carcinoma of the lung.

Despite our applying current, traditional, advocated, and revered oncologic principles for treatment of carcinoma of the lung and employing earlier and earlier diagnosis, more and more radical anatomic resections, and more comprehensive use of chemotherapy and irradiation, the incidence of death from this neoplasm has continued to rise astronomically. At present, it is the number one cause of cancer death in both men and women.

The recently evolving field of molecular biology has begun to challenge and even dispute some inviolate oncologic principles that have been the foundation for our cancer surgery:

1. *Early diagnosis improves survival.* Intuitively, this statement seems valid, but there is no scientific evidence supporting this premise.[3]
2. *Meticulous, intricate, anatomic dissection of tissue planes can remove all tumor and improve survival.* It is commonly known and universally accepted that carcinoma of the lung neither respects nor confines itself to anatomic planes. It recklessly and arrogantly grows through them without restraint. Thoracic surgeons have remained impervious to this scientifically verified information.
3. *Radical, aggressive resection can benefit survival.* In reality, radical surgery has added more to morbidity and surgical mortality than to improved survival. Survival is similar for stage I disease whether pneumonectomy, lobectomy, or wedge resection is performed.[4–6] Outcome seems to depend more on biology than technique.
4. *Radical lymphadenectomy improves survival.* Actually, the true role of lymph nodes in carcinoma of the lung is not understood. Some investigators imply that resection of lymph nodes may diminish the the effectiveness of the immune system and decrease survival.[7, 8] In fact, radical lymphadenectomy can cause massive tissue damage, injuring the sympathetic-parasympathetic system. This can produce pulmonary vascular spasm, right heart burden, and cardiac arrhythmias. Also, lymphatic channels are divided and disrupted, allowing the possibility for lymph that contains neoplastic cells to flow into an area of reparative tissue, which makes an excellent substrate for the growth of carcinoma. Radical lymphadenectomy has many adverse effects and has not been found to improve survival.[9, 10] Even Dr. Naruke has become more conservative by excluding from radical lymphadenectomy patients who have lesions smaller than 2 cm in size, or patients who have stage I or II disease with negative results on sampling, or patients who are aged.
5. *Meticulous anatomic dissection of the hilar area (isolation-ligation) is the gold standard.* Actually, anatomic hilar dissection opens tissue planes; increases tissue injury; activates the corresponding inflammatory reparative process, which seems to disseminate tumor; disrupts and opens lymphatic channels, spilling malignant cells; increases bleeding; and, on occasion, inadvertently causes injury to pulmonary vessels, necessitating a larger lung resection than initially planned. Although isolation-ligation is a pleasing operation that seems intuitively correct, there is no scientific evidence confirming improved survival with this technique.

There is strong evidence that carcinoma of the lung is much more of a systemic disease than any of us ever imagined in the past.[11] It can be multifocal and usually metastasizes very early. Unfortunately, current diagnostics, such as the computed tomography (CT) scan, are able to define lesions only when they become large enough to be visible. At that time, they are already mature and very late in their cycle of growth. Also, negative CT scans do not imply that microscopic tumor is not present, but, rather, that it cannot be visualized by radiograph. After complete resection of a single, visible, primary tumor, eventual progression and growth of previously undetected, microscopic, multifocal, or metastatic areas of carcinoma are inappropriately and inaccurately designated as a recurrence. Actually, recurrence is an improper use of semantics for these frequently occurring situations and should be discarded in favor of progression of previously undetected and invisible microscopic metastatic or multifocal disease. Once a tumor is completely removed and margins are negative, that particular tumor cannot recur.

Investigations that relate the metastatic potential of the tumor to tissue injury and repair at the time of surgical resection will begin to have a significant and profound impact on techniques that will be used by thoracic surgeons in the future. Tissue injury promotes a cascade of changes that elaborate a multitude of humoral substances, which, in turn, accelerate cellular division and facilitate the inflammatory, reparative process for normal tissue. The magnitude of the initial injury determines the magnitude of the reparative process. Unfortunately, this same inflammatory, reparative process can stimulate, concurrently, malignant cell division and enhance growth and spread of the tumor.[12]

Because the smaller incisions of VATS cause less tissue damage than the larger incision of the thoracotomy, a markedly reduced reparative process would be expected to occur in VATS patients who have malignancies. This, in turn, would have less of an effect on peri-intraoperative tumor growth and could explain the improved survival being reported by surgeons currently performing VATS lobectomy for malignancy. Numerous investigators are studying this fascinating phenomenon by trying to develop a better understanding of the relationship between the processes involved in tissue repair and how they impact on tumor growth.

Sixty years ago, almost every patient died of the local effects of carcinoma of the lung, such as bronchial obstruction, hemorrhage, pulmonary abscess, empyema, and pulmonary and pericardial effusion. Extraordinary contributions by thoracic surgeons through the years have just about eliminated death from these secondary causes. At present, most patients with carcinoma of the lung will die from what could be designated as phase II of the disease, which is metastases.

As practicing thoracic surgeons, it is imperative that we develop a better understanding of the biology and natural history of carcinoma of the lung so that surgical advances continue to be made. In the next millennium, our major efforts must be directed to the enigmatic problems of metastases. We must have a better understanding of this perplexing, unpredictable, and uncontrollable occurrence. In fact, we must determine whether some of our surgical interventions could possibly promote, or even facilitate, metastases. At present, Dr. Naruke and other pioneer VATS surgeons are taking giant steps to help clarify some of these complicated issues and valid concerns.

References

1. Naruke T, Goya T, Tsuchiya R, et al: The importance of surgery to non–small cell lung carcinoma of the lung with mediastinal lymph node metastases. Ann Thorac Surg 46:603–610, 1988.
2. Mountain CF, Greenberg SD, Fraire AE: Tumor stage in non-small cell carcinoma of the lung. Chest 99:1258–1260, 1991.
3. Eddy DM: Screening for lung cancer. Ann Intern Med 111: 232–237, 1989.
4. Kotlyarov EV, Rukosuyev AA: Long-term results and patterns of disease recurrence after radical operations for lung cancer. J Thorac Cardiovasc Surg 102:24–28, 1991.
5. Jackman RJ, Good CA, Clagett OT, et al: Survival rates in peripheral bronchogenic carcinomas up to 4 centimeters in diameter presenting as a solitary pulmonary nodule. J Thorac Cardiovasc Surg 57:1–8, 1969.
6. Read RC, Yoder G, Schaeffer RC: Survival after conservative resection for $T_1N_0M_0$ non–small cell lung cancer. Ann Thorac Surg 49:391–400, 1990.
7. Heys SD, Eremin O: The relevance of tumor draining lymph nodes in cancer. Surg Gynecol Obstet 174:553–540, 1992.
8. Funatsu T, Matsubara Y, Hatakenaka R: The role of mediastinoscopic biopsy in preoperative assessment of lung cancer. J Thorac Cardiovasc Surg 104:1688–1693, 1992.
9. Izbicki JR, Thetter O, Habekost M, et al: Radical systemic mediastinal lymphadenectomy in non–small cell lung cancer: A randomized controlled trial. Br J Surg 81:229–235, 1994.
10. Nakahara K, Fujii Y, Matsumura A, et al: Role of systemic mediastinal dissection in N2 non–small cell lung cancer patients. Ann Thorac Surg 56:331–336, 1993.
11. Pantel K, Izbicki J, Passlick B, et al: Frequency and prognostic significance of isolated tumor cells in bone marrow of patients with non–small cell lung cancer without overt metastases. Lancet 347:651–653, 1996.
12. Reid S, Kaufman M, Murthy S, et al: Perioperative stimulation of residual cancer cells promotes local and distant recurrence of breast cancer. J Am Coll Surg 185:290–306, 1997.

Chapter 19

The Immune Response to Surgery: Conventional and VATS Lobectomy

William S. Walker, H. Ann Leaver, Stewart R. Craig, and Peng Lee Yap

The immune response to surgery involves a complex and incompletely defined series of interactions between the mediators of the acute inflammatory response and humoral and cellular components. We will review these processes and identify differences between conventional open thoracotomy lobectomy and a minimally invasive video-assisted thoracic surgical (VATS) procedure. In doing so, it is important to recognize the limitations that apply to our current understanding of immune mechanisms and to appreciate that associations and changes do not necessarily imply causal relationships or clinical relevance. The potential importance of this area in the context of patients undergoing resection for malignant disease has, however, almost certainly been underestimated in favor of more mechanistic considerations regarding tumor stage and details of surgical approach. It is anticipated that the continuing evolution of our understanding of host immune mechanisms may, in future, afford the opportunity to modify or harness these processes to the best advantage of the patient. Rather than providing detailed referencing for the background material, the reader is referred to three excellent clinical reviews that cover much of this ground in substantial detail and provide comprehensive reference listings.[6, 8, 11] This review will introduce developing areas and advances in the immune response to surgery, with particular reference to minimal access thoracic surgery.

Basic Concepts

Although it is not the purpose of this chapter to discuss immunity in detail, it may be helpful to review briefly some of the elements and mechanisms of the immune system that are involved in immunosurveillance and the host response to malignancy and surgery.

The Immune Response

Immune responses can be innate or adaptive. The former is not antigen specific and is unaltered by repetitive exposure. It is predominantly cell mediated via natural killer (NK; non-T, non-B) cells, phagocytes, and polymorph neutrophils (Table 19–1), although few unusual antigens (e.g., pneumococcal antigen) can directly stimulate immunoglobulin M(IgM) production without being dependent on previous exposure. The adaptive response is based upon lymphocyte proliferation and activation and depends on recognition of the antigenic stimulus. Antibodies (Table 19–2) released by B lymphocytes and T lymphocytes (Table 19–3) cooperate in the immune process. Whereas B cells recognize free antigen, T cells require the antigen to be "presented" to them bound to the surface of other antigen-presenting cells (APC). In reality, these immune response processes are interlinked with monocytes and cytokines, and complement, for example, interacting within and between both.

Cytokines

These molecules are polypeptides produced by lymphocytes, monocytes, granulocytes, eosinophils, and endothelial and synovial cells. They constitute a highly important and constantly expanding group of soluble messenger proteins, which can be divided into two broad categories: proinflammatory and anti-inflammatory. Proinflammatory cytokines have low plasma concentrations and short half-lives of up to 20 minutes. They are largely held in store and bound to endothelial membranes near the site of action, whereas anti-inflammatory cytokines are present in plasma in significant concentrations. These two classes of cytokine are normally in balance. The cytokine grouping incorporates diverse families of molecules, including interleukins (IL), interferons (IFN), chemokines, and adhesion molecules. Functions include promotion or suppression of cell growth and migration, modulation of effector cell activity, and control of vascular permeability. It is difficult to repetitively sample and, therefore, monitor cytokine levels in human organs, although bronchoalveolar lavage does make this reasonably feasible for lung tissue. The chemokines are an important subgroup of inducible secreted proinflammatory cytokines that bind target cell surface receptors and are involved in a variety of immune and inflammatory responses. More than 20 chemokines have been characterized to date, and these molecules are now recognized as important initiators of inflammatory influx. There are two broad functional groups: C-X-C ELR chemokines (which include IL-8 and growth related protein [GRP]) act as neutrophils, chemoattractants, and activators, which induce degranulation and release of enzymes; C-X-C ELR-ve and other chemokines are chemoattractors and activators of monocytes, dendritic cells, T lymphocytes, NK cells, B lymphocytes, basophils, and eosinophils.

Malignancy

Tumor cells may be lysed directly by monocytes, probably stimulated by various cytokines, including tumor necrosis factor (TNF) and gamma interferon (IFN-γ). Tumor cells are also destroyed by NK cells. There may also be important interactivity between cytokines and neoplastic cells. A wide range of cytokines have been shown to be released by various tumor cells and to have effector actions on these cells. Similarly, cytokine release, effector activity, or both occur in normal cells in association with malignancy (Table

Table 19–1. Cells Involved in Immune Mechanisms

Cell	Function
Neutrophils	Respond to chemotactic signals from infection or tissue damage; phagocytose bacteria and destroy cellular debris; more efficient if target coated with antibody, complement, or both; influenced by cytokines; capable of antibody-dependent, cell-mediated toxicity
Macrophages	Monocytes in bloodstream colonize various organs as tissue macrophages; secrete a large number of substances that influence: Acute phase response to injury Hemopoiesis (leukocytes) Tissue repair and remodelling Hemostasis Act as antigen presenter Can directly kill microorganisms and tumor cells Capable of antibody-dependent, cell-mediated toxicity
Eosinophils	Release anti-inflammatory histaminases
Mast cells	Basophils in blood and tissue mast cells; release chemotactic agents and inflammatory mediators, including: Histamine, tryptase, leukotrienes, prostaglandins and thromboxanes Receptors for IgE Responsible for hypersensitivity and parasitic immunity
Fibroblasts	Secrete cytokines
B Cells	Produce antibodies; have various subtypes (see Table 19–2)
T Cells	Interact with phagocytic cells to enhance microbial killing; recognize and destroy cells infected with virus; assist with control of B-cell development and antibody production; have various subtypes (see Table 19–3)
Natural killer	Large granulated lymphocytic like cells; can recognize and destroy some cells transformed by viral infection or malignancy, either by direct contact or via antibody-dependent, cell-mediated toxicity

Table 19–2. Antibody Subclasses and Functions

Type	Functions	Relative Plasma Concentration	Characteristics
IgG	Opsonization Complement fixation (IgG1, IgG3) Toxin neutralization Second response	75	4 subclasses: IgG1, IgG2, IgG3, IgG4 Placental transfer Distributed throughout extracellular fluid Half life: 3–4 weeks
IgM	Opsonization Complement activation Agglutination	7–10	Predominantly intravascular Half life: 5 days
IgE	Attaches to mast cells' release of histamine; immediate hypersensitivity reactions	<1	
IgA	Secreted by epithelia Neutralizes intraluminal antigen	10–15	2 subclasses: IgA1, IgA2 Half life: <6 days
IgD	Uncertain	<1	Located on surface of immature B lymphocyte

IgG, IgM, IgE, IgA, IgD = immunoglobulin G, M, E, A, and D, respectively; IgG1, IgG2, IgG3, IgG4 = subclasses of immunoglobulin G; IgA1, IgA2 = subclasses of immunoglobulin A.

Table 19–3. T Lymphocyte Subclasses and Function

Type	CD Designation	Action
T-helper 1 (TH1)	CD4	Interacts with phagocytic cell to enhance microbial killing*
T-helper 2 (TH2)	CD4	Assists with control of B cell development and antibody production*
T-cytotoxic (Tc)	CD8	Recognition and destruction of cells infected with virus†
T-suppressor (Ts)	CD8	Details of suppression unknown

*Requires antigen presented on Major Histocompatibility Complex (MHC) Class II molecules (HLA-D) of Antigen Presenting Cells (APC), i.e., macrophages and B cells.

Activation of T-helper 1 cells requires antigen on APC + Il-; activation leads to mitosis + Il-2 production and expression of Il-2 receptor on cell surface leading to proliferation and secretion of various cytokines.

An antigen recognized and re-expressed by B cells stimulates T-helper 2 cell production of Il-4, which initiates B cell proliferation and sensitization to other stimulatory cytokines.

†Recognize antigen presented on the MHC Class I molecules of all nucleated cells.

19–4). Furthermore, many cytokines are subject to neurohumoral influences and TNF-α, IL-1, and IL-6 have been shown to stimulate the hypothalamus-pituitary axis synergistically. The detailed mechanisms of host defense against tumors are incompletely characterized, but these issues may have relevance to patients undergoing major surgery in the context of malignant disease.

The Effects of Surgery

Major surgery is associated with adverse effects on immunity. These are derived from various mechanisms, including neuroendocrine interactions and stress hormone production; serum factors, such as protein degradation products, complement derived proteins and complement activation; disturbances in leukocyte cell numbers and function; and alterations in immune mediators, such as cytokines and eicosanoids and the proapoptotic mediator fatty acid synthetase (FAS).[9] The most obvious consequence of surgery is tissue trauma, but adverse effects are compounded and modified by changes associated with anesthesia and transfusion (Fig. 19–1). These may be considered separately for convenience, but, as with all aspects of the immune system, it is important to recognize that these distinctions are artificial, and that, in reality, the net effect is the result of multiple interactive processes.

Table 19–4. Cytokine Interactions Documented in Association With Various Human Tumors With Particular Reference to Pulmonary Neoplasms

Cell Type	Cytokines Effectors	Cytokine Released
Macrophage	GM-CSF, IFN-γ, IL-1, IL-2, IL3, IL-4, IL-7, IL-10, TGF-β, TNF-α, FAS, VEGF, M-CSF	EGF, GM-CSF, G-CSF, IFNα, IL-1, IL-6, IL-12, MIP, PDGF, M-CSF, TNF-α
Fibroblast	FGF, GRO-α, IL-1, TNF-α	IL-6, IL-8, MIP-Iα, IFN-β, GM-CSF, G-CSF, M-CSF
NK Cell	FGF, IL-1, IL-2, IL-4, IL-6, IL-7, IL-12, IFN-α, TNF-α, TGF-β, FAS	GM-CSF, IFN-γ, TNF-α, IL-4
Endothelial cell	IL-1, TNF, IFN-γ, IL3, GM-CSF, bFGF, TGF, IL-4, IL-6, IL-8, IL-10, IL-13, EGF, VEGF, IP-10	IL-1, IL-6, IP-10, GM-CSF, G-CSF, M-CSF, PDGF, FGF, IFN-α, TGF-β, IP-10, MCP, GRO-α, RANTES
T lymphocytes	IFN-γ, IL-1, IL-2, IL-4, IL-6, IL-7, IL-8, IL-12, MCP-1, MCP-2, MCP-3, RANTES, FAS	IFN-γ, IL-2, IL-3, IL-5, IL-3, IL-4, IL-6, TNF-α, TNF-β, IL-12, MIP, GM-CSF, TGF-β
Neutrophil	GM-CSF, G-CSF, IFN-γ, IL-1, IL-3, IL-8, IL-10, GRO-1α, TNFα, TNF-β, MIP-2, GM-CSF	IL-2, IL-3, IFN-γ, IL-5, IL-6, IL-8, G-CSF, GM-CSF, MIP-1, TNF-α, TGF-β
Neoplastic cells (lung)	IFn-α, IFN-γ, IL-1, IL-2, IL-3, IL-4, PDGF, HGF	FGF, TGF-α, IL-1, IL-6, IL-8

(TNF = tumor necrosis factor; IL = interleukin, VEGF = vascular endothelial cell growth factor; TGF = transforming growth factor; CSF = colony stimulating factor; IFN = interferon; FGF = fibroblast growth factor; GRO = growth-related protein; HGF = hepatocyte growth factor, MIP = macrophage inflammatory protein; EGF = epidermal growth factor, IP-10 = chemokine; NAP-2 = neutrophil-activating peptide-2; MIP-Iα = chemokine.)

Data from Leaver HA, Yap PL: Cytokines and growth factors. In Prowse C. (ed): Plasma and recombinant blood products in therapy New York, John Wiley & Sons, 1992.

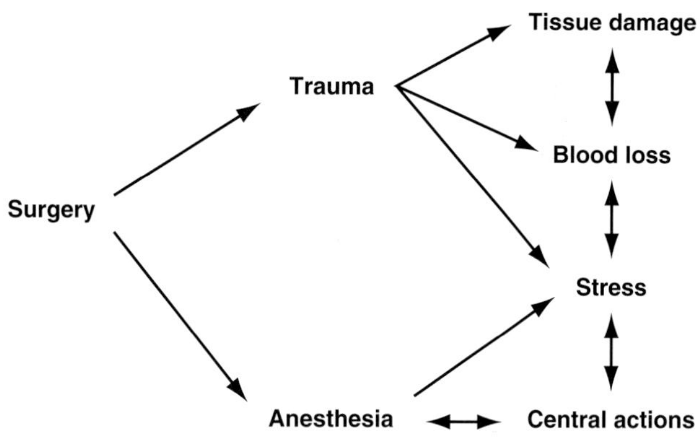

Figure 19–1. Interactive processes initiating immune mechanisms in major surgical procedures.

Tissue Trauma

Tissue trauma initiates a profound sequence of changes that occur both at the local tissue level and as a systemic response. Local events (Fig. 19–2) are initiated by the activation of several cascades, including the complement, kinin-kallikrein, and clotting-fibrinolysis systems. These processes initiate the classic inflammatory response, with consequent increase in capillary permeability, chemotaxis of neutrophils and monocytes, and attraction of macrophages. Cytokines are released locally, notably, IL-1 and IL-6, TNF, and granulocyte macrophage colony stimulating factor (GM-CSF). Systemic effects (Fig. 19–3) include complement activation with elevation of acute phase proteins, notable C-reactive protein and IL-6, and release of leukotrienes and prostaglandins (eicosanoids). The numbers of polymorphs and monocytes increase in peripheral blood, but microbicidal and phagocytic activity decrease while lymphocyte levels drop, returning to normal within about 7 days following surgery. These cells also exhibit abnormalities in intracellular metabolic activity as measured by production of reactive oxygen intermediates, and also show decreased responses to mitogens, antigens, and allogeneic cells during, and up to several days after, major surgery. Decreased immunoglobulin levels may partly be accounted for by hemodilution, catabolism, and protein loss into tissues, but our own data show that this effect occurs after major thoracic surgery in parallel with deliberate postoperative fluid restriction. Shock, an infrequent but definite complication of surgery, further amplifies these deleterious effects, presumably because of the combined effects of circulatory disturbance, volume replacement agents, regional hypoperfusion, and hypothalamic interactions.

Anesthesia

Anesthesia has the potential to affect immune function in several ways. Anesthetic agents of all types at higher than normal concentrations in vitro directly produce dose-dependent inhibition of neutrophil, monocyte, and lymphocyte function. Interaction with the neuroendocrine system may induce changes, and a variety of drugs given during anesthesia have been shown to affect the immune system (Table 19–5). The significance of many of these effects in clinical practice is uncertain, but neutrophil chemotaxis and microbicidal activity, lymphocyte counts, and immunoglobulin levels are all decreased by clinical anesthesia.

Transfusion

Blood transfusion has significant and detrimental effects on immune function—an outcome that has been used deliberately in preparation for renal transplantation. Changes noted include decreased lymphocyte blastogenesis and decreased NK cell activity with increased T suppressor activity. Increased infection rates and impaired long-term survival after resection of malignancy have been noted with blood transfusion as compared to nontransfused patients. Unfortunately, there are many confounding factors that make it difficult to control these observations, such as the severity of surgery and the fact that transfusion is more likely with extensive or emergency surgery and in high-risk patients. Use of white-cell-depleted or filtered donor blood greatly reduces the immunosuppression effect, but plasma transfusions are also detrimental to long-term sur-

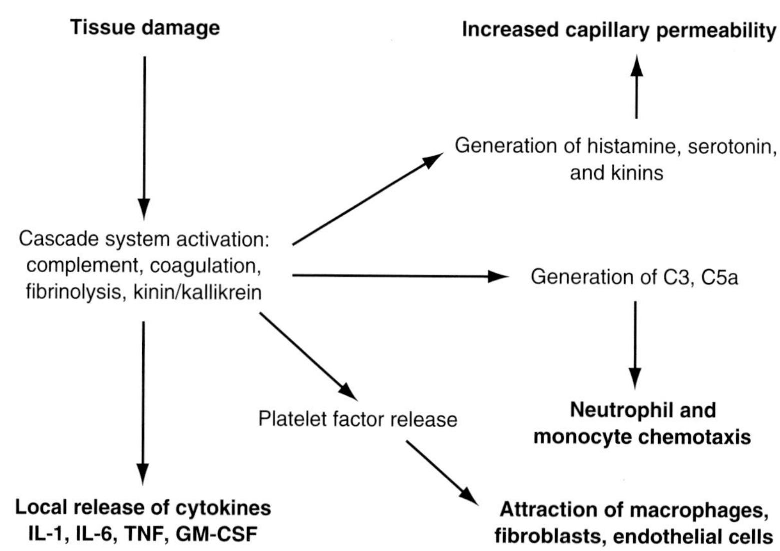

Figure 19–2. Immunologic effects of surgery: The local response.

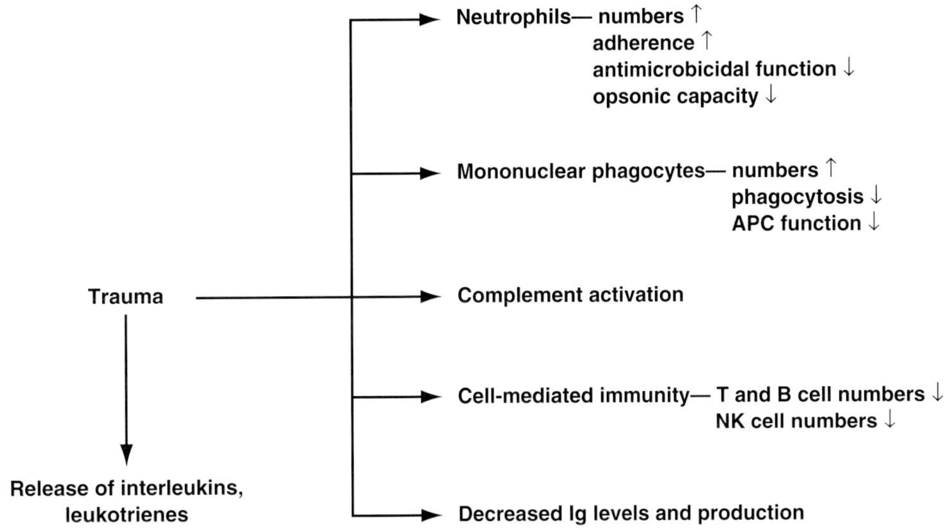

Figure 19–3. Immunologic effects of surgery: The systemic response.

vival, suggesting that part of the effect may be due to products that leak from white cells during storage. Autologous blood is better than donor blood, but it can still cause decreased NK cell counts, and recurrence rates after surgery for cancer appear similar regardless of the transfusion product used. An increased risk of new cancer occurrence has been described in transfused patients for between 3 and 9 years after transfusion. In general, it may be best to avoid transfusion in the context of malignant disease, and, if it must be used, to give washed red-cell concentrate. It may also be better to wait for 48 hours following surgery before transfusing, so as to avoid adding the effects of transfusion during the period of maximum postoperative immunosuppression.

Comparison Between Open and Minimal Access Thoracic Surgery

Minimal access surgery is associated with reduced tissue trauma and would seem intuitively likely to reduce stress hormone production and have fewer adverse effects on immune function. This has been confirmed to some extent in studies comparing laparoscopic and open abdominal surgery, in which the laparoscopic approach was associated with reduced stress responses (glucose, cortisol, prolactin, beta-endorphin, epinephrine, norepinephrine, dopamine, C-reactive protein, and IL-6),[3, 5, 10, 12] and less immune depression as measured by T-cell proliferation[2] and neutrophil hypochlorous acid production.[1] Major thoracic surgical procedures are commonly undertaken for malignant disease when, theoretically at least, it should be advantageous to have as little adverse impact on immune competence as possible. We have, therefore, studied the relative effects on immune function of an open thoracotomy approach and a VATS approach to pulmonary lobectomy.

The data presented in summary form in this section relate to a prospective, randomized, comparative study, which will be reported in detail elsewhere. In brief, 41 patients were randomly allocated to undergo open or VATS pulmonary lobectomy. The open thoracotomy approach employed a standard limited lateral thoracotomy with division of the latissimus but preservation of the serratus, trapezius, and rhomboid muscles. VATS lobectomy was performed by the video endoscopic hilar dissection technique, which included a 5-cm submammary intercostal

Table 19–5. Examples of Interactions Between Various Drugs and the Aspects of the Immune System

Drug Type	Effect
Adrenergic agents	Inhibit protein phosphorylation with reduced triggering of adhesion molecules; inhibit monocyte adherence and spreading; inhibit TNF-α production
Heparin	Inhibits neutrophil adhesion and binding to adhesion molecules
Thiopentone	Reduces neutrophil polarization; increases production of TNF-α; increases IL-4
Intralipid agents	Reduce neutrophil chemotaxis
Propofol	May inhibit B lymphocyte proliferations in ill patients; reduces neutrophil polarization and chemotaxis; increases helper T cell counts; inhibits postphagocytic respiratory burst; increases production of TNF-α, IFN-γ, and IL-4.
Opioid agents	Chemotaxic for neutrophils in vitro and stimulate superoxide production
Nonsteroidal anti-inflammatory agents	Increase TNF-α production; improve macrophage APC activity
Phosphodiesterase inhibitors	Inhibit TNF-α production

access incision, but rib retraction was not employed. Our operative technique remains largely as originally published,[15] although there have been minor modifications with increasing experience.[13] Blood samples were taken preoperatively and at multiple time intervals until 7 days after surgery for white cell counts and analysis of stress proteins and immunoglobulin. Fresh samples were used to determine the metabolic activity of various white cell types. Mean neutrophil and monocyte oxidative activity was analyzed by flow cytometry using the probe 2′,7′ dichlorofluorescin diacetate and compared with the mean values obtained from control leucocytes. White cell numbers were determined by flow cytometry using OKT48/8/3 murine monoclonal antibodies.

For convenience, the data may be considered and the results summarized under three headings:

1. Humoral immune responses
2. Acute phase cytokine and immunologic responses
3. Cellular immune responses

Humoral Immune Responses

Immunoglobulin (IgG, IgM, IgA) levels and complement product (C3, C4) concentrations fell significantly after either form of surgery, but the magnitude of the fall was less marked with a VATS approach. A high correlation between postsurgical changes in the individual components of humoral immunity indicated a possible common clearance mechanism induced by surgery.

Acute Phase Cytokine and Immunologic Responses

Comparison by analysis of variance (ANOVA) between the open and the VATS groups demonstrated significant differences in levels of C-reactive protein, IL-6, TNF, and cortisol after surgery. Reactive oxygen intermediate (ROI) production was significantly ($P<0.03$) elevated in neutrophils of open cases but not VATS cases at 48 hours (Fig 19–4). ROI production increased in both groups in monocytes, but more significantly (open surgery: $P<0.00006$; VATS: $P<0.05$), and to a greater degree, in the open group (Fig 19–5) compared with the VATS group (21% vs 13.2%). The magnitude of increase in ROI production by open case phagocytes may be disadvantageous for two reasons. First, activation of phagocyte reactive oxygen causes

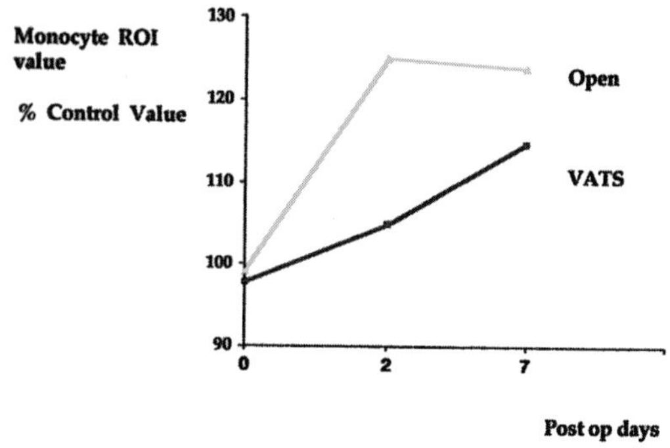

Figure 19–5. Reactive oxygen intermediate (ROI) generation in monocytes of patients undergoing conventional (open; n = 53) and video-assisted (VATS; n = 57) major pulmonary resection (preoperative values at time = 0).

vascular injury, vasoconstriction, and the generation of vasoactive compounds, such as peroxynitrite. Second, hyperactivated cells may respond less appropriately to stimuli, so that an effector arm of the immune system involved in immunosurveillance may not respond as effectively to local stimuli, such as the generation of antiproliferative signals around cancer cells.

Cellular Immune Responses

Leukocyte numbers were compared with presurgical values and oxidative rate with contemporary healthy donor controls. Significant ($P<0.0001$ at day 2; $P<0.0046$ at day 7) decreases in lymphocyte numbers and oxidative activity were noted after surgery, but the VATS approach was associated with less disturbance of absolute T cell levels (Fig 19–6) and better preservation of the CD4/CD8 ratio at 2 days (Fig 19–7). NK cell counts were also less suppressed in the VATS group at 7 days. Increased lymphocyte oxidative metabolism was suppressed in the thoracotomy group at 48 hours compared with the VATS group. There was a greater correlation as judged by comparison

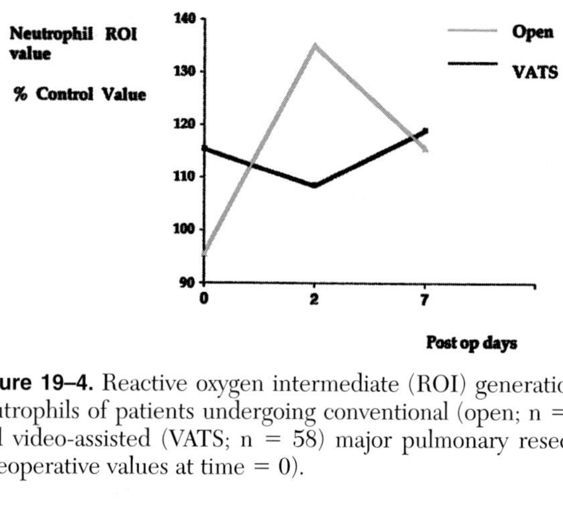

Figure 19–4. Reactive oxygen intermediate (ROI) generation in neutrophils of patients undergoing conventional (open; n = 53) and video-assisted (VATS; n = 58) major pulmonary resection (preoperative values at time = 0).

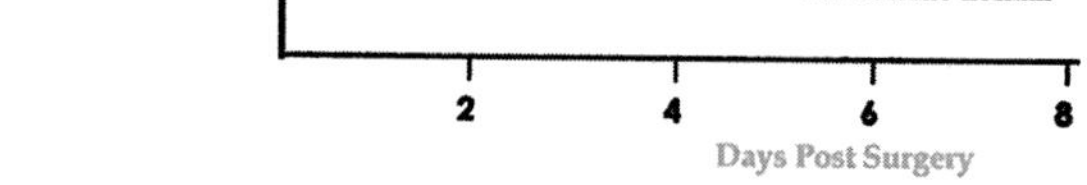

Figure 19–6. Absolute T cell numbers in patients undergoing conventional (open) and video-assisted (VATS) major pulmonary resection. The lower limit of the normal reference range is drawn as a horizontal bar demonstrating that VATS T cell counts remain close to the "normal" range limit compared with the marked fall in open case counts (preoperative values at time = 0). (From Giorgi JA, Kessan AM, Chou CC: *In* Rose NR, ed: Manual of Clinical Laboratory Immunobiology, 4th ed. American Society for Microbiology, Washington, DC, 1992.)

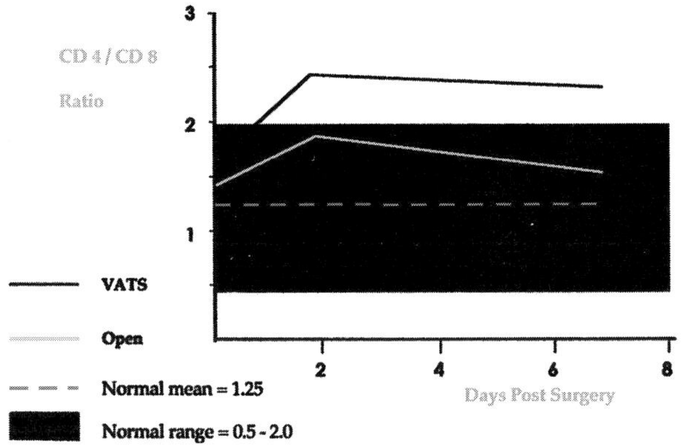

Figure 19–7. CD4/CD8 ratios after conventional (open) and video-assisted (VATS) major pulmonary resection (preoperative values at time = 0).

between Pearson correlation coefficients in a linear network analysis between changes in leukocyte numbers and activity in the VATS group at 48 hours, indicating less immunosuppression with the VATS approach.

In summary, when compared with open lobectomy, VATS lobectomy is associated with:

- Less adverse falls in immunoglobulin and complement levels
- Reduced disturbance of acute phase associated cytokines, indicators, products, and mediators (all of which act as regulators of cellular immunity)
- Better preservation of lymphocyte numbers and function

Conclusion and Discussion

Our studies suggest that a VATS approach to pulmonary lobectomy offers an operative strategy that is less traumatic and less detrimental to immune function than open resection. It remains to be seen to what extent these differences may translate into an observable clinical effect. We[14] and others[4, 7] have noted that, far from compromising survival, a VATS approach offers results in stage I bronchogenic carcinoma cases that are at least equal to those obtained with open lobectomy, and the trend may, indeed, be toward improved survival. It is also worth noting that, taken overall, results for resection of bronchogenic carcinoma by conventional thoracotomy have changed little in 30 years. Failure occurs at a distant site in more than two thirds of all recurrences, which indicates that radical surgery directed at local clearance is conceptually invalid, because most cancers that recur are likely to be metastatic at initial presentation. The ultimate outcome of resection must, therefore, be strongly influenced by host immunity. Minimizing immune disturbance at the time of resection by the use of a VATS approach may offer a simple and cheap method for preserving host immunity and optimizing long-term survival. A further point in favor of a VATS approach in the context of immune function is the low blood loss and, hence, low blood and volume expander requirement, which is associated with this form of resection.

Summary Points

- The immune response to surgery involves interactions between the mediators of the acute inflammatory response and humoral and cellular components. Innate immunity is not antigen specific and is predominantly cell mediated via natural killer (NK; non-T, non-B) cells, phagocytes, and polymorph neutrophils. Adaptive immunity depends on recognition of the antigenic stimulus by lymphocytes. While B lymphocytes recognize free antigen, T lymphocytes require the antigen to be "presented" to them bound to other antigen-presenting cells.
- Cytokines are soluble messenger proteins that can be divided into two broad categories, proinflammatory and anti-inflammatory. The cytokine family includes interleukins, interferons, chemokines, and adhesion molecules. Functions include promotion or suppression of cell growth and migration, modulation of effector cell activity, and control of vascular permeability. Many cytokines are subject to neurohumoral influence and may interact with the hypothalamus-pituitary axis. Cytokines are integral to the immune process and alterations in their levels have profound effects.
- Immune responses, both humoral and cellular, are impaired after tissue trauma, administration of anesthetic drugs, and transfusion of blood products.
- Tumor cells may be destroyed by monocytes and NK cells. Cytokines are released by various tumor cells and have effector actions on these cells. They also are released by, or have effector activity on, normal cells in association with malignancy.
- VATS lobectomy is associated with less systemic upset and better preservation of immune function than conventional open thoracotomy lobectomy as demonstrated by a smaller fall in Ig levels and decreased C-reactive protein, IL-6, TNF, and cortisol levels. Cellular immunity is better preserved with more normal phagocyte and lymphocyte metabolic activity and better maintenance of lymphocyte counts.
- VATS lobectomy may offer an immunologically superior surgical strategy for major pulmonary resection in the context of malignant disease.

References

1. Carey PD, Wakefield CH, Thayeb A, et al: Effects of minimally invasive surgery on hypochlorous acid production by neutrophils. Br J Surg 81:557–601, 1994.
2. Griffith J, Everitt N, Curley P, et al: Laparoscopic versus "open" cholecystectomy: Reduced influence upon immune function and the acute phase response. Surg Endosc 7:123(abstr), 1993.
3. Lefebvre G, Thirion AV, Vaulthier-Brouzes D, et al: Laparoscopic surgery versus laparotomy: Comparative analysis of stress markers. J Gynecol Obstet Biol Reprod 21:507–511, 1992.
4. Lewis RJ, Caccavale RJ, Sisler G, et al: One hundred video-assisted thoracic surgical simultaneously stapled lobectomies without rib spreading. Ann Thorac Surg 63:1415–1422, 1997.
5. Mealy K, Gallagher H, Barry M, et al: Physiological and metabolic responses to open and laparoscopic cholecystectomy. Br J Surg 79:1061–1064, 1992.

6. McBride WT, Armstrong MA, McBride SJ: Immunomodulation: An important concept in modern anaesthesia. Anaesthesia 51: 465–473, 1996.
7. Naruke T: Thoracoscopic surgery for small, non small-cell lung cancer. Is video assisted lobectomy an adequate treatment? Data presented at the IVth International Symposium on Thoracoscopy and Video Assisted Thoracic Surgery, São-Paulo, May, 1997. Pneumol 23:S17 (abstr), 1997.
8. Nielsen HJ: Detrimental effects of perioperative blood transfusion. Br J Surg 82:582–587, 1995.
9. Oka M, Hirazawa K, Yamamoto K, et al: Induction of Fas-mediated apoptosis on circulating lymphocytes by surgical stress. Ann Surg 223:434–440, 1996.
10. Roumen RW, Meurs PA, Kuypers H, et al: Serum interleukin-6 and C-reactive protein responses in patients after laparoscopic or conventional cholecystectomy. Eur J Surg 158:541–544, 1992.
11. Salo M: Effects of anaesthesia and surgery on the immune response. Acta Anaesthesiol Scand 36:201–220, 1992.
12. Vander Velpen G, Penninckx F, Kerremans R, et al: Interleukin-6 and coagulation-fibrinolysis after laparoscopic and conventional cholecystectomy. Surg Endosc 8:1216–1220, 1994.
13. Walker WS: Major pulmonary resection. *In* Walker WS (ed): Video Assisted Thoracic Surgery. Oxford, ISIS Medical Media (in press).
14. Walker WS: VATS lobectomy: The Edinburgh Experience. Semin Thorac Surg 10:291–299, 1998.
15. Walker WS, Carnochan FM, Pugh GR: Thoracoscopic pulmonary lobectomy: Early operative experience and preliminary clinical results. J Thorac Cardiovasc Surg 106:1111–1117, 1993.

COMMENTARY

Anthony P. C. Yim

Mr. Walker and his associates are to be congratulated on their fine work in investigating the immune and cytokine responses in patients who underwent conventional versus VATS lobectomy in a prospective, randomized manner. Because of the multitude of factors that are known to affect the body's immune and cytokine responses (e.g., anesthesia, transfusion, medications), standardization of all these factors in clinical trials may not be easy. Nonetheless, this should not undermine the important nature of this study. There have been many clinical papers on video-assisted thoracic surgery (VATS), but so far, very few studies have focused on the basic science. Because the survival figures after VATS lobectomy for early stage lung cancer have been shown to compare favorably with the conventional approach, elucidation of the mechanism behind this improved survival will have a profound impact on our understanding and management of intrathoracic oncology.

Chapter 20

Video-Assisted Thoracic Surgical Non–Rib-Spreading Simultaneously Stapled Lobectomy

Ralph J. Lewis and Robert J. Caccavale

A new technique known as video-assisted thoracic surgical non–rib-spreading simultaneously stapled lobectomy (VATS(*n*)SSL) has proved to be very beneficial for 200 consecutive patients. Ninety-three males and 107 females, ranging in age from 20 to 92 years, underwent 47 right upper lobectomies (RULs), 18 right middle lobectomies (RMLs), 46 right lower lobectomies (RLLs), 52 left upper lobectomies (LULs), 26 lower lobe lobectomies (LLLs), 9 RUL-RML procedures, and 2 RML-RLL procedures, for 171 primary neoplasms, 7 metastatic tumors, and 22 benign lesions. Operating times averaged 79.5 minutes, and hospitalization averaged 3.07 days. No patient received a transfusion. There was no bronchopleural fistula, surgical mortality, or port implantation. Tumors ranged from 1 cm to 9 cm and averaged 3.44 cm. Seven to 18 lymph nodes were removed from each patient, and bronchial stumps averaged 4 to 5 mm. Thirteen percent of patients had a minor complication, and all recovered completely. Fourteen percent of patients who had malignancies have died of metastases. Long-term survival for neoplasms has been similar to that with open, traditional techniques. Pain, recovery, and cost have been markedly reduced. This large, successful experience with VATS(*n*)SSL is beginning to confirm its validity and numerous benefits.

Our Experience

For more than 8 years, we have been performing video-assisted thoracic surgery (VATS) procedures.[1–3] Many thoracic surgeons agree that this technique is very useful and beneficial for benign problems, and it has found broad and successful applications in this specific area.

Initially, the oncologic efficacy of VATS was questioned, and its use for malignancy was vigorously criticized and debated by some thoracic surgeons. On the basis of our experience, we have found it to be very rewarding for patients with lung carcinoma.[4, 5, 6, 7]

During the past decade, there has been a spate of significant and important technologic advances in the field of general thoracic surgery. This has resulted in re-evaluation and, on occasion, modification of various traditional techniques. Because of numerous demonstrable patient benefits derived from VATS, we began to search for an approach for facilitating lobectomy that would combine VATS and other new and emerging methods and technologies. This different but advantageous technique for lobectomy, which has been used successfully for 6 years, is called VATS non–rib-spreading simultaneously stapled lobectomy (VATS(*n*)SSL).[8, 9]

Our first VATS lobectomy was performed on September 9, 1991, using the isolation-ligation technique. Subsequently, all VATS lobectomies were performed using this technique until August 27, 1992. At that time, isolation-ligation was discontinued in favor of simultaneous stapling; however, some surgeons in our group rejected VATS and continued to use a traditional open isolation-ligation technique for lobectomy. Therefore, initially, the technique used for lobectomy on our service was not dependent upon patient selection but rather was determined by the specific preference of the individual surgeon performing the operation, regardless of the anatomy, body habitus, or physiology of the patient. At present, all surgeons on our thoracic surgical service use VATS(n)SSL as the procedure of choice for lobectomy.

Between August 27, 1992, and May 29, 1997, 200 consecutive VATS(*n*)SSL procedures were performed. In every planned VATS(*n*)SSL, the hilum was ligated successfully by the technique of simultaneous stapling.

Technique

The patient is placed in the supine position under general anesthesia, and a double-lumen, left Mallinckrodt broncho-catheter tube (Critical Care, St. Louis, MO) is placed. A complete bronchoscopy is performed using the pediatric scope. The position of the double-lumen tube is confirmed for single-lung ventilation and is taped in place (Fig. 20–1). The patient is placed in the lateral thoracotomy position. To provide better access to the intrathoracic structures, the intercostal spaces are widened further by separating the table and inflating a plastic bag beneath the contralateral part of the chest (Fig. 20–2). After the chest is prepared and draped antiseptically, four incisions are made, in a quadrilateral or rectangular configuration, in the anterior and posterior intercostal spaces (Fig. 20–3). The incisions average 2 to 3 cm in length except for the cephalic anterior incision. This incision averages 4 to 5 cm in length and is made where the intercostal space is widest. This enables retrieval of the specimen through the anterior space without spreading the ribs. The incisions are made sharply through the skin and subcutaneous tissue; however, the muscles are separated in the direction of their fibers. The parietal pleura is opened bluntly, allowing a finger to probe the thoracic cavity, and the intrathoracic area is palpated for adhesions. The scope is inserted and the intrathoracic contents are carefully visualized and examined for any involvement of the visceral or parietal pleura by the disease process. The

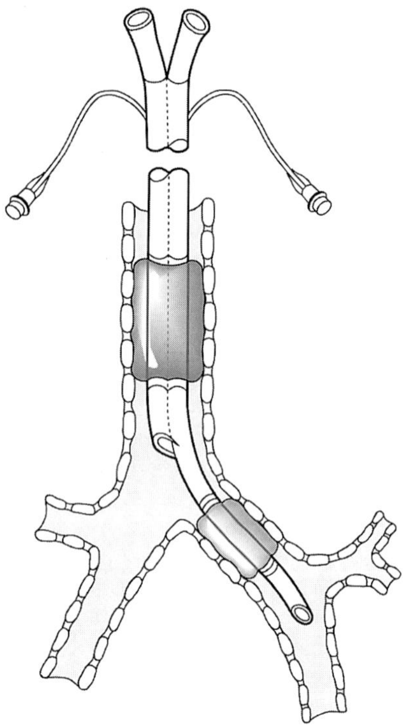

Figure 20–1. Double-lumen tube in position for single-lung ventilation.

lobe to be resected is identified, and the lesion is palpated and localized (Fig. 20–4).

Lower Lobectomy

In general, if a lower lobe is to be excised, the inferior pulmonary ligament is dissected and the inferior pulmonary vein is skeletonized. Any lymph nodes in this area are excised. The parietal pleura of the posterior mediastinum is then opened widely, and all structures are identified. In the right hemithorax, this includes the esophagus and the azygos vein. Dissection is continued to the paratracheal area, and stations #3, #4, #7, #8, and #9 are carefully evaluted, and all identifiable lymph nodes are excised. The hilar structures are skeletonized. The superior segment of the lower lobe is identified, and the posterior portion of the fissure is completed by use of the Endopath EZ 45 stapler (Ethicon Endosurgery, Cincinnati, OH). The anterior mediastinum is then opened and fully dissected; the pulmonary artery, the superior pulmonary vein, and the inferior pulmonary vein are identified. On the left side, stations #5 and #6 are dissected and evaluated, and any visible lymph nodes are removed.

More specifically, for a right lower lobectomy, the fissure is completely opened by sharp and blunt dissection and the vessels are identified. Again, any lymph nodes within the fissure can be resected. Because of magnification provided by the endoscope, nodes as small as 1 or 2 mm can be identified and removed. After skeletonizing the right inferior pulmonary vein, the major fissure is completed, by use of the EZ 45 stapler (Fig. 20–5). A No. 18 red rubber catheter is inserted through the widened ante-

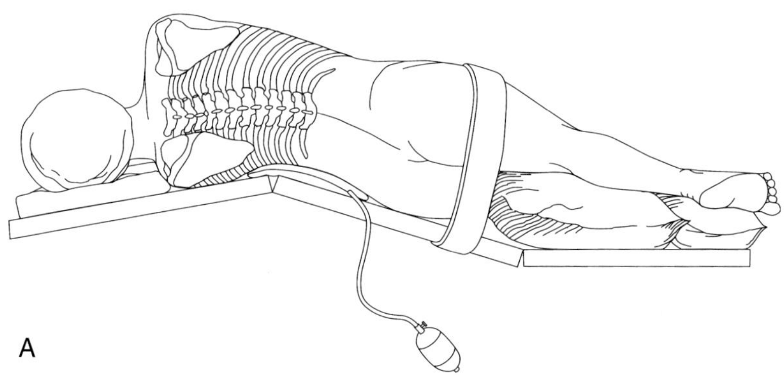

A

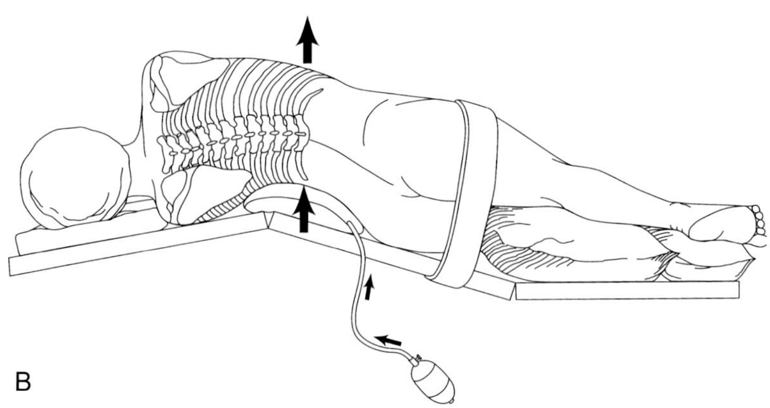

B

Figure 20–2. *A,* Deflated bag beneath chest. *B,* Bag inflated to widen intercostal spaces.

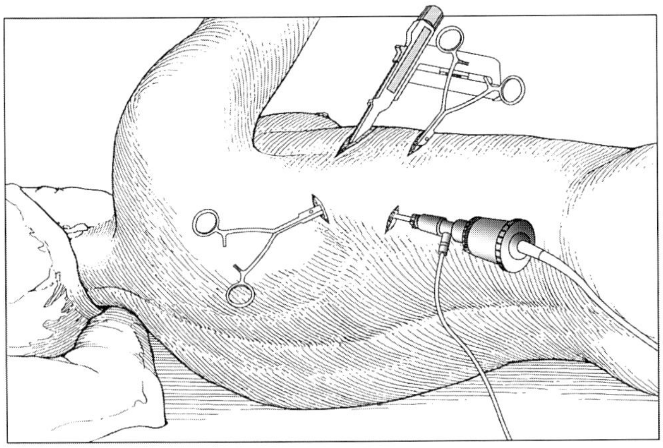

Figure 20–3. Four incisions between ribs in quadrilateral configuration.

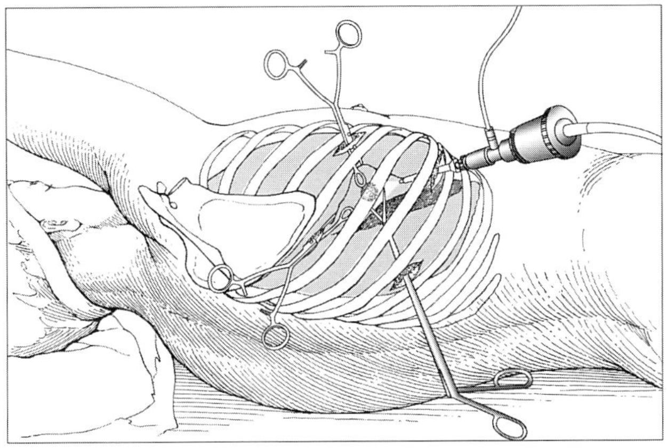

Figure 20–4. Scope and instruments inserted between ribs.

rior cephalic intercostal space and looped around the hilum of the right lower lobe. The lobe is grasped by a VATS clamp (Thoramet, Warsaw, IN) and retracted to better demarcate its hilar structures (Fig. 20–6). The flared end of the catheter is pushed onto the anvil of a TL 60 stapler (Ethicon Endosurgery), and the stapler is carefully inserted through the widened, anterior intercostal space. This is done in a gentle manner so as not to bruise the ribs. By means of the red rubber catheter, all the structures of the base of the lobe are carefully guided between the jaws of the stapler (Fig. 20–7). The red rubber catheter is removed, and the pin of the stapler is closed, encompassing all of the hilar structures of the right lower lobe in their normal anatomic configuration (Fig. 20–8). The stapler jaws are closed between 1.5 and 2.5 mm of the staple length, depending on the thickness of the bronchus. Once this has been accomplished, the stapler is opened, removed, and reloaded. The integrity of the lobar hilar staple line is evaluated. In similar fashion, the red rubber catheter is once again looped around the base of the lobe and pushed onto the anvil of the reloaded TL 60 stapler. This stapler is again brought into the chest through the anterior incision and carefully placed around the base of the lobe. The stapler is positioned between stations 2 and 3 mm above the first staple line, and the stapler is fired. This gives four separate staple lines.

It is imperative to perform two separate firings of the stapler, because bleeding can result from a single application of the stapler. The first application of the stapler should seal the bronchus without crushing it. This may not be tight enough to prevent oozing from the vessels, because this application is intended mainly for bronchial closure. The second application ensures hemostasis, because it is closed tightly distal to the first staple line. A scalpel is used to excise the lobe from the surface of the stapler. Back-bleeding can occur. Once the lobe is free, it is positioned away from the stapler. The stapler is slowly opened and removed (Fig. 20–9). If there is oozing from the staple line, the specific site can be readily grasped with a right-angle clamp and restapled. Bleeding should not occur if the staplers are properly applied. The stump is carefully evaluated, and once it appears to be satisfactorily closed, the lobe is placed in a plastic bag and removed through the widened anterior incision without spreading the ribs. If the tumor is too large to pass through the interspace easily, the lobe is sectioned inside the plastic bag to form segments or smaller pieces. These can be arranged in single file and pass easily between the ribs.

Upper Lobectomy

The upper lobes are resected in a fashion similar to that for the lower lobes. The mediastinum is dissected, exposing the upper lobe bronchus. On the left, the fissure can be

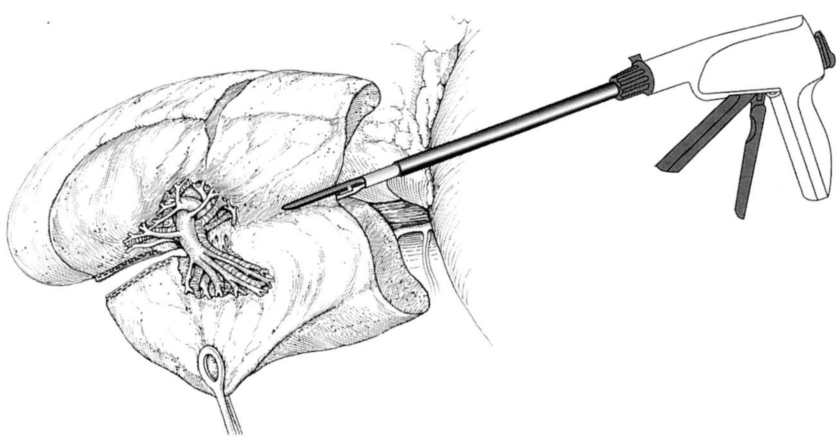

Figure 20–5. In the right lung the fissure has been divided between the right upper lobe and the superior segment of the right lower lobe. The fissure has been opened, exposing the vessels of the right lower lobe, and it is being completed using the EZ 45 stapler.

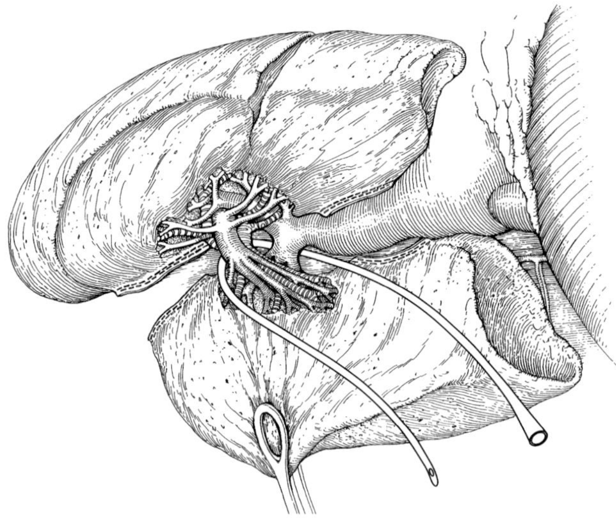

Figure 20–6. Hilar structures of the right lower lobe are looped by a No. 18 red rubber catheter; a VATS clamp elevates and separates the lobes.

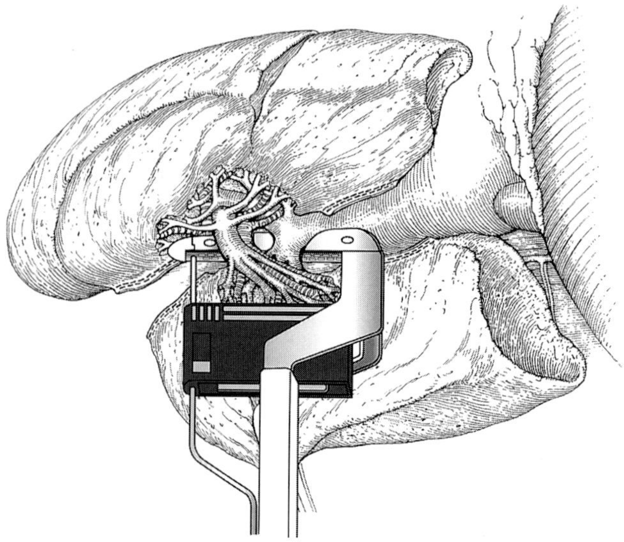

Figure 20–8. The hilar structures are seen in their normal anatomic configuration between the jaws of the TL 60 stapler; the pin is down.

completed by stapling with the EZ 45 stapler. On the right, the minor fissure is frequently absent or only partially developed. To complete the minor fissure, the right superior pulmonary vein is exposed and skeletonized. Usually, there is a bifurcation that delineates the veins to each lobe, permitting the upper lobe veins to be demarcated from those to the middle lobe (Fig. 20–10). The EZ 45 stapler is positioned with its anvil in the bifurcation, so as to cut in the direction of any visible vestige of the minor fissure. The anvil of the stapler is situated above the bronchi and the pulmonary arteries to the middle and lower lobes. These structures remain outside the field to be cut and stapled (Fig. 20–11). The fused right upper and right middle lobes are pulled into the jaws of the EZ 45 stapler. The stapler is lined up with a small remnant of the minor fissure, which is generally present posteriorly (Fig. 20–12). Two firings of the stapler are usually required to open the full length of the minor fissure anteriorly. After the fissure is opened, the pulmonary arteries to the middle and lower lobes are identified. Commonly, these are located at the posterior angle of the middle lobe. If necessary, the posterior portion of the fissure is completed by using the EZ 45 stapler. Once the base of the lobe is skeletonized and freely mobile, the No. 18 red rubber catheter is passed through the wide anterior intercostal space, making a loop around the base of the lobe. The TL 60 stapler is used in the same manner as for resection of a lower lobe. Two individual staple firings are performed, and the lobe is excised from the stapler.

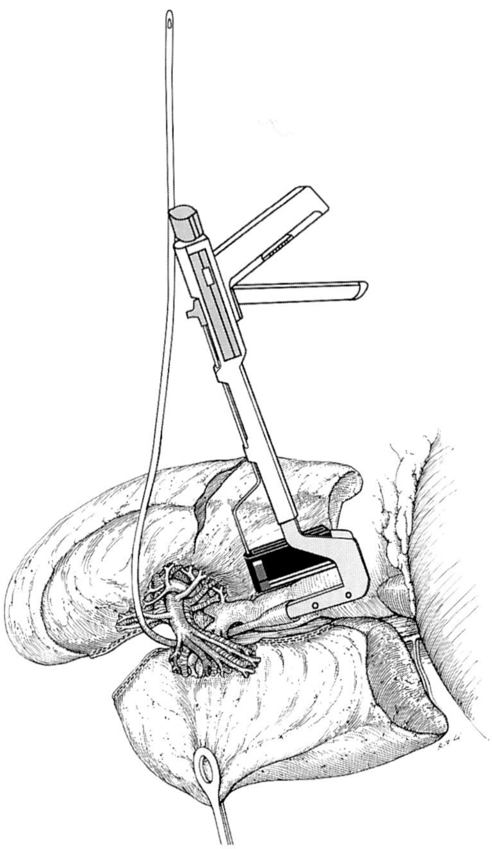

Figure 20–7. The red rubber catheter is used to guide the hilar structures of the right lower lobe between the jaws of the stapler.

Bilobectomy

Occasionally, a bilobectomy is required on the right. After dissecting the mediastinum and exposing all the hilar structures, the posterior and anterior portions of the major fissure are completed using the EZ 45 stapler. The No. 18 red rubber catheter is looped around the base of the right upper and middle lobes. Two firings of the TL 60 stapler facilitate resection of both lobes simultaneously. This is similar to a left upper lobectomy in which the lingula (left middle lobe) and the left upper lobe are resected concurrently.

A right middle and right lower lobectomy may, on occasion, require a slight modification of the technique. If the

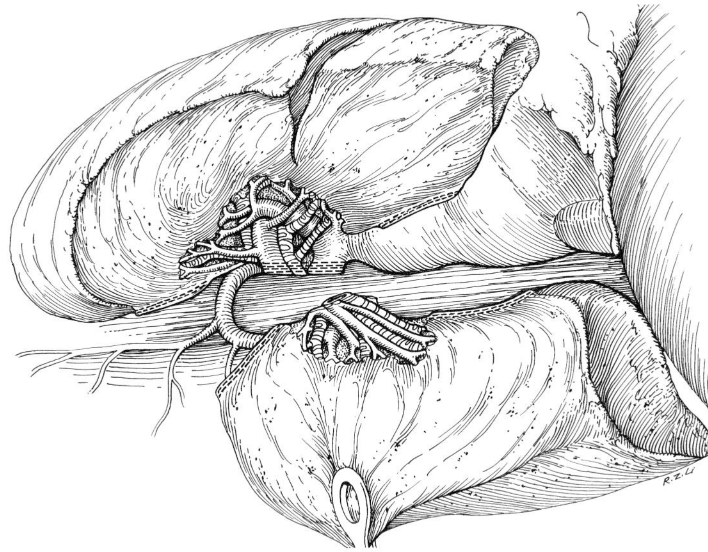

Figure 20–9. The right lower lobe is resected. There are four lines of staples on the proximal bronchus resulting from two separate applications of the stapler.

lesion is in the bronchus intermedius, the right upper lobe bronchus and bronchus intermedius must be exposed in the posterior mediastinum. The bronchus intermedius can be dissected free of the surrounding tissue, stapled very close to its juncture with the right upper lobe bronchus, and then divided. The minor fissure is developed as previously discussed for a right upper lobectomy.

The bilobectomy can be completed by passing a No. 18 red rubber catheter through the minor fissure and around the remaining vascular structures, which now consitute the base of both lobes. This smaller pedicle helps to position the TL 60 stapler properly. In this instance, only the vessels are stapled, because the bronchus has already been divided. After two separate firings, which ensure adequate hemostasis of the vessels, the lobes are excised from the stapler. Each of these lobectomies is preceded by a meticulous and complete dissection of each nodal station.

When the chest wall is very thick and muscular or instrumentation is inadequate, the technique is modified to a "hybrid" method. A 5-cm segment of the fourth or fifth rib is removed between the anterior and posterior axillary lines. Using this incision without spreading the ribs, instruments can be introduced into the thorax more appropriately and safely. Visualization is still accomplished by using the endoscope. The other ports, in combination with this new incision, facilitate dissection and resection in these very rare cases (i.e., in two patients).

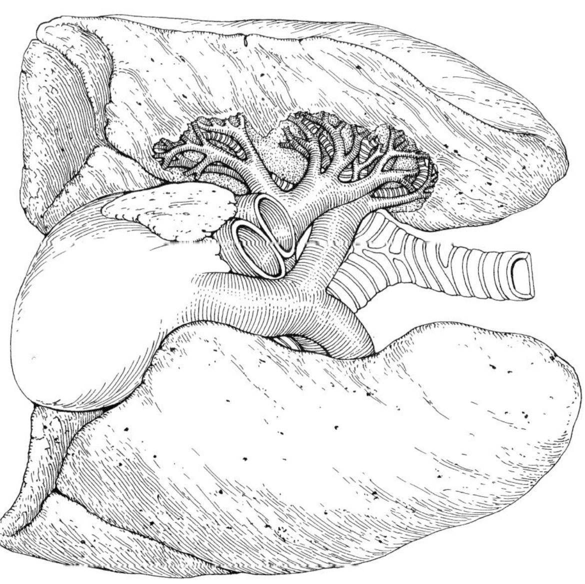

Figure 20–10. A bifurcation of the right superior pulmonary vein demarcates the right upper lobe veins from the right middle lobe veins.

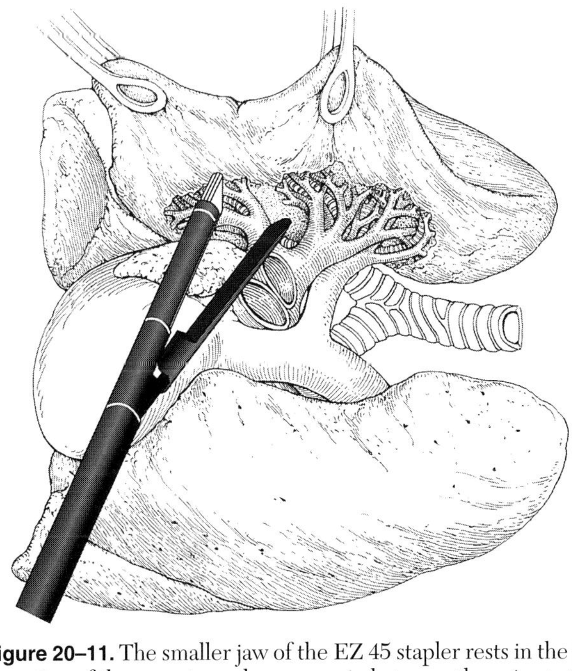

Figure 20–11. The smaller jaw of the EZ 45 stapler rests in the bifurcation of the superior pulmonary vein between the veins to the right upper lobe and the right middle lobe. The pulmonary arteries and bronchi to the right middle and lower lobes rest below the smaller jaw of the linear stapler and are protected. A small vestigial groove of the absent minor fissure can be seen.

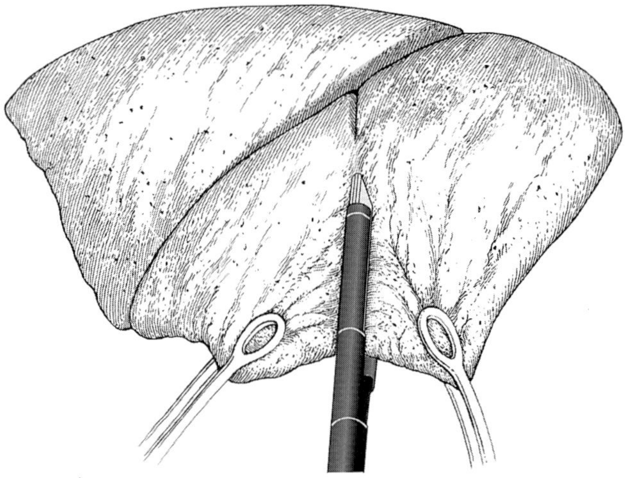

Figure 20–12. The fused right upper and middle lobes are pulled between the jaws of the EZ 45 stapler. The stapler is pointed toward a small remnant of the minor fissure posteriorly. It is fired to complete the minor fissure.

Closure of the Incision

Following removal of the lobe or lobes, the chest is filled with warm saline solution, and the lung is expanded and inspected for air leaks. A small stab wound is made in the lateral lower chest to accommodate a single No. 20 Silastic chest tube, which is positioned in the apex of the thorax under direct visualization by using the video monitor. The chest tube is then sutured to the skin using a No. 0 black silk suture. All wounds are closed using No. 3-0 Vicryl sutures (Ethicon, Somerville, NJ) to the muscle and subcutaneous tissue. A No. 4-0 Monocryl suture (Ethicon) is run continuously in the subcuticular layer to close the skin (Fig. 20–13). Dressings are not used. The chest tube is connected to an underwater seal, and the patient is extubated in the operating room and transferred to the recovery room.

Results

Study Population. Two hundred consecutive patients underwent VATS(*n*)SSL for benign or malignant disease. They ranged in age from 20 to 92 years, with an average age of 66.5 years. There were 93 males and 107 females who had 171 primary lung malignancies, 7 metastatic tumors, and 22 benign lesions (Fig. 20–14). The primary malignant lesions comprised 131 adenocarcinomas, 30 squamous cell carcinomas, 5 large cell carcinomas, 4 carcinoid tumors, and 1 lymphoma. There were 7 metastatic lesions, of which 4 were attributed to the colon, and 1 each to renal, uterine, and melanoma origins. The tumor size of the metastatic lesions ranged from 2 cm to 6 cm, with an average of 3.1 cm, and all these patients are at present alive following resection. Twenty-two benign lesions required lobectomy because of their size or location deep within the lobe, namely, 1 hamartoma, 1 sequestration, 5 giant bullae, 1 organizing pneumonia, 1 *Aspergillus*-related cavitation with a fungus ball, 12 granulomata, and 1 bronchogenic cyst. The average size of the solid benign lesions was 4.6 cm.

Bronchoscopy. The bronchoscopic appearance was visually and cytologically negative in 194 patients. In 6 patients, lesions were identified in segmental bronchioles. Postoperatively, every bronchial margin was microscopically negative for tumor. When mediastinal lymph nodes were enlarged on the computed tomographic scan (<1 cm), or metastasis was suspected, mediastinoscopy was performed. Fifty-eight of these patients, who had a presumed metastatic malignancy, underwent a mediastinoscopy; however, all lymph node biopsies were negative. Lobectomy was not performed for any patient who had a positive result on mediastinoscopy. During VATS exploration, which preceded lobectomy, ipsilateral nodal stations #2, #3, #4 (#5 and #6 on the left), #7, #8, #9, #10, #11, and #12 were carefully explored. Usually, 7 to 18 nodes were able to be excised from the hilar area and the mediastinum. All nodes were negative in 154 patients who had primary malignant disease. Thirteen patients who had a primary malignancy had N1 disease, and 4 patients had N2 nodes (Fig. 20–15).

Operating Times. The average time was 79.5 minutes and ranged from 40 to 150 minutes. For the first 100 cases, the operating time averaged 90.9 minutes, but this decreased to 68 minutes for the second 100 patients. The average

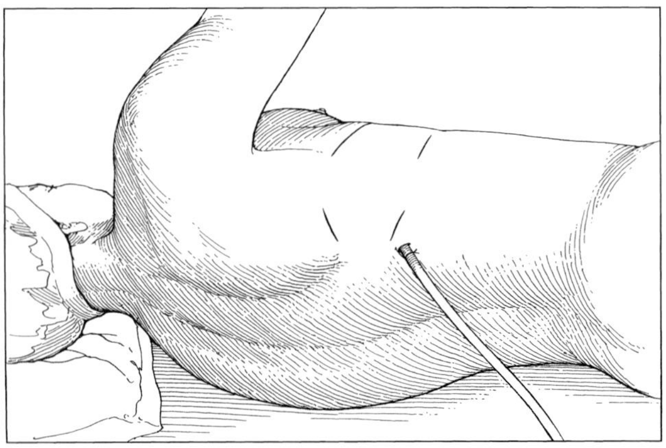

Figure 20–13. The wound closed with subcuticular sutures. No dressings are applied. A single No. 20 chest tube is in place.

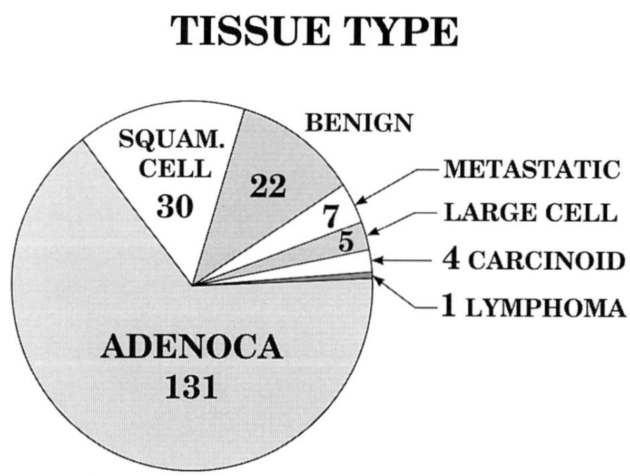

Figure 20–14. Various tissue types of lesions resected by lobectomy.

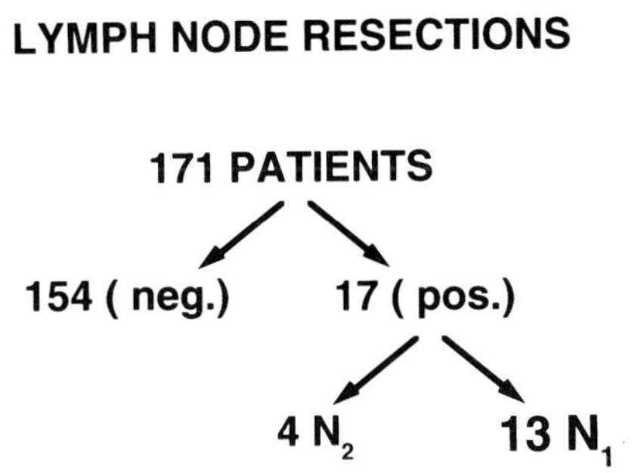

Figure 20–15. Pathologic staging of nodes resected.

length of stay for the 200 patients was 3.07 days—3.50 days for the first 100 and 2.63 days for the second 100. No patient received a blood transfusion, and blood loss was always estimated at less than 100 ml. No patient developed a bronchopleural or bronchovascular fistula. No neoplasm developed at any port site. There was no surgical mortality (Table 20–1).

Types of Procedures. All lobes, or combinations of lobes, were able to be resected satisfactorily by using simultaneous stapling. There were 47 right upper lobectomies, 18 right middle lobectomies, 46 right lower lobectomies, 52 left upper lobectomies, 26 left lower lobectomies, 9 right upper lobectomy–right middle lobectomy procedures, and 2 right middle lobectomy–right lower lobectomy procedures (Fig. 20–16). Bilobectomies were performed if the lesion involved the fissure or was close to the lobar bronchus. Postoperative bronchoscopy consistently revealed bronchial stumps of 4 to 5 mm. The average tumor size for all malignancies was 3.44 cm and the range was from 1.0 to 9.0 cm, i.e., 1.0 cm in 1 patient, 1.5 cm in 16 patients, 2.0 cm in 19 patients, 2.5 cm in 8 patients, 3.0 cm in 53 patients, 3.5 cm in 13 patients, 4.0 cm in 30 patients, 4.5 cm in 5 patients, 5.0 cm in 20 patients, 5.5 cm in 1 patient, 6 cm in 4 patients, 8 cm in 6 patients, 9 cm in 2 patients.

Complications. These comprised minor air leaks in 14 patients, mild subcutaneous emphysema in 2 patients, chest wall bleeding in 1 patient, pneumonia in 3 patients, cardiac arrhythmias in 2 patients, transient cerebrovascular accidents (CVAs) in 3 patients, and inflammation of the chest tube site in 1 patient. The overall complication rate was 13%, and all patients made a complete recovery (Table 20–2). The 14 patients who had air leaks had an average length of stay of 3.05 days and were discharged with Heimlich valves. The average length of time until chest tube removal following hospital discharge was 4 days.

Table 20–1. Average Results in 200 Consecutive Patients

	1st 100 Patients	2nd 100 Patients	Average
OR time	90.9 min	68.0 min	79.5 min
LOS	3.50 days	2.63 days	3.07 days
Fistula (BPF)	0	0	0
Transfusion	0	0	0
Port implantation of tumor	0	0	0
Surgical mortality	0	0	0

OR = operating room; LOS = length of stay; BPF = bronchopleural fistula.

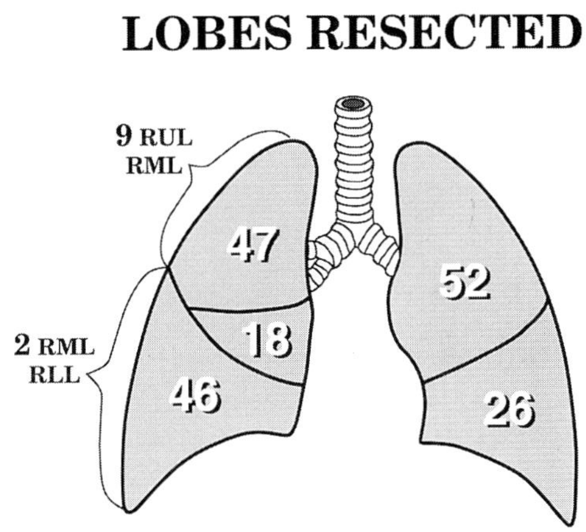

Figure 20–16. Various lobes or combinations resected. RUL = right upper lobe; RML = right middle lobe; RLL = right lower lobe.

Stages. In this series, 171 patients had primary neoplasms and were staged preoperatively as follows: 85 patients at stage I, 85 patients at stage II, and 1 patient at stage IIIa. The stage IIIa patient received preoperative adjuvant therapy for N2 disease biopsied during mediastinoscopy. Postoperative staging changed the classifications to 73 patients at stage I, 85 patients at stage II, 7 patients at stage IIIa, and 6 patients at stage IV (Table 20–3). Determination was made according to the International Staging System.[10]

Follow-up

Patients have been followed from 12 to 69 months, with a mean of 34 months. A total of 31 patients have died, but 7 of these deaths were unrelated to their neoplasms (that is, 4 myocardial infarctions, 1 renal failure, 1 cerebrovascular accident, and 1 alcoholism-related aspiration pneumonia).

Primary neoplasms were the cause of death in 24 patients. Survival for this group of patients ranged from 5 to 38 months, with an average duration of 16.8 months following curative resection. Patients who died had 16 adenocarcinomas and 8 squamous cell carcinomas, involving 5 RULs, 1 RML, 8 RLLs, 9 LULs, and 1 LLL. Six of these patients had N1 nodes, 3 had N2 nodes, and 15 had nega-

Table 20–2. Complications (13%)

Type	No. Patients
Air leak (minor)	14 (3.1 days)
Chest wall bleed	1
Pneumonia	3
Cardiac arrhythmias (transient)	2
CVA (transient)	3
Inflamed chest tube site	1

CVA = cerebrovascular accident.

Table 20–3. Stage of Neoplasm

	Preoperative	Postoperative
Stage I	85	73
Stage II	85	85
Stage IIIa	1	7
Stage IV	0	6

tive nodes. Malignant cells were identified in the vascular system of the resected lobe in 12 patients who died as a result of their malignancy. Preoperatively, 13 patients were at stage I, 10 patients were at stage II, and 1 patient was at stage IIIa. The stage IIIa patient received preoperative adjuvant therapy for N2 nodes diagnosed preoperatively by mediastinoscopy. Postoperatively, this changed to 7 patients at stage I, 12 patients at stage II, 3 patients at stage IIIa, and 2 patients at stage IV. Death was caused by metastases in all patients (i.e., 5 brain, 1 bone, 3 liver, 13 multifocal, and 2 bilateral pulmonary metastases). No patient died because of local disease (Table 20–4).

At this time, 6 patients who underwent a primary carcinoma resection for a cure have manifested a clinical tumor. In this group of patients, there were 4 adenocarcinomas, 1 squamous cell carcinoma, and 1 lymphoma. The tumors range in size from 1.5 to 5 cm with an average size of 2.8 cm. Four patients had neoplastic cells in the vascular system of the resected lobe, 1 patient had positive N1, and 1 patient had positive N2 nodes found on postoperative examination. Preoperatively, 5 patients were at stage I, and 1 patient was at stage II. Postoperatively, this changed to 3 patients at stage I, 2 patients at stage IIIa, and 1 patient at stage IV. The average time for tumor manifestation was 12 months postoperatively. A tumor has been identified in the bone of 3 patients, in the brain of 1 patient, and with a diffuse spread in 2 patients (Table 20–5).

At present, 141 patients who had a resected primary tumor are alive and well without any evidence of neoplasms.

Historical Evolution of Lobectomy

Currently, we are performing VATS for most lung-related, intrathoracic problems requiring surgical intervention (i.e., pleurectomy, decortication, chest wall resection, segmentectomy, and lobectomy). One of the most common and beneficial procedures performed by thoracic surgeons is lobectomy. This complex resectional technique is not new, because it was first performed intentionally in the late 1800s by means of a mass ligation method.[11] Interestingly, during the early 1900s, an isolation-ligation technique was developed for lobectomy; however, the outcomes were appalling.[12, 13] A morbidity of 100% could be anticipated, and a mortality of 50% was acceptable. These poor results

Table 20–4. Clinical Findings in the 24 Patients Who Died of Progression of Primary Lung Cancer

Gender	11M 13F	
Age	54 yr to 92 yr, mean = 72 yr	
Lobes Resected	5 RUL, 1 RML, 8 RLL, 9 LUL, 1 LLL, 0 bilobe	
Tumor Size	1.5 to 9 cm, mean = 3.8 cm	
Pathology	16 adenocarcinoma, 8 squamous cancer	
Nodal Malignancy	15 neg, 9 pos (6 N1, 3 N2)	
Vascular Malignancy	(+) in 12, (−) in 12	
Bronchial	Margin 24 neg	
Stage	PREOP I 13 II 10 IIIa 1	POSTOP I 7 II 12 IIIa 3 (N2) IV 2 (multifocal)
Survival	5 to 38 mo, mean = 16.8 mo	
Location of Metastases Causing Death	5 Brain 1 Bone 13 Multiorgan	3 Liver 2 Bilateral pulmonary
Critical Findings	2 visceral pleura ulcer, 2 multifocal disease 1 preoperative adjuvant therapy, 1 lung cancer and breast cancer	

RUL = right upper lobe; RML = right middle lobe; RLL = right lower lobe; LUL = left upper lobe; LLL = left lower lobe.

Table 20–5. Postoperative Tumor Manifestation (Recurrence*)

GENDER	AGE† (yr)	PATHOLOGY	SIZE‡ (cm)	MALIGNANCY Nodal	Vascular	STAGE	SITE	FINDING
F	68	Adeno	1.5 1.8	(+)	(+)	I → IV	Bone	Multifocal
M	73	Adeno	3	(−)	(+)	I → I	Bone	Ulcerating visceral pleura
F	62	Adeno	2.5	(+)	(+)	I → IIIa	Brain	Ulcerating visceral pleura
M	82	Adeno	1.5	(−)	(−)	I → I	Bone	Ulcerating visceral pleura
F	58	Squamous	5	(−)	(+)	II → IIIa	Diffuse	Chest wall invasion
F	65	Lymphoma	3	(−)	(−)	I → I	Diffuse	Systemic

* Average time to recurrence postoperatively was 12 months.
† Mean 68 yr.
‡ Mean 2.8 cm.

were attributed mainly to the technique of isolation-ligation. At that time, in an attempt to improve these poor outcomes, surgeons began to return to an earlier method for lobectomy, which they designated mass ligation.[14]

During the early era of lobectomy, almost all resections were performed for advanced bilateral bronchiectasis or tuberculosis. The operations were staged procedures that could require 3 to 6 months to complete. We must remember that our current techniques and technologies were not available to those surgeons. Patients received almost no preoperative evaluation, because recognition and knowledge of comorbid conditions were still in their embryonic stages. Cardiopulmonary physiology was poorly understood. Sophisticated diagnostic tests, such as computed tomography (CT) scan, pulmonary function tests (PFTs), cardiac catheterization, and arterial blood gases (ABGs), had not yet been discovered or developed. Many patients who had nearly terminal pulmonary infections, or who had cardiac or other serious comorbid problems, such as renal or hepatic deficiencies, were treated with the available crude and traumatic surgical procedures. Trained anesthesiologists did not yet exist. Endotracheal tubes, positive-pressure ventilation, oxygen, arterial lines, cardioscopes, blood transfusions, and antibiotics had not yet been discovered. Monitoring during the operation usually consisted of an occasional measurement of the blood pressure and pulse.Heavy sedation and local anesthetic blocks were used, and some operations were performed with the patient breathing spontaneously. Surgeons at that time believed coughing could spread infection, and, of even more importance, coughing disturbed them and made the operation more difficult, so the cough reflex was abolished by the liberal use of narcotics.

Early Technique of Lobectomy

Usually three to four ribs had to be resected to attain adequate exposure. The chest was packed with large amounts of gauze in anticipation of adhesions, which would "wall off" the infected area. Further dissection and packing were repeated over a period of months for each patient. When the surgeon was convinced that the viable portion of lung was now adequately protected by a wall of scar tissue, and that resection could be accomplished without spreading infection, the diseased lobe was removed. Paradoxical respiration or pneumothorax resulting from air leaks was not yet understood, so, obviously, chest tubes were not employed. During these staged approaches, purulent material was usually massaged into the "down," or contralateral lung, because the gross and traumatic interventions were completed as quickly as possible. If the other lung was not already infected preoperatively, it was almost certain to be infected postoperatively.

For those patients who had the mental and physical stamina to survive all of these debilitating, painful, and traumatic treatments, a lobectomy was eventually performed. A technique called mass ligation, or tourniquet lobectomy, had evolved. Althouth there were many variations of this method, and surgeons had numerous preferences, the most common practice was to place a large, coarse tourniquet, or a crushing clamp, around a fibrotic, edematous hilum, which was enveloped by engorged, suppurative lymph nodes. Following strangulation of the entire hilum by the tourniquet, the lobe was removed rapidly without clamping the distal bronchus. This maneuver invited purulent material to exude into the chest cavity. Proximally, the individual hilar structures protruding beyond the clamp or tourniquet were ligated separately, but, usually, a coarse continuous suture was employed. The clamp or tourniquet was then removed, and a second continuous suture was placed through the devitalized, ischemic crushed area. Obviously, wound healing was severely jeopardized. Postoperatively, intensive care units, monitoring, supportive modalities, ventilators, blood, oxygen, antibiotics, and portable radiographs—just to name a few of the supportive technologies we use routinely—were not available to surgeons. Patients were returned from the operating room to an open communal ward, and they received minimal or—more commonly—no postoperative care when compared with our current standards.[15–17]

Because many patients died postoperatively of uncontrollable infection, these pioneering surgeons advised against any type of isolation-ligation technique. It was their inherent fear that opening hilar tissue planes to expose each structure would facilitate the spread of infection.[18] However, the few patients who did not die of massive infection usually died of pulmonary or cardiac failure, hemorrhage, or shock.

Despite these very poor results, which could be attributed mainly to a lack of knowledge and the rudimentary techniques and technologies of that era, these pioneering surgeons must be admired, and even complimented, for their brilliant innovations and, on occasion, successful outcomes. It was their genius that allowed them to achieve any success at all in such a debilitated, terminally ill group of patients. Mass ligation was logical and valid, but it was unsuccessful because of the underlying diseases of tuberculosis and bronchiectasis, absence of antibiotics, poor patient selection, ignorance of chest physiology and anesthesia techniques, and lack of supportive modalities. Moreover, the surgical application of the technique was crude and very traumatic. The technique was used without an understanding of the fundamentals of tissue survival and preservation. Bronchopleural fistula remained a major problem of lobectomy, not because of mass ligation, but because of inadequate knowledge, poor preparation, lack of operative sophistication, absence of supportive modalities, and minimal postoperative care. It is amazing that any bronchial resection during that era succeeded.

Revival of the Isolation-Ligation Technique

Because of the recurring problem of bronchopleural fistula, Blades and Kent stimulated renewed interest in the isolation-ligation technique in 1940 at the annual meeting of the American Association for Thoracic Surgery.[19] They proposed it as a method for reducing the high incidence of bronchopleural fistula. Although their series included only 10 patients, 6, or 60%, of these patients developed a bronchopleural fistula postoperatively. Obviously, isolation-ligation by itself did not in any way reduce the incidence of fistula formation; however, the meticulous and intricate dissection of individual hilar struactures and anatomic planes, which it required, fascinated and appealed to many surgeons. It was quickly adopted and applied in all patients requiring a lobectomy. Interestingly, during this period of time, and concurrent with the revival of the isolation-ligation technique, antibiotics were discovered.

The incidence of tuberculosis and bronchiectasis began to decline precipitously because of better methods of sanitation and the availability of antibiotics. Also, many other advances were being made simultaneously in thoracic surgery. Patients in need of surgery were much better evaluted and prepared. They became good operative risks. The edematous, infected, fibrotic bronchi of tuberculosis and bronchiectasis were slowly being replaced by the healthy, noninfected, sufficiently vascularized bronchi of patients with carcinoma. As experience accumulated and anesthesia improved, surgical procedures became safer and better tolerated. In this setting, closure of the healthy, noninfected bronchus resulted in a marked decrease in the occurrence of bronchopleural fistulae, despite the method used. Inexplicably, most surgeons attributed this major improvement primarily to the edifying "clean" resections that could be accomplished with use of the isolation-ligation technique. Apparently, it was not perceived by them, or even by contemporary surgeons of today, that the decreasing incidence of bronchopleural fistula was really related to the profound advances and beneficial changes that were occurring concomitantly in the field of thoracic surgery. Without any documented scientific evidence or confirmation of improved results, isolation-ligation was accepted and adamantly and persuasively advocated by all thoracic surgeons as the standard technique for lobectomy. To attribute the excellent current results of surgical resection for lobectomy entirely to the technique of isolation-ligation would be erroneous and without a scientific basis.

Support and Evidence for Simultaneous Stapling

During the evolution of lobectomy, various ligation techniques have been employed. The Russian literature contains voluminous experimental and clinical information confirming the feasibility and successful outcome of using a single staple line to encompass and ligate all of the structures of the hilum.[20] For the resection of extensively fibrotic, calcific, tuberculous disease, in which the structures of the hilum could not be isolated, we would occasionally, in the past, cross-clamp the entire hilum. After excising the lobe, all of the hilar structures would be ligated simultaneously by running two separate continuous suture lines. There was no surgical mortality, and no patient developed a bronchopleural fistula resulting from the use of this technique. This was safer and more rewarding than attempting an isolation-ligation resection, which had a reported surgical mortality of 27.6%, and a complication rate of 55.2%, in a similar group of patients when the procedure was performed by experienced surgeons at the Mayo Clinic.[21] Because of similarly poor results described by other surgeons, Utley has recommended that simultaneous ligation of all hilar structures be performed when there is a dense, fibrotic, ligneous hilum.[22] In fact, simultaneous stapling of all pulmonary vessels during lobectomy or pneumonectomy has proved to be safe and has been used for many years without any recognized adverse effects.[23]

It should be recalled that clamping and resection anywhere in the body contorts, compresses, and strangulates tissue as arteries and veins are ligated together. Nowhere is this more definitively demonstrated than during a routine wedge resection of lung tissue, in which there is compression, distortion, and overlapping of pulmonary arteries, veins, and bronchioles, which are all simultaneously stapled together. Despite the vast number of wedge resections that have been performed worldwide, vascular or bronchial fistulae resulting from this acceptable procedure have not been reported and have not been a problem.

VATS(*n*)SSL should not be equated with the technique of mass ligation that was practiced and described during the early years of lobectomy. There is a profound difference. VATS(*n*)SSL is a safe, simultaneous ligation of healthy, vascularized, noninfected hilar structures, which are maintained in their normal, anatomic configuration. This distinction has been confirmed by the excellent results attained during the past 8 years in over 300 patients who have undergone lobectomy using this technique. Also, the VATS procedure does not involve a large wedge resection, because a true lobectomy is determined by the length of the remaining bronchial stump. Bronchoscopy performed following VATS(*n*)SSL has consistently corroborated a proximal bronchial stump of 4 to 5 mm, which is similar to our open resections. Because most surgeons are conventional, traditional, and conservative in their philosophical and technical approach to surgical procedures, it is understandable that they are usually reluctant to embrace any innovative surgical technique. Most surgeons wait for data to confirm significant beneficial results and only minimal adverse effects before they attempt to modify their comfortable, convenient, basic techniques and embark on a new, disquieting surgical approach. This is an admirable surgical quality, because we all perform irreversible work; however, to procrastinate far beyond the validation period of a new and efficacious technique denies deserved benefits and advantages to patients.

VATS Versus Isolation-Ligation Resection

Our initial VATS lobectomies, dating back to September 1991, were performed using traditional, accepted, and advocated isolation-ligation techniques.[24] Although this method has been satisfactory for performing lobectomy in the open thoracotomy, isolation-ligation, in our experience, was inefficient, cumbersome, awkward, and even potentially dangerous for VATS. Using old, conventional techniques for new evolving technologies can conceivably cause problems and even impact adversely upon beneficial and safe outcomes. Inexplicably, isolation-ligation has been called the gold standard by surgeons, even though no special advantages can be attributed to it, and no scientific evidence supports this designation. Isolation-ligation has a recognized inherent morbidity and mortality, especially for the elderly. It adds to the operative time and can lead to blood loss. Inadvertent vessel injury during dissection, can, on occasion, necessitate larger pulmonary resections than initially planned. No oncologic benefits can be confirmed; on the other hand, tumor dissemination from opening tissue planes is a real possibility. What is most significant, in our experience, is that long-term survival rates are similar, whether isolation-ligation or simultaneous stapling is used for resection of malignancies.[9, 25–28] Interestingly, en bloc resections have always been strongly advocated and adamantly supported by oncologic surgeons for resection of malignancies. Therefore, VATS(*n*)SSL fully conforms to the stringent oncologic principles of en bloc resection by sealing all lymphatic channels, blood vessels, and tissue planes. Dissection employing isolation-ligation can result in open, draining lymphatics pumping malignant cells into an area of reparative tissue. This type of tissue has been identified as a fertile substrate for promoting the growth of malignant cells, and this sequence of events can impact upon the eventual long-term survival of patients following resection of pulmonary malignancy.[29, 30] Overall survival statistics for clean isolation-ligation resections, as reported in the literature, have not been gratifying, since there is overall 5-year survival of only 40%.[31] Because carcinoma neither respects nor confines itself to anatomic tissue planes, a careful, intricate, meticulous dissection of these same tissue planes appears to be frivolous and without scientific justification for enhancing survival. Rather, it is possible that opening these tissue planes to perform a radical lymphadenectomy may have an adverse effect on long-term survival by enhancing the spread of tumor.[32–34]

Benign Lesions

The technique of VATS(*n*)SSL has been excellent for treatment of benign diseases. Patients who underwent resection for such entities as sequestration, giant bullae replacing the lobe, *Aspergillus*-related abscess with fungus ball, congenital infected pulmonary cysts, and large, deep-seated hamartomas all made rapid, uneventful, and complete recoveries. Their average length of hospital stay was 2.07 days, and all patients were fully recovered within 14 days after surgery. In many of our 22 patients, the benign nature of the disease was diagnosed and fully appreciated preoperatively; nevertheless, lobectomy was still required, because lesions were very large or deep within the lobe and could not be removed by wedge resection. A few were suspected to be carcinoma, and even crossed the fissure, necessitating a bilobectomy. The average size of the solid lesions was 4.6 cm. In retrospect, every one of these patients would have had a lobectomy, even if thoracotomy had been performed and the chest had been opened.

Oncologic Advantages of VATS

Our application of VATS(*n*)SSL for carcinoma conforms to all advocated oncologic principles. We have never supported radical lymph node resection as a curative procedure, because there has never been any scientific evidence confirming improved survival.[35–38] Rather, there is current information that radical lymph node resection could have an adverse effect upon outcomes.[32, 34] It is of interest that surgical mortality and major complications have been attributed directly to the surgical technique of radical lymphadenectomy.[39] So, without any defined benefits for the patient, one must seriously question the reasons for performing this type of radical surgery. In fact, there is now evidence that nodal dissection may not always be indicated for pulmonary lesions smaller than 2 cm.[34, 40] Our approach, using VATS, has been to resect or biopsy all identifiable nodes from the fissures, the hilum, and the mediastinum for their prognostic value. Every attempt is made to avoid operating on patients who have positive N2 nodes because long-term survival is so poor.[41–43] On our service, meticulous preoperative evaluation—which can include CT scan, cervical and parasternal mediastinoscopy, percutaneous needle biopsy of mediastinal nodes, and VATS excision and frozen section of lymph nodes preceding lobectomy—has drastically reduced the number of patients with N2 disease subjected to lobectomy.[9] The added magnification of VATS allows even the smallest nodes (1 to 2 mm) in fissures, or attached to vessels, to be resected. Many of these could be overlooked if conventional open techniques and the naked eye are used. If N2 disease is confirmed during the preliminary VATS exploration, lobectomy is not performed.

Patients who undergo only VATS nodal evaluation are minimally traumatized, so most of them can be discharged from the hospital on the same day as their surgery. Because VATS is much more convenient for the patient and causes much less physical and mental disability than an open thoracotomy, we do not feel obligated or pressured to resect lung tissue when N2 nodes are found, as has been suggested by some surgeons who perform open thoracotomy.[35]

Every bronchoscopy was visually and cytologically negative, except in 6 patients who had an obvious neoplasm in a segmental bronchus. If a tumor is visualized in a segmental bronchus, VATS(*n*)SSL can still be satisfactorily performed. However, if the lesion is in a lobar bronchus, we modify our VATS technique, resecting the bronchus separately to attain the shortest possible stump. All cervical mediastinoscopies were negative for malignancy in this series. Any patient who had a positive N2 node was excluded from resection, because a cure was no longer feasible by our criteria.

We have had very extensive experience with cervical and parasternal mediastinoscopy, dating back to 1965, and we have performed approximately 4000 of these procedures. We no longer routinely perform mediastinoscopy, because VATS lymphadenectomy is far superior and is now our procedure of choice to identify lymph nodes within the thorax. The entire mediastinum can be more completely and thoroughly evaluated with VATS. As mentioned, when positive N2 nodes are encountered, lobectomy is not done. Currently, in this situation, a parietal pleurectomy with talc insufflation is performed to avoid the possibility of recurrent, malignant pleural effusions in the future. If fluid is noted within the pericardial sac, a pericardial window is made at the same time.

Aspects of VATS Lobectomy

Four separate incisions in a quadrilateral or box shape are made for all lobectomies. The anterior cephalic incision is placed at the widest anatomic intercostal space. After being placed in a bag, the entire lobe and tumor can be removed satisfactorily through this wide area without spreading the ribs. These four incisions enhance visibility and maneuverability, because the scope and the instruments can be positioned as needed, and each of the various ports is used. Also, the surgeon and the assistant can work with both hands.

Operating times have been markedly reduced, averaging 79.5 minutes per lobectomy. During the operation, no problems have been caused by arrhythmias, hypotension, hypoxia, or bleeding, and no patient in the entire series has received a transfusion. Blood loss has averaged an estimated 100 ml per patient. Our anesthesiologists state that they can administer much smaller dosages of anesthetic drugs for patients undergoing VATS compared with those required in similar patients undergoing thoracotomy. This lighter level of anesthesia has been very satisfactory and, possibly, could account for the early and vigorous recovery of these patients. All patients are awakened and extubated in the operating room following VATS(*n*)SSL. Because they are able to breathe spontaneously so early after surgery, ventilators have not been necessary. Local infiltration of anesthetics or epidural blocks are not used, and postoperative pain is well controlled by non-narcotic analgesics (e.g., Toradol 30 mg), which are given for 1 to 3 days. In our experience, VATS has been less traumatic and less painful for patients than the conventional thoracotomy. We have found the bone-sparing incision of VATS to be much more beneficial than the muscle-sparing incision of thoracotomy.[44, 45]

After a brief period of time in the recovery room, the patient is transferred to a regular hospital floor, where routine nursing care is provided. After VATS lobectomy, patients have not needed any special type of postoperative care (monitoring, intensive care unit, pulmonary floor). Even patients who had preoperative comorbid conditions experienced rapid and uneventful recovery. Medical consultations are now practically nonexistent, because postoperative arrhythmias, atelectasis, hypoxia, infections, and the like have not been a problem. Many patients request discharge on the second postoperative day. The average length of hospital stay following a VATS lobectomy is currently 2.6 days, and return to preoperative activity levels, which includes return to work, occurs within 7 to 14 days. Elderly patients who have compromised cardiac and pulmonary systems have found VATS lobectomy extremely beneficial. These older patients have emphysema with persistent distention of the lungs, resulting in decreased elasticity and compliance; a fragile chest wall caused by osteoporosis of the ribs; a more rigid, fixed osseous thoracic cage because of arthritis; and weakened, atrophic chest wall muscles. These changes, which are commonly associated with the aging process, necessitate a greater work effort from the patient to generate the forces needed for respiration. Thirty-seven patients were 75 years of age or older. Eleven of them were in their 80s, and 1 patient was 92 years old. The average length of stay for this elderly, frail group was 2.5 days. Each patient made a complete and uneventful recovery, even though 7 of them had been rejected for lobectomy by other institutions because of comorbid conditions, which were interpreted as making them too high a risk.

Nine patients in this series had previous contralateral, open, conventional thoracotomies for pulmonary resection. Each patient affirmed that VATS was less painful, more convenient, and better tolerated, and that VATS allowed them to make a much quicker and more complete recovery. In our experience, patients have been reluctant to undergo a second open thoracotomy, but none has complained about a second VATS operation.

When the first 100 patients were compared with the second 100 patients, operating times decreased by 24.9%, and length of hospital stay decreased by 25.2%. It is to be expected that the initial outcomes from any new technique will continue to improve as experience increases and skills become more refined.

Contraindications

As experience is acquired, fewer and fewer contraindications to VATS lobectomy can be identified. Dense adhesions are no longer an indication to convert to an open chest procedure. In fact, adhesions in the apex or costophrenic angles can be approached ideally and more easily lysed because of the extraordinary access and magnification afforded by VATS. In this series, no patient required conversion to an open technique because of adhesions, hemorrhage, or unfavorable anatomy. Commonly, the minor fissure is incomplete in many patients, but it can be developed anatomically by using the divisions of the right superior pulmonary vein. In 6 patients, bilobectomies were necessary because lesions either crossed the fissure or were in close proximity to another lobar bronchus;

therefore, 4 patients underwent RUL-RML and 2 patients underwent RML-RLL. Usually, the other lobes do not present any particular or unique problems for resection. Two patients had very thick, muscular chest walls. Currently available instrumentation could not reach the hilar area, so a hybrid or modified approach was used. The hybrid incision includes resection of 5 cm of rib from the lateral chest wall. This facilitates access for instruments. However, visibility is still achieved by using the thoracoscope alone. Working through the new incision and the remaining ports, resection can be accomplished satisfactorily. Adequate maneuverability and access to all intrathoracic structrures has been accomplished by this approach for patients who have very thick chest walls, and complex resections have been able to be performed without spreading the ribs. Although we have used this approach for only 2 VATS lobectomies, it has been employed successfully for most VATS pneumonectomies. Despite resection of a segment of rib, if spreading is avoided or kept to a minimum, the patient makes an easy, expeditious recovery with a marked reduction in pain.

Neoplastic Outcomes Following VATS(*n*)SSL

For the resection of cancer, VATS(*n*)SSL has proved to be a superb oncologic operation, which adheres to all accepted principles and criteria. To perform this procedure efficiently and safely, the surgeon must have a complete and detailed knowledge of lung anatomy and its variations. The luxury of dissection by "creeping" forward and exposing anatomy in a piecemeal fashion is not conceded to any surgeon performing VATS(*n*)SSL. One hundred seventy-one patients at our institution have had primary carcinoma of the lung resected, and every bronchial margin was microscopically negative for neoplasm. Thirteen patients had N1 nodes, and 4 patients had microscopically positive N2 nodes found postoperatively after examination by the pathologist. Preoperatively, all patients except one were placed at stage I or stage II. The one patient who was at stage IIIa was enrolled in a protocol recommending preoperative adjuvant therapy because of confirmed N2 nodes at mediastinoscopy. After pathologic examination of the postoperative specimens, staging was upgraded to include stage IV for some patients. No patient in the entire series had a port or chest wall implantation, and there was no isolated recurrence limited only to the operated side. Implantation does not seem to occur from merely touching tumor cells to normal tissue. There is evidence that implantation is much more complex and dependent upon the biology and genetic composition of the tumor.[46, 47]

Some of the patients who died as a result of their primary pulmonary malignancy had neoplastic characteristics that would seem to signal a poor prognosis, such as positive lymph nodes, vascular invasion, or multifocal disease in the resected lobe. In other patients who died, no distinguishing features of their neoplasm present postoperatively could have been used to predict metastases or an early demise. The current anatomic staging systems do not always correlate accurately or consistently with anticipated outcomes for patients undergoing a curative resection for carcinoma of the lung. We hope future staging systems that incorporate pathophysiologic and biologic components of the tumor will allow more valid predictions for survival.[48]

At present, 6 patients have manifested new foci of tumors. Usually, these are designated as recurrences. In reality, once the primary tumor is completely excised, that particular tumor cannot recur. Probably, these new sites of tumor were already present as microscopic metastases or new, microscopic primary tumors, neither of which could be detected earlier because of currently inadequate diagnostic techniques. In fact, all so-called recurrent tumors in this group of patients have presented as distant metastases (that is, 2 in the bone, 2 in the brain, 2 with multiorgan foci).

Of interest, 7 patients who had a single metastasis to the lung from a distant site are still alive.

The present survival rates for lobectomy in primary carcinoma of the lung appear to be similar whether VATS(*n*)SSL or an open conventional resection is performed. If survival is indeed the same, VATS lobectomy must be considered the procedure of choice because of confirmed decreased acute and chronic pain, shorter length of hospital stay, quicker recovery, reduced costs, and overwhelming patient satisfaction compared with the open conventional thoracotomy.

Complications

Complications were few in number and minor in nature. The overall complication rate for VATS(*n*)SSL was 13%. Many of these patients were elderly and had advanced emphysema, marginal cardiac status, and numerous other comorbidities. Excluding patients with minor air leaks, almost all of whom had their chest tubes removed within 7 days following the surgical procedure, the overall complication rate was only 6%. All of these patients recovered expeditiously and uneventfully. Bronchopleural fistula did not occur in any patient, and there was no surgical mortality. These findings compare favorably with published reports for traditional open techniques.[49, 50]

Currently, VATS(*n*)SSL is our procedure of choice for any patient needing a lobectomy. At this time, our only contraindication is a large obstructive hilar lesion. Lung tumors invading one or two ribs of the chest wall can be approached and resected more efficiently from within the thoracic cavity by using VATS. The extent of the tumor involving the ribs can be delineated with better precision by the scope, and the involved ribs can be resected more accurately and with less effort with use of the intrathoracic approach. Only a tumor with appropriate margins is resected, so resection of extraneous and unnecessary normal tissue can be avoided. Moreover, patients can make a remarkable recovery and can be physically ready for discharge on the second postoperative day. As surgeons' experience and skills improve, larger tumors are being resected. The largest tumor removed to date was 9 cm in diameter. It was placed in a plastic bag and divided into segments inside the bag while still in the chest. After the segments were aligned in single file, the tumor was removed easily through the wide anterior incision without spreading the ribs. Using this method, large tumors can be removed. In this series, there were two 9-cm tumors and six 8-cm tumors removed in this manner without spreading the ribs.

Cost Effectiveness of VATS(*n*)SSL

For many thoracic surgeons, the concept of stapling all the hilar structures together simultaneously has been difficult to accept. Most surgeons continue to associate simultaneous stapling with mass ligation and the associated inherent complications that occurred for a multitude of reasons in the past. Even some surgeons within our own group rejected this technique when it was first proposed and continued to perform open, conventional isolation-ligation lobectomies. During the latter part of 1994, we found an ideal opportunity to compare costs for major pulmonary resections between VATS and open techniques. This permitted an equitable and fair comparison, because surgeons from the same group, working in the same hospital, assisted by the same anesthesiologists and nurses, were performing similar pulmonary resections for the same pathology using two different procedures. We found that there was an overall reduction in costs of 51% favoring VATS when compared with open thoracotomy.[51] Since that time, all surgeons in our group have become strong advocates of VATS(*n*)SSL, and currently, all use this technique as their procedure of choice.

There is an ongoing debate among thoracic surgeons concerning the proper sequence of ligation of the hilar structures. Should the bronchus, pulmonary artery, or vein be ligated first to ensure compliance with oncologic principles?[52] Use of VATS(*n*)SSL makes this an invalid argument, because all the structures are ligated simultaneously in their normal anatomic configuration. It is an en bloc cancer resection.

Through the years, we have learned that if VATS is to be performed efficiently, expeditiously, and safely, a team approach—similar to that developed by cardiac surgeons—must be established. The surgeons should have advanced training; basic inherent technical skills for videoscopic operations; an adequate fund of knowledge; an appropriate temperament and attitude for new technologic approaches to surgery; and a strong desire to lead a team dedicated to advancing the quality, spectrum, and comprehensiveness of VATS resections. Trained operating room personnel and dedicated anesthesiologists are mandatory. Surgeons who perform an occasional VATS procedure assisted by inexperienced, peripherally interested operating room personnel, by anesthesiologists who possess only rudimentary knowledge and skills in utilizing double-lumen endotracheal tubes; and by surgical assistants unfamiliar with VATS techniques will have frequent complications, less than optimal results, higher costs, and an abundance of stress and frustration. Many years ago, it was demonstrated that when interested, dedicated cardiac surgeons and operating room personnel worked together as a team in a center with a sufficient volume of cases to ensure the frequent performance of cardiac operations, the procedure became more efficient and successful, and excellent outcomes were attained. This same philosophy must be applied to VATS if progress is to continue.

Because of the multitude of patient benefits that have resulted from VATS, these procedures should no longer be considered experimental by thoracic surgeons. In fact, there is no longer any valid scientific reason or moral justification for performing every lobectomy via the access technique of the open traditional thoracotomy.

Conclusion

The procedure known as VATS(*n*)SSL is not a modified method of mass ligation but instead constitutes a new surgical technique facilitating lobectomy. It is safe, expeditious, and less traumatic and debilitating than a traditional thoracotomy. Overall costs are markedly reduced, and patient acceptance and satisfaction have been extraordinary. All current oncologic principles are observed during resection, and the survival rate of patients who have primary lung neoplasms compares favorably with that in traditional resections. Hemorrhage, bronchopleural fistula, bronchial stump recurrence, and port implantation have not occurred. Pain, hospitalization, and time away from preoperative activity levels are significantly reduced by this method. It is exceedingly beneficial for fragile, elderly, debilitated, and high-risk patients who have significant comorbidity. Even young patients who are reluctant to undergo a formal, traditional thoracotomy accept VATS(*n*)SSL.

As skills improve and experience accumulates, VATS(*n*)SSL may become the procedure of choice for lobectomy. Currently, there is no justification for performing the traditional open thoracotomy for all lobectomies.

References

1. Lewis RJ, Caccavale RJ, Sisler GE: Special report: Videoendoscopic thoracic surgery. N J Med 88:473–475, 1991.
2. Lewis RJ, Caccavale RJ, Sisler GE, et al: One hundred consecutive patients undergoing video-assisted thoracic operations. Ann Thorac Surg 54:421–426, 1992.
3. Lewis RJ: Perspectives in the evolution of video-assisted thoracic surgery. Chest Surg Clin North Am 3:207–213, 1993.
4. Lewis RJ: The role of video-assisted thoracic surgery for cancer of the lung: Wedge resection to lobectomy by simultaneous stapling. Ann Thorac Surg 56:762–768, 1993.
5. Yim APC: Routine video-assisted thoracoscopy prior to thoracotomy. Chest 109:1099–1100, 1996.
6. Lewis RJ, Caccavale RJ, Sisler GE, et al: Video-assisted thoracic surgical resection of malignant lung tumors. J Thorac Cardiovasc Surg 104:1679–1687, 1996.
7. Yim APC, Ko K, Chau W, et al: Video-assisted thoracoscopic anatomic lung resections. Chest 109:13–17, 1996.
8. Lewis RJ: Simultaneously stapled lobectomy: A safe technique for video-assisted thoracic surgery. J Thorac Cardiovasc Surg 109:619–625, 1995.
9. Lewis RJ, Caccavale RJ, Sisler GE, et al: 100 video-assisted thoracic surgical simultaneously stapled lobectomies without rib spreading. Ann Thorac Surg 63:1415–1421, 1997.
10. Mountain CF, Greenberg SD, Fraire AE: Tumor stage in non-small cell carcinoma of the lung. Chest 99:1258–1260, 1991.
11. Gluck T: Experimenteller beitrag zur frage der lung extirpation. Berl Klin Wochenschr 18:645, 1881.
12. Davies HM: Recent advances in the surgery of the lung and pleura. Br J Surg 1:228–258, 1913.
13. Babcock WW: The operative treatment of pulmonary tuberculosis. JAMA 50:1263–1265, 1908.
14. Robinson S: The surgery of bronchiectasis. Surg Gynecol Obstet 24:194–215, 1917.
15. Heuer G: The development of lobectomy and pneumonectomy in man. J Thorac Surg 3:560, 1934.
16. Sarot I: Practical points in lobectomy. J Thorac Surg 8:300–308, 1939.
17. Eggers C: Lobectomy for carcinoma of the lung. J Thorac Surg 4:211, 1934.

18. Lilienthal H: Extirpation of right lower lobe for septic bronchitis. Ann Surg 61:103–105, 1915.
19. Blades B, Kent E: Individual ligation technique for lower lobe lobectomy. J Thorac Surg 10:84–101, 1940.
20. Amosov NM, Berezovsky KK. Pulmonary resection with mechanical suture. J Thorac Cardiovasc Surg 41:325–335, 1961.
21. McGovern EM, Trastek VF, Pairolero PC, et al: Completion pneumonectomy: Indications, complications and results. Ann Thorac Surg 46:141–146, 1988.
22. Utley JR: Completion pneumonectomy and thoracoplasty for bronchopleural fistula and fungal empyema. Ann Thorac Surg 55:672–676, 1993.
23. Gaskin RJ, Bergmann M: Pneumonectomy by "en masse" stapling of hilar vessels. Ann Thorac Surg 19:242–247, 1975.
24. Lewis RJ, Sisler GE, Caccavale RJ: Imaged thoracic lobectomy: Should it be done? Ann Thorac Surg 54:80–83, 1992.
25. Humphrey EW, Smart CR, Winchester DP, et al: National survey of the patterns of care for carcinoma of the lung. J Thorac Cardiovasc Surg 100:837–843, 1990.
26. Nesbitt JC, Putnam JB, Walsh GL, et al: Survival in early-stage non-small cell lung cancer. Ann Thorac Surg 60:466–472, 1995.
27. Williams DE, Pairolero PC, Davis CS, et al: Survival of patients surgically treated for Stage I lung cancer. J Thorac Cardiovasc Surg 82:70–76, 1981.
28. The Ludwig Lung Cancer Study Group: Patterns of failure in patients with resected stage I and stage II non-small cell carcinoma of the lung. Ann Surg 205:67–71, 1987.
29. Yokoi K, Miyazawa N, Imura G: Isolated incisional recurrence after curative resection for primary lung cancer. Ann Thorac Surg 61:1237–1239, 1996.
30. Kim YH, Yun YH: Metastasis of lung carcinoma to proximal femur after hip implant. Orthop Rev 15:534–539, 1986.
31. Lee JS, Hong WK: Prognostic factors in lung cancer. N Engl J Med 327:47–48, 1992.
32. Heys DS, Eremin O: The relevance of tumor draining lymph nodes in cancer. Surg Gynecol Obstet 174:533–540, 1992.
33. Kotlyarov EV, Rukosuyev AA: Long-term results and patterns of disease recurrence after radical operations for lung cancer. J Thorac Cardovasc Surg 102:24–28, 1991.
34. Funatsu T, Matsubara Y, Ikeda S, et al: Pre-operative mediastinoscopic assessment of N factors and the need for mediastinal lymph node dissection in T_1 lung cancer. J Thorac Cardiovasc Surg 108:321–328, 1994.
35. Goldstraw P, Manna MG, Kaplan D, et al: Surgical management of non-small cell lung cancer with ipsilateral mediastinal node metastasis (N_2 disease). J Thorac Cardiovasc Surg 107:19–28, 1994.
36. Mehran RJ, Deslauriers J, Piraux M, et al: Survival related to nodal status after sleeve resection for lung cancer. J Thorac Cardiovasc Surg 107:576–583, 1994.
37. Orringer MD: Editorial on "occult cervical nodal metastases in esophageal cancer: Preliminary results of three-field lymphadenectomy." J Thorac Cardiovasc Surg 113:538–539, 1996.
38. McKneally NF: Invited comment: The importance of surgery to non-small cell carcinoma of lung with mediastinal lymph node metastases. Naruke T, Goya T, Tsuchiya R. Ann Thorac Surg 46:609–610, 1988.
39. Naruke T, Goya T, Tsuchiya R: The importance of surgery to non-small cell carcinoma of lung with mediastinal lymph node metastases. Ann Thorac Surg 46:603–610, 1988.
40. Asamura H, Nakayama H, Kondo H, et al: Lymph node involvement, recurrence and prognosis in resected small peripheral non-small cell carcinomas: Are these carcinomas candidates for video-assisted lobectomy? J Thorac Cardiovasc Surg 111:1125–1134, 1996.
41. Nakahara K, Fujii Y, Matsumura A: Role of systemic mediastinal dissection in N_2 non-small cell lung cancer patients. Ann Thorac Surg 56:331–336, 1993.
42. The Canadian Lung Oncology Group: Investigation for mediastinal disease in patients with apparently operable lung cancer. Ann Thorac Surg 60:1382–1389, 1995.
43. Nakanishi R, Osaki T, Nakanishi K: Treatment strategy for patients with surgically discovered N_2 stage IIIa non-small cell lung cancer. Ann Thorac Surg 64:342–348, 1977.
44. Yim APC, Ho JKS: Minimizing chest wall trauma in video-assisted thoracic surgery. J Thorac Cardiovasc Surg 109:1255–1256, 1995.
45. Landreneau RJ, Pigula F, Luketich JD, et al: Acute and chronic morbidity difference between muscle-sparing and standard lateral thoracotomies. J Thorac Cardiovasc Surg 112:1246–1250, 1996.
46. Jewell WR, Romsdahl MM: Recurrent malignant disease in operative wounds not due to surgical implantation from the resected tumor. Surgery 58:806–809, 1965.
47. Lewis RJ, Caccavale RJ, Sisler GE, et al: Does VATS favor seeding of carcinoma of the lung more than a conventional operation? Int Surg 82:127–130, 1997.
48. Harpole DH, Richards WG, Herndon JE II, et al: Angiongenesis and molecular biologic substaging in patients with stage I non-small cell lung cancer. Ann Thorac Surg 61:1470–1476, 1996.
49. Ginsberg R, Hill L, Eagan R, et al: Modern thirty-day operative mortality for surgical resections in lung cancer. J Thorac Cardiovasc Surg 86:654–658, 1983.
50. Samura H, Naruke T, Tsuchiya R, et al: Bronchopleural fistulas associated with lung cancer operations. J Thorac Cardiovasc Surg 104:1456–1464, 1992.
51. Lewis RJ, Caccavale RJ, Sisler GE, et al: Is video-assisted thoracic surgery cost-effective for major pulmonary resections? NJ Med 93:35–41, 1996.
52. Grismer JT, Read CR: Evolution of pulmonary resection techniques and review of the bronchus first method. Ann Thorac Surg 60:1133–1137, 1995.

COMMENTARY

John R. Benfield

The technique of simultaneously stapled lobectomy flies in the face of conventional wisdom. Had I been asked in the past about the advisability of using this method, I would have cautioned against it with the expectation that there would be an unacceptable incidence of bronchopleural fistula and perhaps bronchovascular fistula. I would have predicted an inordinately high local recurrence rate. My concern about fistula would have been based on the history of mass ligation methods. I have attributed a good technical outcome of lobectomy at least partially to precise, clean separation of the bronchovascular structures; conversely, I have believed that extraneous tissue around the closure of major structures impairs healing. My worry about local recurrence would have come from my reliance on palpation for assessing the size and extent of neoplasms and a prediction that the proposal for using video-assisted thoracic surgery (VATS) would severely limit this important feature of lobectomies for the treatment of cancer.

The facts in this chapter suggest that I have been worrying too much. Neither bronchopleural nor bronchovascular fistulae occurred as a result of VATS procedures, and the incidence of local recurrence was quite acceptable, albeit that mean follow-up is currently only 34 months, because the VATS simultaneously stapled lobectomy approach is still relatively new.

What is new about this procedure? The length of the incision is not really new, because four of the documented incisions totaled 10 to 14 cm, and many traditional thoracotomies do not require longer incisions. The adaptation of incisions to the body build of individual patients is not new, because, when the chest wall is thick, rib segments are removed. Only the enhanced visual exposure that results from the magnification provided by telescopes, the avoidance of intercostal nerve trauma, and the loss of direct palpation capability are new.

The reported results are superb. How many thoracic surgeons can equal outcomes that include mean operating times of 80 minutes without any transfusions, and blood loss that was "always less than 100 ml" I cannot say that my patients regularly do not need time in the intensive care unit or that they require postoperative analgesics for only 1 to 3 days. It is remarkable that ". . . no patient was converted to an open technique because of adhesions, hemorrhage, or unfavorable anatomy." Every bronchial margin was microscopically free of tumor. In evaluating these results, I cannot help but wonder how many lobectomies were done by the author and his associates by conventional open thoracotomy during the study period. The facts that have been made available leave the possibility that the authors are good at selecting patients for VATS lobectomy, and the implication that VATS lobectomy is the method of choice could be misleading.

Lewis says, "Trained operating room personnel and dedicated anesthesiologists are mandatory. Surgeons who perform an occasional VATS procedure assisted by inexperienced, peripherally interested operating room personnel . . . will have frequent complications, less than optimal results, higher costs, and an abundance of stress and frustration." I transpose this advice into the real setting of general thoracic surgery, which is most often done in community hospitals where lobectomies are uncommon operations. In such settings, VATS lobectomy is apt to be far less safe and effective than in an environment that provides the team Lewis suggests. In short, the privilege to undertake VATS lobectomy should be granted to teams and not only to individual surgeons.

Change is hard to accept when it seeks to replace conventional wisdom, particularly when the proposal for change includes elements of a less satisfactory past. Lewis has presented impressive and important evidence to support VATS simultaneously stapled lobectomy. It works well when done by him in his environment, in part because it is being done by individuals who have had decades of experience with conventional lobectomy methods. I believe it would not work well today in the average environment in which thoracic surgery is done, and I hope that future generations of thoracic surgeons will still be able to prepare themselves to do VATS lobectomies with adequate experience in opening the chest to feel the lung and that they will appreciate the three-dimensional aspects of thoracic anatomy.

COMMENTARY

F. Griffith Pearson

The technique of video-assisted, minimal-access lobectomy with simultaneous stapling of the hilar structures (arteries, veins, and bronchus) is conceptually completely original and is totally unfamiliar to the traditional pulmonary surgeon of today. As the authors note in their historical review of the topic, mass ligation of the lobar or pulmonary hilum was reported decades ago during the early experience with lung resection for pulmonary tuberculosis and cancer. Using modern technology and video-assisted imaging, Dr. Lewis has developed a series of simple but ingenious innovations for the expeditious removal of one or more lobes of the lung. He reports a large experience with 200 patients managed since 1991. He discusses the improved performance achieved with experience by comparing the operating times and hospital length of stay for the first 100 patients and the succeeding 100 cases. Nevertheless, even the early experience is impressive, with a relatively short mean length of hospital stay, no mortality, and no disabling morbidity.

The technical features of the procedure are described in detail and include innovations such as positioning the patient to increase the interspace between the ribs on the operative side, the use of a catheter to guide the anvil of the stapler to encircle the hilum of the lobe, the use of four lines of staples to avoid bleeding and air leaks, and the postoperative use of a single No. 20 chest drain. The results achieved in these 200 patients—171 of whom were operated on for primary cancer of the lung—are impressive. Surgery has been performed on all lobes on both sides, and the cases include 6 patients in whom a bilobectomy was necessary. The mean operating time for all cases was 79 minutes, and the average length of hospital stay ws 3.07 days. There were no deaths and no bronchopleural fistulae, and minor air leaks occurred in only 7% of cases (14 patients). No patient required a transfusion, and it appears that narcotic analgesics were used rarely, if ever.

With a mean follow-up of 34 months (with a range of 12 to 69 months), there have been 31 deaths, of which 24 were due to recurrence of the primary cancer. None of these deaths was due to recognized local recurrence! All cancer deaths were caused by hematogenous metastases. At the time the report was made, there were 6 additional patients who were alive and who had recurrent tumor, all resulting from distant metastases. These results do suggest that the survival after this type of lobectomy is in the same range as the expected survival when standard techniques of resection for primary lung cancer are used. The absence of local recurrence is remarkable, although the follow-up in many of these patients may be relatively short. The absence of local recurrence may also reflect the case selection: The authors note that a contraindication to this technique of lobectomy is the recognition of a tumor proximal to the segmental level on bronchoscopy. Indeed, they report very few patients in whom the primary tumor was visible on bronchoscopy in this series. Finally, the authors have conducted a thorough and thoughtful review of the literature, dating back to the earliest attempts at lobectomy for both benign and malignant disease. They recognize that their recommendations for mass ligation using limited-access techniques are heretical to a majority of today's thoracic surgeons. Indeed, a recent report by Michael Mack and associates in the Annals of Thoracic Surgery (64:211–15, 1997) concludes that video-assisted techniques for pulmonary resection in patients who have lung cancer appear to have significant limitations and are still in evolution. I too have been skeptical, and generally negative, about the role of minimal-access, video-assisted techniques for surgical resection of primary lung cancer. Lobectomy and pneumonectomy are broadly accepted as the appropriate procedures for all stages of resectable disease. I share a common concern that VATS resection does not permit palpation in the mediastinum or hilum of the lung. I am skeptical regarding the complete nodal exposure and sampling achieved with VATS, and I believe that small but abnormal scirrhous nodes would easily be overlooked. Having made this statement, however, I cannot argue with the oustanding results obtained by Drs. Lewis and Caccavale: no mortality, minimal morbidity, and no recognized instance of clinical local recurrence in 171 consecutive resections for primary cancer of the lung.

During the past few years, I have heard Dr. Ralph Lewis present his experience and arguments in favor of the video-assisted approach that he has developed. My judgment has always been clouded by an immediate aversion to the technique of mass ligation of the hilar structures. After completing a detailed review of the technical features described in this chapter, along with the exceptionally good results, I find myself much less certain of my previous solid skepticism.

Chapter 21

Resection for Pulmonary Metastases

Joseph B. Zwischenberger and Scott K. Alpard

In selected patients who meet specific criteria, resection of multiple pulmonary metastases is currently the recognized standard of care, with long-term survival (>5 years) expected in up to one third of patients. Since the late 1980s, video-assisted thoracic surgery (VATS) has realized an expanded role in the diagnosis and management of solitary pulmonary metastasis; moreover, VATS may be valuable in selected patients who have more than one pulmonary metastasis. At the time of presentation, an isolated pulmonary nodule does not necessarily represent the systemic or untreatable spread of a primary neoplasm. An isolated pulmonary nodule must first be diagnosed as a metastasis, a primary neoplasm, or other primary pathology.

The resection of a pulmonary metastasis was first reported in the late 1800s[1–3] and described for the first time in 1927, and again in 1930.[4, 5] By 1939, one of the first long-term survivors of pulmonary metastasectomy was reported by Barney and Churchill[6] in a patient with hypernephroma. The patient subsequently survived for 23 years following resection.

Pathology

Neoplastic growth, mechanism of spread, and location of metastases are determined by tumor biology and host resistance. Pulmonary metastases can occur by hematogenous, lymphatic, or aerogenous spread, or through direct invasion. Pulmonary involvement of extrathoracic sites most commonly arises from hematogenous dissemination.[7] Multiple or individual tumor cells may be filtered by the lungs or adhere to the underlying capillary endothelium. While most of the tumor cells are destroyed, those that escape detection within the pulmonary capillary bed become seeds of metastatic disease. The number and size of tumor emboli are directly correlated with the development of pulmonary disease.[8] Tumor emboli can be viewed radiographically, but filling pulmonary capillaries are occasionally confused with diffuse infiltrative processes, such as infection or edema.[9] Tumor cells can also travel by lymphatics, occupying a discrete position or diffusely involving the entire lung, as seen in lymphangitic metastases of breast carcinoma or other metastatic adenocarcinomas. Lymphangitic spread is a result of hematogenous metastases extending from the capillaries to the lymphatics, or arising secondary to retrograde lymphatic spread from abdominal nodal groups to hilar and mediastinal nodes.

Endobronchial metastases are generally secondary to direct bronchial metastasis or parenchymal or mediastinal lymph node metastasis with direct bronchial extension[10, 11]—most frequently, renal cell and breast carcinoma—followed by colon and thyroid cancer. As the metastasis grows, direct extension into other structures may occur. Aerogenous spread of the tumor from one site within the bronchus to another rarely occurs, and, depending on histology, can be indistinguishable from multiple sites of primary bronchial carcinoma. Other routes of pulmonary metastasis may include bronchial artery spread and spread from transbronchial aspirations.[10–12]

Symptoms

Most metastatic lesions are peripherally located, and diagnosis is routinely made on chest radiographs. Because of the peripheral or subpleural location of pulmonary metastases, patients are rarely (<5%) symptomatic before a diagnosis is made. When symptomatic, patients complain of dyspnea, pain, cough, hemoptysis, or wheezing. Dyspnea may be caused by endobronchial obstruction, parenchymal replacement, pleural effusion, or lymphatic invasion. When the onset of dyspnea is acute, contributing factors may include hemorrhage into a lesion, hemorrhage into the pleural space, or pneumothorax (thought to be due to tumor necrosis), erosion into a bronchus, or formation of a bullous lesion that eventually ruptures).[13] Endobronchial lesions may also be obstructing and may result in dyspnea, hemoptysis, or both. Lymphangitic carcinomatosis, most commonly associated with carcinomas of the stomach, breast, prostate, and pancreas, leads to debilitating dyspnea caused by loss of lung compliance out of proportion with the radiologic findings.[12, 14] Chest pain, when present, reflects the development of parietal pleural metastases or direct chest wall involvement. The majority of patients who are symptomatic at presentation do not have resectable disease.

Diagnosis

Diagnostic imaging is the key to identifying a patient in whom the primary site is controlled, yet whose metastatic disease is confined to the lung in areas that are technically amenable to resection. The standard chest radiograph is the most cost-effective screening tool for pulmonary metastases, but it is also the least sensitive and specific. Follow-up chest radiographs demonstrate pulmonary parenchymal changes consistent with a parenchymal mass lesion. The diverse appearance of metastases includes solitary or multiple nodules, well-circumscribed or diffuse opacities, and miliary or massive manifestations. Metastases are most commonly found in the peripheral one third of the lung fields, usually at the lung bases, and this is consistent with hematogenous spread of the tumor via the pulmonary circulation.[7] Choriocarcinoma is an exception, because its metastatic distribution is found in the posterior portion of the upper lobes.[15, 16] The most common presentation of pulmonary metastases is well-circumscribed spherical nodules unassociated with linear densities.[17]

Computed tomography (CT) is the imaging modality of

choice for the detection or exclusion of pulmonary metastases, having replaced conventional chest radiography and linear tomography.[17–19] On CT, pulmonary metastases appear well circumscribed and lack artifacts from the pulmonary vasculature (twinkling star sign).[20] Pleural and subpleural lesions are more easily detected on CT, and, when contrast enhancement is used, CT surpasses conventional techniques by approximately 10^3.[21] CT remains costly and still has limitations. It rarely detects lung lesions greater than 3 mm in diameter and occasionally misses larger lesions, whereas central lesions may be obscured by the pulmonary vasculature. Gains in sensitivity provided by CT are not accompanied by an increase in specificity. To exclude malignancy, CT relies on the presence of calcification within the lesion,[22] and CT is capable of diagnosis in only 63% of benign lung masses.[23] Use of CT to guide needle aspiration biopsies, however, has greatly enhanced our ability to distinguish benign from malignant nodules.

Conventional CT is potentially flawed by artifacts produced by breathing and by misregistration (the space between the slices) of adjacent slices, because each axial slice is acquired during a separate breath-hold. Spiral acquisition CT (SACT) or spiral CT overcomes several disadvantages of conventional CT, because continuous rotation of the radiograph tube and continuous transport of the patient through the scanner allow rapid acquisition of CT data.[24, 25] Misregistration is an additional occurrence with CT and may result in failure to detect lesions as large as 1.5 cm in diameter.[26] Within the scanned volume, SACT provides complete contiguity of slices, improving diagnostic accuracy and reducing the need for repeat scans.[27]

Spiral CT as an imaging modality for pulmonary metastasectomy appears to yield more detail than standard CT. In most cases, pulmonary metastases are spheric, multiple, bilateral, and located peripherally in the middle and lower lung fields.[28] In a prospective study involving 104 patients who had extrathoracic malignancy and suspected pulmonary metastases, Collie and associates[27] concluded that SACT is the technique of choice for assessing pulmonary metastases. Other groups[28–30] also reported that SACT performed significantly better than conventional CT in regard to the number of metastases detected. The ability of SACT to detect more metastases than conventional CT is of importance only if the accuracy of clinical staging is improved to the degree that treatment may be altered.[30–32] Many think spiral CT may allow site-specific strategies for resection, especially when minimally invasive techniques are attempted.

Anatomically based imaging techniques (chest radiography [CXR], CT, spiral CT) are still tissue-nonspecific, so an interest has developed in assessing chest masses with biochemical imaging. A number of radiotracers with varying specificities can be used, but most continue to be prohibitively expensive for use in routine diagnostic study. These include radiotracers that reflect tumor blood flow (Tc-99m-HMPAO), tumor-seeking characteristics (Ga-67-citrate or T1-201-chloride), or high rates of glucose utilization [F-18]2-fluoro-2-D-deoxyglucose (FDG). High-resolution positron emission tomography (PET) with FDG is a technique that can usually distinguish benign from malignant processes.[33, 34] The current applications of PET in oncology include characterizing tumor lesions, differentiating recurrent disease from treatment effects, tumor staging, evaluating the extent of disease, and monitoring therapy.[35] Assessing tumor metabolism by using PET with FDG takes advantage of the enhanced glucose uptake observed in neoplastic cells.[36] This imaging technique produces high-quality tomographic images reflective of the metabolic characteristics of imaged tissue. When lung neoplasms were shown to utilize glucose,[37] PET with FDG was used to diagnose, stage, restage, assess treatment response, and evaluate solitary pulmonary nodules in lung cancer.[38]

In assessing the resectability of pulmonary metastases, PET may prove particularly useful in excluding other sites of metastatic disease. Monitoring the therapeutic response of thoracic neoplasms also continues to be a challenge. Persistent parenchymal density after resection, as shown by CT, does not always imply malignancy. Additionally, PET is a useful technique for evaluating possible residual malignancies.[39] Another significant benefit of FDG-PET in evaluating chest masses is its high negative predictive value.[40, 41] Biochemical imaging may improve sensitivity, but as yet it is not anatomically precise enough to guide strategic planning of metastasectomy.

Treatment

Most patients who have metastatic solid tumors present with multiple metastatic sites or unresectable pleural or pulmonary metastases, so resection of pulmonary metastases confers no survival advantage. Surgical resection of all visible or palpable metastases is indicated when there is control of the primary tumor and metastases are confined to the lungs. A management algorithm for suspected pulmonary metastases is proposed in Figure 21–1.

Surgery

In patients who have technically resectable pulmonary metastases, control of the primary cancer, absence of extrathoracic metastases, and complete resection of all palpable metastases are associated with improved long-term survival relative to treatment-related risk, almost regardless of histology. Pulmonary metastasectomy can also be useful in restaging disease, providing prognostic information, dictating further treatment, or providing adjuvant treatment following chemotherapy. Surgical approaches and resection techniques for pulmonary metastases include median sternotomy, trans-sternal bilateral (clamshell) thoracotomies, posterolateral thoracotomy, and video-assisted thoracic surgery (VATS).[42, 43] The choice of approach depends on the individual patient, tumor histology, number of lesions, location of nodules, and laterality of the disease. If all metastases are resected, patient survival is not influenced by the choice of incisions; however, each approach is associated with various advantages and disadvantages (Table 21–1). To preserve as much lung as possible and provide adequate margins, abnormal lesions are resected while the lung is inflated, if exposure allows. When more extensive resection is necessary, segmentectomy or lobectomy may be required[7] (Table 21–2). Some thoracic surgeons advocate VATS as a combined diagnostic

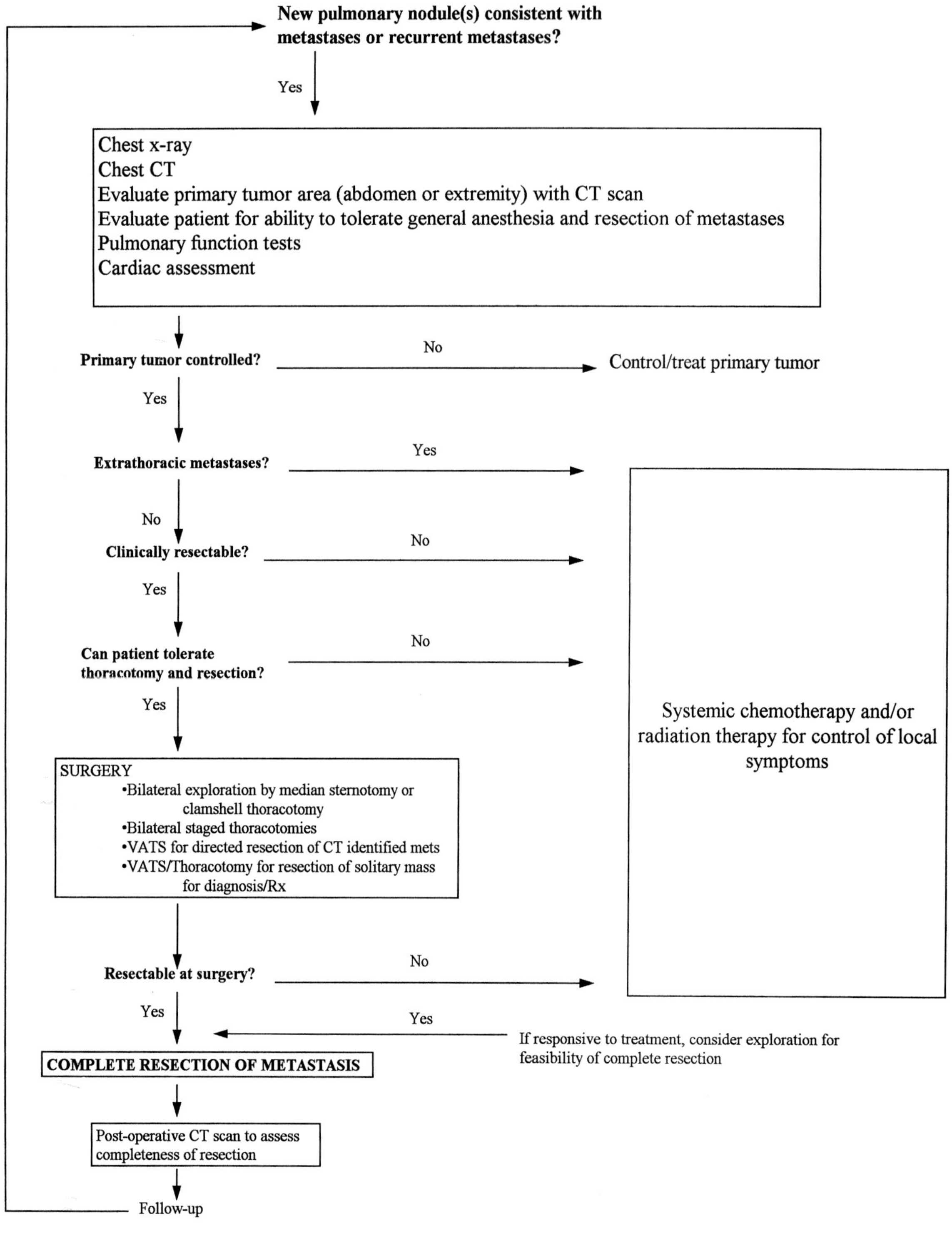

Figure 21–1. Management algorithm for suspected pulmonary metastases. mets = metastases.

and therapeutic modality because of the perceived decrease in morbidity and mortality.

Median Sternotomy

Median sternotomy is the preferred surgical approach for pulmonary metastasectomy.[44–47] This procedure is recommended for initial exploration and resection in patients who have multiple unilateral or bilateral nodules, or in those who have pulmonary metastases from osteogenic or soft tissue sarcomas. Median sternotomy allows single-stage exploration and resection of disease in both hemithoraces and provides the opportunity to find metastases undetected by preoperative radiographic studies. A double-lumen endotracheal tube is recommended as an aid to exposure and palpation. The sternum is separated and the lung mobilized by dividing the inferior pulmonary ligament and any pleural adhesions. The lungs are sequen-

Table 21–1. Advantages and Disadvantages of Surgical Incisions for Resection of Pulmonary Metastases

Median Sternotomy	
Advantages	Bilateral thoracic explorations with one incision Decreased pain
Disadvantages	Exposure impaired for: Posterior and medial lesions (near hilum) Left lower lobe in patients with obesity, congestive heart failure, or chronic obstructive pulmonary disease (increased thoracic anteroposterior diameter)
Posterolateral Thoracotomy	
Advantages	Familiar approach to the hemithorax Excellent exposure
Disadvantages	Only one hemithorax may be explored per incision Muscles usually divided (except for muscle-sparing technique) Increased pain
Video-Assisted Thoracic Surgery (VATS)	
Advantages	Excellent visualization of pleural surfaces Minimal morbidity and discomfort May identify pleural studding, malignant effusions, etc.
Disadvantages	Unable to visualize metastases within the lung parenchyma Unable to bimanually palpate lung Learning curve Increased length of procedure Potential for increased costs (↑ operating room time, ↑ equipment cost, versus ↓ length of stay)

tially deflated and palpated, metastases are identified and resected to maximize remaining lung parenchyma, and the deflated lung is reinflated.

Many surgeons reinflate the lung before wedge resection of the metastases to minimize resection of functional parenchyma. Now, endoscopic stapling and cutting devices that have reticulating heads also simplify wedge resection of metastases. Left lower lobectomies can be performed, but the overlying heart makes this approach more difficult. The left lower lobe can be exposed by using gentle traction on the pericardium and rotation of the table toward the surgeon. The left lower lobe is elevated by placing surgical packs posterior to the hilum of the deflated lung, as well as using an internal mammary artery retractor to facilitate exposure. Previous sternal irradiation is an absolute contraindication to median sternotomy because of poor wound healing. Relative contraindications include morbid obesity and chest-wall involvement. Postoperative morbidity of sternotomy and thoracotomy is reviewed in Table 21–3.

Table 21–2. Type of Resection in 729 Patients With Pulmonary Metastases Undergoing 843 Operations*

Resection	No. Patients	%
Wedge resection	478	56
Segmental resection	102	13
Lobectomy/bilobectomy	228	27
Sleeve resection	22	
Double sleeve resection	12	
Pneumonectomy	21	2
Sleeve pneumonectomy	2	
Exploratory thoracotomy	5	1
Mediastinal metastasectomy (without lung tissue)	9	1
Total	843	100

*Data from Vogt-Moykopf I, Krysa S, Bulzebruck H, et al: Surgery for pulmonary metastases: The Heidelberg experience. Chest Surg Clin North Am 4:85–112, 1994.

Posterolateral Thoracotomy

Posterolateral thoracotomy, a familiar approach for pulmonary resection of lung cancer, is a recommended technique for unifocal and selected unilateral pulmonary metastases.[48] Although thoracotomy may improve the exposure for those metastases located posterior to or near the hilum on the left side,[46] the surgeon is limited to one hemithorax, and bilateral thoracotomies would rarely be performed at the same operation; instead, staged thoracotomies would be necessary to accomplish bilateral exploration.

Extended Thoracotomy

Bilateral anterior thoracotomies with transverse sternotomy (clamshell), or unilateral thoracotomy with partial or complete median sternotomy (hemi-clamshell) have recently been suggested for pulmonary metastasectomy. These approaches not only facilitate bilateral exploration, lower lobe exposure, and detection of hemithorax exten-

Table 21–3. Postoperative Morbidity and Surgical Approach*

Type of Morbidity	Median Sternotomy (N = 330)	Lateral Thoracotomy (N = 198)
Secondary thoracotomy	10 (3%)	6 (3%)
Hemorrhage	10 (3%)	8 (4%)
Empyema	9 (3%)	1 (1%)
Bronchopleural fistula	3 (1%)	4 (2%)
Respiratory insufficiency	17 (5%)	2 (1%)
Pulmonary embolism	1 (1%)	—
Suction by bronchoscopy	17 (5%)	8 (4%)
Wound infection	6 (2%)	3 (2%)
Paresis of phrenic nerve	5 (2%)	4 (2%)
Paresis of recurrent nerve	5 (2%)	3 (2%)

*Data from Vogt-Moykopf I, Krysa S, Bulzebruck H, et al: Surgery for pulmonary metastases: The Heidelberg experience. Chest Surg Clin North Am 4:85–112, 1994.

sion of mediastinal disease but also allow exposure of the mediastinum, the pericardium, the pleura, and the lung.[49] Exposure is improved, but these incisions require sacrifice of the internal mammary artery and potentially cause more discomfort.

Video-Assisted Thoracic Surgery (VATS)

In the 1990s, advances in endoscopic surgical instrumentation and refinements in VATS provided surgeons the ability to perform VATS parenchyma-sparing wedge resections for peripheral lung lesions. Results with these procedures were similar to those achieved by open approaches. Because pulmonary metastases are located in the lung periphery and are immediately subpleural,[50] they are often amenable to VATS. The first report of a thoracoscopic pulmonary metastasectomy described use of the Nd : YAG laser to resect a solitary focus of metastatic renal cell carcinoma.[51] In 1993, Dowling and associates[52] reported the first series of VATS for metastasectomy. Following these reports, McCormack and associates[53] retrospectively compared the efficacy of conventional CT and plain CXR in identifying lesions found at open thoracotomy. The authors concluded that standard imaging techniques do not identify all lung metastases adequately. Therefore, surgical approaches that preclude manual palpation of the lung should not be used for therapeutic metastasectomy. In 1995, Liu and associates[54] concluded that VATS was ideal for diagnostic and therapeutic metastasectomy. However, only immediate postoperative results were used in this study. Landreneau and associates[55] reported minimal morbidity and no mortality in 61 patients who underwent 85 thoracoscopic pulmonary resections.

Advantages and benefits claimed for VATS metastasectomy include decreased pain, shorter hospital stay, and more rapid recovery. Complications, while rare, include atelectasis, pneumonia, air leak lasting more than 1 week, and failure to resect all metastases, leaving positive margins or pleural seeding with extraction of the metastasis.[21, 48] Nodules that cannot be visualized intraoperatively because they are too small or too far from the pleural surface may require localization by a CT-guided hook wire to permit thoracoscopic excision similar to needle localization for breast biopsies.[56] Landreneau and associates[57] reported results of 155 VATS resections in patients who had a history of cancer and new indeterminate pulmonary nodules. A solitary nodule representing a metastatic focus was found in 10 of these patients, who had neither evidence of local recurrence of their primary malignancy or any other site of metastatic disease. Extrapulmonary sites of systemic metastasis were found in 4 of the 10 patients after VATS, whereas the other 6 patients were without recurrence. Yim and associates[58] recommended that VATS not be used for therapeutic metastasectomy because of the high rate of early recurrence following this procedure. In 1996, McCormack and associates[59] reported a prospective study involving 18 patients in whom median sternotomy detected up to double the number of metastases predicted by CT scan. McCormack concluded that therapeutic metastasectomy should incorporate open approaches allowing bimanual palpation of the entire lung.

Currently, VATS remains a popular tool for diagnosing, staging, and treating solitary pulmonary nodules, including potential metastases.[60, 61] Unfortunately, metastases within the lung parenchyma may be undetectable by VATS, which visualizes only the visceral pleura, so usefulness for complete resection is limited. VATS precludes bimanual palpation of the lungs for lesions not identified on the surface or localized by CT scan. VATS as a diagnostic or therapeutic tool, or both, has also been used to assist median sternotomy. In this setting, VATS offers increased exposure by visualizing the retrocardiac left lower lobe.[62] Therefore, VATS seems most applicable in diagnosing metastases,[52] increasing exposure in the setting of median sternotomy,[62] or staging the extent of metastases.[60, 61]

Radiation Therapy

Radiation therapy is most widely used for palliation of symptoms in patients who have advanced unresectable disease. Baeza and associates[63] reported on 62 patients treated with whole-lung irradiation for pulmonary metastases caused by tumors of various histologic types. On CXR, 34% had complete or more than 50% reduction in pulmonary metastases, 26% had no change, and 18% showed progression of disease.

Patient Selection

The most important factors in selecting patients for pulmonary metastasectomy include control of the primary tumor, ability to resect all metastatic disease, no extrathoracic metastases, and sufficient cardiopulmonary reserve for the planned resection.[64] Patients who experience long-term survival following pulmonary metastasectomy usually have a limited number of pulmonary nodules, long tumor doubling times, and long disease-free intervals.[64] Complete surgical resection, however, is crucial to achieve long-term survival.

There is wide variability in the characteristics of pulmonary metastases from different primary neoplasms and in the subsequent survival of patients who have these metastases. To help define the association of pulmonary metastases with postresection survival, preoperative indicators should be compared in patients who have the same type of primary tumor. Various prognostic factors related to specific tumors are reviewed in Table 21–4.

Resectability

The most important prognostic indicator, as well as the most constant single variable reflecting prolonged post-thoracotomy survival, is complete resectability of pulmonary metastases. Extrapulmonary disease (e.g., regional lymph nodes, pericardium, parietal pleura) is a known negative prognostic indicator. If all metastases can be resected, if morbidity can be kept low, and if pulmonary parenchyma is conserved, palliation and prolonged survival may be achieved.[65, 66] In all solid tumors, the inability to perform complete resection at the time of thoracotomy predicts a shortened and limited post-thoracotomy survival along with an unfavorable risk-benefit ratio.

Location and Stage of the Primary Tumor

The specific anatomic location of the primary tumor does not usually influence postresection survival. Whereas the initial or primary stage may suggest the biologic aggressiveness of the tumor, survival in patients who have a more advanced stage of primary neoplasms may not differ from that in patients who have an earlier stage of the disease if the primary tumor is completely resected. Negative nodal status has been predictive of improved postresection survival for patients who have breast cancer.[67] Although not confirmed in later studies,[68] improved post-thoracotomy survival has been linked to Dukes stage A colorectal carcinoma (5-year survival rate of 37.5%) as compared with Dukes stage C (5-year survival rate of 15%).[69]

Number of Metastases Resected

Patients who have fewer metastases found and resected at thoracotomy experience longer post-thoracotomy survival than patients who have numerous metastases. In osteogenic sarcoma, increased survival has been associated with 4 or fewer nodules resected at thoracotomy.[70] A more favorable outcome was associated with Ewing's sarcoma when fewer than 4 nodules were resected.[71] A favorable outcome was predicted with soft tissue sarcoma if fewer than 16 nodules were resected at thoracotomy.[72] A single nodule in patients who had colorectal metastasis correlated with prolonged survival.[68] The number of nodules resected did not influence survival in patients who had breast cancer,[73] renal cell carcinoma,[64] or melanoma.[75]

Disease-Free Interval (DFI)

The disease-free interval (DFI) is determined from the time of resection of the primary tumor to the time at which (pulmonary) metastases are detected. A short DFI may represent a tumor with greater virulence and a poor prognosis, in which metastases can be multiple and experience rapid growth. A long DFI may correlate with longer postresection survival in a less biologically aggressive tumor. In patients who have renal cell carcinoma,[76] soft tissue sarcoma,[77] colorectal cancer[78] osteogenic sarcoma,[79] or breast carcinoma,[73] a DFI of greater than 12 months is associated with prolonged survival following thoracotomy. The longer the DFI, the greater the chance for successful treatment of metastases[43, 45, 80]; however, others have not found the DFI to be a significant prognostic indicator.[72, 81]

Nodules (Preoperative)

The debate over the prognostic value of the number of nodules found on preoperative radiographic studies continues. While the number and size of nodules on preoper-

Table 21–4. Prognostic Factors Dependent on Primary Tumor†

	Patient		Lung Metastasis			Resection	
Primary Tumor	Age	Sex	Number	DFI	Lymph Node	Type	Radicality
Breast carcinoma	NS	NS	*	*	*	NS	NS
Testicular carcinoma	NS	NS	NS	NS	NS	NS	*
Hypernephroma	NS	NS	*	*	NS	NS	NS
Colorectal carcinoma	NS	NS	*	NS	NS	NS	NS
Osteosarcoma	*	NS	*	NS	NS	NS	NS
Soft tissue sarcoma	NS	NS	NS	NS	NS	NS	*

NS = not significant; * = significant; DFI = disease-free interval.

†Data from Vogt-Moykopf I, Krysa S, Bulzebruck H, et al: Surgery for pulmonary metastases: The Heidelberg experience. Chest Surg Clin North Am 4:85–112, 1994.

ative studies is thought by many to carry important prognostic information (indicating the biologic aggressiveness of the tumor), others disagree with their prognostic value, because nodule number is commonly underestimated.[82] Patients who have sarcoma have shown significant improvement in survival associated with the number of nodules seen preoperatively.[45, 70–72, 83] This correlation between improved survival and nodule number has not been found in patients who have melanoma[84] or renal cell carcinoma.[81]

Tumor Doubling Time

Based on observations made by Collins,[85] Joseph and associates[86] first described selecting patients for pulmonary metastasectomy using tumor doubling time (TDT), which is determined by measuring the same metastasis (the most rapidly growing nodule) on similar studies, such as serial CXRs. To calculate TDT, a mathematical formula may be used:

$$\text{Tumor doubling time} = \frac{\text{time between first and second measurements} \times 0.231}{\ln(\text{second diameter} \div \text{first diameter})}$$

All metastases do not grow at the same rate. Therefore, errors in calculating TDT can occur. The biologic nature of the metastases may be indirectly revealed by TDT and, therefore, influence postresection survival, because a short TDT is associated with decreased survival after metastasectomy.[86, 87] We prefer to resect metastases when they are detected and avoid follow-up CXR to determine doubling times.

Age and Gender

Age and gender should not be considered prognostic factors beyond their usual influence on post-thoracotomy survival as determined by cardiopulmonary conditioning.

Although many authors have reported that various prognostic factors play a role in patient survival, Robert and associates[88] reported that survival was not related to DFI, multiple lung metastases, or recurrent tumors following a first or second procedure. This report encompasses 276 patients who underwent curative removal of metastatic disease, with survival rates of 69% and 48% at 2 years and 5 years, respectively.

Results

Critical analysis of results and assessment of factors that influence survival depend on the careful evaluation of patients who have homogeneous tumor histology, stages, and selection criteria. Analysis of outcome has been difficult, because natural history and survival following metastasectomy may vary widely. In 1991, the International Registry of Lung Metastases was established to assess long-term results of pulmonary metastasectomy.[89] The initial report included 5206 cases. Following complete resection, survival rates at 5, 10, and 15 years were 36%, 26%, and 22%, respectively. The report concluded that the best prognosis was for resection of metastatic germ cell tumors, whereas resection of metastatic melanoma had the worst prognosis. Table 21–5 provides a comprehensive bibliography by primary tumor histology.

Osteogenic Sarcoma

The lung is the major site of metastases in patients who have osteogenic sarcoma and is involved in 80% of all relapses in this disease.[65] Before the development of effective chemotherapy, more than 90% of patients who had osteogenic sarcoma died of pulmonary metastases. The strongest predictor of increased survival remains the ability to render the patient free of disease at resection of pulmonary metastasis. In addition, chemotherapy following resection of the primary tumor can improve the disease-free survival rate as well as alter the pattern of pulmonary recurrence.[65] Coupling aggressive surgical resection and chemotherapy has significantly impacted the salvage rates for patients with osteogenic sarcoma.[80, 90–94] Before this aggressive approach to pulmonary disease, the 5-year survival rate for these patients was reported to be as low as 17%.[95] Salvage rates have since more than doubled, with patients now experiencing 5-year survival rates of 35 to 40%,[7] justifying aggressive surgical treatment for initial and recurrent pulmonary metastases.[96, 97]

Long-term follow-up has been reported following aggressive pulmonary metastasectomy.[98] However, during the second decade of follow-up, a significant number of 10-year survivors developed secondary malignancies.

Soft Tissue Sarcoma

Most soft tissue sarcoma metastases occur in the lung within the first 2 years following initial diagnosis.[99] Pulmonary resection offers the only possibility for cure, because most of these tumors are resistant to chemotherapy. Five-year survival rates of 18% to 35% have been reported following metastasectomy.[72] Various factors have been suggested to correlate with increased survival, including 4 or fewer nodules, a DFI of greater than 12 months, the ability to render the patient free of disease at the time of operation, and tumor doubling times greater than 40 days. The number of metastases resected did not correlate with survival in those patients who were rendered completely disease free.[45] Sufficient lung function and reserve are the only limiting factors in resection.[21]

Ewing's Sarcoma

Ewing's sarcoma is the second most common childhood bone tumor, following osteogenic sarcoma. The most common site of metastases at presentation, as well as the most common site of initial relapse, is the lung. Lanza and associates[71] reported a 5-year survival rate of 15% and a post-thoracotomy median survival time of 28 months in patients rendered disease free who underwent thoracotomy for pulmonary metastases. In those patients not rendered disease free, post-thoracotomy median survival time was 12 months. No patient was alive 22 months following thoracotomy. Resection of fewer than 4 malignant nodules correlated with increased survival.

Table 21–5. Survival Following Pulmonary Metastasectomy

Investigator	Year	No. Patients	5-Year Survival Rate (%)
Osteogenic Sarcoma			
Martini et al [96]	1971	22	29
Marcove et al [133]	1975	22	31
Giritsky et al [93]	1978	19	57.8 (3 yr)
Putnam et al [70]	1983	39	40
Belli et al [34]	1989	20	37
Carter et al [94]	1991	25	20
Snyder et al [92]	1991	21	39
Beattie et al [98]	1991	22	18 (19 yr)
Skinner et al [135]	1992	247	41
Saltzman et al [136]	1993	26	39
Inoue et al [137]	1996	22	33.9
Renal Cell Carcinoma			
Morrow et al [116]	1980	30	24
Jett et al [76]	1983	44	27
Mountain et al [104]	1984	20	54
Dernevick et al [113]	1985	33	21
Vogt-Moykopf et al [80]	1988	42	42
Schott et al [114]	1988	39	32.7
Roberts et al [117]	1989	33	24
di Silverio et al [118]	1991	17	35
Pogrebniak et al [81]	1992	23	60
Fourquier et al [115]	1997	50	44
Breast Carcinoma			
Schlappack et al [67]	1988	50	12
Goya and Tsuchiya [101]	1990	23	50
Lanza et al [73]	1992	44	50
Staren et al [102]	1992	33	36
Friedel et al [138]	1994	90	27
McDonald et al [139]	1994	60	37.8
Morone et al [140]	1996	12	11
Simpson et al [141]	1997	17	62
Head and Neck Cancer			
Redina et al [142]	1986	6	66.7 (3 yr)
Mazer et al [143]	1988	44	43
Finley et al [129]	1992	20	29
Wedman et al [128]	1996	21	59
Colorectal Cancer			
McCormack and Attiyeh [69]	1979	35	22
Mansel [144]	1986	66	38
Brister et al [78]	1988	27	21
Goya and Tsuchiya [101]	1990	85	44.3
McAfee et al [68]	1992	139	30.5
Maebeya et al [145]	1993	14	25.7
Yano et al [121]	1993	27	41.1
Zapatero et al [146]	1994	13	23
Csekeo et al [147]	1995	25	28
Girard et al [148]	1995	65	27
Otani et al [149]	1995	31	32
van Halteran et al [150]	1995	38	43
Regnard et al [151]	1995	101	21
Saito et al [153]	1996	19	39
Okumura et al [153]	1996	159	40.5
Soft Tissue Sarcoma			
Martini et al [154]	1978	102	26
Creagan et al [155]	1979	112	29
Putnam et al [72]	1984	67	30

Table continued on following page

Table 21–5. Survival Following Pulmonary Metastasectomy *Continued*

Investigator	Year	No. Patients	5-Year Survival Rate (%)
Jablons et al [45]	1989	68	25
Casson et al [156]	1992	58	25.8
Levenback et al [157]	1992	45	43
Gadd et al [158]	1993	78	23 (3 yr)
Robinson et al [159]	1994	40	70
Bouros et al [160]	1906	255	38
Melanoma			
Cahan et al [161]	1973	12	33
Mathisen et al [162]	1979	86	21
Thayer et al [163]	1985	18	11.1
Wong et al [164]	1988	47	25
Gorenstein et al [75]	1991	56	25
Harpole et al [165]	1992	98	20
Karakousis et al [166]	1994	39	14
Tafra et al [167]	1995	106	27
Gynecologic Neoplasms			
Fuller et al [168]	1985	15	36
Matsukuma et al [169]	1989	35	36
Levenback et al [157]	1992	45	43

Breast Cancer

Although 20% of breast cancer patients die of isolated pulmonary metastases, lung involvement in breast cancer is a common indicator of widespread metastatic disease. New pulmonary nodules in the setting of breast cancer are difficult to evaluate, just as it is difficult to distinguish "adenocarcinoma" in the lungs as either breast metastases or a primary lung carcinoma. In a patient who has a history of breast cancer, a solitary nodule in the lung has a greater than 50% chance of being a primary bronchogenic carcinoma and only a 33% chance of being a lung metastasis.[100] Surgical resection of isolated pulmonary metastases resulting from breast cancer has resulted in 5-year survival rates of 14 to 50%. In 1990, Goya and Tsuchiya[101] reported a 5-year survival rate of 50% in 23 patients who had breast cancer and who underwent metastasectomy. Staren and associates[102] then reported on 63 patients who had isolated lung metastases in whom the 5-year survival rate following pulmonary resection was 36%. Again, 50% of patients who presented with adenocarcinoma in the lung were found to have new primary tumors unrelated to previous breast cancer. In those who had pulmonary metastases as a result of breast cancer, wedge resection with 1- to 2-cm margins was reported as adequate. Complete lymph node dissection was unnecessary unless the lymph nodes were obviously enlarged. Provided that the metastases were isolated to the lung, no differences in the type of resection, DFI, or number of metastases were found. Surgical resection has also resulted in a significantly increased survival rate compared with that for patients treated medically,[102–104] with a postresection 5-year survival rate of approximately 35%. Although a beneficial role for the surgical resection of isolated pulmonary metastases arising from breast tissue has been implied, it remains difficult to separate surgery's contribution from that of chemotherapy, because combination therapy is almost invariably used.

Germ Cell Tumors

Germ cell tumors comprise 95% of all testicular cancers. With multidisciplinary therapy, a cure rate of 85% has been reported for disseminated testicular tumors.[105] The goal of surgery, considered second-line therapy following curative cisplatin-based combination chemotherapy, is complete resection of any residual tumor and complete remission. Mediastinal lymphadenectomy should be included at the time of resection.[106] Surgical resection provides cytoreduction as well as histologic evaluation of tumor nodules, helping to direct further therapy.

Renal Cell Carcinoma

Renal cell carcinoma accounts for approximately 3% of all adult malignancies, with distant metastases present in 30% of patients at diagnosis. The lung is the most common site of metastasis arising from renal cell carcinoma and is the site of occurrence in 50 to 60% of patients.[107] Renal cell carcinoma is a tumor that has no known effective chemotherapy or radiation therapy regimen. Libby and associates[108] reported on simultaneous renal cell carcinoma with pulmonary primary tumors. Formal anatomic resection is recommended for each of these neoplasms. With use of interleukin-2 (IL-2) preceding metastasectomy, Kim and Louie[109] reported a decrease in the size of the metastasis and a reduction in the primary tumor, allowing complete resection. Survival was not affected by the number of lesions or the DFI. When metastases were isolated to the lung, Goya and Tsuchiya[101] reported a 40% 5-year survival rate in patients who had renal cell carcinoma. At present, 50 to 75% of patients who have renal cell carcinoma present with or develop pulmonary metastases.[110] The behavior of this cancer is unpredictable, and spontaneous disease regression has been reported. The efficacy of pulmonary metastasectomy for renal cell carcinoma has been reported, with 5-year survival rates ranging from 21 to 60%.[80, 81, 104, 111–118] Many of these studies, however, include metastasectomy from other sites in addition to the lung.

Colorectal Carcinoma

Although the lung is the most frequent site of extra-abdominal metastases in colorectal carcinoma,[119] only 1% of patients who have this disease present with isolated pulmonary metastases as the first site of recurrence. Control of the primary site is an important prognostic factor for these patients.[73, 120, 121] Following curative resection, pulmonary metastases were seen in 10 to 20% of patients,[122] and isolated pulmonary metastases were found in 2 to 4% of these patients.[123, 124] In most cases, metastasectomy is possible because colorectal metastases in the lung are few in number and slow growing. The 5-year survival rate after metastasectomy is 25 to 42%.[120, 123–125] Following pulmonary metastasectomy, the lung is the most common site of recurrence.[123, 125] In selected patients who have recurrent pulmonary metastases, resection has been suggested.[73, 125] McCormack and associates[124] reported 10-year results of lung resection for colorectal metastasis. Outcome was not found to be significantly altered by the DFI, the number of nodules, or the status of the primary tumor. Resection offers the only possibility of long-term survival in patients who have isolated pulmonary metastases, and, in the absence of effective chemotherapy for metastatic colorectal cancer, these patients should be considered for resection. In a patient who has a history of colorectal cancer, adenocarcinoma in a solitary pulmonary nodule could be metastasis or a primary lung cancer. A lobectomy and lymph node dissection should be performed if histology is uncertain.

Head and Neck

Patients who have head and neck primary tumors have late-appearing second primary lesions, because 15% present with additional primary tumors, either in the airway or the upper digestive system. Therefore, patients who appear after head and neck resection with a new lesion in the lung are first approached for possible cure of a second primary tumor.[126] All lesions (second primaries or metastatic) should be treated by surgical resection, because surgery provides the best possible cure.[127] In this subgroup of patients, anatomic resection (i.e., lobectomy), rather than just wedge resection for metastases arising from head and neck tumors, is recommended. The first site of recurrence of all head and neck cancers, except those of the lip, tonsil, and adenoid, is the lung.[7] Wedman and associates[128] reported on 138 patients who had cancer of the head and neck and who developed pulmonary metastases. Pulmonary metastasectomy was performed in 21 patients, and 18 of these patients (86%) had complete resection. The 5-year survival rate in the metastasectomy group was 59% versus 4% in the group not undergoing surgical resection. The most important predictor of post-thoracotomy survival is rendering the patient disease free. Improved long-term survival has also been linked to the presence of only one malignant pulmonary nodule, locoregional primary control, and a disease-free interval of 1 year.[129]

Melanoma

Resection of pulmonary metastases arising from melanoma was first described in 1936.[130] Pulmonary metastases are the second most common site of spread in melanoma,[75] and have been reported in 11% of patients in whom respiratory failure is the most common cause of death.[75] Unfortunately, distant metastases are often multiple and widespread. Wedge resection of palpable disease has demonstrated that solitary nodules respond much better than multiple nodules.[126] Tafra and associates[131] reported on 106 patients who had a 5-year survival rate of 27% following pulmonary metastasectomy of melanoma. In patients who have pulmonary metastases arising from melanoma, surgical resection should be aggressively considered. No chemotherapy regimen has proven consistently efficacious, and those that are used have limited value and associated high morbidity.

Minimally Invasive Thoracic Surgery (MITS) Survey

Members of the Minimally Invasive Thoracic Surgery Core Group were surveyed (n = 8) regarding video-assisted metastasectomy. Table 21–6 shows how often (per year) VATS metastasectomy is performed and the indications for VATS metastasectomy. The group of VATS enthusiasts disagreed as to whether VATS was primarily diagnostic (1 nodule) or therapeutic (2 nodules). Neither supported VATS for multiple (>2) nodules. The responses were evenly divided (4 yes and 4 no) as to whether spiral

Table 21–6. Minimally Invasive Thoracic Surgery (MITS)

MITS Survey (n = 8)

How Many Times a Year Do You Perform Metastasectomy?

	Mean	*Range*
No. metastasectomy (total)	6	4–10
No. via VATS	2	0–5
No. open thoracotomy	1	0–3
No. median sternotomy	3	0–5
VATS Metastasectomy: No. of Potential Metastases Identified by CT Scan		
One	4	
Two	4	
Three	—	
Four	—	
Unlimited	—	
? Bilateral VATS at same anesthesia	Yes 2	No 6

CT improved the chance for complete resection; 2 respondents estimated that tumor is left behind in 0 to 25% of cases, whereas 1 respondent indicated that the number was between 25 and 50%.

Conclusion

Surgical resection of pulmonary metastases remains the best method of local control to render the patient disease free. Surgery attempts to control the biologic sequelae of the primary malignancy through mechanical removal, but it does not change the fundamental biology of metastases. Regardless of the primary tumor histology, resectability is the most important factor associated with potential long-term survival. Complete resection of pulmonary metastases is associated with long-term or disease-free survival in 20 to 25% of patients, in contrast to unresectable metastases. Treatment of pulmonary metastases continues to improve as we await the results of various clinical studies examining improved adjuvant therapies directed at biologic and molecular events in the neoplastic cell's life cycle.

References

1. Weinlechner: Wien Med Wochenschr 20:1882.
2. Weinlechner: Wien Med Wochenschr 32:1892.
3. Kronlein RU: Ueber Lungenchirirugie. Berl Klin Wochenschr 9:129–132, 1884.
4. Divis G: Ein Beitrag zur operativen Behandlung der Lunggenschwultse. Acta Chir Scand 62:329, 1927.
5. Torek F: Removal of metastatic carcinoma of the lung and mediastinum: Suggestions as to technique. Arch Surg 21:1416–1424, 1930.
6. Barney JD, Churchill ED: Adeno-carcinoma of the kidney with metastasis to the lungs treated by pulmonary resection. J Urol 42:269–276, 1939.
7. Pass HI: Treatment of metastatic cancer to the lung. *In* De Vita V, Hellman S, Rosenberg S (eds): Principles and Practice of Oncology. Philadelphia, JB Lippincott, 1993, pp 2186–2200.
8. Liotta LA, Saidel MG, Kleinerman J: The significance of hematogenous tumor cell clumps in the metastatic process. Cancer Res 36:889–894, 1976.
9. Dwyer AJ, Reichert CM, Woltering EA, et al: Diffuse pulmonary metastasis in melanoma: Radiographic-pathologic correlation. AJR Am J Roentgenol 143:983, 984, 1984.
10. Berg HK, Petrelli NJ, Herrera L, et al: Endobronchial metastasis from colorectal carcinoma. Dis Colon Rectum 27:745–748, 1984.
11. Shapshay SM, Strong MS: Tracheobronchial obstruction from metastatic distant malignancies. Ann Otol Rhinol Laryngol 91:648–651, 1982.
12. Janower ML, Blennerhassett JB: Lymphangitic spread of metastatic cancer to the lung. A radiologic-pathologic classification. Radiology 101:267–273, 1971.
13. Libshitz HI, North LB: Pulmonary metastases. Radiol Clin North Am 20:437–451, 1982.
14. Schwarz MI, Waddell LC, Dombeck DH, et al: Prolonged survival in lymphangitic carcinomatosis. Ann Intern Med 71:779–783, 1969.
15. Wagner D: Trophoblastic cells in the blood stream in normal and abnormal pregnancy. Acta Cytol 12:137–139, 1968.
16. Hendin AS: Gestational trophoblastic tumors metastatic to the lung. Radiologic-clinical correlations. Cancer 53:58–61, 1984.
17. Pass HI, Dwyer A, Makuch R, et al: Detection of pulmonary metastases in patients with osteogenic and soft-tissue sarcomas: The superiority of CT scans compared with conventional linear tomograms using dynamic analysis. J Clin Oncol 3:1261–1265, 1985.
18. Kreel L: Computer tomography of the thorax. Radiol Clin North Am 16:575–584, 1978.
19. Sones PJ Jr, Torres WE, Colvin RS, et al: Effectiveness of CT in evaluating intrathoracic masses. AJR Am J Roentgenol 139:469–475, 1982.
20. Kuhns LR, Borlaza G: The "twinkling star" sign: An aid in differentiating pulmonary vessels from pulmonary nodules on computed tomograms. Radiology 135:763, 764, 1980.
21. Chen PW, Pass HI: Indications for resection of pulmonary metastases. *In* Baue AE, Geha AS, Hammond GL, et al (eds): Glenn's Thoracic and Cardiovascular Surgery, 6th ed. Stamford, CT: Appleton & Lange, 1996, pp 499–510.
22. Siegelman SS, Zerhouni EA, Leo FP, et al: CT of the solitary pulmonary nodule. AJR Am J Roentgenol 135:1–13, 1980.
23. Siegelman SS, Khouri NF, Leo FP, et al: Solitary pulmonary nodules: CT assessment. Radiology 160:307–312, 1986.
24. Kalender WA, Seissler W, Klotz E, et al: Spiral volumetric CT with single-breath-hold technique, continuous transport, and continuous scanner rotation. Radiology 176:181–183, 1990.
25. Vock P, Soucek M, Daepp M, et al: Lung: Spiral volumetric CT with single-breath-hold technique. Radiology 176:864–867, 1990.
26. Krudy AG, Doppman JL, Herdt JR: Failure to detect a 1.5 centimeter lung nodule by chest computed tomography. J Comput Assist Tomogr 6:1178–1180, 1982.
27. Collie DA, Wright AR, Williams JR, et al: Comparison of spiral-acquisition computed tomography and conventional computed tomography in the assessment of pulmonary metastatic disease. Br J Radiol 67:436–444, 1994.
28. Kauczor HU, Hansen M, Schweden F, et al: Computerized tomography in diagnosis of lung metastases: Improvement with the spiral technique. Radiologe 34:569–575, 1994.
29. Costello P, Anderson W, Blume D: Pulmonary nodule: Evaluation with spiral volumetric CT. Radiology 179:875–876, 1991.
30. Remy-Jardin M, Remy J, Giraud F, et al: Pulmonary nodules: Detection with thick-section spiral CT versus conventional CT. Radiology 187:513–520, 1993.
31. Davis SD: CT evaluation for pulmonary metastases in patients with extrathoracic malignancy. Radiology 180:1–12, 1991.
32. Chalmers N, Best JJ: The significance of pulmonary nodules detected by CT but not by chest radiography in tumour staging. Clin Radiol 44:410–412, 1991.
33. Kubota K, Matsuzawa T, Fujiwara T, et al: Differential diagnosis of lung tumor with positron emission tomography: A prospective study. J Nucl Med 31:1927–1932, 1990.
34. Strauss LG, Conti PS: The applications of PET in clinical oncology. J Nucl Med 32:623–648, 1991.
35. Hoh CK, Schiepers C, Seltzer MA, et al: PET in oncology: Will it replace the other modalities? Semin Nucl Med 27:94–106, 1997.
36. Duhaylongsod FG, Lowe VJ, Patz EF Jr, et al: Detection of primary and recurrent lung cancer by means of F-18 fluorodeoxyglucose positron emission tomography (FDG PET). J Thorac Cardiovasc Surg 110:130–140, 1995.
37. Nolop KB, Rhodes CG, Brudin LH, et al: Glucose utilization in vivo by human pulmonary neoplasms. Cancer 60:2682, 2689, 1987.
38. Gupta NC, Frank AR, Dewan NA, et al: Solitary pulmonary nodules: Detection of malignancy with PET with 2-[F-18]-fluoro-2-deoxy-D-glucose. Radiology 184:441–444, 1992.
39. Kim EE, Chung SK, Haynie TP, et al: Differentiation of residual or recurrent tumors from post-treatment changes with F-18 FDG PET. Radiographics 12:269–279, 1992.
40. Itoh K, Takekawa H, Tsukamoto E, et al: Single photon emission computed tomography using ^{201}Tl chloride in pulmonary

nodules: Comparison with ^{67}Ga citrate and ^{99m}Tc-labeled hexamethylpropyleneamine-oxime. Ann Nucl Med 6:253–260, 1992.

41. Hubner KF, Buonocore E, Singh SK, et al: Characterization of chest masses by FDG positron emission tomography. Clin Nucl Med 20:293–298, 1995.
42. Johnston MR: Median sternotomy for resection of pulmonary metastases. J Thorac Cardiovasc Surg 85:516–522, 1983.
43. Roth JA, Pass HI, Wesley MN, et al: Comparison of median sternotomy and thoracotomy for resection of pulmonary metastases in patients with adult soft-tissue sarcomas. Ann Thorac Surg 42:134–138, 1986.
44. Urschel HC Jr, Razzuk MA: Median sternotomy as a standard approach for pulmonary resection. Ann Thorac Surg 41:130–134, 1986.
45. Jablons D, Steinberg SM, Roth J, et al: Metastasectomy for soft tissue sarcoma. Further evidence for efficacy and prognostic indicators. J Thorac Cardiovasc Surg 97:695–705, 1989.
46. Pogrebniak HW, Pass HI: Initial and reoperative pulmonary metastasectomy: Indications, technique, and results. Semin Surg Oncol 9:142–149, 1993.
47. Pastorino U, Valente M, Gasparini M, et al: Median sternotomy and multiple lung resections for metastatic sarcomas. Eur J Cardiothorac Surg 4:477–481, 1990.
48. Lanza LA, Putnam JB Jr: Resection of pulmonary metastases. *In* Roth JA, Ruckdeschel JC, Weisenburger TH (eds): Thoracic Oncology, 2nd ed. Philadelphia: W.B. Saunders, 1995, pp 569–589.
49. Bains MS, Ginsberg RJ, Jones WG II, et al: The clamshell incision: An improved approach to bilateral pulmonary and mediastinal tumor. Ann Thorac Surg 58:30–33, 1994.
50. Crow J, Slavin G, Kreel L: Pulmonary metastasis: A pathologic and radiologic study. Cancer 47:2595–2602, 1981.
51. Dowling RD, Wachs ME, Ferson PF, et al: Thoracoscopic neodymium:yttrium-aluminum-garnet laser resection of a pulmonary metastasis. Cancer 70:1873–1875, 1992.
52. Dowling RD, Keenan RJ, Ferson PF, et al: Video-assisted thoracoscopic resection of pulmonary metastases. Ann Thorac Surg 56:772–775, 1993.
53. McCormack PM, Ginsberg KB, Bains MS, et al: Accuracy of lung imaging in metastases with implications for the role of thoracoscopy. Ann Thorac Surg 56:863–866, 1993.
54. Liu HP, Lin PJ, Hsieh MJ, et al: Application of thoracoscopy for lung metastases (comments). Chest 107:266–268, 1995.
55. Landreneau RJ, Hazelrigg SR, Ferson PF, et al: Thoracoscopic resection of 85 pulmonary lesions. Ann Thorac Surg 54:415–420, 1992.
56. Shah RM, Spirn PW, Salazar AM, et al: Localization of peripheral pulmonary nodules for thoracoscopic excision: value of CT-guided wire placement. AJR Am J Roentgenol 161:279–283, 1993.
57. Landreneau RJ, Mack MJ, Hazelrigg SR, et al: The role of video-assisted thoracic surgery in thoracic oncological practice. Cancer Invest 13:526–539, 1995.
58. Yim AP, Lin J, Chan AT, et al: Video-assisted thoracoscopic wedge resections of pulmonary metastatic osteosarcoma: Should it be performed? Aust N Z J Surg 65:737–739, 1995.
59. McCormack PM, Bains MS, Begg CB, et al: Role of video-assisted thoracic surgery in the treatment of pulmonary metastases: Results of a prospective trial. Ann Thorac Surg 62:213–217, 1996.
60. Kodama K, Doi O, Higashiyama M, et al: Surgical management of lung metastases. Usefulness of resection with the neodymium:yttrium-aluminum-garnet laser with median sternotomy. J Thorac Cardiovasc Surg 101:901–908, 1991.
61. Miller DL, Allen MS, Trastek VF, et al: Videothoracoscopic wedge excision of the lung. Ann Thorac Surg 54:410–414, 1992.
62. Hazelrigg SR, Naunheim K, Auer JE, et al: Combined median sternotomy and video-assisted thoracoscopic resection of pulmonary metastases. Chest 104:956–958, 1993.
63. Baeza MR, Barkley HT Jr, Fernandez CH: Total-lung irradiation in the treatment of pulmonary metastases. Radiology 116:151–154, 1975.
64. Rusch VW: Pulmonary metastasectomy. Current indications. Chest 107:322S–331S, 1995.
65. Goorin AM, Shuster JJ, Baker A, et al: Changing pattern of pulmonary metastases with adjuvant chemotherapy in patients with osteosarcoma: Results from the multiinstitutional osteosarcoma study. J Clin Oncol 9:600–605, 1991.
66. Rosen G, Caparros B, Huvos AG, et al: Preoperative chemotherapy for osteogenic sarcoma: Selection of postoperative adjuvant chemotherapy based on the response of the primary tumor to preoperative chemotherapy. Cancer 49:1221–1230, 1982.
67. Schlappack OK, Baur M, Steger G, et al: The clinical course of lung metastases from breast cancer. Klin Wochenschr 66:790–795, 1988.
68. McAfee MK, Allen MS, Trastek VF, et al: Colorectal lung metastases: Results of surgical excision. Ann Thorac Surg 53:780–785, 1992.
69. McCormack PM, Attiyeh FF: Resected pulmonary metastases from colorectal cancer. Dis Colon Rectum 22:553–556, 1979.
70. Putnam JB Jr, Roth JA, Wesley MN, et al: Survival following aggressive resection of pulmonary metastases from osteogenic sarcoma: Analysis of prognostic factors. Ann Thorac Surg 36:516–523, 1983.
71. Lanza LA, Miser JS, Pass HI, et al: The role of resection in the treatment of pulmonary metastases from Ewing's sarcoma. J Thorac Cardiovasc Surg 94:181–187, 1987.
72. Putnam JB Jr, Roth JA, Wesley MN, et al: Analysis of prognostic factors in patients undergoing resection of pulmonary metastases from soft tissue sarcomas. J Thorac Cardiovasc Surg 87:260–268, 1984.
73. Lanza LA, Natarajan G, Roth JA, et al: Long-term survival after resection of pulmonary metastases from carcinoma of the breast. Ann Thorac Surg 54:244–247, 1992.
74. Pogrebniak HW, Roth JA, Steinberg SM, et al: Reoperative pulmonary resection in patients with metastatic soft tissue sarcoma. Ann Thorac Surg 52:197–203, 1991.
75. Gorenstein LA, Putnam JB, Natarajan G, et al: Improved survival after resection of pulmonary metastases from malignant melanoma. Ann Thorac Surg 52:204–210, 1991.
76. Jett JR, Hollinger CG, Zinsmeister AR, et al: Pulmonary resection of metastatic renal cell carcinoma. Chest 84:442–445, 1983.
77. Roth JA, Putnam JB Jr, Wesley MN, et al: Differing determinants of prognosis following resection of pulmonary metastases from osteogenic and soft tissue sarcoma patients. Cancer 55:1361–1366, 1985.
78. Brister SJ, de Varennes B, Gordon PH, et al: Contemporary operative management of pulmonary metastases of colorectal origin. Dis Colon Rectum 31:786–792, 1988.
79. Pastorino U, Valente M, Gasparini M, et al: Lung resection as salvage treatment for metastatic osteosarcoma. Tumori 74:201–206, 1988.
80. Vogt-Moykopf I, Bulzebruck H, Merkle NM, et al: Results of surgical treatment of pulmonary metastases. Eur J Cardiothorac Surg 2:224–232, 1988.
81. Pogrebniak HW, Haas G, Linehan WM, et al: Renal cell carcinoma: Resection of solitary and multiple metastases. Ann Thorac Surg 54:33–38, 1992.
82. Pass HI, Donington JS: Metastatic cancer to the lung. *In* De Vita VT Jr, Hellman S, Rosenberg SA (eds): Cancer Principles and Practice of Oncology, 5th ed. Philadelphia: Lippincott-Raven, 1997, pp 2536–2551.
83. Meyer WH, Schell MJ, Kumar AP, et al: Thoracotomy for pul-

monary metastatic osteosarcoma. An analysis of prognostic indicators of survival. Cancer 59:374–379, 1987.

84. Pogrebniak HW, Stovroff M, Roth JA, et al: Resection of pulmonary metastases from malignant melanoma: Results of a 16-year experience. Ann Thorac Surg 46:20–23, 1988.
85. Collins VP, Loeffler RK, Tivey H: Observations on growth rates of human tumors. Am J Roentgenol 76:988–1000, 1956.
86. Joseph WL, Morton DL, Adkins PC: Prognostic significance of tumor doubling time in evaluating operability in pulmonary metastatic disease. J Thorac Cardiovasc Surg 61:23–32, 1971.
87. Takita H, Edgerton F, Karakousis C, et al: Surgical management of metastases to the lung. Surg Gynecol Obstet 152:191–194, 1981.
88. Robert JH, Ambrogi V, Mermillod B, et al: Factors influencing long-term survival after lung metastasectomy. Ann Thorac Surg 63:777–784, 1997.
89. The International Registry of Lung Metastases: Long-term results of lung metastasectomy: Prognostic analyses based on 5206 cases. J Thorac Cardiovasc Surg 113:37–49, 1997.
90. Marion J, Burgers V, Breur K, et al: Role of metastasectomy without chemotherapy in the management of osteosarcoma in children. Cancer 45:1664–1668, 1980.
91. Pastorino U, Valente M, Santoro A, et al: Results of salvage surgery for metastatic sarcomas. Ann Oncol 1:269–272, 1990.
92. Snyder CL, Saltzman DA, Ferrell KL, et al: A new approach to the resection of pulmonary osteosarcoma metastases. Results of aggressive metastasectomy. Clin Orthop 270:247–253, 1991.
93. Giritsky AS, Etcubanas E, Mark JB: Pulmonary resection in children with metastatic osteogenic sarcoma: Improved survival with surgery, chemotherapy, and irradiation. J Thorac Cardiovasc Surg 75:354–362, 1978.
94. Carter SR, Grimer RJ, Sneath RS, et al: Results of thoracotomy in osteogenic sarcoma with pulmonary metastases. Thorax 46:727–731, 1991.
95. Marcove RC, Mike V, Hajek JV, et al: Osteogenic sarcoma under the age of twenty-one. A review of one hundred and forty-five operative cases. J Bone Joint Surg Am 52:411–423, 1970.
96. Martini N, Huvos AG, Mike V, et al: Multiple pulmonary resections in the treatment of osteogenic sarcoma. Ann Thorac Surg 12:271–280, 1971.
97. Shah A, Exelby PR, Rao B, et al: Thoracotomy as adjuvant to chemotherapy in metastatic osteogenic sarcoma. J Pediatr Surg 12:983–990, 1977.
98. Beattie EJ, Harvey JC, Marcove R, et al: Results of multiple pulmonary resections for metastatic osteogenic sarcoma after two decades. J Surg Oncol 46:154–155, 1991.
99. Vezeridis MP, Moore R, Karakousis CP: Metastatic patterns in soft-tissue sarcomas. Arch Surg 118:915–918, 1983.
100. Casey JJ, Stempel BG, Scanlon EF, et al: The solitary pulmonary nodule in the patient with breast cancer. Surgery 96: 801–805, 1984.
101. Goya T, Tsuchiya R: Surgical resection of metastatic neoplasms of the lung. Gan To Kagaku Ryoho 17:771–776, 1990.
102. Staren ED, Salerno C, Rongione A, et al: Pulmonary resection for metastatic breast cancer. Arch Surg 127:1282–1284, 1992.
103. McCormack PM, Martini N: The changing role of surgery for pulmonary metastases. Ann Thorac Surg 28:139–145, 1979.
104. Mountain CF, McMurtrey MJ, Hermes KE: Surgery for pulmonary metastases. A 20-year experience. Ann Thorac Surg 38:323–330, 1984.
105. Anyanwu E, Krysa S, Buelzebruck H, et al: Pulmonary metastasectomy as secondary treatment for testicular tumors. Ann Thorac Surg 57:1222–1228, 1994.
106. Toth L, Bodrogi I, Baki M, et al: Thoracic surgery of testicular cancer patients. Eur J Surg Oncol 19:609–613, 1993.
107. Lim DJ, Carter MF: Computerized tomography in the preoperative staging for pulmonary metastases in patients with renal cell carcinoma. J Urol 150:1112–1114, 1993.
108. Libby DM, Altorki NK, Gold J, et al: Simultaneous pulmonary and renal malignancy. Chest 98:153–156, 1990.
109. Kim B, Louie AC: Surgical resection following interleukin 2 therapy for metastatic renal cell carcinoma prolongs remission. Arch Surg 127:1343–1349, 1992.
110. Cozzoli A, Milano S, Cancarini G, et al: Surgery of lung metastases in renal cell carcinoma. Br J Urol 75:445–447, 1995.
111. Katzenstein AL, Purvis R Jr, Gmelich J, et al: Pulmonary resection for metastatic renal adenocarcinoma: Pathologic findings and therapeutic value. Cancer 41:712–723, 1978.
112. Mayo P, Saha SP, McElvein RB: Long-term survival after resection of multiple pulmonary metastases from adenocarcinoma of the kidney. South Med J 74:1161, 1162, 1981.
113. Dernevik L, Berggren H, Larsson S, et al: Surgical removal of pulmonary metastases from renal cell carcinoma. Scand J Urol Nephrol 19:133–137, 1985.
114. Schott G, Weissmuller J, Vecera E: Methods and prognosis of the extirpation of pulmonary metastases following tumor nephrectomy. Urol Int 43:272–274, 1988.
115. Fourquier P, Regnard JF, Rea S, et al: Lung metastases of renal cell carcinoma: Results of surgical resection. Eur J Cardiothorac Surg 11:17–21, 1997.
116. Morrow CE, Vassilopoulos PP, Grage TB: Surgical resection for metastatic neoplasms of the lung: Experience at the University of Minnesota Hospitals. Cancer 45:2981–2985, 1980.
117. Roberts DG, Lepore V, Cardillo G, et al: Long-term follow-up of operative treatment for pulmonary metastases. Eur J Cardiothorac Surg 3:292–296, 1989.
118. di Silverio F, Facciolo F, D'Eramo G, et al: Surgery of pulmonary metastases from renal and bladder carcinoma. Scand J Urol Nephrol Suppl 138:215–218, 1991.
119. Turk PS, Wanebo HJ: Results of surgical treatment of nonhepatic recurrence of colorectal carcinoma. Cancer 71:4267–4277, 1993.
120. Saclarides TJ, Krueger BL, Szeluga DJ, et al: Thoracotomy for colon and rectal cancer metastases. Dis Colon Rectum 36:425–429, 1993.
121. Yano T, Hara N, Ichinose Y, et al: Results of pulmonary resection of metastatic colorectal cancer and its application. J Thorac Cardiovasc Surg 106:875–879, 1993.
122. Gilbert JM, Jeffrey I, Evans M, Kark AE: Sites of recurrent tumour after "curative" colorectal surgery: Implications for adjuvant therapy. Br J Surg 71:203–205, 1984.
123. Smith JW, Fortner JG, Burt M: Resection of hepatic and pulmonary metastases from colorectal cancer. Surg Oncol 1:399–404, 1992.
124. McCormack PM, Burt ME, Bains MS, et al: Lung resection for colorectal metastases. 10-year results. Arch Surg 127:1403–1406, 1992.
125. Mori M, Tomoda H, Ishida T, et al: Surgical resection of pulmonary metastases from colorectal adenocarcinoma. Special reference to repeated pulmonary resections. Arch Surg 126:1297–1301, 1991.
126. Krasna MJ: Thoracoscopic management of metastatic lesions to the lung. *In* Brown WT (ed): Atlas of Video-Assisted Thoracic Surgery. Philadelphia, W.B. Saunders, 1994, pp 209–216.
127. Lefor AT, Bredenberg CE, Kellman RM, et al: Multiple malignancies of the lung and head and neck. Second primary tumor or metastasis? Arch Surg 121:265–270, 1986.
128. Wedman J, Balm AJ, Hart AA, et al: Value of resection of pulmonary metastases in head and neck cancer patients. 18:311–316, 1996.
129. Finley RK III, Verazin GT, Driscoll DL, et al: Results of surgical resection of pulmonary metastases of squamous cell carcinoma of the head and neck. Am J Surg 164:594–598, 1992.

130. Arce MJ: Pneumonectomie totale (le tampon-drainage en chirurgie endothoracique). Mem Acad Chir 62:1412–1416, 1936.
131. von Segesser LK, Weiss BM, Pasic M, et al: Temporary lung support using an intravascular gas exchanger. Thorac Cardiovasc Surg 40:121–125, 1992.
132. Vogt-Moykopf I, Krysa S, Bulzebruck H, Schirren J: Surgery for pulmonary metastases: The Heidelberg experience. Chest Surg Clin North Am 4:85–112, 1994.
133. Marcove RC, Martini N, Rosen G: The treatment of pulmonary metastasis in osteogenic sarcoma. Clin Orthop 111:65–70, 1975.
134. Belli L, Scholl S, Livartowski A, et al: Resection of pulmonary metastases in osteosarcoma. A retrospective analysis of 44 patients. Cancer 63:2546–2550, 1989.
135. Skinner KA, Eilber FR, Holmes EC, et al: Surgical treatment and chemotherapy for pulmonary metastases from osteosarcoma. Arch Surg 127:1065–1070, 1992.
136. Saltzman DA, Snyder CL, Ferrell KL, et al: Aggressive metastasectomy for pulmonic sarcomatous metastases: A follow-up study. Am J Surg 166:543–547, 1993.
137. Inoue K, Yamamoto R, Nishiyama N, et al: Prognostic factors of resected pulmonary metastases of osteogenic sarcoma. Nippon Kyobu Geka Gakkai Zasshi 44:1065–1069, 1996.
138. Friedel G, Linder A, Toomes H: The significance of prognostic factors for the resection of pulmonary metastases of breast cancer. Thorac Cardiovasc Surg 42:71–75, 1994.
139. McDonald ML, Deschamps C, Ilstrup DM, et al: Pulmonary resection for metastatic breast cancer. Ann Thorac Surg 58:1599–1602, 1994.
140. Morone G, Meriggi F, Forni E: Surgical treatment of pulmonary metastasis from breast carcinoma. Personal contribution and considerations on the experience in the literature. Ann Ital Chir 67:833–836, 1996.
141. Simpson R, Kennedy C, Carmalt H, et al: Pulmonary resection for metastatic breast cancer. Aust N Z J Surg 67:717–719, 1997.
142. Rendina EA, de Vincentiis M, Primerano G, et al: Pulmonary resection for metastatic laryngeal carcinoma. J Thorac Cardiovasc Surg 92:111–117, 1986.
143. Mazer TM, Robbins KT, McMurtrey MJ, et al: Resection of pulmonary metastases from squamous carcinoma of the head and neck. Am J Surg 156:238–242, 1988.
144. Mansel JK, Zinsmeister AR, Pairolero PC, et al: Pulmonary resection of metastatic colorectal adenocarcinoma. A ten year experience. Chest 89:109–112, 1986.
145. Maebeya S, Miyoshi S, Suzuma T, et al: Surgical resection of pulmonary metastases from colorectal cancer. Kyobu Geka 46:503–506, 1993.
146. Zapatero J, Flandes J, Lago J, et al: Prognostic factors in pulmonary metastases from colorectal cancer. Respiration 61:280–282, 1994.
147. Csekeo A, Orban K, Agocs L, et al: Surgical treatment of pulmonary metastases from colorectal tumors. Orv Hetil 136:235–238, 1995.
148. Girard P, Baldeyrou P, Grunenwald D: Lung metastases from colorectal cancer: Results of surgery. Presse Med 24:1028–1032, 1995.
149. Otani Y, Kondo T, Saito R, et al: Surgical treatment of metastatic lung tumor from colorectal cancer. Kyobu Geka 48:735–740, 1995.
150. van Halteren HK, van Geel AN, Hart AA, et al: Pulmonary resection for metastases of colorectal origin. Chest 107:1526–1531, 1995.
151. Regnard JF, Nicolosi M, Coggia M, et al: Results of surgical treatment of lung metastases from colorectal cancers. Gastroenterol Clin Biol 19:378–384, 1995.
152. Saito H, Kikuchi T, Matsunaga Y, et al: Surgical resection of pulmonary metastases from colorectal cancer. Kyobu Geka 49:909–911, 1996.
153. Okumura S, Kondo H, Tsuboi M, et al: Pulmonary resection for metastatic colorectal cancer: Experiences with 159 patients. J Thorac Cardiovasc Surg 112:867–874, 1996.
154. Martini N, McCormack PM, Bains MS, et al: Surgery for solitary and multiple pulmonary metastases. N Y State J Med 78: 1711–1714, 1978.
155. Creagan ET, Fleming TR, Edmonson JH, et al: Pulmonary resection for metastatic nonosteogenic sarcoma. Cancer 44: 1908–1912, 1979.
156. Casson AG, Putnam JB, Natarajan G, et al: Five-year survival after pulmonary metastasectomy for adult soft tissue sarcoma. Cancer 69:662–668, 1992.
157. Levenback C, Rubin SC, McCormack PM, et al: Resection of pulmonary metastases from uterine sarcomas. Gynecol Oncol 45:202–205, 1992.
158. Gadd MA, Casper ES, Woodruff JM, et al: Development and treatment of pulmonary metastases in adult patients with extremity soft tissue sarcoma. Ann Surg 218:705–712, 1993.
159. Robinson MH, Sheppard M, Moskovic E, et al: Lung metastasectomy in patients with soft tissue sarcoma. Br J Radiol 67:129–135, 1994.
160. Bouros D, Papadakis K, Siafakas N, et al: Natural history of patients with pulmonary metastases from uterine cancer. Cancer 78:441–447, 1996.
161. Cahan WG: Excision of melanoma metastases to lung: Problems in diagnosis and management. Ann Surg 178:703–709, 1973.
162. Mathisen DJ, Flye MW, Peabody J: The role of thoracotomy in the management of pulmonary metastases from malignant melanoma. Ann Thorac Surg 27:295–299, 1979.
163. Thayer JO Jr, Overholt RH: Metastatic melanoma to the lung: Long-term results of surgical excision. Am J Surg 149:558–562, 1985.
164. Wong JH, Euhus DM, Morton DL: Surgical resection for metastatic melanoma to the lung. Arch Surg 123:1091–1095, 1988.
165. Harpole DH Jr, Johnson CM, Wolfe WG, et al: Analysis of 945 cases of pulmonary metastatic melanoma. J Thorac Cardiovasc Surg 103:743–748, 1992.
166. Karakousis CP, Velez A, Driscoll DL, et al: Metastasectomy in malignant melanoma. Surgery 115:295–302, 1994.
167. Tafra L, Dale PS, Wanek LA, et al: Resection and adjuvant immunotherapy for melanoma metastatic to the lung and thorax. J Thorac Cardiovasc Surg 110:119–128, 1995.
168. Fuller AF Jr, Scannell JG, Wilkins EW Jr: Pulmonary resection for metastases from gynecologic cancers: Massachusetts General Hospital experience, 1943–1982. Gynecol Oncol 22: 174–180, 1985.
169. Matsukuma K, Miyake M, Iino H, et al: Surgical management of pulmonary metastasis from carcinoma of the uterine cervix. Nippon Sanka Fujinka Gakkai Zasshi 41:1911–1915, 1989

COMMENTARY

Stephen R. Hazelrigg

This represents a very comprehensive coverage of the topic of pulmonary metastases. The issue of video-assisted thoracic surgery (VATS) resection of metastases for therapeutic purposes remains the main area of controversy. The concern with VATS is that nodules may be missed and may result in lower cure rates. There is no evidence that a nodule that is missed and later resected results in impaired long-term survival, and, in fact, there are data pertaining to soft tissue sarcomatous metastases that show no difference if nodules were resected at a later date.[1] As imaging technology improves, the risk of not identifying a nodule preoperatively will be less, making VATS resection less controversial. With spiral CT scans, we have used VATS for resection of solitary lung metastases for therapeutic purposes.

Reference

1. Roth JA, Putnam JB Jr, Wesley MN, et al: Differing determinants of prognosis following resection of pulmonary metastases from osteogenic and soft tissue sarcoma patients. Cancer 55:1361–1366, 1985.

COMMENTARY

Ugo Pastorino

In this article, Drs. Zwischenberger and Alpard provide a very comprehensive update on the subject, with an extensive review of the literature as well as a large series of cases from their own group. I agree with most of their statements concerning patient selection, surgical approach, and results achieved in the treatment of various primary tumors.

The overall picture of pulmonary metastasectomy indicates that permanent cure can be achieved in about one third of cases, but the interpretation of individual series is often difficult because of tumor heterogeneity and the evolution of surgical eligibility since the late 1970s. These elements justify the apparent inconsistency of data on prognostic factors. In this respect, the International Registry of Lung Metastases, by pooling more than 5000 cases with extensive follow-up, has clarified in a definitive way that the disease-free interval (DFI), the number of lesions, and the completeness of resection are significant independent predictors of patient outcome, and the combination of anatomic (number, resectability) and biologic (DFI) elements has resulted in a simple and innovative system of classification into four groups. This classification has proven effective in assessing prognosis of all tumor types (with the sole exception of testicular cancer) in very much the same way as has tumor-node metastasis (TNM) evaluation. It is also clear that such prognostic factors cannot be used to select candidates for surgery, although, in melanoma, the presence of two unfavorable factors (multiple lesions and short DFI) confers a very poor life expectancy (8% 5-year survival, median 13 months).

Although the efficacy of lung metastasectomy has never been confirmed by controlled clinical trials, but has relied only on cumulative evidence of long-term survival (in comparison with unresected cases), favorable results have been invariably linked to the same oncologic guidelines applied to the treatment of primary malignancies. These include careful preoperative and intraoperative assessment of the extent of disease, complete resection with safe surgical margins, and preservation of as much functional parenchyma as possible. In addition, intensive follow-up has been adopted to rescue some of the patients with limited intrathoracic relapse.

The concept of minimally invasive surgery through video-assisted thoracoscopy has been perceived by some as a revolutionary approach that could justify a revision of oncologic principles. In my view, the surgical approach of the future should continue to be instrumental in the achievement of the main oncologic goals and not vice versa.

In pulmonary metastases, even more than in primary lung tumors, preoperative staging is inaccurate. Although the nodal component of the disease is less critical in metastatic disease, the assessment of the exact number of metastases, their location, and the optimal volume of resection requires careful palpation of the lung, in both inflated and deflated states.

As an example, in the experience of the International Registry, the overall accuracy of radiologic assessment in terms of number of lung metastases was 61%, being underestimated in 25% of cases and overestimated in 14%. However, in patients who had bilateral surgical exploration, the number of radiologic metastases was accurate in only 37% of cases and underestimated in 39%. One could argue that the largest discrepancy applies to multiple lesions; however, even in presumed solitary metastases, the accuracy of radiologic staging was still only 82%. Spiral computed tomography (CT) is expected to improve preoperative assessment, but it is not clear to what extent higher sensitivity may improve surgical performance, because the chances of false-positive lesions increase proportionally. As demonstrated by McCormack,[1] surgical exploration via thoracotomy allowed resection of additional metastases in 56% of patients whose lesions were undetected by previous thoracoscopy. There may still be debate on the clinical relevance of early resection of radiologically occult metastases, as well as on bilateral screening of patients who have unilateral disease. What is certain, however, is that these two questions should be answered by prospective clinical trials (thoracotomy versus thoracoscopy and bilateral versus unilateral exploration) before denying a patient the possible benefit of being rendered disease free with a one-stage complete resection.

Different techniques of resection can be applied to adapt to the specific condition of each patient. The procedures include wedge resection with mechanical staplers; precision resection with diathermy, argon beam, or YAG laser; and anatomic resection of segment, lobe, or whole lung. For volumes smaller than a segment, precision resections (i.e., cutting out a uniform layer of 5 to 10 mm of normal lung tissue around the nodule) may adapt better to the shape and location of metastatic deposits, thus resulting in a better preservation of the lung. Moreover, avoidance of metal staples facilitates radiologic follow-up and prevents occurrence of artifacts mimicking relapse at CT scanning. As a matter of fact, in the last few years, I have gradually abandoned the use of mechanical staplers for multiple metastasectomies, and the option of performing carefully tailored resections represents another reason to prefer limited thoracotomy to thoracoscopy.

As far as the morbidity and mortality of different surgical approaches are concerned, any claims of a putative advantage of video-assisted thoracoscopy should rely on randomized trials in which similar patients and procedures are compared. Such evidence is scanty if one looks at the very few randomized studies performed in benign disease (e.g., pneumothorax, emphysema). In the Registry data, the mortality after complete resection was 0.8% overall, and 0.5% in the subset of solitary lesions of less than 2 cm in diameter treated by sublobar resection.

On the other hand, if one wishes to compare thoracoscopy with open approaches for unilateral procedures, then muscle-sparing thoracotomies should be considered the gold standard. Such a conservative approach combines a small skin incision with full preservation of major thoracic muscles (i.e., latissimus, pectoralis, serratus) and their nerves, but still permits palpatory inspection, complex lung resections, and bronchoplastic procedures. In our group, we have been using anterior or lateral muscle-sparing thoracotomies for many years and for most thoracic operations, including metastasectomy when median sternotomy was not indicated.

In conclusion, lung metastasectomy is a potentially curative treatment with predictable outcome whenever complete resection is achieved. I agree with Dr. Zwischenberger that, given the present knowledge, video-assisted thoracoscopy is only acceptable for diagnostic purposes, but not as a valid therapeutic alternative to well-established techniques. Prospective randomized trials are the appropriate instrument to assess the relative efficacy of thoracoscopic metastasectomy (combined with spiral CT) versus that of muscle-sparing thoracotomy or sternotomy, in terms of cure rates (>5 years), mortality, morbidity, pulmonary function, and quality of life.

Reference

1. McCormack PM, Bains MS, Begg CB, et al: Role of video-assisted thoracic surgery in the treatment of pulmonary metastases: Results of a prospective trial. Ann Thorac Surg 62: 213–217, 1996.

Section IV

The Mediastinum

Chapter 22

Videomediastinoscopy

Paul De Leyn and Toni Lerut

Surgical exploration of the mediastinum was first developed by Harken and associates.[1] A Jackson laryngoscope was inserted into the mediastinum through a supraclavicular incision, and lymph node biopsy specimens were taken. These surgeons thought that the presence of involved mediastinal lymph nodes would preclude successful resection of the cancer. More than 40 years later, their reasoning still proves to be valid. The prognostic importance of the level and extent of nodal involvement has led to the development of a thoracic lymph node map, which is important not only prognostically but also therapeutically. Cervical mediastinoscopy through a pretracheal suprasternal incision was developed by Carlens[3] in Sweden, and subsequently popularized by Pearson and associates in North America.[19] Although mediastinoscopy is used mainly as an invasive staging method for patients who have non–small cell lung cancer (NSCLC), it can also be used in the diagnosis of lymphoma, sarcoidosis, and mediastinal tumors.

Rationale for Performing Staging of the Mediastinum in Patients Who Have Non–Small Cell Lung Cancer

Lymph node involvement is a very important prognostic factor in NSCLC without distant metastases. Patients who do not have metastatic lymph nodes (N0 disease) or who have only intrapulmonary or hilar node involvement (N1 disease) are generally considered for straightforward resection. However, those who have ipsilateral (N2) or contralateral (N3) metastatic mediastinal lymph nodes—so-called locally advanced disease—are usually not considered for primary surgical treatment.

When ipsilateral mediastinal nodes are involved, results of primary surgery are disappointing. Pearson and associates[19] reported on 79 patients who were operated on despite the presence of positive nodes proven by mediastinoscopy. This group represents a carefully selected subset of patients, and those who had extracapsular spread or involvement of high paratracheal nodes were excluded from surgery. The complete resectability rate was 64%, and the overall 5-year survival rate was 9%. One can assume that, if thoracotomy was undertaken in all patients having positive mediastinoscopy findings, the 5-year survival rate would have been extremely low. A more recent study from Funatsu and associates[7] confirms this finding. They operated on 117 patients who had positive findings on mediastinoscopy. In 26 patients (22.2%), no resection could be performed. Curative resection was achieved in 13 patients (11.1%), whereas in 78 patients (66.7%), the resection was not curative. The 5-year survival rate of the 92 patients undergoing resection (excluding the 26 exploratory thoracotomies) was 6%. When the survival figures of a surgical procedure parallel the natural history of a disease, it is difficult to recommend the procedure to patients.

Several phase II[2, 9, 15, 23] and two phase III studies[20, 21] suggest that induction chemotherapy increases both the resectability and the long-term survival of patients who have N2 disease. In such a setting, it becomes increasingly important to identify these patients before resection. Moreover, in comparing surgical and nonsurgical combined modality treatments, it is of paramount importance that the clinical staging be as accurate as possible.

In a prospective randomized study at the M.D. Anderson Cancer Center,[21] 60 patients who had stage IIIa disease (according to the Union Internationale Contre Cancer [UICC] classification, 1988) were randomly assigned to receive either six cycles of neoadjuvant chemotherapy and surgery, or surgery alone. The estimated 2- and 3-year survival rates were 60% and 56%, respectively, for the neoadjuvant chemotherapy group versus 25% and 15%, respectively, for those who had surgery alone. One of the pitfalls of this study was that it included patients who had microscopically proven N2 disease as well as patients with T3N0M0 disease. The latter group is known to have a far better prognosis.

In our own experience,[25] we have prospectively studied 39 consecutive patients who had pathologically proven N2 NSCLC. They were treated with three cycles of vindesine-fosfamide-Platinol (VIP) induction. The response rate to chemotherapy was 59% (95% confidence interval 34–75%). Surgical exploration was performed only on those patients who had at least a partial clinical response. The complete resection rate was as high as 95%. The mediastinal nodes were negative (downstaging) in 9 of the 19 resection specimens, with 2 complete pathologic responses. The median survival time of all patients was 19 months, with a projected 2-year survival rate of 49%. Several of these patients had unfavorable prognostic characteristics with respect to clinical and biologic findings, tumor location, and extent of disease. Before we used this induction scheme, we had operated on only 19 patients who had N2 disease proven by mediastinoscopy over a period of 9 years. These patients constituted a rigorously selected group. The median survival time in these strictly selected patients was only 12 months, with a 2-year survival rate of 21%.

These data reiterate that incomplete resection results in poor survival in patients who have N2 disease and that induction chemotherapy improves the results. Therefore, staging of the mediastinum is of paramount importance in patients with NSCLC.

The mediastinum can be staged invasively by cervical mediastinoscopy, left anterior mediastinotomy, extended cervical mediastinoscopy, or thoracoscopy. Noninvasive methods include computed tomography (CT) and position emission tomography (PET). In the first part of this chapter, we describe in detail the technique of mediastinoscopy and the role of extended cervical mediastinoscopy, left anterior mediastinotomy, and thoracoscopy. In the second part, we compare the results of cervical mediastinoscopy with noninvasive staging methods such as CT and PET.

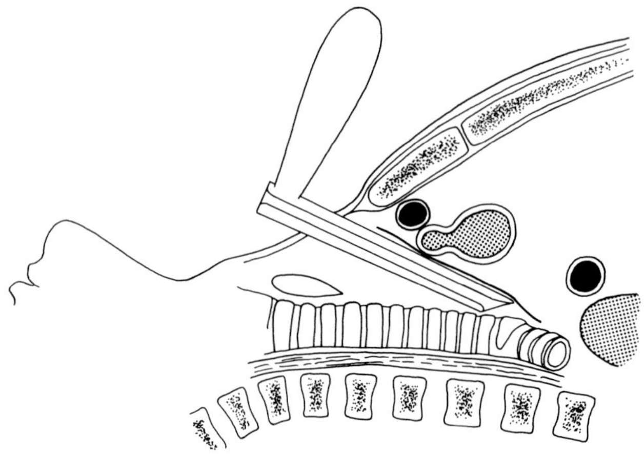

Figure 22–1. The neck of the patient is extended. The mediastinoscope is advanced through a suprasternal notch incision in the pretracheal space.

Invasive Staging Methods

Cervical Mediastinoscopy: Operative Technique

Mediastinoscopy is performed with the patient under general anesthesia. The endotracheal tube is positioned at the left corner of the mouth. The neck is extended. A small transverse cervical incision is made approximately one finger's breadth above the manubrium. The pretracheal muscles are separated vertically in the midline to expose the anterior surface of the trachea. The thyroid isthmus is retracted superiorly, and the tracheal surface is exposed just below the isthmus. At this point, one should avoid dissecting downward into the mediastinum. It is easier to incise the pretracheal fascia just below the isthmus and then carry down the dissection onto and close to the anterior surface of the trachea. The surgeon's index finger is advanced along the pretracheal plane, and the mediastinum is carefully palpated for the presence of nodal disease. This palpation is of extreme importance, because pretracheal nodes are more easily palpated than visualized. The finger is withdrawn and the mediastinoscope is advanced (Fig. 22–1). The plane in front of the mediastinoscope is developed with the use of blunt dissection, using a metal sucker through the channel of the mediastinoscope. Small bleeding vessels can be coagulated. One has to be very careful with coagulation at the left paratracheal side because of the presence of the left recurrent nerve. Bleeding at this side is best handled with a hemostatic gauze introduced through the mediastinoscope. To avoid major complications, it is important to visualize anatomic landmarks, such as the azygos vein, the right and left main bronchi, and the right pulmonary artery, before actual biopsies are taken. When major bleeding occurs, packing is the first thing to do. Packing for at least 10 minutes causes most—even dramatic—bleeding to stop. Through the mediastinoscope, vascular clips can be placed easily. If packing and vascular clips have no effect, right thoracotomy (for bleeding of the azygos vein, caval vein, or right pulmonary artery) or median sternotomy (for bleeding from the aorta or innominate artery and vein) may be necessary.

Using cervical mediastinoscopy (Fig. 22–2), the following nodal stations (according to the Mountain/Dresler modification[17] from the Naruke/ATS-LCSG map [see Chapter 24]) can be sampled: the highest mediastinal nodes (level 1), left and right upper paratracheal nodes (levels 2L and 2R), left and right lower paratracheal nodes (levels 4L and 4R), and subcarinal nodes (level 7). The posterior subcarinal nodes, paraesophageal nodes (level 8), inferior pulmonary ligament nodes (level 9), subaortic nodes (level 5), and para-aortic nodes (level 6) cannot be biopsied using standard cervical mediastinoscopy.

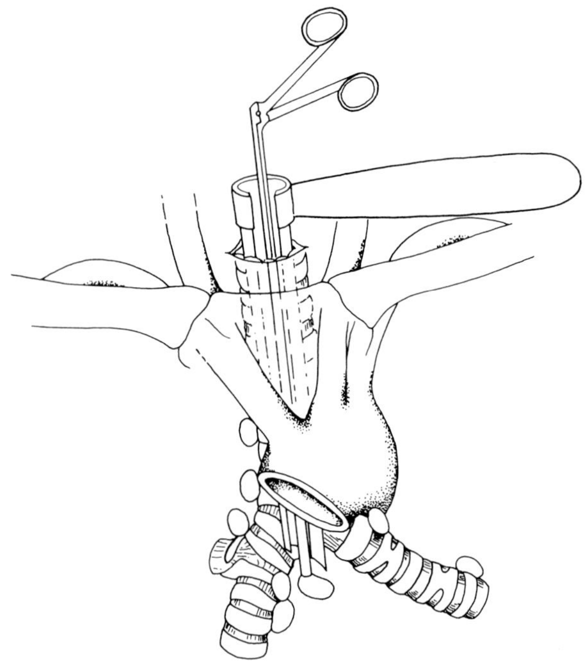

Figure 22–2. The left and right paratracheal, pretracheal, and subcarinal nodes can be biopsied easily.

Cervical Mediastinoscopy: Complications

Cervical mediastinoscopy is a low-risk procedure. In experienced hands, cervical mediastinoscopy has no mortality and a morbidity rate as low as 2.3%.[13] Although it can be performed as an outpatient procedure,[1] we prefer to keep the patient in the hospital for one night. The most serious complication is severe hemorrhage. The incidence of bleeding necessitating immediate thoracotomy varies in the literature between 0.01% and 0.6%. Other major complications are injury of the esophagus, damage to the recurrent laryngeal nerve (usually the left), and pneumothorax. In a 20-year period, we performed more than 4000 cervical mediastinoscopies. There was no hospital mortality. Major bleeding requiring immediate intervention occurred in four patients. Injury to the esophagus was seen in one patient, in whom the mediastinum was drained through the mediastinoscopy incision, and this fistula dried up after a few days of conservative treatment.

Video-Assisted Mediastinoscopy: Enhancing Proven Technology

The development of videoscopic and video-assisted technology has opened new perspectives in surgical practice. A mediastinoscope was designed to enable videoscopic recording of mediastinoscopy (Fig. 22–3). Because the working channel of the mediastinoscope remains unchanged, the surgical procedure can be performed under direct vision as usual, but the built-in optics can be connected to a video camera, allowing simultaneous video recording and viewing on a TV monitor.

The advantages are the following:

1. The operation can still be performed under direct vision, even when the telescope is inserted and a video camera is connected. However, the magnified image on the screen offers a highly detailed image (Fig. 22–4). As a result, a more accurate and extensive dissection is possible. With some experience, the subcarinal nodes can be completely dissected with the esophagus open to visualization.
2. Classic mediastinoscopy is a difficult procedure to teach, because the working channel is narrow. With direct and simultaneous video recording on a TV monitor, several people can follow the operation. Thus, this technique offers greater teaching capabilities.
3. Mediastinoscopy is accepted worldwide as a key procedure for the staging of lung cancer. However, there seems to be great variation in the way that biopsies are sampled. Videotaping the surgical procedure may result in greater accuracy of judgment during clinicopathological discussions.
4. Widespread international use of videotaped mediastinoscopy may lead to better understanding and standardization of this procedure.

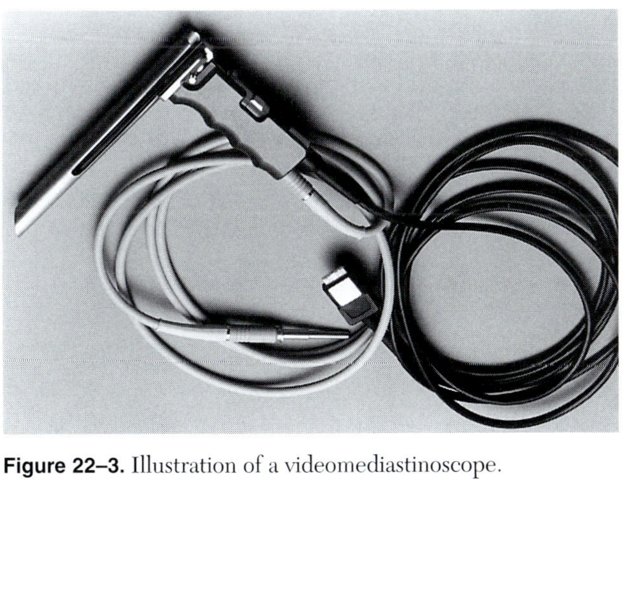

Figure 22–3. Illustration of a videomediastinoscope.

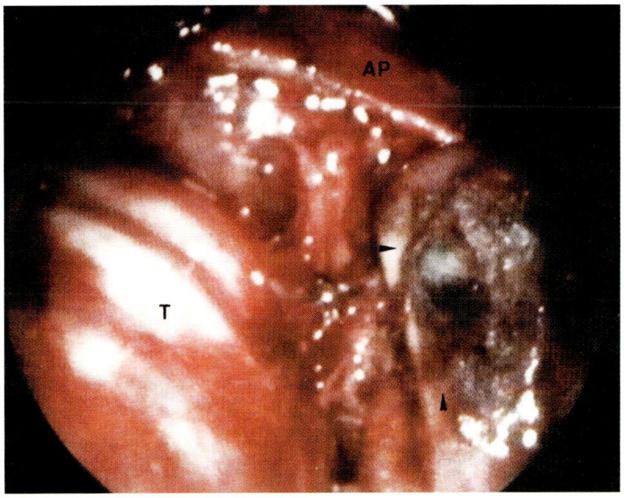

Figure 22–4. A view on videomediastinoscopy illustrating the right paratracheal lymph node. T = trachea; AP = first branch of right pulmonary artery; arrows indicate the margin of the right paratracheal lymph node.

Many simple thoracoscopic procedures (for assessment of pneumothorax, pleural effusion, early empyema) can be performed by means of non–video-assisted thoracoscopy.[24] The advantages are the use of a single incision and the simplicity of the procedures. The disadvantage is the lack of visibility. The videomediastinoscope has light optics built into its framework. As a result, more complex thoracoscopic procedures can be performed using this scope. At our institution, all thoracic sympathectomies and some dissections of the mammary artery coronary artery bypass graft (CABG) are performed with this instrument.

Extended Cervical Mediastinoscopy

For left upper lobe tumors, the subaortic nodes (level 5) and para-aortic nodes (level 6) are frequently involved. These nodes cannot be biopsied by routine cervical mediastinoscopy. Ginsberg and associates[8] described a technique to explore these levels through the cervical incision. After the cervical mediastinoscopy is complete, blunt dissection is performed between the innominate and carotid arteries, and the mediastinoscope is introduced above the aortic arch. In experienced hands, this technique has a high level of accuracy and minimal morbidity.[8, 12]

Left Anterior Mediastinotomy

Another surgical technique is the anterior mediastinotomy. This technique was originally described by McNeil and Chamberlain.[16] It can be used to biopsy mediastinal masses, but in patients who have lung cancer, it is performed to sample the subaortic and para-aortic nodes, which are inaccessible by cervical mediastinoscopy. The original technique involves a vertical parasternal incision, for excising the second cartilage. Because of better wound healing and better cosmetic results, a transverse incision over the second intercostal space, without removing the rib cartilage, is more often used. As we discuss later, these nodal levels are easily reached by left thoracoscopy, with better visibility and fewer wound complications. At present, left anterior mediastinotomy is less frequently used than thoracoscopy for staging of these nodal levels.

Thoracoscopy

Mediastinal nodes can also be sampled through thoracoscopy. Although there are indications for thoracoscopic sampling of mediastinal nodes (see Chapter 25), cervical mediastinoscopy remains the procedure of choice, especially for the higher mediastinal levels (1, 2, and 4). Cervical mediastinoscopy has an extremely low morbidity. Higher mediastinal nodes are easily reached by cervical mediastinoscopy, and, moreover, contralateral mediastinal nodes can also be biopsied. Thoracoscopy should be reserved for the particular indications. Cervical mediastinoscopy can be technically impossible, as in cases of previous laryngectomy, large goiter, and previous mediastinoscopy in patients who have received neoadjuvant chemotherapy. In such cases, thoracoscopic nodal sampling can be performed. The lower mediastinal nodes (posterior subcarinal and paraesophageal) are difficult to sample by cervical mediastinoscopy. If there is a strong suspicion of involvement at the nodal levels (e.g., on PET scan), thoracoscopy can be performed (after negative cervical mediastinoscopy). The subaortic nodes (level 5) and para-aortic nodes (level 6) cannot be reached by routine cervical mediastinoscopy. Although Ginsberg described a technique to biopsy these nodes through an extended cervical mediastinoscopy,[8] this technique is not widely used. These nodes can be biopsied easily by left anterior mediastinotomy or left thoracoscopy. We prefer to use left thoracoscopy for this purpose. Potential advantages are better visibility (especially of the left phrenic nerve), less wound infection (when early irradiation is necessary), and a better cosmetic result.

Noninvasive Staging Methods

Mediastinoscopy and CT Scanning

In the late 1970s, CT was introduced and used as a noninvasive method for staging of the mediastinum. Nodes may be enlarged because of inflammation, and we now know that only 50% of enlarged nodes seen on CT scan are actually positive.[6] In these cases, surgical staging should be performed to confirm histologic nodal involvement. Although small lymph nodes may contain metastatic deposits of clinical importance, many centers use CT findings as their selection criteria to perform cervical mediastinoscopy in patients who have NSCLC. They believe that the false-negative rate of CT findings in these patients is so low that thoracotomy can be performed without mediastinoscopy. There are no large series analyzing the value of cervical mediastinoscopy in the absence of enlarged mediastinal nodes on CT scan. A study by Goldstraw and associates[10] evaluated 13 patients who had normal mediastinum and hilum on CT scan. Mediastinoscopy in all these cases was negative. They concluded that the finding of a normal mediastinum on preoperative CT allows the surgeon to avoid a preoperative mediastinal surgical exploration. In a retrospective study from our institution,[5] cervical mediastinoscopy was performed on 235 consecutive patients who had potentially operable NSCLC and small nodes on CT scan. Nodes were considered to be small when their largest cross-sectional diameter was less than 15 mm. In 47 patients (20%), the cervical mediastinoscopy was positive. In 16 of these patients (34%), more than one level was involved and in 45% of the patients (N = 21), the N2 disease was extranodal. Forty-two patients presented with a T1N0 lesion. Cervical mediastinoscopy findings were positive in 9.5% of these patients. In T2N0 patients, the overall incidence of positive were mediastinoscopy findings was 17.7%. For T3N0 and T4N0 lesions, cervical mediastinoscopy findings were positive in 31.2% and 33.3% of the cases, respectively. Because of these findings, we adopted the policy of performing invasive mediastinal staging in every patient who has potentially operable NSCLC.

Mediastinoscopy and PET Scanning

Using the mechanisms of glucose metabolism, PET is able to make "biologic" images of tissues. Lung tumor cells have a much higher rate of glycolysis in comparison with non-neoplastic cells, and an increased cellular uptake of glucose is possibly caused by an increased number of transport proteins. The altered glucose metabolism is visualized by the radio-labeled glucose analogue [^{18}F]fluoro-2-deoxy-D-glucose (FDG). The same uptake mechanism as occurs in glucose takes place in FDG, but the latter is trapped metabolically in the cell after phosphorylation by hexokinase. The accumulation of FDG in neoplastic cells is scanned by the PET camera, and high-resolution images are generated for the diagnosis and staging of neoplasms.

The FDG-PET scan has been found to be very accurate in differentiating between benign and malignant pulmonary nodules. In rather small groups of patients, other authors have found that PET scanning is between 93 and 100% accurate in predicting mediastinal involvement in NSCLC. In a prospective study of 690 lymph node stations in 68 patients,[26] the accuracy of the PET scan was 94%, with a sensitivity of 93% and a specificity of 95%. The negative predictive value was as high as 99%. Because of the very high negative predictive value, we do not perform cervical mediastinoscopy in patients who have negative hilar or mediastinal nodes on PET scan. Although the positive predictive value of the PET scan is high (86%), we recommend performing surgical mediastinal staging in patients who have positive mediastinal nodes. This enables patients who have false-positive results to undergo straightforward resection. In our population of patients with NSCLC, false-positive findings are mainly found in those with pneumoconiosis. Although digital fusion images distinguish hilar from mediastinal nodes, we perform mediastinoscopy, even if only the hilar nodes are involved on PET scan. Since the introduction of the PET scan in the clinical staging of NSCLC in our hospital, we perform one third fewer mediastinoscopies for this indication. As the PET scan becomes more widely used in the staging of other carcinomas (e.g., colon, stomach, lymphoma), we are increasingly consulted to perform surgical mediastinal staging for patients who have solitary positive mediastinal findings.

Conclusion

A very important prognostic factor in patients who have NSCLC is the involvement of mediastinal nodes. Results of primary surgery in patients who have preoperatively diagnosed ipsilateral mediastinal nodes (N2), or contralateral mediastinal nodal disease (N3), are disappointing. Neoadjuvant chemotherapy seems to significantly prolong survival in this group of patients. Classic imaging (CT, magnetic resonance imaging) has low accuracy, with a positive predictive value of 50% and a negative predictive value of 80%. All patients who have enlarged nodes[3] (1 cm at their shortest axis or 1.5 cm at their maximal cross-sectional diameter) should undergo surgical staging, because nearly half of these nodes prove to be benign. Because of its low negative predictive value, CT alone should not be used to select patients (who have no or small nodes on CT scan) for primary resection without mediastinoscopy. Cervical mediastinoscopy has an extremely low rate of morbidity and a very high level of accuracy. Because of this, cervical mediastinoscopy plays a key role in the staging of patients who have NSCLC. Before we had PET scan, all patients who had potentially operable NSCLC underwent cervical mediastinoscopy in our department. For the exploration of the subaortic nodes (level 5) and para-aortic nodes (level 6), left anterior mediastinotomy or left thoracoscopy could be used. In detecting diseased mediastinal nodes in NSCLC, the PET scan has proved to have a very high sensitivity. When findings on PET scanning of the mediastinum are negative, we do not perform invasive staging. Although the specificity is also high, false-positive results are possible (especially in patients who have pneumoconiosis), and a positive mediastinal finding on PET scan should always be confirmed by invasive mediastinal staging. Because of its low morbidity, high accuracy, and low cost, mediastinoscopy remains the most important staging procedure for these patients. Video-assisted mediastinoscopy is a refinement of the existing technique and results in a higher visibility, which in turn allows better dissection and better teaching capabilities. These positive achievements may eventually lead to a more uniform use of this extremely important staging procedure.

References

1. Bonadies J, D'Agostino RS, Ruskis AF, et al: Outpatient mediastinoscopy. J Thorac Cardiovasc Surg 106:686–688, 1993.
2. Burkes RL, Ginsberg RJ, Shepherd FA, et al: Induction chemotherapy with mitomycin, vindesin, and cisplatinum for stage III unresectable non–small-cell lung cancer: Results of the Toronto phase II trial. J Clin Oncol 10:580–586, 1992.
3. Carlens E: Mediastinoscopy: A method for inspection and tissue biopsy in the superior mediastinum. Dis Chest 36:343–352, 1959.
4. De Leyn P, Schoonooghe P, Deneffe G, et al: Surgery for non-small cell lung cancer with unsuspected metastasis to ipsilateral mediastinal or subcarinal nodes (N2 disease). Eur J Cardiothorac Surg 10:649–655, 1996.
5. De Leyn P, Vansteenkiste J, Cuypers P, et al: Role of cervical mediastinoscopy in staging of non-small cell lung cancer without enlarged mediastinal lymph nodes on CT scan. Eur J Cardiothorac Surg 12:706–712, 1997.
6. Dillemans B, Deneffe G, Verschakelen J, et al: Value of computed tomography and mediastinoscopy in preoperative evaluation of mediastinal nodes in non-small cell lung cancer. Eur J Cardiothorac Surg 8:37–42, 1994,
7. Funatsu T, Matsubaru Y, Hatakenaka R, et al: The role of mediastinoscopic biopsy in preoperative assessment of lung cancer. J Thorac Cardiovasc Surg 104:1688–1695, 1992.
8. Ginsberg RJ, Rice TW, Goldberg M, et al: Extended cervical mediastinoscopy. A single procedure for bronchogenic carcinoma of the left upper lobe. J Thorac Cardiovasc Surg 94:673–678, 1984.
9. Ginsberg RJ: Multimodality therapy for stage IIIA (N2) lung cancer. Chest 103:356S–359S, 1993.
10. Goldstraw P, Kurzer M, Edwards D: Preoperative staging of lung cancer: Accuracy of computed tomography versus mediastinoscopy. Thorax 38:10–15, 1983.
11. Harken DE, Black H, Clauss R, et al: A simple cervicomediastinal exploration for tissue diagnosis of intrathoracic disease. N Engl J Med 251:1041–1044, 1954.
12. Lopez L, Varela A, Freixinet J, et al: Extended cervical mediastinoscopy: Prospective study of fifty cases. Ann Thorac Surg 57:555–558, 1994.
13. Luke WP, Pearson FG, Todd TRJ, et al: Prospective evaluation of mediastinoscopy for assessment of carcinoma of the lung. J Thorac Cardiovasc Surg 91:53–56, 1986.
14. Martini N, Flehinger BJ: The role of surgery in N2 lung cancer. Surg Clin North Am 67:1037–1049, 1987.
15. Martini N, Kris MG, Flehinger BJ, et al: Preoperative chemotherapy for stage IIIa (N2) lung cancer: The Sloan-Kettering experience with 136 patients. Ann Thorac Surg 55:1365–1374, 1993.
16. McNeil TM, Chamberlein JM: Diagnostic anterior mediastinotomy. Ann Thorac Surg 2:532–539, 1966.
17. Mountain CF, Dressler CM: Regional lymph node classification for lung cancer staging. Chest 111:1718–1723, 1997.
18. Naruke T, Suemasu K, Ishikawa S: Lymph node mapping and curability at various levels of metastasis in resected lung cancer. J Thorac Cardiovasc Surg 76:832–837, 1978.
19. Pearson FG, Delarue NC, Ilves R, et al: Significance of positive superior mediastinal nodes identified at mediastinoscopy in patients with resectable cancer of the lung. J Thorac Cardiovasc Surg 83:1–11, 1982.
20. Rosell R, Gomez-Codina J, Camps C, et al: A randomized trial comparing preoperative chemotherapy plus surgery with surgery alone in patients with non-small-cell lung cancer. N Engl J Med 330:153–158, 1994.
21. Roth JA, Fossella F, Komaki R, et al: A randomized trial comparing perioperative chemotherapy and surgery with surgery alone in resectable stage IIIA non-small-cell lung cancer. J Natl Cancer Inst 86:673–680, 1994.
22. Schirren J, Cuénoud P-F, Bülzebruck H, et al: Chirurgie du carcinome bronchique avec envahissement nodulaire mediastinal. Ann Chir 48:852–861, 1994.

23. Shepherd FA: Induction chemotherapy for locally advanced non-small cell lung cancer. Ann Thorac Surg 55:1585–1592, 1993.
24. Urschel JD: Current applications of nonvideo thoracoscopy. Int Surg 82:131–133, 1997.
25. Vansteenkiste JF, De Leyn PR, Deneffe GJ, et al: Vindesine-ifosfamide-platinum (VIP) induction chemotherapy in surgically staged IIIA-N2 non-small cell lung cancer: A prospective study. Ann Oncol 9:261–267, 1998.
26. Vansteenkiste JF, Stroobants SG, De Leyn PR: Lymph node staging in non-small cell lung cancer with FDG-PET-scan: A prospective study on 690 lymph node stations. J Clin Oncol 16:2142–2149, 1998.

COMMENTARY

Anthony P. C. Yim

Staging plays a crucial role in the management of primary lung cancer, and mediastinoscopy is an established technique. Identification of mediastinal nodal disease changes subsequent management strategy. Videomediastinoscopy as advocated by the authors represents a refinement and improvement of an established technique that allows an enlarged image of high resolution to be projected on the video monitor. As the authors point out, it has proved to be an invaluable tool for teaching, and perhaps eventual standardization of this technique. In addition, we have also found the videoscope to be useful for other procedures, such as subxiphoid pericardial window.

Chapter 23

Diagnostic Thoracoscopy for Mediastinal Masses

Tiziano De Giacomo, Erino Angelo Rendina, Federico Venuta, and Giorgio Furio Coloni

The mediastinum is the site of a wide spectrum of benign and malignant diseases, providing a great diagnostic and therapeutic challenge to surgeons.

Although a reasonable differential diagnosis can be made on the basis of clinical history, physical examination, and radiologic workup, in most cases the precise nature of mediastinal lesions cannot be determined without histologic examination of the tissue. The ideal diagnostic approach should allow the physician to obtain the correct histologic diagnosis with minimal trauma to the patient. A number of techniques are currently employed for the diagnosis of mediastinal diseases, varying with the size and location of the lesion. These techniques range from fine needle aspiration biopsy (FNA) to open thoracotomy. Video-assisted thoracoscopy (VAT) represents a potentially advantageous route for biopsy and resection of thoracic lesions. An excellent exposure of the operative field with minimal surgical trauma is achieved by VAT, and thus we employ this modality extensively in the diagnosis and treatment of mediastinal diseases.

General Principles

The mediastinum is the middle section of the thoracic cavity, lying between the mediastinal pleura on either side. It extends anteriorly from the jugular notch to the xiphoid process, and posteriorly from the first to the eleventh vertebral bodies. Superiorly, it is in direct communication with the neck; inferiorly, it is limited by the diaphragm, and anteriorly, by the sternum.

Many arbitrary divisions of the mediastinum have been proposed to allow an organized approach to mediastinal lesions.[4, 9, 34] For our purposes, it seems easy and satisfactory to subdivide the mediastinum into three compartments:

Anterior Mediastinum. This area is bounded anteriorly by the sternum and posteriorly by the anterior surfaces of the great vessels and the pericardium.

Middle Mediastinum. This area is limited posteriorly by the esophagus and laterally by the mediastinal pleura.

Posterior Mediastinum. Included in this area are the esophagus and paravertebral structures.

The majority of lesions developing in the anterior mediastinum are lymphomas, thymic lesions, and germ cell tumors; less common diseases are of vascular, mesenchymal, or thyroidal origin. In the middle mediastinum, primary or secondary lymphadenopathy and enterogenic cysts represent the more frequently occurring lesions. Neurogenic tumors and enteric cysts predominate in the posterior mediastinum. Mesenchymal tumors are rare but can occur in any of the three compartments (Table 23–1).

Most mediastinal lesions can be identified on the standard chest radiograph (CXR), including anteroposterior and lateral views, and this is one of the most important diagnostic tests in the evaluation of mediastinal masses.[13, 25] Computed tomography (CT) scan provides additional fundamental information about the exact location and characteristics of the lesion (i.e., density, homogeneity, vascular nature), as well as its radiologic behavior (i.e., infiltration, encapsulation, compression) toward the surrounding structures.[1, 41] Magnetic resonance imaging (MRI) can supply additional information. This can be used to depict the mediastinum in both the coronal and sagittal planes and allows excellent visualization of the aortic root, the aortopulmonary window, the subcarinal space, the brachial plexus, and the spinal cord. MRI is particularly useful in the evaluation of involvement of vascular or spinal structures by posterior mediastinal tumors.[7, 21]

Nuclear medicine studies and positron emission tomography (PET) are rarely required in the evaluation of mediastinal masses, but, in selected cases, these techniques can be helpful in providing better characterization of the lesion and better follow-up after treatment.[29, 33, 35, 37] Serum levels of numerous biochemical markers may be altered in association with mediastinal diseases: α-fetoprotein (αFP), β-human chorionic gonadotropin (βHCG), catecholamines, and thyroid and parathyroid hormones are investigated in selected cases when clinically indicated. Approximately 10% of mediastinal seminomas are accompanied by elevated levels of βHCG, usually not greater than 100 ng/ml. Higher levels suggest the presence of nonseminomatous elements in the tumor.[12] The serum αFP level is always normal in pure mediastinal seminoma. If this marker is elevated, the tumor is likely to contain nonseminomatous elements. Very high levels of βHCG and αFP (>500 ng/ml) are usually associated with malignant nonseminomatous germ cell tumors, and biopsy confirmation is often unnecessary for starting the appropriate treatment.

In the past, a major surgical approach was recommended for almost all mediastinal lesions for resection, biopsy, debulking, or both when excision proved impossible. At present, major surgery is not indicated for all lesions, and the modern approach to the treatment of mediastinal tumor is often multidisciplinary. This makes histologic confirmation of the diagnosis of paramount importance in determining the best therapeutic protocol. With the advances in neoadjuvant treatment, some mediastinal tumors that were previously considered unresectable and as conferring a poor prognosis can now be approached with preoperative chemotherapy, irradiation, or both, followed by surgical resection.

Table 23–1. Common Tumors and Cysts of the Mediastinum

Anterior Mediastinum	Middle Mediastinum	Posterior Mediastinum
Thymic neoplasms and cysts	Lymphomas	Neurogenic tumors
Lymphomas	Enterogenic cyst	Enteric cyst
Germ cell tumors	Mesothelial cyst	Lymphomas
Ectopic or aberrant thyroid	Metastatic lymphadenopathy	Mesenchymal tumors
Mesenchymal tumors	Granulomatous adenopathy	
Parathyroid adenoma		
Vascular masses (angiomas, lymphangiomas, aneurysms)		

At present, standard histologic examination routinely involves immunohistochemistry, immunofluorescence tests, and on occasion, electron microscopy. Frozen sections should be used extensively to obtain a preliminary diagnosis and to judge whether the tissue sample is sufficient for a detailed histologic analysis.[16] When possible, the surgeon should incise the tumor rather than use the biopsy forceps, to avoid crushing artifacts during removal of the specimen. In addition, the use of electrocautery must be limited to the base of the specimen until the diagnosis is achieved. Among the various surgical procedures for mediastinal biopsy, VAT offers the opportunity of obtaining accurate samples of mediastinal lesions with minimal surgical trauma.

Diagnostic Surgical Techniques

Fine Needle Aspiration

A safe and easy procedure, fine needle aspiration (FNA) can be very helpful for cytologic diagnosis of metastatic carcinomas of the mediastinum. However, in other tumors, such as lymphoma, this procedure is often inconclusive, and definitive diagnosis calls for histologic examination of a larger amount of tissue.[15, 43] Furthermore, some tumors are surrounded by an intensely inflammatory process, which makes the diagnosis difficult even when large specimens are obtained.

Mediastinoscopy

This procedure, first described by Carlens in 1959, remains the procedure of choice for biopsy of paratracheal lesions. Extended mediastinoscopy, as suggested by Ginsberg and associates,[10] allows access to the anterior compartment of the mediastinum for biopsy of the aortopulmonary window and prevascular nodal stations. This approach has not been extensively used because of the limited view and the risk of injury to the great vessels. Video mediastinoscopy is currently in use, and many believe it improves visibility and facilitates dissection (see Chapter 22).

Anterior Mediastinotomy

As first described by Chamberlain in 1965, this is a safe and widely used approach[8, 24] for diagnosis of mediastinal masses. It provides a limited field of view and is often complicated by opening the pleural space. We still use anterior mediastinotomy for anterior mediastinal masses that strictly adhere to or infiltrate the anterior chest wall, so that the procedure can be accomplished under local anesthesia.[30]

Video-Assisted Thoracoscopy

This approach allows excellent visualization of the mediastinum from a lateral point of view. In addition, the entire hemithorax can be explored for visceral, pleural, or diaphragmatic lesions. Advanced endoscopic instruments permit visually guided biopsy or resection of lesions in all mediastinal compartments.[17, 23, 27, 30]

Thoracotomy and Partial or Total Sternotomy

These procedures should be employed for diagnostic purposes only when results with other procedures are inconclusive or when such procedures are not feasible.

Thoracoscopic Surgical Technique

For diagnosis of mediastinal diseases, VAT is usually performed with the patient under general anesthesia and using double-lumen tracheal intubation. In selected cases, VAT can be accomplished using deep sedation and local anesthesia with the patient breathing spontaneously. This approach is indicated for simple procedures and for patients who have severe medical problems and in whom paralysis and tracheal intubation are highly risky or contraindicated (e.g., patients who have a large mediastinal mass with airway compression or poor cardiorespiratory status).*

The patient is placed in the lateral decubitus position, and prepared and draped as for standard thoracotomy. Rotation of the operative table and use of the Trendelenburg and reverse Trendelenburg positions can be helpful in lung retraction for providing better exposure of the operative field (Fig. 23–1). Usually two or three trocars are employed, with the scope placed at the midaxillary line in the sixth or seventh intercostal space. We currently employ a 10-mm, zero-degree thoracoscope with an operative channel. After exploration of the chest cavity, the mediastinal

*Editor's note: We do not advise using VAT under local anesthesia for this group of patients.

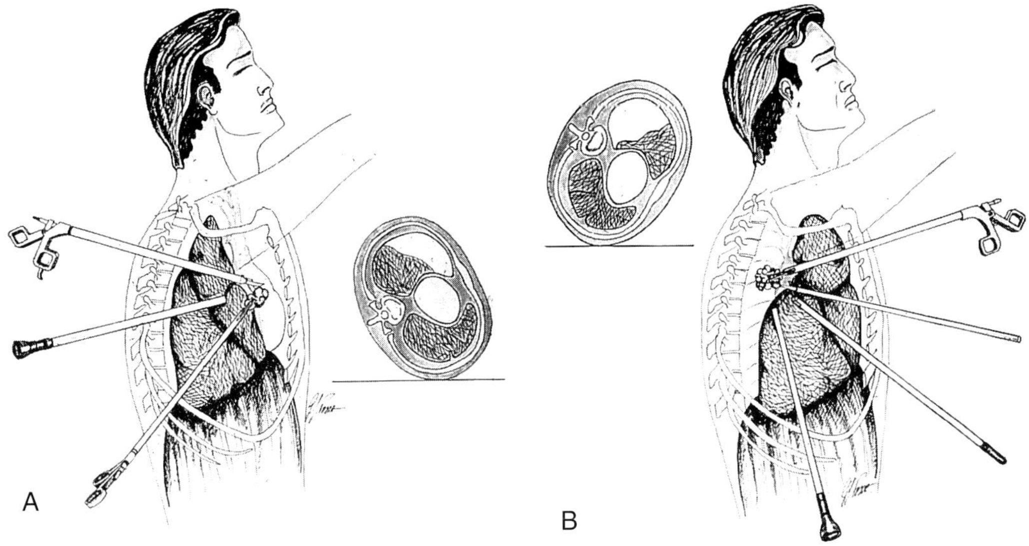

Figure 23–1. Thoracoscopic approach to the mediastinum. Patient is placed in the lateral decubitus position. *A*, Anterior rotation of the operative table; *B*, posterior rotation of the table is helpful in lung retraction for better exposure of the operative field.

lesion is identified and biopsied. Extensive use of intraoperative frozen section examination is employed to assess the adequacy of the specimen. Simultaneous pericardial and pleural biopsy can be performed on the lung. Pleural and pericardial effusions can be treated with pleurodesis and by creating a pericardial window, respectively (Fig. 23–2). On completion of the procedure, a chest tube is left in place and usually removed on the first postoperative day. Postoperative hospital stay is usually 24 to 48 hours. Nonsteroidal anti-inflammatory medications are often helpful for pain control.

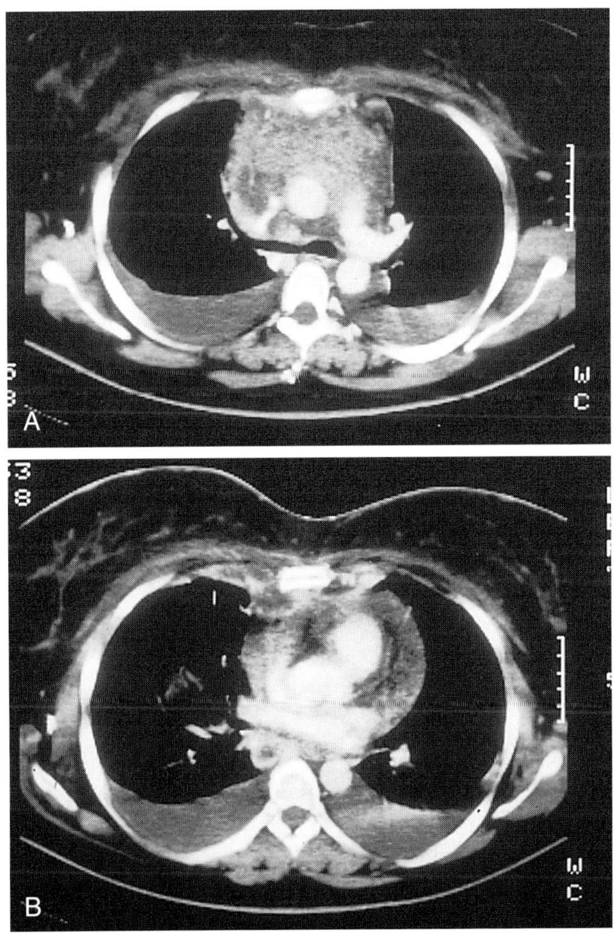

Figure 23–2. Computed tomography (CT) scan of a patient with mediastinal lymphoma and both pleural and pericardial effusion. *A*, At the level of the carina, a large, extensive, infiltrating mass is evident. A bilateral pleural effusion can also be seen. *B*, At a lower level, pericardial effusion can be observed. A left-sided thoracoscopy allowed diagnostic biopsy of the primary tumor, creation of a pericardial window, and ipsilateral drainage of the effusion with pleural biopsy.

Anterior Mediastinum

The differential diagnosis of anterior mediastinal masses includes lymphomas, thymic neoplasms, mesenchymal tumors, and germ cell tumors. Less common diseases are substernal goiters, cysts, metastatic cancers, and vascular lesions. The role of surgery in lymphoma is primarily to obtain a positive histologic diagnosis by biopsy. Only in very rare cases of isolated mediastinal lymphoma can one justify a complete surgical resection.[31] A large amount of tissue is required for a definitive diagnosis, and FNA is usually inadequate. The thoracic surgeon may also occasionally be asked to obtain a biopsy of a persistent or an intrathoracic mass that recurs after treatment (Fig. 23–3) to assess response. In these cases, the surgical approach can present some technical problems.

At the primary site of disease, the marked reduction of the neoplastic mass and the reactive fibrosis induced by chemotherapy and radiation therapy make the dissection difficult, and it is mandatory to resect and examine as much tissue as possible to rule out any residual focus of malignancy. Furthermore, these patients may have multiple lesions, and it is necessary to employ an approach that allows the surgeon to reach all of them.

Thoracoscopy provides a large specimen and, when required, allows simultaneous pleural and lung biopsy, pericardial window or biopsy, and pleurodesis.[5] Well-

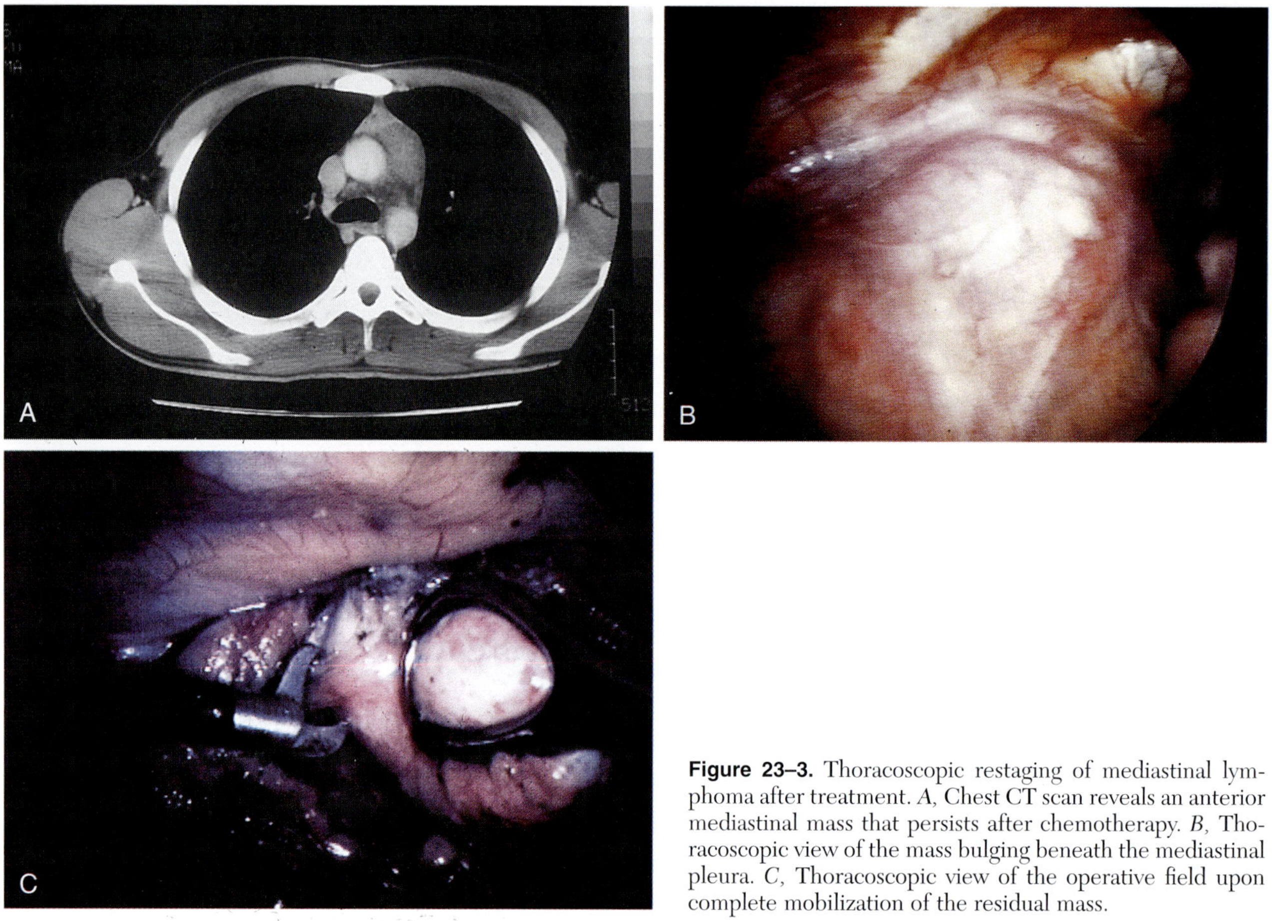

Figure 23–3. Thoracoscopic restaging of mediastinal lymphoma after treatment. *A,* Chest CT scan reveals an anterior mediastinal mass that persists after chemotherapy. *B,* Thoracoscopic view of the mass bulging beneath the mediastinal pleura. *C,* Thoracoscopic view of the operative field upon complete mobilization of the residual mass.

encapsulated anterior mediastinal masses that are suspected of being thymomas on the basis of preoperative imaging can be removed without histologic confirmation[18, 36, 44] (Fig. 23–4). Thymic masses that appear to be advanced or invasive should be treated with preoperative chemotherapy after histologic confirmation. In this subset of patients, VAT is very helpful because it provides histologic diagnosis and accurate evaluation of the extent of the disease.[39]

We believe that VAT is superior to anterior mediastinotomy as a diagnostic approach to anterior mediastinal masses. The excellent visualization of the thoracic cavity and mediastinal structures permits safe dissection and easy biopsy. In addition, the entire thoracic cavity can be simultaneously assessed for visceral, pleural, or diaphragmatic tumor implants, as well as pleural effusion and associated parenchymal lesions. Anterior mediastinotomy should be reserved for lesions that infiltrate the intercostal muscle of the anterior chest, or for a very large mass that results in severe airway compression, making paralysis, tracheal intubation, and curarization difficult and dangerous. Such biopsies can be performed using local anesthesia (Fig. 23–5).

Middle Mediastinum

The majority of lesions that develop in the middle mediastinum are either benign cystic masses (bronchogenic or mesothelial cysts) or lesions arising from lymphatic tissue (i.e., lymphomas, granulomatous inflammatory processes, sarcoidosis, metastatic carcinomas). Cervical mediastinoscopy is the procedure of choice to assess paratracheal lesions, and VAT should play a role only in selected cases when lesions involving other structures (e.g., lung, pleura, pericardium) must be evaluated simultaneously. Thoracoscopic diagnosis and resection of mediastinal cystic lesions are usually very feasible, and thus a more invasive approach can be avoided.[14, 22, 26] The role of VAT in lung cancer staging is discussed in a subsequent section of this chapter.

Posterior Mediastinum

Posterior mediastinal masses include enterogenic cysts and neurogenic tumors, both of which are almost always benign in adults. Lymphoma can also arise in this compartment. Neurogenic tumors stem from the nerve sheath (i.e., neurilemoma, neurofibroma, and neurosarcoma), from autonomic nervous structures (i.e., ganglioneuroma, neuroblastoma, ganglioneuroblastoma), and from paraganglia (i.e., pheochromocytoma and chemodectoma). Usually, FNA is inconclusive because of the relative acellularity of these lesions. Radiologic workup in most cases can suggest the diagnosis, and thoracoscopy or open thoracotomy is employed to confirm the diagnosis and to perform resection.[19] Posterior mediastinal lymphadenopathy can be easily visualized and biopsied by VAT (Figs. 23–6 and 7).

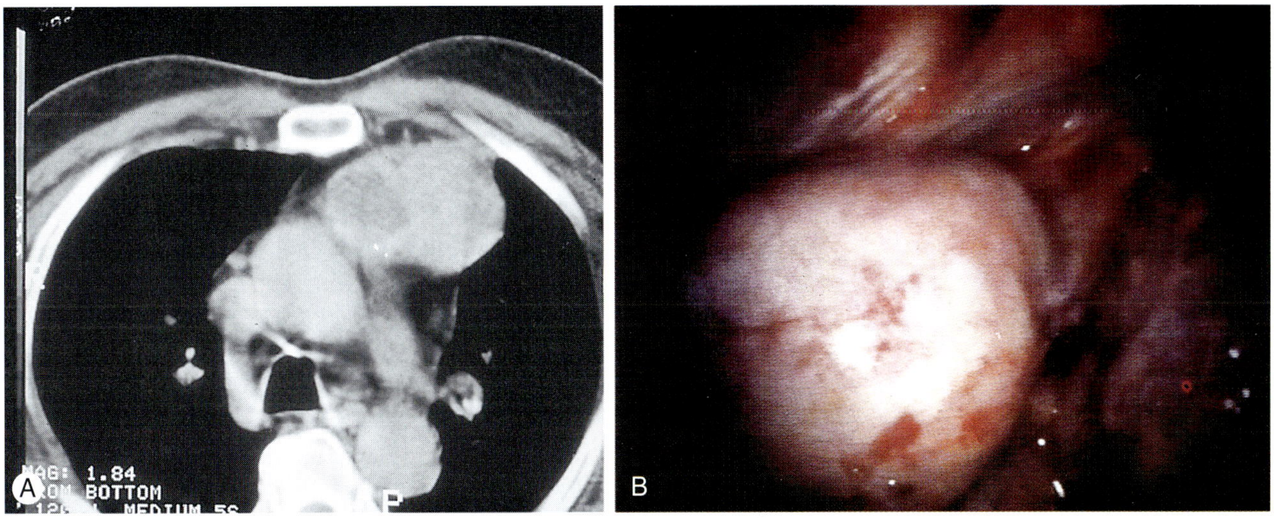

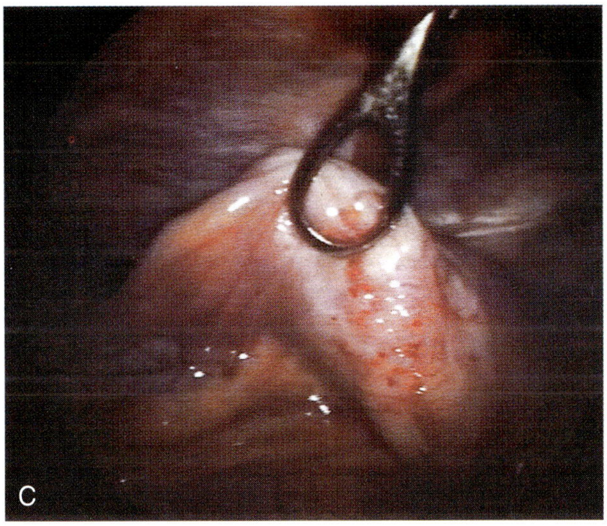

Figure 23–4. Thymoma. *A*, Computed tomography (CT) scan suggests a well-encapsulated stage I thymoma. *B*, The thoracoscopic view of the lesion confirms the absence of infiltration. *C*, VAT demonstrates clear dissection planes.

Lung Cancer Staging

Lung cancer staging often requires both noninvasive and invasive procedures to assess the extent of tumor involvement accurately. With the evolution of neoadjuvant therapy, some lesions previously considered unresectable are now treated with chemotherapy and radiation followed by surgical resection. Accurate pathologic staging is mandatory for a proper selection of patients to be included in a neoadjuvant treatment protocol. This allows appropriate

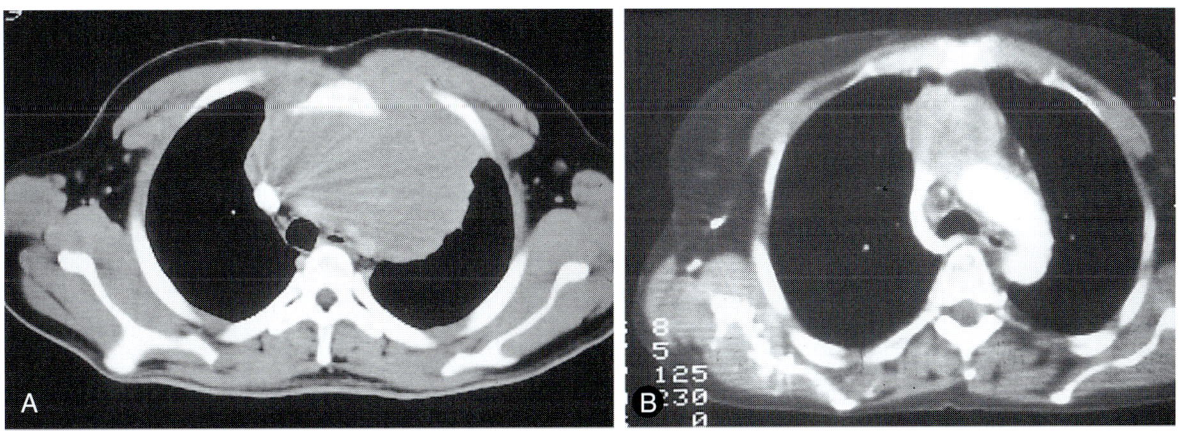

Figure 23–5. *A*, Chest computed tomography (CT) scan shows a large mass in the anterior mediastinum that infiltrates the chest wall. This is a good indication for anterior mediastinotomy under local anesthesia. *B*, CT evidence of extensively infiltrating mediastinal mass not adherent to the anterior chest wall; VAT is preferable to anterior mediastinotomy.

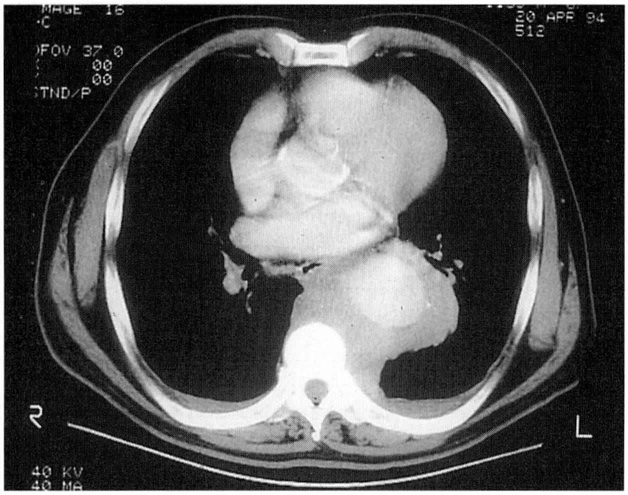

Figure 23–6. Diagnostic thoracoscopy for posterior mediastinal tumors. Computed tomography (CT) scan of the chest demonstrates an infiltrating large mass surrounding the descending aorta. Thoracoscopy revealed non-Hodgkin's lymphoma.

clinical stratification to standardize inclusion criteria, which leads to valid and reproducible post-treatment results. The role of VAT is limited but specific as an adjunct to other procedures in lung cancer staging.[32, 40] The staging system for lung cancer is based on the evaluation of the extension of the primary tumor (T), the involvement of regional lymph nodes (N), and the presence of distant metastases (M).

In the evaluation of T status, VAT can have a specific role in patients who have locally advanced lung cancer. Unresectable disease can be identified without the need for exploratory thoracotomy. As diagnostic procedures, CT and MRI scans are notoriously inaccurate in the confirmation of local invasion, because of the many false-positive and false-negative results (sensitivity = 43% and specificity = 74%).[11] Atelectasis is a common cause of misjudging mediastinal invasion on CT and MRI scans. Thoracoscopy allows the surgeon to assess tumor adherence to, and invasion of, mediastinal structures. Sometimes, VAT is not able to provide visualization of the entire area of involvement, especially when multiple adhesions or a big tumor is present. In our experience,[6] VAT yielded accurate staging in 90% of patients who had preoperative symptoms suggestive of mediastinal invasion.

Thoracoscopy also plays an important role in the evaluation of pleural involvement.[45] The diagnostic accuracy in this situation increases to 100%. In all cases of lung cancer with pleural effusion and negative preoperative cytology, VAT should be performed. In our experience, VAT demonstrated pleural involvement in 6 of 10 patients who had cytologically negative pleural effusion.[6]

Mediastinal nodal status is a major determinant of survival in patients who have lung cancer. Differentiation between N0 and N1 disease is not really important in the resectability decision, and VAT usually cannot supply information about these nodal stations without lung dissection. Evaluation of mediastinal nodes by CT is principally based on size, with nodes larger than 1 cm in diameter considered malignant. There is 88.7% specificity on CT, with a sensitivity of only 71%.[29, 42] Often, it is possible to find metastatic disease in small nodes (<1 cm), and this is especially true in patients who have adenocarcinoma.

The most common cause of false-positive mediastinal nodes during noninvasive staging is benign hypertrophic lymphadenopathy resulting from postobstructive pneumonia. False-positive nodes are also more frequent in patients who have T3 disease. Gauging the size of lymph nodes is suboptimal as a criterion because of the high rate of false-negative (10 to 20%) lesions, and, thus, we believe that histologic evaluation is mandatory. Cervical mediastinoscopy continues to be the best procedure for assessing mediastinal node status.[3, 38] It allows the surgeon to access paratracheal nodal stations bilaterally. A unilateral procedure, such as VAT, is unable to reach lymph nodes at levels 1, 2, and 3, which could be assessed easily by mediastinoscopy. On the other hand, VAT can play an adjunctive role in the evaluation of specific nodal stations not accessible by mediastinoscopy, such as posterior subcarinal[20] and pulmonary ligament nodes (levels 8 and 9) (Fig. 23–8). After negative mediastinoscopy, a thoracoscopic approach seems justified only when CT suggests bulky adenopathy in these stations, and this procedure may confirm N2 disease, which would contraindicate surgical resection.

In M1 disease VAT can be useful for excisional biopsy of secondary lung lesions in the same or the contralateral thoracic cavity. Overt lesions can be either second primary tumors or represent metastatic spread to the lung parenchyma from a primary bronchogenic cancer. Thus, VAT can be useful in identifying M1 disease.

We believe that VAT is preferable to anterior mediastinotomy or extended cervical mediastinoscopy for the

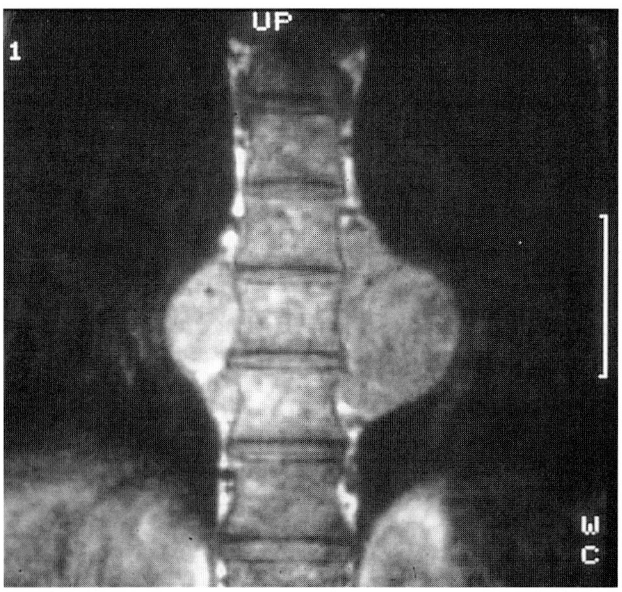

Figure 23–7. Diagnostic thoracoscopy for posterior mediastinal tumors. Magnetic resonance imaging (MRI) scan demonstrates bilateral paravertebral masses. Thoracoscopic biopsy revealed extramedullary hematopoietic tissue.

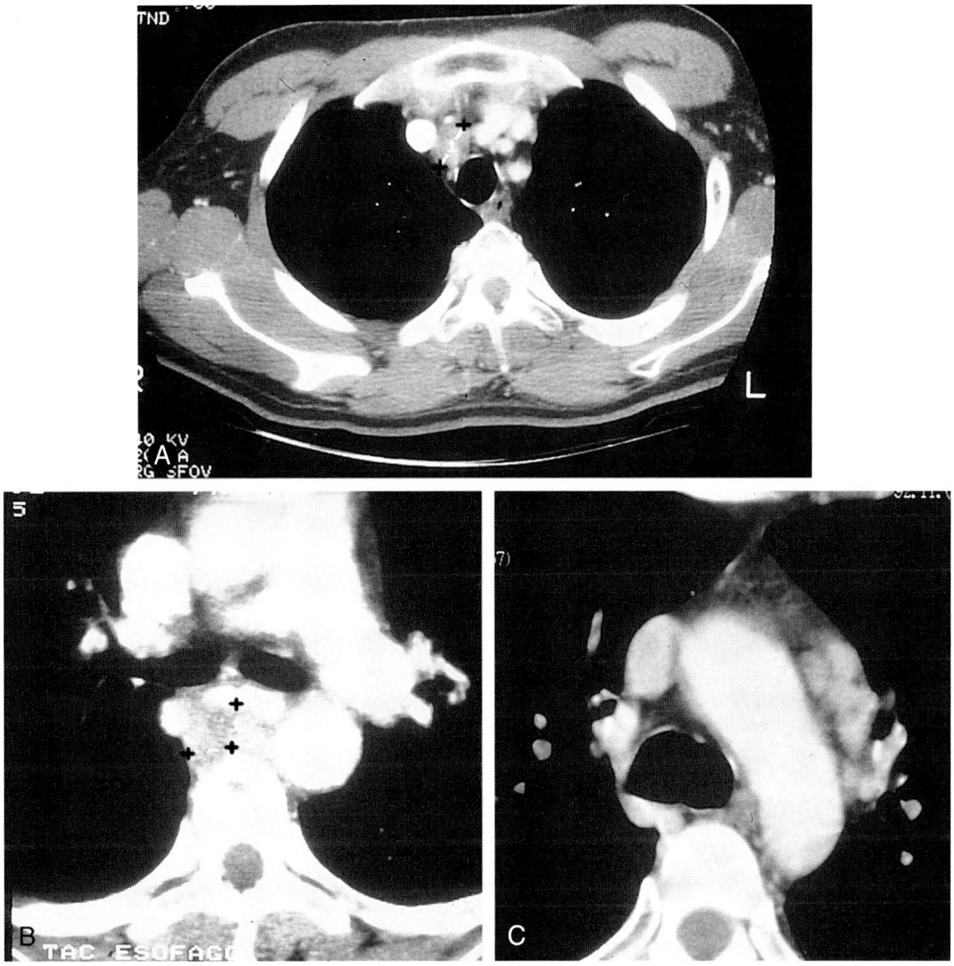

Figure 23–8. Role of thoracoscopy in the evaluation of mediastinal nodes. *A*, Computed tomography (CT) evidence of enlarged paratracheal lymph nodes. Biopsy should be accomplished by cervical mediastinoscopy. *B*, Chest CT scan showing posterior mediastinal nodes compressing and displacing the esophagus, easily accessible by thoracoscopy. *C*, CT demonstration of preaortic lymphadenopathy. Thoracoscopy proved adequate for safe dissection and biopsy.

evaluation of the preaortic and aortopulmonary window nodes (levels 5 and 6).

Conclusion

VAT has a limited but specific role in lung cancer staging. Direct visualization and histologic evidence of local invasion from the primary tumor can be obtained. It provides an excellent way to assess pleural involvement and allows simultaneous performance of talc pleurodesis when needed. Mediastinoscopy remains the procedure of choice for evaluating the status of the mediastinal nodes, because it allows bilateral exploration. In our opinion, however, thoracoscopy is preferable to anterior mediastinotomy and extended cervical mediastinoscopy for assessing the status of nodes at levels 5 and 6 as well as subcarinal and posterior mediastinal nodes not accessible during other procedures.

Invasive surgical procedures, such as thoracotomy and sternotomy, should be employed for biopsy or staging purposes only when other, less invasive techniques are not feasible.

References

1. Brown K, Aberle DR, Batra P, et al: Current use of imaging in the evaluation of primary mediastinal masses. Chest 98:466–473, 1990.
2. Carlens E: Mediastinoscopy: A method of inspection and tissue biopsy in the superior mediastinum. Chest 36:343, 1959.
3. Coughlin M, Deslauriers J, Beaulieau M, et al: Role of mediastinoscopy in the pretreatment staging of patients with primary lung cancer. Ann Thorac Surg 40:556–560, 1985.
4. Davies DV, Coupland RE (eds): The respiratory system. *In* Gray's Anatomy: Descriptive and Applied. London, Longmans, Green and Co, 1958.
5. De Giacomo T, Rendina EA, Venuta F, et al: Video-assisted thoracoscopic surgery in patients previously treated for intrathoracic lymphoma. J Thorac Cardiovasc Surg 112:1108, 1109, 1996.
6. De Giacomo T, Rendina EA, Venuta F, et al: Thoracoscopic staging of IIIB non-small cell lung cancer before neoadjuvant therapy. Ann Thorac Surg 64:1409–1411, 1997.
7. Dooms GC, Higgins CB: The potential of magnetic resonance imaging for the evaluation of thoracic arterial disease. J Thorac Cardiovasc Surg 92:1088–1095, 1986.
8. Elia S, Cecere C, Giampaglia F, et al: Mediastinoscopy vs ante-

rior mediastinotomy in the diagnosis of mediastinal lymphoma: A randomized trial. Eur J Cardiothorac Surg 6:361–365, 1992.

9. Fraser RG, Paré JAP, Paré PD, et al: The normal chest (the mediastinum). *In* Fraser RG, Paré JAP, Paré PD, et al (eds): Diagnosis of Diseases of the Chest. Philadelphia, WB Saunders, 1988, pp 107–120.
10. Ginsberg RJ, Rice TW, Goldberg M, et al: Extended cervical mediastinoscopy—the best procedure for staging left upper lobe tumors. J Thorac Cardiovasc Surg 94:673, 1978.
11. Glazer HS, Kaiser LR, Anderson DJ, et al: Indeterminate mediastinal invasion in bronchogenic carcinoma: CT evaluation. Radiology 173:37–42, 1989.
12. Hainsworth JD, Greco FA: General features of malignant germ cell tumors and primary seminomas of the mediastinum. *In* Shields TW (ed): Mediastinal Surgery. Malvern, PA, Lea & Febiger, 1991, pp 211–218.
13. Harris GJ, Harman PK, Trinkle JK, et al: Standard biplane roentgenography is highly selective in documenting mediastinal masses. Ann Thorac Surg 44:238–241, 1987.
14. Hazelrigg SR, Landreneau RJ, Mack MJ, et al: Thoracoscopic resection of mediastinal cysts. Ann Thorac Surg 56:659–660, 1993.
15. Herman SJ, Holub RV, Weisbrod GL, et al: Anterior mediastinal masses: Utility of transthoracic needle biopsy. Radiology 180: 167–170, 1991.
16. Juttner FM, Fellbaum C, Popper H, et al: Pitfalls in intraoperative frozen section histology of mediastinal neoplasms. Eur J Cardiothorac Surg 4:584–586, 1990.
17. Kern JA, Daniel TM, Tribble CG, et al: Thoracoscopic diagnosis and treatment of mediastinal masses. Ann Thorac Surg 56:92–96, 1993.
18. Landreneau RJ, Dowling RD, Castillo WM, et al: Thoracoscopic resection of an anterior mediastinal tumor. Ann Thorac Surg 54:142–144, 1992.
19. Landreneau RJ, Dowling RD, Ferson PF. Thoracoscopic resection of a posterior mediastinal neurogenic tumor. Chest 102: 1288–1290, 1992.
20. Landreneau RJ, Hazelrigg SR, Mack MJ, et al: Thoracoscopic mediastinal lymph node sampling: Useful for mediastinal lymph node stations inaccessible by cervical mediastinoscopy. J Thorac Cardiovasc Surg 106:554–558, 1993.
21. Levitt RG, Glazer HS, Roper CL, et al: Magnetic resonance imaging of mediastinal and hilar masses: A comparison with CT. Am J Roentgenol 145:9–14, 1985.
22. Lewis RJ, Caccavale RJ, Sisler GE: Imaged thoracoscopic surgery: A new technique for resection of mediastinal cysts. Ann Thorac Surg 53:318–320, 1992.
23. Mai J, Loddenkamper R, Brandt HJ: Diagnostic thoracoscopy in mediastinal space-occupying lesions. Pneumologie 43:122–125, 1989.
24. McNeill TM, Chamberlain JM: Diagnostic anterior mediastinotomy. Ann Thorac Surg 2:532, 1966.
25. Moore EH: Radiologic evaluation of mediastinal masses. Chest Surg Clin N Am. 2:1–22, 1992.
26. Naunheim KS, Andrus CH: Thoracoscopic drainage and resection of giant mediastinal cyst. Ann Thorac Surg 55:156–158, 1993.
27. Naunheim KS: Video thoracoscopy for masses of the posterior mediastinum. Ann Thorac Surg 56:657–658, 1993.
28. Park HM, Tarver RD, Siddiqui AR, et al: Efficacy of thyroid scintigraphy in the diagnosis of intrathoracic goiter. Am J Roentgenol 148:527–529, 1987.
29. Patterson GA, Ginsberg RJ, Poon PY, et al: A prospective evaluation of magnetic resonance imaging, computed tomography and mediastinoscopy in the preoperative assessment of mediastinal node status in bronchogenic carcinoma. J Thorac Cardiovasc Surg 94:679–684, 1987.
30. Rendina EA, Venuta F, De Giacomo T, et al: Comparative merits of thoracoscopy, mediastinoscopy and mediastinotomy for mediastinal biopsy. Ann Thorac Surg 57:992–995, 1994.
31. Ricci C, Rendina EA, Venuta F, et al: Surgical approach to isolated mediastinal lymphoma. J Thorac Cardiovasc Surg 99: 691–695, 1990.
32. Rusch VW, Bains MS, Burt ME, et al: Contribution of videothoracoscopy to the management of the cancer patient. Ann Surg Oncol 1:94–98, 1994.
33. Shapiro B, Sisson J, Kalff V, et al: The location of middle mediastinal pheochromocytomas. J Thorac Cardiovasc Surg 87: 814, 1984.
34. Shields TW: The mediastinum and its compartments. *In* Shields TW (ed): Mediastinal Surgery. Malvern, PA, Lea & Febiger, 1991, pp 3–5.
35. Spies WG: Radionuclide studies of the mediastinum. *In* Shields TW (ed): Mediastinal Surgery, Malvern, PA, Lea & Febiger, 1991, pp 50–61.
36. Sugarbaker DJ: Thoracoscopy in the management of anterior mediastinal masses. Ann Thorac Surg 56:653–656, 1993.
37. Valk PE, Pounds TR, Hopkins DM, et al: Staging non-small cell lung cancer by whole-body positron emission tomographic imaging. Ann Thorac Surg 60:1573–1582, 1995.
38. Van Schil PEY, Van Hee RHGG, Shoofs ELG: The value of mediastinoscopy in preoperative staging of bronchogenic carcinoma. J Thorac Cardiovasc Surg 97:240–243, 1989.
39. Venuta F, Rendina EA, Pescarmona EO, et al: Multimodality treatment of thymoma. A prospective study. Ann Thorac Surg 64:1585–1592, 1997.
40. Wain JC: Video-assisted thoracoscopy and the staging of lung cancer. Ann Thorac Surg 56:776–778, 1993.
41. Waller DA, Rees MR: Computed tomography of the chest in the preoperative assessment of mediastinal tumors—does it improve surgical management? J Thorac Cardiovasc Surg 39: 158–161, 1991.
42. Webb WB, Gatsonis C, Zerhouni E, et al: CT and MR imaging in staging non-small cell bronchogenic carcinoma: Report of the Radiologic Diagnostic Oncology Group. Thorac Radiol 178: 705–713, 1991.
43. Weisbrod GL: Percutaneous fine needle biopsy of the mediastinum. Clin Chest Med 8:27–41, 1987.
44. Yim APC: Video-assisted thoracoscopic management of anterior mediastinal masses. Preliminary experience and results. Surg Endosc 9:1184–1188, 1995.
45. Yim APC: Routine video-assisted thoracoscopy prior to thoracotomy. Chest 109:1099–1100, 1996.

Chapter 24

Thoracoscopic Staging for Intrathoracic Malignancy

Joshua R. Sonett and Mark J. Krasna

The importance of accurate cancer staging is well described and accepted. Precise staging, as described by the American Joint Committee on Cancer (AJCC) and the International Union Against Cancer (IUAC), allows more accurate prognostication and prediction of survival, treatment planning, evaluation of results of treatment, exchange of information on cancer treatment, and investigation of experimental treatments.[2] This concept of cancer care has clearly facilitated the treatment of patients with thoracic malignancies and led to new and accepted paradigms in their surgical and medical treatment. Staging is not just used to predict prognosis; it is now an essential element in the planning treatment of all thoracic malignancies. Because treatment strategies and prognoses vary depending on the stage at the time of presentation, the need for complete and accurate pathologic staging has become more clearly defined. Accurate staging of thoracic malignancies begins with noninvasive techniques; however, definitive diagnosis and final staging still depend on pathologic specimens. In the development of staging in lung cancer, the concept of surgical staging of thoracic malignancies was pioneered by Carlens and associate[6, 13] and promulgated by Pearson.[37] These pioneers established mediastinoscopy as a well-accepted and important adjunctive diagnostic tool by proving its accuracy compared with noninvasive staging. Although noninvasive—and even percutaneous and endobronchial—techniques have been used and continue to improve, many patients still have suboptimal clinical staging compared with final pathologic staging. Until recently, the final determination of the true pathologic stage was made by direct surgical exploration at the time of the intended resection. With the advent and refinement of thoracoscopy, most thoracic malignancies can be accurately diagnosed and staged with minimal morbidity before treatment is begun.

Diagnosis of Malignancy

Thoracoscopy has a well-defined role in the diagnosis of pleural effusions and parenchymal masses, and it may be considered the initial staging procedure for these lesions. The efficacy of thoracoscopy in diagnosing pleural effusions is well described; it is the procedure of choice for recurrent undiagnosed pleural effusions.[5, 31, 41] With the use of an operating thoracoscope (Fig. 24–1), pleural visualization, biopsy, and talc poudrage can all be performed with a single small incision. Thoracoscopy as well may be used to make an effective diagnosis of an indeterminate pulmonary lesion.[19, 23, 29] However, its role versus percutaneous needle biopsy is a source of continuous debate. In patients who have no significant surgical risks and in whom definitive anatomic lung resection is planned, diagnosis by thoracoscopy before resection is cost effective and efficient. The specimen should always be removed in a protected bag to prevent inadvertent seeding of the thoracoscopic port site. This approach may also allow the surgeon to evaluate the pleura for unsuspected metastases or proceed with a video-assisted thoracic surgery (VATS) anatomic pulmonary resection. However, for a high-risk patient undergoing surgery in whom general anesthesia should be avoided, or for a patient whose undiagnosed mass is thought to be benign by radiologic criteria, a percutaneous needle biopsy may be effective in diagnosing benign or malignant lesions. At the University of Maryland, undiagnosed parenchymal lung lesions have been definitively diagnosed as benign or malignant 83% of the time.[44, 45] For this reason, it is our practice to stage patients selectively, by thoracoscopy or percutaneous needle biopsy according to the nature of the lesion and the condition of the patient. Lesions that are not definitively diagnosed by percutaneous biopsy, or those that are too small to biopsy accurately, are either directly removed by thoracoscopy or with the aid of computed tomography (CT) scan needle localization[46](Fig. 24–2).

Staging: Known Malignancy

Lung Cancer

The treatment and prognosis of non–small-cell lung cancer (NSCLC) are dependent on the stage at the time of presentation. The modern staging system, based on the pioneering work of Naruke and Mountain,[32, 36] is now used routinely in the treatment management of patients who have lung cancer. The components of TNM staging are tumor size and extension or proximity to other mediastinal structures (T stage), lymph node status (N stage) in the hilum and mediastinum, and absence or presence of metastatic disease (M stage) (Table 24–1). A combination of noninvasive, percutaneous, endobronchial, and surgical techniques may be used to define the accurate stage of each patient clinically and pathologically. Although treatment of each patient is individualized, generally accepted staging protocols proceed on a logical course from noninvasive to invasive until satisfactory staging has been accomplished. Indications for the use of thoracoscopic staging are listed in Table 24–2, and can be defined in terms of TNM staging.[10]

The presence of positive mediastinal or hilar lymph nodes, as described by the AJCC and the IUAC, is perhaps the most significant independent predictor of survival in

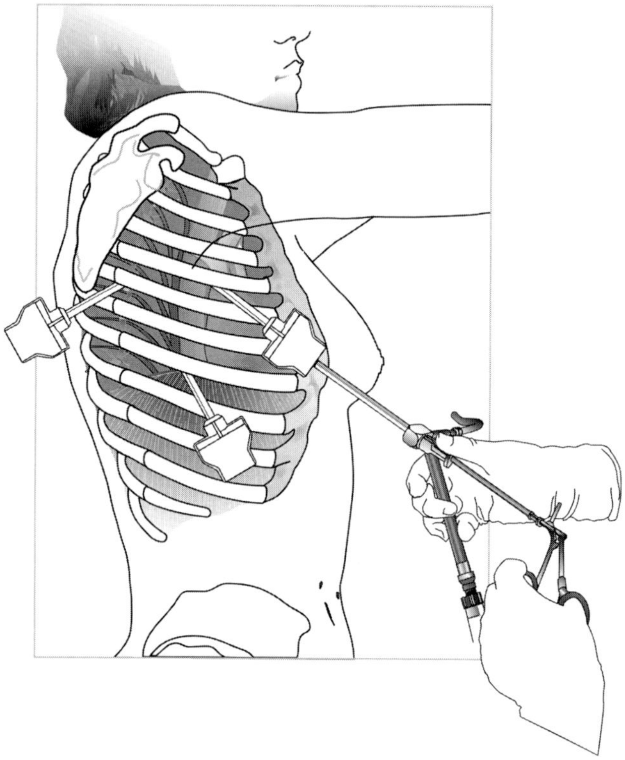

Figure 24–1. Patient position for thoracoscopic exploration.

Table 24–1. Staging System for Lung Cancer

Definitions

Primary Tumor (T)

TX Primary tumor cannot be assessed or tumor cannot be proven by presence of malignant cells in sputum or bronchial washings without visualization by imaging or bronchoscopy

T0 No evidence of primary tumor

Tis Carcinoma in situ

T1 Tumor <3 cm

T2 Tumor with any of the following features of size or extent:
- Invades the visceral pleura
- Associated with atelectasis or obstructive pneumonitis that extends to the hilar region but does not involve the entire lung

T3 Tumor of any size that directly invades any of the following:
- Mediastinum
- Heart
- Great vessels
- Trachea
- Esophagus

Lung Stage Groupings

Occult	TX	N0	M0
IA	T1	N0	M0
IB	T2	N0	M0
IIA	T1	N1	M0
IIB	T2	N1	M0
	T3	N0	M0
IIIA	T1	N2	M0
	T2	N2	M0
	T3	N1	M0
	T3	N2	M0
IIIB	Any T	N3	M0
	T4	Any N	M0
IV	Any T	Any N	M1

NSCLC. The lymph node staging map (Fig. 24–3), now widely known and accepted, clearly defines anatomic landmarks that differentiate hilar nodes (N1, nodes 10–13, double digit) from mediastinal nodes (N2, nodes 1–9, single digit). The presence of N2 or N3 (contralateral mediastinal nodes) dramatically changes both prognosis and treatment options. The presence of lymph nodes greater than 1 cm on CT scan increases the probability of malignant adenopathy; however, only 65% of these lymph nodes are pathologically positive for malignant cells (88% if the lymph nodes are greater than 1.5 cm).[48] For this reason, definitive pathologic diagnosis of mediastinal adenopathy

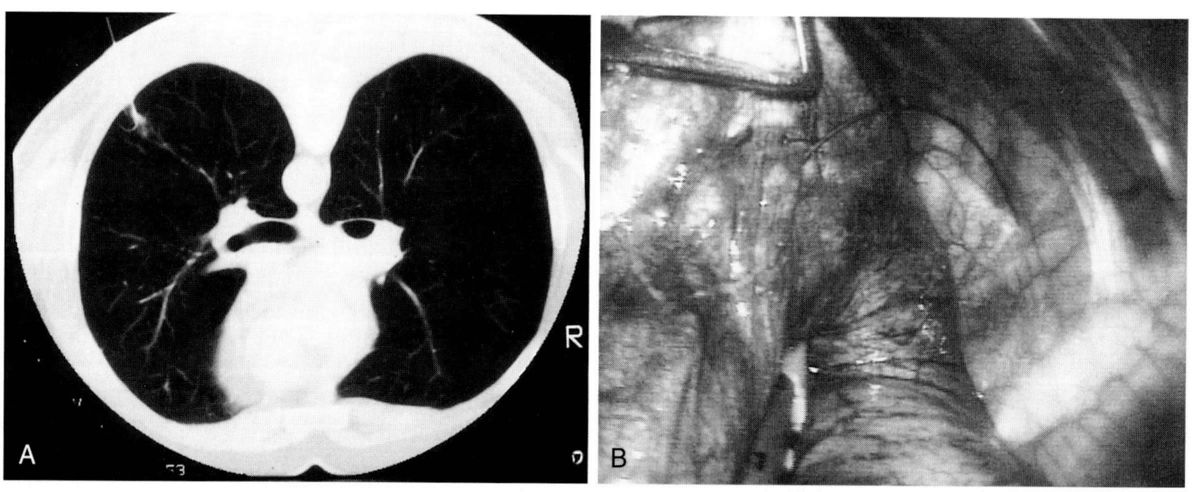

Figure 24–2. Needle localization of subcentimeter pulmonary nodule by *A*, computed tomography and *B*, thoracoscopy.

Table 24–2. Indications for Video-Assisted Thoracic Surgery (VATS) Staging of Lung Cancer

Nodal Status	
	>1 cm aortopulmonary window lymph node (levels 5, 6) >1 cm post-subcarinal lymph node (level 7), negative at mediastinoscopy >1 cm mediastinal adenopathy: not able to perform mediastinoscopy (status post tracheostomy, status post mediastinoscopy, severe cervical kyphosis)
Tumor Status	
	Rule out aortic invasion Rule out tracheal or superior vena cava invasion Rule out pleural studding or malignant pleural effusion Diagnose unknown pulmonary lesion
Metastasis (M) Status	
	Diagnose ipsilateral or contralateral synchronous pulmonary lesions
Routine	
	? VATS in all patients with negative cytology or minimal pleural effusion

is indicated before significant treatment planning can be finalized.

Although percutaneous biopsy of selective lymph nodes can be attained by CT or transbronchial biopsy, mediastinoscopy ensures the most complete staging of both unilateral and contralateral lymph nodes, helping to define Stage IIIA versus IIIB disease. Despite its low morbidity and efficacy, mediastinoscopy is limited in its ability to access the A-P window (levels 5 and 6) or the posterior subcarinal lymph nodes (level 7), and by its inability to access inferior pulmonary ligament adenopathy. Although extended mediastinoscopy, as described by Ginsberg,[12] may technically allow the surgeon to biopsy levels 5 and 6 lymph nodes, the procedure may add increased morbidity secondary to manipulation of the great vessels, especially in elderly cancer patients. At present, video-assisted mediastinoscopy provides improved optics and visibility at the time of mediastinoscopy. These advantages clearly enhance the quality of the field of dissection and provide an opportunity to teach residents; however, the technique does not add any new capabilities in terms of sampling recognized nodal stations. Finally, mediastinoscopy may be cumbersome or impossible in patients who have had a previous mediastinoscopy, or who have a tracheostomy or severe cervical kyphosis.

Thoracoscopic lymph node staging as an adjunct to mediastinoscopy for evaluation of A-P window lymph nodes has been well described and evaluated by Nakanishi.[35, 36] Thoracoscopy offers advantages over parasternal mediastinotomy in its improved visualization of the A-P window and its ability to examine the entire hemothorax. The use of thoracoscopy to sample an ipsilateral suspicious adenopathy, at levels 5 and 6, immediately before performance of thoracotomy has been prospectively studied by Ishidi[16] and Ghosn[11] and found to have 100% concordance (17 patients) and 92% concordance (27 patients), respectively. These data substantiate the use of VATS as a staging procedure that can be performed in conjunction with mediastinoscopy, or, if need be, as the primary minimally invasive staging technique.

The ability of VATS to stage mediastinal lymph nodes accurately may be particularly applicable in the setting of positive adenopathy and neoadjuvant therapy previously documented by mediastinoscopy. Results of neoadjuvant trials to date indicate that patients who have persistent malignant adenopathy after neoadjuvant therapy have a worse survival rate compared with that of patients who had complete regression of their adenopathy.[43] However, repeat mediastinoscopy carries increased morbidity and markedly decreased sensitivity. For these reasons, postneoadjuvant staging by thoracoscopy may be particularly useful. Although persistent malignant adenopathy may not contraindicate definitive resection, it may allow more accurate decisions to be made in regard to additional therapy or resection. Future prospective trials, which will better define the role of thoracoscopy in restaging patients who have completed neoadjuvant therapy, are currently being formulated.[8] In this way, patients who are complete pathologic responders could be offered surgical resection, whereas those who have residual disease could consider additional therapy.

Thoracoscopy is particularly useful in ruling out unresectable T4 invasion in primary lung cancer and T3 invasion in very high risk patients. CT scanning may indicate aortic or chest wall abutment, but it is only 50% accurate in all but the worst cases in predicting direct involvement.[14] Thoracoscopy may thus either avoid an unnecessary thoracotomy or downstage a patient to a resectable stage by showing no direct tumor spread. Thoracoscopy is also an excellent tool for identifying unsuspected pleural metastasis and for possibly avoiding an exploratory thoracotomy.

The routine use of thoracoscopy has been prospectively evaluated in five studies (Table 24–3). In these studies, thoracoscopy was used preoperatively in all patients who were clinically staged as resectable. Of a total of 596 patients, 41 (7%) were found to have unresectable disease and were thus able to avoid exploratory thoracotomy.[3, 26, 39, 47, 51] Although this may not indicate an absolute role for the *routine* use of thoracoscopy, it certainly encourages its early use in patients who have advanced disease or a likelihood of unresectability.

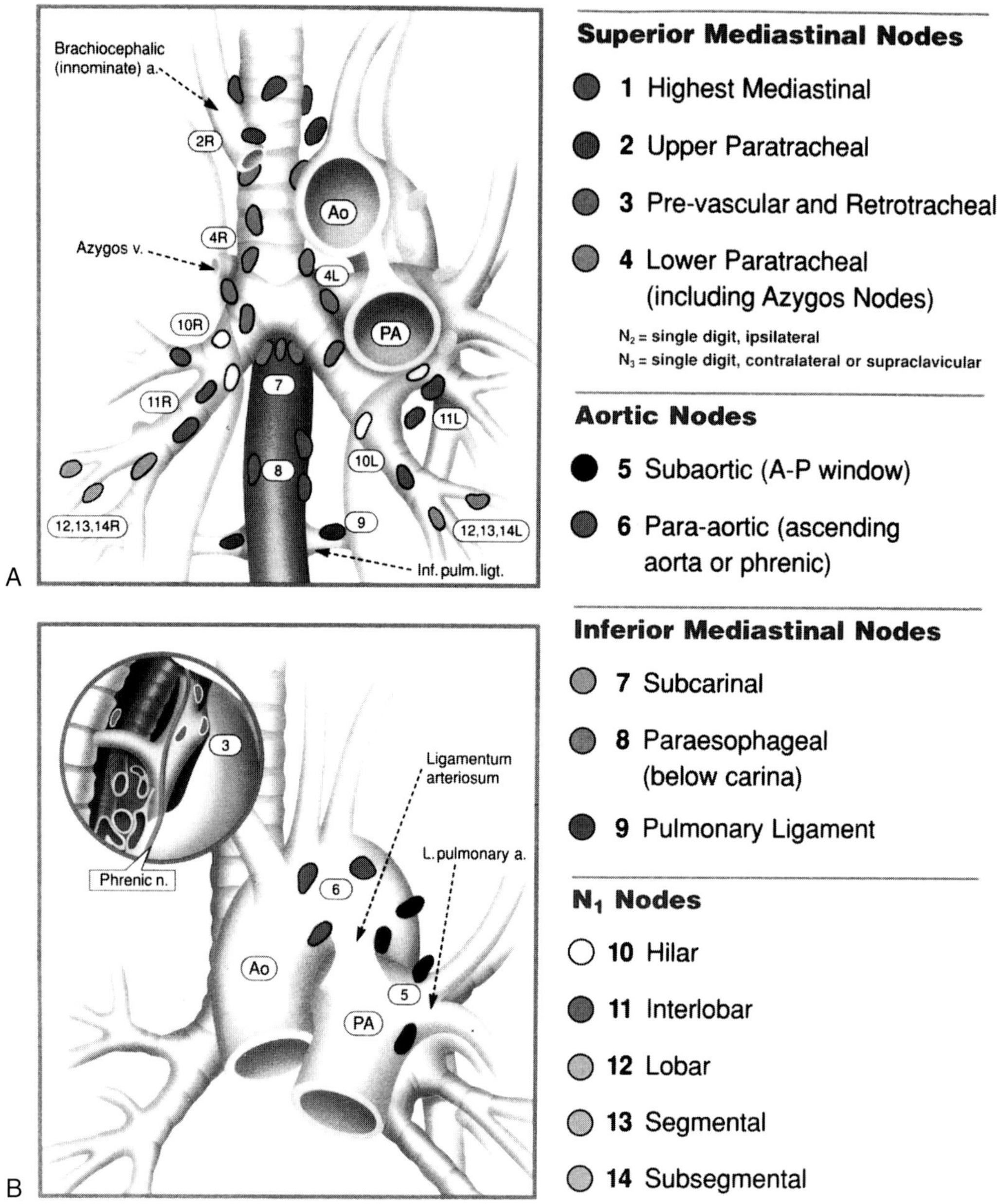

Figure 24–3. *A*, Lung cancer map showing aortopulmonary and *B*, lateral projections.

Finally, thoracoscopy may help define M stage in patients who have questionable satellite lesions in the ipsilateral lobe or lesions in the contralateral node. This allows clinical decisions to be made preoperatively regarding the treatment of these patients who have either intrapulmonary metastases or synchronous primary lung cancer.

Table 24–3. Routine Use of Video-Assisted Thoracic Surgery (VATS) Exploration in All Lung Cancer Patients Who Have Potentially Resectable Lesions

Author	No. Patients	Inoperable (%)	Institution
Asamura et al	116	4.3	National Cancer Center, Japan
Roviaro et al	286	5.7	University of Milan, Italy
Loscertales et al	151	11.9	University Virgen Macerena, Spain
Wain	43	5.0	Massachusetts General Hospital, USA
Yim	63	3.3	Chinese University of Hong Kong

Esophageal Cancer

The AJCC Staging System for esophageal carcinoma is well accepted as a guide for prognosis and as a tool for outcome comparison studies. It is also increasingly accepted as a guide for treatment options and use of multimodality therapy. As treatment options may vary according to stage, and dosing of radiation therapy may vary depending on the extent of malignant adenopathy, the importance of accurate pathologic staging of esophageal cancer has become more pronounced. The current IUAC and AJCC esophageal staging systems (Table 24–4) are based on the TNM staging system. Primary grading of a tumor is based on depth, penetration through the anatomic layers of the esophagus (T1–T3), and possible invasion of adjacent organs (T4). Nodal staging is based on the early work of Akiyama[1] and is now internationally defined by the nodal staging map (Fig. 24–4).[7] The presence and extent of malignant adenopathy have been found to be the best predictors of prognosis in patients with esophageal cancer.[9, 42] Because noninvasive methods are relatively poor predictors of malignant adenopathy, and mediastinoscopy has poor access to the majority of esophageal lymph node stations,[33] thoracoscopy may be ideally suited to define the pathologic stage of esophageal carcinoma.[20, 25, 30, 45]

The feasibility and accuracy of thoracoscopic lymph node staging in esophageal carcinoma were defined by studies at the University of Maryland[18] and subsequently validated in multi-institutional trials.[21] Thoracoscopy has been found to have a 100% positive predictive value, and, more importantly, when combined with laparoscopy it has a 93% negative predictive value.[21, 27] Currently, CT scan can be expected to be only 60% effective in predicting malignancy in enlarged lymph nodes, and is, basically, ineffective in predicting micrometastases. Similarly, endoscopic ultrasound (EUS) has a high positive predictive value (60–70%), especially when combined with endoscopic biopsy, but a low negative predictive value of malignant lymph nodes without gross enlargement.

The precise pathologic staging of lymph nodes, even when not enlarged, is important, because it can dramatically alter the therapeutic options of the patient. A patient who does not have early systemic dissemination (malignant adenopathy) may be offered primary resection and so may avoid the possible complications and morbidity of preoperative chemotherapy and radiation therapy. Additionally, in patients with proven malignant adenopathy, complete and accurate lymph node staging may allow more precise delivery of radiation therapy. Suntharalingam and associates have reported on limiting the field, and thus the potential toxicity of preoperative radiation, to a definitively staged tumor mass and malignant adenopathy rather than the entire esophagus. This approach has enabled delivery of directed radiotherapy with a lower integral dose, fewer side effects, and equivalent response rates.[22]

In addition to defining lymph node status, thoracoscopy is an excellent tool for definitively diagnosing direct invasion of the aorta or lung. Both CT and EUS are excellent predictors of tumor depth (T), but they may not accurately predict minimal T4 status. Abutment without pathologic invasion is also difficult to ascertain by noninvasive methods. Thoracoscopy can be used definitively to separate and define abutment without invasion, as well as rule in direct invasion. Exact definition of presence or absence of T4 invasion may prevent a noncurative exploratory thoracotomy or allow resection of a tumor judged to be unresectable by noninvasive staging.

Thoracoscopy staging can also be used to define pulmonary lesions that may represent early metastasis. A small pulmonary lesion may be detected on CT scan or, more recently, positron-emission tomography (PET) scan, and can be resected for diagnosis by thoracoscopy.[28] Gross

Table 24–4. Staging System for Esophageal Cancer

Definitions

Primary Tumor (T)

TX	Primary tumor cannot be assessed
T0	No evidence of primary tumor
Tis	Carcinoma in situ
T1	Tumor invades lamina propria or submucosa
T2	Tumor invades muscularis propria
T3	Tumor invades adventitia
T4	Tumor invades adjacent structures

Regional Lymph Nodes (N)

NX	Regional lymph nodes cannot be assessed
N0	No regional lymph node metastasis
N1	Regional lymph node metastasis

Distant Metastasis (M)

MX	Distant metastasis cannot be assessed
M0	No distant metastasis
M1	Distant metastasis

Tumors of the Lower Thoracic Esophagus

M1a	Metastasis in celiac lymph nodes
M1b	Other distant metastasis

Tumors of the Midthoracic Esophagus

M1a	Not applicable
*M1b	Nonregional lymph nodes, other distant metastases, or both

Tumors of the Upper Thoracic Esophaqus

M1a	Metastasis in cervical nodes
M1b	Other distant metastasis

Stage Grouping

I	T1	N0	M0
IIA	T2	N0	M0
	T3	N0	M0
IIB	T1	N1	M0
	T2	N1	M0
III	T3	N1	M0
	T4	Any N	M0
IV	Any T	Any N	M1
IVA	Any T	Any N	M1a
IVB	Any T	Any N	M1b

Modified from American Joint Committee on Cancer, Task Force on Esophagus. Mountain CF, Chairman. Carcinoma of the esophagus. *In* Beahrs OH, Meyers M (eds): Manual for Staging of Cancer. Philadelphia: JB Lippincott, 1983:61.

* For tumors of the midthoracic esophagus, use only M1b, because these tumors with metastasis in nonregional lymph nodes and those with metastasis in other distant sites have an equally poor prognosis.

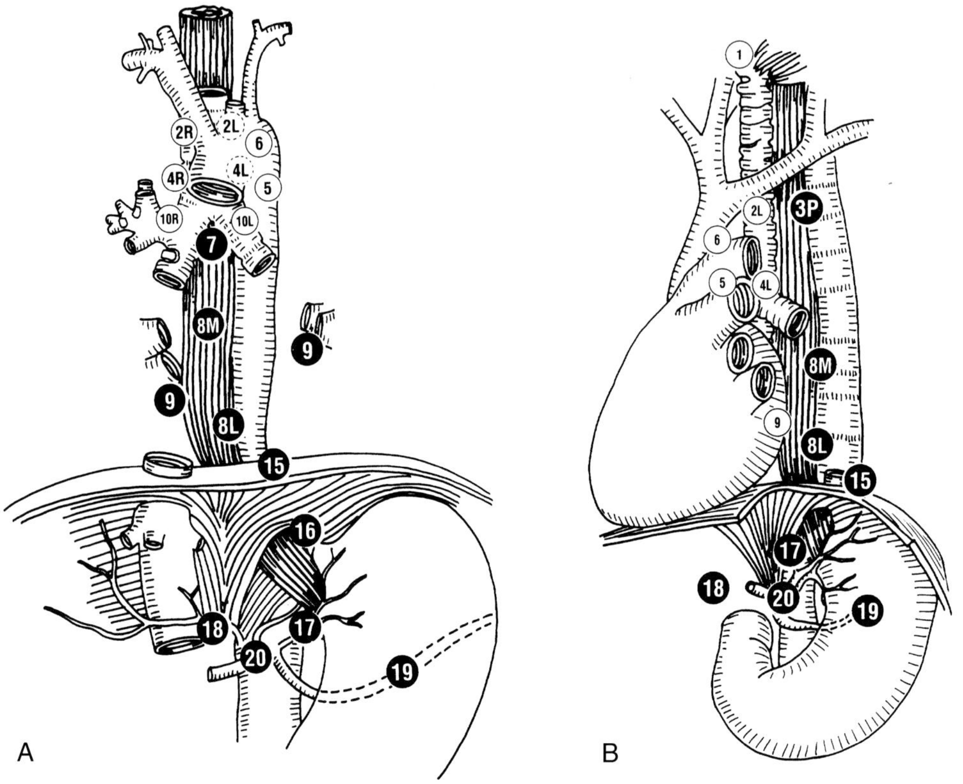

1	Supraclavicular nodes	Above suprasternal notch and clavicles
2R	Right upper paratracheal nodes	Between intersection of caudal margin of innominate artery with trachea and the apex of the lung
2L	Left upper paratracheal nodes	Between top of aortic arch and apex of the lung
● 3P	Posterior mediastinal nodes	Upper paraesophageal nodes, above tracheal bifurcation
4R	Right lower paratracheal nodes	Between intersection of caudal margin of innominate artery with trachea and cephalic border of azygos vein
4L	Left lower paratracheal nodes	Between top of aortic arch and carina
5	Aorto-pulmonary nodes	Subaortic and para-aortic nodes lateral to the ligamentum arteriosum
6	Anterior mediastinal nodes	Anterior to ascending aorta or innominate artery
● 7	Subcarinal nodes	Caudal to the carina of the trachea
● 8M	Middle paraesophageal lymph nodes	From the tracheal bifurcation to the caudal margin of the inferior pulmonary vein
● 8L	Lower paraesophageal lymph nodes	From the caudal margin of the inferior pulmonary vein to the esophagogastric junction
● 9	Pulmonary ligament nodes	Within the inferior pulmonary ligament
10R	Right tracheo-bronchial nodes	From cephalic border of azygos vein to origin of RUL bronchus
10L	Left tracheo-bronchial nodes	Between carina and LUL bronchus
● 15	Diaphragmatic nodes	Lying on the dome of the diaphragm, and adjacent to or behind its crura
● 16	Paracardial nodes	Immediately adjacent to the gastroesophageal junction
● 17	Left gastric nodes	Along the course of the left gastric artery
● 18	Common hepatic nodes	Along the course of the common hepatic artery
● 19	Splenic nodes	Along the course of the splenic artery
● 20	Celiac nodes	At the base of the celiac artery

Figure 24–4. Esophageal cancer map showing *A*, anteroposterior and *B*, lateral projections, and definitions.

pleural invasion and pleural implantation may also be diagnosed easily by thoracoscopy.

Mesothelioma

The treatment of malignant mesothelioma has historically been thought of in nihilistic terms, with virtually no long-term survivors. However, the fact that this is a pleural tumor makes it perhaps the most ideally suited to be diagnosed and staged thoracoscopically. A new staging system for malignant mesothelioma, which was proposed by the International Mesothelioma Interest Group (IMIG), has recently been agreed upon and accepted internationally (Table 24–5).[40] The most important aspects of staging early mesothelioma are definitive tissue diagnosis and thoracoscopic exploration of the pleural cavity. Progress in defining the tumor status thoracoscopically and relating it to prognosis can be directly attributed to the extensive work of Boutin.[5]

Given the nature of mesothelioma to seed incisional sites, it is important to plan a thoracoscopic approach that may be directly excised at the time of definitive resection

Table 24–5. New International Staging System for Diffuse Malignant Pleural Mesothelioma

Definitions

T1	Tumor limited to the ipsilateral parietal surface, including mediastinal and diaphragmatic pleura No involvement of the visceral pleura T1b tumor involves the ipsilateral parietal surface, including mediastinal and diaphragmatic pleura Scattered foci of tumor also involve the visceral pleura
T2	Tumor involves each of the ipsilateral pleural surfaces (i.e., parietal, mediastinal, diaphragmatic, and visceral pleura) with at least one of the following features: Involvement of diaphragmatic muscle Confluent visceral pleural tumor (including the fissures), or extension of tumor from visceral pleura into the underlying pulmonary parenchyma
T3	Describes locally advanced but potentially resectable tumor. Tumor involves all of the ipsilateral pleural surfaces (i.e., parietal, mediastinal, diaphragmatic, and visceral pleura), with at least one of the following features: Involvement of the endothoracic fascia Extension into the mediastinal fat Solitary, completely resectable focus of tumor extending into the soft tissues of the chest wall Non-transmural involvement of the pericardium
T4	Describes locally advanced, technically unresectable tumor. Tumor involving all of the ipsilateral pleural surfaces (parietal, mediastinal, diaphragmatic, and visceral pleura) with at least one of the following features: Diffuse extension or multifocal masses of tumor in the chest wall, with or without associated rib destruction Direct transdiaphragmatic extension of tumor to the peritoneum Direct extension of tumor to the contralateral pleura Direct extension of tumor to one or more mediastinal organs Direct extension of tumor into the spine Tumor extending through to the internal surface of the pericardium with or without a pericardial effusion; or tumor involving the myocardium
N	Lymph nodes
NX	Regional lymph nodes cannot be assessed
N0	No regional lymph node metastases
N1	Metastases in the ipsilateral bronchopulmonary or hilar lymph nodes
N2	Metastases in the subcarinal or ipsilateral mediastinal lymph nodes, including the ipsilateral internal mammary nodes
N3	Metastases in the contralateral internal mammary, ipsilateral, or contralateral supraclavicular lymph nodes
M	Metastases
MX	Presence of distant metastases cannot be assessed
M0	No distant metastasis
M1	Distant metastases present

Staging

Stage I	Ia	T1aN0M0
	Ib	T1bN0M0
Stage II		T2N0M0
Stage III		Any T3M0
		Any N1M0
		Any N2M0
Stage IV		Any T4
		Any N3
		Any M1

(Fig. 24–5). Complete surgical staging of mesothelioma may also include mediastinoscopy for additional nodal staging and laparoscopy to rule out transdiaphragmatic tumor extension. Clear definition and treatment of the early stages of this disease, rather than diagnosis and palliation of its advanced stages, may result in curative treatments instead of nihilistic palliation.

Other Malignancies

Thoracoscopic staging has been described in the treatment planning of recurrent squamous cell cancer of the larynx. In one study, thoracoscopy was used prospectively to evaluate three patients who had stomal recurrence before undergoing major reoperative surgery. In two of the three patients, thoracoscopy identified tumor invasion of the great vessels; these patients were spared an exploratory operation.[48] Thoracoscopy has also been described for restaging recurrent Hodgkin's disease in the chest and for defining and diagnosing unknown mediastinal masses.[38] VATS exploration of these lesions may facilitate removal of a greater quantity of tissue for diagnosis and may also allow definitive resection. The thoracoscopic approach to these lesions must be individualized, and the placement of second and third access ports should be based on thoracoscopic localization of the lesion.

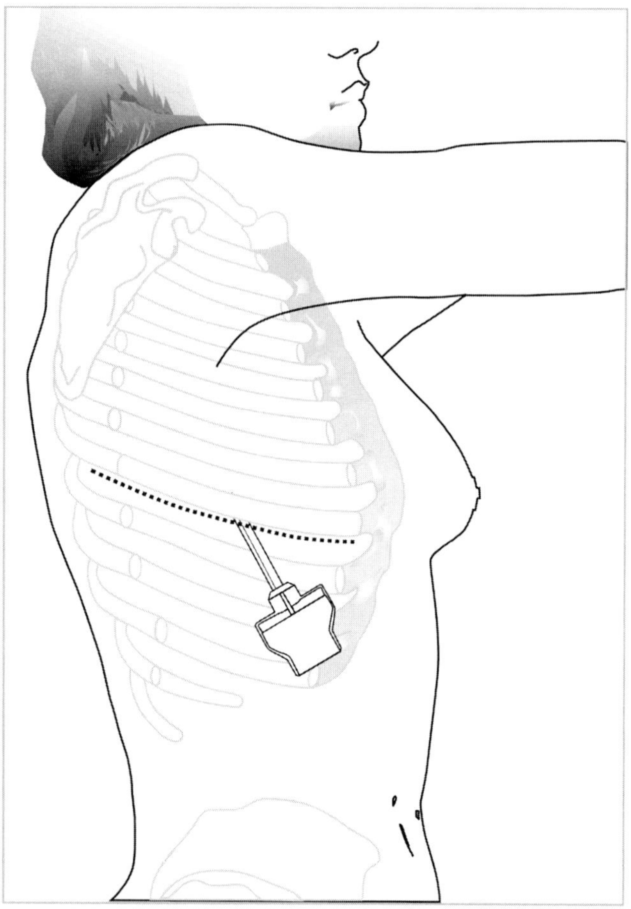

Figure 24–5. Mesothelioma setup and port placement (in seventh intercostal space).

Thoracoscopic Ultrasound

The use of ultrasound probes has been extended to intraoperative thoracoscopy.[15] Hida and associates used this technique to obtain accurate visualization of 100% of 13 malignant nodules, but they were unable to visualize three nonmalignant nodules. This technique may be useful in the future as an adjunct to endoscopic ultrasound in esophageal staging. The full potential of this evolving technology is yet to be appreciated, but it may ultimately improve our ability to detect small paryenchymal nodules and periesophageal lymph nodes.

Thoracoscopic Techniques

The techniques of thoracoscopic staging are well described[17, 19, 24] and are consistent with routine thoracoscopic techniques. In general, thoracoscopic ports should be placed along future incision sites and as anteriorly as possible to take advantage of wider rib interspaces. When staging lung carcinoma, a single thoracoscopic port should be chosen with the aid of the operating thoracoscope (Fig. 24–6) to rule out malignant pleural effusion or pleural implants. If mesothelioma is a possibility, the single port should be placed in the seventh intercostal space (ICS) so that resection may be performed if the patient should require an extrapleural pneumonectomy. The port incision can be used as a chest tube site and, if needed, additional ports can be placed in line with a potential thoracotomy incision. For more extensive staging, such as sampling

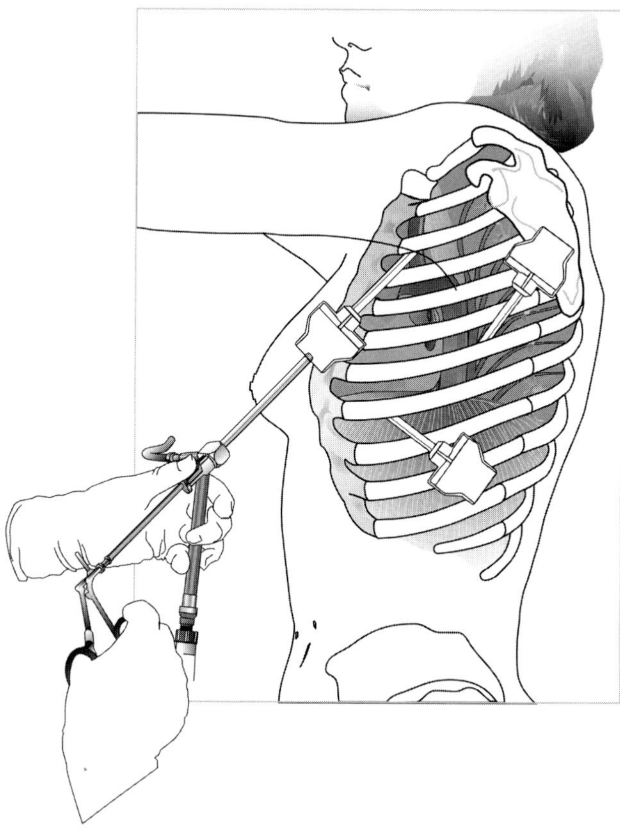

Figure 24–6. Setup for left thoracoscopic lung cancer staging.

levels 5 and 6 lymph nodes (A-P window), the classic triangular orientation of ports should be maintained. Exploration using this configuration may also allow mobilization of the lung from the aorta to rule out T4 disease. When applied to the A-P window, the "port triangle" or "baseball diamond" configuration may be placed somewhat more anteriorly and superiorly (Fig. 24–7) to improve access to the superior portion of the thorax.

The techniques of staging esophageal carcinoma are similar to those used in staging lymph nodes for lung cancer. Complete lymph node sampling is technically simpler if performed in the right hemithorax, but it may be performed from the left side if specific pathologic questions, such as A-P window adenopathy or aortic arch invasion, need to be addressed. Similarly, if nondiagnosed pulmonary lesions are present, their diagnosis can be made at the time of lymph node sampling, and this decision determines the use of the right or left hemithorax. Because esophageal dissection mandates dissection from the apex of the chest to the esophageal hiatus, it is important to have video monitors at both the head and the feet (Fig. 24–8). The angle of the camera is changed as the dissection proceeds from the thoracic inlet to the esophageal hiatus, and the orientation of the field changes to a more caudad view. Dissection proceeds more efficiently if a forward view is maintained at all times to avoid mirror orientation. In this way, viewing the superior and then the inferior monitors helps maintain orientation. The use of an operating thoracoscope is strongly encouraged, because

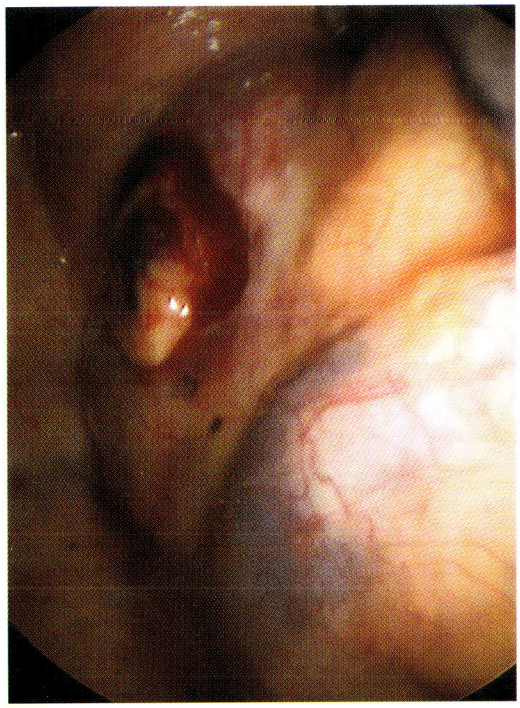

Figure 24–7. "Port triangle" or "baseball diamond" configuration applied to A-P window.

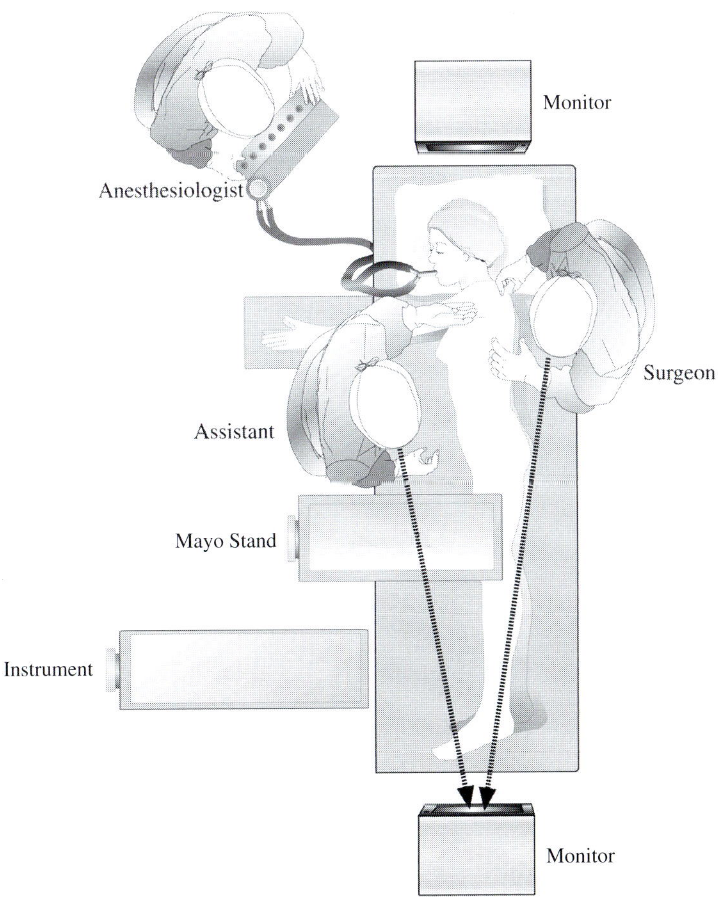

Figure 24–8. Setup for right thoracoscopic esophageal cancer staging.

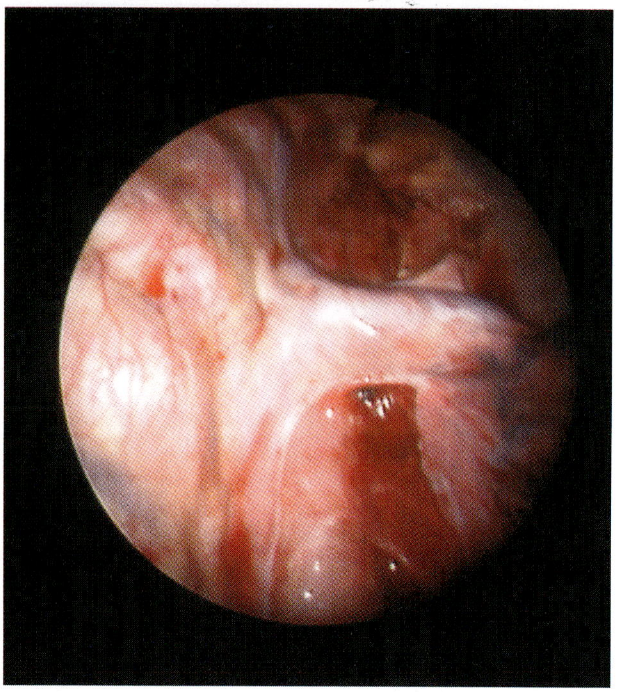

Figure 24–9. Esophageal lymph node sampling of level 2, 4, and 10 nodal stations.

this facilitates mobilization and dissection and allows another port to be used for retraction or mobilization. The use of CO_2 inflation may also facilitate decompression of the lung and improve visibility of the esophageal hiatus by depressing the diaphragm. This can be done safely with low flows and low pressures.[50] Staging of lymph nodes is best performed in a systematic fashion, with sampling of nodal stations as defined by the AJCC lymph node staging map and directed by identifying suspicious lymph nodes on preoperative CT or EUS. It is not sufficient merely to view lymph node regions that appear normal; even normal-sized nodes, which could harbor metastatic tumor deposits, should be biopsied (Fig. 24–9).

Summary

Complete and accurate staging of all thoracic malignancies is important for active treatment issues, prognosis, and comparison of outcome studies. Accurate preoperative staging may facilitate such decisions as proceeding directly to surgery, incorporating neoadjuvant therapy, or avoiding unnecessary exploratory surgery. Thoracoscopic staging has been documented as safe and effective, and it may be used as an adjunct to radiologic and endoscopic staging if final pathologic questions remain in doubt. The importance of accurate staging should not be underestimated, and proper staging to help guide treatment should be considered the standard of care.

References

1. Akiyama H, Tsurumaru M, Kawamura T, et al: Principles of surgical treatment for carcinoma of the esophagus. Ann Thorac Surg 194:438–446, 1981.
2. American Joint Committee on Cancer, Task Force on Esophagus. Mountain CF, Chairman: Carcinoma of the esophagus. *In* Beahrs OH, Meyers M (eds): Manual for Staging of Cancer. Philadelphia: JB Lippincott, 1983:61.
3. Asamura H, Nakayma H, Kondo H, et al: Thoracoscopic evaluation of histologically/cytologically proven or suspected lung cancer: A VATS exploration. Lung Cancer 16:183–190, 1997.
4. Boutin C, Astoul P, Seitz B: The role of thoracoscopy in the evaluation and management of pleural effusions. Lung 168:1113–1121, 1990.
5. Boutin C, Rey F, Gouvernet J, et al: Thoracoscopy in pleural malignant mesothelioma: A prospective study of 188 consecutive patients. Part 2: Prognosis and staging. Cancer 72:394–404, 1993.
6. Carlens E: Mediastinoscopy. Dis Chest 36:343, 1959.
7. Casson AG, Inculet RI, Zankowicz, et al: Lymph node mapping for resectable carcinoma of the esophagus. A guide for thoracic surgeons. Bristol-Myers Squibb Company, Princeton, New Jersey, 1992.
8. CALGB: A phase II trial of VATS restaging of mediastinal lymph nodes. (DeCamp M: Personal Communication, 1998.)
9. Ellis Jr FH, Watkins Jr E, Krasna MJ, et al: Staging of carcinoma of the esophagus and cardia: A comparison of different staging criteria. J Surg Oncol 52:231–235, 1993.
10. Ferguson M, Olak J, CALGB Thoracic Surgery Sub-committee: CALGB Thoracic Procedures Manual.
11. Ghosn P, Rabbat A, Gariepy G: "Staging" thoracique par videothoracoscopie: Nouvelle technique. Ann Chir 48:773–776, 1994.
12. Ginsberg RJ: Extended cervical mediastinoscopy: A single staging procedure for bronchogenic carcinoma of the left upper lobe. Thorac Cardiovasc Surg 94:673, 1987.
13. Harken DE, Black H, Clauss R, et al: A simple cervicomediastinal exploration for tissue diagnosis of intrathoracic disease. N Engl J Med 251:1041–1044, 1954.
14. Heelan R, Martini N, Westwt JW, et al: Carcinoma involving the hilum and mediastinum: computed tomographic and magnetic resonance evaluation. Radiology 156:111, 1985.
15. Hida Y, Kato H, Nishibe T, et al: Value of intraoperative intrathoracic ultrasonography during video-assisted thoracoscopic pulmonary resection. Surg Laparosc Endosc 6:472–475, 1996.
16. Ishida T, Ishii T, Yamazaki K, et al: Thoracoscopic limited resection of bronchogenic carcinoma in patients over the age of 80. Int Surg 81:237–240, 1996.
17. Krasna MJ: Introduction to thoracoscopic surgery: Indications, basic techniques and instrumentation. *In* Cuschieri A, MacFadyen BV (eds): Seminars in Laparoscopic Surgery. Philadelphia, WB Saunders 3:201–210, 1996.
18. Krasna MJ, Flowers JL, Attar S, et al: Combined thoracoscopic/laparoscopic staging of esohageal cancer. J Thorac Cardiovasc Surg 111:800–807, 1996.
19. Krasna MJ, McLaughlin JS: Efficacy and safety of thoracoscopy for diagnosis and treatment of intrathoracic disease: The University of Maryland experience. Surg Laparosc Endosc 4:182–188, 1994.
20. Krasna MJ, McLaughlin JS: Thoracoscopic lymph node staging for esophageal cancer. Ann Thor Surg 56:671–674, 1993.
21. Krasna MJ, Reed C, Jaklitsch MT, et al: Thoracoscopic staging of esophageal cancer: A prospective multiinstitutional trial. Ann Thorac Surg 60:1337–1340, 1995.
22. Krasna MJ, Sonett JR, Suntharalingam M, et al: The role of thoracoscopic staging in trimodality therapy for esophageal cancer. Proceedings of OESO, 5th World Congress, 1996.
23. Landreneau RJ, Hazelrigg SR, Ferson P: Thoracoscopic resection of 85 pulmonary lesions. Ann Thorac Surg 54:415, 1992.
24. Landreneau RJ, Mack MJ, Hazelrigg SR, et al: Video-assisted thoracic surgery: Basic technical concepts and intercostal approach strategies. Ann Thorac Surg 54:800–807, 1992.
25. LoCicero J: Laparoscopy/thoracoscopy for staging: II. Prether-

apy nodal evaluation in carcinoma of the esophagus. Semin Surg Oncol 9:56–58, 1993.
26. Loscertales J, Garcia Diaz F, Jimenez Merchan R, et al: Valoracion de la resecabilidad del cancer de pulmon mediante videotoracoscopia exploradora. Arch Bronconeumol 32:275–279, 1996.
27. Luketich JD, Schauer P, Landreneau R, et al: Minimally invasive surgical staging is superior to endoscopic ultrasound in detecting lymph node metastases in esophageal cancer. J Thorac Cardiovasc Surg 114:817–823, 1997.
28. Luketich JD, Schauer PR, Meltzer CC, et al: role of positron emission tomography in staging esophageal cancer. Ann Thorac Surg 64:765–769, 1997.
29. Mack MJ, Arnoff R, Acuft T, et al: Present role of thoracoscopy in the diagnosis and treatment of diseases of the chest. Ann Thorac Surg 54:403–408, 1992.
30. McKenna RJ: Minimally invasive surgery for pulmonary and esophageal tumor. Semin Surg Oncol 10:411–416, 1994.
31. Menzies R, Charbonneau M: Thoracoscopy for the diagnosis of pleural disease. Ann Intern Med 114:271–276, 1991.
32. Mountain CF: A new international staging system for lung cancer. Chest 89 (suppl):225S–233S, 1986.
33. Murray G, Wilcox B, Starek P: The assessment of operability of esophageal carcinoma. Ann Thorac Surg 23:393, 1977.
34. Nakanishi R, Mitsudomi T, Osaki T: Combined thoracoscopy and mediastinoscopy for the evaluation of mediastinal lymph node metastasis in left upper lobe lung cancer. J Thorac Cardiovasc Surg 35:347–349, 1994.
35. Nakanishi R, Yasumoto K: Combined thoracoscopy and mediastinoscopy for mediastinal lymph node staging of lung cancer. Int Surg 81:359–361, 1996.
36. Naruke T, Goya T, Tsuuchiya R, et al: Prognosis and survival in resected lung cancer based on the new international staging system. J Thorac Cardiovasc Surg 96:440, 1988.
37. Pearson FG: Mediastinoscopy: A method of biopsy in the superior mediastinum. J Thorac Cardiovasc Surg 49:11, 1965.
38. Rendina EA, Venuta F, DeGiacomo T, et al: Comparative merits of thoracoscopy, mediastinoscopy, and mediastinotomy for mediastinal biopsy. Ann Thorac Surg 57:992–995, 1994.
39. Roviaro GC, Varoli F, Rebuffat C, et al: Videothoracoscopic operative staging for lung cancer. Int Surg 81:252–254, 1996.
40. Rusch VW, Members of the International Mesothelioma Interest Group: A proposed new international TNM staging system for malignant pleural mesothelioma. Chest 108:1122–1128, 1995.
41. Sharma S, D'Cruz A: Thoracoscopy in the diagnosis of pleural effusion of ambiguous etiology. J Surg Oncol 48:133–135, 1991.
42. Skinner DB, Little A, Ferguson MK, et al: Selection of operation for esophageal cancer based on staging. Ann Thorac Surg 204:391–401, 1986.
43. Sugarbaker D, Herndon J, Kohnman L, et al: Results of cancer and leukemia group B protocol 8935: A multiinstitutional phase II trimodality trial for stage IIIA (N2) non–small-cell lung cancer. J Thorac Cardiovasc Surg 109:473–485, 1995.
44. Sugarbaker DJ, Jaklitsch MT, Liptay MJ: Thoracoscopic staging and surgical therapy for esophageal cancer. Chest 107(6 suppl):218S–223S, 1995.
45. Templeton PA, Krasna MJ: Use of gadolinium enhanced MRI to evaluate for airway invasion in patients with esophageal carcinoma. (Abstract). Presented at Radiological Society of North America, 1994.
46. Templeton P, Krasna MJ: Needle/wire lung nodule localization for thoracoscopic resection. Chest 104:953–954, 1993.
47. Wain JC: Video-assisted thoracoscopy and the staging of lung cancer. Ann Thorac Surg 56:776–778, 1993.
48. Wax MK, Garnett JD, Graeber G: Thoracoscopic staging of stomal recurrence. Head Neck 17:409–413, 1995.
49. Whittesey D: Prospective computed tomographic scanning in the staging of bronchogenic cancer. J Thorac Cardiovasc Surg 95:876, 1988.
50. Wolfer RD, Krasna MJ, Hasnain JU, et al: Hemodynamic effects of carbon dioxide insufflation during thoracoscopy. Ann Thorac Surg 58:404–408, 1994.
51. Yim APC: Routine video-assisted thoracoscopy prior to thoracotomy. Chest 109:1099–1100, 1996.

COMMENTARY

Manson Fok

This is a thoughtful discussion of the role of thoracoscopic staging in intrathoracic malignancies. My concern and reservation about using this procedure for esophageal cancer is that significant mobilization and dissection of the mediastinum is required to access the T-staging of the tumor properly, as well as to achieve precise biopsy of its various lymph nodes from cranial to caudal regions. The procedure itself, therefore, may have inherent risks of causing inadvertent bleeding or mediastinal injuries to vital organs, which would affect subsequent definitive treatment. After such extensive mediastinal exploration, subsequent resection of the tumor would be difficult because of adhesions, especially if resection by thoracoscopy were contemplated. Risk of injury to other structures, such as the recurrent laryngeal nerve, would also be increased. Although the information yielded by thoracoscopic staging is important and perhaps highly accurate, its role is chiefly to establish accurate data for selecting patients to participate in clinical trials of preoperative adjuvant therapies. The decision to perform resection remains multifactorial, and resection for palliation is still widely accepted. This often allows good candidates who have borderline resectability to be given the benefit of the doubt, because currently available alternative, nonsurgical therapies for the treatment of this disease are insufficient.

Chapter 25

Mediastinal Cysts

Mitchell J. Magee, Stephen R. Hazelrigg, and Theresa M. Boley

The first case report of a mediastinal cyst (bronchogenic cyst) was published by Meyer in 1859.[16] Overall, mediastinal cysts are uncommon, accounting for approximately 10% of all radiographically detected mediastinal masses.[23] Mediastinal cystic lesions may arise from numerous sources, including lymphangiomas (cystic hygromas), meningoceles, thymic cysts, parathyroid cysts, pericardial cysts, pancreatic cysts, thoracic duct cysts, hydatid cysts, teratomatous cysts, and foregut cysts (bronchogenic, esophageal, and neurenteric). Mediastinal cysts are reported to represent 18 to 25% of all primary mediastinal mass lesions. Bronchogenic cysts and pericardial cysts are the most common types.[5, 6, 7, 11, 21]

The mediastinum is most frequently divided into three compartments: anterior (or anterosuperior), middle, and posterior. Cysts are less commonly found in the anterior mediastinum when compared with the other two mediastinal compartments. Of all anterior mediastinal masses, cysts constitute only 7%, and they often arise from the cervical region, usually from substernal thyroid goiters. Thyroid cysts can be identified as such by iodine enhancement, and their management is dictated more by the solid thyroid component than the presence of a cyst.[1, 21] These will not be discussed further in this review. Primary cysts are the most common lesion found in the middle mediastinum and represent 60% of all masses in this compartment. Middle mediastinal cysts are usually bronchogenic or pericardial.[3, 5, 6, 7, 21] Cysts represent the second most common posterior mediastinal mass, with foregut cysts predominating.[5, 7, 21] Foregut cysts include bronchogenic, esophageal, and neurenteric cysts, and are collectively more common in children than adults. Foregut cysts constitute approximately 10% of all pediatric mediastinal masses.[14]

Although malignant transformation of mediastinal cysts has been reported, it is rare. The histopathologic types of the few reported cases of malignancy include adenocarcinoma, squamous cell carcinoma, leiomyosarcoma, and large cell anaplastic carcinoma.[11]

Types of Mediastinal Cysts

The most common cystic lesions of the mediastinum are identified by their origin and grouped for discussion below in order of their frequency of occurrence.[23] The unique features of each of these histologic types of cysts will be discussed, followed by a more uniform proposed approach to management.

Bronchogenic Cysts

Bronchogenic cysts account for 10 to 15% of all primary mediastinal masses,[21] and are most commonly found in the middle or posterior mediastinum, but they may occur in any of the mediastinal compartments.[7, 23] Bronchogenic cysts arise from abnormal budding of the bronchial tree.[14, 23] Bronchogenic cysts appear radiographically as round or oval masses, molding themselves to surrounding structures.[23] They are uniformly dense and may contain a rim of calcification. Grossly, they may be unilocular, septated, or multiple; they have thin fibrous walls and are filled with milky mucoid or gelatinous material. Microscopically, bronchogenic cysts are lined with a ciliated pseudostratified columnar mucus-secreting epithelium.[14, 23] Smooth muscle or cartilage may be seen within the fibrous cyst wall in 70 to 80%.[23] There are rare reports of associated leiomyosarcoma or adenocarcinoma.[23] Mediastinal bronchogenic cysts arise early in gestation and usually do not communicate with the tracheal bronchial tree.[7, 14, 19, 23] Bronchogenic cysts are located more peripherally within the lung parenchyma, arise later during gestation, and often have a patent bronchial communication.[14]

Bronchogenic cysts are seen over a wide age range, from childhood to middle adulthood, but occur most often in the first three decades of life.[6, 23] Most reported bronchogenic cysts have been in the pediatric age group, in which they are often seen as life-threatening emergencies, with airway obstruction resulting in atelectasis, air trapping, and respiratory distress.[2, 16] Infection superimposed on fever is the most frequent mode of presentation in pediatric cases beyond infancy.[14] The majority of bronchogenic cysts in older children and adults were previously thought to be asymptomatic.[23] More recent reports show that the majority of bronchogenic cysts in adults are eventually symptomatic.[8] Acute inflammatory changes and ulcerations of the cyst wall may develop, with compression of adjacent mediastinal structures. Dense adhesions to adjacent organs may complicate surgical excision.[8] One reported series identified the majority (67%) of mediastinal bronchogenic cysts as either symptomatic or complicated at the time of surgical extirpation. The majority of patients had multiple, progressive symptoms. Common symptoms included chest pain (61%), cough, dyspnea, and fever.[21] Standard posteroanterior (PA) and lateral chest radiographs usually adequately demonstrate the location of the cyst, its size, density, and contours, as well as its relationship to adjacent mediastinal structures.[6] Computed tomography (CT) scan has been proposed as the single most important diagnostic procedure for carinal bronchogenic cyst, and, with added contrast, it should confirm the nonvascular nature of the mass. Other diagnostic measures, such as esophagography, sonography, and echocardiography, can be helpful but are usually unnecessary.[6, 8]

Pericardial Cysts

Pericardial cysts are uncommon, benign, developmental anomalies that represent 7% of all mediastinal masses, and may be found in approximately 1 in 100,000 persons.[1, 4, 13, 18]

They result from failure of one or more fetal lacunae to coalesce into the pericardial coelom.[9] The cyst wall is composed of connective tissue, with collagen and elastic fibers that are lined with a single layer of mesothelial cells. Lymphocytes, plasma cells, and calcifications can be seen. They commonly appear multilocular, but most are unilocular and contain clear, water-like fluid.[1, 4, 9] Cysts that communicate with the pericardial space are more properly termed true pericardial diverticula.[9, 23] There have been no reports of malignant change.[23]

Pericardial cysts are typically discovered as an incidental finding on a routine chest radiograph, appearing as a round, discrete mass abutting both the diaphragm and the anterior chest wall along the heart border (Fig. 25–1).[1, 4, 9, 23] Fifty to 70% of cysts are found in the right cardiophrenic angle, approximately 25% are along the left heart border, and the remainder are found more superiorly in the anterior or posterior mediastinum.[1, 4, 23] Although pericardial cysts are considered a congenital anomaly, most patients present in middle adult life without any symptoms or physical findings.[1, 4, 9] As many as one third may have associated symptoms, most commonly chest pain, dyspnea, or cough.[1, 9] These cysts usually remain unchanged in size or slowly enlarge over a period of many years. Rare reported complications include torsion of the cyst; sudden death after a stress test; atrial fibrillation treated effectively by removal of the cyst; and spontaneous hemorrhage into the cyst, resulting in cardiac tamponade.[4] Although plain chest radiographs are usually sufficient for diagnosis, echocardiogram and thoracic CT scan may be helpful in confirming the cyst (Fig. 25–2).[1, 9] The differential diagnosis includes Morgagni's foramen, diaphragmatic hernia, enlarged pericardial fat pad, diaphragmatic tumors, cardiac tumors, pleural and pulmonary masses, or other mediastinal masses.[1, 4]

Enteric Cysts

Enteric cysts arise from cellular rests of the developing foregut. They are lined with mucosal epithelium and usually secrete squamous, columnar, or gastric mucus. A variably thick fibromuscular wall often consists of two layers of smooth muscle The presence of parietal cells may rarely result in acid secretion with erosion of the cyst wall and perforation. Malignant transformation has not been reported.[16, 23] These cysts usually present in children as a rounded or irregularly shaped posterior mediastinal mass, which may be uniform or loculated. Simple mediastinal enteric cysts tend to be larger and more posterior than bronchogenic cysts. They may be associated with a variety of symptoms depending on their composition. The presence of concomitant vertebral anomalies, such as hemivertebra or spina bifida anomalies, necessitates evaluation for an intraspinal mass. Of neurenteric cysts located within the mediastinum, 90% are located posteriorly, with approximately two thirds on the right side superior to the tracheal carina.[14, 23]

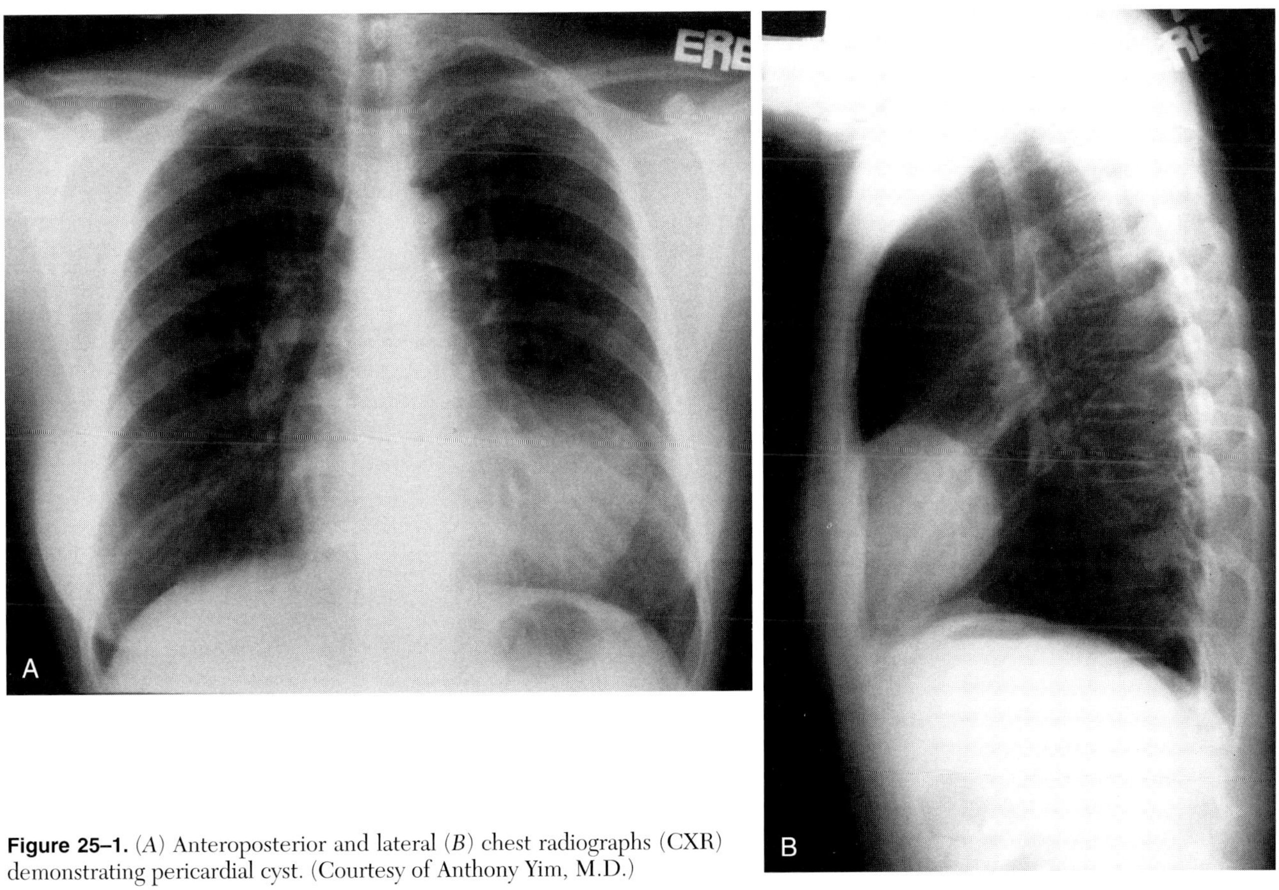

Figure 25–1. (*A*) Anteroposterior and lateral (*B*) chest radiographs (CXR) demonstrating pericardial cyst. (Courtesy of Anthony Yim, M.D.)

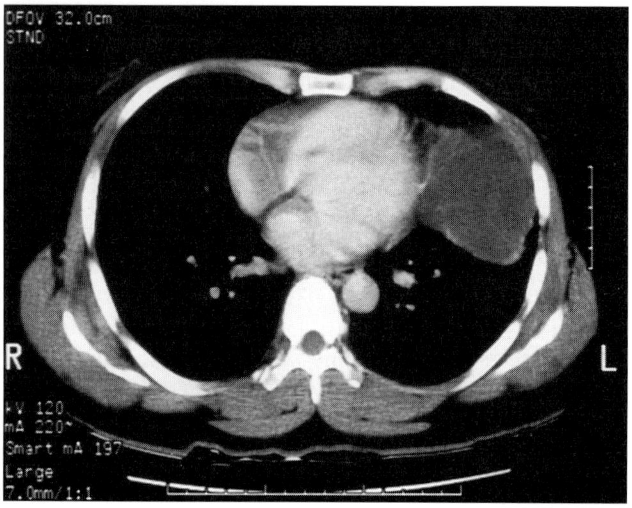

Figure 25–2. CT scan demonstrating pericardial cyst. (Courtesy of Anthony Yim, M.D.)

Thymic Cysts

Thymic cysts represent only 1% of all mediastinal tumors and 5% of all mediastinal cysts.[15, 20] True thymic cysts are congenital lesions derived from embryonal thymic tissue and account for 78% of all cysts of the thymus. Acquired thymic cysts have been recognized to coexist in patients with mediastinal Hodgkin's disease and in patients having undergone previous thoracic surgery. Thymic cysts have a smooth fibrous capsule and may be multilocular, with contents varying from clear and watery to turbid or hemorrhagic. An inconstant epithelial lining may be squamous, cuboidal, columnar, or a mixture, and many cysts contain only degenerative debris without an epithelial lining. The presence of cholesterol granulomas is generally unique to thymic cysts and an unusual finding in other mediastinal cystic lesions. Malignant degeneration has been reported but is extremely rare. Thymic cysts usually present in the second to fifth decades of life as an asymptomatic, smooth, uniformly dense, circumscribed mass in the anterosuperior mediastinum.[15, 20, 23]

Parathyroid Cysts

Parathyroid cysts are rare. They are usually located in the neck, with only 10% located in the mediastinum. Only 38 mediastinal parathyroid cysts have been reported in the world literature. The thymus and inferior parathyroid glands are both derived from the third pharyngeal pouch; therefore, thymic elements may be found in the wall of parathyroid cysts. The cysts usually present as an asymptomatic mass in the fourth to seventh decades of life. Hormonally functional parathyroid cysts probably result from cystic degeneration of a hyperfunctioning adenoma.[7, 17]

Treatment

The options available for treatment of patients who have mediastinal cysts include observation, percutaneous or transbronchial fine needle aspiration, mediastinoscopy for aspiration or biopsy, and resection by mediastinoscopy, thoracoscopy, or thoracotomy. Swanson and associates reported the first successful surgical treatment of a mediastinal cyst in 1928. The cyst was aspirated and the cavity ablated by sclerosis with formaldehyde and Dakin's solution. This technique has not been consistently successful.[3, 10]

The natural history of incidentally found asymptomatic mediastinal cysts is not known. If the diagnosis is certain based on diagnostic studies and the patient is an asymptomatic adult, observation may be appropriate, particularly if operative risks are increased by comorbid disease. Serial radiographic follow-up with intervention only for suspected malignancy, symptoms, or associated infection, compression, or enlargement has been proposed by some.[10, 11, 22] Cysts in children should probably be removed when they are identified, because they do not regress spontaneously and they occupy space needed for normal growth and development. The arguments favoring early surgical intervention in adults include the small risk of malignant degeneration, uncertainty in diagnosis, the unknown risk of developing future symptoms or complications, and the risk of increased surgical complications related to growth or scarring when future signs or symptoms necessitate surgical intervention.

The utility of percutaneous, transbronchial, or mediastinoscopic needle aspiration is limited. Needle aspiration alone allows decompression of the cyst and examination of its contents for evidence of malignancy, but this procedure is associated with an ill-defined risk of recurrence.[19] Aspiration of the cyst followed by injection of a sclerosant, such as tetracycline, hypertonic saline, or ethanol, to destroy the epithelial lining may decrease but not eliminate the risk of recurrence seen with aspiration alone. This technique is contraindicated when an air-fluid level within the cyst suggests communication with the airway. Pericardial cysts have been reportedly treated effectively by percutaneous aspiration and cyst injection under fluoroscopic guidance with no evidence of recurrence of the cysts on 3-year follow-up. For cysts adjacent to the proximal tracheal bronchial tree, mediastinoscopy may allow partial, or, rarely, complete, removal of the cyst wall, allowing more complete histologic evaluation.

Mediastinal cysts often represent ideal lesions for resection by minimally invasive techniques. Surgical excision offers the advantages of complete and definitive treatment, elimination of the mediastinal mass and prevention of any potential complications, relief of symptoms when present, and histologic evaluation.[1] Video-assisted thoracoscopic surgery offers a safe and effective approach to the surgical management of mediastinal cysts. Standard general anesthesia with selected one-lung ventilation is performed, and the patient is placed in a full lateral decubitus position. Tilting the table so that the patient is placed a more prone position for posterior mediastinal cysts, and in the opposite direction toward a more supine position for anterior lesions, may improve exposure. Similarly, the Trendelenburg position may be useful for relatively caudal masses, and reverse Trendelenburg for superior mediastinal cysts. A 10-mm 0-degree rigid thoracoscope is placed through the fourth or fifth intercostal space along the posterior axillary line. Following collapse of the ipsilateral lung and initial exploration, instruments—usually endoscopic grasping forceps and reticulating endoscopic scis-

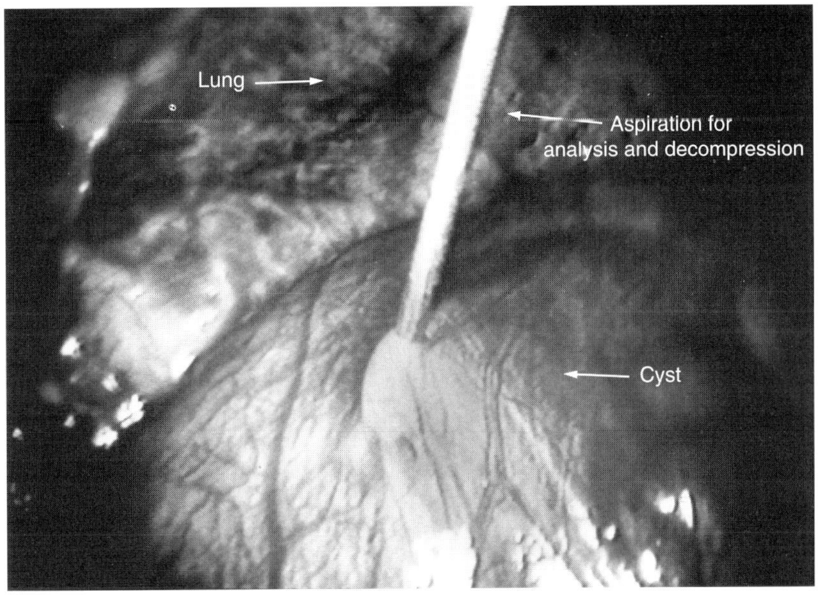

Figure 25–3. Aspiration of pericardial cyst. (Courtesy of Anthony Yim, M.D.)

sors—are introduced through the second or third intercostal space in the posterior axillary line, and through the fifth or sixth intercostal space in the anterior axillary line. A triangle is thus created with the thoracoport sites as the corners and the cyst projected near the center. The parietal pleura is incised and dissected from the surface of the cyst. Under thoracoscopic visual guidance, percutaneous aspiration of the cyst contents allows for decompression and ease of manipulation of the cyst for resection and eventual removal through a port site.[24] Aspirated fluid may be sent for culture or cytology if clinically indicated (Fig. 25–3). A stab incision at the site of the percutaneous aspiration may be used to introduce forceps to grasp and maneuver the cyst during dissection; this frees one of the thoracoport sites for a retractor, if necessary. Using blunt and sharp dissection, the cyst is separated from the pleura, adjacent surrounding mediastinal structures, or pericardium. The phrenic nerve must be clearly identified and spared from injury (Fig. 25–4). Complete removal of the cyst can be achieved in most patients. Tissue planes are usually well preserved and distinct, making dissection straightforward for benign lesions. Ill-defined tissue planes, suggesting invasion and possible malignancy, warrant consideration of open resection.[24]

Total excision is the primary aim, and every effort should be made to remove the entire cyst to prevent recurrence. However, complete excision of cysts that are intractably adherent to adjacent vital structures is technically difficult and generally not advisable. When the cyst cannot be removed completely, partial excision with cautery destruction of the epithelial mucosal lining is an acceptable alternative.[7, 8, 9, 12, 19]

Operative time generally does not exceed 1 hour, and the endotracheal tube is routinely removed in the operat-

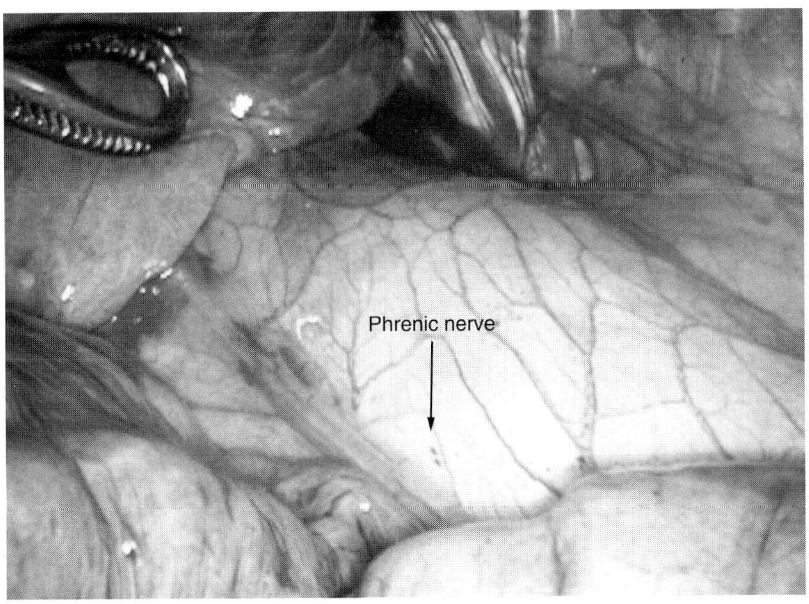

Figure 25–4. The phrenic nerve must be carefully identified and preserved.

ing room. Intraoperative intercostal nerve blocks using bupivacaine at the thoracoport sites may help facilitate postoperative pain control. Unless the lung is inadvertently injured, patients can be managed without a chest tube. Our standard practice has been to place a small tube through one of the partially closed thoracoport sites for draining any residual fluid, blood, or air. This is removed within several hours so that recovery and hospital discharge are not delayed. Uncomplicated procedures require less than 24 hours in hospital. Recurrence has not been reported with follow-up limited to 6 months.

References

1. Abad C, Rey A, Feijóo J: Pericardial cyst surgical resection in two symptomatic cases. J Cardiovasc Surg 37:199–202, 1996.
2. Bailey PV, Tracy T, Connors RH, et al: Congenital bronchopulmonary malformations: Diagnostic and therapeutic considerations. J Thorac Cardiovasc Surg 99:597–603, 1990.
3. Bolton JWR, Shahian DM: Asymptomatic bronchogenic cysts: What is the best management? Ann Thorac Surg 53:1134–1137, 1992.
4. Borges AC, Gellert K, Dietel M: Acute right-sided heart failure due to hemorrhage into a pericardial cyst. Ann Thorac Surg 63:845–847, 1997.
5. Cohen AJ, Thompson L, Edwards F, et al: Primary cysts and tumors of the mediastinum. Ann Thorac Surg 51:378–386, 1991.
6. Davis RD, Oldham HN, Sabiston DC: Primary cysts and neoplasms of the mediastinum: Recent changes in clinical presentation, methods of diagnosis, management, and results. Ann Thorac Surg 44:229–237, 1987.
7. Downey RJ, Cerfolio RJ, Deschamps C, et al: Mediastinal parathyroid cysts. Mayo Clin Proc 70:946–950, 1995.
8. Estrera AS, Landay MJ, Pass LJ: Mediastinal carinal bronchogenic cyst: Is its mere presence an indication for surgical excision? South Med J 80:1523–1526, 1987.
9. Ferguson M: Thoracoscopic management of pericardial disease. Semin Thorac Cardiovasc Surg 5:310–315, 1993.
10. Ginsberg RJ, Atkins RW, Paulson DL: A bronchogenic cyst successfully treated by mediastinoscopy. Ann Thorac Surg 13:266–268, 1972.
11. Gotti G, Haid MM, Volteranni L, et al: Letter to the Editor: Unusual malignancy in the wall of a mediastinal cyst. J Thorac Cardiovasc Surg 106:1233, 1234, 1993.
12. Gourin A, Garzon A, Rosen Y, et al: Bronchogenic cysts: Broad spectrum of presentation. NY State J Med 76:714–719, 1976.
13. Gürlek A, Dagalp AZ, Özyurda Ü: A case of multiple pericardial hydatid cysts. Int J Cardiol 36:366–368, 1992.
14. Haddon MJ, Bowen A: Bronchopulmonary and neurenteric forms of foregut anomalies. Radiol Clin North Am 29:241–254, 1991.
15. Klaveren RJ, Festen J, Lacquet LK, et al: Letter to the Editor: A symptomatic thymic cyst in the middle mediastinum. J Thorac Cardiovasc Surg 107:1169–1171, 1994.
16. Koonz AR: Congenital cysts of the lung. Bull Johns Hopkins Hosp 37:340–361, 1925.
17. Landau O, Chamberlain DW, Kennedy RS, et al: Mediastinal parathyroid cysts. Ann Thorac Surg 63:951–953, 1997.
18. LeRoux BT: Pericardial coelomic cysts. Thorax 14:27–35, 1959.
19. Miller DC, Walter JP, Guthaner DF, et al: Recurrent mediastinal bronchogenic cyst: Cause of bronchial obstruction and compression of superior vena cava and pulmonary artery. Chest 74:218–220, 1978.
20. Sirivella S, Gielchinsky I, Parsonnet V: Mediastinal thymic cysts: A report of three cases. J Thorac Cardiovasc Surg 110:1771, 1772, 1995.
21. St.-Georges R, Deslauriers J, Duranceau A, et al: Clinical spectrum of bronchogenic cysts of the mediastinum and lung in the adult. Ann Thorac Surg 52:6–13, 1991.
22. Terry PB: William Tell and technology. Chest 88:486, 487, 1985.
23. Wick MR: Mediastinal cysts and intrathoracic thyroid tumors. Semin Diagn Pathol 7:285–294, 1990.
24. Yim APC: Video-assisted thoracoscopic resection of anterior mediastinal masses. Int Surg 81:350–353, 1996.

COMMENTARY

Anthony P. C. Yim

In experienced hands, video-assisted thoracic surgery (VATS) provides a viable approach to resection of a variety of benign mediastinal cysts. As the authors point out, thoracoscope-guided needle aspiration for decompressing a cyst (if the content is thin) may facilitate subsequent dissection and mobilization. Preservation of the phrenic nerve is of paramount importance. Placement of a fiberoptic scope in the esophagus helps to identify this structure in a difficult dissection. For most benign cysts, the surrounding tissue plane is generally well preserved, so gentle blunt dissection with a dental pledget generally facilitates mobilization. On the other hand, suspicion of tissue-plane invasion calls for conversion to an open technique for completing the resection. Planned conversion should never be regarded as a defeat but rather a display of good clinical judgment.

Chapter 26

Transcervical Approach to the Thymus

Hon Chi Suen and Joel D. Cooper

History of Transcervical Thymectomy

Thymectomy was originally performed via the transcervical route, mainly for patients with thyrotoxicosis. In 1912, Sauerbruch[22] performed a transcervical thymectomy on a patient who had myasthenia gravis and severe hyperthyroidism, with subsequent improvement of myasthenic symptoms. Von Haberer[24] reported 40 transcervical thymectomies in 1917, only one of which was performed for myasthenia gravis. The symptoms of myasthenia gravis also improved in this patient after transcervical thymectomy. Blalock[2] was the first surgeon to perform a successful thymectomy in a young woman who had a thymoma and severe myasthenia gravis. He used the partial sternotomy approach, splitting the sternum from the suprasternal notch to the right third intercostal space. Because of the improvement of myasthenic symptoms, he was encouraged to perform thymectomy for myasthenia gravis alone. By 1944, he had accumulated experience from 20 cases of thymectomy for myasthenia gravis, and he emphasized that the best results were obtained in patients who had illness of short duration and who underwent complete thymectomy.[3] In 1955, Keynes[13] reported a series of 260 thymectomies using the median sternotomy approach. The transcervical approach was reintroduced by Akakura,[1] Crile,[8] and Carlens[6] in the 1960s. This approach was associated with less surgical morbidity, but it did not always result in complete thymectomy. In 1984, Henze[10] reported that removal of residual thymic tissue in patients who had persistent myasthenic symptoms after transcervical thymectomy could result in improvement of symptoms. Cooper,[7] in 1988, described an improved technique of transcervical thymectomy that provided better exposure and facilitated complete thymectomy.

Indications for Transcervical Thymectomy

We perform transcervical thymectomy primarily for patients who have myasthenia gravis unaccompanied by a thymoma. In patients who have a thymoma, the transsternal approach is the preferred method. Occasionally, in elderly or frail patients who have a stage I thymoma on computed tomography (CT) scan, the transcervical route is used. Transcervical thymectomy has also been used successfully to remove ectopic intrathymic hyperfunctional parathyroid tumors.[23]

Technique of Transcervical Thymectomy

The technique of transcervical thymectomy has changed little since it was described by Cooper in 1988.[7] Preoperatively, the patient is informed of the possible need for median sternotomy if an unsuspected thymoma is found, or if the surgeon is concerned about the exposure because of the patient's habitus. However, conversion to the transsternal approach has been required in fewer than 1% of cases.

The patient is positioned supine with the vertex of the head resting at the very top end of the operating table. An inflatable bag is placed underneath the shoulders to extend the neck. An intravenous line is placed in a right forearm vein, because the venous return from the right brachiocephalic vein is not hindered by the occasional compression of the innominate vein during dissection. On the left arm, a blood pressure cuff is placed, because the innominate artery is occasionally compressed during dissection, making blood pressure recording from the right arm unreliable. An arterial line is not used routinely. An endotracheal tube is brought out through the left corner of the mouth and angled down toward the table. Eye protectors are placed.

The neck and the anterior chest are prepared with antiseptic solution, and a 4-cm curved collar incision is made between the sternomastoid muscles, with the midpoint of the incision about 2 cm above the sternal notch. Subplatysmal skin flaps are raised down to the sternal notch and up to the level of the thyroid cartilage. The strap muscles are separated in the midline and the cleidocleido ligament is incised down to the sternal notch to improve exposure. The upper poles of the thymus gland are found lying immediately superficial to the inferior thyroid veins and subjacent to the posterior surface of the strap muscles. The thymic gland is surrounded by an outer capsule, and within this capsule, the gland is removed by dissection from surrounding areolar tissue. The left superior pole is mobilized first. A "peanut" dissector is very helpful in developing the correct tissue plane during this part of the procedure. The thyrothymic ligament at the highest point of the superior pole is divided between ligatures, with the ligature on the superior pole of the thymus left long for traction. The right upper pole is similarly dissected free, and a ligature is left long for traction on the most superior aspect.

The two upper poles usually come together in the midline just above the sternal notch, anterior to the innominate vein. On occasion, one pole (usually the left) may pass posterior to the innominate vein, whereas the other pole is in the usual position, superficial to the vein. When the upper poles have been fully mobilized and found to pass anterior to the innominate vein, the surgeon's index finger is passed between the sternum (posterior to the divided cleidocleido ligament) and the thymus gland to separate the anterior surface of the thymus gland bluntly from the sternum. The superior poles are then retracted forward, and the posterior portions of the gland are dissected free down to the innominate vein. The venous drainage pattern is highly variable but usually consists of two midline veins draining into the innominate vein. They are ligated and divided under direct vision. However, additional venous drainage to the left internal mammary vein and the superior vena cava is common.

One of the authors, Dr. Cooper, developed a special, narrow, right-angle retractor (Cooper thymectomy retractor, Pilling Co., Fort Washington, PA) (Fig. 26–1), which is passed behind the sternal notch and attached to the Poly-Tract apparatus for upward traction of the sternum. The surgeon and the surgical assistant simultaneously lift up the retractor to partially suspend the patient from the manubrium. Another assistant then tightens the screw on the retractor with a wrench. The bag underneath the shoulders is then deflated, allowing the shoulders and the thoracic spine (and, thus, the mediastinum) to fall backward in relation to the sternum, improving access through the thoracic inlet. With the use of a headlight and magnification loupes, the anterior mediastinum can be well visualized, with the surgeon seated on a stool at the head of the table (Fig. 26–2). The transcervical approach could be supplemented by the use of a telescope and video-assisted thoracic surgery (VATS) instruments through the cervical incision, if desired, but this has not been necessary in our experience except to demonstrate the procedure to observers.

After division of the thymic veins, dissection can be carried along the posterior surface of the thymus gland, anterior to the innominate vein. The gland is separated from the pericardium by sharp dissection over the anterior surface of the ascending aorta. When there is dense adhesion, a piece of pericardium may be removed in continuity with the gland.

Each of the lower poles is then dissected free, using both sharp and blunt dissection. Usually, the mediastinal pleura can be separated from the thymus gland by blunt dissection, but, if adherent, a portion of the pleura can be taken with the thymus gland by sharp dissection. Great care should be taken not to injure the phrenic nerves. We have found it advantageous to dissect the right lower pole first, followed by the posterior surface of the gland, and, finally, the left lower pole. Particular care is needed in dissecting the aortopulmonary window, often the site of additional lobes or extension of the gland. Meticulous dissection must be performed to ensure a complete thymectomy but yet avoid injury to the phrenic nerves. Figures 26–3 and 26–4 are examples of operative specimens obtained with the transcervical approach.

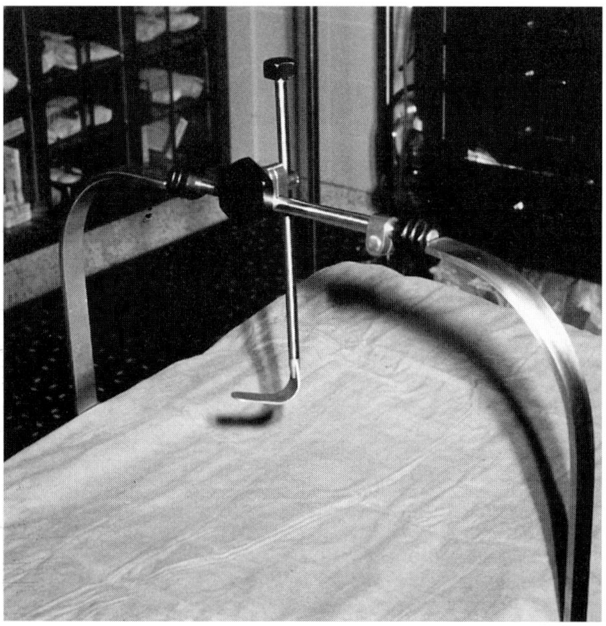

Figure 26–1. Right-angle retractor that is positioned behind the manubrium to place upward traction on the sternum. (From Cooper JD, Al-Jilaihawa AN, Pearson FG, et al: An improved technique to facilitate transcervical thymectomy for myasthenia gravis. Ann Thorac Surg 45:243, 1988, with permission.)

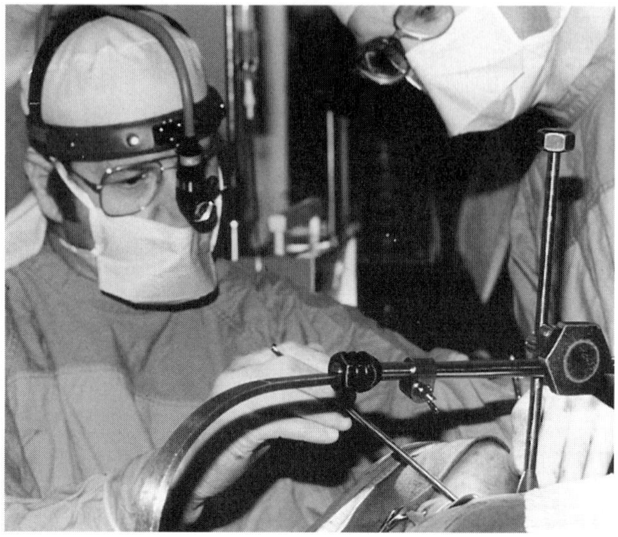

Figure 26–2. The surgeon, equipped with a headlight and seated on a stool at the head of the table, performs transcervical thymectomy.

After thymectomy is performed, the mediastinum is carefully inspected to ensure hemostasis. A red rubber catheter is inserted into the mediastinum and brought out through the incision during closure of the wound to evacuate as much air as possible. The catheter is removed after sustained manual inspiration is achieved and while the last knot of the platysmal closure is being tied. No chest tube is required, even when the pleura has been widely opened or excised. The skin is closed with a fine, continuous, subcuticular, absorbable suture. Figure 26–5 illustrates the technique of transcervical thymectomy.

Results

In 1988, Cooper and associates[7] reported the results of transcervical thymectomy in 65 patients who had myasthenia gravis and who were operated on between 1977 and 1986. Patients who had thymoma were excluded. The age range was 14 to 55 years (mean = 27 years) and the gender distribution was 50 females (76.9%) and 15 males (24.1%).

There were no major complications and no patient required blood transfusion. There was no phrenic nerve paralysis and no patient required tracheostomy. Only a few patients required postoperative percutaneous aspiration of pleural air. None required tracheal intubation for

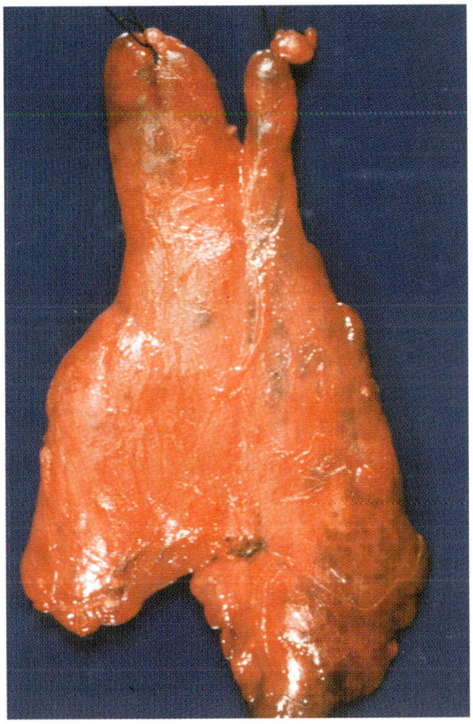

Figure 26–3. A large thymus, weighing 50 g, removed through the transcervical route.

more than 6 hours after transcervical thymectomy. There was one wound infection and one postpericardiotomy syndrome.

At the time of the 1988 report, all patients had been followed for a minimum of 1 year (median = 3.5 years). Four years after thymectomy, one patient died of pneumonia, likely related to bulbar weakness. A second patient died 5 years after operation of viral pneumonia apparently unrelated to myasthenia.

The patients were staged pre- and postoperatively using the modified Osserman classification[19]:

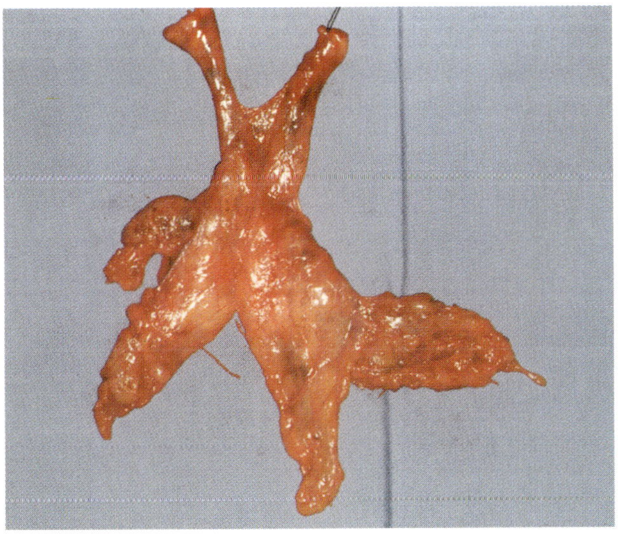

Figure 26–4. This transcervical thymectomy specimen has an extra lobe at the aortopulmonary window.

- 0—Asymptomatic
- 1—Ocular signs and symptoms only
- 2—Mild generalized weakness
- 3—Moderate generalized weakness, bulbar dysfunction, or both
- 4—Severe generalized weakness, respiratory dysfunction, or both

Preoperatively, 64 (98%) of the patients had generalized weakness; 25 (38%) had mild generalized weakness; and 39 (60%) had moderate or severe weakness. The mean clinical grade dropped from 2.7 before thymectomy to 0.5 at the last follow-up before the 1988 report. Ninety-five percent of the patients improved by one or more grades postoperatively, with 86% improving by two or more grades. Five percent of patients had no improvement, but no patient's condition deteriorated. At the time of the last follow-up, 85% of the patients had no generalized weakness. Thirty-three patients (52%) had complete remission (i.e., no symptoms and no need for medication).

The long-term clinical outcome (mean follow-up period after thymectomy of 8.4 years) in 52 of the previous 65 patients was recently reported by Bril and associates. These 52 patients ranged in age from 14 to 50 years, with a mean age of 28.5 years. Thirty-seven (71.2%) were female and 15 (28.8%) were male. The mean Osserman grade decreased from the preoperative value of 2.7 to 0.4 at the last follow-up. Most patients (90.4%) improved at least one grade, and 82.7% had minimal or no residual symptoms. Complete remission was present in 44.3%.

Only 25 of the 65 patients in the original report returned for follow-up at 5 years. Compared with the return rates in other reported series, significantly fewer patients returned for follow-up ($P < .001$; odds ratio = 11.38) in the transcervical group. The complete remission rate at the last follow-up in the 30 patients who were not seen for follow-up for more than 5 years was 50%, which is higher than the 44.2% rate for all patients. This suggests that patients lost to follow-up at 5 years likely have at least as good a result as those available for long term follow-up assessment.

To date, the senior author has performed more than 200 transcervical thymectomies for myasthenia gravis with similarly good results.

Discussion

It is generally accepted that complete removal of the thymus gland is essential to achieve the optimal rate of remission. Re-exploration and removal of residual retained thymus gland has been reported to result in improvement of myasthenic symptoms in cases of incomplete thymectomy. Therefore, the goal of thymectomy for myasthenia gravis should be complete thymectomy through the least invasive approach.

Jaretzki[11] demonstrated that the distribution of thymic tissue in the mediastinum and neck can be highly variable in location. Masaoka[15] identified the occasional presence of thymic tissue in extra-anatomic mediastinal locations. These ectopic remnants are identifiable only microscopically in mediastinal fat and are of uncertain significance in the outcome of thymectomy for myasthenia gravis. Re-

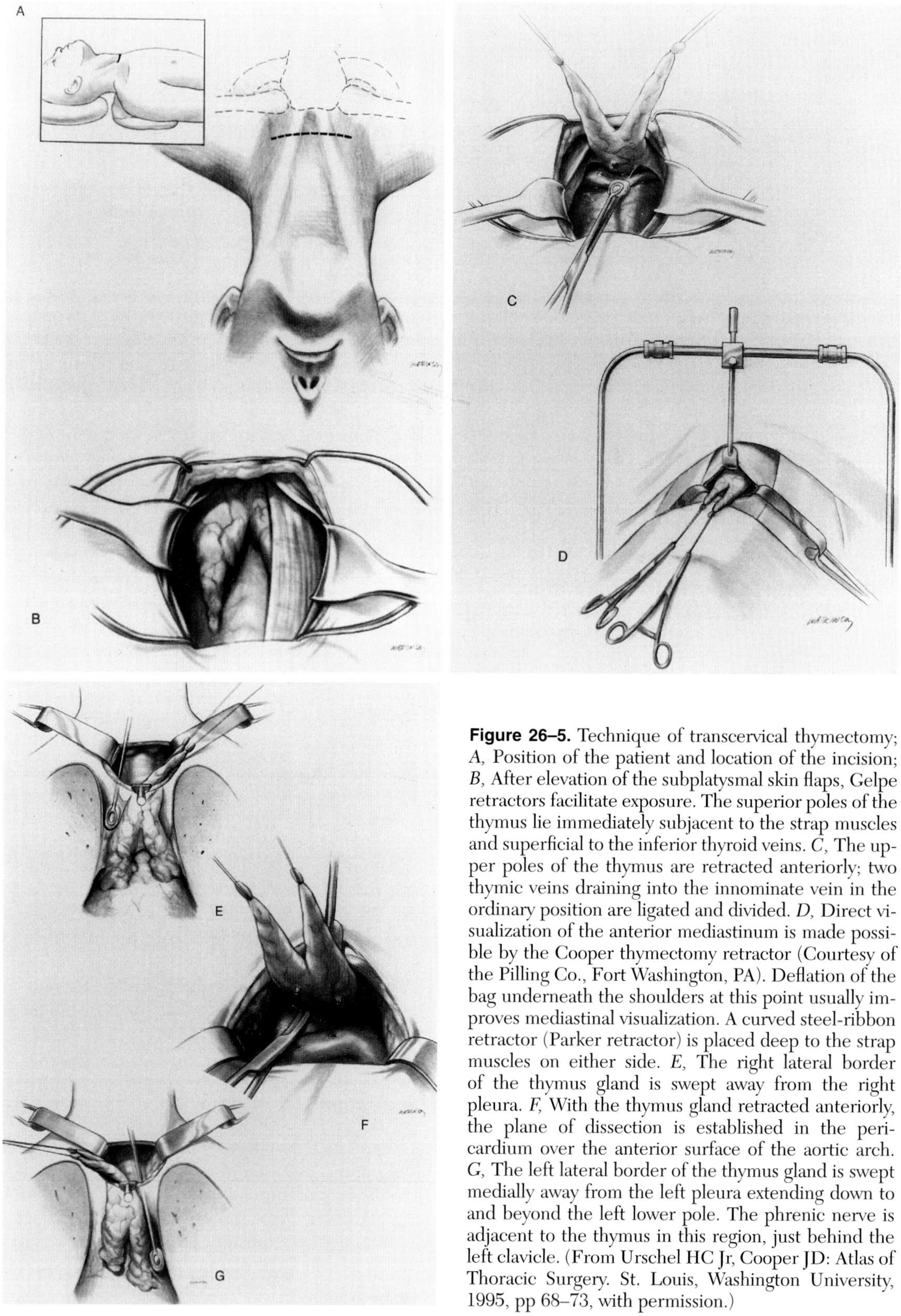

Figure 26–5. Technique of transcervical thymectomy; *A*, Position of the patient and location of the incision; *B*, After elevation of the subplatysmal skin flaps, Gelpe retractors facilitate exposure. The superior poles of the thymus lie immediately subjacent to the strap muscles and superficial to the inferior thyroid veins. *C*, The upper poles of the thymus are retracted anteriorly; two thymic veins draining into the innominate vein in the ordinary position are ligated and divided. *D*, Direct visualization of the anterior mediastinum is made possible by the Cooper thymectomy retractor (Courtesy of the Pilling Co., Fort Washington, PA). Deflation of the bag underneath the shoulders at this point usually improves mediastinal visualization. A curved steel-ribbon retractor (Parker retractor) is placed deep to the strap muscles on either side. *E*, The right lateral border of the thymus gland is swept away from the right pleura. *F*, With the thymus gland retracted anteriorly, the plane of dissection is established in the pericardium over the anterior surface of the aortic arch. *G*, The left lateral border of the thymus gland is swept medially away from the left pleura extending down to and beyond the left lower pole. The phrenic nerve is adjacent to the thymus in this region, just behind the left clavicle. (From Urschel HC Jr, Cooper JD: Atlas of Thoracic Surgery. St. Louis, Washington University, 1995, pp 68–73, with permission.)

tained thymus, when found at re-exploration, always consists of grossly missed lobes or typical extensions into the mediastinum rather than hypertrophy of microscopic, extra-anatomic foci, which would not have the normal shape, location, and capsular investment always found. Therefore, the need to remove all mediastinal fat, just because there may be occasional microscopic remnants, is doubtful.

Transcervical thymectomy appears to be the most minimally invasive way to perform thymectomy. Through a single 4-cm incision in the lower neck, the entire thymus gland can be visualized directly and removed with low morbidity. No drainage tube of any sort is needed postoperatively, and more than 90% of patients are discharged by the second day after surgery (median postoperative stay is 1 day). Return to complete activity with no restriction occurs within 3 to 4 days. There is no chance of development of poststernotomy complications (e.g., sternal drainage, sternal infection, difficult future sternotomy). It is noteworthy that in 1997, Bulkley and associates reported on a large series of 202 trans-sternal thymectomies for myasthenia gravis in which operative morbidity was 33%.[5] All these factors make early thymectomy through the transcervical approach appealing and acceptable to patients and neurologists. However, transcervical thymectomy may be the most technically demanding way of performing a thymectomy, and we do not recommend this method to the occasional surgeon.

For a minimally invasive procedure to succeed, it has to produce the same results as, or even better results than, conventional procedures. We have compared our results with those of several published series. The Duke University series,[18] in which the sternotomy approach was used, was similar size (55 patients), composed of patients who had a minimal follow-up of 1 year, and covered a similar period of time (1979–1985). But, unlike our series of 65 consecutive thymectomies, the Duke study was a retrospective, selective study, excluding all patients who received prednisone or azathioprine preoperatively. Although our patients had slightly more severe disease as a group, the improvement after surgery was essentially identical (Table 26–1).

We have also compared our results with those of Jaretzki's maximal thymectomy,[12] which involves a combination of median sternotomy and cervical incision with en bloc thymectomy and anterior mediastinal exenteration, including mediastinal pleura from the level of the thoracic inlet to the diaphragm, pericardiophrenic fat pad, and all accessible mediastinal fat. Table 26–2 shows that the two series have similar results. The incidence of complete remission following thymectomy was also similar in the two series.

We agree that complete remission rate is the best indicator for comparisons between different series. Table 26–3 is a comparison of complete remission rates for different thymectomy approaches, and no major difference is observed between different series.

The use of VATS has been proposed as a new approach to thymectomy,[14] the main reason being its superior cosmesis. We maintain that a large series with long follow-up demonstrating equivalent complete remission rates when compared with currently accepted approaches (transsternal and transcervical) is needed before VATS can be promoted as an acceptable form of thymectomy for myasthenia gravis. Before this gold standard is met, new approaches should be evaluated only prospectively in specialized centers.

While we are awaiting the long-term results of VATS in thymectomy, we can identify a number of potential disadvantages of this method that do not occur with the transcervical approach. Thymectomy using VATS requires placement of a double-lumen endotracheal tube and an arterial line for one-lung anesthesia. The larger double-lumen endotracheal tube causes more trauma to the vocal cords and may result in a higher incidence of postoperative aspiration in patients who have bulbar symptoms. The phrenic nerve on the side opposite the instrumentation side may not be easy to identify, making the phrenic nerve prone to damage. The right VATS approach limits the ability of performing an extensive dissection of tissue in the aortopulmonary window, and, therefore, risks incomplete thymectomy. The left superior thymic pole descends pos-

Table 26–1. Comparison of Results Obtained From Toronto General Hospital and the Duke University Series

Variable	TGH (N = 65)	Duke (N = 55)
Patients receiving preop medical therapy (%)	94	62
Mean preop grade	2.7	2.5
Mean follow-up grade	0.5	0.5
Patients receiving prednisone on follow-up (%)*	44	45
Improvement of ≥ 1 grade (%)	95	92
Improvement of ≥ 2 grades (%)	86	71
No improvement (%)	5	7
Deterioration	0	1
Postoperative deaths	0	1
Patients with no generalized weakness at last follow-up (%)	85	80

* Excludes patients receiving prednisone preoperatively.
TGH = Toronto General Hospital.
Modified from Olanow CW, Wechsler AS, Sirotkin-Roses M, et al: Thymectomy as primary therapy in myasthenia gravis. Ann NY Acad Sci 505:595, 1987, with permission; From Cooper JD, Al-Jilaihawa AN, Pearson FG, et al: An improved technique to facilitate transcervical thymectomy for myasthenia gravis. Ann Thorac Surg 45:242, 1988, reprinted with permission from The Society of Thoracic Surgeons.

Table 26–2. Comparison of Results Obtained From Toronto General Hospital and Columbia-Presbyterian Series

Variable	TGH (N = 65)	Columbia-Presbyterian (N = 72)
Mean preop grade*	2.7	3.0
Mean follow-up (yr)	3.6	3.4
Mild cases (%)	40	20
Complete remission (%)	52	46
Asymptomatic (%)		
±Anticholinesterase	63	79
±Prednisone, immunosuppressive drugs	88	90
No improvement (%)	5	4

* Excludes grade 5 patients.
TGH = Toronto General Hospital; complete remission = no weakness, no treatment.
Modified from Jaretzki A, Younger DS, Penn AS, et al: "Maximum" thymectomy for myasthenia gravis: Surgical anatomy, operative technique, and results. J Thorac Cardiovasc Surg 95:747, 1988, with permission; From Cooper JD, Al-Jilaihawa AN, Pearson FG, et al: An improved technique to facilitate transcervical thymectomy for myasthenia gravis. Ann Thorac Surg 45:244, 1998, reprinted with permission from The Society of Thoracic Surgeons.

Table 26–3. Comparison of Complete Remission Rates for Transcervical, Trans-sternal, and Extended Thymectomy

Reference	Surgical Approach	Duration of Follow-up (yr)	Complete Remission Rate (%)
Bril et al,[4] 1998	Transcervical	8.4	44.2
Masaoka et al,[16] 1996	Extended	5.0	45.8
DeFilippi et al,[9] 1994	Transcervical	5.0	43.0
Papatestas et al,[21] 1987	Trans-sternal	10.0	32.0
Papatestas et al,[20] 1981	Trans-sternal	5.0	24.0
Papatestas et al,[20] 1981	Transcervical	5.0	24.0
Jaretzki et al,[12] 1988	Maximal	3.3	46.0
Mulder et al,[17] 1989	Trans-sternal	3.6	36.0

From Bril V, Kozic J, Ilse WK, et al: Long-term clinical outcome after transcervical thymectomy for myasthenia gravis. Ann Thorac Surg 65:1521, 1998, reprinted with permission from The Society of Thoracic Surgeons.

terior to the innominate vein in about 5% of patients, and could pose difficulty to the VATS approach. Pre-existing pleural adhesions preclude the VATS approach. Finally, VATS is associated with a 10 to 15% incidence of chronic pain resulting from intercostal nerve trauma, a complication not associated with transcervical thymectomy.

In summary, transcervical thymectomy is the most minimally invasive approach with a proven long-term excellent remission rate for myasthenia gravis. It has minimal morbidity, requires a short hospital stay, and returns the patient to the preoperative state quickly. However, it is more difficult to learn, and it is not recommended for the occasional surgeon.

References

1. Akakura I: Mediastinoscopy. Presented at the XIth International Congress of Bronchoesophagology, Hakone, Japan, 1965.
2. Blalock A, Mason MF, Morgan HJ, et al: Myasthenia gravis and tumors of the thymic region. Report of a case in which the tumor was removed. Ann Surg 110:544, 1939.
3. Blalock A: Thymectomy in the treatment of myasthenia gravis: Report of twenty cases. J Thorac Cardiovasc Surg 13:316, 1944.
4. Bril V, Kojic J, Ilse WK, et al: Long-term clinical outcome after transcervical thymectomy for myasthenia gravis. Ann Thorac Surg 65:1520, 1998.
5. Bulkley GB, Bass KN, Stephenson GR, et al: Extended cervicomediastinal thymectomy in the integrated management of myasthenia gravis. Ann Surg 226:324, 1997.
6. Carlens E, Johansson L, Olsson P: Mediastinoscopy auxiliary to thymectomy by the cervical route. Bronches 17:408, 1967.
7. Cooper JD, Al-Jilaihawa AN, Pearson FG, et al: An improved technique to facilitate transcervical thymectomy for myasthenia gravis. Ann Thorac Surg 45:242, 1988.
8. Crile G Jr: Thymectomy through the neck. Surgery 59:213, 1966.
9. DeFilippi VJ, Richman DP, Ferguson MK: Transcervical thymectomy for myasthenia gravis. Ann Thorac Surg 57:194, 1994.
10. Henze A, Biberfeld P, Christensson B, et al: Failing transcervical thymectomy in myasthenia gravis: An evolution of transsternal re-exploration. Scand J Thorac Cardiovasc Surg 18:235, 1984.
11. Jaretzki A, Wolff M: "Maximum" thymectomy for myasthenia gravis: Surgical anatomy and operative technique. J Thorac Cardiovasc Surg 96:711, 1988.
12. Jaretzki A. Younger DS, Penn AS, et al: "Maximum" thymectomy for myasthenia gravis: results. J Thorac Cardiovasc Surg 95: 747, 1988.
13. Keynes G: Investigations into thymic disease and tumor formation. Br J Surg 62:499, 1955.
14. Mack M, Landreneau RJ, Yim AP, et al: Results of video-assisted thymectomy in patients with myasthenia gravis. J Thorac Cardiovasc Surg 112:1352, 1996.
15. Masaoka A. Nagaoka Y, Kotake Y: Distribution of thymic tissue in the anterior mediastinum: Current procedures in thymectomy. J Thorac Cardiovasc Surg 70:747, 1975.
16. Masaoka A. Yamakawa Y, Niwa H, et al: Extended thymectomy for myasthenia gravis patients: A 20 year review. Ann Thorac Surg 62:853, 1996.
17. Mulder DG, Graves M, Herrmann C: Thymectomy for myasthenia gravis: Recent observations and comparisons with past experience. Ann Thorac Surg 48:551, 1989.
18. Olanow CW, Wechsler AS, Sirotkin-Roses M, et al: Thymectomy as primary therapy in myasthenia gravis. Ann NY Acad Sci 505:595, 1987.
19. Osserman KE, Genkins G: Studies in myasthenia gravis: Review of twenty year experience in over 1200 patients. Mt Sinai J Med 38:497, 1971.
20. Papatestas AE, Genkins G, Kornfeld P: Comparison of the results of the transcervical and transsternal thymectomy in myasthenia gravis. Ann NY Acad Sci 377:766, 1981.
21. Papatestas AE, Genkins G, Kornfeld P, et al: Effects of thymectomy in myasthenia gravis. Ann Surg 206:79, 1987.
22. Schumacher ED, Roth J: Thymektomie bei cenem Fall von Morbus Basedowii mit Myasthenie. Mitt a. d. Grenzgeb d. Med. u. Chir. 25:746, 1912.
23. Wells SA Jr, Cooper JD: Closed mediastinal exploration in patients with persistent hyperparathyroidism. Ann Surg 214:555, 1991.
24. Von Haberer A: Zur klinischen Bedeutung der Thymus Druese. Arch Klin Chir 109:193, 1917.

Chapter 27

Partial Sternotomy Approach to the Thymus

José Ribas Milanez de Campos, Luiz Tarcisio B. Filomeno, Paulo E. Marchiori, and Fabio B. Jatene

Myasthenia gravis (MG) is an autoimmune disease of neuromuscular transmission characterized by weakness and fatigability of the voluntary muscles. The exact pathogenetic mechanism behind this, however, has remained unclear.

The most noticeable clinical symptom is rapid fatigue of the voluntary muscles, which can be brought on by exercise, fever, emotion, or the use of drugs that block the neuromuscular junction. The most frequently involved muscle groups are the extrinsic ocular muscles; the muscles involved in facial expression, chewing, and swallowing; the muscles supporting the head; and the proximal muscles of the limbs. Some other groups are rarely or irregularly affected, including the diaphragm, the intercostals, and the intrinsic ocular muscles. The characteristic feature of MG is variability in the strength of affected muscles rather than a generalized tiredness. It varies from day to day, with weakness generally getting worse toward the evening. Short-term weakness is often due to physical exertion, but the emotional state could also affect its manifestation. Affected muscles lose further strength if contraction is maintained or repeated (*pathologic fatigability*).

The diagnosis of MG is made clinically, based on the history and physical examination. It can be further confirmed by electromyography, radiography, and computed tomography (CT) scans of the chest, serologic tests for anti-acetylcholine receptor antibody and anti–striated muscle antibodies, tests using short-acting anticholinesterase, pulmonary function tests, and other tests for pathologies associated mainly with the thyroid.

Indications for Thymectomy

In our unit, thymectomy is indicated for practically all patients diagnosed with MG, except in the following cases:

1. During the initial stage, when spontaneous remission is still possible (usually within the first year of onset).
2. In patients younger than 12 years of age, in whom thymectomy is generally deferred on the basis of the understanding that the thymus may be important for immunologic development at an early age. Surgery is indicated only when clinical symptoms cannot be controlled with medication, including steroids.
3. In patients aged 55 or older treated clinically with good results. CT scans of the chest and anti–striated muscle antibody studies are essential in this group, however, because they can suggest a thymoma requiring surgical resection. Surgery is also indicated for patients who fail medical therapy.

In our experience, the purely ocular form of MG is rare. In the majority of cases, a good history and a complete physical examination often reveal weakness in other muscle groups, especially using the aforementioned supplementary tests.

Preoperative Management

If only motor symptoms are present without any bulbar involvement, the patient is prepared with the minimal dose of anticholinesterase drugs necessary for normal activities. All patients with bulbar symptoms are also given corticosteroids, with increasing doses up to 80 mg/day over a minimum of 3 weeks on an outpatient basis. Some patients require hospitalization a few days before surgery because of intensification of their myasthenic symptoms.

Patients with severe clinical symptoms, including those with respiratory failure requiring mechanical ventilation, are initially treated in the intensive care unit with anticholinesterase drugs, corticosteroids, immunosuppressants, and some with plasmapheresis. They undergo thymectomy only when they demonstrate a significant clinical improvement. Patients with marked symptoms and those requiring mechanical ventilation have rarely been operated on.[1] Preoperative pulmonary function tests can select out patients who require more extensive preparation: vital capacity below 70%, forced expiratory volume in 1 second below 50%, maximal voluntary ventilation below 50%, Haebish index less than 5.*

The volume flow curve generally shows a flattened "myasthenic pattern" because the muscle contraction is inadequate to achieve maximal flow.[3] MG may affect both inspiratory and expiratory muscles in almost all patients with all clinical forms of the disease. Evaluating respiratory function preoperatively is necessary to prevent respiratory complications following thymectomy. In patients with MG, vital capacity is usually low, total lung capacity tends to be normal, and residual volume is normal or elevated. Vital capacity is reduced because of both inspiratory and expiratory muscle weakness. This pattern is similar to the changes found in patients with laryngeal, tracheal, and/or large bronchial stenosis. This finding in MG patients suggests eventual fatigue of the laryngeal muscles.

Surgical Technique

The thymus, embryologically derived from the third branchial pouch, is a cervicothoracic structure extending from the inferior border of the thyroid gland to the level of

*Haebish index: maximal voluntary ventilation − forced vital capacity / forced vital capacity (MVV − FVC / FVC).[2]

the fourth costal cartilage. A partial sternotomy provides a direct and adequate surgical approach to the gland. If necessary, it can be modified by extending it caudad to a total sternotomy or cephalad by adding a transverse component at the base of the neck. The patient is placed in the supine position with a pad under the shoulders. A vertical midline incision is made on the skin, starting 2 cm below the suprasternal notch up to the level of the fourth intercostal space (Fig. 27–1). The incision is carried down through the subcutaneous tissue to expose the upper sternal border, presternal fascia, and muscle, which are incised down to and through the sternal periosteum. The superior mediastinum in the midline, above the manubrium, is dissected bluntly with the finger to clear the areolar mediastinal tissue away from the posterior surface of the sternum. The bone of the manubrium is divided with a Lebsche knife or a compressed-air or electric-powered saw in a downward direction. The entire manubrium and upper part of the sternal body down to the fourth intercostal space are divided. Lateral and progressive retraction of the two halves of the sternum is accomplished with a Finochietto spreader (Fig. 27–2). The thymus gland (characteristically gray-pink in color) is then exposed and dissected, with excision of the gland and all the surrounding fat (yellow tissue), starting from the base of the thyroid superiorly and the phrenic nerves laterally, up to the lower pericardium (Fig. 27–3). Grasping with a tissue clamp (Duval or Babcock) permits the appropriate elevating tension for easy dissection of the thymus from the underlying structures. The dissection can also be started from below and progress upward, in the same extracapsular plane. An effort is made to push the mediastinal pleura laterally, trying to avoid rupturing the pleura. If this occurs, the defect can be repaired with sutures. In the posterolateral dissection of the thymus, extreme care is taken not to damage the phrenic nerve, because diaphragmatic palsy can be a major postthymectomy management problem. The thymic bed is then carefully inspected to ensure hemostasis, to confirm that all the thymic tissue has been removed, and to verify the integrity of the pleural spaces (Fig. 27–4). Bleeding from the sternal edges is managed with cautery and bone wax. Drainage of the anterior mediastinum is provided by

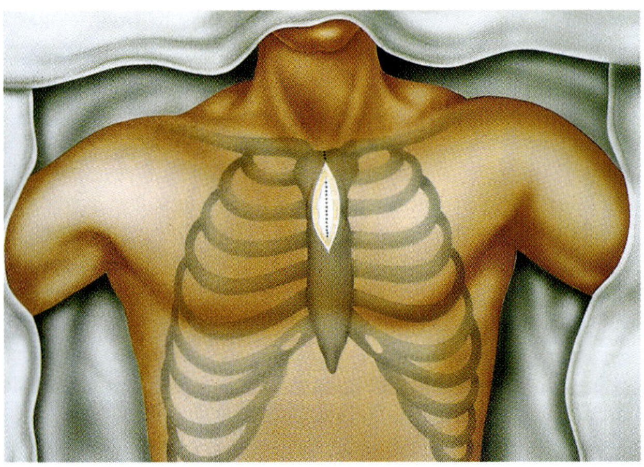

Figure 27–1. With the patient in the supine position, the skin incision is made from 2 cm below the suprasternal notch up to the fourth intercostal space.

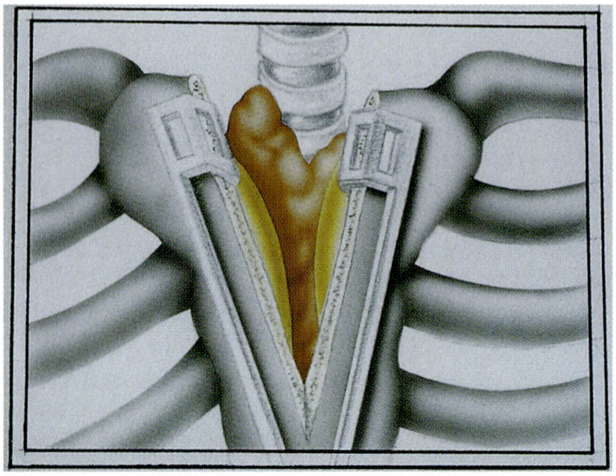

Figure 27–2. After a sternum-splitting incision, the two halves of the sternum are retracted laterally with a Finochietto spreader. The thymus gland is then exposed.

a suprasternal Hemovac-type suction catheter. Approximation of the sternum is accomplished with two or three 4–0 stainless steel wires placed through or around the sternum in each intercostal space. The subcutaneous and skin layers are closed with absorbable sutures. The skin is closed with intradermal sutures and reinforced by a Steri-strip dressing.

Postoperative Management

Successful management of these patients requires close cooperation among the neurologist, thoracic surgeon, anesthetist, nurses, and physiotherapists. Patients are awakened immediately after the operation and managed in

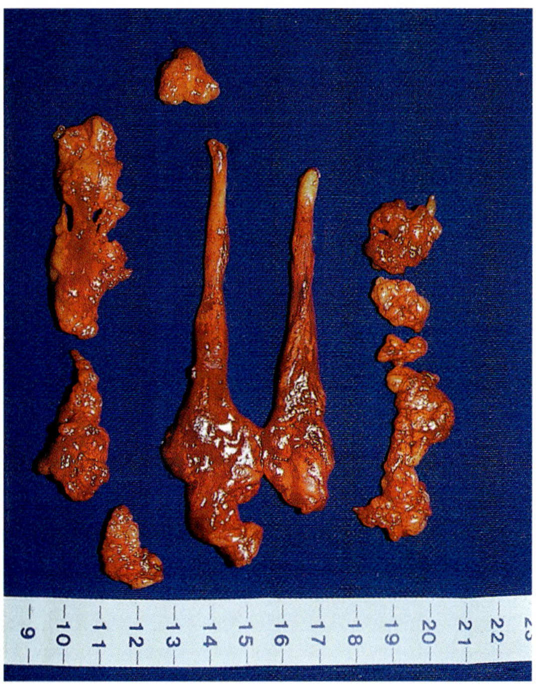

Figure 27–3. The resected thymus gland and the surrounding fat tissue.

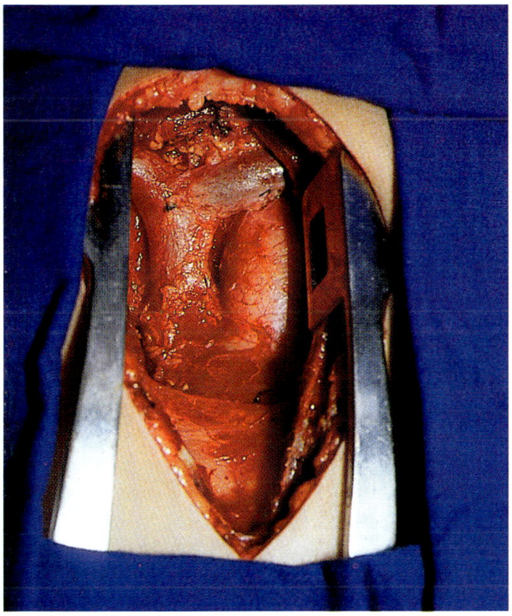

Figure 27–4. The anterior mediastinal thymic bed is carefully inspected to ensure hemostasis, the totality of the thymectomy, and the integrity of the pleural spaces.

an intensive care unit for the first 24 hours. After discharge, they are returned to the neuromuscular clinic for long-term follow-up and to be evaluated at intervals of 3 to 6 months. The postoperative management protocol we use is as follows:

- Early extubation—in the operating room.
- First postoperative day: reduction of anticholinesterase drugs to half.
- At 24 hours: removal of the mediastinal drain.
- Continue the same dose of corticosteroid therapy until the third week, then reduction by 5 mg/wk until 10 to 20 mg/d is attained.
- Immunosuppression with cytotoxic drugs and plasmapheresis is used only in severe cases with continued symptoms and/or resistance to corticosteroid therapy.
- Antibiotics (cephalothin) is continued for 7 days postoperatively.
- Outpatient follow-up in the neurology unit for control and adjustment of medication based on symptoms.

Results

During the last 45 years, 1150 patients with MG were managed and followed up at our institution: 150 with the congenital form, 110 with thymomas, and 890 with the acquired type (immunologic). The series includes 473 patients operated on using the previously described technique from 1973 to 1998. The sex distribution revealed a predominance in women (almost 70%), and the mean age was 34.3 years.

The clinical staging of these 473 patients by Osserman's classification is detailed in Table 27–1. The clinical status corresponds to the most recent exacerbation of the disease before the operation, which was performed on an elective basis whenever possible. The period of follow-up ranged from 1 month to 25 years. The mean follow-up was 7.3 years. The clinical outcome for all operated patients is summarized in Table 27–2. Pathologic examination of the surgical specimens revealed the following: 69% follicular hyperplasia, 17% thymic atrophy, and 14% normal thymus.

There were no operative or hospital deaths. There were no phrenic or recurrent nerve injuries in this patient population. There were 11 late deaths, which were unrelated to the procedure. No patient required reoperation. Of the four patients who required ventilatory support after surgery, three were treated with plasmapheresis. All patients improved after the operation. One patient developed osteomyelitis in the sternum, and five experienced subcutaneous fluid collection. There was no residual pneumothorax or hemothorax in this series.

Table 27–1. Preoperative Patient Distribution According to Osserman's Classification (N = 473)

	Stage	No. of Patients
I	Ocular	34
IIA	Generalized mild	123
IIB	Generalized moderately severe	203
III	Acute severe	96
IV	Late severe	17

Discussion

The technique of surgical removal of the thymus gland is controversial, but the benefit of thymectomy as part of the treatment for MG has been demonstrated repeatedly since the initial observations of Blalock and colleagues in 1939.[4] In the untreated myasthenic population, the incidence of crisis is 2.8% a year; in thymectomized patients or those treated with corticosteroids, it is 0.8% a year (personal communication and experience of our neurology unit).

Patient selection for operation remains ill defined and controversial. Our surgical approach of partial median sternotomy with the goal of removing all thymic and perithymic tissue was consistently applied in each instance. This approach allows excellent visualization of the thymus gland, its vascular attachments, and perithymic tissues. The borders of extracapsular plane resection are the thy-

Table 27–2. Postoperative Outcome in 473 Patients Who Underwent Thymectomy Through Partial Sternotomy

Outcome	No. of Patients	Percentage
Complete remission*	60	12.7
Significant improvement†	295	62.3
Mild improvement‡	83	17.5
No response	35	7.4

*Asymptomatic, off all medications.

†Few symptoms and dosage of preoperative medication decreased by more than half.

‡Reduction of symptoms and dosage of preoperative medication decreased by less than half.

roid gland superiorly, between the phrenic nerves laterally, and the pericardial sac and adjacent mediastinal pleura inferiorly. All visible anterior mediastinal fat was excised with the thymus.

The use of the transcervical route for thymectomy remains controversial, despite its effectiveness in selected patients.[5, 6] The initial motivation for using this approach was that it is less invasive, requires a shorter hospitalization, and has a lower perioperative morbidity compared with the trans-sternal approach. On the other hand, more radical *"maximal"* thymectomy has been advocated by others but this approach remains unpopular among surgeons performing thymectomy.[7, 8] It has recently gained some support owing to the superior complete remission rate associated with this approach and reports of residual thymic tissue or thymoma following transcervical resections.[9, 10]

There has been no prospective controlled trial in which patients were randomized to receive either operation or medical therapy. The reasons for the lack of controlled, prospective studies may be the low incidence of MG in the general population, the life-threatening nature of the disease, and the long period necessary to obtain adequate and useful follow-up data on the outcome of therapy.

A retrospective study comparing patients with or without thymectomy and with or without corticosteroids in similar groups based on sex, duration of illness, and clinical stage did not show a statistical difference in the clinical course.[11] Nevertheless, the thymectomy group showed a marked reduction in the use of anticholinesterase drugs and corticosteroids, thus avoiding the side effects of these medications.

Nowadays, improvements in anesthesia, perioperative care, and surgical instruments and techniques have markedly reduced operative morbidity and mortality. Our results demonstrate that thymectomy by partial sternotomy for MG patients without thymoma was an effective therapeutic modality in 355 cases (75%) in our series. It is impossible to separate the importance of surgery from that of medical treatment, but our combined program has been shown to be a safe and effective approach to the management of this condition.

ACKNOWLEDGMENTS

The authors would like to thank Professor Jose Lamartine de Assis and Professor Nagib Curi for invaluable assistance in the evaluation and treatment of these patients and in the preparation of the manuscript.

References

1. Masaoka A, Yamakawa Y, Niwa H, et al: Extended thymectomy for myasthenia gravis patients: A 20 year review. Ann Thorac Surg 62:853–859, 1996.
2. Saraiva PAP, Assis JL, Leitao FBP, et al: Anesthesie pour thymectomie trans-sternale dans la myastenie grave. Sem Hop Paris 59:3373–3377, 1983.
3. Assis JL: Neuroimunologia. *In* Melaragno F, Naspitz CK (eds): Miastenia Grave. São Paulo, Sarvier, 1982, pp 97–136.
4. Blalock A, Mason MF, Morgan HJ, Riven SS: Myasthenia gravis and tumors of the thymic region: Report of a case in which the tumor was removed. Ann Surg 110:544–559, 1939.
5. DeFilippi VJ, Richman DP, Ferguson MK: Transcervical thymectomy for myasthenia gravis. Ann Thorac Surg 57:194–197,1994.
6. Bril V, Kojic J, Ilse WK, Cooper JD: Long-term clinical outcome after transcervical thymectomy for myasthenia gravis. Ann Thorac Surg 65:1520–1522, 1998.
7. Jaretzki A, Penn AS, Younger DS, et al: "Maximal" thymectomy for myasthenia gravis. J Thorac Cardiovasc Surg 95:747–757, 1988.
8. Masaoka A, Nagaoka Y, Kotake Y: Distribution of thymic tissue at the anterior mediastinum. J Thorac Cardiovasc Surg 70:747–753, 1975.
9. Henze A, Biberfeld P, Christensson B, et al: Failing transcervical thymectomy in myasthenia gravis. Scand J Thorac Cardiovasc Surg 18:235–238, 1984.
10. Austin EH, Olanow CW, Wechsler AS: Thymoma following transcervical thymectomy for myasthenia gravis. Ann Thorac Surg 35:548–550, 1983.
11. Assis JL: Tratamento. In Melaragno F, Naspitz CK (eds): Miastenia Grave. São Paulo, Sarvier, 1990, pp 223–253.

Chapter 28

VATS Approach to the Thymus*

Anthony P. C. Yim and Mohammad Bashar Izzat

Myasthenia gravis (MG) is an autoimmune disorder of the postsynaptic nicotinic acetylcholine receptor, and is characterized by weakness and fatigability of voluntary muscles.[1] The ocular muscles are frequently involved, rendering ptosis and diplopia the most common mode of presentation.[2] Anticholinesterase drugs have been used to treat MG for over half a century, and since the 1960s, corticosteroids and other immunosuppressive agents have clearly improved the prognosis of myasthenic patients. Thymectomy, first introduced by Alfred Blalock in the 1930s for the treatment of MG, has also become an established therapeutic option.[3] However, despite the fact that the condition has been recognized for over a century, many controversies still remain over the diagnosis, natural history, and therapy. Regarding thymectomy, there is uncertainty whether old-onset patients, or those with ocular symptoms only, should be operated upon.[4–9]

Currently, the most common surgical approach to thymectomy is via a median sternotomy. Other techniques—notably, the transcervical approach, and the more radical approach, which combines median sternotomy with a transcervical incision—have their advocates. Video-assisted thoracic surgery (VATS) provides an alternative approach that has several advantages over the others. This chapter presents our technique of VATS thymectomy, discusses the perioperative management in our institution, and describes our criteria for patient selection and reports on our intermediate results.

Our Current Practice

The average annual incidence of MG in Hong Kong is 4 per million population with a female to male ratio of 1.6 : 1.[2] In our hospital, since 1985, we have adopted a policy of offering thymectomy—as soon as possible after the diagnosis is established—to all patients younger than 70 years of age who have generalized MG, and to selected patients who have ocular myasthenia. It is vital that thoracic surgeons work closely with neurologists and anesthetists to achieve the optimal result.

Preoperative Management

The weakness that stems from MG affects voluntary muscles, including those involved in respiration, so that patients are at risk of developing postoperative respiratory failure. If bulbar palsy is present, patients may also develop aspiration pneumonia. Medical treatment has its own complications. Anticholinesterase treatment increases vagal tone, enchances oral secretion, and potentiates laryngeal spasm. Prolonged steroid use can result in electrolyte imbalance and increased susceptibility to infections.

Before elective surgery, it is important that distribution and severity of muscle weakness are carefully assessed. Respiratory function and nutritional status should also be documented and medical treatment optimized. Patients who have severe weakness may require preoperative plasmapheresis, together with steroid and anticholinesterase therapy. Admission to the intensive care unit for ventilatory support is indicated for patients who are already in respiratory failure, but it is not necessary to wait until the patient is extubated before surgery can proceed. Intravenous imunoglobulin is an alternative to plasmapheresis, but there is no clear evidence that one is better than the other.[10, 11] The patient should be warned of the possibility of postoperative ventilation. The operation is usually arranged as the first case on the elective list. Premedication is prescribed as appropriate, but respiratory depressant drugs are avoided. Stress doses of steroids may be required.

Intraoperative Management

Anesthesia Considerations

General anesthesia via left-sided, double-lumen endobronchial tube is employed. Patients are induced with propofol 2 mg/kg and fentanyl 2 μg/kg. Intubation can usually be achieved without muscle relaxants. Pretreatment of the tracheobronchial tree with local anesthetics facilitates intubation.[12] Proper positioning of the endobronchial tube is confirmed by the fiberoptic bronchoscope after intubation and reconfirmed after positioning. Selective one-lung ventilation to the left lung is essential to the operation.

Hypoxemia during one-lung ventilation is usually caused by shunting of blood. When this is encountered, the position of the double-lumen endobronchial tube and hemodynamic stability should be confirmed. A low level of continuous positive airway pressure (CPAP) applied to the collapsed right lung may improve saturation. Applying positive end expiratory pressure (PEEP) to the ventilated lung can also raise oxygen saturation during one-lung ventilation.[13]

Anesthesia is maintained with isoflurane 1-2%, 60% nitrous oxide in oxygen, and a single bolus of morphine 0.1 mg/kg. Ventilation is controlled to achieve normocapnia. Patients who have MG are usually more susceptible to the neuromuscular blocking effect of volatile anesthetics,[14] so nondepolarizing muscle relaxants are usually not required.[15, 16]

Patients who have MG are usually very sensitive to nondepolarizing muscle relaxants.[17–19] If muscle relaxation is

* Adapted from Yim APC, Kay R, Izzat MB, et al: Video-assisted thoracoscopic thymectomy for myasthenia gravis. Semin Thorac Cardiovasc Surg 11:65–73, 1999.

necessary during the course of anesthesia, a reduced dose of an intermediate-acting, nondepolarizing muscle relaxant should be used followed by a carefully titrated intravenous infusion. Monitoring neuromuscular transmission is mandatory to adjust the dose of muscle relaxant and to ensure complete reversal of neuromuscular blockade after surgery.[20]

There is routine monitoring and continuous display of an electrocardiogram, noninvasive blood pressure, pulse oximetry, end-tidal carbon dioxide, airway pressure, ventilatory volume, inspired oxygen, and neuromuscular transmission. An arterial line and a ventral venous catheter for invasive pressure monitoring may be required for coexisting medical conditions.

Surgical Considerations

Surgical Anatomy of the Thymus

The thymus weighs between 10 and 35 g at birth, and it grows to between 20 and 50 g at puberty; after that, it slowly involutes to between 5 and 15 g in an adult.[21] With the process of involution, the thymic parenchyma is gradually replaced by fibroadipose tissue. The fully developed gland is bilobed, but its exact shape is largely molded by the adjacent structures. It occupies the anterior mediastinum with the superior horns often extending into the neck, lying deep to the sternothyroid. The body of the gland is related anteriorly to the sternum and the upper four costal cartilages; posteriorly to the pericardium, the ascending aorta, the brachiocephalic veins, and the superior vena cava, and laterally to the mediastinal pleura. Its relationship with the veins is of great surgical importance. The fibrous capsule of the thymus blends in with the pretracheal fascia. The arterial supply is derived from branches of the internal mammary artery and venous drainage through two or three tributaries to the left brachiocephalic vein.

Surgical Technique

Under general anesthesia with selective one-lung ventilation, the patient is placed in the full left lateral decubitus position and the table is flexed at 30 degrees, just inferior to the level of the nipples, for opening up the upper intercostal spaces.[22] We advocate a right-sided approach. An incision is made just in front of the tip of the scapula, along the posterior axillary line, for the insertion of a zero-degree telescope (Fig. 28–1). Instrument ports are usually placed in the third intercostal space, midaxillary line, and at the fifth or sixth intercostal space, anterior axillary line (see Fig. 28–1). Additional ports are made for lung retraction as necessary.[23] In young female patients, the instrument ports can be placed strategically over the submammary fold for cosmetic consideration (Figures 28–2A and B).

The entire hemithorax is carefully examined, with particular attention to the mediastinum. The right phrenic nerve is identified and carefully preserved throughout the dissection. We advocate the use of conventional thoracic instruments, such as a sponge-holding forceps.[24] The right inferior horn of the thymus can be identified where it drapes over the pericardium. The mediastinal pleura over the free edge of the right inferior thymic horn is sharply incised. The thymus can then be lifted up and bluntly dis-

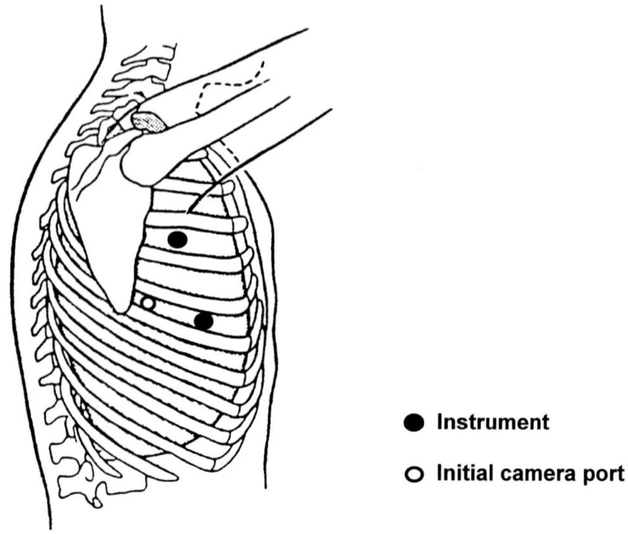

Figure 28–1. Diagram showing positions of camera and instrument ports approaching thymus. (From Yim APC, Kay RLC, Izzat MB, et al: Video-assisted thoracoscopic thymectomy for myasthenia gravis. Semin Thorac Cardiovasc Surg 11:65–73, 1999.)

sected off the underlying pericardium, extending onto the aorta in a cephalad manner until the left brachiocephalic vein is exposed. We have found it helpful to apply deliberate and gentle traction on the thymus, and to use a dental pledget for gentle, blunt dissection. The thymic venous tributaries (usually two or three) draining into the left brachiocephalic vein can be identified, clipped (Endoclip, Autosuture, United States Surgical Corporation), and divided (Fig. 28–3). It is important to obtain vascular control before attempting further manipulation of the thymus. Dissection is then carried behind the sternum. With gentle traction on the thymus, using a sponge-holding forceps,[24] the left inferior horn can be identified and likewise dissected up to the thymic isthmus. The most difficult part of the operation is to dissect the superior horns. In most cases, the right internal mammary vein is divided to facilitate exposure. With gentle and deliberate inferior traction on the thymus, the superior horns can be carefully dissected free of their fascial attachments. The left superior horn may occasionally pass behind, instead of in front of, the brachiocephalic vein, and this anatomic variation has to be anticipated. (We have encountered this in one case, and thoracoscopic dissection was successfully accomplished.) The thymus as a free specimen can then be removed in a plastic bag through the most anterior port, as the intercostal space is wider anteriorly. Following thymectomy, the anterior mediastinal soft tissue, including the pericardial fat, is separately removed. The specimen is inspected for completeness of resection (Fig. 28–4A–E). In small children who have hyperplastic thymus, we have found it useful to retract part of the gland via an anteriorly placed wound. This maneuver creates more room for further dissection.

The thymic bed is inspected for hemostasis and completeness of resection. The brachiocephalic veins should be skeletonized and the junction to form the superior vena cava should be clearly visible (Fig. 28–5). Chest drainage is optional. The lung is reinflated under direct vision and a layered closure of the stab wounds completes the operation.

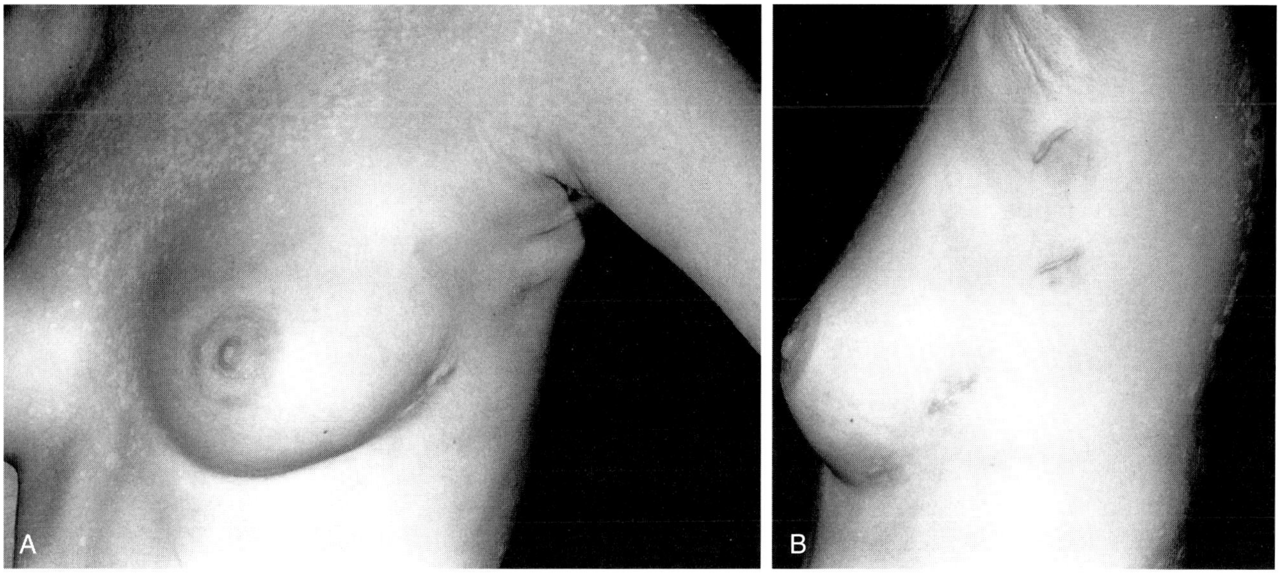

Figure 28–2. *A, B.* Postoperative view of a young female patient, showing the port positions. The lower ports are placed strategically in the submammary fold. (From Yim APC, Kay RLC, Izzat MB, et al: Video-assisted thoracoscopic thymectomy for myasthenia gravis. Semin Thorac Cardiovasc Surg 11:65–73, 1999.)

Results

In our institution, we have attempted 25 VATS thymectomies. Three were not related to MG. One was converted to a lateral thoracotomy because of bleeding. Therefore, 21 thoracoscopic thymectomies were successfully carried out for MG (9 males ranging in age from 9 to 75 years, with a mean age of 35.2). The final pathologies included 3 cases of thymoma, 9 of hyperplastic thymus, 4 of atrophic thymus, and 5 of normal thymus. There was no surgical mortality. The median hospital stay was 3 days. Preoperatively, 3 patients were in stage I, 10 in stage IIa, 2 in stage IIb, 4 in stage III, and 2 in stage IV, according to the modified Osserman and Genkins classification[25] (Table 28–1). After a mean period of 31 months (range 2 to 48 months), 2 patients were in complete remission (class I), 14 patients were asymptomatic on decreased medication (class II), 3 patients had symptomatic improvement on decreased medication (class III), 1 patient had no change in symptoms (class IV), and 1 patient had worsening of symptoms (class V), according to the classification by DeFilippi and associates.[26]

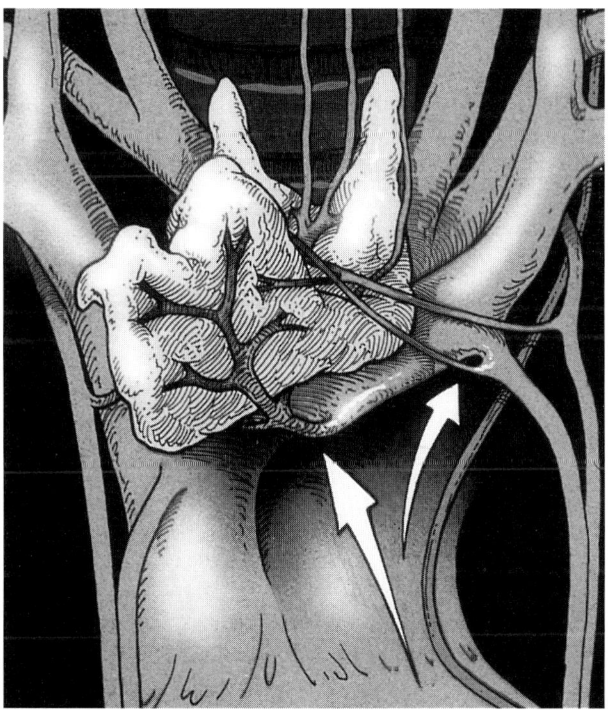

Figure 28–3. After identification of the left brachiocephalic vein, the thymic venous tributaries and arterial branches *(arrows)* are clipped and divided. (From Mack MJ, Landreneau RJ, Yim AP, et al: Results of VATS thymectomy in patients with myasthenia gravis. J Thorac Cardiovasc Surg 112:1352–1360, 1996, with permission.)

The patient in class V was an elderly man who presented with purely ocular symptoms when he was 73 years old. However, within 1 year, his symptoms progressed to involve the bulbar muscles. At this point, he was referred for surgery. Thoracoscopic thymectomy was performed and an atrophic thymus was removed without complication. Postoperatively, his symptoms never improved, and after 8 months, he developed acute respiratory failure leading to death within 2 days of admission. This was clearly a case of thymectomy failure, which was related not to any particular surgical approach, but to the unpredictable natural history in patients who have late-onset MG.[6, 8] He represented the only death in our series.

Complications resulting from surgery were relatively few. We had 1 patient who required conversion to a lateral thoracotomy for control of bleeding from a short but wide venous stump on the left brachiocephalic vein. In addition, we had 1 patient who had Down syndrome who developed postoperative pneumonia and required prolonged ventilation and a tracheostomy.

Although our patient numbers are too small for a multivariant analysis, we observed the same trend we reported

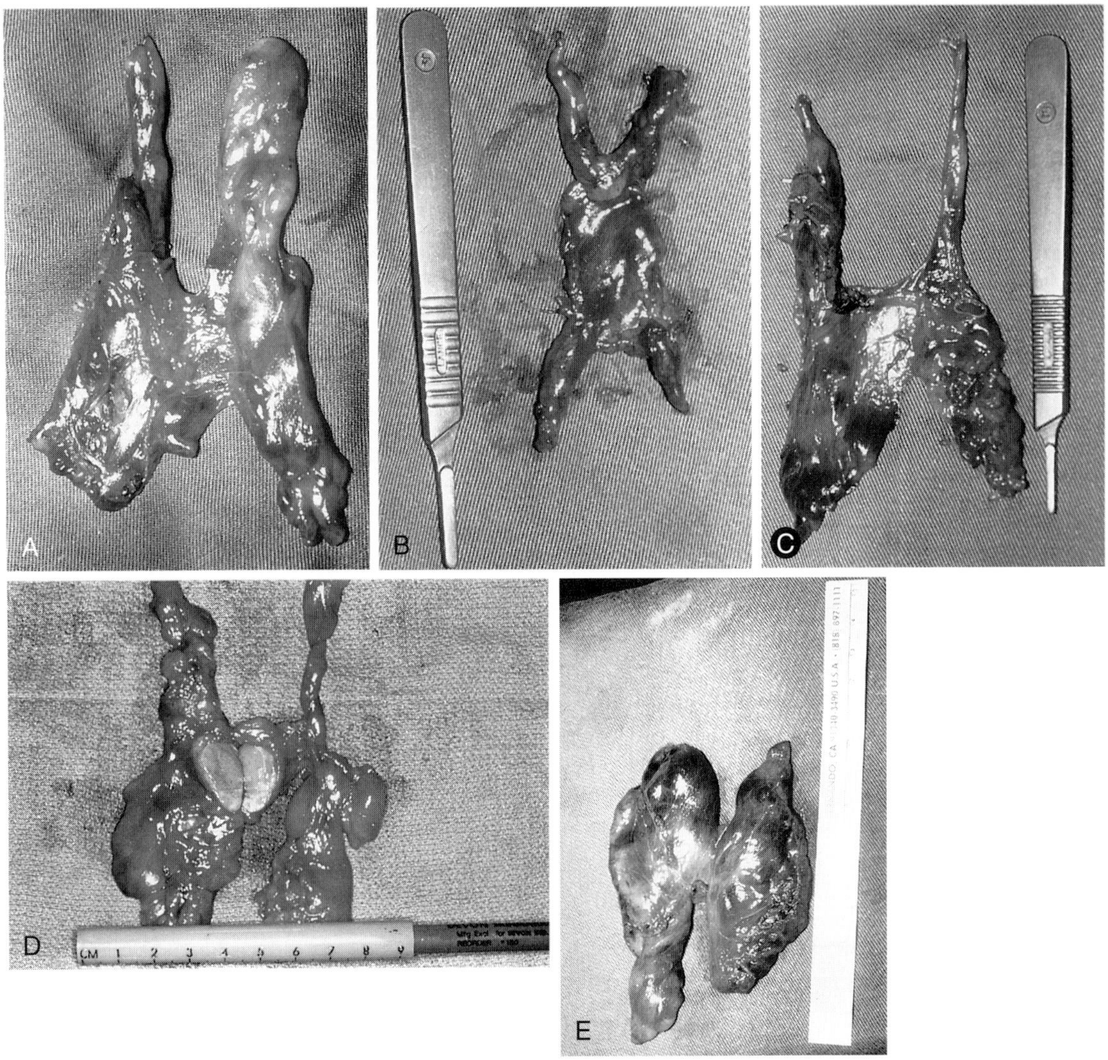

Figure 28–4. Examples of complete extracapsular thymectomy by the VATS approach. The specimens (A–E) vary in shape and size, but the upper and lower poles are clearly identified in each case. Specimen D shows a thymus containing a 2-cm thymoma. (From Yim APC, Kay RLC, Izzat MB, et al: Video-assisted thoracoscopic thymectomy for myasthenia gravis. Semin Thorac Cardiovasc Surg 11:65–73, 1999.)

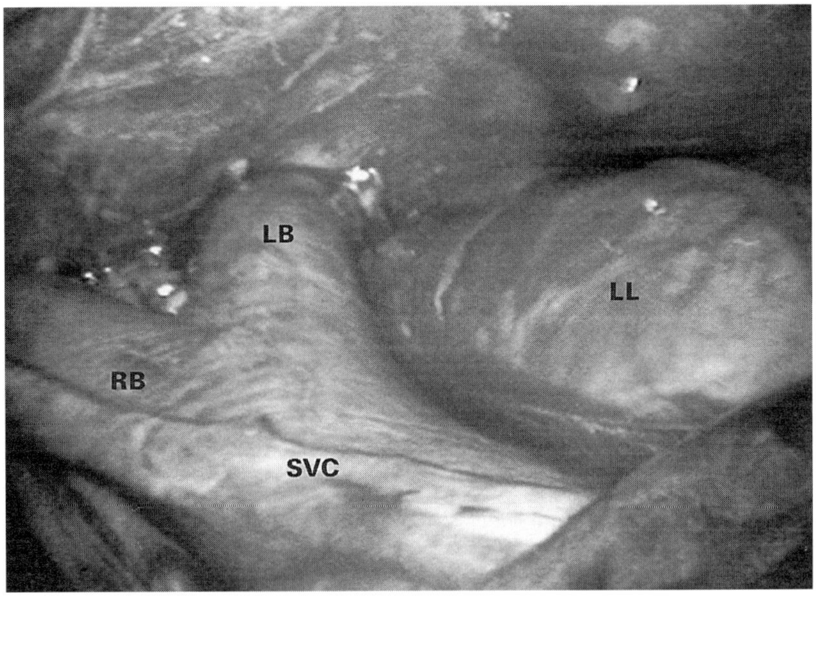

Figure 28–5. Thoracoscopy view following thymectomy, showing complete removal of the gland and clear visualization of the venous anatomy. (RB = right brachiocephalic vein, LB = left brachiocephalic vein, SVC = superior vena cava, LL = left lung.) (From Yim APC, Kay RLC, Izzat MB, et al: Video-assisted thoracoscopic thymectomy for myasthenia gravis. Semin Thorac Cardiovasc Surg 11: 65–73, 1999.)

Table 28–1. Modified Osserman and Genkins Classification of Myasthenia Gravis (MG)

Stage I	Ocular myasthenia gravis: involvement restricted to extraocular muscles
Stage IIa	Mild generalized MG: generalized weakness without respiratory muscle involvement
Stage IIb	Moderately generalized MG: more severe generalized involvement, bulbar symptoms common and relative sparing of respiratory muscles
Stage III	Acute fulminating MG: Rapid onset (within 6 months) of respiratory muscle involvement
Stage IV	Late severe MG: severe symptoms which have progressed for more than 2 years after onset of ocular or mild generalized MG

From Mack MJ, Landreneau RJ, Yim AP, et al: Results of VATS thymectomy in patients with myasthenia gravis. J Thorac Cardiovasc Surg 112:1352–1360, 1996.

previously[9, 27]: That patients who had mild generalized MG and those found to have thymic hyperplasia benefited most from surgery.

Discussion

Many uncertainties remain over the optimal treatment of MG. For surgeons who have an interest in thymectomy, controversies exist over patient selection and surgical techniques. Regarding patient selection, arguments have been put forward not to operate on ocular symptoms alone, because ocular MG is not only less likely to respond to thymectomy, but also carries a better prognosis compared with generalized MG. On the other hand, it has been shown that between 30 and 70% of patients who have initial ocular symptoms will eventually develop generalized myasthenia.[4, 5] It is on that basis that we advised some of our patients to have surgery, even though their presentation was purely ocular. We have also performed thymectomies for a few patients who found their ocular symptoms extremely disabling.

It is also debatable whether elderly patients with late-onset MG should be operated upon.[6, 8] In our institution, we normally do not recommend thymectomy to patients who are older than 70 years of age.[9] The patient (aged 75) who died following thymectomy, as we discussed previously, was a notable exception. Surgery was recommended because of progression of disease despite increased medication. Unfortunately, thymectomy did little to help. This underscores the uncertainties in the natural history for this group of patients.

Apart from patient selection, the best surgical approach to thymectomy remains controversial. The available options include median sternotomy with or without a transverse cervical extension, partial sternotomy, the transcervical approach, and VATS approach. Regardless of technique, it is generally agreed that thymectomy for MG should be complete. The Columbia-Presbyterian group[28] advocated maximal thymectomy. This procedure involves a combination of median sternotomy with cervical incision to achieve en bloc thymectomy and anterior mediastinal exenteration, including the mediastinal pleura from the level of the thoracic inlet to the diaphragm, the pericardial fat pad, and all the mediastinal fat. Despite this radical approach, however, when compared with sternotomy alone[29] or the transcervical approaches, results in terms of clinical improvement did not appear to be significantly different.[30]

The VATS approach is similar to the transcervical approach in that both are associated with minimal chest wall trauma, low postoperative morbidity, short hospital stay, and, perhaps more importantly, improved patient acceptance for surgery earlier in the disease, compared with the trans-sternal approach. However, VATS has additional advantages over the conventional transcervical approach in that visibility is much better and there is no crowding of instruments through a single access site. The thymus, being largely an anterior mediastinal structure, can be more directly approached through the chest than through the neck. Video assistance provides a wide, magnified operative field. We believe that by examining the thymic beds and the resected specimens,[23] we are performing the same operation thoracoscopically as is performed by the trans-sternal approach.

But even among the surgeons performing VATS thymectomy, there is controversy over the exact technique, and, in particular, whether the thymus should be approached from the left or the right. Mineo and associates[31] in Rome advocate a left-sided approach and the use of the pneumomediastinum to facilitate dissection. On the other hand, we advocate the right-sided approach for the following reasons[32, 33]: first, the superior vena cava, easily identified from the right, provides a clear landmark for further dissection of the innominate veins; second, the confluence of the two innominate veins to form the superior vena cava is a very difficult area to dissect well and can be more easily accomplished from the right side; third, from the ergonomic standpoint, it is easier for right-handed surgeons performing VATS to start at the inferior poles and work cephalad from the right side. The ultimate surgical goal of thymectomy is to remove the gland and the anterior mediastinal tissue completely. Which side to approach remains largely the surgeon's preference, which is ultimately influenced by his experience and training.

We have shown that in our institution, patients who underwent thoracoscopic thymectomy had a significantly lower analgesic requirement and shorter hospital stays than a historical group who underwent trans-sternal thymectomy.[23] The collective experience of 33 patients from four centers (Columbia Hospital in Dallas, University of Pittsburgh, Southern Illinois University, and our own) was analyzed.[27] Clinical improvement was seen in 88% of the patients who underwent thoracoscopic thymectomy. Our meta-analysis, compared with nine published series performed by other approaches, showed no difference in clinical improvement following thymectomy between series[27] (Table 28–2 and Fig. 28–6). Since completion of that study, our results, even though they are still intermediate, continue the early trends.

Concerns have been raised regarding using the VATS approach for thymoma, with[16] or without associated MG.[39] We are careful in restricting this technique to small,

Table 28–2. Comparison of VATS With Other Surgical Approaches for Thymectomy

Series	Technique	Mean Follow-Up (Month)	No. in Complete Remission	No. Improved
Jaretzki et al,[28] 1988 (n = 95)	TS + TC	40	36 (37.9%)	88 (92.6%)
Lennquist et al,[34] 1990 (n = 30)	TS + TC	50	6 (20%)	29 (96.7%)
	Total TS + TC (n = 30)		42 (33.6%)	117 (93.6%)
First et al,[35] 1994 (n = 46)	TS	75	13 (28.2%)	40 (87%)
Hatton et al,[36] 1989 (n = 52)	TS	46	14 (28%)	30 (57.7%)
Nussbaum et al,[37] 1992 (n = 84)	TS	51	20 (41.7%)	45 (93.8%)
Mulder et al,[38] 1989 (n = 84)	TS	36	30 (35.7%)	67 (79.8%)
Kay et al,[9] 1994 (n = 36)	TS	49	12 (24.5%)	26 (72.2%)
	Total TS (n = 266)		89 (33.5%)	208 (78.2%)
Cooper et al,[30] 1988 (n = 65)	TC	41 (median)	34 (52.3%)	62 (95.4%)
DeFlilippi et al,[26] 1994 (n = 53)	TC	51	9 (17%)	43 (81.1%)
	Total TC (n = 118)		43 (36.4%)	105 (89%)
Mack et al,[27] 1996 (n = 33)	VATS (n = 33)	23	6 (18.2%)	29 (87.9%)

TS = trans-sternal; TC = transcervical; TS + TC = combined trans-sternal + transcervical;

completely encapsulated thymoma (Masaoka[40] stage I). Clinical judgment is of paramount importance in thymic surgery, and any sign of tissue plane invasion mandates conversion to an open dissection.[24]

Conclusion

Thoracoscopic thymectomy represents a new, viable alternative approach for patients who have MG. We prefer a right-sided approach, because visibility of the venous anatomy is essential for dissection. Our own, as well as collective, experience so far shows that this approach produces results at least as favorable as other conventional surgical techniques. By minimizing chest-wall trauma, the thoracoscopic approach not only causes less postoperative pain and a shortened hospital stay, but it may lead to wider acceptance of earlier thymectomies by MG patients and their neurologists. The true role of this approach in thoracic surgery, however, awaits long-term follow-up.

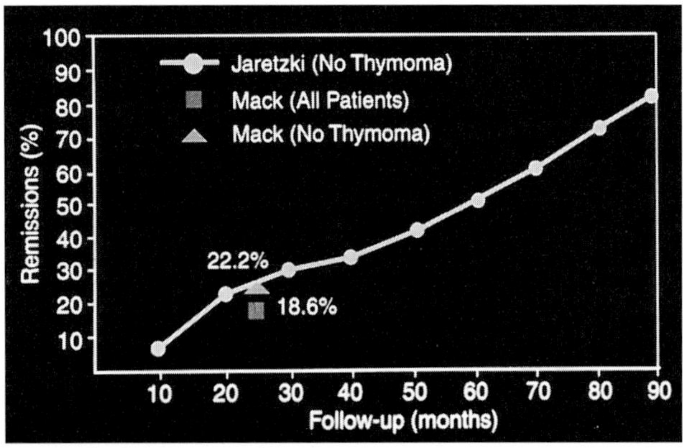

Figure 28–6. Remission rates for myasthenia gravis (MG). Comparison of collective experience of VATS thymectomy at 2 years (18.6%) with Jaretzki series (24%) of maximal thymectomy. If the patients who have thymoma are eliminated from the VATS series, the remission rate rises to 22.4% at 2 years. (From Mack MJ, Landreneau RJ, Yim AP, et al: Results of VATS thymectomy in patients with myasthenia gravis. J Thorac Cardiovasc Surg 112: 1352–1360, 1996, with permission.)

ACKNOWLEDGMENT

The authors are grateful to Alex Fung for his editorial assistance.

References

1. Drachman DB: Myasthenia gravis. N Engl J Med 330:1797–1810, 1994.
2. Yu YL, Hawkins BR, Ip MS, et al: Myasthenia gravis in Hong Kong Chinese. Epidemiology and adult disease. Acta Neurol Scand 86:113–119, 1992.
3. Hagen JA, Patterson GA: Surgery of myasthenia gravis. *In* Pearson FG, Deslauriers J, Ginsberg RJ, et al (eds): Thoracic Surgery. New York, Churchill Livingstone, 1995.
4. Sommer N, Sigg B, Melms A, et al: Ocular myasthenia gravis: Response to long term immunosuppressive treatment. J Neurol Neurosurg Psychiatr 62:156–162, 1997.
5. Oosterhuis HJ: The natural course of myasthenia gravis: A long term follow up study. J Neurol Neurosurg Psychiatr 52:1121–1127, 1989.
6. Donaldson DH, Ansher M, Horan S, et al: The relationship of age to outcome in myasthenia gravis. Neurology 40:786–790, 1990.
7. Schumm F, Wiethölter H, Fateh-Moghadam A, et al: Thymectomy in myasthenia with pure ocular symptoms. J Neurol Neurosurg Psychiatr 48:332–337, 1985.
8. Lanska DJ: Indications for thymectomy in myasthenia gravis. Neurology 40:1828, 1829, 1990.
9. Kay R, Lam S, Wong KS, et al: Response to thymectomy in Chi-

nese patients with myasthenia gravis. J Neurol Sci 126:84–87, 1994.

10. Cosi V, Lombardi M, Piccolo G, Erbetta A: Treatment of myasthenia gravis with high-dose intravenous immunoglobulin. Acta Neurol Scand 84:81–84, 1991.
11. Thornton CA, Griggs RC: Plasma exchange and intravenous immunoglobulin treatment of neuromuscular disease. Ann Neurol 35:260–268, 1994.
12. Chan MTV, Ng SK, Low JM: Letter: A non muscle-relaxant technique for video-assisted thoracoscopic thymectomy in myasthenia gravis. Anaesth Intens Care 23:256–257, 1995.
13. Benumof JL: Conventional and differential lung management of one-lung ventilation. *In* Benumof JL (ed): Anesthesia for Thoracic Surgery, 2nd ed, Philadelphia, WB Saunders, 1995.
14. Nilsson E, Muller K: Neuromuscular effects of isoflurane in patients with myasthenia gravis. Acta Anaesthesiol Scand 34: 126–131, 1990.
15. El-Dawlatly AA, Ashour, MH: Anaesthesia for thymectomy in myasthenia gravis: A non-muscle-relaxant technique. Anaesth Intens Care 22:458–460, 1994.
16. Rowbottom SJ: Isoflurane for thymectomy in myasthenia gravis. Anaesth Intens Care 17:444–447, 1989.
17. Smith CE, Donati F, Bevan DR: Cumulative dose-response curves for atracurium in patients with myasthenia gravis. Can J Anaesth 36:402–406, 1989.
18. Nilsson E, Meretoja OA: Vecuronium dose-response and maintenance requirements in patients with myasthenia gravis. Anesthesiology 73:28–32, 1990.
19. Paterson IG, Hood JR, Russell SH, et al: Mivacurium in the myasthenic patient. Br J Anaesth 73:494–498, 1994.
20. Baraka A: Anaesthesia and myasthenia gravis. Can J Anaesth 39:476–486, 1992.
21. Bannister LH: Thymus. *In* Peter L. Williams: Gray's Anatomy, 38th ed. Edinburgh, Churchill Livingstone, 1995, pp 1423–1431.
22. Yim AP: Minimizing chest wall trauma in Video Assisted Thoracic Surgery. J Thorac Cardiovasc Surg 109:1255–1256, 1995.
23. Yim APC, Kay RLC, Ho JKS. Video-Assisted Thoracoscopic Thymectomy for Myasthenia Gravis. Chest 108:1440–1443,1995.
24. Yim APC: Cost containment strategies in video assisted thoracoscopic surgery—an Asian perspective. Surg Endosc 10: 1198–1200, 1996.
25. Osserman KE, Genkins G: Studies in myasthenia gravis: review of a 20-year experience in over 1200 patients. J Mt Sinai Hosp 38:497–537, 1971.
26. DeFilippi VJ, Richman DP, Ferguson MK: Transcervical thymectomy for myasthenia gravis. Ann Thorac Surg 57:194–197, 1994.
27. Mack MJ, Landreneau RJ, Yim AP, et al: Results of VATS thymectomy in patients with myasthenia gravis. J Thorac Cardiovasc Surg 112:1352–1360, 1996.
28. Jaretzki A, Penn AS, Younger D, et al: "Maximal" thymectomy for myasthenia gravis. J Thorac Cardiovasc Surg 95:747–757, 1988.
29. Olanow CW, Wechsler AS, Sirotkin-Roses M, et al: Thymectomy as primary therapy in myasthenia gravis. Ann NY Acad Sci 505:595–606, 1987.
30. Cooper JD, Al-Jilaihawa AN, Pearson FG, et al: An improved technique to facilitate transcervical thymectomy for myasthenia gravis. Ann Thorac Surg 45:242–247, 1988.
31. Mineo TC, Pompeo E, Ambrogi V, et al: Adjuvant pneumomediastinum in thoracoscopic thymectomy in myasthenia gravis. Ann Thorac Surg 62:1210–1212, 1996.
32. Mack M: Reply to letter by Mineo TC, Pompeo E, Ambrogi V. Video-Assisted Thoracoscopic Thymectomy. From the right or from the left? J Thorac Cardiovasc Surg 114:517, 1997.
33. Yim APC: Letter: Thoracoscopic Thymectomy: Which side to approach? Ann Thorac Surg 64:584, 1997.
34. Lennquist S, Andaker L, Lindvall B, et al: Combined cervicothoracic approach in thymectomy for myasthenia gravis. Acta Chir Scand 156:53–61, 1990.
35. First WH, Thirumalai S, Doehring CB, et al: Thymectomy for the myasthenia gravis patient: Factors influencing outcome. Ann Thorac Surg 57:334–338, 1994.
36. Hatton PD, Diehl JT, Daly BDT, et al: Transsternal radical thymectomy for myasthenia gravis: A 15-year review. Ann Thorac Surg 47:838–840, 1989.
37. Nussbaum MS, Rosenthal GJ, Samatha FJ, et al: Management of myasthenia gravis by extended thymectomy with anterior mediastinal dissection. Surgery 112:681–688, 1992.
38. Mulder DG, Graves M, Hermann C: Thymectomy for myasthenia gravis: Recent observations and comparisons with past experience. Ann Thorac Surg 48:551–555, 1989.
39. Landreneau RJ, Dowling RD, Castillo WM, et al: Thoracoscopic resection of an anterior mediastinal tumor. Ann Thorac Surg 54:142–144, 1992.
40. Masaoka A, Monden Y, Nakahara K, et al: Follow up study of thymoma with references to their clinical stages. Cancer 48: 2485–2492, 1981.

COMMENTARY

Alfred Jaretzki III

These presentations (Chapters 26, 27, and 28) give excellent descriptions of three minimally invasive operations for resection of the thymus in the treatment of nonthymomatous myasthenia gravis (MG) as well as data on the results that appear to support the use of these techniques.

To decide whether these are the operations of choice, there are two questions that must be answered. Do these minimally invasive procedures remove all of the thymus that surgical-anatomic studies have demonstrated to be present? And, whether these procedures remove all of the thymus or not; is complete resection necessary? Although the clinical results should supply the answers to these questions, the interpretation of the available data is often misleading.

Why is interpretation of data misleading? The problem stems from the lack of uniform standards and misuse of statistics.[1] Multiple and conflicting classifications of disease severity, grading systems, and definitions of terms are used. "Remission" may include the use of immunosuppressive therapy, and although "improvement" is used as a comparative measure of response, levels of improvement at this time are imprecise without quantitation. Patients who have thymoma are often included in the analysis, and thus results are unpredictably skewed. And, perhaps most importantly, the data are frequently analyzed improperly.

Recognizing these deficiencies, the importance of a common language, and the need for appropriate analysis of the data, the Medical Advisory Board of the Myasthenia

Gravis Foundation of America, Inc., established a Thymectomy Task Force to develop a set of guidelines.[2] It is anticipated that their report will be completed and circulated by the end of 1999. When these guidelines become available and are employed, including the use of multi-institutional, risk-adjusted, prospective studies with the data centrally stored and appropriately monitored, it should become easier to determine the relative value of the various surgical techniques.

Do these techniques remove all of the thymus? I don't think so. Surgical anatomic studies have demonstrated that the thymus is much more extensive than described in these reports (Fig. 28A–1). A photograph of a typical specimen removed by transcervical–trans-sternal maximal thymectomy illustrates that maximal resections remove what has been described anatomically (Fig. 28A–2). In contrast, the illustrations and photographs of the specimens removed by these minimally invasive procedures indicate that these techniques produce incomplete resections. Since as little as two grams of residual thymus have been demonstrated to be symptomatic and their removal therapeutic,[3] the amount of thymus overlooked by these minimally invasive techniques appears to be significant.

Is it necessary to remove all the thymus? I think so. The evidence supporting the desirability of achieving a truly total thymectomy, or as nearly total as is surgically possible, is based upon the few Life Table Analysis comparisons available and comparison of crude data corrected for length of follow-up.

The data in Life Table Analysis of remissions indicate that the answer to whether all of the thymus should be removed is yes. The Kaplan-Meier Life Table Analysis technique is the analysis of choice.[4] Hazard rates are also acceptable. Remission, strictly defined, is the most reliable determinant in evaluating the results of thymectomy. When the remission rates in a series of a now recognized limited resection are compared with an extensive resection using Life Table Analysis, a direct relationship between the extent of resection and the results is clearly defined (Fig. 28A–3). The difference is striking and supports the premise that the more aggressive the resection, the better the results.

Crude rates corrected for mean length of follow-up also indicate that all of the thymus should be removed. A direct relationship between extent of resection and results is demonstrated and clearly lends credibility to the observation that the more extensive the resection, the better the results (Fig. 28A–4). Accordingly, these data support the view that minimally invasive procedures do not produce results equivalent to the more aggressive resections and that these resections are incomplete.

Uncorrected crude rates are unreliable and misleading, and use of these data in evaluating these patients should be universally discontinued. The length of follow-up postoperatively is an important factor in evaluating the results of any treatment for MG. Uncorrected crude rates do not correct for length of follow-up. Unfortunately, the majority of the thymectomy literature (including my earlier reports) and all the tables in these reports use only uncorrected

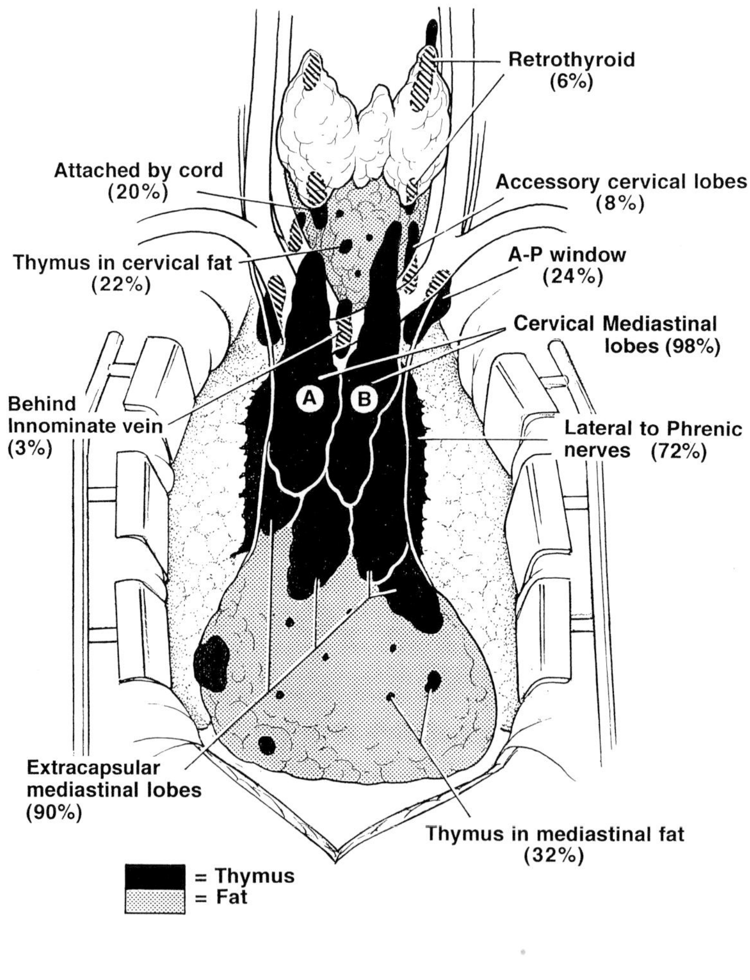

Figure 28A–1. Composite anatomy of the thymus. The illustration is based on surgical-anatomic studies of 50 consecutive transcervical–trans-sternal maximal thymectomies for myasthenia gravis (MG). (Black = thymus; gray = fat which may contain islands of thymus and microscopic thymus). The frequencies (percentages of occurrence) of the variations are noted. There was thymic tissue outside the confines of the cervical-mediastinal lobes (*A*, *B*) in the neck in 32% of the specimens, in the mediastinum in 98%. The maximal thymectomy technique is required to ensure complete removal of these variations. (From Jaretzki A III: Thymectomy for myasthenia gravis: An analysis of the controversies regarding technique and results. Neurology 48 (Suppl): S52–S63, 1997, with permission.)

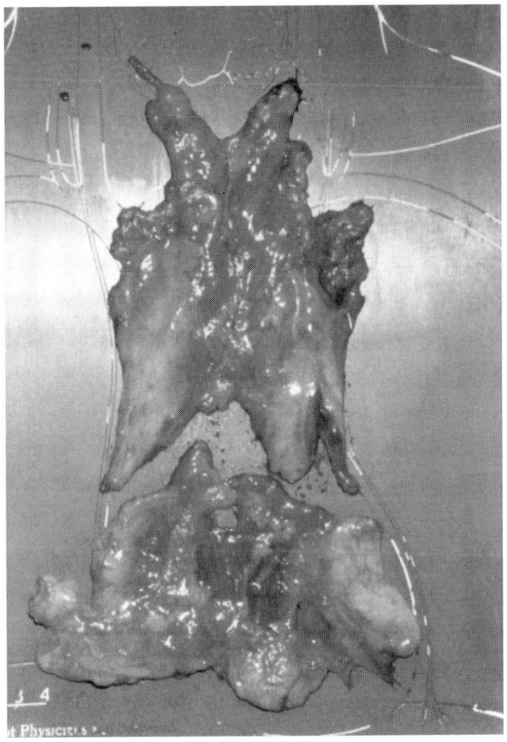

Figure 28A–2. Photograph of the typical transcervical-transsternal maximal thymectomy specimen. The specimen consists of the en bloc resected cervical and mediastinal thymus, suspected thymus, and pretracheal and anterior mediastinal fat, from thyroid isthmus to diaphragm, with adherent mediastinal pleural sheets bilaterally. The specimen was divided *after* removal to indicate the division between the grossly visable thymus and the inferior anterior mediastinal fat.

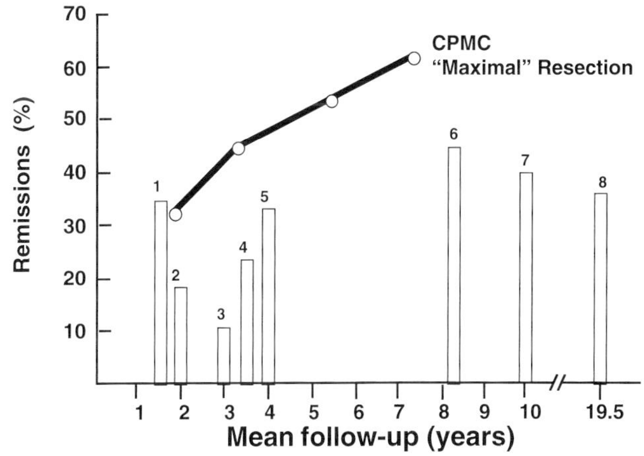

Figure 28A–4. Comparison of Crude Remission Rates Corrected for Mean Follow-up. This analysis indicates that the more aggressive the resection, the better the results; that the extended trans-sternal resection comes closest to the maximal procedure, and that the transcervical–trans-sternal maximal thymectomy results are superior to the other resectional techniques. The remission rates for the Columbia-Presbyterian Medical Center (CPMC) maximal thymectomy are recorded at 2, 3 1/2, 5 1/2, and 7 1/2 years. The bars represent reported thymectomy remissions rates at mean follow-up indicated by the following: #1-Maximal(Ashour); #2-Video-assisted Thoracic Surgery (VATS) [Mack]; #3-Basic Transcervical (series of 2); #4-Standard Trans-sternal (series-of-4); #5-Extended Trans-sternal (series of 4); #6-Extended Transcervical (9); #7-Standard Trans-sternal (MGH); #8-Standard Trans-sternal (Mayo). All data, except for Bar #6, are referenced in the original publication. (From Jaretzki A III: Thymectomy for myasthenia gravis: An analysis of the controversies regarding technique and results. Neurology 48 (Suppl): S52–S63, 1997, with permission.)

crude data. When the uncorrected crude data in these reports are compared with crude data corrected for length of follow-up, as in Figure 28A–4, it becomes clear that the uncorrected data give incorrect information.

Data should not be "mixed." Crude data, crude data corrected for mean length of follow-up, Life Table Analysis

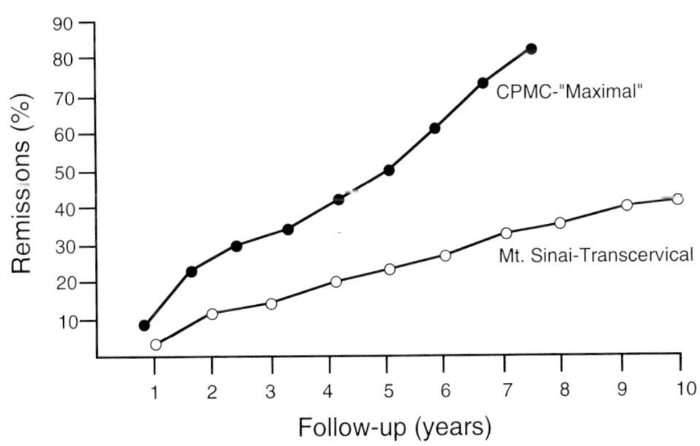

Figure 28A–3. Comparative Life Table Analysis remission rates. Columbia-Presbyterian Medical Center (CPMC) maximal thymectomy[3] is compared with Mt. Sinai basic transcervical thymectomy[8] for patients who have MG without thymoma. The difference is striking. At 7.5 years, the rates are 81% vs. 32%. (From Jaretzki A III, Cooper J, Mulder DG, et al: Symposium: Thymectomy for myasthenia gravis. Contemp Surg 34:65–86, 1989.)

data, and other types of analysis are also erroneously compared in the thymectomy literature. Such comparisons are invalid. Figure 28–6 is such an example, and, accordingly, the comparison is invalid.

Should the mediastinal fat be excised? I think so. It has been suggested that it is not necessary to remove microscopic foci of the thymus and, therefore, not necessary to include in the resection all the mediastinal fat defined in Figure 28A–1, which is removed by maximal thymectomy. Extracapsular masses of thymic tissue, which usually have a gross appearance of fat, may lie at the periphery of the mediastinal fat resection and clearly need to be removed. Moreover, examination of our specimens after reoperations on patients who have had transcervical and standard trans-sternal thymectomies revealed in a number of instances, in addition to missed encapsulated lobes, gross unencapsulated thymus, suggesting the possibility of regeneration. If the meta-analysis using crude data corrected for length of follow-up proves to be valid, the need for the more complete resection will be confirmed.

The following recommendations should be considered in evaluating the role of these minimally invasive procedures:

1. Reserve judgment regarding the role of these minimally invasive resectional procedures in the treatment of MG. They are not as complete as the more extensive procedures, and at this time, the evidence suggests that the results are not comparable.

2. If a videoscopic technique is to be employed, the video-assisted thoracoscopic extended thymectomy (VATET) technique[5, 6] is suggested. This procedure, includes a formal neck dissection and bilateral thoracoscopic approaches, thereby removing the accessory thymic tissue in the neck and giving good bilateral mediastinal exposure.
3. In the resection of thymic neoplasms (regardless of size, lack of preoperative evidence of invasion, or presence of myasthenia gravis), the evidence suggests, as summarized by Lovelace,[7] that any approach that circumvents a complete sternotomy should not be used. These tumors require wide local resection to avoid seeding and late recurrence. Complete removal of all thymic tissue to treat patients who have MG (or prevent its occurrence) is also indicated.
4. Regardless of the approach, injury to the phrenic and recurrent laryngeal nerves must be avoided. Injury to these structures, especially in a patient who has MG, can be devastating.
5. Surgery for the patient who has MG requires excellent preoperative preparation with reversal of oropharyngeal and respiratory muscle weakness, using therapy other than cholinesterease inhibitors alone.
6. In future analysis of the results of thymectomy, it is recommended that the guidelines of the Thymectomy Task Force of the Myasthenia Gravis Foundation of America be followed. The universal use of these guidelines should help resolve the confusion that now exists.

References

1. Jaretzki A III: Thymectomy for myasthenia gravis: An analysis of the controversies regarding technique and results. Neurology 48(Suppl):S52–S63, 1997.
2. Jaretzki A III, Barohn RJ, Ernstoff RM, et al: Thymectomy Task Force of the Medical Advisory Board of the Myasthenia Gravis Foundation of America. Ann Thorac Surg 64:1311, 1997.
3. Jaretzki A III, Penn AS, Younger DS, et al: "Maximal" thymectomy for myasthenia gravis: Results. J Thorac Cardiovasc Surg 95:747–757, 1988.
4. Kaplan EL, Meier P: Nonparametric estimation from incomplete observations. J Am Stat Assoc 53:457–481, 1958.
5. Novellino L, Longoni M, Spinelli L, et al: "Extended" thymectomy, without sternotomy, performed by cervicotomy and thorascopic technique in the treatment of myasthenia gravis. Int Surg 79:378–381, 1994.
6. Scelsi R, Ferro MT, Scelsi L, et al: Detection and morphology of thymic remnants after video-assisted thoracoscopic thymectomy (VATET) in patients with myasthenia gravis. Int Surg 81:14–17, 1996.
7. Lovelace RE, Younger DS: Myasthenia gravis with thymoma. Neurology 48(Suppl):S76–S81, 1997.
8. Papatestas AE, Genkins G, Kornfield P, et al: Effects of thymectomy in myasthenia gravis. Ann Surg 206:79–88; 1987.
9. Bril V, Kojic S, Ilse W, et al: Long-term clinical outcome after transcervical thymectomy for myasthenia gravis. Ann Thorac Surg 65:1520–1522, 1998.

COMMENTARY

Michael J. Mack

The previous insightful commentary, written by a physician who is acknowledged to be one of the world's foremost experts on the role of thymectomy in myasthenia gravis, deserves careful consideration and analysis. Dr. Jaretzki outlines the problems appropriately and makes judgments about the evidence in support of each technique. He offers an assessment of difficult-to-evaluate data and makes recommendations regarding video-assisted thoracic surgery (VATS) as it applies to thymectomy. With some of these recommendations I wholeheartedly agree, and with some I respectfully disagree. The goal of thymectomy by any approach should be removal of all *gross* thymic tissue. There is a recognized wide variability in size, number, and location of lobes in the mediastinum and neck area, all of which should be resected en bloc. It is true that lack of clinical improvement has been associated with incomplete resection; moreover, reoperation and resection of a "missed" grossly identifiable lobe or thymic remnant has resulted in clinical improvement, even when as little as 2 g of tissue are found. Although it is also true that microscopic remnants of thymic tissue have been identified in detailed anatomic descriptions by Masaoka[1] in extra-anatomic mediastinal locations, it has not been demonstrated that these microscopic foci are clinically relevant.

Myasthenia gravis is a disease of significant variability in its natural course, and no randomized controlled trial has ever been performed that has documented the benefit of thymectomy compared with medical therapy, nor is such a trial likely to be done. We are, therefore, left with trying to sort out the results of a number of published series conducted by different techniques, all of which have negligible mortality and minimal morbidity for clinical response outcome analysis. Each series has individual data recording severity of disease, duration of preoperative symptoms, demographic composition (including mean age and gender), and duration of follow-up. All of these variables are known to affect outcomes. Additionally, the parameters used in different series to describe disease severity as well as clinical improvement vary widely, again confounding meaningful analysis. In the presence of all these factors, it is impossible to make a definitive assessment and statements regarding outcome efficacy.

Experience with VATS thymectomy is limited and there does not yet exist extensive data regarding long-term results. Although our remission rate (88%) is comparable with those of published series of thymectomy performed by other techniques,[2] our complete response rate is lower (18.2%), appropriately raising concerns regarding incomplete resection. However, because the mean follow-up time is short—29 months—and because the complete remission rate continues to improve up to 5 years after thymectomy, we anticipate that more of our patients will achieve complete remission. In addition, a significant number of our patients were older than 50 years (N = 7), and in this age group thymectomy is known to be less effective than in younger patients; however, it is incumbent upon us to demonstrate equivalent results in more patients with longer follow-up.

We agree with Dr. Jaretzki's assessment that the degree of resection by VATS is not as extensive as by the extended transthoracic or the maximal combined transthoracic and transcervical techniques. We also agree with his assessment that VATS thymectomy is more complete than either the standard trans-sternal approach or the standard or extended transcervical approach. However, as mentioned earlier, the clinical relevance of this remains to be determined. Even the most radical resections result in only a 50% complete response rate, leading one to believe that patient selection and disease variability significantly affect surgical outcomes.

Although morbidity is a minor concern with all approaches, the VATS approach is clearly less invasive than the trans-sternal and maximal techniques, and I submit that this is true for the transcervical approach also. The VATS approach is clearly the most cosmetically acceptable of all techniques, and although critics argue that cosmesis should be at best a minor factor in choosing an approach, this is clearly a major factor for some patients, especially young women, who represent a significant number of patients who have the disease. It is hoped that a less invasive approach that does not compromise the degree of resection will lead to more rapid acceptance by patient and neurologist, and that this acceptance would lead to earlier intervention in the course of the disease, which is known to lead to better outcomes.

I disagree that the addition of a cervical incision to VATS is to be recommended. The cervical area is well visualized and accessed by a VATS-only approach, especially when an adjuvant pneumomediastinum is added. I also do not feel that a limited encapsulated stage 1 thymoma is a contraindication to the VATS approach. We are able to perform the same resection by VATS as by the trans-sternal approach (wide local), and placement of excised tissue in an endoscopic bag before extraction obviates any concerns about tumor seeding. Additionally, we have had neither phrenic nor recurrent laryngeal nerve injury, nor am I aware of any reports of such.

I do agree with following the guidelines of the Thymectomy Task Force of the Myasthenia Gravis Foundation of America in future outcome analysis. Adherence to these guidelines should help resolve some of the confusion that exists when opinion prevails over objectivity. We look to Dr. Jaretzki to provide continuing leadership in this field.

References

1. Masaoka A, Monden Y, Seike Y, et al: Reoperation after transcervical thymectomy for myasthenia gravis. Neurology 32;83–85, 1982.
2. Mack MJ, Landreneau RJ, Yim AP, et al: Results of VATS thymectomy in patients with myasthenia gravis. J Thorac Cardiovasc Surg 112:1352–1360, 1996.
3. Jaretzki A III, Barohn R, Kaminski H, et al: Thymectomy Task Force of the Medical Advisory Board of the Myasthenia Gravis Foundation of America. Ann Thorac Surg 1997;64:1311.

COMMENTARY

Toni Lerut

For several decades, three accepted approaches of thymectomy for myasthenia gravis have been in use (i.e., the trans-sternal approach with maximal tissue clearance, the trans-sternal approach with partial sternotomy, and the transcervical approach). There is, however, no consensus as to which approach is the best. The reasons for this lack of unanimity are threefold. First, all three procedures seemingly offer equal long-term results, and it is really not known whether every thymocyte needs to be removed. Second, extended long-term follow-up is required to judge the final results. Third, there are simply too few patients to set up large controlled, randomized trials to evaluate the value of each of the three techniques.

The recent introduction of the thoracoscopic approach creates new perspectives, but in the meantime, this new technique also fuels the debate about which is the preferred surgical access. Skeptics question the completeness of thymectomy when performed by video-assisted thoracic surgery (VATS), particularly when the procedure involves the cervical excision of the gland.

This criticism is enhanced by the existing controversy over which approach—left or right—is preferable. Some groups even use a combined VATS and cervical approach or perform thymectomy through bilateral VATS dissection.

This controversy clearly illustrates the fact that the VATS approach is still surrounded by some doubt regarding its usefulness. Further long-term results are needed before neurologists will accept the widespread application of VATS for thymectomy.

What then makes the VATS approach so attractive? Claims that VATS patients have less consumption of pain medication and shorter hospital stays are noted to be the most obvious advantages. These advantages, however, are relative and probably not significant, because most patients who undergo transcervical thymectomy or thymectomy through a partial sternotomy can generally be discharged after 2 to 4 days. Moreover, the VATS approach has its own set of potential complications, and, occasionally, disabling postthoracoscopy intercostal neuralgia does occur.

Perhaps a more important advantage is cosmesis. Patients who have myasthenia gravis, especially women, seem to be particularly averse to the presence of a scar on the neck or, even more, over the proximal part of the sternum. In my opinion, treatment of patients who have myasthenia gravis is one of the very few indications in which cosmesis is an acceptable argument for performing minimally invasive surgery, such as VATS thymectomy. This consideration was taken into account in our own decision to favor a VATS approach for thymectomy in the treatment of myasthenia gravis.

Data for a total of 31 thymectomies for treatment of patients with myasthenia gravis have been collected and analyzed. These patients were operated on in two university institutions (both universities were in Rome, and the surgeons were Drs. Mineo and Leuven). Myasthenia was clinically staged according to a modified Osserman classification: classes I (N = 6), II (N = 13), III (N = 10), and IV (N = 2). Intentional extended thymectomy was always pursued to completely remove both thymic gland and mediastinal fatty tissue as potential sites of ectopic thymic islets. Postoperatively, reduction of pyridostigmine dosage, remission rate, improvement rate, and change in Osserman class were recorded at 3, 6, 12, and 24 months. One patient required conversion to median sternotomy. Operative complications included transient ventricular arrhythmia in three patients. Mean operative time was 143 minutes. Histopathologic diagnoses included 9 lymphofollicular hyperplasias and 4 encapsulated thymomas. Neither mortality nor major morbidity occurred postoperatively. Mean hospital stay was 5.4 days. Mean follow-up was 29.7 months. At 24 months, use of pyridostigmine decreased from a mean of 302 to 200 mg/day, mean Osserman class decreased from 2.2 to 0.9 (analysis of variance $P < 0.05$), whereas remission and improvement rates calculated by the Kaplan-Meer method were 31% (N = 8) and 90% (N = 27), respectively. The results are similar to those of historical control subjects who were treated with open surgery.

A major issue is the continued treatment of patients who did not respond after thymectomy. Occasionally, favourable reports of redo surgery have been published, but they are too few for any conclusions to be drawn as to the level of completeness of the previous thymectomy and the status of the surrounding thymic tissue. At present, little is known about redo surgery after VATS thymectomy, including findings at surgery and patient outcomes. Perhaps a more aggressive position in regard to redo surgery, using a classic open approach for those who do not respond to VATS surgery is warranted, and this will provide more information about whether VATS thymectomy is indeed as complete a procedure as open surgery.

A word of caution is required regarding the author's attitude toward thymectomy for thymoma, even when restricting the indication to small and well-encapsulated Masaoka stage I cases. Masaoka staging is pathologic analysis. Therefore, only the pathologist is able to tell whether the tumor is really completely encapsulated. Converting to an open operation when signs of tissue plane invasion are discovered is a dangerous procedure that carries the risk of microscopic tumor seeding during the operation. Complete resection is the only chance for cure of this condition; therefore, no treatment that jeopardizes the patient's outcome should be accepted.

In conclusion, VATS thymectomy offers an attractive dimension to the spectrum of treatment modalities for myasthenia gravis. The technique is safe, but remaining doubts related to the completeness of the resection require further clarification through analysis of long-term outcomes and findings at the time of redo surgery, when indicated. Obviously, VATS thymectomy should be performed by surgeons familiar with open surgery, and premature widespread application may jeopardize the future of this approach. For patients who have thymoma, aggressive radical resection through an open approach remains the treatment of choice and offers the best chance for cure.

Chapter 29

Posterior Mediastinal Masses

Jeanne M. Lukanich, Raphael Bueno, and David J. Sugarbaker

During the 1990s, the utility of videothoracoscopy and minimally invasive techniques in both the diagnosis and treatment of intrathoracic lesions has rapidly evolved and become well established.[9] We review posterior mediastinal masses and their treatment and focus on minimally invasive techniques that can be and have been strategically applied for diagnosis and definitive therapy.

Posterior Mediastinal Masses

Classification

Posterior mediastinal masses are located in the posterior mediastinal compartment, which is composed of the paravertebral sulci and the extreme dorsal portion of the central or visceral compartment, located posterior to the trachea and the heart (Fig. 29–1). Twenty-six percent of all mediastinal tumors are located in the posterior mediastinum,[7] making it the second most common anatomic location for mediastinal masses. The vast majority of posterior mediastinal tumors in adults are benign, but statistically there is a greater chance of malignancy with decreasing age of the patient or very advanced age.[12] Neurogenic tumors and primary cysts constitute the major pathologic entities of the posterior mediastinum, although numerous others have been reported.[8, 15, 22, 29, 31]

Neurogenic tumors make up the most common group of posterior mediastinal masses (Table 29–1) and account for 20 to 30% of all mediastinal masses.[1, 39] They are slightly more common in females than in males and occur with equal frequency in both paravertebral sulci. Most neurogenic tumors are discovered in the upper half of the chest. They can be further divided into categories based on the neural tissue of origin and also classified into benign and malignant counterparts. Neurilemomas and malignant schwannomas compose approximately 55% of neurogenic tumors.[14] Ganglioneuromas and ganglioneuroblastomas arise from sympathetic ganglion nerve cells in adults; they account for 30 to 35% of neurogenic posterior mediastinal tumors. Neurofibromas represent approximately 10% of neurogenic tumors. They contain both a nerve sheath and nerve cell components.[1, 30] Tumors of paraganglionic origin are rare.[12] Less than 10% of all neurogenic posterior mediastinal tumors are malignant in adults.

Mediastinal cysts compose the other common group of posterior mediastinal masses (Table 29–2).[7] The vast majority of mediastinal cysts are benign. They arise principally from secretory cells of the esophagus, respiratory tract, and pericardium or from the thoracic duct or spinal meninges. Bronchogenic cysts are the most prevalent and account for 60% of mediastinal cysts.

A variety of other types of tumors compose the last major group of posterior mediastinal masses (Table 29–3).[41] Benign and malignant lymph nodes, although more common in the anterior and middle mediastinum, may present as posterior mediastinal masses.[19, 39, 43] It should also be remembered that other entities in proximity to the posterior mediastinum may protrude into or abut the posterior mediastinum, mimicking a true posterior mediastinal mass.

Clinical Presentation

The clinical presentation of a posterior mediastinal mass is variable, and as many as 50 to 70% are found incidentally.[19] Approximately half of these lesions are asymptomatic. As the majority of the series published in the literature group all mediastinal masses together, large series restricted to posterior mediastinal masses and their symptoms are not available when clinical presentations are categorized. Symptoms on presentation depend on the type of mass and its malignant potential.[6, 7] When present, symptoms are vague, but can generally be divided into the following categories: pain, compressive symptoms, infectious complications, and systemic effects.

Size

The size of the mass generally correlates with the severity of pain when pain is present. In general, larger mediastinal masses are associated with greater pain. The exact location of the mass in the posterior mediastinum, however, is the most important predicator of pain. Pain is often described as back or upper extremity pain, but can vary greatly. A rostrally situated mass may cause a general feeling of fullness. More caudally, pain is usually localized and can range from very mild to severe. Pain may have a radicular quality, especially if the mediastinal mass involves or impinges on nerve roots.[19] Pain may also be caused by direct invasion into malignant masses, but erosion can occur in large benign masses as well.[6, 12] Commonly invaded structures include the bony spine, the chest wall, the pleura, and adjacent nerves or ganglia.

Compression

Mechanical compressive symptoms are more common in children than in adults[12, 39] and generally fall into four categories: esophageal, vascular, airway, and spinal. Esophageal compression occurs by virtue of the proximity of the esophagus to a lesion in the posterior mediastinum, and translates into dysphagia, and, rarely, complete obstruction.[3] Vascular compression may involve the vena cavae, especially the superior vena cava, and, occasionally, the subclavian and azygos veins. Vascular compression is almost exclusively venous and may present as lower extremity or upper extremity isolated swelling or as a more gen-

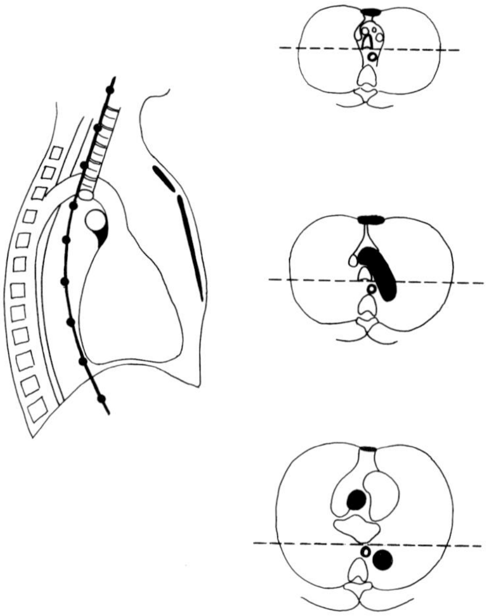

Figure 29–1. Posterior mediastinum. Cross-sectional illustration demonstrates the boundary of the posterior mediastinum at various levels. Note that this boundary moves anteriorly as the superior mediastinum is approached.

eralized superior vena cava syndrome. Superior vena cava syndrome is most likely to occur in the setting of a malignant superior posterior mediastinal mass in the presence of fixation.[6, 39] Airway distortion caused by posterior mediastinal masses is more common in infants and children than in adults. Cough and dyspnea may be present,[6] and the patient's position may exacerbate symptoms. Stridor caused by a posterior mediastinal masses is rare. Spinal cord compression may result in pain or focal neurologic deficits. Horner's syndrome may occur, especially if the posterior mediastinal mass is located superiorly in the thorax.[19] Paraplegia has been reported. Diaphragmatic paralysis may occur from either pressure or direct phrenic nerve invasion.[10]

Infection

Infectious symptoms arising from posterior mediastinal masses may be the result of compression of an airway owing to a benign mass, generally a mediastinal cyst,[40] with postobstructive pneumonitis. Fever and leukocytosis are frequent. Infection may lead to a general septic state with manifestations of lethargy, bacteremia, and, rarely, multiorgan dysfunction. Neurogenic tumors rarely cause infectious complications unless they are massive.

Systemic Evidence

Systemic evidence of posterior mediastinal masses may be found with both benign and malignant masses, but it is more commonly in the latter disease processes.[39] Malignant neurogenic tumors are often associated with constitutional symptoms, such as general malaise and fever. Neurofibromas often occur in association with von Recklinghausen's disease, a hereditary condition characterized by multiple neurofibromas and other tumors of fibroblastic origin. Systemic manifestations in this disease can vary greatly, from limited benign cutaneous lesions to seizures and mental retardation. It is important to recognize von Recklinghausen's disease, because of the risk of malignant degeneration in these neurogenic tumors.[1]

Neurogenic tumors of paraganglionic origin may be chemically active and generate systemic symptoms. These symptoms are similar to those of active pheochromocytoma and include paroxysmal or persistently recalcitrant hypertension, tachycardia, headache, diabetes mellitus, and hypermetabolism.[12, 39] Neuroblastoma, an aggressive malignant tumor of the autonomic nervous system that occurs in infants and young children, often causes symptoms attributable to mechanical compression or pain caused by metastatic disease.[20] Acute cerebellar ataxia with opsoclonus or chaotic nystagmus has been described. These abnormal eye movements are the result of immune complex production.[39]

Cystic posterior mediastinal masses rarely cause systemic symptoms but may be associated with generalized or systemic disorders. Neuroenteric cysts are seen predominantly in infants who have congenital abnormalities of the bony spine, spinal canal, or alimentary tract as a result of embryologic developmental dysfunction.[39]

Lymphomas of the posterior mediastinum, although much less common than neurogenic tumors or mediastinal cysts, often exhibit systemic manifestations that are well known to most clinicians. Fever, fatigue, weight loss, night sweats, and pruritus are quite common, and their presence or absence must always be documented during investigation of a posterior mediastinal mass. Chronic anemia or dysproteinemia syndromes have been described in patients who have benign mediastinal lymph node hyperplasia (Castleman's disease).[19]

Table 29–1. Posterior Mediastinal Masses: Group 1 (Neurogenic Tumors)

Origin	Benign	Malignant
Nerve sheath	Neurilemoma	Malignant schwannoma
Autonomic ganglia	Ganglioneuroma	Ganglioneuroblastoma
		Neuroblastoma
Nerve sheath and nerve cell	Neurofibroma	Neurofibroma
Sympathetic nerve	Pheochromocytoma	Malignant pheochromocytoma
Parasympathetic nerve	Paraganglioma	Malignant paraganglioma
Neuroectodermal stem cell		Small cell (Askin's tumor)

Table 29–2. Posterior Mediastinal Masses: Group 2

Cysts
Bronchogenic cyst
Cystic hygroma
Enteric duplication cyst
Meningocele
Neurenteric cyst
Pericardial cyst
Thoracic duct cyst

Patient Evaluation

The workup for posterior mediastinal masses involves a number of modalities. The importance of an accurate history and physical examination cannot be overemphasized. They provide the foundation on which other diagnostic studies are based. Some posterior mediastinal masses are associated with specific syndromes, whereas others produce systemic effects; therefore, the presence or even absence of physical findings may affect the differential diagnosis. Information from the history and physical examination should be used to narrow the differential diagnosis. Further workup can be directed toward the most likely diagnoses. Previous operations may provide clues to diagnosis on history. Special attention to adenopathy should be given to all lymph-node–bearing regions during physical examination. A complete neurologic evaluation is mandatory for posterior mediastinal masses and may identify spinal involvement of neurogenic tumors.

Chest Roentgenography (CXR)

Commonly, chest roentgenography (CXR) suggests or confirms a posterior mediastinal mass. A mediastinal mass can often be localized to the posterior mediastinum on standard posterior and anterior (PA) and lateral CXRs. These radiographs provide information on tumor size, density, bilaterality, the presence of calcification, and other associated thoracic processes or abnormalities, such as bony involvement.

Table 29–3. Posterior Mediastinal Masses: Group 3

Other Tumors	
Benign	**Malignant**
Castleman's disease	
	Chordoma
Ectopic extramedullary hematopoietic tissue	Extramedullary plasmacytoma
Fibroma	Fibrosarcoma
Hemangioepithelioma	
Lipoma	Liposarcoma
Lymph nodes	Lymphoma
Rare infections	
Teratoma	
Tumors arising outside of the mediastinum and projecting into the posterior mediastinum	

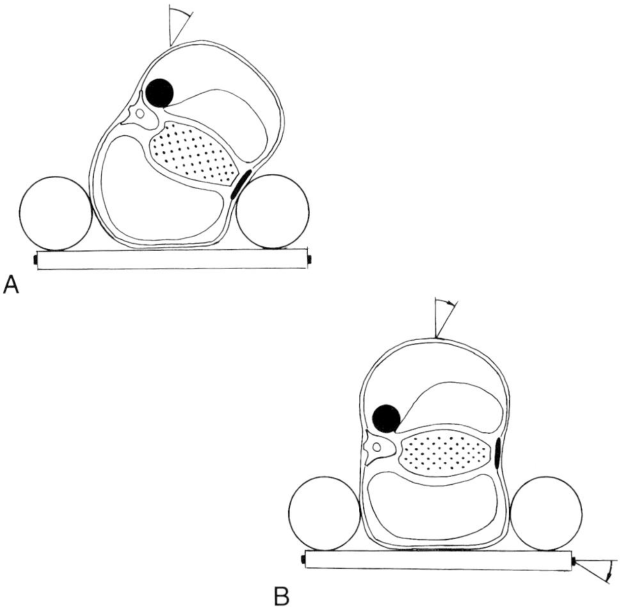

Figure 29–2. Videothoracoscopic positioning for resection of a posterior mediastinal mass. *A*, Extreme lateral decubitus position; *B*, lateral decubitus position with rotation of the operating table.

Computed Tomography (CT)

Scanning of the thorax by CT is the preferred imaging modality for the mediastinum in general. Because CT scanning is readily available and easily interpreted by radi-

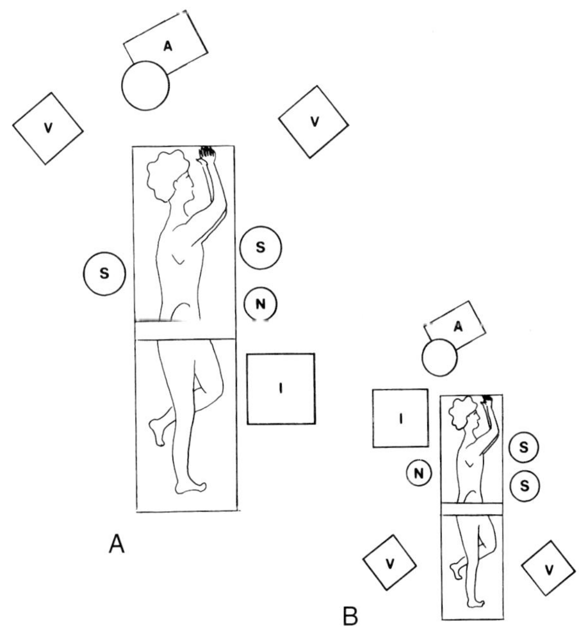

Figure 29–3. Operating room layout. *A*, Mass located in upper hemithorax; *B*, mass located in inferior hemithorax. Indicators: A = anesthesia, V = videothoracoscopy monitor, S = surgeon, N = scrub nurse or scrub technician, I = instrument table.

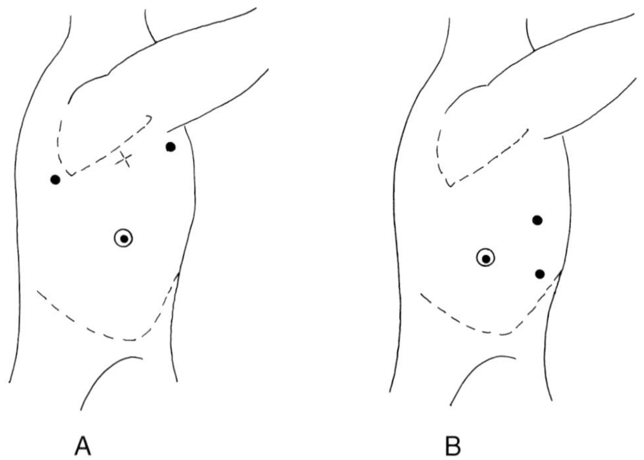

Figure 29–4. Port positioning for videothoracoscopic resection of a posterior mediastinal mass. *A*, Mass located in superior hemithorax; *B*, mass located in inferior hemithorax. Indicators: bull's-eye = initial camera port, X = alternative working port.

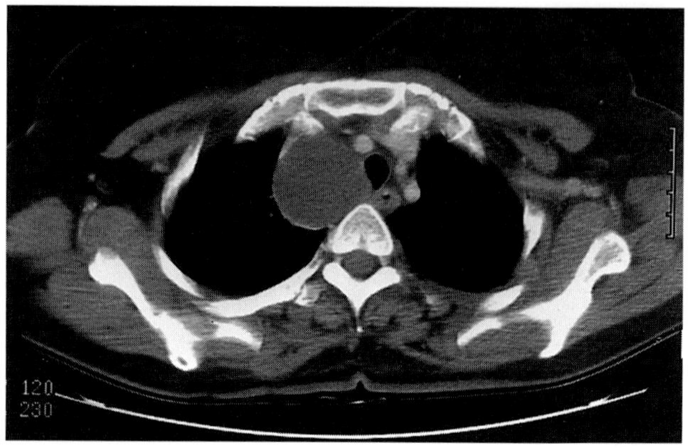

Figure 29–6. Computed tomography scan corresponding to Figure 29–5, showing a representative cross-sectional image of this bronchogenic cyst.

ologists and thoracic surgeons, it is the gold standard for the evaluation of a posterior mediastinal mass.[23] With posterior mediastinal masses, the information provided by this modality includes exact location, density with identification of the cystic component, tumor extension or invasion, relationships with other surrounding structures, and other associated intrathoracic abnormalities. Finally, this modality is beneficial in planning surgical resection.

Nuclear Scanning

Nuclear scanning for posterior mediastinal masses provides little additional information in the workup of posterior mediastinal masses. Thallium scanning is rarely useful for neurogenic tumors or cystic masses. Occasionally, it is used as an adjunct study in lymphoma, but it is neither sensitive nor specific for that disease. Bone scanning is occasionally obtained to document bony spine or rib involvement, because this may affect further workup, tumor staging, or the surgical approach.[19] This information is often available from the CT scan and the CXR alone. Bony abnormalities remote from the mass, however, may significantly alter the working diagnosis of a mediastinal mass. Paragangliomas and pheochromocytomas have a propensity to spread to the bone. A metaiodobenzylguanidine (MIBG) scan detects neuroblastoma and pheochromocytomas,[19, 23] because the diagnostic compound is a precursor of epinephrine. Technetium-99 pertechnate scans can be used to identify gastric mucosa in enteric cysts.[23]

Magnetic Resonance Imaging (MRI)

Magnetic resonance imaging (MRI) is a more recent radiologic modality that is rarely required in the evaluation of a posterior mediastinal mass. Little additional information is obtained in addition to that garnered from CT scanning. Occasionally, MRI may be useful when the mass is located in the extremes of the hemithorax, or closely associated with the aortic arch. MRI has the capability of confirming or ruling out vascular involvement, or identifying vascular abnormalities posing as posterior mediastinal masses. Rarely, the arterial feeding vessel of a pulmonary sequestration may be identified. Scanning with MRI is also

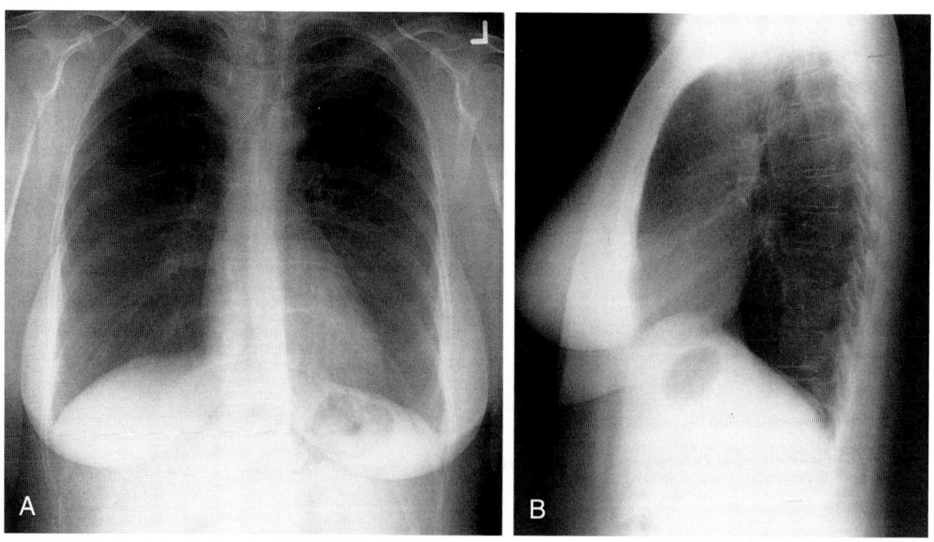

Figure 29–5. *A*, Posteroanterior and *B*, lateral radiographs of a 49-year-old woman demonstrating a mediastinal mass located in the superior aspect of the right hemithorax.

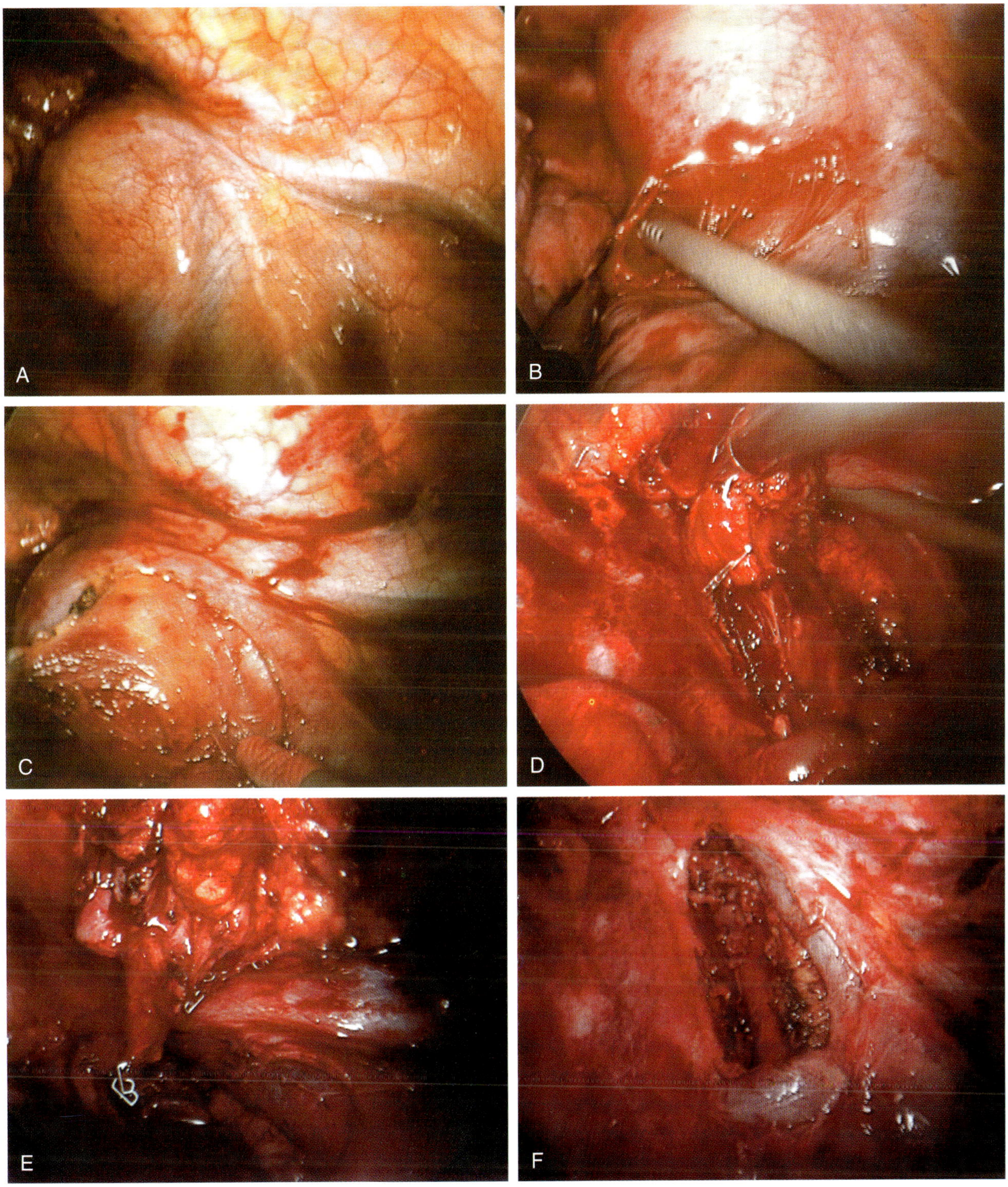

Figure 29–7. Videothoracoscopic resection of a benign posterior mediastinal cyst. *A,* In situ cyst: Note the proximity of the azygos vein inferiorly and the draping of the superior vena cava with the phrenic nerve over the cyst anterosuperiorly. *B,* Division of the pleura at the posterior edge of the cyst by means of endoscopic scissors followed by blunt dissection of the cyst with a mounted sponge. *C,* Cyst freed circumferentially from surrounding tissues. The superior vena cava is well mobilized. *D,* Blunt dissection of the cyst out of the mediastinum. Cyst is decompressed. Attachments remain superiorly. *E,* View of the cyst following stapled division of the cyst wall at the thoracic inlet. *F,* Bed of the mediastinal cyst following excision. The superior vena cava and azygos vein are clearly demonstrated.

performed to identify spinal involvement in neurogenic tumors suspicious for being "dumbbell" tumors.[12, 23, 34]

Other Imaging Modalities

Other imaging studies may occasionally be indicated. Barium swallow can define the relationship of a posterior mediastinal mass to the esophagus. Esophageal ultrasound (EUS) can be used to delineate leiomyomas and some enteric cysts.[2, 3, 23, 30] Rarely, angiography may be needed to define a vascular lesion.

Fine needle aspiration (FNA) biopsy with radiologic guidance is an extremely useful modality in the workup of a posterior mediastinal mass.[7, 19, 35] In the case of a solid mass, a diagnosis of neural tumor or lymphoma can often be made. Neurogenic tumors may be difficult to characterize in detail because of low cellularity and similarities in appearance between types.[23] Lymphomas are now often subtyped with FNA by using monoclonal antibodies.[23] Biopsy diagnosis by FNA of extramedullary hematopoiesis has been described.[11] As is always the case, the ability to make a diagnosis is dependent on the experience of the cytopathologist, but the literature supports this modality in making confident diagnoses. With cystic masses, FNA may be used to temporize surgical intervention by decompression, but typically they recur. Aspiration of all infected cysts allows microbiologic evaluation so that antimicrobial treatment can be specifically directed.[32]

Serum biochemical markers are of limited use in the workup of posterior mediastinal masses. Catecholamines and their degradation products may be elevated in pheochromocytoma.[19, 42] Ferritin may be elevated in neuroblastoma or ganglioneuroblastoma.[23]

Videothoracoscopy

Diagnostic Thoracoscopy

Simple diagnostic thoracoscopy for posterior mediastinal masses is uncommon, but, nonetheless, it should be in the armamentarium of thoracic surgeons. Diagnostic thoracoscopy should be used selectively and undertaken only when other, less invasive, procedures prove nondiagnostic. The merits of the procedure are wide views of the mediastinum, the ability to take multiple biopsy specimens with frozen section confirmation or guidance, and the ability to obtain concurrent biopsies of lung parenchyma and pleural abnormalities.[13, 33] Inspection with incisional or excisional biopsy is most appropriate for posterior mediastinal lymphadenopathy in which a diagnosis of lymphoma is suspected.[32, 43] Small, solid, well-circumscribed tumors should be excised completely at the initial setting if a tissue diagnosis has not yet been made. Cystic masses should be recognized on radiologic workup before thoracoscopy is performed, thereby shifting the procedure from a diagnostic to a therapeutic modality. Occasionally, patients who have large posterior mediastinal masses, or masses juxtaposed to significant anatomic structures, may benefit from diagnostic thoracoscopy before the appropriate surgical approach for resection is chosen.[36]

Therapeutic Thoracoscopy

The mainstay of therapy for posterior mediastinal masses is resection or excision; on occasion, aspiration or unroofing is indicated. Minimally invasive videothoracoscopic counterparts to standard open procedures have now been performed safely,[2, 4, 10, 13, 16, 17, 24, 26, 29, 32, 37] and widespread development of these techniques is under way.

Since 1991, reports of thoracoscopic treatments of nearly every type of posterior mediastinal mass have become commonplace in the medical literature. Resection of neurogenic tumors; esophageal leiomyoma; and benign lymph node hyperplasia, resection, or drainage of bronchogenic cysts and various other treatments of disease entities have been described.[2, 4, 5, 16, 21, 22, 24, 25, 27, 32, 36, 37] In patients who are medical candidates for thoracoscopy, videothoracoscopic resection of a well-defined and well-circumscribed posterior mediastinal mass should be considered.

Age

Age is not a contraindication for thoracoscopic resection of a posterior mediastinal mass if the patient's general medical and cardiopulmonary status allow general anesthesia with single-lung ventilation.[9] However, the age of the patient is important in decision-making regarding the malignant potential of individual posterior mediastinal lesions. At present, general use of thoracoscopic resection cannot be recommended for the treatment of malignant posterior mediastinal masses, because these techniques are not easily accomplished with invasive tumors. Open thoracotomy remains the standard approach for cancer operations and likely offers the highest chance of cure.

Size

Size of a posterior mediastinal mass is important and should be considered while planning an attempt at thoracoscopic resection. An extremely large solid tumor

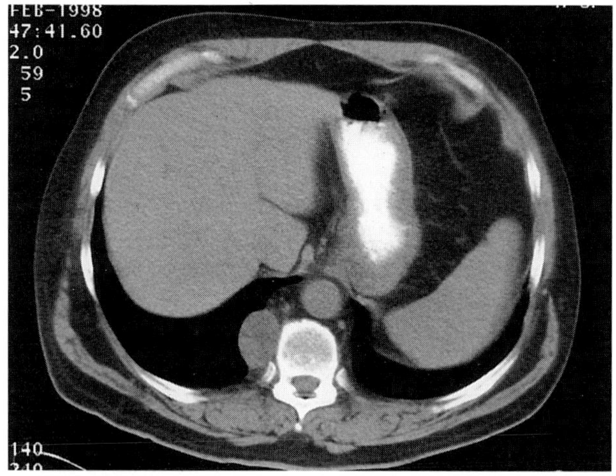

Figure 29–8. Computed tomography scan of a 60-year-old man, demonstrating an asymptomatic posterior mediastinal neurogenic tumor in the lower right hemithorax.

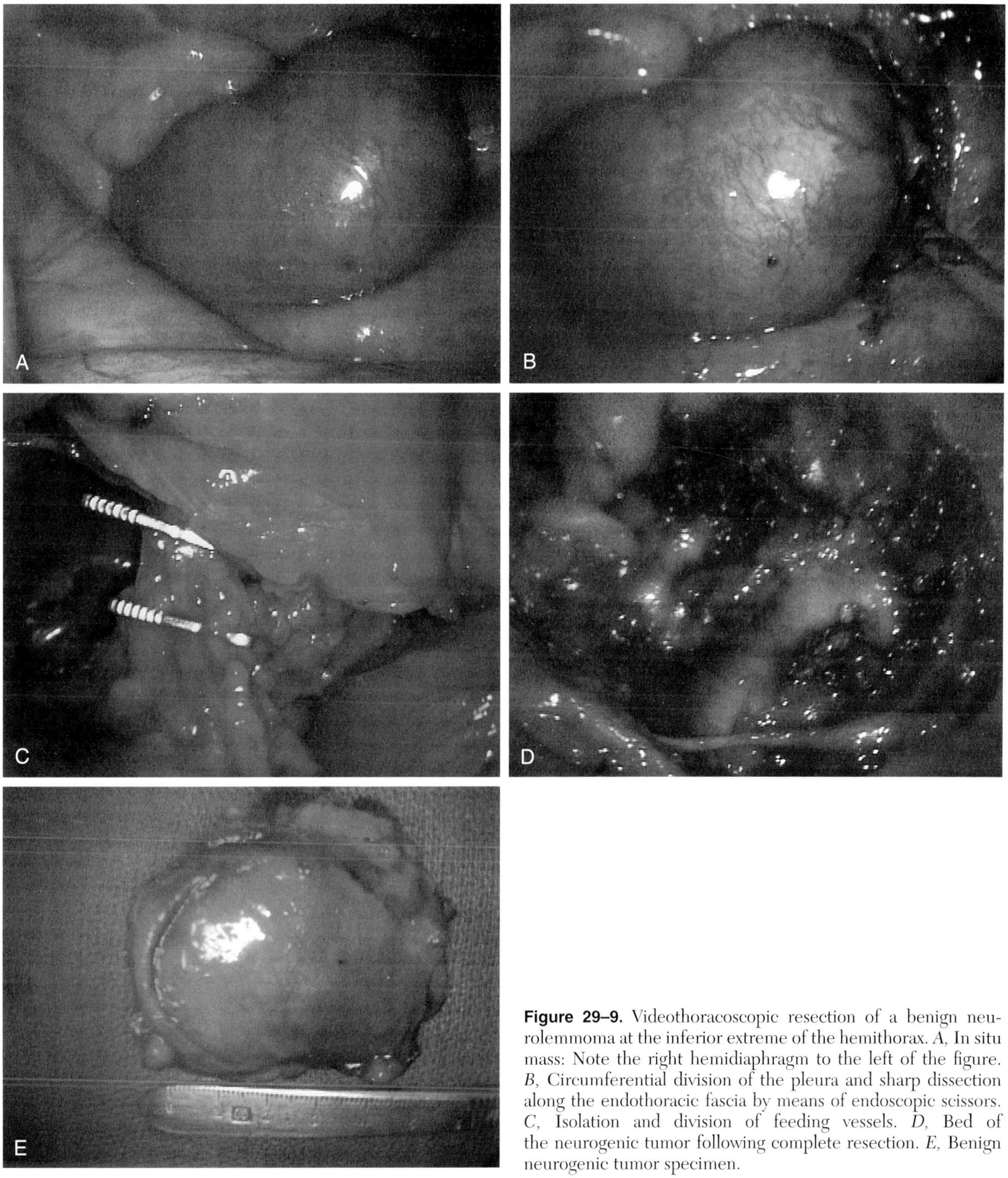

Figure 29–9. Videothoracoscopic resection of a benign neurolemmoma at the inferior extreme of the hemithorax. *A,* In situ mass: Note the right hemidiaphragm to the left of the figure. *B,* Circumferential division of the pleura and sharp dissection along the endothoracic fascia by means of endoscopic scissors. *C,* Isolation and division of feeding vessels. *D,* Bed of the neurogenic tumor following complete resection. *E,* Benign neurogenic tumor specimen.

may prove difficult to resect thoracoscopically[4] because exposure and retraction are limited by present instrumentation and the confines and anatomy of the bony thorax. Solid masses of even moderate size and cystic masses resected without intraoperative drainage will require a utility thoracotomy for removal, and the procedure should be carefully thought out during the planning process.[35, 36]

Location

Exact location of a posterior mediastinal mass may make thoracoscopic resection difficult, because of proximity of surrounding structures or difficulty with visualization and exposure. Lesions at the extremes of the hemithorax may prove difficult to resect safely, although new instrumentation and the placement of additional ports for exposure

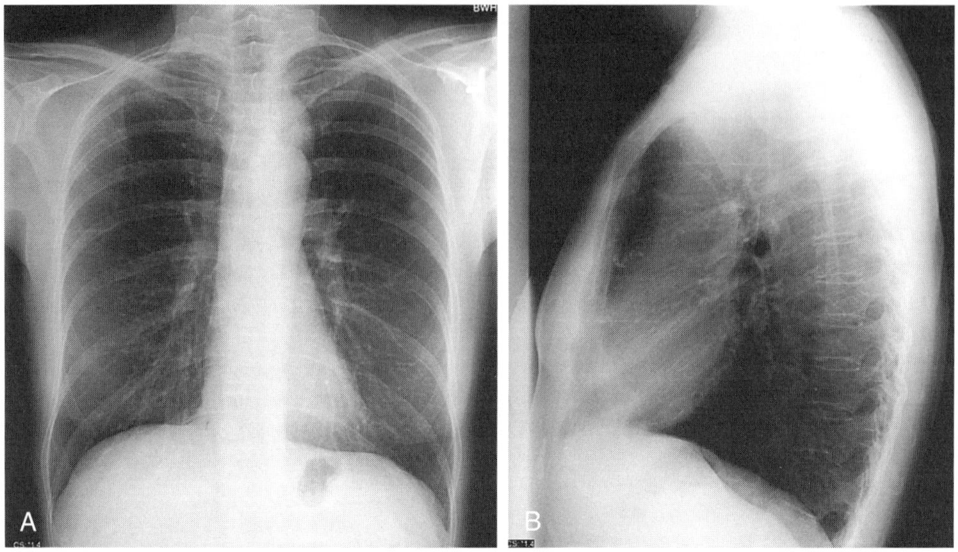

Figure 29–10. *A*, Posteroanterior and *B*, lateral chest radiographs of a 63-year-old woman demonstrating a left-sided posterior mediastinal mass abutting the aortic arch.

may improve thoracoscopic resectability.[32] Solid masses near the aortic arch also present similar challenges.

Contraindications

Other contraindications to thoracoscopic resection are dependent on diagnosis. Neurogenic tumors that have a high likelihood of malignancy (those in children younger than 16 years of age) or that extend through the vertebral foramina or into the intradural space should be excluded from consideration for treatment by thoracoscopic resection alone.[18] Large infected cysts should also be excluded from attempts at thoracoscopic resection if the risk of pleural contamination in a given patient is considered substantial.[16]

All patients undergoing attempted thoracoscopic resection of posterior mediastinal masses should be asked to sign consent for possible thoracotomy, and the implications of this procedure should be discussed preoperatively.[31] The surgeon should remain cognizant that the videothoracoscopic approach should achieve as complete a resection as that obtained with the standard open approach. The procedure should be converted to a thoracotomy if this is not technically possible.

Videothoracoscopic Technique

Contraindications

The preoperative evaluation for thoracoscopic resection of a posterior mediastinal mass should be identical to that obtained before thoracotomy is performed. Contraindications for thoracoscopic resection of a posterior mediastinal mass include pleural symphysis and the inability of the patient to tolerate single-lung ventilation.[21] As mentioned, videothoracoscopic resection is also generally contraindicated in the case of a known malignant posterior mediastinal mass.[35]

Procedural Details

Placement of a thoracic epidural catheter is commonly performed preoperatively at our institution. The patient is then brought to the operating room and, under general anesthesia, intubated with a double-lumen endotracheal tube that allows single-lung ventilation. An orogastric tube is passed. The appropriate lung is collapsed. The patient is placed in a lateral decubitus position. The patient may be rotated slightly more anteriorly than the classic posi-tion for posterolateral thoracotomy (Fig. 29–2*A*), or the operating table is rotated to achieve this position (Fig. 29–2*B*).[16, 21, 22, 25, 28, 35] The patient is prepared and draped as for thoracotomy. Two video monitors are placed on either side of the patient's shoulders to provide the optimal view for all members of the surgical team

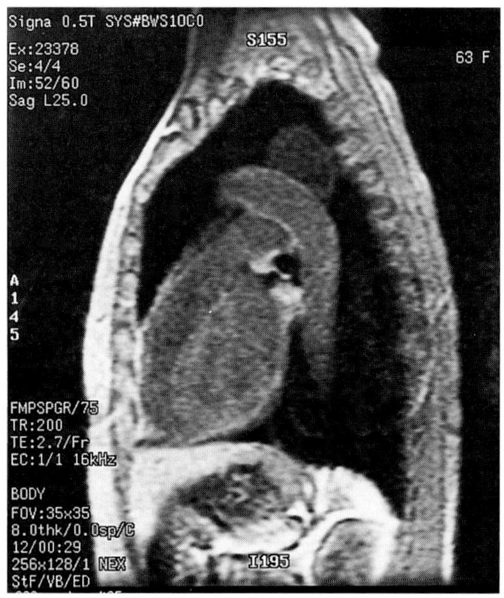

Figure 29–11. Magnetic resonance image corresponding to Figure 29–10 confirms the cystic nature of this mass and distinctly delineates it from the aortic arch.

(Fig. 29–3*A*). On rare occasions, the monitors may be positioned on either side of the patient's knees if the mass is located extremely inferiorly within the he1x, necessitating viewing through a camera port located more cephalad to it (Fig. 29–3*B*). In this way, the area of interest is maintained between the surgeon and the video monitor, and thereby normal orientation is preserved.[21, 31]

The first port, which allows introduction of the thoracoscope, is typically inserted in the midaxillary line in the sixth, seventh, or eighth intercostal space, based on the site of the posterior mediastinal mass, through a 1-cm incision.[25, 31] Initial entry into the chest is performed bluntly with a finger for safety.[38] Local adhesions are bluntly mobilized. A 30-degree thoracoscope generally provides excellent visibility in all regions of the hemithorax and is our thoracoscope of choice. After the mass has been identified, two or three additional 1-cm operating incisions are positioned to create the best convergence on the mass. In general, convergence is obtained in one of two ways. Upper posterior mediastinal masses are typically approached via working ports placed anteriorly and posteriorly in the usual triangular configuration, most often in the fourth, fifth, or sixth intercostal spaces (Fig. 29–4*A*).[25, 27, 28] These incisions are placed far enough apart to prevent encroachment of instruments and the thoracoscope.[21] Lower posterior mediastinal masses should be approached via two anteriorly placed port sites (Fig. 29–4*B*).[16] Spinal needles may be passed transthoracically to identify optimal port position before making incisions. Thought should be given to the creation of these sites, especially with a view toward utility minithoracotomy to facilitate the removal of noncompressible masses if necessary. Utility thoracotomy also allows the insertion of conventional instruments not yet available in thoracoscopic models, and for emergency access.[36] Occasionally, another incision or stab wound to facilitate retraction of the lung may be necessary and can be placed near the thoracoscope port.

If the posterior mediastinal mass is believed to be cystic, aspiration by means of a long spinal needle through one of the working ports under direct thoracoscopic visualization is often helpful, because it facilitates grasping and manipulation of the cyst and expedites removal.[16, 22, 32, 35] Whenever fluid is aspirated, a specimen should be sent for culture and Gram's stain analysis.

The parietal pleura immediately next to the mass may be divided by using endoscopic scissors or a hook cautery, taking care to avoid injury to important nearby structures.[16, 22, 24] Retraction of the mass is performed by means of a smooth or toothed grasper as indicated.[27] Retraction thereby allows a combination of sharp dissection with scissors and blunt dissection with mounted sponges to mobilize the mass gradually from surrounding structures.[35] Small vessels (<2 mm) may be cauterized, whereas larger vessels are clipped with endoscopic clip appliers. Nerve trunks or intercostal bundles intimate with the mass may also be ligated with clips and divided with endoscopic scissors.[24, 28]

Solid posterior mediastinal masses are circumferentially dissected to remove the mass in its entirety. With neurogenic tumors, sharp dissection is often required to develop a well-defined plane between the mass and the endothoracic fascia, whereas blunt dissection can be used to create a plane between underlying mucosa in esophageal leiomyoma.[2, 21] Major blood supply to neurogenic tumors is often pedicled and should be clipped and divided.[35]

Cystic posterior mediastinal masses should also be removed completely, if possible. However, extrathoracic extension or cyst adherence to vital structures may make this dissection hazardous and necessitate alternative measures to complete resection.[16, 32] Simple developmental cysts may be unroofed only, with resection of a portion of the wall for pathologic examination.[27] Once circumferentially mobilized, cyst extensions may either be stapled or clipped, then divided proximally. Recurrence of cysts treated in this manner is uncommon. Cyst wall adherent to vital structures has also been left intact and the mucosa cauterized.[16]

Completing the Procedure

After complete resection of the posterior mediastinal mass, an endoscopic bag should be used to remove all lesions,[30, 44] thereby preventing contamination of trocar incisions with malignant cells should the mass prove to be a cancer at final pathologic diagnosis, or with microorganisms should the mass prove to be infected. Hemostasis of the tumor bed is achieved, and a careful evaluation for any chylous leak made. Chest tube drainage is established through the most inferior working port site. Extra holes may be created in the chest tube by using a rongeur to facilitate complete drainage of the hemithorax. Lung reinflation is confirmed by direct thoracoscopic viewing. The thoracoscope is subsequently removed, and the remaining incisions are closed anatomically. The chest tube is maintained per usual protocol, but most often can be removed within 24 hours.

Complications

Complications of videothoracoscopic resection of posterior mediastinal solid tumors and cysts have been reported, but, in general, they are in type and incidence similar to complications of corresponding open procedures. These complications are addressed in detail elsewhere, but primarily include intraoperative bleeding, postoperative bleeding requiring repeat thoracoscopy for treatment, and conversion to open procedures.[16] Therapeutic videothoracoscopy has compared favorably with open thoracotomy for posterior mediastinal masses with respect to postoperative length of stay, pain control, and return to work.[4]

Figures 29–5 to 29–11 show examples of posterior mediastinal masses recently treated videothoracoscopically at our institution. No intraoperative or postoperative complications were encountered in these patients. All of these entities demonstrated benign pathology. There were no conversions to open procedures.

Summary

Videothoracoscopy has evolved rapidly since the late 1980s. Multiple reports have documented its utility and safety in the diagnosis and treatment of posterior mediastinal masses, including neurogenic tumors, mediastinal cysts, esophageal leiomyomata, and paravertebral abscesses. Whereas thoracoscopic intervention may be viewed as less invasive than standard diagnostic and therapeutic procedures, the potential benefits and risks should be considered on an individual basis before its recommendation.

References

1. Azarow KS: Primary mediastinal masses. J Thorac Cardiovasc Surg 106:67, 1993.
2. Bardini R, Segalin A, Ruol LA, et al: Videothoracoscopic enucleation of esophageal leiomyoma. Ann Thorac Surg 54:576, 1992.
3. Bonavina L, Pavanello M, Baisi A, et al: Mediastinal cyst involving the oesophagus: Diagnosis and results of surgical treatment. Eur J Surg 162:703, 1996.
4. Bousamra M, Haasler GB, Patterson GA, et al: A comparative study of thoracoscopic vs open removal of benign neurogenic mediastinal tumors. Chest 109:1461, 1996.
5. Brusset A, Bonnette P, Hatahet Z, et al: Single lung transplantation for pulmonary lymphangiomyomatosis. Unexpected need for extracorporeal circulation. Chest 107:278, 1995.
6. Cohen AJ, Thompson L, Edwards FH, et al: Primary cysts and tumors of the mediastinum. Ann Thorac Surg 51:378, 1991.
7. Davis RD Jr, Oldham NH Jr, Sabiston DC Jr: Primary cysts and neoplasms of the mediastinum; Recent changes in clinical presentation, methods of diagnosis, management, and results. Ann Thorac Surg 44:229, 1987.
8. De Montpreville VT, Dulmet EM, Chapelier AR, et al: Extramedullary hematopoietic tumors of the posterior mediastinum related to asymptomatic refractory anemia. Chest 104:1623, 1993.
9. DeCamp MM Jr, Jaklitsch MT, Mentzer SJ, et al: The safety and versatility of video-thoracoscopy: A prospective analysis of 895 consecutive cases. J Am Coll Surg 181:113, 1995.
10. Feo CF, Chironi G, Porcu A, et al: Videothoracoscopic removal of a mediastinal teratoma. Am Surg 63:459, 1997.
11. Fielding JR, Owens M, Naimark A: Intrathoracic extramedullary hematopoiesis secondary to B_{12} and folate deficiency: CT appearance. J Comput Assist Tomogr 15:308, 1991.
12. Goldberg M, Burkes RL: Current management of mediastinal tumors. Oncology (Huntingt) 8:99, 1994.
13. Gossot D, Toledo L, Fritsch S, et al: Mediastinoscopy vs thoracoscopy for mediastinal biopsy; results of a prospective nonrandomized study. Chest 110;1328, 1996.
14. Grillo HC, Mathisen D: Combined approach to 'dumbbell' intrathoracic and instraspinal tumors. Ann Thorac Surg 36:402, 1983.
15. Hargreaves HK, Wright TC Jr: A large functioning parathyroid lipoadenoma found in the posterior mediastinum. Am J Clin Pathol 76:89, 1981.
16. Hazelrigg SR, Landreneau RJ, Mack MJ, et al: Thoracoscopic resection of mediastinal cysts. Ann Thorac Surg 1993; 56: 659.
17. Hazelrigg SR, Nunchuch SK, LoCicero J, et al: Video Assisted Thoracic Surgery Study Group Data. Ann Thorac Surg 56:1039, 1993.
18. Heltzer JM, Krasna MJ, Aldrich F, et al: Thoracoscopic excision of a posterior mediastinal dumbbell tumor using a combined approach. Ann Thorac Surg 60:431, 1995.
19. Hoffman OA, Gillespie DJ, Aughenbaugh GL, et al: Primary mediastinal neoplasms (other than thymoma). Mayo Clin Proc 68:880, 1993.
20. Jean A: Effet de lesions localisées du bulbe rachidien sur le stade oesophagien de la deglutition. J Physiol Paris 64:507, 1972.
21. Kaiser LR: Video-assisted thoracic surgery. Ann Surg 220:720, 1994.
22. Kern JA, Daniel TM, Tribble CG, et al: Thoracoscopic diagnosis and treatment of mediastinal masses. Ann Thorac Surg 56:92, 1993.
23. Kohman LJ: Approach to the diagnosis and staging of mediastinal masses. Chest 103(Suppl):328S, 1993.
24. Landreneau RJ, Dowling RD, Ferson PF: Thoracoscopic resection of a posterior mediastinal neurogenic tumor. Chest 102: 1288, 1992.
25. Landreneau RJ, Mack MJ, Hazelrigg SR, et al: The role of video-assisted thoracic surgery in thoracic oncologic practice. Cancer Invest 13:526, 1995.
26. Landreneau RJ, Nawarawong W, Boley TM, et al: Intrathoracic goiter: Approaching the posterior mediastinal mass. Ann Thorac Surg 52:134, 1992.
27. Lewis RJ, Caccavale RJ, Sisler GE: Imaged thoracoscopic surgery: A new thoracic technique for resection of mediastinal cysts. Ann Thorac Surg 53:318, 1992.
28. Mack MJ: Thoracoscopy and its role in mediastinal disease and sympathectomy. Semin Thorac Cardiovasc Surg 5:332, 1993.
29. Mack MJ, Aronoff RJ, Acuff TE, et al: Present role of thoracoscopy in the diagnosis and treatment of diseases of the chest. Ann Thorac Surg 54:403, 1992.
30. Miller JI, Jr: Mediastinum. In Levine BA, Copeland EM III, Howard RJ, et al (eds): Current Practice of Cardiothoracic Surgery, New York, Churchill Livingstone, 1994, p 21.
31. Naunheim KS: Video thoracoscopy for masses of the posterior mediastinum. Ann Thorac Surg 56:657, 1993.
32. Naunheim KS, Andrus CH: Thoracoscopic drainage and resection of a giant mediastinal cyst. Ann Thorac Surg 55:156, 1993.
33. Rendina EA, Venuta F, De Giacomo T, et al: Comparative merits of thoracoscopy, mediastinoscopy, and mediastinotomy for mediastinal biopsy. Ann Thorac Surg 57:992, 1994.
34. Ricci C, Rendina EA, Venuta F, et al: Diagnostic imaging and surgical treatment of dumbbell tumors of the mediastinum. Ann Thorac Surg 50:586, 1990.
35. Roviaro G, Rebuffat C, Varoli F, et al: Videothoracoscopic excision of mediastinal masses: Indications and technique. Ann Thorac Surg 58:1679, 1994.
36. Roviaro GC, Rebuffat C, Varoli F, et al: Major thoracoscopic operations: Pulmonary resection and mediastinal mass excision. Int Surg 81:354, 1996.
37. Schwarz CD, Puschmann R, Eckmayr J, et al: Videoendoscopic removal of a mediastinal cyst. Chest 105;1254, 1994.
38. Shields TW: The significance of ipsilateral mediastinal lymph node metastasis (N2 disease) in non-small cell carcinoma of the lung. A commentary. J Thorac Cardiovasc Surg 99:48, 1990.
39. Shields TW: Primary lesions of the mediastinum and their investigation and treatment. *In* Shields TW (ed): General Thoracic Surgery, 4th ed. Baltimore, Williams & Wilkins, 1994, p 1724.
40. St. Georges R, Deslauriers J, Duranceau A, et al: Clinical spectrum of bronchogenic cyst of the mediastinum and lung in the adult. Ann Thorac Surg 52:6, 1991.
41. Strollo DC, Rosado-de-Christenson ML, Jett JR: Primary mediastinal tumors: Part II. Tumors of the middle and posterior mediastinum. Chest 112:1344, 1997.
42. Sugarbaker DJ: Introduction: Multimodality therapy of chest malignancies update. Chest 103(Suppl):327S, 1993.
43. Suzuki T, Suzuki S, Kamio Y, et al: Mediastinal tuberculous lymphadenitis diagnosed and treated by thoracoscopy. Thorac Cardiovasc Surg 45:140, 1997.
44. Walsh GL, Nesbitt JC: Tumor implants after thoracoscopic resection of a metastatic sarcoma. Ann Thorac Surg 59:215, 1995.

COMMENTARY

Stephen R. Hazelrigg

When evaluating an adult patient with a posterior mediastinal mass, there are several important pieces of information I try to obtain:

1. Careful review of the CT scan is conducted to exclude intraspinal involvement ("dumbbell lesion"). If there remains doubt, we obtain an MRI scan, which usually yields the final answer. All dumbbell lesions are resected with the assistance of neurosurgery.
2. An inspection is performed to determine whether there is any suspicion of lymphoma. Although this is more common in the middle and anterior mediastinal masses, it may occur in the posterior location. This is the one instance in which fine needle biopsy (FNB) may be valuable for posterior mediastinal masses.
3. An examination is made to uncover any suspicion of pheochromocytoma or ganglioneuroblastoma. These lesions are rare in the adult population; however, their catecholamine release intraoperatively may produce significant problems if unexpected. The MIBG scan, as noted in the chapter, can provide the diagnosis as well as the preoperative testing of catecholamines.

After determining that these lesions are not "dumbbell," lymphoma, or pheochromocytoma, we recommend video-assisted thoracic surgery (VATS) as the preferred method of resection. The majority of these patients tolerate the resection well and are discharged within 48 hours. Acute pain control is much better with VATS than with thoracotomy. The high lesions must be approached cautiously to avoid injury to surrounding nerve structures, especially the brachial plexus and stellate ganglia (Horner's syndrome).

Chapter 30

Thoracoscopic Sympathectomy and Splanchnicectomy

Tadasu Kohno and Shinichi Takamoto

There are two thoracic sympathectomies: upper and lower. Upper thoracic sympathectomy is indicated for palmar hyperhidrosis, causalgia, Raynaud's disease, and other vascular disorders in the upper extremities. Lower thoracic sympathectomy is useful for relief of intractable upper abdominal pain.

Historical Perspective

In the past, the approaches used for surgical thoracic sympathectomy included the cervical or supraclavicular, transaxillary, dorsal, and transthoracic routes. However, until thoracoscopic electrocautery sympathectomy became popular, these approaches caused excessive morbidity in patients. Therefore, thoracic sympathetic nerve blocks or other medical modalities were often chosen as preferred alternatives for these conditions. The minimally invasive method of thoracoscopy, first described by Kux,[1] offers an acceptable option to patients.

Thoracic sympathectomy was first reported by Alexander in 1889[2] in an epileptic patient. Successful vasomotor involvement in thoracic sympathectomy was first described by Jaboulay in 1899. Janesco and Brunning reported cervical sympathectomy for vascular diseases in 1923, and Royle reported the procedure for Raynaud's diseases and spastic paralysis of the upper limb in 1928.[3] Adson and associates reported a cervical approach for thoracic sympathectomy in the treatment of palmar hyperhidrosis. In 1929,[5] they performed this surgery via a posterior approach, with resection of one or two ribs; resection was revived by Cloward in 1969.[6]

Transthoracic sympathectomy was first reported by Atkins in 1949.[7] This procedure had the disadvantages of chest tube insertion, painful incisions, and unattractive cosmetic results, which caused dissatisfaction in up to 29%[8] of patients. Kux in 1951[1] first described thoracoscopic sympathectomy as a new therapeutic approach.

There are three procedures currently performed for both upper and lower thoracoscopic surgical thoracic sympathectomies. Two of these procedures require general anesthesia, with or without split-lung ventilation. The third procedure can also be performed under local anesthesia.

The upper thoracic sympathectomy involves separation or resection of the second, third, and sometimes fourth thoracic sympathetic ganglia. For the first procedure, the patient is placed in the full lateral position, and, in many cases, three trocar sites are necessary. For the second procedure, the patient is placed in a semi-sitting position, and one 7-mm trocar incision is made. The third procedure is performed with the patient in a semi-sitting position, and one 3-mm trocar incision and one needle puncture are made. Each of these procedures is described in this chapter.

In the lower thoracic sympathectomy, the lower level of the chain and the greater and lesser splanchnic nerves are separated to control pain in patients who have uncontrolled severe upper abdominal pain caused by chronic pancreatitis or an upper abdominal malignancy (e.g., pancreatic carcinoma, gastric cancer). Approximately 85% of pain fibers run through the sympathetic system. The fibers usually arise in the area between the fifth and the tenth thoracic sympathetic ganglia to the greater splanchnic nerve and in the area between the ninth and eleventh thoracic ganglia to the lesser splanchnic nerve. This procedure is also described in this chapter.

There is a 25 to 33% incidence of familial hyperhidrosis reported.[9, 10] The pathophysiology of palmar hyperhidrosis is not clear, but the hyperactivity of the sympathetic nerve caused by mental stress may be related to the excessive sweating.

Anatomy of the Thoracic Sympathetic Chain

The thoracic sympathetic ganglia rest against the heads of the ribs. The first thoracic ganglion is usually fused with the inferior cervical ganglion to form the stellate ganglion (cervicothoracic ganglion). The next ganglion, which rests on the head of the second rib, is called the second thoracic ganglion. Each of the thoracic ganglia corresponds numerically to the number of a rib (Fig. 30–1). The thoracic sympathetic chain runs posterior to the parietal pleura.

In some cases, one or more accessory sympathetic fibers, known as Kuntz fibers, are found lateral to the thoracic sympathetic chain. Kuntz fibers communicate with the sympathetic system and must be treated at the same time (see Fig. 30–5). This accessory fiber (or fibers) may be the cause of inadequate operation or recurrence of symptoms.

The uppermost rib seen on the back side is usually the second rib. The second rib has an intercostal muscle on its upper side, whereas the first rib does not. This helps in differentiating the first from the second rib. If a long needle is inserted at the second intercostal space and the midclavicular line; the place is easy to identify from the outside, and focusing on the needle with a thoracoscope is a quick and easy confirmation of the number of the rib.

The greater splanchnic nerve is formed by branches from the fifth to the tenth thoracic ganglia and runs medial to the thoracic sympathetic chain. The lesser splanchnic nerve is formed by the fibers from the ninth to the

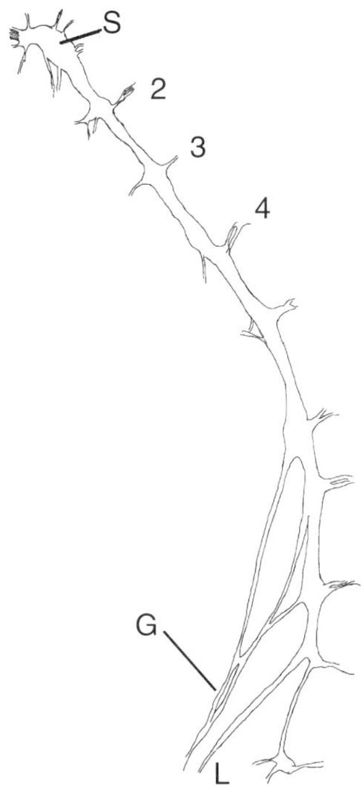

Figure 30–1. Anatomy of the left thoracic sympathetic chain (S = stellate ganglion), 2: 2nd thoracic sympathetic ganglion 3: 3rd thoracic sympathetic ganglion, 4: 4th thoracic sympathetic ganglion, G: greater splanchnic nerve, L: lesser splanchnic nerve.

The first thoracic sympathetic ganglion is usually fused with the inferior cervical ganglion to form the stellate ganglion (cervicothoracic ganglion). Injuring this ganglion is the cause of Horner's syndrome.

eleventh thoracic ganglia and also runs medial to the thoracic sympathetic chain (see Fig. 30–1).

Indications and Patient Selection

Upper Thoracic Sympathectomy

The most common indication for thoracic sympathectomy is either palmar or axillary hyperhidrosis, or both, regardless of the approach. Hyperhidrosis is a pathologic condition characterized by excessive sweating for normal thermoregulation, with an extraordinarily low palmar temperature. The excessive sweating may occur in any part of the body, and is mainly associated with mental stress. However, the most troublesome manifestations of this condition occur on the hands, arms, and axillae. Usually, patients range in age from the teen years to the 30s, but the symptom may appear in early childhood and persist throughout adult life. Hyperhidrosis is not a life-threatening condition, but it markedly impedes the patient's social and professional activities. The most cumbersome problems occur when patients engage in such activities as shaking hands, writing, typing, using a camera or cellular phone, or playing with a video game.

Raynaud's syndrome and Buerger's disease in the upper extremities are also indications for upper thoracic sympathectomy. The patients referred for this surgery have, in most cases, failed medical therapy. Sometimes these patients have already undergone vascular reconstruction.

Other vascular disorders that are indications for this operation are critical ischemia, ulceration, and rest pain despite thorough medical treatment. However, for these indications, the effect of thoracic sympathectomy may not last long,[17] probably because of denervation hypersensitivity of the blood vessels, progression of the disease, and intense vasomotion.

Vasospasm and vascular occlusive diseases in the arms and palmar region have been reported to improve after thoracic sympathectomy.[16] However, the long-term benefit is not clear.[17]

Lower Thoracic Sympathectomy and Splanchnicectomy

The indication for lower thoracic sympathectomy and splanchnicectomy is uncontrolled upper abdominal pain. Generally, patients are suffering from chronic pancreatitis or upper abdominal malignancy. Usually, they have tried various combinations of oral analgesia or celiac plexus block guided by computed tomography (CT). When these treatments are unsuccessful, surgery is indicated.

Technique

Upper Thoracic Sympathectomy

The three methods of performing thoracoscopic thoracic sympathectomy require the same video endoscopic surgical equipment as used in regular thoracoscopic surgery and the same commercially available endoscopic surgical instruments. The only difference is in the scope used. Any type of camera controller, xenon light source, monitors, or video cassette recorder (VCR) used in endoscopic surgery is acceptable for all these procedures.

Three-Trocar Method. This is currently a conventional method in thoracoscopic thoracic sympathectomy.

The main advantages of this procedure are that it enables resection of the thoracic sympathetic nerve—particularly for histologic confirmation—and lysis of adhesions around the trocar site and the nerve. With this procedure, it is also possible to skeletonize the second and third ganglia thoracic sympathetic trunk. The disadvantages are the need for general anesthesia with one-lung ventilation and at least three trocar incisions to perform this procedure.

For bilateral procedures, repositioning of the patient is another time-consuming factor. General anesthesia with split-lung ventilation is used for this procedure. The patient is placed in the full lateral position.

Usually, a 3- to 10-mm diameter thoracoscope can be used, according to the surgeon's preference. It is the authors' preference that, for the right-sided procedure, the primary surgeon should stand at the back side of the patient if the surgeon is right-handed. The first trocar incision, with a length of 3 to 10 mm for the scope, should be made at the fourth intercostal space and the anterior axillary line. Inspection of the chest cavity should be the next step. If there are some adhesions around the trocar site or the apex of the lung, adhesiolysis must be performed. When no adhesion is present, two 3- to 5-mm trocars are placed at the midaxillary line in the third and fourth intercostal spaces. Usually, the uppermost rib seen on the back side is the second rib. If there is any doubt about the number of the rib, insert a long needle at the second intercostal space and the midclavicular line, as mentioned above. This point is easily identified from outside the body, and the rib should be counted to confirm the number. Then the parietal pleura is opened over the sympathetic nerve from the second to the third ribs, with an electrode or a pair of endoscopic scissors. The nerve is then resected (Fig. 30–2). If the patient has coexisting axillary hyperhidrosis, the nerve should be resected to the fourth rib. If bleeding is negligible and no procedure is performed on the lung, no chest tube is usually necessary. The skin incisions are closed either by stitches or tape, according to the length of the incision.

For the bilateral procedure, repositioning of the patient is necessary. The intrathoracic procedure is performed in basically the same fashion as on the first side.

One-Trocar Method. This approach is now a relatively widely accepted procedure.

The main advantages are the need for only a one-trocar incision, 7 to 10 mm in length, and no need to reposition patient for bilateral procedures. The disadvantages are that the surgeon cannot maneuver independently of the visual field, the thoracic sympathetic nerve cannot be resected, adhesions will be difficult to lyse, and general anesthesia, with or without one-lung ventilation, is necessary.

The patient should be placed approximately in a 45-degree semi-sitting position (Fig. 30–3). General anesthesia should be administered with or without one-lung ventilation. One 7- to 10-mm trocar incision should be made at the third intercostal space and the anterior axillary line for a resectoscope (Fig. 30–4). Following the trocar placement, the scope should be inserted to look for adhesions. If a dense or broad adhesion is found, the possibility of changing the approach must be considered. If there is no or a very slight adhesion found, 200 to 800 ml of carbon dioxide (CO_2) is insufflated into the chest cavity, according to the size of the patient. During the CO_2 insufflation, the apical region should be monitored carefully by the scope to guard against an excessive amount of CO_2. The CO_2 insufflation provides an excellent visual field for performing the procedure. With the electrode of the resectoscope hooked to an electrocautery system—usually with a power of 15 to 25 watts—the second and third ganglia thoracic sympathetic chain should be ablated and severed at the rib. For axillary hyperhidrosis, additional separation of the thoracic sympathetic nerve at the fourth rib is necessary. In some cases there is an accessory sympathetic fiber called a Kuntz fiber, lateral to the main sympathetic nerve (Fig. 30–5). This accessory fiber must be divided as well. After completion of the procedure, the CO_2 in the chest cavity should be sucked out and hemostasis should be checked. Then the skin incision is closed. Usually, no chest tube is necessary.

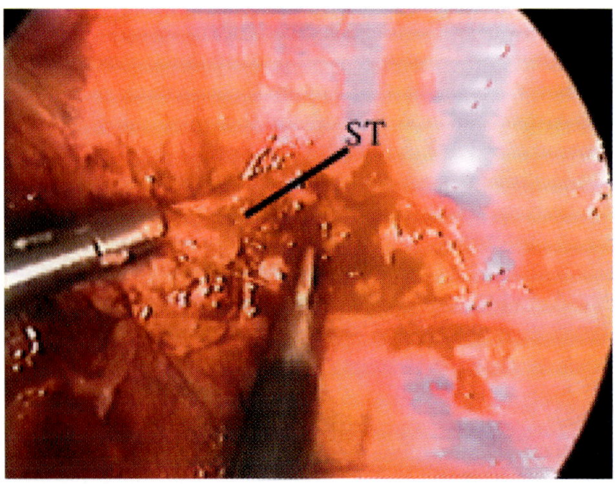

Figure 30–2. Resection of the thoracic sympathetic trunk (ST = sympathetic trunk). The upper thoracic sympathetic trunk is held with a grasper and separated from the surrounding tissue.

For the contralateral procedure, the primary surgeon simply needs to go to the other side of the patient. The procedure itself is the same.

Instead of an electrocautery, a laser device can also be used for this procedure.[18]

Two-Trocar Method. The main advantages of this procedure are the need for only one 3-mm trocar incision with one needle puncture, the ability of the surgeon to maneuver independently of the scope, and avoidance of repositioning the patient for the bilateral procedure. Other advantages of this procedure are the possibility of using local anesthesia with spontaneous ventilation—which means the procedure can be performed in an outpatient setting—and the capability of performing an intraoperative sweat test using a perspiration meter to confirm the success of the surgical intervention. Such a test is impossible to conduct with the patient under general anesthesia. However, the disadvantages include inability to resect the sympathetic chain and to lyse adhesions.

The patient is placed approximately in a 45-degree semi-sitting position (see Fig. 30–3). General anesthesia is not always mandatory. For local anesthesia, about 3 ml of 0.5 to 1.0% procainamide is injected subcutaneously at the third intercostal space and the midaxillary line following premedication with an intramuscular injection of either 2.5 mg of midazolam or 15 mg of pentazocine. An incision of about 3 mm should be made at this point, followed by a 3-mm trocar with a stopcock (Fig. 30–6) insertion. A 2.7- to 3.0-mm scope is inserted to see whether there are any adhesions around the trocar site or the apex. When adhesions are present around the trocar incision or around the apex of the lung, changing the approach may be a better option. If no adhesion is found, 200 to 800 ml of CO_2 is then put into the chest cavity from the CO_2 insufflator while the cavity is observed with the scope in order to insufflate only enough CO_2 to perform the procedure. A 14-G needle is inserted at the midclavicular line and the second intercostal space after local anesthesia is injected. A 23-G papillary thyroid carcinoma (PTC) needle with a length of 20 cm is put through the 14-G needle and about 7 to 10 ml of local anesthesia (i.e., 0.5 to 1.0% procainamide) is injected around the sympathetic nerve at the second and third ribs. Patients usually feel only somewhat cold on the back during administration of this local anesthesia. An electrode (Fig. 30–7) is then placed through the 14-G needle.

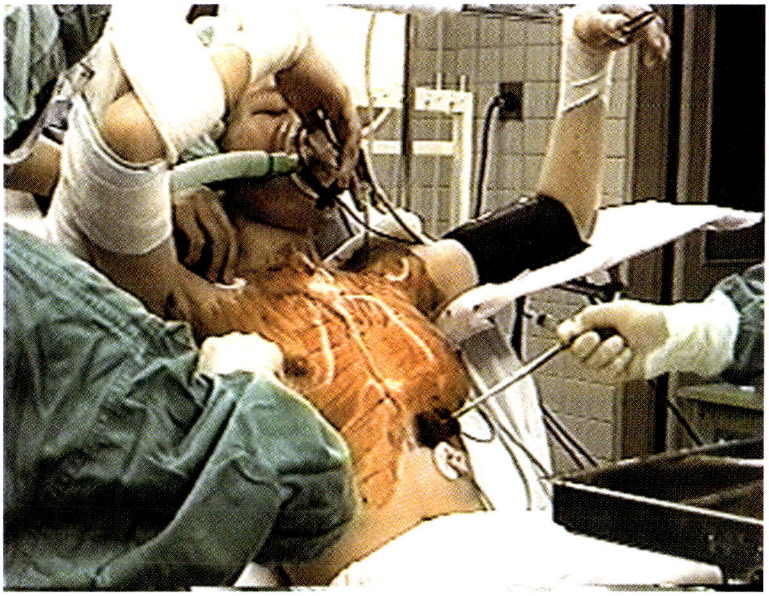

Figure 30–3. This 40- to 60-degree semi-sitting position, with the patient's arms up, provides the surgeon an excellent view of the upper thoracic sympathetic nerve. Repositioning the patient is not necessary for the bilateral procedure.

The sympathetic nerve, as well as the accessory fiber (Kuntz fiber), should be divided at the rib by the electrode with a power of 15 to 25 watts. Patients usually do not feel any pain during the ablation of the nerve fiber. Sometimes, patients may feel some dyspnea if an excessive amount of air or CO_2 gets into the chest cavity through the 14-G needle. Suctioning out the excessive air or CO_2 is a simple and easy solution. After inspection for hemostasis, with a suction probe that goes through the 14-G needle (see Fig. 30–7), the CO_2 is sucked out of the cavity. The incisions are closed with tape and without any stitches. Usually, no chest tube is necessary.

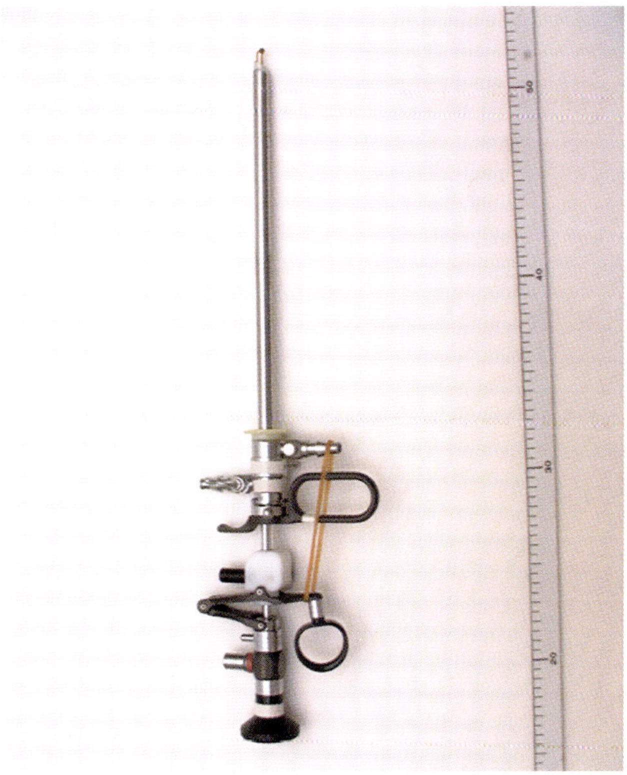

Figure 30–4. The resectoscope has a working channel through which an electrode is passed. This scope has been used extensively by urologists and gynecologists.

Lower Thoracic Sympathectomy and Splanchnicectomy

This procedure is indicated for patients who have uncontrollable upper abdominal pain. The same variation of approaches is employed in thoracoscopic splanchnicectomy and lower thoracic sympathectomy. The left-sided procedure should be considered first, because, in many cases, the organs that cause pain are located in the left upper abdomen, and the left-sided intervention alone may be adequate.[11] The right-sided intervention is considered only when the left-sided procedure is insufficient.

The patient is placed in the full lateral position for all these approaches. Anesthesia can range from local anesthesia with normal ventilation to general anesthesia with one-lung ventilation. Insufflation with CO_2 can be used in single-lumen intubation or local anesthesia procedures.

The advantage of using general anesthesia with one-lung ventilation and resection of the nerve fiber is that it is a currently available technique and its efficiency has already been evaluated. Also, full-lung collapse provides an excellent visualization of the lower thoracic cavity.

The advantage of using local anesthesia is the capability of performing an intraoperative evaluation of the effect of the procedure.

There are surgical techniques for splanchnicectomy. Although the nerve resection method is an evaluated procedure, the necessity of resecting the splanchnic nerve has not yet been clarified. Separation and cautery ablation of the fiber may be sufficient.[11] The three-trocar-site method, the one-trocar method, and the two-puncture method described for the upper thoracic sympathectomy can be used for this procedure.

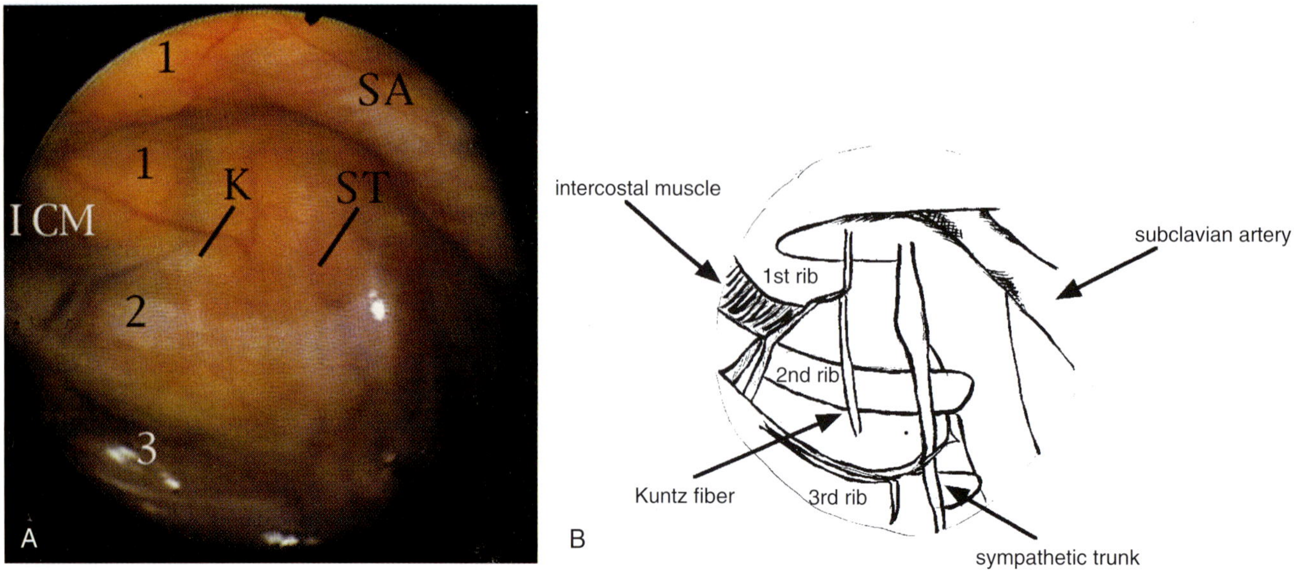

Figure 30–5. Kuntz fiber, the thoracic sympathetic trunk, and the surrounding structure (SA = subclavian artery, ST = sympathetic trunk, K = Kuntz fiber, ICM = first intercostal muscle, 1 = first rib, 2 = second rib).
The Kuntz fiber runs lateral to the thoracic sympathetic trunk. It is well identified with careful observation.

Results

Upper Thoracic Sympathectomy

For a patient who has hyperhidrosis, the effect of dry hands is immediate. In the patient undergoing this procedure under local anesthesia, we monitor the amount of sweat with a perspiration meter and the temperature of the hand intraoperatively. We even give an intraoperative mental stress test (i.e., calculating or memorizing and repeating numbers), to see the effect. The effects of a dry hand and rising palmar temperature occur when a local anesthesia is given around the sympathetic nerve.

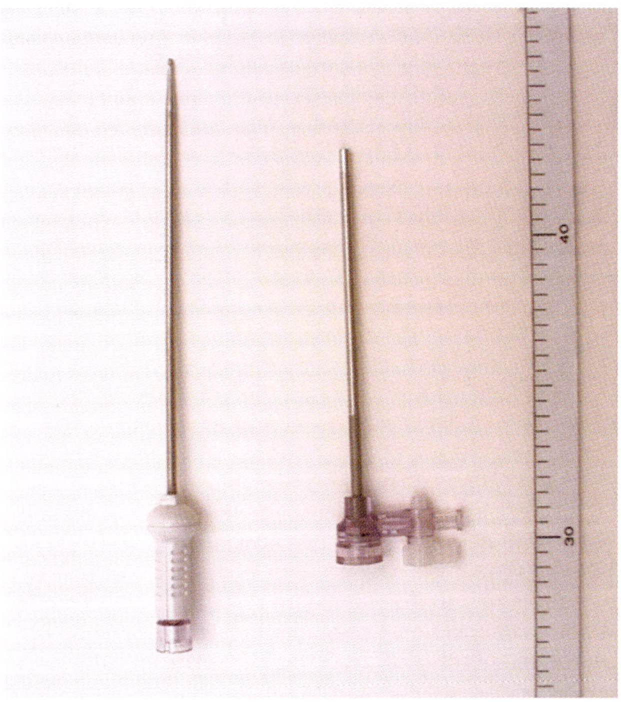

Figure 30–6. A 3-mm diameter trocar with a stopcock. This trocar (Access needle, Ethicon, Cincinnati, OH) has a valve and a stopcock. An instrument or scope with a diameter up to 3 mm can pass through this scope.

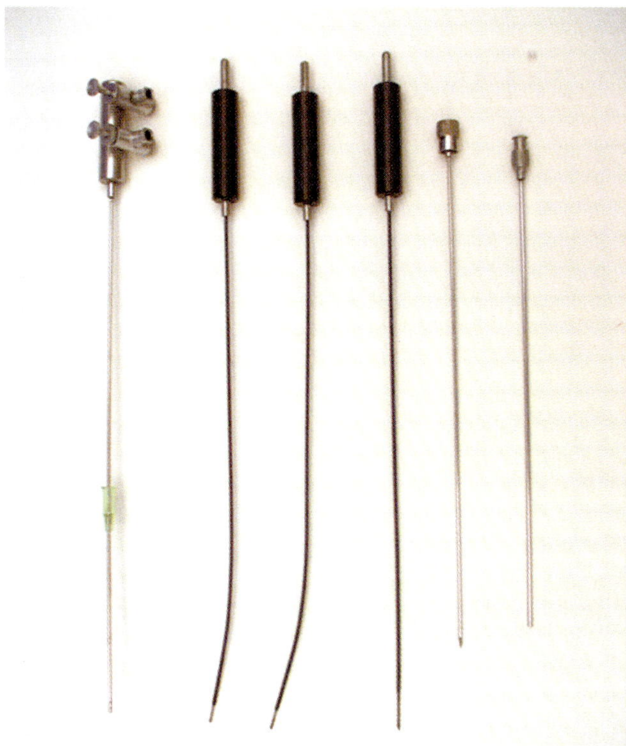

Figure 30–7. Instruments that have a diameter of 1.7 mm (MIST) can pass through a 14-G needle. The irrigation/suction probe goes through the needle. The two instruments on the right, a trocar and an obturator, were specially made for these instruments.

A concern for this procedure is whether the effect of dry hand is long lasting or not. In our series, the longest follow-up has been 50 months, and we have had no recurrence so far. It is suspected that missed accessory fibers may cause recurrence.

The positive effects achieved by this surgery for vascular disorders, however, do not last long. In our series of operations for Raynaud's or Buerger's disease in the upper limb, the effect lasted for only about 2 years. The reason for this is not clear. However, the vascular disorder may progress and may cause recurrence in a relatively short period.

The patient's satisfaction is usually excellent. The side effect of the procedure is compensatory sweating on the back and around the abdomen and thigh when a mental stress test is given. Theoretically, this compensatory sweating could happen to every patient. It is reported that this sweating was seen in 37 to 75% of patients.[12] The amount of compensatory sweating differs from patient to patient. How the patient feels about the compensatory sweating also depends on the patient. The issue of compensatory sweating is addressed on the preoperative informed consent form. Other possible morbidities are pneumothoracies, bleeding, allodynia, and Horner's syndrome. Allodynia is a kind of dysesthesia, which appears as an irritable and sometimes painful reaction to a non-noxious stimulus to normal skin. It is usually seen around the arms. Allodynia may be caused by an accidental intercostal nerve injury. We had no mortality and no serious morbidity in any patients who have undergone this procedure.

Lower Thoracic Sympathetic Nerve Resection

Usually, the effect of pain relief is achieved immediately after surgery. Complete pain relief is reported in 60 to 100% of patients suffering from upper abdominal intractable pain. The long-term results are difficult to obtain and often academic, because many of the patients who need this procedure are at the end stage of malignancy.

No serious complication has been reported to our knowledge. In our series, some slight gastrointestinal complications—diarrhea or constipation—were the only patient complaints.

Summary

It is true that surgical sympathectomy is an established technique that provides relief from symptoms. Oseco[13] reported more than 1600 thoracic sympathetic nerve blocks with a success rate of 70%, whereas Byrne[14] reported endoscopic thoracic sympathectomy with a success rate of 92%. However, palmar hyperhidrosis is not a life-threatening condition. If the procedure is extensive and may give patients serious morbidity, only a few patients will choose surgical intervention. We must refine our technique so that the procedure can be done in a day surgery setting in order to offer an attractive option to patients who have palmar hyperhidrosis. The single-puncture technique reported by Claes and Gothberg[15] has been a widely accepted procedure. However, we have experienced awkwardness in performing this procedure when we want to move the electrode while keeping the visual field stable. Sometimes, the electrode has moved through the working channel of the resectoscope out of the visual field at a point when we still have to coagulate. We think this is unsafe, and we have now changed to using one small scope and a 14-G needle puncture. Again, because palmar hyperhidrosis is not a life-threatening condition, the procedure must have minimal mortality or serious morbidity. In many surgical operations, the cosmetic factor is the last to be considered. However, for this kind of condition, particularly in a young female patient, cosmesis must be considered as one of the important aspects of the procedure.

Three techniques have been described. Each approach has some advantages and disadvantages. Surgeons must pick a method according to their preference.

However, the double-puncture technique is the authors' preference. This method enables coagulation of the sympathetic trunk with a stable visual field. It also requires the smallest skin incision.

Even though thoracoscopic thoracic sympathectomy is a simple procedure, the surgeon must be familiar with thoracoscopic surgical manipulation before attempting this operation.

References

1. Kux E: The endoscopic approach to the vegetative nervous system and its therapeutic possibilities. Dis Chest. 20:139–147, 1951.
2. Byrne J, Walsh TN, Hederman WP: Thoracoscopic sympathectomy. *In* Gossot D (ed): Surgical Thoracoscopy, New York, Springer, 1993, pp 93–98.
3. Royle ND: Sympathecic trunck section: A new operation for Raynaud's disease and spastic paralysis of the upper limb. Med J Aust 2:436–439, 1928.
4. Adson AW, Craig WM, Brown GE: Essential hyperhidrosis cured by sympathetic ganglionectomy and trunk resection. Arch Surg 31:794–798, 1935.
5. Adson AW, Brown GE: Raynaud's disease of the upper extremity: Successful treatment by resection of sympathetic cervicothoracic and 2nd thoracic ganglia and intervening trunk. JAMA 92:444–447, 1929.
6. Cloward RB: Hyperhidrosis. J Neurosurg 30:545–551, 1969.
7. Atkins HJB: Per axillary approach to the stellate and upper thoracic sympathetic ganglia. Lancet 2:1152–1154, 1949.
8. Sternberg MO, Bakkman S, Kott J, et al: Transaxillary thoracic sympathectomy for primary hiperhidrosis of the upper limbs. World J Surg 6:458–463, 1982.
9. Orteu CH, McGregor LM, Rustin MHA: Recurrence of hyperhidrosis after endoscopic transthoracic sympathectomy—Case report and review of the literature. Clin Exp Dermatol 20:230–233, 1995.
10. Drott C, Claes G: Hyperhidrosis treated by thoracoscopic sympathectomy. Cardiovasc Surg 4:788–790, 1996.
11. Noppen M, Meysman M, D'Haese J, et al: Thoracoscopic splanchnicolysis for the relief of chronic pancreatitis pain; Experience of a group of pneumonologists. Chest, 113:528–531, 1998.
12. Edmondson RA, Bannerjee AK, Rennie JA: Endoscopic transthoracic symathectomy in the treatment of hyperhidrosis. Ann Surg 215:289–293, 1992.
13. Oseko K: Endoscopic thoracic sympathetic nerve ablation. J B Orthop 8:131–134, 1995.

14. Byrne J, Walsh TN, Hederman WP: Endoscopic transthoracic electrocautery of the sympathetic chain for palmar and axillary hyperhidrosis. Br J Surg 77:1046–1049, 1990.
15. Claes G, Gothberg C: Endoscopic electrocautery of the thoracic sympathetic chain. Scand J Plast Reconstr Hand Surg 21:29–33, 1993.
16. Koman LA, Smith BP, Pollock FE Jr, et al. The microcirculatory effects of peripheral sympathectomy. J Hand Surg Am 20:709–717, 1995.
17. Lau H, Cheng SW: Burger's disease in Hong Kong: A review of 89 cases. Aust NZ J Surg 67:264–269, 1997.
18. Kao MC: Video endoscopic sympathectomy using a fiberoptic CO_2 laser to treat palmar hyperhidrosis. Neurosurgery 30:131–135, 1992.

COMMENTARY

Dominique Gossot

As written by the authors at the end of the chapter, "Each approach has some advantages and disadvantages. Surgeons must pick a method according to their preference". It is indeed one of the features of thoracoscopic sympathectomy that many different techniques (using different positioning and different instrumentation) have been described, all with equally satisfactory results.

We agree with the authors that the one-puncture technique, although appealing, has the major limitation of giving a limited maneuvering possibility. It is also almost impossible to resect the sympathetic chain, except if using an ureteroscope loop, as proposed by Claes and Drott.[1]

With regard to the two-puncture technique as described by the authors, we think that the inability to resect the sympathetic nerve might be a shortcoming of the method. There is no doubt that the immediate result must be as good as that achieved by complete nerve resection. However, we have recently shown that a limited sympathectomy that preserves the main trunk but only divides the rami communicantes leads to more relapses than a conventional resection.[2] Although these findings have not been published, it seems that the experience of other authors[3] supports the fact that limited T2 resection leads to recurrence. The possibility of neural regeneration from the ganglions might occur if the main trunk has been preserved and only coagulated. We hope that Drs. Kohno and Takamoto will report the long-term results of this procedure.

We still use a three-port technique with the patient in the lateral position. After having used different positions (supine, semi-sitting, prone), we came back to the lateral position because of better control in case of an unexpected intraoperative problem, such as oozing, bleeding from an intercostal vein, or the necessity of freeing adhesions. Now that miniaturized instrumentation is available, the cosmetic result is excellent. We use a 5-mm scope and 2 microinstruments (3 mm). No stitches are necessary and the entry sites are simply closed with Steri-Strips. Contrary to the authors, we prefer to leave a small-diameter chest tube in place for a few minutes. We have tried not to use a chest tube, but have experienced some cases of pneumothorax requiring drainage.

Discussion about technical details can be endless. The main issue with thoracoscopic sympathectomy is to select the indication with great care. As mentioned by Drs. Kohno and Takamoto, the results of sympathectomy for vascular disorders are usually disappointing. Only patients who have severe disease and failure of medical therapy should be operated on. With regard to hyperhidrosis, only those patients who have followed adequate medical therapy and iontophoresis should be referred to the surgeon. They must be made clearly aware of the possible side effects, especially compensatory sweating. As demonstrated recently by Drs. Andrews and Rennie, there is no predictive factor for compensatory sweating, and it is more common than usually reported.[4] Clear communication to the patient about this side effect may avoid dissatisfaction and disappointment for patients and surgeons alike.[5]

References

1. Drott C, Güthberg G, Claes G: Endoscopic transthoracic sympathectomy: An efficient and safe method for the treatment of hyperhidrosis. J Am Acad Dermatol 33:78–81, 1995.
2. Gossot D, Toledo L, Fritsch S, et al: Thoracoscopic sympathectomy for upper limb hyperhidrosis: Looking for the right operation. Ann Thorac Surg 64:975–978, 1997.
3. Bonjer HJ, Hamming JF, duBois NAJJ, et al: Advantages of limited thoracoscopic sympathectomy. Surg Endosc 10:721–723, 1996.
4. Andrews BT, Rennie JA: Predicting changes in the distribution of sweating following thoracoscopic sympathectomy. Br J Surg 84:1702–1704, 1997.
5. Herbst F, Plas EG, Függer R, et al: Endoscopic thoracic sympathectomy for primary hyperhidrosis of the upper limbs: A critical analysis and long-term results of 480 operations. Ann Surg 220:86–90, 1994.

Chapter 31

Laparoscopic Antireflux Surgery

Kenric M. Murayama and Keith S. Naunheim

Gastroesophageal reflux is a common physiologic event that causes symptoms in roughly 40 million adult Americans.[1–3] In most normal adults, the reflux episodes are transient and do not constitute a disease. Gastroesophageal reflux becomes pathologic when it causes signs and symptoms of tissue injury in the esophagus, oropharynx, or respiratory tract. Interestingly, reflux has been recognized as a clinically significant disease process only since the mid-1930s.[4] In patients with gastroesophageal reflux disease (GERD), insufficient resting lower esophageal sphincter (LES) pressures are frequently the cause. The majority of reflux episodes (70 to 100%) in normal adults occur during a phenomenon known as transient lower esophageal sphincter relaxation (TLESR).[5]

It was not until 1951 that Allison, who is credited with initiating the modern era of antireflux surgery, described an operation to treat GERD, addressing his belief that the gastroesophageal junction must be returned to its normal intra-abdominal location.[4, 6] Before that time, surgical treatment of GERD focused on reduction of the hiatal hernia and closure of the crura, with generally poor results. In 1956, Rudolf Nissen performed the first fundoplication to treat GERD,[7] and although several antireflux operations have been developed since that time, the Nissen fundoplication remains the standard by which other antireflux operations are measured. Recently, the application of advanced laparoscopic techniques in antireflux operations has revolutionized the role of surgery in the treatment of GERD.[7–12] Patients are being referred for surgery at an ever-increasing rate, and this renewed interest has stimulated novel research that contributes to our understanding of the pathophysiology of GERD.[12–15]

Although this chapter focuses primarily on the laparoscopic treatment options for GERD, it is important to first discuss the manifestations of the disease and the patient evaluation process. Only then can reasonable recommendations be made regarding the implementation of surgical and nonsurgical treatment options.

Pathophysiology

Most patients with GERD have an acidic refluxate, and the degree of mucosal injury is largely dependent on the concentration of the acid and the time of exposure to it.[1] GERD patients usually have normal rates of acid secretion, but some part of the esophageal defense mechanism is inadequate. There are three components to the esophageal defense mechanism: anatomic antireflux barriers, luminal clearance mechanisms, and tissue resistance factors.[16–19] Antireflux barriers limit the exposure of the esophagus to refluxate. The LES, intra-abdominal segment of the esophagus, esophageal hiatus, phrenoesophageal ligament, and acute angle of His all contribute to the normal physiologic barrier to reflux by maintaining the high-pressure zone at the gastroesophageal junction.[16] Factors contributing to normal luminal clearance, which limits the duration of exposure to gastric refluxate, include gravity and normal esophageal peristalsis.[17] It has been demonstrated that normal esophageal peristalsis can compensate for significant acid reflux by rapid clearance of the esophagus.[18]

Although antireflux barriers and luminal clearance mechanisms minimize the duration of contact between refluxate and esophageal mucosa, the total contact time is approximately 1 to 2 hours per day, even in the majority of normal individuals.[19] Remarkably, reflux symptoms occur in a minority of these people, and complications of GERD in an even smaller number. Normal tissue resistance to injury is now recognized as the third component of protection against GERD and consists primarily of the intrinsic structure and function of mucosal elements,[17] a collection of complex processes beyond the scope of this chapter. Unfortunately, long-standing GERD frequently damages the mucosa and its protective mechanisms, leading to a cycle that is difficult to reverse and eventually results in continued mucosal injury.[18]

Clinical Presentation

The clinical manifestations of GERD depend largely on the anatomic site of injury, and a distinction is made between typical and atypical disease symptoms. *Typical GERD* relates to esophageal manifestations, and *atypical GERD* applies to nonesophageal manifestations, primarily upper aerodigestive and respiratory symptoms.[20, 21] The most common presentation of typical GERD is reflux esophagitis, defined as recurrent esophageal symptoms (e.g., heartburn) and/or mucosal injury with associated inflammation. The frequency and severity of heartburn attacks do not always correlate with the degree of mucosal injury seen endoscopically.[21]

Patients with GERD frequently complain of regurgitation of partially digested food, a bitter or acidic taste in the mouth, or water brash. Some patients with reflux esophagitis complain of atypical chest pain resembling pain of cardiac origin. Prolonged GERD can lead to a variety of other typical complaints; for example, dysphagia can result from disordered esophageal motility secondary to recurrent injury and inflammation. Alternatively, the appearance of dysphagia to solid foods may indicate the presence of a complication of GERD, such as an esophageal stricture or carcinoma.

Not infrequently, GERD patients present with atypical symptoms caused by laryngopharyngeal reflux with damage to the oropharynx, larynx, or respiratory tract.[20–24] Interestingly, patients with atypical GERD may have few, if any, typical symptoms, despite significant upright daytime reflux.[20, 25] Complaints of a sore throat, chronic earache, recurrent sinusitis, globus pharyngeus, and poor dentition may all be indicators of oropharyngeal GERD.[20, 21] Injury to the larynx and/or respiratory tract by the refluxate can manifest as hoarseness, halitosis, chronic cough, bronchitis, wheezing, asthma, and aspiration pneumonia.[22–24]

As knowledge is gained about atypical GERD, it becomes increasingly evident that it is a complex, multifactorial disease whose manifestations may be caused not just by direct exposure to the refluxate but by vagal reflex pathways as well. For example, laryngopharyngeal reflux with aspiration of acid into the airway may cause asthma-like symptoms, but bronchospasm can also be elicited by esophageal acidification without direct airway contamination.[22]

Diagnostic Evaluation

When a patient is suspected of having GERD, the health care provider has several responsibilities. First, and most importantly, the clinician must suspect reflux as the cause of the presenting signs and symptoms, a particularly difficult diagnosis in patients with atypical GERD. Typical reflux symptoms are common, and usually no further evaluation is undertaken, but a trial of lifestyle changes (Table 31–1) and first-line medications (see section on Medical Therapy) is implemented. Second, the presence of reflux must be not only proved but also demonstrated to be pathologic by documenting a correlation between symptoms and reflux events. Third, the severity of tissue injury must be assessed, because this often serves as a guide to treatment selection. Finally, esophageal and LES function must be evaluated to determine whether the normal antireflux barriers and luminal acid clearance mechanisms are impaired. A variety of tests and procedures are available (Table 31–2), but the evaluation of patients suspected of having significant GERD can be streamlined to the following studies in most situations.[12, 13, 21, 25, 26]

Twenty-four-hour continuous esophageal pH monitoring is a common method both for establishing pathologic gastroesophageal reflux and for determining a correlation with symptoms. A patient-activated event marker correlates reflux events (defined as pH <4) with symptoms, activity, and body position.[21, 25] Basic parameters measured are the total number of reflux episodes, total number of episodes longer than 5 minutes, and total time that esophageal pH is less than 4.[21, 25] Patients with typical reflux symptoms and erosive esophagitis may not need to have a pH study, as almost all have acid reflux.[12]

Esophageal manometry evaluates esophageal motility and adequacy of LES function, two components of the normal esophageal defense mechanism. Esophageal peristalsis and clearance are compromised in a significant number of patients with GERD.[18] Manometry can identify peristaltic abnormalities and, in some cases, may identify a concomitant disorder (e.g., scleroderma). Preoperative identification of significant abnormal esophageal motility should serve as a "red flag" for the surgeon, who must be certain that creation of a 360-degree fundoplication will not result in "surgical achalasia."[27] Thirty to 50% of patients with gastroesophageal reflux have a normal LES pressure (10 to 30 mm Hg).[21, 28] A low LES pressure in patients with GERD is associated with a high failure rate of medical therapy and may predict which patients will re-

Table 31–1. Lifestyle Modifications for Gastroesophageal Reflux Disease Patients

Elevate head of bed 6 in.
Minimize tobacco use
Minimize excessive alcohol consumption
Reduce dietary fat and meal size
Have last oral intake 4–6 hr before bedtime
Lose weight
Avoid the following foods
- Chocolate
- Carminatives (spearmint, peppermint)
- Coffee (caffeinated and decaffeinated)
- Tea
- Cola beverages
- Tomato and citrus juices

Avoid the following drugs, if possible
- Anticholinergics
- Theophylline
- Diazepam
- Narcotics
- Calcium channel blockers
- β-agonists
- Progesterone
- α-antagonists

From Orlando RC: Reflux esophagitis. *In* Yamada T (ed): Textbook of Gastroenterology, vol 1, 2nd ed. Philadelphia, JB Lippincott, 1995, p 1214.

Table 31–2. Studies for Assessing Gastroesophageal Reflux Disease (GERD)

Document Presence of Gastroesophageal Reflux

Barium esophagram/upper gastrointestinal series
Standard acid reflux test
24-hr continuous esophageal pH monitoring
Biliary reflux monitoring
Radionuclide scintiscanning

Assess Correlation of Gastroesophageal Reflux With Symptoms

Bernstein's acid perfusion test
24-hr continuous esophageal pH monitoring
Acid suppression therapy trial

Assess Mechanisms of GERD

Barium esophagram/upper gastrointestinal series
Esophageal manometry
Gastric emptying scan
Scintigraphic reflux study

Assess Complications of GERD

Upper endoscopy
- Esophagogastroduodenoscopy with esophageal biopsy
- Laryngoscopy
- Bronchoscopy

Barium esophagram

lapse after cessation of medical therapy.[14, 29] Patients with low LES pressures are most likely to benefit from an antireflux operation.

Upper endoscopy is the best technique to assess the extent of esophageal mucosal injury related to GERD. Common findings cover the spectrum from normal-appearing to Barrett's epithelium and include erythema, edema, erosions, ulcerations, and strictures. Endoscopic biopsy is essential to document the histology of abnormal-appearing mucosa. Even normal-appearing mucosa should be biopsied, because histologic evidence of chronic esophagitis may be observed by a trained pathologist. All patients with suspected gastroesophageal reflux who have failed conservative first-line therapy should undergo endoscopy to evaluate the mucosa before initiation of intensive, physician-guided therapy (Fig. 31–1).[4]

Laryngoscopy should be performed in patients presenting with upper airway symptoms consistent with those seen in atypical GERD. Erythema and edema of the cricoarytenoid folds and the posterior aspect of the true

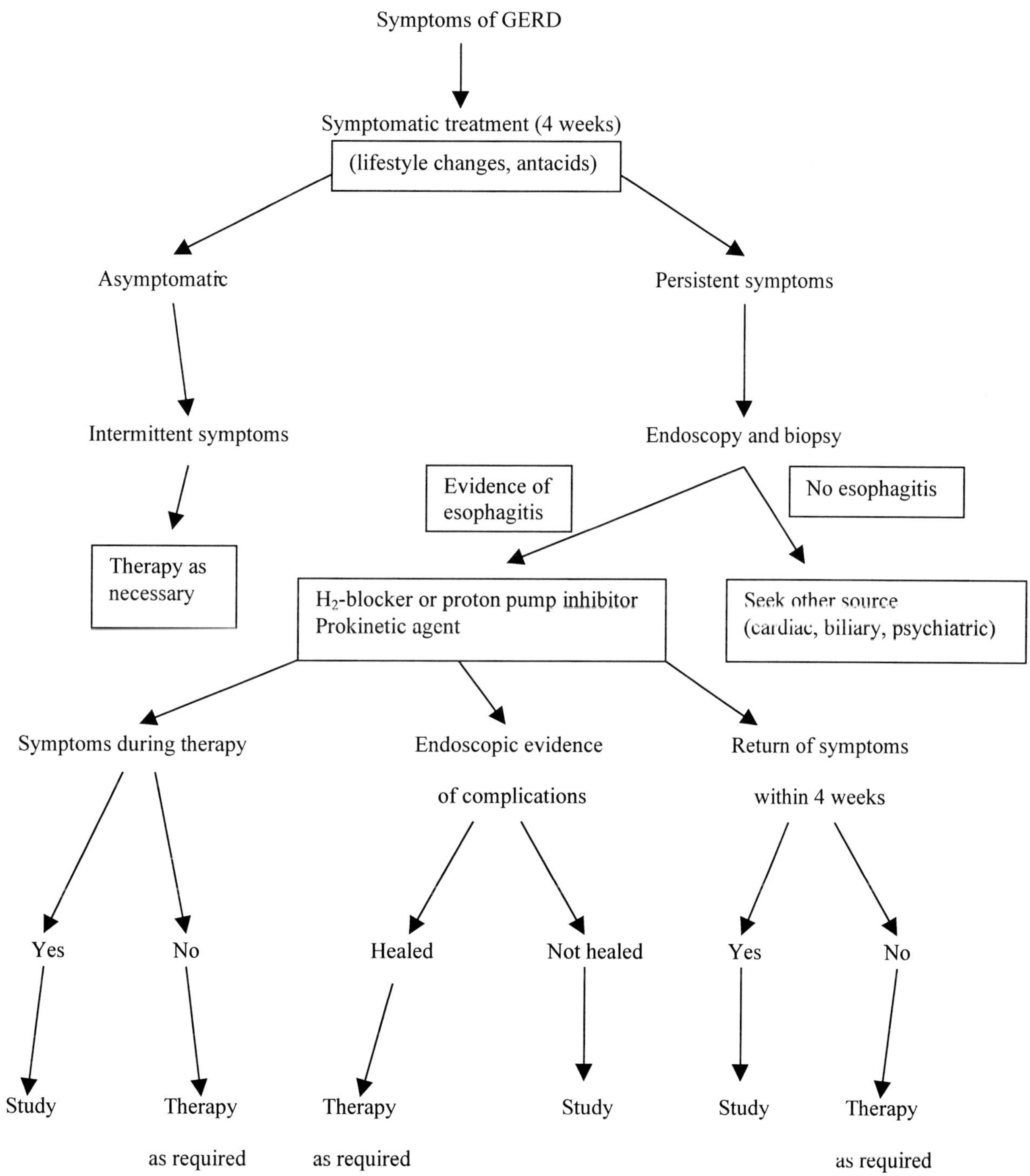

Figure 31–1. Algorithm for evaluation of patients with gastroesophageal reflux disease. (From Bremner RM, Bremner CG, Peters JH, et al: Fundamentals of antireflux surgery. *In* Peters JH, DeMeester TR [eds]: Minimally Invasive Surgery of the Foregut. St. Louis, Quality Medical Publishing, 1994, p 119.)

vocal cords are the most common findings, but patients may also have mucosal ulcerations or vocal cord granulomas.[21, 24] Approximately 50% of patients with symptoms of laryngopharyngeal reflux have abnormal laryngoscopic examinations.[30]

Barium swallow is frequently performed early in the evaluation process of patients presenting with upper gastrointestinal symptoms, but it is not an essential component of the workup. If a large hiatal hernia is suspected, a barium swallow may be helpful in evaluating for the presence of a foreshortened esophagus. Unfortunately, barium swallow is relatively insensitive for GERD and motility abnormalities.

Patients with symptoms of GERD may initially be managed with lifestyle changes and nonprescription antacid therapy. Lifestyle modifications effectively reduce GERD symptoms in many patients, cost little, and in many cases improve the quality of life (see Table 31–1).[17] If this initial phase of therapy fails to control symptoms, an endoscopy should be performed to assess the presence or absence of a hiatal hernia and esophagitis before initiation of aggressive therapy.[4] For patients with atypical symptoms, laryngoscopy should be undertaken as well. Once the suspicion of esophagitis secondary to GERD has been confirmed, the second phase of medical therapy may be instituted. If patients have symptoms while on therapy, develop complications of GERD, or have recurrence of symptoms within 4 weeks of cessation of therapy, further evaluation should be performed to quantify the amount and determine the mechanisms of reflux.

Medical Therapy

The goals of medical therapy for patients with GERD are elimination of symptoms and prevention of long-term mucosal injury and resultant complications. The first phase of treatment is the institution of lifestyle changes and nonprescription antacid therapy. Although compliance is difficult for many patients, lifestyle modifications must be recommended, and every effort must be made to adhere to these guidelines. Physician-directed therapy is governed by the severity of symptoms and mucosal injury and whether therapy is for acute alterations or for maintenance.[21] Patients with symptoms of GERD and no evidence of mucosal injury may be treated medically, with the principal goal being symptom relief. When mild or early mucosal injury is present, patients should have a trial of an H_2-receptor antagonist and, possibly, a prokinetic agent. If severe mucosal injury or intractable symptoms are present, a proton pump inhibitor should be substituted for the H_2-receptor antagonist. Regardless of the degree of injury, the goal of medical therapy is healing of the mucosa, with scheduled endoscopic re-evaluation after 2 to 3 months of intensive medical therapy. If mucosal injury persists or if symptoms remain intractable, antireflux surgery should be considered and the appropriate preoperative evaluation undertaken.

Surgery should also be considered if a patient develops complications. The two most common and significant esophageal complications of GERD are acid-peptic strictures and Barrett's esophagus. Acid-peptic strictures of the esophagus can occur with prolonged mucosal injury and should be biopsied and dilated as part of the initial management once the diagnosis of GERD is made. Recurrence of a stricture on intensive medical therapy or inability to fully dilate a stricture is an indication for surgery.

Barrett's esophagus is diagnosed by the presence of glandular, columnar epithelial cells extending more than 2 to 3 cm proximal from the gastroesophageal junction. Endoscopically, the characteristic feature of the metaplastic mucosa is a color change to a more velvety, richer pink appearance. A defective LES is identified in more than 90% of patients with Barrett's esophagus, but in only 46% of patients with uncomplicated esophagitis.[31, 32] About 10% of patients with reflux esophagitis have endoscopic evidence of Barrett's esophagus, although the range is wide among various studies.[33] In patients with GERD, Barrett's esophagus is more common in white men older than age 40 years. The diagnosis is made by upper endoscopy with systematic mucosal biopsies.[33] Although it is well accepted that Barrett's esophagus is a premalignant process, the exact incidence and prevalence of esophageal cancer in these patients are uncertain.[34] Our strategy for management of patients with Barrett's esophagus is shown in Table 31–3. The role of antireflux surgery in patients with low-grade dysplasia and the role of esophagectomy in patients with high-grade dysplasia are controversial. The factors promoting the progression of dysplasia to carcinoma and the time frame in which this occurs are unknown.[34] Presently, when low-grade dysplasia is present, we recommend aggressive medical therapy if the patient has not been treated and laparoscopic antireflux surgery if low-grade dysplasia is present in spite of maximal medical therapy. Once Barrett's esophagus is present, data suggest that neither operative nor nonoperative therapy will promote regression of the mucosal changes or prevent development of carcinoma.[35, 36]

Surgical Therapy

Historically, hiatal hernia surgery and surgery for the treatment of GERD are intimately intertwined. In fact, reflux was not recognized as a clinically significant disease

Table 31–3. Management of Patients With Barrett's Esophagus

No Signs of Dysplasia

Surveillance endoscopy with biopsies
Intensive medical therapy
Antireflux surgery if intractable symptoms or complications

Low-Grade Dysplasia

Surveillance endoscopy with biopsies every 6–24 mo
Intensive medical therapy
Antireflux surgery if intractable symptoms or complications

High-Grade Dysplasia

Esophagectomy or frequent endoscopic evaluation

Carcinoma in Situ

Esophagectomy

until the 1930s, and the association between GERD and esophagitis was not recognized until the late 1940s.[4] It was not until 1951 that Allison first coined the term *reflux esophagitis* and designed one of the earliest known operations for this problem. His procedure focused on the misplaced stomach and consisted of reduction of the stomach into the abdomen, its fixation to the abdominal wall, and closure of the diaphragmatic crura.[6] Although he recognized that the gastroesophageal junction must have an intra-abdominal location, he erroneously assumed that simple anatomic repair of the hernia would correct GERD. This same lack of appreciation of GERD as a separate disease entity resulted in the development by other surgeons of several anatomic operations that repaired the hernia but had generally poor functional results.

It was not until Nissen's report describing fundoplication that the current era of antireflux surgery was born.[37] Nissen's operation emphasized use of a fundoplication to create a functional valve and restore an effective LES. Although the Nissen fundoplication was clearly effective in eliminating gastroesophageal reflux,[29] its role in the management of patients with significant GERD was less than might have been expected. Generally, only patients with significant complications of GERD were referred for surgery in the 1970s and 1980s.[10] There were two main reasons for the seeming lack of interest in surgical treatment of GERD: (1) the widespread use of histamine receptor antagonists and, more recently, proton pump inhibitors effectively eliminated symptoms of GERD in a majority of patients and resulted in healing of esophagitis in many; and (2) patients and referring physicians believed that antireflux operations were associated with significant morbidity and poor outcome.

The role of surgery in the management of patients with GERD is being redefined. The single most important reason has been the widespread application of laparoscopic techniques to antireflux operations in general and to the Nissen fundoplication in particular. Since Dallemagne and colleagues' first report of nine successful laparoscopic Nissen fundoplications,[9] thousands have been performed, with generally excellent results. In addition, the study by Spechler demonstrated that surgery was more effective than medical therapy for the treatment of symptoms and esophagitis in patients with complicated GERD.[38] Although this information was not necessarily novel, it reinforced the concept that antireflux surgery was effective in treating patients with complicated GERD, and, with the addition of laparoscopic techniques, the revolution was under way.

The ensuing years have resulted in a continued evolution of the management strategy for patients with GERD. The indications for surgical and, more specifically, laparoscopic treatment of GERD are broadening. Chronic medical therapy for GERD has several shortcomings: (1) expense of long-term proton pump inhibitor therapy, (2) frequent recurrence of disease after cessation of therapy, (3) noncompliance in patients with few symptoms who have complications of GERD (e.g., stricture, ulceration, or metaplasia), and (4) unknown consequences of long-term acid suppression therapy. These factors have resulted in young patients with significant GERD being referred with increasing frequency for laparoscopic antireflux surgery. Young patients who respond to medical therapy for GERD and are faced with lifelong reliance on therapy are being considered earlier for surgery because of the increased availability and validation of laparoscopic antireflux operations.

Laparoscopic Treatment

Indications. The indications for laparoscopic treatment of GERD are shown in Table 31–4. It is important to recognize that the indications for laparoscopic antireflux operations, as for all other laparoscopic operations, should be no different from those for the same procedure performed through a standard operative approach. If complications of GERD have developed despite optimal medical therapy, surgery should be recommended. Patients with persistent symptoms despite adequate medical management are also candidates, as are those who are unable to maintain an optimal drug regimen owing to medication intolerance or noncompliance. Finally, patients who are managed on constant medical therapy but who do not wish to subject themselves to the bother and expense of lifelong medication and lifestyle and diet modification may also be considered candidates for surgery.

Contraindications. Contraindications for laparoscopic treatment of GERD are shown in Table 31–4. Although previous major upper abdominal surgery has been a relative contraindication to laparoscopic antireflux surgery, improvements in equipment and surgical technique have facilitated performance in this situation, and cases must

Table 31–4. Indications and Contraindications for Laparoscopic Antireflux Operations

Indications

Symptomatic gastroesophageal reflux disease (typical and atypical)
- Refractory to maximal medical therapy
- Noncompliant patient
- Medical therapy intolerance

Complications of gastroesophageal reflux disease
- Mucosal ulcerations refractory to medical therapy
- Esophageal stricture
- Recurrent aspiration pneumonia
- Chronic laryngopharyngeal complications
- Barrett's metaplasia (early)*

Contraindications

Absolute

Contraindication to surgery in general
- Cannot tolerate general anesthesia
- Uncorrectable coagulopathy

Foreshortened esophagus

Relative

Previous significant upper abdominal surgery
- Gastric resection
- Liver resection—left lobe
- Splenectomy or history of splenic trauma

*Controversial.

be considered individually. A failed antireflux operation performed either via a laparotomy or through minimally invasive techniques does not necessarily preclude an attempt at revision or redo of the fundoplication laparoscopically. However, such a reoperation should not be undertaken lightly and should be attempted only by surgeons well versed in laparoscopic antireflux procedures after re-evaluation of the recurrent GERD. Significant esophageal dysmotility is a contraindication to performing a Nissen fundoplication; however, a partial fundoplication can be performed in this situation. The current recommendation for patients with proven foreshortened esophagus and GERD is performance of an esophageal lengthening procedure in combination with an antireflux operation. The most commonly performed lengthening procedure is the Collis gastroplasty, which is frequently performed transthoracically.[4] A combined laparoscopic and right thoracoscopic approach has recently been described to allow the combined Collis-Nissen procedure to be performed using only minimally invasive techniques.[39] If this procedure provides clinical results equivalent to those achieved with the open method, foreshortened esophagus may not be a contraindication to a laparoscopic approach in the future.

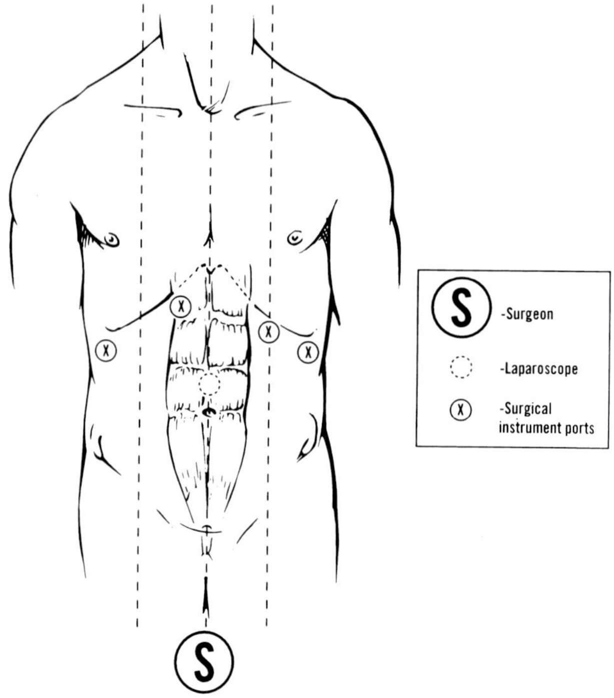

Figure 31–2. Surgical port placement. Exact locations can and should be modified according to patient body habitus and intra-abdominal anatomy.

Surgical Strategy. The principal goals of any antireflux operation are to correct the hiatal hernia, if present, and to return a 3- to 5-cm length of esophagus into the peritoneal cavity and fix it within the abdomen. Hiatal hernia correction usually requires reduction of the stomach and a portion of the esophagus into the abdominal cavity, as well as crural closure to narrow the hiatal defect. Maintaining a length of esophagus within the abdomen is commonly accomplished by performing a full (360-degree) or partial (180- to 270-degree) fundoplication.

All laparoscopic antireflux procedures are performed under general anesthesia, and our preference is to place the patient in the lithotomy position, although the straight supine position is an option. The lithotomy position permits the surgeon to stand between the legs of the patient, which are cradled in stirrups or positioned on modified fracture tables. A nasogastric or orogastric tube and Foley catheter should be placed before the operation to avoid injury to the stomach and bladder. The reverse Trendelenburg table position is essential to maximize exposure to the area of the esophageal hiatus and the lower mediastinum. Measures should be taken to ensure that patients, particularly heavy ones, will not slide down the operating table when this position is used. This is achieved by using either a surgical "bean bag" or "thigh slings" (bath towels loosely wrapped around the upper thigh and the bar of the stirrups).

For all laparoscopic antireflux operations, we use at least five operating ports, as demonstrated in Figure 31–2. Standard carbon dioxide insufflation is used, and surgeon preference determines whether open or closed initiation of pneumoperitoneum is utilized. We place the supraumbilical port first, 2 to 3 fingerbreadths superior to the umbilicus, and use this port for the laparoscope. The port in the right anterior axillary line is used for placement of the liver retractor, and the left anterior axillary line port is used for retraction of the stomach and other first assistant maneuvers. The right subxiphoid and left subcostal ports are used by the operating surgeon. It is essential that every surgeon performing these procedures be facile in two-handed surgical techniques, intracorporeal suturing, and management of esophageal, gastric, and splenic injuries. Although many antireflux operations and modifications exist, the most commonly performed procedures are described here.

Laparoscopic Nissen Fundoplication

Technique. The operation begins with retraction of the left lobe of the liver against the left hemidiaphragm using an atraumatic retractor (Fig. 31–3). It is not necessary and can be counterproductive to take down the diaphragmatic connections to the liver. The first assistant uses an atraumatic grasper, such as an endoscopic Babcock clamp, to retract the stomach inferiorly. The gastrohepatic omentum is divided using either electrosurgical cautery or the harmonic scalpel (Ethicon Endo-Surgery, Inc., Cincinnati, OH) beginning near the incisura angularis and extending superiorly toward the phrenoesophageal ligament (see Fig. 31–3). An aberrant left hepatic artery is present in up to 25% of cases and should be identified and preserved.[40] Although it can make dissection of the right crus and retroesophageal window more difficult, the operation can usually be completed without division of this vessel. The right crus can usually be visualized after division of the gastrohepatic omentum is completed (see Fig. 31–3). Care should be exercised to avoid injuring the caudate lobe of the liver, which should be just to the patient's right of the right crus. Dissection of the space between the right crus and the esophagus can be initiated at this time, entering the lower mediastinal fat. Occasionally, small venous

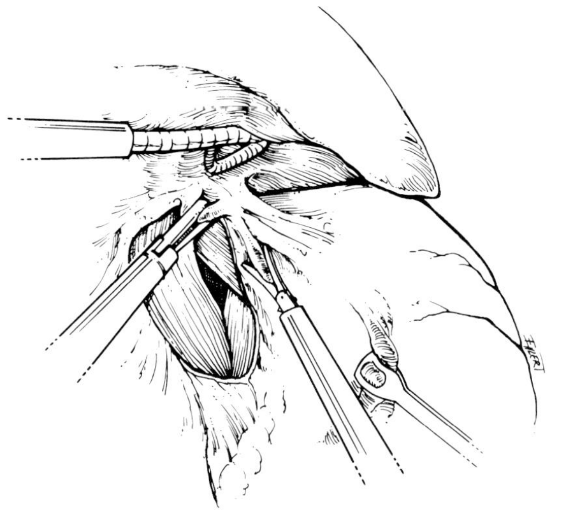

Figure 31–3. Visualization of the right crus of the diaphragm after dissection of the gastrohepatic omentum. An atraumatic retractor is used to elevate the left lobe of the liver. The stomach is retracted caudad with an atraumatic clamp such as a Babcock grasper.

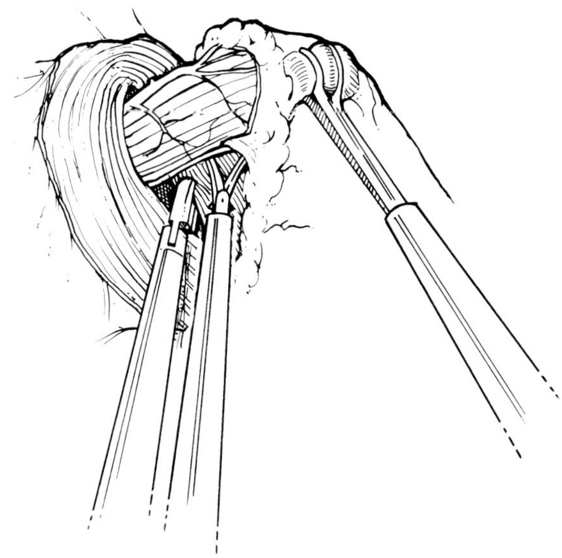

Figure 31–4. The retroesophageal window is opened using blunt and sharp dissection. The proximal stomach is retracted anteriorly and to the patient's left to facilitate exposure of the retroesophageal window.

branches to the distal esophagus may be present and can be coagulated.

Attention is turned toward the phrenoesophageal ligament, completing dissection over the esophagus toward the left crus. The cardia of the stomach is retracted inferiorly, and the left crus is dissected completely free from all attachments to the distal esophagus and cardia, essentially completing anterior and lateral mobilization of the distal esophagus and gastroesophageal junction. The left vagus nerve can be visualized adherent to the anterior distal esophagus.

The distal esophagus is retracted to the patient's left, and the critical retroesophageal window is created approaching from the patient's right (Fig. 31–4). In general, this can be performed using blunt dissection with coagulation of obvious vessels, provided the left crus has been dissected free from all attachments to the esophagus and cardia. Special care must be taken to ensure that the dissection is not entering the lower mediastinum or the left pleural space by limiting dissection to the anteroinferior surface of the left crus. Once the retroesophageal window is opened completely, a blunt grasper can be placed through it carefully to avoid injury to the spleen. A Penrose drain (1 in. wide, 6 in. long) is grasped and brought through the window and is subsequently used for atraumatic retraction of the distal esophagus. Using the Penrose drain for retraction allows further dissection and visualization of the crura down to their origin.

At this point in the operation, the gastric decompression tube is removed and a bougie is placed transorally. We prefer a 52- to 56-French, tapered, mercury-weighted bougie, but the specific size and bougie type are up to the surgeon. Every surgeon undertaking laparoscopic antireflux procedures must ensure that the person placing the bougie has some experience with this procedure, because the risk of esophageal and gastric perforation is highest during this maneuver. Once the bougie is safely in the proper location, the size of the hiatal closure is estimated and the bougie is retracted back into the distal esophagus. The right and left crura are brought together using a heavy (at least 2–0) nonabsorbable suture material. Usually, we place two to four crural closure sutures, which, if tied too tightly, can tear or cause necrosis of the crus (Fig. 31–5). At completion of the crural closure, we recommend replacement of the bougie across the hiatus to ensure that the closure is of the proper tightness.

The two steps remaining are completion of the fundoplication and division of the short gastric vessels (SGVs). Although the debate regarding the necessity of SGV division continues, we believe that this maneuver is essential to minimize the risk of postoperative dysphagia. Most sur-

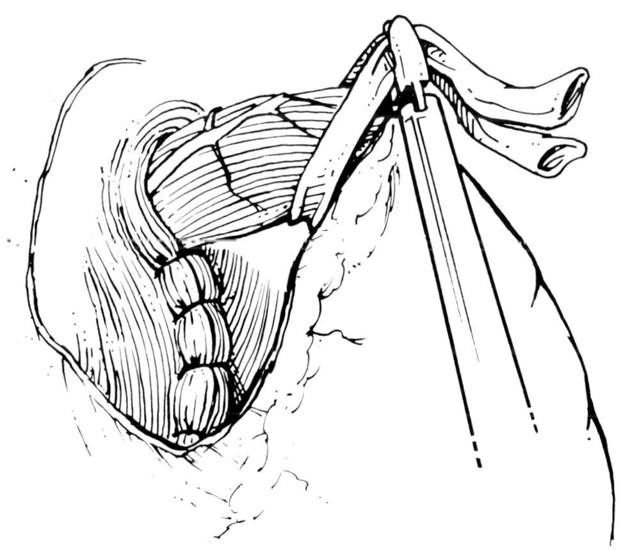

Figure 31–5. A Penrose sling is placed through the retroesophageal window to facilitate atraumatic retraction of the gastroesophageal junction. Two to four crural closure stitches are placed, also facilitated by retraction with the Penrose sling.

geons divide the SGVs before completion of the fundoplication to ensure that the wrap will be loose enough to minimize dysphagia. This can be simply performed by retraction of the stomach to the patient's right by the surgeon and elevation of the gastrosplenic omentum by the first assistant. The gastrosplenic omentum can be divided between surgical clips, but we prefer the simple technique using the harmonic scalpel, which does not require dissection and individual ligation or clipping of the SGVs. Division of these vessels begins at the mid–greater curvature of the stomach and proceeds proximally until all SGVs are divided. Fundoplication can be completed in most patients without prior division of SGVs, and if it is performed first, fundoplication may actually facilitate SGV division by retracting the stomach away from the spleen and placing tension on the gastrosplenic omentum.

Fundoplication is completed by placing an atraumatic grasper (e.g., Babcock clamp) through the retroesophageal window from the patient's right. We do not routinely exclude the right vagus nerve from fundoplication, because the necessity of this maneuver is not certain.[41] The fundus of the stomach is grasped and passed through the retroesophageal window (Fig. 31–6). At this point, the bougie is placed across the gastroesophageal junction again, and the fundoplication is pulled together. The fundus of the stomach is passed back and forth through the window to ensure that the window is large enough and that proper locations of the fundus are being used for the wrap. Two to four fundoplication sutures are placed, as shown in Figure 31–7. We prefer a heavy (at least 2–0) nonabsorbable suture material and do not routinely use pledgets. Each suture includes a generous bite of esophagus in addition to the gastric bites to the left and right of the esophagus. These sutures can be placed with the bougie left in position, and special care is taken to avoid inclusion of the left vagus in the sutures. The sutures for the completed Nissen fundoplication, shown in Figure 31–8, should be located in the right anterior quadrant relative to the esophagus.

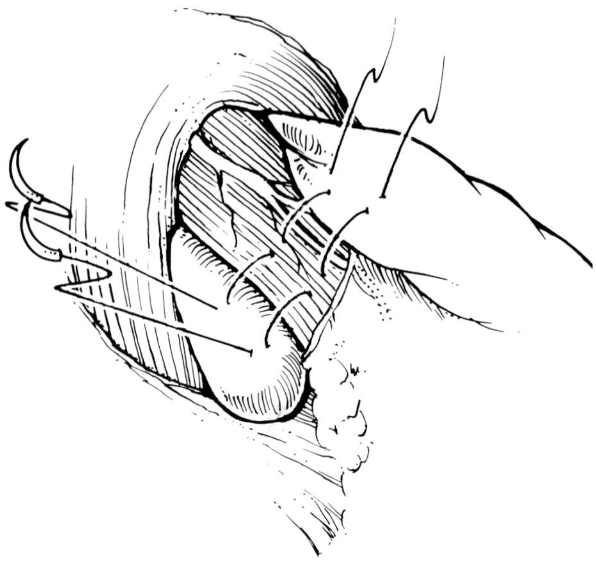

Figure 31–7. A fundic wrap 1.5 to 2 cm in length is created using two or three nonabsorbable sutures. Care is taken to exclude the anterior trunk of the vagus nerve.

Upon completion of the operation, the bougie is withdrawn, hemostasis is ensured, and a nasogastric tube is replaced. An antiemetic is given by anesthesia before waking the patient to avoid early nausea and emesis, decreasing the risk of early crural disruption.

Results. Laparoscopic Nissen fundoplication has rapidly become the standard of care for the surgical treatment of GERD in the years since Dallemagne's first report. Although there was no prospective, randomized trial leading to this widespread acceptance, several studies have demonstrated that laparoscopic Nissen fundoplication is

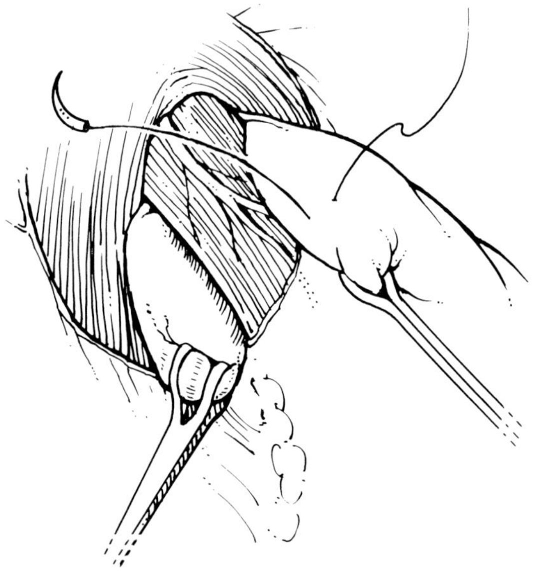

Figure 31–6. The fundus of the stomach is passed through the retroesophageal window, and the fundoplication is begun after ensuring that the wrap will not be too tight nor under excessive tension.

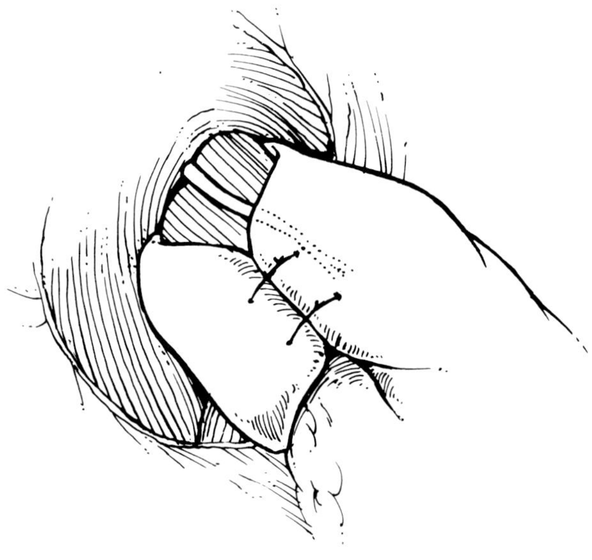

Figure 31–8. Appearance of the completed Nissen fundoplication. The sutures should be located over the right anterior quadrant of the esophagus.

effective at eliminating significant reflux and that it can be done safely and cost-effectively with results similar to those achieved by the open operative approach. Peters and colleagues[13] found in a series of 81 patients that symptom resolution after laparoscopic Nissen fundoplication was similar to that after the open approach.

Patient satisfaction, postoperative dysphagia, gas bloat, and recurrence of reflux are important aspects of the postoperative assessment in patients who have undergone an antireflux procedure. Patient satisfaction is generally high, because all medication can be stopped postoperatively and quality of life is improved. Persistent dysphagia has been reported in up to 21% of patients after Nissen fundoplication, but this has been decreased significantly by shortening the fundic wrap to 1.5 cm long.[29, 42] Prolonged gas bloat is seen in approximately 8% of patients and persistent dysphagia in 3 to 8%, but satisfactory results are reported by greater than 85% of patients undergoing Nissen fundoplication.[8, 42, 43]

The efficacy of the laparoscopic approach for Nissen fundoplication has been well documented. Pitcher and colleagues[11] reported that the early (<4 week) dysphagia rate was 34% but decreased significantly thereafter to 7%, comparing favorably with the rate for the open procedure. Gas bloat was not a major problem in their series of 68 patients, but increased flatulence occurred in 10% after laparoscopic Nissen fundoplication. Similarly, Peters and colleagues[13] noted no statistical difference in postoperative dysphagia when comparing patients undergoing laparoscopic (6.2%) vs. open (8.1%) Nissen fundoplication and found similar satisfaction in the two groups of patients. Laparoscopic Nissen fundoplication is a safe operation with a cumulative morbidity of 6 to 25% and a cumulative mortality rate less than 0.1%.[1] Interestingly, complications common to open Nissen fundoplication such as splenectomy, pneumonia, atelectasis, and wound infection are unusual with the laparoscopic approach.[1]

One of the more controversial issues regarding laparoscopic Nissen fundoplication has been whether the SGVs should be divided. Many authors strongly recommend division of these vessels to decrease the incidence of postoperative dysphagia, and DeMeester and colleagues advocated routine division of the SGVs during open Nissen fundoplication.[29] Unfortunately, most reports addressing this issue are anecdotal, and surgeon practice is based on personal experience. The Rossetti-Hell modification of the Nissen fundoplication does not entail short gastric artery division, it creates a fundic wrap primarily from the anterior wall of the stomach. An early report by Geagea[44] suggested that the results of a laparoscopic Rossetti fundoplication were similar to those of Nissen fundoplication. However, Hunter and colleagues prospectively compared patients undergoing laparoscopic Nissen fundoplication, Rossetti-Hell fundoplication, and Toupet fundoplication and reported a significantly higher rate of postoperative dysphagia with the laparoscopic Rossetti-Hell operation.[45] Recently, a prospective, double-blind, randomized trial comparing laparoscopic Nissen fundoplication with and without SGV division was reported.[46] The authors of that study found no significant differences in dysphagia rates and patient satisfaction between the two groups, suggesting that SGV division is not necessary to prevent dysphagia.[46] In actuality, the importance of SGV division during Nissen fundoplication is still uncertain and may be unrelated to postoperative dysphagia. The most prudent recommendation at this time is that surgeons who perform laparoscopic antireflux surgery perform the operation they are most comfortable with through the open approach. Our preference is to divide the SGVs routinely using the harmonic scalpel, performing a traditional Nissen fundoplication.

Rattner and Brooks compared open and laparoscopic Nissen fundoplication and evaluated patient satisfaction, cost, and efficacy.[47] The authors were able to demonstrate a faster implementation of clear liquid intake, return to work, and return to full function in the laparoscopic group; however, patient satisfaction was similar in both groups. In addition, laparoscopic Nissen fundoplication was associated with significantly lower total costs than the open approach.

Interestingly, the study by Rattner and Brooks emphasized the importance of patient expectations and personality.[47] Similarly, Watson and colleagues studied a group of 77 patients undergoing laparoscopic Nissen fundoplication who had completed an illness behavior questionnaire.[48] High scores for "affective" and "hypochondriacal" behavior were associated with poor satisfaction with the surgical outcome.[48] Therefore, it is essential to identify and educate patients with unrealistic expectations and to adequately prepare patients for results that may be less than perfect.

Laparoscopic Toupet Fundoplasty

Partial fundoplication can play a role when the patient's esophageal motility is abnormal. Advanced laparoscopic surgeons must have these operations in their armamentarium in the event that 360-degree fundoplication is not possible or is contraindicated (e.g., in conjunction with a laparoscopic Heller myotomy for treatment of achalasia). The Toupet fundoplasty is the most frequently performed partial fundoplication. The laparoscopic approach for this procedure has gained widespread acceptance in Europe and is advocated by some surgeons in the United States.[49] The initial operation described by Andre Toupet in 1963 was a 180-degree posterior fundoplasty with sutures apposing the fundic wrap to the crura posteriorly and to the esophagus anteriorly.[50] Concerns about the inadequacy of this fundoplasty in preventing gastroesophageal reflux led to a modification in which the wrap encompassed 270 degrees of the esophageal circumference.[51]

Technique. The operation begins similarly to the laparoscopic Nissen fundoplication. The patient is placed in either the lithotomy position or the straight supine postion, and all port placements are the same as for the laparoscopic Nissen fundoplication. The gastrohepatic omentum is opened, and the phrenoesophageal ligament is divided to expose the crura and the gastroesophageal junction. The large retroesophageal window is created, and the fundus of the stomach is brought through this window. As shown in Figure 31–9, three intracorporeal sutures (2–0 nonabsorbable) are placed between the posterior aspect of the fundic wrap and the right crus, followed by three sutures

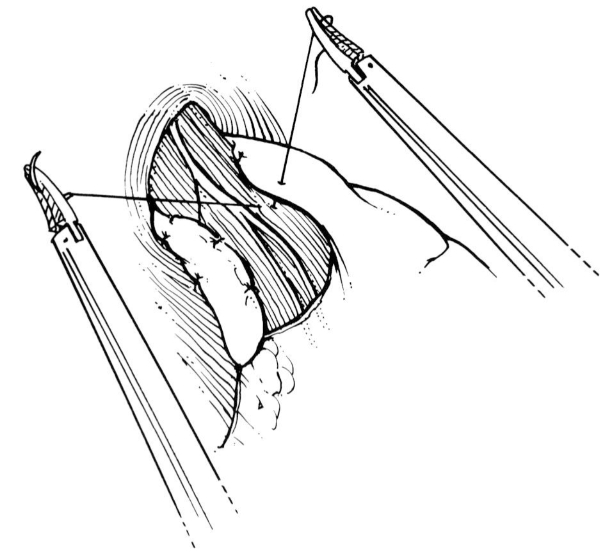

Figure 31–9. Laparoscopic Toupet posterior partial fundoplasty. Adequate purchase of esophageal musculature ensures nondehiscence of the fundoplasty.

placed between the anterior aspect of the fundic wrap and the right anterolateral wall of the esophagus. Often an apical stitch can be placed that incorporates the fundic wrap, right crus, and esophagus. An esophageal bougie (50 to 56 French, tapered, mercury weighted) is placed at this time. This dilates the esophagus and allows more accurate suture placement to ensure that the fundoplasty encompasses 270 degrees of the esophageal circumference. Subsequently, the fundus to the left of the esophagus is sutured in similar fashion with three posterior sutures fixing it to the left crus and three sutures to the left-anterior aspect of the esophagus to complete the operation.

Results. A randomized trial in Sweden compared open Toupet fundoplasty to open Nissen fundoplication and found that the modified Toupet procedure was durable over time and prevented GERD as well as the Nissen fundoplication and had fewer side effects.[52] The laparoscopic Toupet fundoplasty has been reported to have a lower incidence of postoperative dysphagia compared with the laparoscopic Nissen fundoplication.[49]

Laparoscopic Dor Fundoplasty

The Dor partial fundoplasty is a 180-degree anterior wrap that was initially described three decades ago but has not gained widespread acceptance.[50] The operation does not require extensive dissection of the esophageal hiatus and results in minimal exposure of the distal esophagus. Concern over whether an adequate segment of intra-abdominal esophagus is created to prevent GERD has limited the application of the Dor anterior fundoplasty.

Technique. The operation begins similarly to the laparoscopic Nissen fundoplication and Toupet fundoplasty. However, the gastrohepatic omentum does not need to be opened, and only a limited amount of the phrenoesophageal ligament needs to be dissected to identify the right and left crura. The anterior fundus of the stomach is grasped with a Babcock clamp and rotated toward the patient's right. If there is no tension on the stomach, the fundus is sutured to the right crus using a 2–0 nonabsorbable suture material. In general, two sutures are used to secure the fundus to the right crus and two sutures are placed to secure the fundus to the anterior esophagus (Fig. 31–10). Subsequently, the mercury-weighted, tapered 50- to 56-French bougie is placed to ensure that a 180-degree anterior fundoplasty is performed, and two sutures are used to transfix the fundus to the left crus.

Results. The principal use of this procedure has been to buttress repairs of anterior, distal esophageal perforations or as an adjunct to Heller myotomy to minimize postoperative reflux. In the latter situation, the operation is performed in the same fashion, except the right and left crural sutures also incorporate a bite of the cut edge of esophageal musculature and thus may serve to keep the myotomy open. The comparative efficacy of the Dor fundoplasty as an antireflux operation has never been studied.

Laparoscopic Hill Repair

The Hill repair was introduced as an alternative to the standard Nissen fundoplication and the Belsey Mark IV partial fundoplication. The operation has not enjoyed widespread acceptance for a variety of reasons, including questions about the validity of the anatomy described and the reproducibility of results in the hands of other surgeons.[53] When performed by properly trained surgeons, the Hill repair as an antireflux operation appears to provide acceptable results.[53] In 1994, Hill and colleagues[53] reported on the first 40 patients undergoing laparoscopic Hill repair. Ninety-seven percent of patients experienced control of reflux, and 92% reported subjective improvement. Unfortunately, early postoperative dysphagia seems to be a problem with the laparoscopic Hill repair as well, although the actual incidence is uncertain. Because of the

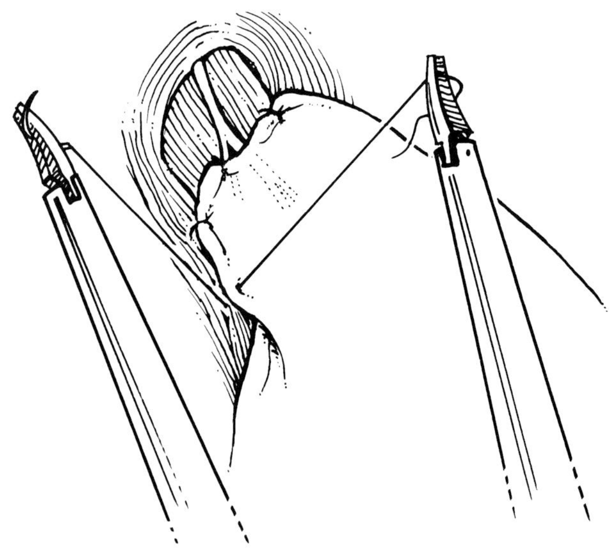

Figure 31–10. Laparoscopic Dor anterior partial fundoplasty. Special care must be taken to avoid suture incorporation of the anterior vagus nerve.

skepticism associated with the open Hill repair, use of the laparoscopic approach to the Hill repair has been limited.

Complications of Laparoscopic Fundoplication

Complications of laparoscopic antireflux operations fall into several categories. The most obvious complications occur intraoperatively and include hemorrhage, technical difficulty, and esophageal or gastric perforation. Significant intraoperative hemorrhage occurs infrequently but is most often the result of splenic trauma or bleeding from the SGVs during division. Collet and Cadiere reported two cases of intraoperative hemorrhage out of 758 laparoscopic antireflux operations.[54] In general, bleeding can be managed laparoscopically, but it should not be allowed to persist to the point where transfusion is considered. SGV division has been greatly facilitated by the harmonic scalpel, which minimizes the need to dissect each individual vessel before division. In addition, the coagulative effect of the instrument seems to be better than surgical clips for preventing hemorrhage in our experience.

Intraoperative technical difficulties leading to conversion to an open procedure are generally related to the patient's body habitus or internal anatomy. Large amounts of intra-abdominal fat, particularly in the lesser omentum, gastrosplenic ligament, and epiphrenic fat pad, can make dissection and identification of normal structures difficult. Additionally, a large hiatal hernia, particularly a paraesophageal hernia, can easily disorient even an experienced surgeon and lead to esophageal perforation or pleural injury.

Perforation of the esophagus or stomach is the greatest fear of every surgeon performing laparoscopic antireflux procedures. Perforation occurs either during dissection of these structures or during passage of the bougie. Schauer and colleagues reviewed 364 laparoscopic Nissen fundoplications performed by 14 surgeons and found evidence of 17 perforations.[55] They were able to identify three mechanisms leading to the 17 perforations: improper dissection of the retroesophageal window, improper passage of the bougie, and suture pull-through postoperatively. Ten of the 17 perforations (3% of the total number of patients) occurred during dissection of the retroesophageal window and in general were the result of inadequate exposure, due to either excessive fat or large hiatal hernia. Prevention of this complication is best accomplished by careful dissection and a clear understanding of the borders of the retroesophageal window (Fig. 31–11). Dissection of the window is most difficult when a paraesophageal hernia is present. Trus and colleagues reviewed 76 cases of laparoscopic repair of paraesophageal hernia and found that 5 (7%) visceral perforations occurred during dissection.[56]

Passage of the bougie intraoperatively is potentially dangerous and can lead to visceral perforation even in the open operative setting. Schauer and colleagues found that 4 of 17 perforations occurred during bougie passage.[55] Lowham and colleagues found 11 cases of bougie perforation in 1620 laparoscopic foregut operations.[57] There are several factors that can lead to this complication: (1) inexperienced anesthesia personnel passing the dilator; (2) downward traction on the gastroesophageal junction, leading to angulation of this area, predisposing the dilator to perforate the anterior esophagus or stomach (Fig. 31–12); and (3) anterior angulation of the esophagus after crural closure, leading to posterior perforation of the distal esophagus with bougie passage. The surgeon must ensure that the person passing the bougie is experienced with the technique (i.e., well-lubricated bougie, anterior elevation of the mandible, and gentle rotation of the bougie as it passes) and knows when to stop (i.e., when the bougie meets unusual resistance).[55, 57] As the bougie is passed, it is essential to continuously watch and scrutinize its passage into the stomach, taking special care to create no angulation at the gastroesophageal junction.

Repair of a small esophageal or gastric perforation can be accomplished laparoscopically, but if the injury is large or if an esophageal injury appears to be relatively craniad, it is more prudent to convert to an open repair. Allowing an esophageal tear to progress into the mediastinum during a laparoscopic repair is ill advised.

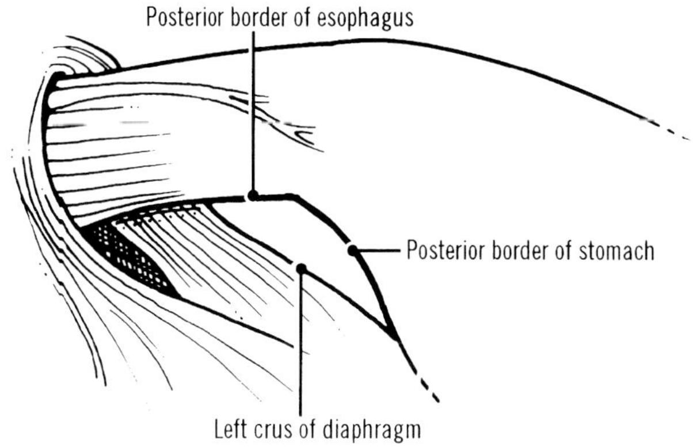

Figure 31–11. Borders of the retroesophageal window include (1) posterior border of the distal esophagus, (2) posterior aspect of the proximal stomach, and (3) left crus of the diaphragm.

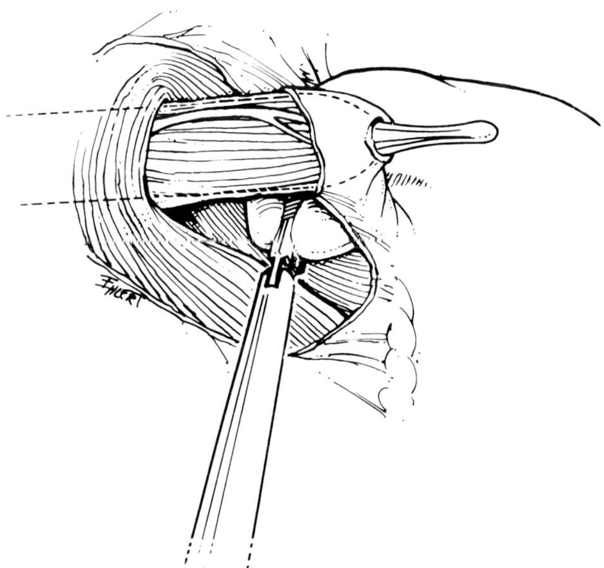

Figure 31–12. Any anterior displacement of the gastroesophageal junction during passage of the bougie can predispose to anterior perforation of the esophagus or stomach.

The second group of complications has been touched on previously and includes functional postoperative problems such as dysphagia, gas bloat, increased flatulence, and chest pain. Pitcher and colleagues demonstrated that the most frequent postoperative symptom is dysphagia (Table 31–5).[11] The authors inquired about a variety of symptoms before and after the 4-week postoperative point and found significant symptomatic improvement after 4 weeks. These functional complications are most frequently associated with Nissen fundoplication but can occur with any antireflux procedure.

The final group of complications consists of intraoperative technical errors that result in failure of the antireflux repair. The three most common are misplacement of the fundoplication, delayed breakdown of the wrap, and herniation of the wrap into the chest. The most frequent mistake is a misplaced fundoplication in which the fundic wrap is actually sutured around the proximal stomach instead of the distal esophagus—the so-called gastro-gastric wrap. This can occur when a tubular stomach is mistakenly identified as the distal esophagus at the time of surgery but more commonly results from inadequate exposure and dissection of the esophagus. A gastro-gastric wrap may also occur if the fundoplication sutures pull out of the esophagus postoperatively. When this occurs, the fundic wrap may slip down onto the proximal stomach, resulting in a "slipped Nissen."[58] This may occur either because the esophageal "bites" incorporated by the sutures are too small or because an inadequate distal esophageal dissection was performed. The latter error results in an inadequate length of intra-abdominal esophagus and a fundic wrap under tension as the esophagus withdraws up into the chest.

Complete breakdown of the fundoplication may occur and results from either poor suture technique with inadequate purchase of tissues or excessive tension on the sutured tissues. If the SGVs are not divided during a Nissen fundoplication, the sutures for the fundoplication may be under excessive tension, leading to breakdown of the wrap. Inadequate dissection of the epiphrenic fat pad and proximal stomach can result in either increased tightness of the wrap or inadequate placement of sutures into fat rather than viscera.

Finally, herniation of a Nissen wrap into the chest can occur and may lead to dysphagia, chest pain, and even gastric volvulus or necrosis. This may result either from breakdown of the crural closure or from inadequate esophageal dissection, leading to upward traction of the fundoplication, as can happen with foreshortened esophagus.

Table 31–5. Postoperative Complications

Symptom	<4 Weeks		>4 Weeks	
	No. of Patients	Percentage	No. of Patients	Percentage
Dysphagia	24	34	5	7
Gas bloat	2	3	1	1
Flatulence	7	10	6	9
Chest pain	2	3	1	1

Reprinted from Pitcher DE, Curet MJ, Martin DT, et al: Successful management of severe gastroesophageal reflux disease with laparoscopic Nissen fundoplication. (With permission from Excerpta Medica Inc. From Am J Surg 168:547–554, 1994.)

Conclusion

Ultimately, measures of success for any operation are related to outcomes and patient satisfaction. For any laparoscopic operation there is the added measure of comparison to the open version of the operation. As previously discussed, the reported results of laparoscopic antireflux operations, in particular the Nissen fundoplication and Toupet fundoplasty, are similar to or better than the results of the open versions of these operations.

The laparoscopic approach to antireflux surgery has helped revolutionize the management of patients with severe GERD. Thorough diagnostic evaluation and proper patient selection are the first steps to successful laparoscopic surgical management of GERD. Selection of the correct operation is the next critical step, as different clinical situations mandate different procedures (Fig. 31–13). It is essential that surgeons undertaking antireflux surgery understand the pathophysiology of GERD and are able to perform a variety of antireflux procedures via either the laparoscopic or the open approach (laparotomy, thoracotomy), as the situation dictates. Finally, surgeons must develop the expertise and gain the experience necessary for the successful performance of advanced laparoscopic operations such as antireflux procedures. This requires adequate instruction and proctoring until the surgeon becomes proficient with two-handed techniques and intracorporeal suturing. When all these benchmarks are met,

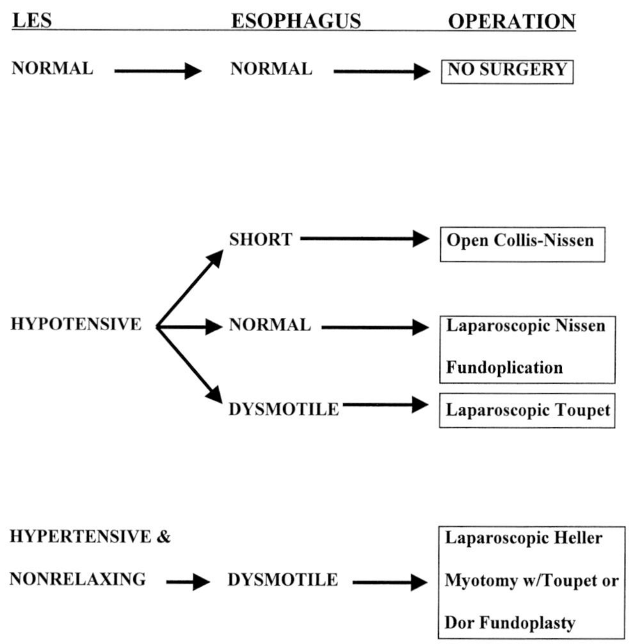

Figure 31–13. Surgical management of disease of the foregut. (From Raiser F, Hinder RA, Kraus MA: Pitfalls in the surgical management of gastroesophageal reflux disease. Contemp Surg 40:189, 1996.)

successful results can be expected in 85 to 90% of patients, with less morbidity and shorter hospital stays than with the open approach. Thus, the laparoscopic approach to antireflux surgery is becoming the standard by which other antireflux therapy is measured.

References

1. McKenzie D, Grayson T, Polk HC: The impact of omeprazole and laparoscopy upon hiatal hernia and reflux esophagitis. J Am Coll Surg 183:413, 1996.
2. Pellegrini CA: Therapy for gastroesophageal reflux disease: The new kid on the block (Editorial). J Am Coll Surg 180:485, 1995.
3. Heartburn Across America: A Gallup Organization National Survey. Princeton, NJ, Gallup Organization, 1988.
4. Bremner RM, Bremner CG, Peters JH, et al: Fundamentals of antireflux surgery. *In* Peters JH, DeMeester TR (eds): Minimally Invasive Surgery of the Foregut, 1st ed. St. Louis, Quality Medical Publishing, 1994, p 119.
5. Mittal RK, Holloway RH, Penagini R, et al: Transient lower esophageal sphincter relaxation. Gastroenterology 109:601, 1995.
6. Allison PR: Reflux esophagitis, sliding hiatal hernia and the anatomy of repair. Surg Gynecol Obstet 92:419, 1951.
7. Wu JS, Dunnegan DL, Luttmann DR, et al: The influence of surgical technique on clinical outcome of laparoscopic Nissen fundoplication. Surg Endosc 10:1164, 1996.
8. Hinder RA, Filipi CJ, Wetscher G, et al: Laparoscopic Nissen fundoplication is an effective treatment for gastroesophageal reflux disease. Ann Surg 220:472, 1994.
9. Dallemagne B, Weerts JM, Jehaes C, et al: Laparoscopic Nissen fundoplication: Preliminary report. Surg Laparosc Endosc 1:138, 1991.
10. Cuschieri A, Hunter J, Wolfe B, et al: Multicenter prospective evaluation of laparoscopic antireflux surgery. Surg Endosc 7:505, 1993.
11. Pitcher DE, Curet MJ, Martin DT, et al: Successful management of severe gastroesophageal reflux disease with laparoscopic Nissen fundoplication. Am J Surg 168:547, 1994.
12. Hunter JG, Trus TL, Branum GD, et al: A physiologic approach to laparoscopic fundoplication for gastroesophageal reflux disease. Ann Surg 223:673, 1996.
13. Peters JH, Heimbucher J, Kauer WKH, et al: Clinical and physiologic comparison of laparoscopic and open Nissen fundoplication. J Am Coll Surg 180:385, 1995.
14. Costantini M, Zaninotto G, Anselmino M, et al: The role of a defective lower esophageal sphincter in the clinical outcome of treatment for gastroesophageal reflux disease. Arch Surg 131:655, 1996.
15. Sataloff DM, Pursnani K, Hoyo S, et al: An objective assessment of laparoscopic antireflux surgery. Am J Surg 174:63, 1997.
16. Heine KJ, Mittal RK: Crural diaphragm and lower esophageal sphincter as antireflux barriers. Viewpoints Dig Dis 23:1, 1991.
17. Orlando RC: Reflux esophagitis. *In* Yamada T (ed): Textbook of Gastroenterology, vol 1, 2nd ed. Philadelphia, JB Lippincott, 1995, p 1214.
18. Rakic S, Stein HJ, DeMeester TR, et al: Role of esophageal body function in gastroesophageal reflux disease: Implications for surgical management. J Am Coll Surg 185:380, 1997.
19. Schindlbeck NE, Heinrich C, Konig A: Optimal thresholds, sensitivity, and specificity of long-term pHmetry for the detection of gastroesophageal reflux disease. Gastroenterology 93:85, 1987.
20. Koufman J, Sataloff RT, Toohill R: Laryngopharyngeal reflux: Consensus conference report. J Voice 10:215, 1996.
21. Richter JE: Typical and atypical presentations of gastroesophageal reflux disease. Gastroenterol Clin North Am 25:75, 1996.
22. Wetscher GJ, Glaser K, Hinder RA, et al: Respiratory symptoms in patients with gastroesophageal reflux disease following medical therapy and antireflux surgery. Am J Surg 174:639, 1997.
23. Johnson WE, Hagen JA, DeMeester TR, et al: Outcome of respiratory symptoms after antireflux surgery on patients with gastroesophageal reflux disease. Arch Surg 131:489, 1996.
24. Deveney CW, Benner K, Cohen J: Gastroesophageal reflux and laryngeal disease. Arch Surg 128:1021, 1993.
25. Fein M, Hagen JA, Ritter MP, et al: Isolated upright gastroesophageal reflux is not a contraindication for antireflux surgery. Surgery 122:829, 1997.
26. Perdikis G, Lund RJ, Hinder RA, et al: Esophageal manometry and 24-hour pH testing in the management of gastroesophageal reflux patients. Am J Surg 174:634, 1997.
27. Raiser F, Hinder RA, Kraus MA: Pitfalls in the surgical management of gastroesophageal reflux disease. Contemp Surg 49:189, 1996.
28. Richter JE, Castell DO: Gastroesophageal reflux: Pathogenesis, diagnosis, and therapy. Ann Intern Med 97:93, 1982.
29. DeMeester TR, Bonavina L, Albertucci M: Nissen fundoplication for gastroesophageal reflux disease. Ann Surg 204:9, 1986.
30. Koufman JA: The otolaryngologic manifestations of gastroesophageal reflux disease: A clinical investigation of 225 patients using ambulatory 24-hour pH monitoring and an experimental investigation of the role of acid and pepsin in the development of laryngeal injury. Laryngoscope 101:1, 1991.
31. Iascone C, DeMeester TR, Little AG, et al: Barrett's esophagus: Functional assessment, proposed pathogenesis, and surgical therapy. Arch Surg 118:543, 1983.
32. Stein HJ, Hoeft S, DeMeester TR: Reflux and motility pattern in Barrett's esophagus. Dis Esophagus 5:21, 1992.
33. Phillips RW, Wong RKH: Barrett's esophagus: Natural history, incidence, etiology and complications. Gastroenterol Clin North Am 20:791, 1991.
34. Roenberg JC, Fromm D: Barrett's esophagus—adenocarcinoma of the esophagus. *In* Wanebo HJ (ed): Surgery for Gastrointestinal Cancer: A Multidisciplinary Approach, 1st ed. Philadelphia, Lippincott-Raven Publishers, 1997, p 281.
35. Hamilton SR, Hutcheon DF, Ravich WJ, et al: Adenocarcinoma in Barrett's esophagus after elimination of gastroesophageal reflux. Gastroenterology 86:356, 1984.
36. McDonald ML, Trastek VF, Allen MS, et al: Barrett's esophagus: Does an antireflux procedure reduce the need for endoscopic surveillance? J Thorac Cardiovasc Surg 111:1135, 1996.
37. Nissen R: Gastropexy and fundoplication in surgical treatment of hiatus hernia. Am J Dig Dis 6:954, 1961.
38. Spechler SJ: Comparison of medical and surgical therapy for complicated gastroesophageal reflux disease in veterans. N Engl J Med 326:786, 1992.
39. Swanstrom LL, Marcus DR, Galloway GQ: Laparoscopic Collis gastroplasty is the treatment of choice for the shortened esophagus. Am J Surg 171:477, 1996.
40. Edoga JK, Willekes CL: Laparoscopic fundoplication and the aberrant left hepatic artery. Arch Surg 132:448, 1997.
41. Peillon C, Manouvrier J-L, Labreche J, et al: Should the vagus nerves be isolated from the fundoplication wrap? Arch Surg 129:814, 1994.
42. Stein HJ, DeMeester TR, Hinder RA: Outpatient physiologic testing and surgical management of foregut motility disorders. Curr Probl Surg 29:415, 1992.
43. Lerut T: Laparoscopic antireflux surgery: A critical analysis. Personal correspondence.
44. Geagea T: Laparoscopic Nissen-Rossetti fundoplication. Surg Endosc 8:1080, 1994.
45. Hunter JG, Swanstrom L, Waring JP: Dysphagia after laparoscopic antireflux surgery. Ann Surg 224:51, 1996.
46. Watson DI, Pike GK, Baigrie RJ, et al: Prospective double-blind

randomized trial of laparoscopic Nissen fundoplication with division and without division of short gastric vessels. Ann Surg 226:642, 1997.

47. Rattner DW, Brooks DC: Patient satisfaction following laparoscopic and open antireflux surgery. Arch Surg 130:289, 1995.
48. Watson DI, Chan ASL, Myers JC, et al: Illness behavior influences the outcome of laparoscopic antireflux surgery. J Am Coll Surg 184:44, 1997.
49. McKernan JB: Laparoscopic repair of gastroesophageal reflux disease—Toupet partial fundoplication versus Nissen fundoplication. Surg Endosc 8:851, 1994.
50. Swanstrom LL, Hunter JG: Laparoscopic partial fundoplication. *In* Peters JH, DeMeester TR (eds): Minimally Invasive Surgery of the Foregut, 1st ed. St. Louis, Quality Medical Publishing, 1994, p 159.
51. O'Sullivan GC, DeMeester TR, Joelsson BE, et al: Interaction of lower esophageal sphincter pressure and length of sphincter in the abdomen as determinants of gastroesophageal competence. Am J Surg 143:40, 1982.
52. Thor KBA, Silander T: A long-term randomized prospective trial of the Nissen procedure versus a modified Toupet technique. Ann Surg 210:719, 1989.
53. Aye RW, Hill LD, Kraemer SJM, et al: Early results with the laparoscopic Hill repair. Am J Surg 167:542, 1994.
54. Collet D, Cadiere GB: Conversions and complications of laparoscopic treatment of gastroesophageal reflux disease. Am J Surg 169:622, 1995.
55. Schauer PR, Meyers WC, Eubanks S, et al: Mechanisms of gastric and esophageal perforations during laparoscopic Nissen fundoplication. Ann Surg 223:43, 1996.
56. Trus TL, Bax R, Richardson WS, et al: Complications of laparoscopic paraesophageal hernia repair. J Gastrointest Surg 1:221, 1997.
57. Lowham AS, Filipi CJ, Hinder RA, et al: Mechanisms and avoidance of esophageal perforation by anesthesia personnel during laparoscopic foregut surgery. Surg Endosc 10:979, 1996.
58. Peters JH, DeMeester TR: The lessons of failed antireflux repairs. *In* Peters JH, DeMeester TR (eds): Minimally Invasive Surgery of the Foregut, 1st ed. St. Louis, Quality Medical Publishing, 1994, p 188.

COMMENTARY

Toni Lerut

The numbers of laparoscopic antireflux procedures are rapidly increasing worldwide, but great controversy persists regarding its value in treating gastroesophageal reflux disease (GERD). There is, however, substantial evidence that in experienced centers, the results of laparoscopic antireflux surgery at short-term follow-up match those of open surgery, justifying the choice of minimal access surgery with its related advantages for patients who have the correct indications.

As a result, we have adopted a laparoscopic Nissen-type operation as the standard for uncomplicated GERD. If possible, we prefer to use the Nissen–Rosetti procedure. We try not to divide the short gastric vessels because this may result in excessive reduction of the fundus and the gastric reservoir. To avoid gallbladder dysfunction, the vagal branches to the liver are not divided. Contrary to the practice of the St. Louis group, a bougie is never used because of concern about its preparation and because its use is not considered essential for adequate calibration of the hiatus oesophagei and the wrap.

From a total of 141 interventions, a group of 50 patients who had undergone surgery at least 1 year previously were submitted to a subjective and objective re-evaluation, including a barium swallow endoscopy, manometry, and a 24-hour pH study. Of these patients, 48 (96%) were free of symptoms, 5 (10%) had a pathologic 24-hour pH study, and 5 (10%) had an intrathoracic migration of the fundoplication or one or more reflux episodes as shown by the barrium swallow, but all had a normal 24-hour pH study. Only 1 patient had grade 1 esophagitis as shown by endoscopy.

Overall, complete subjective and objective reflux control was seen in 88% of these patients. In regard to anatomic appearance, 40 patients had a totally successful correction. Adverse effects persisted in 20% of the patients. Dysphagia occurred in 4 patients (8%). Of the 2 patients who had high dysphagia, 1 required myotomy of the cricopharyngeal muscle. The remaining 2 patients had low dysphagia, which was resolved in 1 by a laparoscopic intervention that converted a 360-degree fundoplication to a 270-degree partial fundoplication. More adverse effects were seen after performance of laparoscopic procedures than occurred in our historical series of Belsey repairs, in which only 8.8% of patients experienced adverse effects.

Laparoscopic procedures are now part of the spectrum of techniques available to the surgeon after a thorough investigation of each patient's condition. It is of paramount importance to evaluate by barium swallow whether the cardia is reduced under the diaphragm when the patient is upright. If this is not the case, or if there is a hiatal hernia larger than 5 cm, secondary brachyesophagus should be considered a contraindication to laparoscopic surgery, and a transthoracic procedure should be selected.

Lack of insight into the patient's condition and lack of experience on the part of the surgeon, occasioned by the rapid spread of laparoscopic antireflux surgery throughout the surgical community, are the main causes of the occasionally reported high numbers of complications and short-term failures (as high as 25% in some reports).

Chapter 32

Achalasia

Santiago Horgan and Carlos A. Pellegrini

Achalasia of the esophagus is a disease characterized by a long history of dysphagia, regurgitation of undigested food, and weight loss. These symptoms are caused by inadequate lower esophageal sphincter (LES) relaxation in response to swallows, absence of peristalsis, and high basal pressure at the LES. As a result of poor esophageal emptying, the esophagus dilates progressively to accommodate the food that has not been transferred to the stomach, and, eventually, becomes a large inert sac with a tight distal orifice. The etiology of achalasia is not known; patients who have achalasia have anomalies both of the muscle and the innervation of the esophagus. Of these, the neural component is generally considered to be the most important; indeed, Auerbach's plexus is absent in many patients. In most patients who have achalasia, ganglion cells are not present in the body or in the LES.

The neural alterations described are thought to create an imbalance between cholinergic and noncholinergic stimuli. Indeed, it appears that the lack of relaxation of the LES and the presence of high basal tone are consequences of an alteration in the mediation of LES relaxation normally produced by nitric oxide (NO) and vasoactive intestinal peptide (VIP).[1, 2] These studies have shown that in patients who have achalasia, there is a selective loss of postganglionic inhibitory neurons that contain NO and VIP.

Diagnosis

The diagnosis of achalasia is established by a history of dysphagia and weight loss, and confirmed by typical findings in the diagnostic studies.[3] All patients who have symptoms of achalasia should be evaluated with an esophagogram, manometry, and upper endoscopy. Ultrasound is helpful in some patients.

Esophagogram

An esophagogram is important to evaluate the anatomy of the esophagus; in patients who have achalasia, it shows a smooth tapering of the distal esophagus (bird beak) with dilation of the body (Fig. 32–1). As the disease progresses, the esophagus elongates, eventually acquiring a sigmoid shape typical of patients who have end-stage disease. Esophagograms are valuable in ruling out other diseases known to cause dysphagia, particularly cancer of the esophagus. The study is especially helpful to the surgeon when therapy is being planned, because the width, length, and overall shape of the esophagus determine the kind of procedure to be used.

Manometry

Manometry provides information about relaxation of pressure in the LES and motility in the body of the esophagus. The typical findings are absence of relaxation of the LES in response to swallows, increased basal tone (usually between 30 and 40 mmHg) and absent or minimal evidence of peristalsis. Thus, to make a diagnosis of achalasia on manometry, one has to find absence of peristalsis and either absence of, or some evidence of, defective relaxation of the LES. The total pressure, or the basal tone of the LES, is less important. In fact, it has been found that LES pressure is normal in 40% of patients who have achalasia. The study of the relaxation of the LES and the determination of complete relaxation is difficult; thus, either absent or obviously impaired relaxation is clear in only 70 to 80% of patients. Manometry is the diagnostic gold standard for achalasia, but, in some patients, the diagnosis is also based on clinical findings and data received from upper gastrointestinal series. In addition, it is important to remember that achalasia is not just a disease, but, more correctly, a spectrum of diseases, and that many motility disorders can, over time, evolve into the more typical form of achalasia. Thus, in the early stages of achalasia, patients may have only minimally impaired (and therefore difficult to observe) relaxation of the LES, which becomes evident over time.

Endoscopy

This procedure should be performed in patients who have symptoms of achalasia to rule out cancer or other causes of distal esophageal obstruction. Typical findings are dilation and atony of the esophagus. The mucosa can present esophagitis as a result of fermentation of retained food.

Endoscopic ultrasound is used to evaluate thickening of the esophageal wall in patients for whom the diagnosis of achalasia is questionable.

Radionuclide Measurement

In addition, radionuclide measurement of esophageal emptying may be useful to determine transit time through the esophagus, which is markedly delayed in patients with achalasia. If a good barium swallow is performed, this study is not needed.

Treatment

The treatment of achalasia has been the subject of controversy for many years. Because there is no treatment that can modify poor peristalsis in the body of the esophagus, all therapeutic maneuvers have been directed at decreasing pressure in the LES. There are several options available today to achieve this goal: medical treatment (including drugs and botulinum toxin injections), balloon dilation, and surgery.

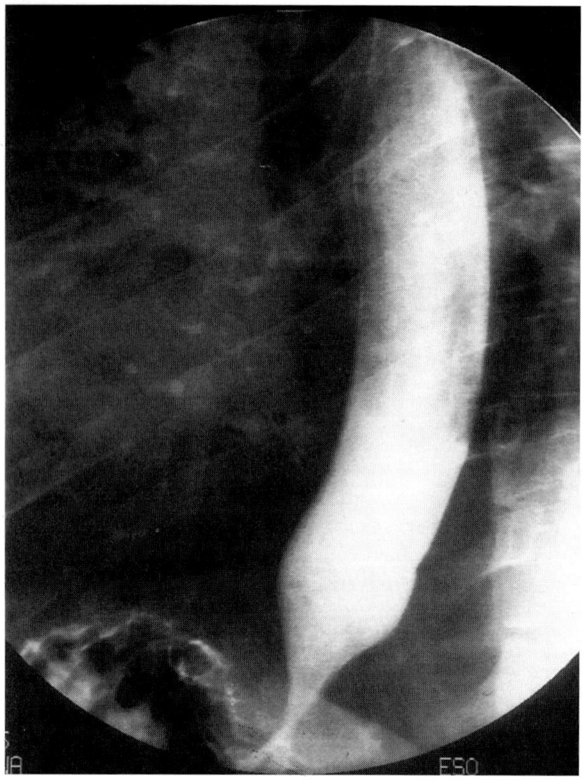

Figure 32–1. Esophagogram in a patient with achalasia.

Medical Treatments

Calcium channel blockers (e.g., nifedipine, verapamil)[4] and nitrates have been used with very little positive effect. This line of treatment should be reserved for patients who are poor candidates for surgery. Botulinum toxin has been used since 1993, when Pasricha and associates[5] showed that botulinum toxin injection in the LES of piglets results in significant reduction of basal pressure. Shortly thereafter, the same group reported their initial experience using botulinum toxin in patients who had achalasia.[6] Their report showed that when injected into the LES, botulinum toxin caused a substantial and sustained reduction of pressure and improved emptying of the esophagus. This sparked considerable enthusiasm in the gastroenterology community, and several groups started to use it as their first choice to treat achalasia.[7–9] This form of treatment is effective in about two thirds of patients initially, but symptoms recur in two thirds of the responders within the first 2 years;[8] thus, injections need to be repeated frequently. This form of therapy should be used primarily in elderly patients who will not be treated with surgery.

Pneumatic Dilation

Pneumatic dilation has been commonly used since the late 1970s as the initial treatment for achalasia. In this procedure, the muscle fibers of the gastroesophageal junction (GEJ) are disrupted as a consequence of the inflated balloon pressure. In 1980, Vantrappen and associates from Belgium reported the largest series of pneumatic dilations.[10] Excellent results (no dysphagia) were obtained in 37.5% of 537 patients and good results (occasional dysphagia of short duration) in 39.5%, thus achieving a 77% success rate. Perforation of the esophagus occurred in 2.6% of patients with a 0.2% mortality rate. Between 1980 and 1990, Ferguson[11] reviewed the results of pneumatic dilation in many centers in the United States, Europe, and South America. His findings confirmed Vantrappen's data. This review included almost 900 patients who were treated with different types of dilators: The overall improvement rate was 71%. More than 16% of patients required subsequent dilations, and 8% required a Heller myotomy. Gastroesophageal reflux disease (GERD) occurred in 27% of patients, with a mortality rate of 0.3%. In the same review, Ferguson also analyzed the results of esophagomyotomies for achalasia, which were performed in centers in the United States and abroad during the same decade. The overall success rate in 1199 patients was 89%. Fewer than 3% of patients required a second operation, and the incidence of GERD was 10%. The mortality rate was 0.3%.

Only one prospective randomized study has been performed to date to compare pneumatic dilation with the Heller myotomy. In 1989, Csendes and associates from Chile published the results of their trial (mean follow-up 62 months), which included 81 patients, 39 of whom were treated by dilation via a Mosher bag and 41 by surgery.[12] Overall results were good in 65% of patients after one or more dilations and in 95% of patients after myotomy, thus showing a major difference in outcome in favor of surgery. Birgisson and associate[13] reported that in their experience, symptoms of achalasia were relieved with only 1 dilation in 58% of patients; 2 dilations in 26% of patients; and 3 dilations in 16% of patients. In their 9 years of experience using Rigiflex dilators, 8 perforations (7%) occurred in more than 115 dilations. Six of the perforations occurred with use of the 3.5-cm dilator, one with the 3.0-cm dilator, and one with the 4.0-cm dilator.

These results suggest that surgical treatment has an advantage over dilation: A myotomy performed under direct vision is able to relieve the obstruction more precisely, more often, and with fewer complications than the blind rupture of the muscle fibers obtained by dilation. However, in spite of better results, surgical treatment generally has been considered a second line of treatment, to be used only in patients who have failed or suffered complications of dilation. The pain of surgical incision, postoperative disability associated with long recovery time, and cost of hospitalization have been the arguments commonly used in favor of pneumatic dilation as the initial treatment for achalasia. However, minimally invasive techniques make it possible today to obtain the results of surgery with much less discomfort, a shorter hospital stay and a shorter recovery period.

Current Minimally Invasive Techniques for Esophageal Myotomy

In 1991, stimulated by the excellent results obtained with laparoscopic cholecystectomy, we decided to apply minimally invasive techniques to the treatment of achalasia. We started performing the Heller myotomy thoracoscopically with good results, minimal postoperative pain, and shorter hospital stay.[14, 15]

We observed that a large number of patients treated

thoracoscopically were developing symptoms of reflux after the myotomy, so we decided to make a surgical approach to these patients through the abdomen. The laparoscopic myotomy, first described by Cuschieri in 1991,[16] has several advantages over the thoracoscopic technique. First, the anesthesia is easier to administer, because a double-lumen tube is not needed; second, the myotomy can be performed more easily through the abdomen; third, the myotomy can clearly be extended into the stomach (decreasing the chances of ending with an incomplete myotomy); fourth, a partial fundoplication can be added to avoid postoperative reflux; and, last, the absence of a chest tube decreases postoperative pain.

Currently, our indications for thoracoscopic myotomies are for use in patients who have a recurrence after a previous laparoscopic myotomy, patients who have diffuse esophageal motor disorders, and patients who have nutcracker esophagus. The laparoscopic approach is our treatment of choice in patients who have achalasia.

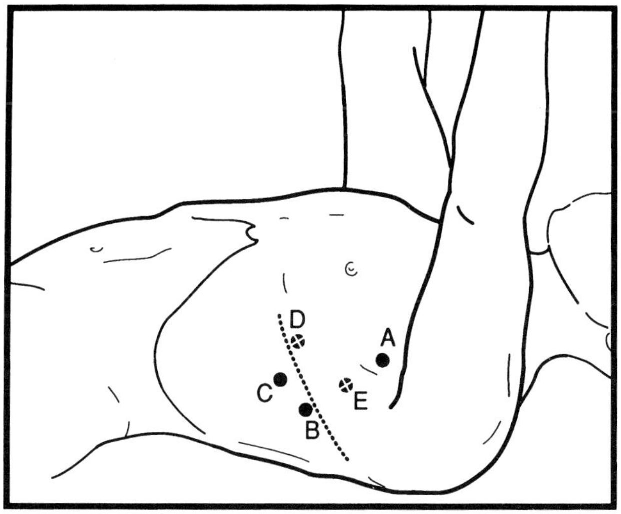

Figure 32–2. Thoracoscopic myotomy: Port placement.

Thoracoscopic Approach

Operative Techniques

Our current operative technique is similar, with small modifications, to that originally reported by us in 1991. After induction of general endotracheal anesthesia and double-lumen tracheal intubation, a 52 French lighted bougie is placed transorally inside the esophagus. This bougie plays a key role during the thoracoscopic Heller myotomy; at the beginning of the procedure, it facilitates identification of the esophagus by transillumination. Subsequently, it helps gauge the depth of penetration of instruments and manipulation of the esophagus. An endoscope is used once the myotomy has been performed, which allows an accurate assessment of the appropriate length of the myotomy. If the myotomy is too short, dysphagia will persist; if it is too long (>0.5 to 1.0 cm into the gastric wall), gastroesophageal reflux will occur.

The patient is positioned in the right lateral decubitus position, and five 10-mm ports are introduced into the left side of the chest, as shown in Figure 32–2. After upward retraction of the left lung, the inferior pulmonary ligament is divided. Aided by the transillumination of the endoscope (Fig. 32–3) or the lighted bougie, the esophagus is easily identified in the groove between the pericardium and the aorta. Once the esophagus has been identified and exposed, the myotomy is subsequently carried down through the longitudinal and circular layers by use of a 90-degree angled hook. When the submucosal plane is reached, the myotomy is extended upward and downward by use of the hook cautery or the bipolar scissors (Fig. 32–4), and the muscle is opened by application of gentle traction on the longitudinal muscle.

The lowest part of the myotomy represents the most delicate part of the procedure. It is crucial to the outcome, and it is also the most difficult part of the operation, because it is at this level that the muscle layers are less clearly identified and the mucosa is thinner, making the risk of perforation higher. In our original series, we had 3 such perforations among 24 patients; 2 were repaired by an open technique and 1 by thoracoscopic suturing.

When the myotomy is complete, the edges of the muscle layers are separated by blunt dissection, so that about 40% of the circumference of the mucosa becomes visible. The operation is completed by insertion of a chest tube through the lowest trocar site. This operation is usually accomplished in 2 to 3 hours; blood loss is minimal, and recovery is rapid.

Laparoscopic Myotomy

This operation is performed under general anesthesia, with the patient placed in the semilithotomy and reverse Trendelenburg position. A bean bag is used to maintain the reverse Trendelenburg position safely. Sequential pneumatic stockings are placed on the patient's legs to diminish the risk of venous thrombosis, which is increased by the position and use of positive intraperitoneal pressure for several hours. An orogastric tube is used to deflate the stomach (the tube is pulled after the stomach is inspected and it is not reinserted), and a Foley catheter is inserted to empty the bladder and monitor urine output through the

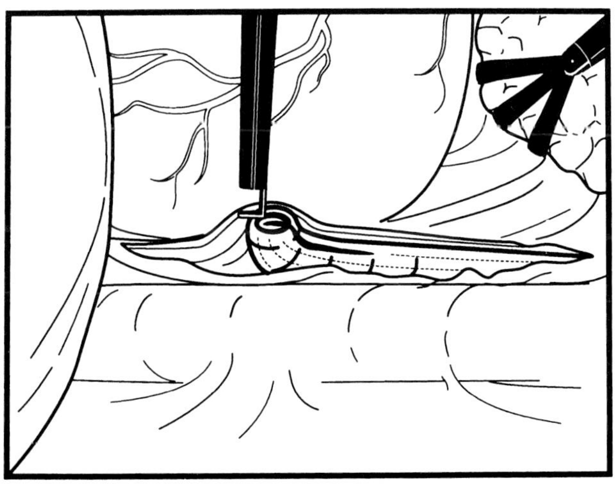
Figure 32–3. Thoracoscopic myotomy: Endoscope exposing esophagus.

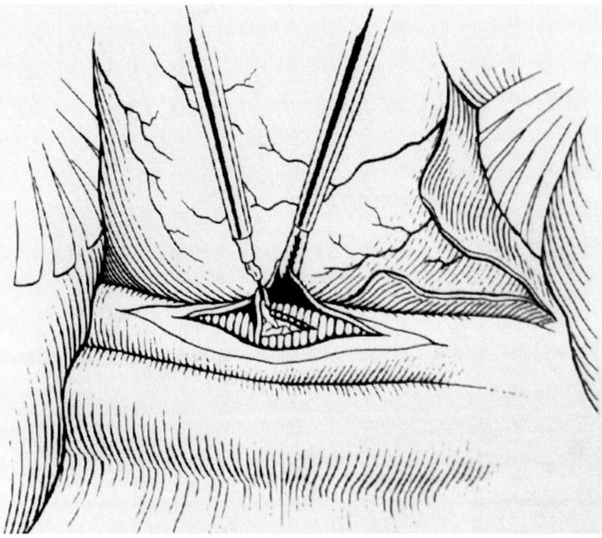

Figure 32–4. Thoracoscopic myotomy: Technique.

operation. The Foley catheter is left in place postoperatively only in patients who are going to receive epidural analgesia after the operation; otherwise, it is removed in the recovery room. The video monitor is placed above the patient's head. The surgeon stands between the legs of the patient and the first assistant stands on the right side. We use a camera holder to support the liver retractor, so a second assistant is not required. If the camera holder is not used, the second assistant stands on the left side of the patient.

Pneumoperitoneum is achieved by use of a Veres needle in the area where the first trocar will be placed. Employment of an open technique to establish pneumoperitoneum is rarely required. Once insufflation is established, the ports are positioned as shown in Figure 32–5. The first

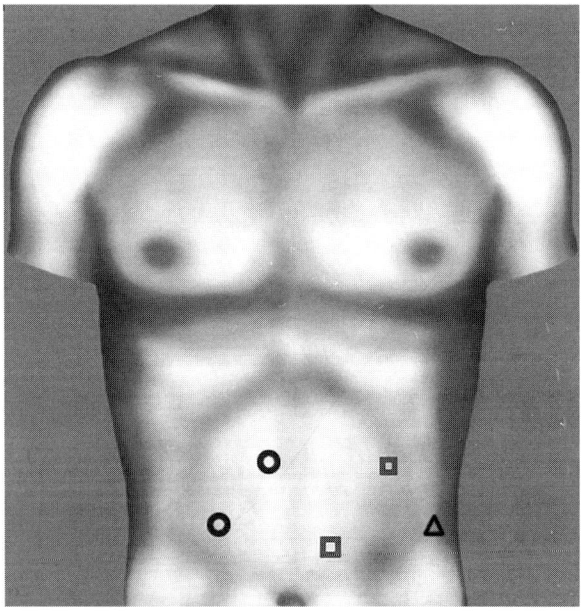

Figure 32–5. Laparoscopic myotomy: Port placement.

port (5/11 mm, used for the camera) is placed with use of the Visiport (U.S. Surgical, Norwalk, CT), because we believe this decreases the chance of injury to a major vessel or the bowel. The camera port is usually positioned 2 cm to the left of the umbilicus and about 10 cm below the costal margin. After a routine laparoscopy of the abdomen has been performed, the remaining ports are placed, depending on the anatomy of the patient. A 5/11-mm port that provides access to instruments held by the surgeon's right hand is placed in the left midclavicular line 1 cm below the costal margin (to avoid subcostal nerve injury) at a 45-degree angle to the camera port. A 5-mm port is inserted in the epigastrium near the midline, directly above the anterior edge of the left lobe of the liver, which provides access to instruments held by the surgeon's left hand. Unless the patient has a very large liver (in which case a 10-mm liver retractor is needed), we prefer to use a 5-mm liver retractor, which is placed through a port positioned where the right anterior axillary line crosses the camera port line. A 5/11-mm port placed at the level of the camera port in the left anterior axillary line provides access to instruments held by the first assistant's right hand.

In the original version of the laparoscopic technique, after adequate exposure of the hiatus was gained by retracting the left lobe of the liver anteriorly, the gastrohepatic ligament was opened and the right crus of the diaphragm dissected. Misidentification of the structures in this area can, however, lead to inferior vena cava injury or transection of the nerve of Latarjet (important for the preservation of adequate gastric emptying). We have found that the left crus can always be easily identified by downward traction of the gastric fundus, and so we start our operation by dissecting the left crus and dividing the gastrohepatic ligament.

To that end, the first assistant is asked to grasp the top of the fundus (or the greater curvature at a convenient point if a large hiatal hernia is present) with a Babcock clamp and pull downward. The peritoneum overlying the left crus of the diaphragm is then opened sharply. The division of the peritoneum continues to the left until the phrenogastric ligament is completely divided. Occasional use of electrocautery may be needed during this step. Dissection is carried down along the left crus and as far as possible toward the upper pole of the spleen. At this point, it is usually easier to choose a point in the greater curvature several centimeters down from the divided phrenogastric attachments, and divide all short gastric vessels going upward until one reaches the previously divided phrenogastric ligament.

We routinely divide all short gastric vessels to mobilize the fundus of the stomach fully. Although we prefer to use the Harmonic scalpel (Ethicon, Inc., Somerville, NJ) to take down the short gastric vessels, clips can also be employed. In the latter case, we recommend that all the vessels be double-clipped, to avoid potential bleeding, which can result from dislodging a clip when manipulating the stomach. When the left crus has been completely dissected and the greater curvature of the stomach is free, the mediastinum may be entered, and the inner side of the left crus can be separated from the left side of the esophagus. Conversely, the decision may be made to continue the division of the peritoneum that overlies the anterior aspect of the hiatus and the phrenoesophageal membrane toward the right until the right crus (at its top) has been exposed. The gastrohepatic ligament, a continuation of the peritoneum that overlies the right crus, is divided from the top of the right crus. The division is extended downward as needed to expose the bottom of the right crus.

Esophageal Mobilization

The esophagus can be approached from the right (with the assistant maintaining downward traction at the cardioesophageal junction) or from the left (with the assistant grasping the fundus and pulling down and to the patient's right). We use the tip of the electrocautery device (having previously retracted the wire) to dissect the esophagus bluntly, pushing it alternatively to the right or the left. A 52 French lighted bougie placed transorally into the esophagus provides a surface over which the esophageal wall can be dissected, and a platform over which the myotomy can be carried out. At this time, the fat pad from the esophageal junction is removed. The anterior vagus is identified and carefully dissected from the esophagus. The myotomy is performed with an L-shaped hook electrocautery mounted at the tip of a suction-irrigation device (Surgiwand, U.S. Surgical, Norwalk, CT).

After marking the area of the muscularis externa that is to be divided with the heel of the electrocautery, the circular layer is identified. Initially, one or two circular fibers are lifted away from the mucosa by placing the tip of the hook electrocautery in the submucosal plane (Figs. 32–6 and 32–7). These fibers are dissected away from the mucosa and divided. The rest of the myotomy is performed following this plane, and the edges are dissected away from each other, also following this plane.

Bleeding can occur close to the mucosa. Gentle pressure instead of coagulation should be applied over the mucosa, and these bleeding points usually stop without any other treatment. We have found that in patients treated with botulinum toxin, the mucosa is difficult to separate from the muscularis propria because the submucosal plane has been lost. Consequently, it is difficult to separate the muscle edges from each other (Figs. 32–8 and 32–9). This difficulty makes the operation longer and the risk of lacerating the mucosa greater.

A Dor fundoplication is routinely added to the myotomy to avoid postoperative reflux.[17] In principle, this operation is the reverse of a Toupet, with the wrap covering the anterior aspect of the distal esophagus and fixed to the edges of the diaphragm (Figs. 32–10 and 32–11). Its main advantage under these circumstances is that the fundus of the stomach covers the exposed mucosa of the esophagus.

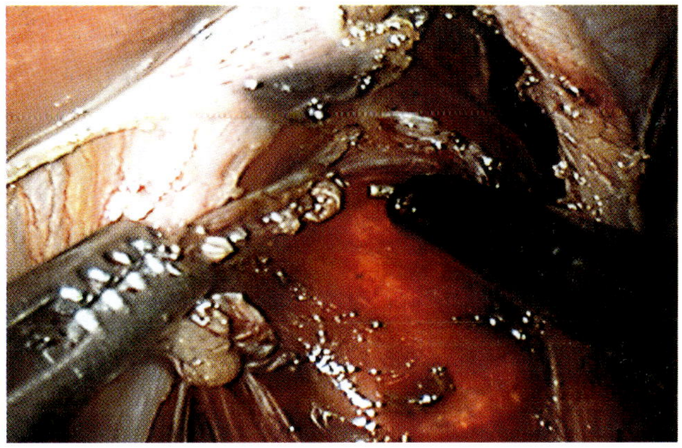

Figure 32–7. Laparoscopic myotomy: Technique.

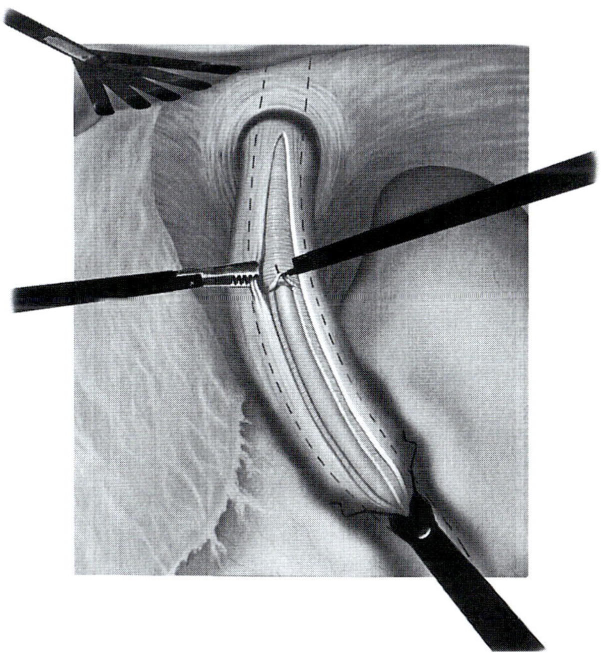

Figure 32–6. Laparoscopic myotomy: Schematic view of technique to perform the myotomy.

Results of Operations

Our initial report showed that thoracoscopic myotomy yielded excellent results in terms of resolution of dysphagia.[14] Because of the high incidence of postoperative reflux

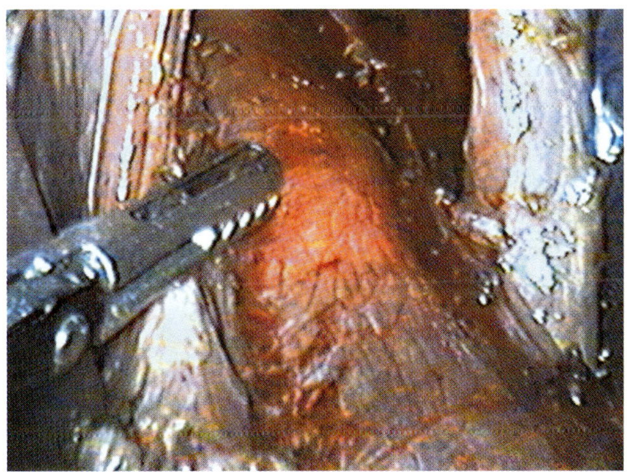

Figure 32–8. Laparoscopic myotomy completed in a patient not treated with botulinum toxin.

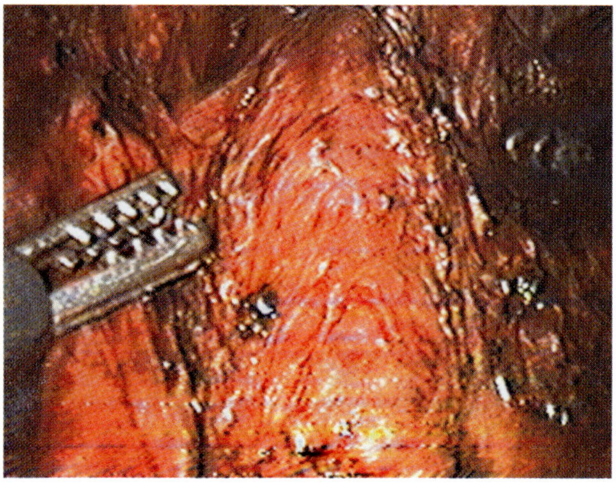

Figure 32–9. Laparoscopic myotomy completed in a patient treated with botulinum toxin.

in these patients, and because the laparoscopic route had become widely used in the treatment of reflux disease, we started the laparoscopic approach in a routine fashion in 1993. The results obtained in the first 57 patients treated by the laparoscopic approach showed that dysphagia was markedly reduced in the great majority of patients, with an average decrease from a 3.8 (on a scale of 0 to 4) preoperatively to a score of 0.7 postoperatively. Regurgitation, the other main symptom in patients with achalasia, decreased from 2.7 (on the same scale) to 0.9 postoperatively (Fig 32–12). These results appear to be maintained over time. Our analysis of patients who have gone beyond 5 years suggests that dysphagia and regurgitation continue to be under control.[18] Our experience since 1995 with the laparoscopic approach has convinced us and others of its advantages: Simple administration of anesthesia, no need for a chest tube, greater ease of performing the antireflux procedure, and relative ease in extending the myotomy into the stomach.

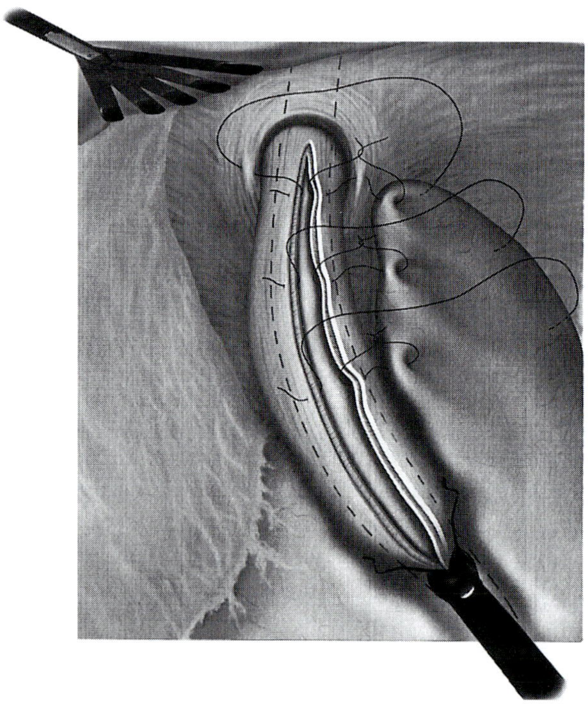

Figure 32–10. Laparoscopic myotomy: Schematic view of the technique to perform a Dor fundoplication.

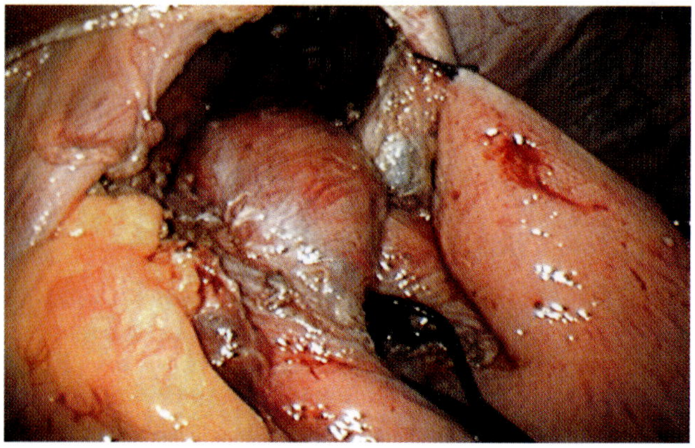

Figure 32–11. Laparoscopic myotomy: Technique for performing a Dor fundoplication.

Our experience is echoed in the current literature. In 1997, Hunter and associates[19] reported on 40 patients, of whom 90% had excellent to good results after laparoscopic myotomy. Of the 6 perforations, all occurred at the gastric end of the myotomy, and all were repaired laparoscopi-

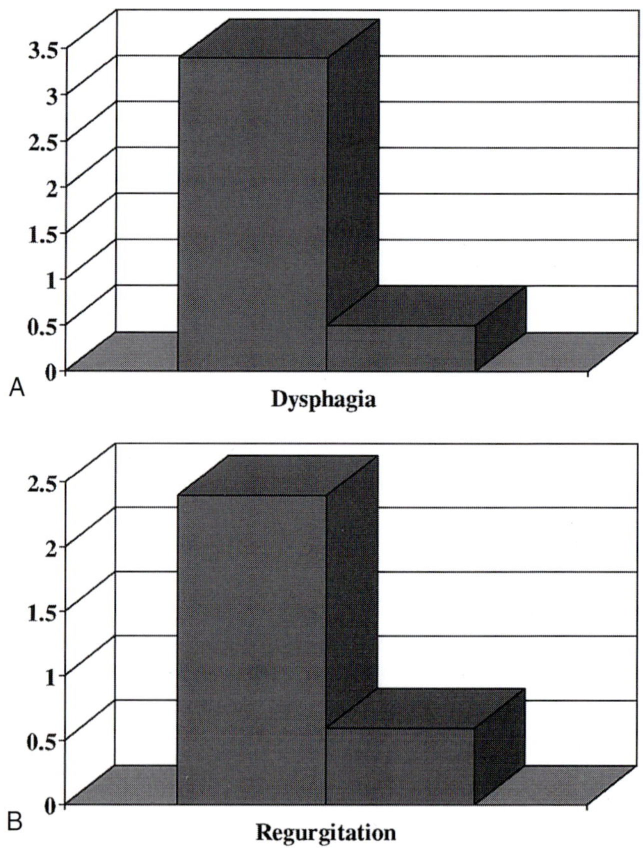

Figure 32–12. *A*, Dysphagia improvement with Heller myotomy. *B*, Regurgitation improvement with Heller myotomy.

cally. The Toupet fundoplication was used in these patients as an antireflux procedure.

In a study completed in 1998, Rosati and associates[20] reported on 61 patients treated laparoscopically with excellent to good results in over 98% of patients, with a mean follow-up period of 21 months (range of 1 to 62 months). Of 7 patients in whom perforation occurred, 5 were repaired laparoscopically; 3 patients were converted to open surgery, and 1 needed a postoperative dilation to relieve persistent dysphagia. Overall, LES pressure diminished from 52 to 27 mm Hg, and barium swallow showed a decrease in esophageal diameter from 52 mm before surgery to 27 mm postoperatively.

Complications

Laceration of the mucosa is the most common complication of laparoscopic myotomy. We have found that perforations occur more frequently in patients treated with botulinum toxin. These perforations, which usually occur at the GEJ, are very small and can be closed laparoscopically using 5/0 silk sutures. The Dor fundoplication provides additional support to the repair.

Residual dysphagia is often the consequence of an incomplete myotomy; this can be avoided by extending the myotomy well into the stomach. We have found that when examined endoscopically, the LES is at least 1 to 2 cm below what the surgeon observes externally as the junction of the stomach and esophagus. For this reason, it is important to extend the myotomy at least 2 cm beyond the place where the GEJ is identified. Intraoperative endoscopy is used to evaluate the completion of the myotomy (Fig. 32–13).

Conclusions

Achalasia is a disorder characterized by the lack of peristalsis in the body of the esophagus and by the absence of relaxation of the LES. The goal of treatment is to decrease the basal tone of the LES, because the motility cannot be recovered. Medical treatment has little or no effect on decreasing the LES pressure, and should, therefore, be used only in patients for whom balloon dilatations or surgical treatment are not valid options.

The use of botulinum toxin has shown good results only in the short term, but has the potential to make a subsequent operation more difficult.

Pneumatic dilation is an appropriate treatment for patients who have achalasia. On the other hand, when perforations occur during dilation, patients usually have to be treated surgically, if this is not done, a stricture can be the final result.

Surgery results in excellent improvement in a high percentage of patients, with a rate of complications similar to that which occurs with pneumatic dilation. When perforations occur during the surgical myotomy, they can almost always be repaired during the same procedure with no change in outcome.

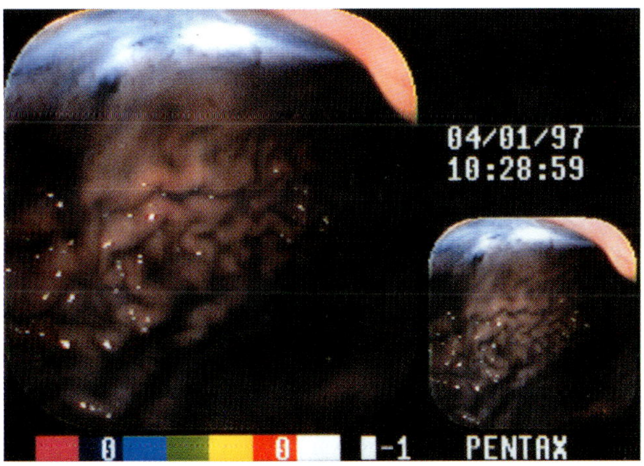

Figure 32–13. Laparoscopic myotomy: Endoscopic view of the completed myotomy. The light of the laparoscope can be observed through the exposed mucosa of the stomach.

References

1. Aggestrup S, Uddman R, Sundler F, et al: Lack of vasoactive intestinal polypeptide nerves in esophageal achalasia. Gastroenterology 84:924–927, 1983.
2. Guelrud M, Rossiter A. Souney PF, et al: The effect of vasoactive intestinal polypeptide on the lower esophageal sphincter in achalasia. Gastroenterology 103:377–382, 1992.
3. Couturier D. Samama J: Clinical aspects and manometric criteria in achalasia. Hepatogastroenterology 38:481–487, 1991.
4. Traube M, Dubovik S, Lange RC, et al: The role of nifedipine therapy in achalasia: Results of a randomized, double-blind, placebo-controlled study. Am J Gastroenterol 84:1259–1262, 1989.
5. Pasricha PJ, Ravich WJ, Kalloo AN: Effects of intrasphincteric botulinum toxin on the lower esophageal sphincter in piglets. Gastroenterology 105:1045–1049, 1993.
6. Pasricha PJ, Ravich WJ, Hendrix TR, et al: Treatment of achalasia with intrasphincteric injection of botulinum toxin. A pilot trial. Ann Intern Med 121:590–591, 1994.
7. Pasricha PJ, Ravich WJ, Hendrix TR, et al: Intrasphincteric botulinum toxin for the treatment of achalasia (see comments) [published erratum appears in N Engl J Med 333:75, 1995]. N Engl J Med 332:774–778, 1995.
8. Pasricha PJ, Rai R, Ravich WJ, et al: Botulinum toxin for achalasia: Long-term outcome and predictors of response. Gastroenterology 110:1410–1415, 1996.
9. Fishman VM, Parkman HP, Schiano TD, et al: Symptomatic improvement in achalasia after botulinum toxin injection of the lower esophageal sphincter. Am J Gastroenterol 91:1724–1730, 1996.
10. Vantrappen G, Hellemans J: Treatment of achalasia and related motor disorders. Gastroenterology 79:144–154, 1980.
11. Ferguson MK: Achalasia: Current evaluation and therapy. Ann Thorac Surg 52:336–342, 1991.
12. Csendes A, Braghetto I, Henriquez A, et al. Late results of a prospective randomised study comparing forceful dilatation and oesophagomyotomy in patients with achalasia (see comments). Gut 30:299–304, 1989.
13. Birgisson S, Richter JE: Achalasia: What's new in diagnosis and treatment? Dig Dis 15(Suppl 1):1–27, 1997.
14. Pellegrini C, Wetter LA, Patti M, et al: Thoracoscopic esophagomyotomy. Initial experience with a new approach for the treatment of achalasia. Ann Surg 216(3):291–296, 1992; discussion 296–299.
15. Pellegrini CA, Leichter R, Patti M, et al: Thoracoscopic

esophageal myotomy in the treatment of achalasia. Ann Thorac Surg 56:680–682, 1993.
16. Shimi S, Nathanson LK, Cuschieri A: Laparoscopic cardiomyotomy for achalasia. J R Coll Surg Edinb 36:152–154, 1991.
17. Dor I, Humbert P, Dor V, Figarella I: L'Interet de la technique midifiee la prévention du réflux apres cardiomyotomie extra muquese de Heller. Mem Acad Chir 88:881–883, 1962.
18. Horgan S, Hudda K, Eubanks T, et al: Does botulinum toxin injection make esophagomyotomy a more difficult operation? Surg Endosc (in press).
19. Hunter JG, Trus TL, Branum GD, et al: Laparoscopic Heller myotomy and fundoplication for achalasia. Ann Surg 225:655–665, 1997.
20. Rosati R, Fumagalli U, Bona S, et al: Evaluating results of laparoscopic surgery for esophageal achalasia. Surg Endosc 12:270–273, 1998.

COMMENTARY

Keith S. Naunheim

The chapter depicts the relatively large experience of Horgan and associates with achalasia patients treated with myotomy via minimally invasive surgical techniques. Their clinical results are indeed excellent and provide a benchmark to which others in the field can aspire. There are some variations in techniques used by other institutions of which the reader should be aware. Not all surgeons in this field completely mobilize the fundus and upper greater curvature of the stomach by dividing all short gastric vessels. The performance of a Dor fundoplication can be undertaken without tension in many patients, without the need for dividing these vessels.

In our own institution, we perform the Dor fundoplication rather than the Toupet, because it has a number of advantages. First, it does not require circumferential dissection of the lower esophagus and the gastroesophageal junction (GEJ). This cuts down not only the operative time but also the risk of perforation when the posterior wall of the esophagus is dissected. In addition, the posterior attachments of the GEJ are not taken down, and the risk of eventual herniation of the partial fundoplication into the chest is decreased. Finally, the anterior fundoplication covers the exposed esophageal mucosa and is, therefore, available to help buttress any mucosal laceration that has been sutured. Our own stitches for the Dor fundoplication include a bite of the stomach, a bite of the esophageal musculature, and a portion of the diaphragm. These three structures are fixed together and the esophageal musculature is retracted laterally toward either edge of the hiatus in an attempt to decrease the risk of the muscle edges healing with resultant dysphagia.

There are many different ways to divide the esophageal musculature once the correct submucosal plane is identified. Most recently, we have been using a Maryland dissector to separate the muscle from the submucosa, followed by muscular division using the Harmonic scalpel. A hooked cautery has the potential for damaging the mucosa with its heel if inadequate upward tension is placed to pull the muscle away from the mucosal layer. The inactive (nonvibrating) limb of the Harmonic scalpel can be placed between the muscle and the submucosa, and, thus, the muscle is divided without any danger of damage to the mucosal layer. Other surgeons have used endoscopic shears, with or without bipolar cautery, to divide this layer.

Although the authors discuss the importance of continuing the dissection onto the stomach, they do not describe the overall extent of the myotomy. In most patients, the lower esophageal sphincter has a length of no more than 2 to 3 cm. It is desirable to extend the myotomy for 1 cm onto the stomach to be certain that a complete myotomy is performed. Taking this into account, as well as the length of the esophageal sphincter, a 5 to 7 cm myotomy is an appropriate length in most patients. This can almost always be achieved with a laparoscopic approach, because the myotomy can be extended up into the mediastinum. The surgeon who abides by these suggestions and those espoused by Horgan and Pelligrini in this chapter is likely to enjoy a success similar to that outlined above.

Chapter 33

Esophageal Leiomyoma, Diverticulum, and Duplication Cyst

Alex G. Little

Although the technological advances that have contributed to the development and evolution of minimally invasive thoracic surgery have added options for the treatment of esophageal leiomyoma, diverticulum, and duplication cyst, they have not changed the indications for or the principles of operative intervention. Indications for operation are based first on an understanding of esophageal pathophysiology and second on the results of an appropriate and sufficient diagnostic evaluation. In addition to surgical technique, this chapter considers the pathophysiology, diagnostic alternatives, and indications for operative therapy of these three entities. The final section presents the minimally invasive surgical techniques that can be used in the management of these conditions.

Esophageal Leiomyoma

These benign tumors arise from the smooth muscle of the esophagus. Although benign tumors of the esophagus are relatively rare, constituting only approximately 5% of all esophageal neoplasms, leiomyomas are by far the most common, representing approximately 67% of all benign tumors.[1] They can occur at any level; however, they are more likely to be found in the lower esophagus than in the upper.

These intramural tumors are solitary, grow slowly if at all, and are eccentrically located within the circular muscle of the esophagus. They are well differentiated and histologically are composed of fusiform cells with eosinophilic and fibrillated cytoplasm. The tumor mass is relatively acellular, and larger tumors are composed of abundant amounts of collagen. Over time, if the tumor enlarges, it can ultimately bulge into the esophageal lumen, causing distortion. However, these tumors do not infiltrate surrounding tissue, so the overlying mucosa is rarely if ever invaded.[1, 2]

Most patients are asymptomatic. Despite infringement into the lumen by the tumor, symptoms of esophageal obstruction are uncommon because of the distensibility of the uninvolved esophagus and are produced only by very large tumors. Therefore, the clinical picture is usually benign, and both odynophagia and dysphagia are unusual. In fact, most leiomyomas are relatively small and are discovered incidentally. When symptoms are present, dysphagia is the most common. Chest discomfort or pain is present in some patients and is described as a squeezing sensation of mild to moderate severity. Although perhaps related to secondary peristaltic waves initiated by the tumor bulk and attempts to pass the tumor, the exact cause of this chest discomfort is unclear, as abnormal esophageal motility patterns in these patients have not been described.

When symptoms lead the patient to seek medical attention, the initial focus may be on the chest discomfort, so the evaluation begins with cardiac investigations. Ultimately, esophageal symptoms stimulate performance of a barium swallow and/or an endoscopic examination. The barium esophagogram appearance, shown in Figure 33–1, is quite distinctive, as the mass has a smooth surface, has distinct margins, and is localized, not circumferential. Perhaps most frequently, however, a leiomyoma is seen on a chest x-ray as a posterior mediastinal mass or is found unexpectedly during performance of esophagoscopy for unrelated symptoms. During endoscopy (which should be performed even if a prior barium study exists, to rule out possible carcinoma or sarcoma), the mucosa is intact, and the appearance is that of an extrinsic mass that narrows the lumen. Endoscopic biopsy should be avoided, as adherence of the tumor to the mucosal injury may complicate a later surgical resection.

Historically, the generally recommended treatment of a clinically identified leiomyoma is surgical.[1, 2] However, the need for operative intervention should be based on symptoms and concerns about future events, including growth and malignant degeneration. Recent experience suggests that in the absence of symptoms, surgical intervention is not an absolute requirement. The report of Glanz and Grunebaum suggests that most of these tumors remain stable in size over time.[3] These authors followed four patients for up to 15 years and identified no change in the size of their tumors. Therefore, a leiomyoma less than 5 cm in size that is truly asymptomatic can be followed, and surgical intervention is not absolutely required. If resection is not performed, occasional barium contrast radiologic or endoscopic examinations should be performed to detect changes such as enlargement or signs of mucosal invasion.

Regarding the malignancy concern, the malignant variant of leiomyosarcoma is an extremely rare esophageal tumor. Further, these sarcomas probably arise primarily rather than develop from previously benign leiomyomas. There are no documented instances of transition from a benign to a malignant tumor. Consequently, the risk of malignant degeneration does not appear to be sufficient to justify routine removal of all leiomyomas.

Esophageal Diverticulum

The near eradication of tuberculosis in the West has eliminated tuberculous mediastinal lymphadenitis and traction diverticula of the esophagus. Therefore, essentially all diverticula of the body of the esophagus are of the pulsion variety and are due to an underlying motility abnormality.[4]

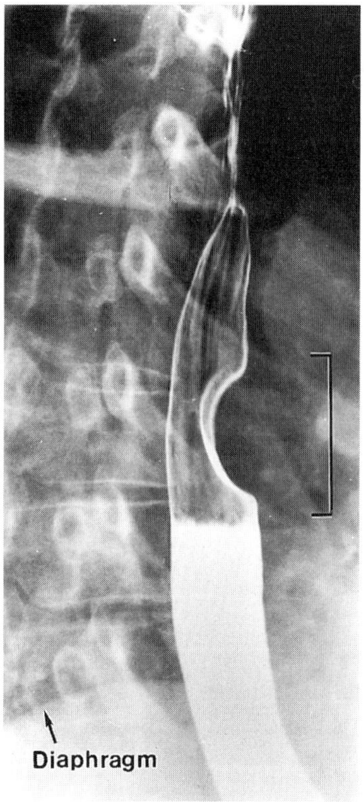

Figure 33–1. This barium contrast esophagogram shows the typical appearance of an esophageal leiomyoma. The tumor is in the mid-esophagus, has a smooth surface, and is not circumferential.

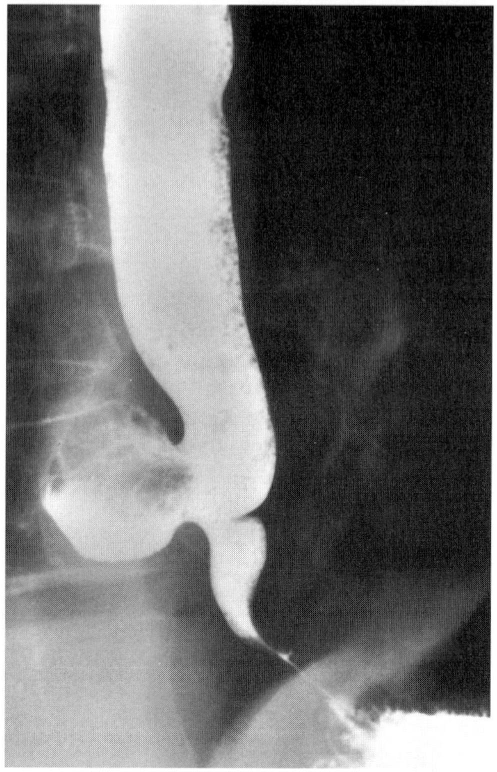

Figure 33–2. This barium swallow examination shows an epiphrenic diverticulum.

The most frequent location for a diverticulum is in the distal esophagus near the gastroesophageal junction—hence the identification as epiphrenic. Occasionally, diverticula are found elsewhere along the body of the thoracic esophagus. Pharyngoesophageal, or Zenker's, diverticulum of the cervical esophagus is not considered in this chapter.

Most patients with esophageal diverticula have symptoms. Typical symptoms are regurgitation; esophageal, not oropharyngeal, dysphagia; and, infrequently, chest pain. Respiratory sequelae of chronic aspiration, including cough, wheezing, and pneumonia, can be present as well.[5] These symptoms, like the diverticulum itself, are manifestations of the motility disturbance. They usually lead to the performance of a barium esophagogram, with findings like those in Figure 33–2. The evaluation is not complete, however, until esophageal manometry has been performed. The manometric or motility abnormalities associated with diverticula are varied and frequently nonspecific and do not fit nicely into the pattern of a known motility disorder. Figure 33–3 shows the motility pattern of a patient with an epiphrenic diverticulum in which the abnormality consists of a forceful and prolonged contraction of the lower esophageal sphincter (LES) following a normal deglutitive relaxation. Table 33–1 documents the range of associated motility abnormalities seen in 10 patients with esophageal diverticula.

Treatment of patients with diverticula is indicated to relieve dysphagia, palliate chest pain, and protect against pulmonary soilage caused by chronic aspiration of regurgitated esophageal contents. Surgical therapy must address the motor disorder or run the risk of persistent dysphagia and regurgitation, as well as diverticulum recurrence, if diverticulectomy alone is performed. This means that esophagomyotomy of the abnormally functioning muscle identified by the manometric examination is essential. If the myotomy crosses the LES, a nonobstructive antireflux procedure such as a Belsey fundoplication should also be performed to protect against development of iatrogenic reflux.

Esophageal Duplication Cyst

Esophageal congenital cysts are created during the embryologic process of separation of the pulmonary tree and the esophagus from their common origin. These cysts are the-

Figure 33–3. This manometric study of the lower esophageal sphincter (LES) of the patient from Figure 33–2 documents that the LES or lower esophageal high-pressure zone (LEHPZ), although having a normal resting pressure, both fails to completely relax with a swallow and exhibits an abnormally sustained contraction following the deglutitive relaxation.

Table 33–1. Manometry Characteristics in 10 Patients With Esophageal Diverticula

	Lower Esophageal Sphincter			Esophageal Body		
Location/Patient No.	Pressure (mm Hg)	Length (cm)	Deglutitive Relaxation Characteristics	Contractions	Pressure (mm Hg)	Duration (sec)
Epiphrenic						
1	—	—	—	Normal peristalsis, occasionally tertiary	110	4.2
2	13	3.3	Complete*	Normal peristalsis	80	—
3	33	3.0	Complete	30% peristaltic, 70% simultaneous	200	>8.0
4	39	5.0	Complete	Occasionally repetitive and synchronous	40	4.5
5	—	—	—	Most simultaneous; no peristalsis	25	4.0
6	8.5	2.0	Complete	Aperistalsis lower ⅓	22	2.0
7	9.6	4.6	Incomplete	20% repetitive, 10% simultaneous	62	4.3
8	—	—	—	100% simultaneous middle and lower esophagus; some peristaltic contractions upper ⅓ of esophagus	15	4.2
Midesophageal						
9	10	2.3	Complete†	Normal peristalsis; occasionally simultaneous lower ⅓	50	
10	17	2.3	Complete	Normal peristalsis; 40% repetitive	120–290	4.5

*Followed by a contraction of 60 mm Hg amplitude.
†Followed by a prolonged (>10 sec) contraction.
The manometric findings in 10 patients with esophageal diverticulum are shown. In patients 1, 5, and 8 the catheter could not be passed through the LES.

oretically separable into three categories: duplications, bronchogenic cysts, and neurenteric cysts. For practicality and because of the difficulty in distinguishing one type of cyst from another, these are considered together as duplication cysts.[6]

Cysts can be found at any location, but the intrathoracic esophagus is a more common location than the cervical esophagus. Cyst size, shape, and degree of connection to the esophagus are all highly variable, although communication with the lumen is uncommon. In adults, most cysts are not associated with symptoms and are found incidentally when a posterior mediastinal mass is identified on a chest x-ray.[6, 7] However, duplications can become infected, can cause dysphagia if they are large enough, and can perforate or bleed if they contain gastric mucosa. In infants, pulmonary compromise can be caused by relatively large cysts, but this is not an issue in adults.

The natural history of esophageal cysts is variable. Malignant degeneration has been reported, but the incidence appears to be quite low, and duplication cysts can be considered benign.[6] However, the possibilities of enlargement, infection, and bleeding suggest that surgical excision is appropriate for most patients.

Minimally Invasive Surgical Techniques

Lesions of the distal esophagus are equally accessible from either the right or the left chest. Approaching from the left side allows performance of a concomitant antireflux procedure if necessary. The right chest is preferable for access to lesions of the mid- and upper esophagus, where the aorta interferes with left-side approaches.

The patient is placed in the lateral decubitus thoracotomy position with the operating table flexed to maximize the intercostal distances. Ventilation of the contralateral lung is continued via a double-lumen endotracheal tube, and the ipsilateral lung is allowed to collapse. Thoracoports are arrayed as depicted in Figure 33–4. The lung is retracted anteriorly to expose the posterior mediastinum. Retraction can be accomplished with a fan-shaped retractor or by grasping and elevating the lung. Exposure is further facilitated by tilting the operating table to lean the patient forward.

As illustrated in Figure 33–5, the parietal pleura overlying the esophagus is grasped, elevated, and incised to gain entry into the posterior mediastinum. The azygos vein is divided between hemoclips or with an EndoGIA stapling device if necessary for exposure of the upper esophagus. Further blunt and sharp dissection suffices to separate the esophagus from the mediastinal fat. It is safer to push gently on the esophagus with a blunt-tipped instrument to provide countertraction than to grasp the easily torn muscle, which, in contrast to the stomach, does not have a serosal cover. When the dissection is between the esophagus and the aorta, the esophageal arteries need to be either clipped or controlled with the harmonic scalpel. If the operation is being performed for a cyst or a leiomyoma, only enough dissection to expose the lesion is necessary. When

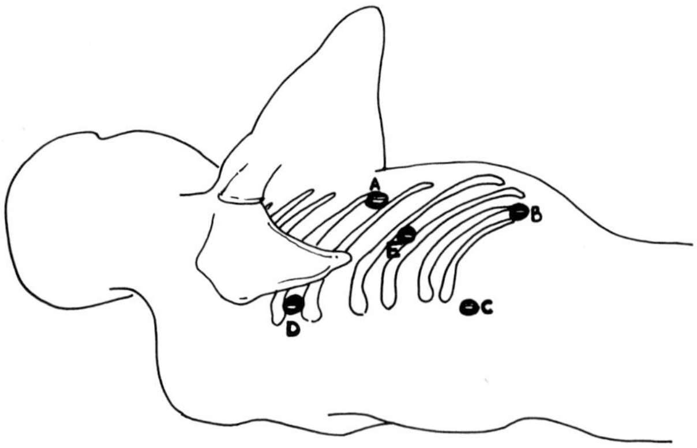

Figure 33–4. Appropriate patient positioning and thoracoport array for minimal access esophageal surgery. Port sites A and B provide access for lung retraction and/or surgical assistance during the procedure. Ports C and D are the major operating locations, and the video camera is placed through port E. Both 0- and 30-degree cameras are used, as required.

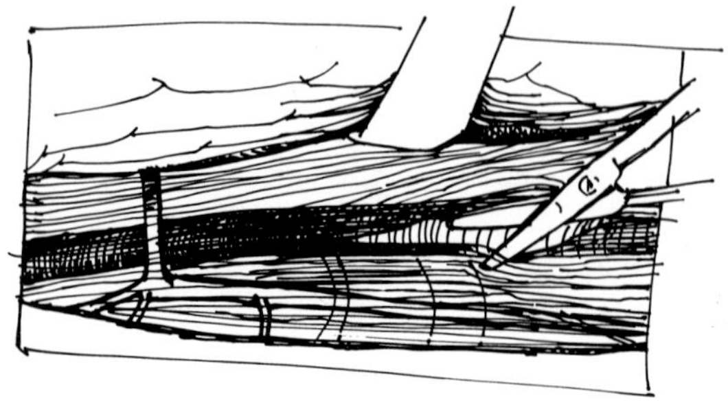

Figure 33–5. With the lung retracted anteriorly, the mediastinal pleura over the esophagus is incised. The esophagus is dissected free from surrounding tissues to the extent necessary to expose the lesion. The azygos vein is divided between hemoclips or with an EndoGIA stapler if necessary to expose the upper esophagus. A right-sided procedure is depicted here, but the technique is essentially the same when a left thoracic approach is chosen.

the operation is necessitated by a diverticulum and motor disorder, it is better to encircle the esophagus with a Penrose drain so that traction can be applied during the myotomy.

After exposure has been gained and the esophagus mobilized (Fig. 33–6), the leiomyoma is dissected from the muscle and mucosa. The tumor can be either grasped directly or lifted by a suspension suture that transfixes the tumor. Invasion of or attachment to the muscle or mucosa does not occur, so the tumor can be separated from them with ease. Electrocautery should not be used for fear of injuring the mucosa. Bleeding from the esophageal muscle is minimal and responds to gentle pressure. A defect is created in the muscular wall of the esophagus by removal of the tumor. This creates the potential for the unsupported mucosa to be distended by esophageal pressure and over time develop into a diverticulum. Therefore, the muscular window or defect should be repaired. A small defect can be covered by suturing the remaining muscle together over it in a transverse orientation. This could produce a narrowing of the lumen if the muscular gap is large, in which case suturing an onlay patch of parietal pleura is preferable.

The operative technique for excision of an esophageal cyst is identical to that for a leiomyoma.[8] However, it is important to remember that cysts occasionally communicate with the esophageal lumen or are adherent to the mucosa because of prior cyst infection. In these instances, it is prudent to unroof the cyst and cauterize its mucosal lining rather than risk extensive damage by attempting to dissect the cyst free of all attachments.

Figure 33–7 shows the stapling of a diverticulum following adequate dissection to expose and identify its neck. Although a transabdominal approach is feasible for a low, epiphrenic diverticulum,[9] the transthoracic technique is required for higher lesions. If the diverticulum is broad based, to guard against narrowing the esophageal lumen, either a large bougie (at least a size 50 French) should be positioned within the esophagus or the stapling effects should be monitored endoscopically. Although not depicted here (other chapters illustrate the technique), an esophagomyotomy of the abnormally functioning esophagus distal to the diverticulum is an integral part of the operation, including an antireflux procedure if the myotomy crosses the gastroesophageal junction.

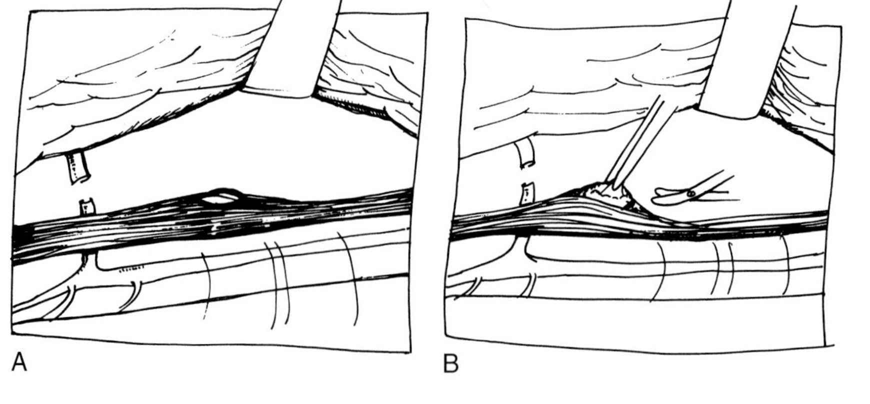

Figure 33–6. *A,* The beginning of the dissection of a leiomyoma from the esophagus. *B,* As the dissection proceeds, the tumor is extracted from its "nest" within the smooth muscle. After complete removal of the tumor, the muscular defect is either closed primarily or reinforced with a patch of parietal pleura.

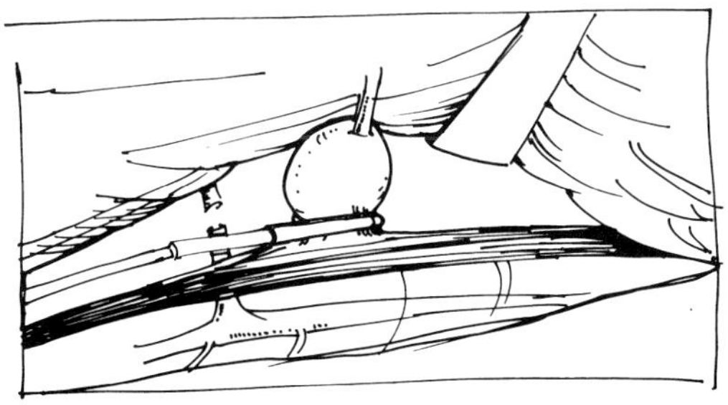

Figure 33–7. Placement of an EndoGIA stapler across the neck of an esophageal diverticulum. Protection against esophageal narrowing is provided either by endoscopic monitoring or by placement of a large dilator within the esophagus during the stapling.

References

1. Schmidt HW, Clagett OT, Harrison EG: Benign tumors and cysts of the esophagus. J Thorac Cardiovasc Surg 41:717–723, 1961.
2. Seremetis MG, Lyons WS, DeGuzman VC, Peabody JW: Leiomyoma of the esophagus. Cancer 38:2166–2175, 1976.
3. Glanz I, Grunebaum M: The radiologic approach to leiomyoma of the esophagus with a long term follow-up. Clin Radiol 28:197–203, 1977.
4. Evander A, Little AG, Ferguson MK, Skinner DB: Diverticula of the mid- and lower esophagus: Pathogenesis and surgical management. World J Surg 10:820–828, 1986.
5. Altorki NK, Sanagawa M, Skinner DB: Thoracic esophageal diverticula. J Thorac Cardiovasc Surg 105:260–264, 1993.
6. Cohen SR, Geller KA, Birns JW, et al: Foregut cysts in infants and children: Diagnosis and management. Ann Otol Rhinol Laryngol 91:622–627, 1982.
7. Salo JA, Ala-Kulju KV: Congenital esophageal cysts in adults. Ann Thorac Cardiovasc Surg 44:135–140, 1987.
8. Lewis RJ, Corravale RJ, Sisler GE: Imaged thoracoscopic surgery: A new thoracic technique for resection of mediastinal cysts. Ann Thorac Surg 53:318–325, 1992.
9. Rosati R, Fumagalli V, Bona S, et al: Diverticulectomy, myotomy, and fundoplication through laparoscopy. Ann Surg 227:174–178, 1998.

COMMENTARY

Keith S. Naunheim

The chapter is well written, concise, and instructive. I entirely agree with Dr. Little's comments regarding indications for surgery in patients with these lesions. Asymptomatic small to medium-sized duplication cysts, diverticula, and leiomyomata do not necessarily require operative intervention. Intermittent surveillance with specific imaging studies should be performed to rule out enlarging lesions, but surgery is not necessarily indicated unless the lesions grow or become symptomatic. In short, the mere presence of these lesions is not an indication for operative intervention.

There are a few technical points that might be added to the chapter. Dr. Little points out that following resection of a leiomyoma, the esophageal mucosa is exposed. It can be difficult to detect small defects in the mucosa that have occurred as a result of tearing during the dissection. I prefer to instill saline within the chest cavity to cover the esophageal mucosa. The nasogastric tube is then placed so that the holes are directly beneath the mucosa, and the anesthesiologist rapidly injects 50 to 100 ml of air into the esophageal lumen, thus distending it and ballooning it out. In this way, small leaks can be identified by the stream of air bubbles and can be repaired.

It should also be pointed out that very large esophageal diverticula may be difficult to approach solely through a thoracoscopic or laparoscopic approach. A joint approach can facilitate removal. A video-assisted thoracic surgery (VATS) approach can be used to dissect out a wall of the diaphragm down to its neck. In a laparoscopic approach, it may be difficult to place the stapler appropriately across the broad neck of a low epiphrenic diverticulum. A subsequent laparoscopic approach can facilitate this maneuver as well as the myotomy with or without a fundoplication.

Finally, Dr. Little's figures depict the performance of the esophageal procedures using both endoscopic and standard scissors and instruments. One must always remember that enlarging a trocar site can be quite useful in allowing the placement of a long standard instrument that may facilitate dissection. Many surgeons feel it is the distraction of ribs rather than the incision of muscles that causes the major discomfort following a thoracotomy, and simply enlarging a trocar site does not necessarily greatly increase the perioperative pain or analgesic requirements.

Chapter 34

Thoracoscopic Esophagectomy With Extended Mediastinal Lymphadenectomy for Cancer

Takashi Akaishi, Iwao Kaneda, and Norio Higuchi

Thoracoscopic esophagectomy as a treatment for malignancy has been described in the literature since 1992. Gossot has reported its feasibility in a porcine experiment,[1] and Cushieri[2] has described clinical experience and established a technical prototype, proposing the use of coaxial scissors, forceps, and other special devices for retracting the esophagus.[3] In San Antonio, Texas, the first international symposium for thoracoscopic surgery was held and the en bloc esophagectomy was proposed.[4] Since then, there has been little doubt of the feasibility of esophagectomy by means of thoracoscopy. However, as surgical experience has accumulated, it appears that the technique has no particular advantages over the conventional open technique.[5–8] Thoracoscopic esophagectomy may have some real benefits, including less postoperative pain and better preservation of pulmonary function.[9] However, these advantages have not been widely recognized.

Extended lymphadenectomy in addition to esophagectomy has the theoretical advantage of improving patients' prognoses. This may be technically difficult with the thoracoscopic approach since vital neurovascular structures have to be preserved in the dissection. This chapter, therefore, provides technical details of the surgical procedure for thoracoscopic esophagectomy in which the esophagectomy is accompanied by an extended lymphadenectomy in the mediastinum, avoiding harmful manipulation that may cause injury to nerves or small blood vessels in the tracheobronchial tree. Subsequently, there is a survey and discussion of worldwide assessment of this modality.

Surgical Indications for Thoracoscopic Esophagectomy

Patients who exhibit primary lesions that do not invade the submucosal layer should be excluded. Experience has shown that no lymph node metastases are usually found in these patients; therefore, endoscopic mucosal resection is a more appropriate treatment. An exclusion criterion should also be applied to patients whose primary lesions are preoperatively suspected of invading the surrounding organs, because there is not yet a thorascoscopic technique for resecting these tumors.

If a patient does not seem to tolerate ventilation of the left lung and collapse of the right lung, the thoracoscopic approach should be abandoned, or an approach in which the patient is placed in a prone position with bilateral lung ventilation might be considered, as Cushieri has recommended.[3]

Operative Procedures

Under general anesthetic and independent lung ventilation, the patient is placed on the left side, the right lung is collapsed, and the left lung is ventilated with 100% oxygen (Fig. 34–1). In almost all cases, one-lung ventilation can be maintained throughout the thoracic part of the surgery without any difficulty, but, occasionally, the anesthesiologist may require bilateral lung ventilation for a couple of minutes to remove phlegm or check the position of the double-lumen intratracheal tube.

The surgeon stands behind the patient. The assistant and the camera operator stand on the other side. Six trocars are applied around the point on the midaxillary line that crosses the fourth intercostal space[9, 10] (Fig. 34–2). The most caudal trocar is placed first, and the adhesion between the parietal and visceral pleura is checked. A telescope angled at 30 degrees is then introduced through this trocar. Looking cranially through the telescope, the following trocars are placed: a midaxillary trocar at the fourth intercostal space, a posterior axillary trocar at the fifth intercostal space, a posterior axillary trocar at the third intercostal space, seen between the latter two, an anterior axillary trocar at the second intercostal space, with telescope turned ventrally, and an anterior axillary trocar at the fourth intercostal space. Care should be taken not to cause bleeding, which necessitates wiping the telescope frequently during the operation. The telescope is moved to the midaxillary trocar at the fourth intercostal space, which enables the entire mediastinal area to be viewed. Cushieri has recommended a prone position for the procedure, because collapsing one lung is not necessary for exposure of the posterior mediastinum.[3]

Optic-Visual System

Thoracoscopic esophagectomy follows the general rules of visual optic systems in thoracoscopy. To provide the correct orientation for surgeons who are facing each other, one of the two images projected on the monitors must be inverted. An inverted image can be achieved by an interface between the two monitors or by actually inverting one of the monitors, unless the image becomes blurred because of a dysfunction of the beam alignment.

Surgical Instruments (Fig. 34–3)

The surgeon uses scissors and grasping forceps during thoracoscopy. Indiscriminate grasping or severing must be avoided. The actions of the assistant play a critical role in this surgery. The assistant surgeon uses many kinds of in-

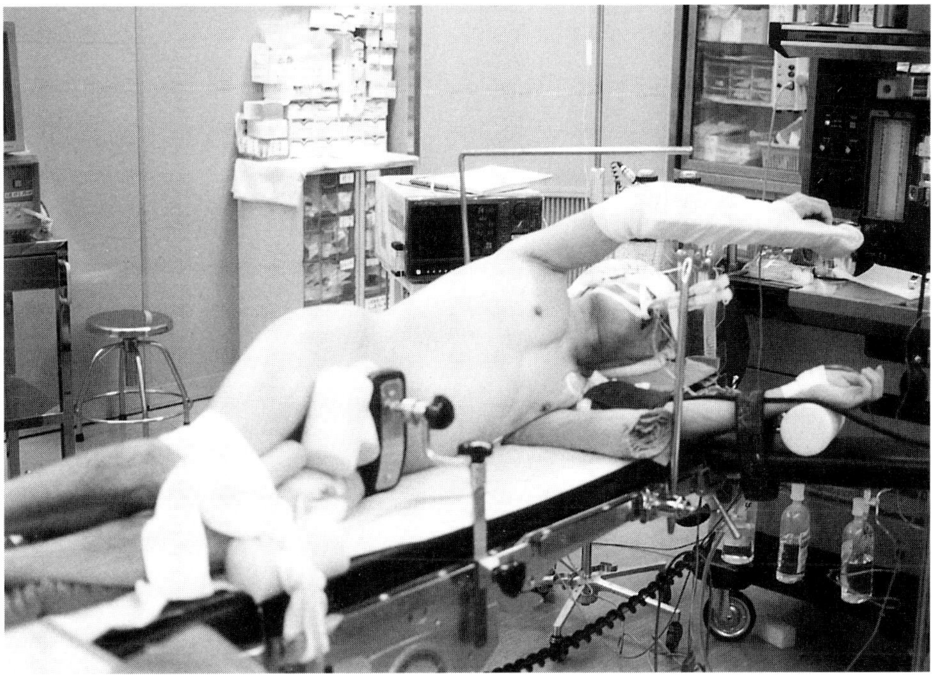

Figure 34–1. The patient is in the left lateral decubitus position with the right hand up. A double-lumen intratracheal tube is set.

struments to secure the operating field for the surgeon. The majority of the assistant's work is devoted to putting countertraction on the esophagus, trachea, or bronchus, using the following devices

- Cherry dissector (Ethicon EndoSurgery, Cincinnati, OH)
- Grasping forceps
- Nerve retractor
- Suction finger

The nerve retractor is a device originally used in laryngeal microsurgery. The suction finger (Atom Co., Tokyo, Japan) was innovated by the authors, who made holes at the top of an intrauterine irrigator. This instrument is not only a surgical aspirator, but it is also used for feeling and dissecting tissue. Its shape resembles that of the surgeon's actual index finger.

Thoracoweb Maneuver

Surgery in the posterior mediastinum requires the lung to be separated from the surgical field. To provide a panoramic view from the thoracic apex to the esophageal hiatus, a running suture should be applied to the mediastinal pleura along the pulmonary ligament, and, after each hook, the suture should be picked up with a device called an EndoClose (AutoSuture Japan, Tokyo, Japan). The suture should then be guided out of the thoracic cage and tied to the forceps, which results in a zigzag pattern in the

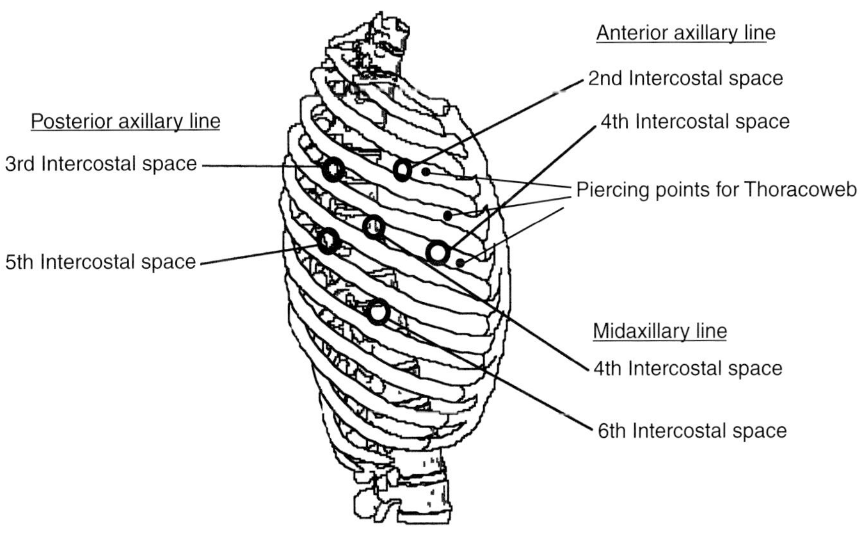

Figure 34–2. Location of trocars and piercing points for Thoracoweb.

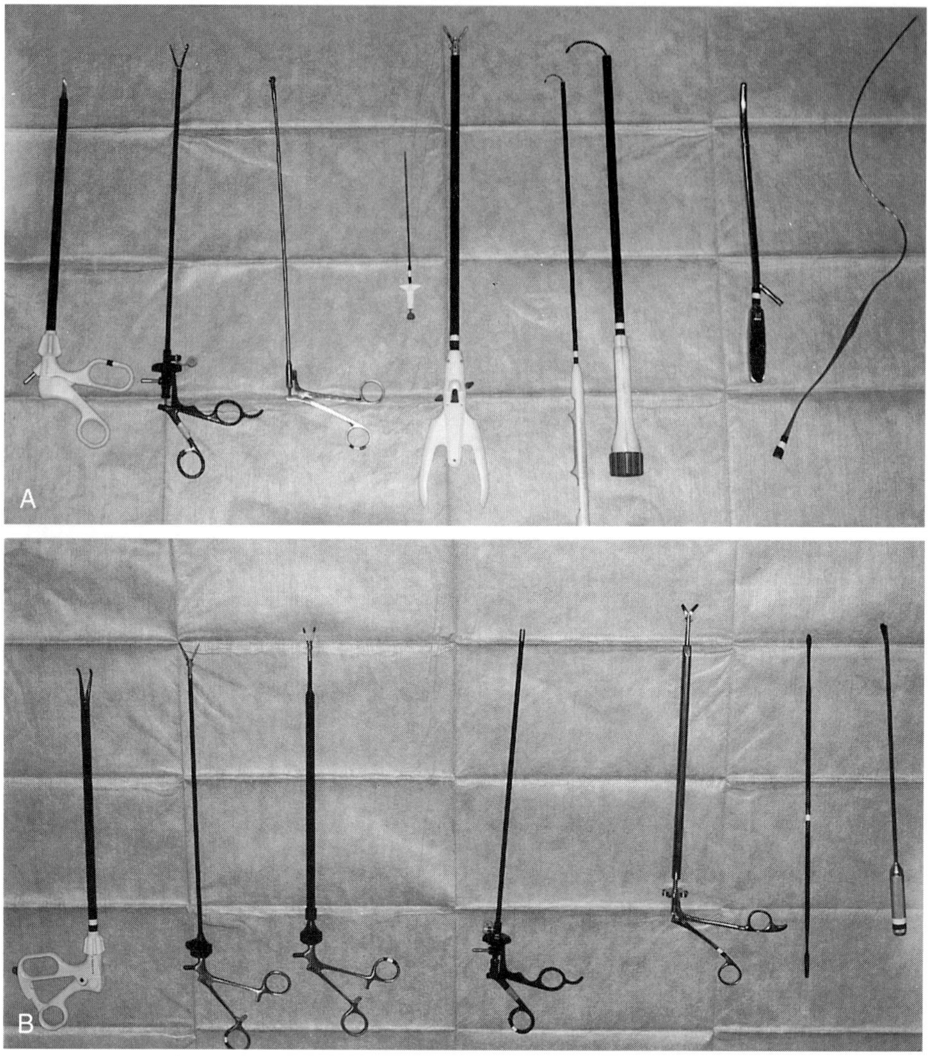

Figure 34–3. Surgical devices. *A,* Left to right: scissors, lymph node forceps, EndoClose, Endo-Stitch, EndoRetract Mini, Suction Finger, staple leader. *B,* Left to right: right-angled forceps, three types of grasping forceps, curved scissors, Sendai Spatula, spatula.

pleural space (Fig. 34–4). This technique is referred to as the Thoracoweb maneuver.[9] The first stitch should be applied to a tendinous part of the right hemidiaphragm to open the cardiophrenic angle. By applying the stitch to this strong point, the chance of breaking the hooked point is reduced. In an earlier series, only the ends of the running suture were pulled out of the thoracic cage.[10] In many cases, stitches were broken. In contrast, the Thoracoweb maneuver allows each stitch to share the tension, thus improving the life of the stitches.

A suture may be hooked to each loop of Thoracoweb outside the rib cage and made into a new loop. The Thoracoweb can be released when the anesthesiologist requires inflation of the collapsed lung. The secondary loops are pulled to retrieve the first loops so that the web can be restored.

Surgical Procedures

Dorsal Aspect of the Esophagus. After the mediastinum is exposed by the Thoracoweb, the endoscopic linear cutter is inserted by using a white cartridge from the trocar of the sixth intercostal space and the azygos arch is divided (Fig. 34–5). The right bronchial artery, which runs beneath the azygos arch, should be preserved to save blood perfusion through the tracheobronchial tree. The assistant should apply suitable countertraction by pulling the esophagus in the ventral direction, providing sufficient room for the surgeon to work between the esophagus and the descending aorta. The surgeon separates the esophagus from the descending aorta by severing the proper esophageal arteries (arteriae oesophagicae propriae).

Particular attention should be paid to preserving the left bronchial arteries that arise around the junction of the aortic arch and the descending aorta[11] (Fig. 34–6). The thoracic duct should also be preserved unless there is evidence of invasion by the tumor or metastatic lymph nodes.

Ventral Aspect of the Esophagus. The assistant should pull the esophagus in the dorsal direction, and the lower lobe of the right lung should be pulled in the ventral direction, thus creating a space between the lung and the esophagus. First the pulmonary veins and pericardium should be exposed, and then the procedure should continue cranially and caudally. In the cranial direction, when

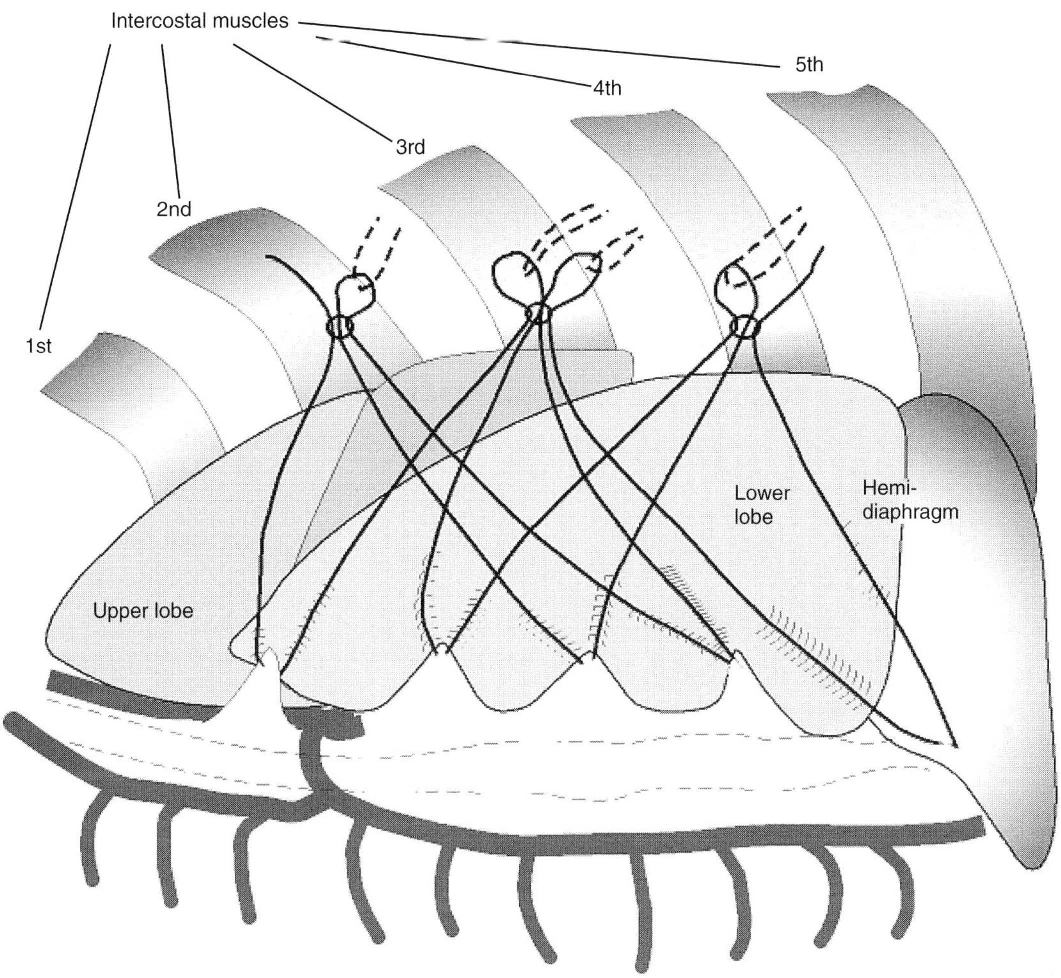

Figure 34–4. Thoracoweb maneuver: Each suture loop is hooked with a ligature (broken lines) when lung inflation is necessary.

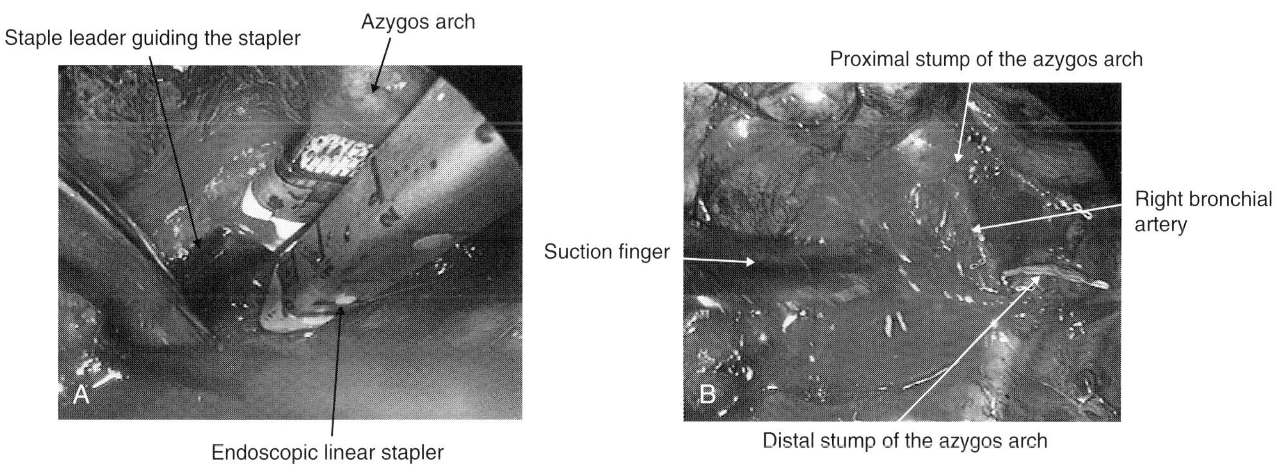

Figure 34–5. *A*, *B*, Dividing the azygos arch: The right bronchial artery should be preserved.

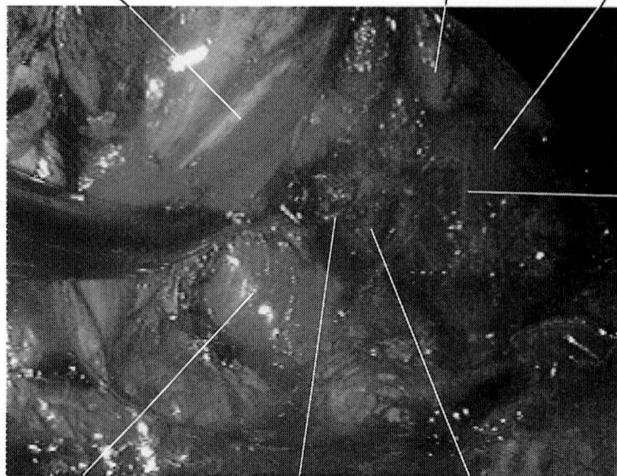

Figure 34–6. Infra-aortic arch lymph nodes with a macroscopic metastasis: Fine left bronchial arteries should be preserved.

the infracarinal lymph nodes are encountered, the dissection should proceed ventral to the nodes. As a result, the bilateral main bronchus is exposed. The lymph nodes should be dissected as they are detached from the bronchi and the bronchial arteries, so that the pulmonary branches of the vagus nerve are the last remaining tissue attached to the nodes. A complete separation should not be performed until the following preparation has been completed.

The trunk of the right vagus nerve should be identified and followed to the gastrointestinal tract branch. The nerve should be divided carefully to ensure preservation of the pulmonary branches (Fig. 34–7). The membranous part of the trachea and the right main bronchus are exposed and followed to the same region of the left main bronchus. The assistant should raise the esophagus by using a retractor inserted along the left man bronchus (Fig. 34–8). This facilitates observation of the left portion of the infracarinal lymph nodes, which are visible from the space between the esophagus and the descending aorta. These lymph nodes should be separated from the bronchus, but the left bronchial artery should be preserved. Finally, the infracarinal nodes are completely separated from the arteries and the nerves. Caudally, the dissection continues up to the esophageal hiatus.

Descending Along the Left Margin. While the assistant raises the esophagus, the gastrointestinal branch of the left vagus nerve should be located and divided. The distal nerve represents the left margin of the lymphadenectomy, and this nerve, as well as the esophagus, should be dissected with the attached nodes caudal toward the diaphragm. Care must be taken not to enter the left pleural cavity.

Superior Mediastinum. Metastases are most frequently found (32%) around the right recurrent laryngeal nerve nodes.[10] The right vagus nerve is followed cranially until it passes between the subclavian artery and the vein (Fig. 34–9). The right recurrent laryngeal nerve should be identified as a branch of the vagus nerve along the right sub-

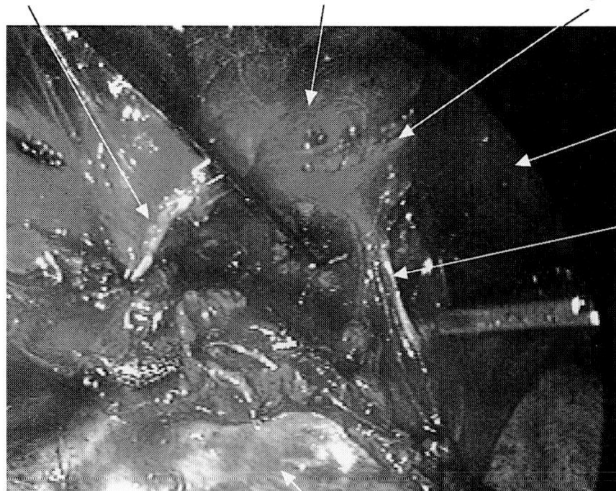

Figure 34–7. Dividing the gastrointestinal branch of the right vagus nerve.

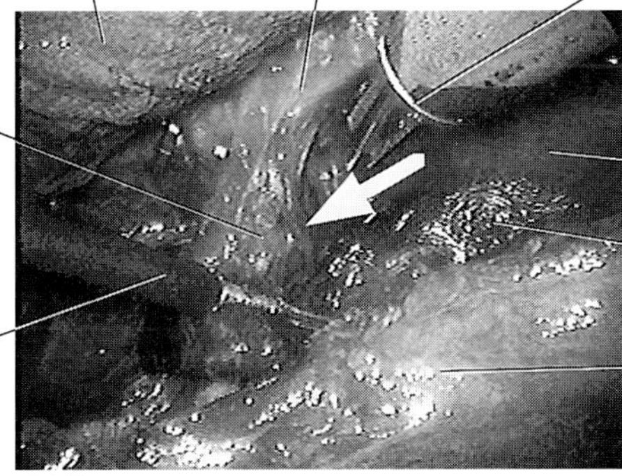

Figure 34–8. Infracarinal lymph nodes: The nodes are everted before being separated from the tracheal bifurcation.

clavian artery. The main trunk of the recurrent nerve is identified, and the surrounding lymph nodes that are attached to the esophagus are removed (Fig. 34–10). The magnified view provided by the thoracoscope is effective. Small scissors, forceps, and a nerve retractor are useful at this point. Adjacent periesophageal soft tissue should also be removed, and this forms the cranial margin of the thoracoscopic procedure.

Dorsal Side of the Esophagus. There are no significant structures except for the thoracic duct that runs from right to left.

The Left Paratracheal Nodes (Fig. 34–11). The esophagus is separated from the membranous part of the trachea. The assistant then raises the left tracheobronchial angle by using the EndoRetract Maxi (AutoSuture, Tokyo, Japan) to draw the esophagus dorsally, thus exposing the left recurrent laryngeal nerve. First, the ladder-like fine nerve branches between the nerve and the trachea should be divided. The left paratracheal lymph nodes then become visible between the nerve and the trachea. The nerve trunk is suspended by the esophagus and not teased until it is separated from the esophagus after the lymphadenectomy is complete.

The esophagus is divided at a cancer-free level by using an endoscopic linear cutter. If the posterior mediastinal route is used for reconstruction, each stump of the esophagus must be connected by using a long suture to retrieve the stomach at the neck.

The abdominal and cervical procedures are identical to the conventional esophagogastrectomy. The patient is placed in a supine position, and the lymphadenectomy is initiated through the upper abdomen in order to create a gastric tube. The stomach is raised to the neck by using any available route, and is then anastomosed with the cervical esophagus.

Two-Stage Esophagectomy. Two-stage (Lewis) esophagectomy is indicated in cases in which abdominal exploration must precede the esophagectomy. For example, the two-stage esophagectomy is indicated if potential lymph node metastases must be checked first in the abdomen, or if cervical exploration is not preferred. It may also be appropriate when the resectability of a tumor located in the caudal third of the thoracic esophagus is uncertain.

After the resectability is ascertained, and the lymphadenectomy in the upper abdomen and the gastric tube formation are completed, the patient is turned to the left lateral decubitus position. The trocar holes are made in the

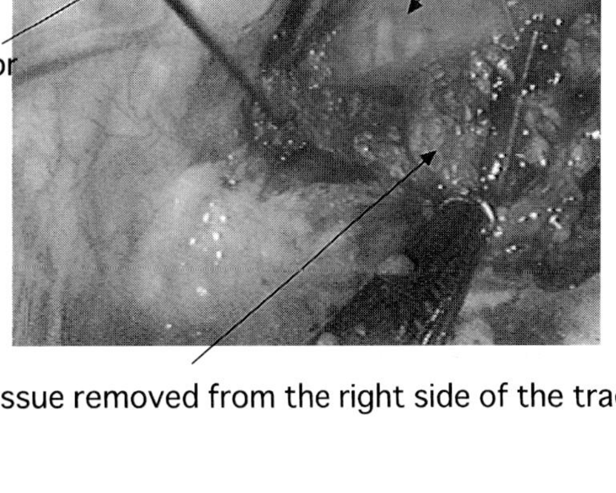

Figure 34–9. Lymphadenectomy along the right side of the trachea: The right vagus nerve is lifted.

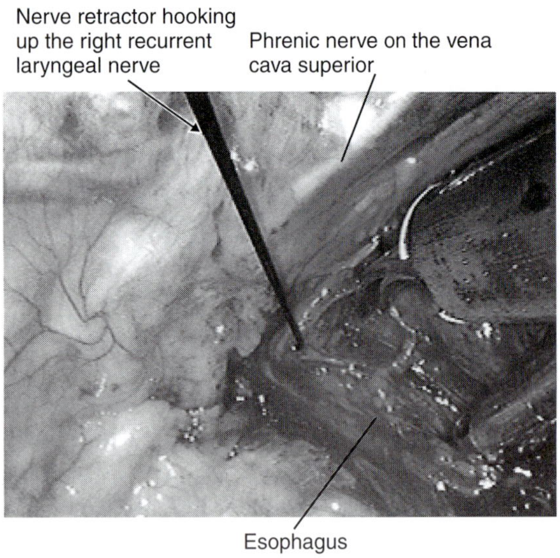

Figure 34–10. Exposing the right recurrent laryngeal nerve on the right subclavian artery.

same manner described previously, except the sixth intercostal hole is used as a 6-cm utility thoracotomy. The device for the pursestring suture is passed through this incision. The head of the anastomosing device is then inserted to the proximal esophagus, the pursestring suture is tied, the gastric tube is pulled out, the shaft of the anastomosing device is dipped into the tip of the gastric tube, the esophagogastrostomy is completed, and the endoscopic stapler is passed through the incision to close the point of entry of the anastomosing device.

Worldwide Review (Table 34–1)

Since 1992, a great deal of clinical experience has been gained in thoracoscopic esophagectomy, and reports have been pessimistic about the outcomes for the procedure. The incidence of pulmonary complications has not been reduced compared with conventional open procedures.[5] The two-stage esophagectomy has also resulted in a 12% in-hospital mortality, and all of these deaths have been

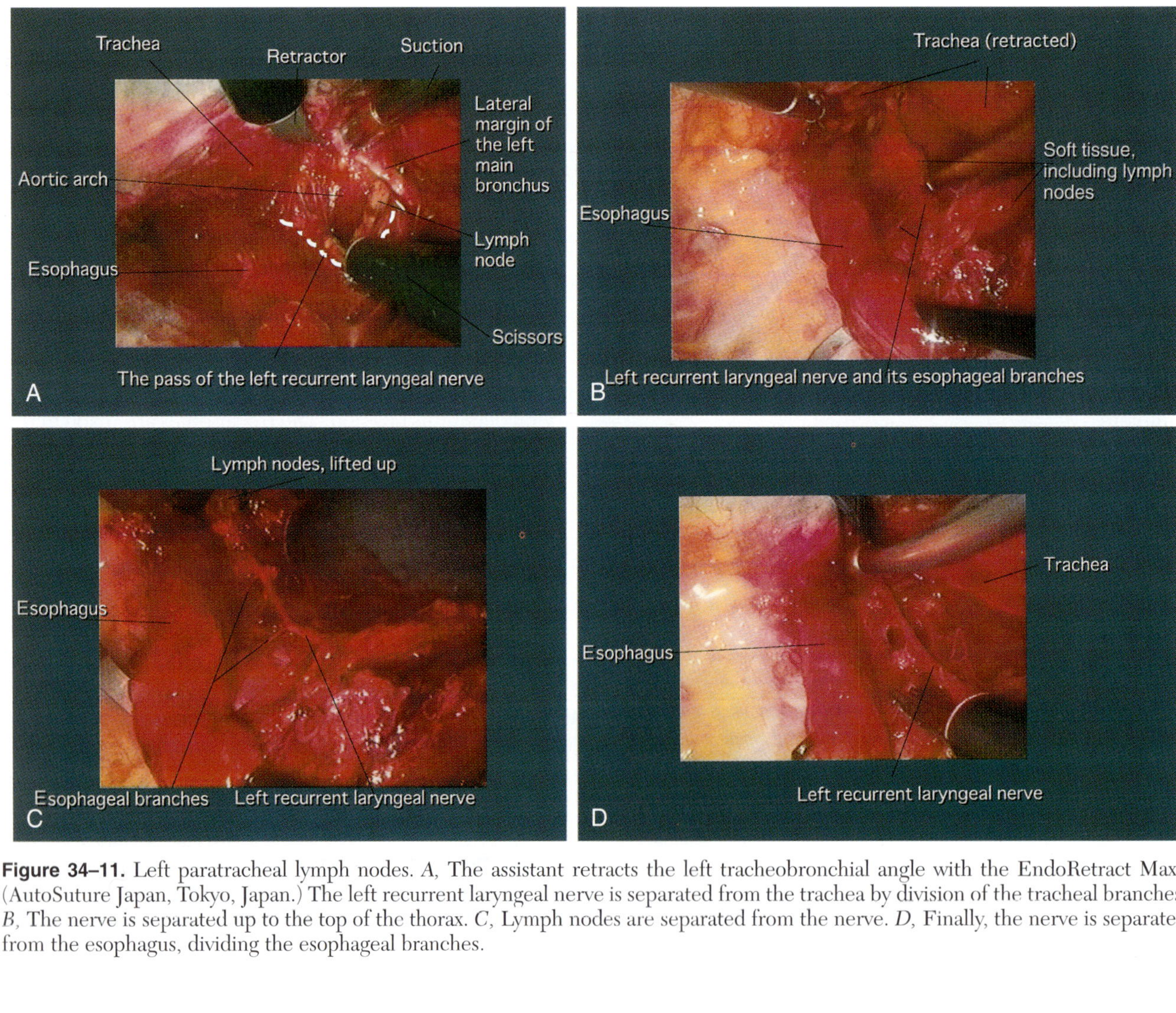

Figure 34–11. Left paratracheal lymph nodes. *A*, The assistant retracts the left tracheobronchial angle with the EndoRetract Maxi. (AutoSuture Japan, Tokyo, Japan.) The left recurrent laryngeal nerve is separated from the trachea by division of the tracheal branches. *B*, The nerve is separated up to the top of the thorax. *C*, Lymph nodes are separated from the nerve. *D*, Finally, the nerve is separated from the esophagus, dividing the esophageal branches.

Table 34–1. Morbidity and Mortality in Thoracoscopic Esophagectomy

Author	Gossot	Robertson	McAnena	Dexter	Akaishi
Complication					
Pulmonary					
Pneumonia	1 (4.2%)	5 (29%)	nd	13 (59%)	3 (7.7%)
Atelectasis	3 (12.5%)	13 (76%)	9 (100%)	nd	5 (12.8%)
Pleural cavity					
Effusion	1 (4.2%)	8 (47%)	1 (11.1%)	2 (9%)	1 (2.6%)
Cardiovascular	nd	nd	nd	4 (18%)	2 (5.1%)
Recurrent nerve paresis	3 (12.5%)	nd	3 (33.3%)	8 (36%)	7 (17.9%)
Anastomotic leak	5 (20.8%)	3 (18%)	0 (0%)	2 (9%)	2 (5.1%)
Case completed	24	17	0	22	39
Case converted	3	5	(1?)	2	0
Hospital death	1 (4.2%)	2 (12%)	0 (0%)	2 (13.5%)	1 (2.6%)*

nd = no description.

* After 3 months, of renal failure as a result of adjuvant chemotherapy.

caused by anastomotic leak.[6] Both regular thoracoscopic esophagectomy and two-stage esophagectomy have a high conversion rate into open thoracotomy, with 3 out of 29 (10.3%), and 5 out of 22 (22.7%) cases reported, respectively, indicating some technical difficulty or inadequate surgical indications.

What Are the Benefits of Thoracoscopic Esophagectomy?

It is well known that conventional thoracotomy produces a decline in postoperative vital capacity. In other words, thoracotomy produces postoperative constrictive pulmonary dysfunction. The incidence of postoperative pulmonary complications is closely related to preoperative vital capacity.[12] Pain relieving treatment during the early postoperative period accelerates recovery, although the vital capacity of patients still stays below preoperative levels.[13–16] In observations over the long term, assessment of the recovery of postoperative vital capacity is still controversial.[9] In our previous study,[16] thoracoscopic esophagectomy was advantageous not only in terms of postoperative pain relief, but also in the long-term recovery of postoperative vital capacity compared with conventional open approaches.

The Role of the Abdominal Procedure in Relation to Postoperative Pulmonary Functions

In spite of the advantages described above, vital capacity still drops in the early postoperative period, especially during the first month. The degree of the drop, however, is less than that observed in open procedures. In the field of laparoscopic cholecystectomy,[17] there have been several reports on the apparent benefits of preserving vital capacity in the early postoperative period. In the field of esophagectomy, Jagot has attempted a laparoscopic mobilization of the stomach, and has reported a minimal reduction in forced vital capacity on the eighth postoperative day.[18] This report predicts that in the near future, laparoscopic procedures will accompany thoracoscopic procedures in carrying out a total endoscopic esophagectomy.

Is the Thoracoscopic Esophagectomy Acceptable for the Surgical Treatment of Esophageal Cancer?

According to Dexter,[7] the cancer-specific survival rate 2 years after surgery is 33%. Law[19] has reported a 62% 2-year survival rate that is comparable with the 63% rate in open thoracotomy patients. The survival rate for patients undergoing thoracoscopic esophagectomy appears to be almost identical to that for patients undergoing open procedures in the same facility. The author's results agree with those described previously. Cancer recurrence at the port site in thoracoscopic esophagectomy is rare, and only one case has been reported.[19]

Conclusions

Until now, thoracoscopic esophagectomy has achieved surgical outcomes comparable with those achieved by conventional open esophagectomy. Summarizing the previous reports, procedures inside the thorax must be refined so that an inherent benefit is achieved in the patient's quality of life.

References

1. Gossot D, Debiolles H, Ghnassia MD, et al: Chirurgie de l'oesophage par thoracoscopie: Étude de faisabilité. Gastroenterol Clin Biol 16:325–327, 1992.
2. Cuschieri A, Shimi S, Banting S: Endoscopic oesophagectomy through a right thoracoscopic approach. J R Coll Surg Edinb 37:7–11, 1992.
3. Cuschieri A: Thoracoscopic subtotal oesophagectomy. Endosc Surg Allied Technol 2:21–25, 1994.
4. Collar J-M, Lengele B, Otte JB, et al: En bloc and standard esophagectomies by thoracoscopy. Ann Thorac Surg 56:675–679, 1993.
5. Gossot D, Cattan P, Fritsch S. et al: Can the morbidity of esophagectomy be reduced by the thoracoscopic approach? Surg Endosc 9:1113–1115, 1995.
6. Robertson GS, Lloyd DM, Wicks AC, et al: No obvious advantages for thoracoscopic two-stage oesophagectomy. Br J Surg 83:675–678, 1996.

7. Dexter SP, Martin IG, McMahon MJ: Radical thoracoscopic esophagectomy for cancer. Surg Endosc 10:147–151, 1996.
8. McAnena OJ, Rogers J, Williams NS: Right thoracoscopically assisted oesophagectomy for cancer. Br J Surg 81:236–238, 1994.
9. Akaishi T, Miyazaki S, Miyata G, et al: Thoracoscopic esophagectomy with extended mediastinal lymphadenectomy as a standard surgical treatment for the esophageal cancer. *In* Topuzlu C, Tekant Y (eds): Joint Euro Asian Congress of Endoscopic Surgery. Bologna, Monduzzi Editore, 1997.
10. Akaishi T, Kaneda I, Higuchi N, et al: Thoracoscopic *en bloc* total esophagectomy with radical mediastinal lymphadenectomy. J Thorac Cardiovasc Surg 112:1533–1540, 1996.
11. Funami, Y, Okuyama, K, Shimada Y, et al: Anatomic study of the bronchial arteries with special reference to their preservation during the radical dissection of the upper mediastinum lymph nodes. Surgery 119:67–75, 1996.
12. Nagawa H, Kobori O, Muto T, et al: Prediction of pulmonary complications after transthoracic oesophagectomy. Br J Surg 81:860–862, 1994.
13. Eng J, Sabanathan S: Continuous extrapleural intercostal nerve block and post-thoracotomy pulmonary complications. Scand J Thorac Cardiovasc Surg 26:219–223, 1992.
14. Bigler D, Møller, J, Kamp-Jensen M, et al: Effect of piroxicam in addition to continuous thoracic epidural bupivacaine and morphine on postoperative pain and lung function after thoracotomy. Acta Anaesthesiol Scand 36:647–650, 1992.
15. Welte M, Haimerl E, Groh J, et al: Effect of interpleural morphine on postoperative pain and pulmonary function after thoracotomy. Br J Anaesthesiol 69:637–639, 1992.
16. Deneuville M, Bisserier A, Regnard JF, et al: Continuous intercostal analgesia with 0.5% bupivacaine after thoracotomy: A randomized study. Ann Thorac Surg 55:381–385, 1993.
17. McMahon AJ, Russell IT, Ramsay G, et al: Laparoscopic and minilaparotomy cholecystectomy: A randomized trial comparing postoperative pain and pulmonary function. Surgery 115: 533–539, 1994.
18. Jagot P, Sauvanet A, Berthoux L, et al: Laparoscopic mobilization of the stomach for oesophageal replacement. Br J Surg 83:540–542, 1996.
19. Law S, Fok M, Chu KM, et al: Thoracoscopic esophagectomy for esophageal cancer. Surgery 122:8–14, 1997.

COMMENTARY

Toni Lerut

Management of carcinoma of the esophagus today is very controversial. Nevertheless, it is still accepted that surgical treatment provides the best chance for cure, provided there is complete tumor removal, that is, a so-called R0 resection. Among the different surgical approaches, transthoracic esophagectomy represents the first choice, because it provides good exposure that allows extended lymphadenectomy. Now, there are several series indicating that extended lymphadenectomy provides significantly better locoregional tumor control and improved cure rates, especially, if it is performed early, in stage I and II carcinomas.

Because of a higher incidence of morbidity, especially pulmonary complications, after transthoracic resection, transhiatal resection has gained popularity, because it appears to decrease pulmonary complications, However, it is not widely accepted as a curative treatment, because it allows only a periesophageal lymphadenectomy. Moreover, it is a blind procedure, so it also carries a higher risk of intraoperative complications, such as bleeding, tracheobronchial tree, and recurrent nerve lesions.

In this respect, a thoracoscopic video-assisted thoracic surgical (VATS) approach offers an interesting alternative, because it combines the advantage of the transhiatal procedure—less pulmonary morbidity—and the advantage of the transthoracic resection—oncologic radicality.

The experience described in this chapter is different from that of other centers in that this is the first group to focus on extended lymphadenectomy, especially along the left recurrent nerve and the brachiocephalic trunk. This dissection is very demanding, requiring the highest technical skills. In this respect, it is important to stress the importance of obtaining sufficient experience (e.g., by going to the pig laboratory), which indeed the authors did before performing the operation on human beings. Such an approach is to be strongly recommended to anyone who has an interest in proceeding with this technique.

The questions to be answered are, of course, whether in humans thoracoscopic esophagectomy matches the intended goals. Clearly, visibility is better and the operation is safer than one performed through a transhiatal approach with blunt dissection. This advantage does recommend it for consideration to those who prefer the transhiatal approach.

From the available world literature, however, it seems that VATS esophagectomy has not really improved reported mortality and morbidity after transhiatal or transthoracic resection. Mortality with VATS varies between 0 and 13%, which is about equal to what can be obtained today with open surgery. Indeed, most centers with experience in this type of surgery now report a mortality rate of less than 5%, even after transthoracic resection. Recurrent nerve palsy after VATS esophagectomy is relatively high, up to 36% in one series, which is higher than what has been reported after transhiatal and, certainly, transthoracic resections. The same can be said for anastomotic leaks, although the authors' series features quite a low incidence, matching the actual leakage rate from most centers with experience in this type of surgery. The main advantage of the VATS approach seems to be a lower incidence of pulmonary complications,especially when compared with transthoracic resection. Nevertheless, the incidence of pulmonary complications is not lower than that after transhiatal resection. The reasons for this are twofold. First, in patients who have chronic obstructive pulmonary disease, which is frequently the case in esophageal carcinoma, the hypoxic pulmonary vasoconstriction reflex may be impaired during unilateral ventilation. This may result in poor compensation for hypoxia. Thoracoscopic mobilization is a time-consuming technique, and most reported series of this approach focus on extensive resections. The mean duration of thoracoscopic surgery is 3 hours or more, enhancing the previously described side effects. Second, as mentioned by the authors, the use of laparotomy to mobilize the stomach may, in part, contribute to pulmonary complications as well.

The most important question, of course, is the oncologic outcome in terms of locoregional tumor control and cure rate. Although port site inoculation has been only occasionally reported, it remains a matter of concern, and it has been reported by more than one author. Thoracoscopic mobilization, because of the lack of bimanual palpation, seems to result in increased manipulation of the esophagus and the tumor. Little or no data are available about R0 resection rates and locoregional recurrence rates.

Moreover, 2-year and 5-year survival rates seem to indicate incomplete tumor and node dissection. Indeed, in the series reported by Dexter, the 2-year survival rate was only 33%, which is far below the result obtained after extended or en bloc transthoracic esophagectomy, which has had 50 to 60% 2-year survival rate being reported frequently, even in stage III disease.

Samartino, in 1997, reported a series of 11 patients, of whom 8 were in stage IIA and IIB. Five patients died between 6 and 24 months, while 3 are alive, but with recurrent disease at follow-up between 4 and 16 months. Again these results are clearly inferior to the actual standards, indicating incomplete resection and, possibly, dissemination secondary to tumor manipulation.

In conclusion, it seems from the available data that thoracoscopic esophagectomy is quite feasible. However, evidence is lacking that this procedure offers a clear advantage over traditional surgery, with the exception of pulmonary complications. The latter instance, however, only applies when compared with the transthoracic approach. From the oncologic point of view, as shown by the authors of this chapter, enlarged lymhadenectomy seems feasible when performed by experienced surgeons. The procedure, however, may be time consuming which jeopardizes its attractiveness.

Longer follow-up and, above all, randomized trials are necessary to prove the oncologic value of this technique. Therefore, this procedure should be reserved only for clinical pilot studies in selected centers that have proven experience in treating carcinoma of the esophagus.

References

Peracchia A, Rosati R, Fumagalli V, et al: Thoracoscopic dissection of the esophagus for cancer. Int Surg 82:1–4, 1997.

Samartino P, Chirletti P, Calcaterra D, et al: Videoassisted transhiatal esophagectomy for cancer. Int Surg 82:406–416, 1997.

COMMENTARY

Dominique Gossot

The main merit of Dr. Akaishi's chapter is to describe a technique that fulfills the criteria of radical esophagectomy. This has not always been the case, neither in our preliminary experience[1] nor in some other reports. The extensive lymph node dissection achieved by Dr. Akaishi demonstrates that minimally invasive thoracic surgery is entering an age of maturity. In our preliminary experience with complex thoracoscopic procedures, the major issue was simply to know whether the technique was feasible. Now that surgeons have more skills and more knowledge, the main issues are twofold:

1. Can an endoscopic technique fulfill the criteria for oncologic surgery?
2. If the technique is feasible, should it be done? In other words, should it be the preferred approach over conventional surgery?

The thoracoscopic technique described by Dr. Akaishi is a true radical esophagectomy with extended lymphadenectomy, because not only lymph nodes around the right recurrent laryngeal nerve are dissected, but also those located on the left lateral aspect of the trachea. One may assume that hemostasis should be thoroughly controlled to avoid troublesome oozing. Some authors have reported similar thoracoscopic extensive lymph node dissection with an average of 20 nodes sampled. However, according to Law and associates[2], a larger number of lymph nodes are removed with open thoracic surgery.

The second issue raised by Dr. Akaishi's chapter is to know whether video-assisted thoracic surgery (VATS) esophagectomy should be the preferred approach. The main rationale for choosing a thoracoscopic rather than an open approach in surgery for esophageal cancer is to try to reduce the high respiratory morbidity of this operation.

The respiratory complication rate of 19%, which we have observed in our series, does not allow us to assert that the thoracoscopic approach gives a major benefit in terms of respiratory morbidity. These results suggest that thoracotomy might be only one of the factors of respiratory morbidity. This is supported by the recent work of Nagawa and associates, who studied the predictive factors of respiratory morbidity after transthoracic esophagectomy.[3] Of the three predictive factors, only one was of respiratory origin, FEV_1; the other two were the presence of liver cirrhosis and the stage of the tumor. The mediastinal trauma resulting from difficult dissection of a large tumor is indeed a potential cause of respiratory complication. This factor is probably not reduced by the endoscopic approach.

As the interest in thoracoscopic esophagectomy seems to decline throughout Europe,[4, 5] there have been a number of recent publications in Japan and Asia, all of which report a more radical resection. Dr. Akaishi's work contributes to answering the question: What is the best approach for surgical treatment of esophageal cancer?

References

1. Gossot D, Fourquier P, Celerier M: Thoracoscopic esophagectomy: Technique and initial results. Ann Thorac Surg 56:667–670, 1993.

2. Law S, Fok M, Chu KM, et al: Thoracoscopic esophagectomy for esophageal cancer. Surgery 122:8–14, 1997.
3. Nagawa H, Kabori, O, Muto T: Prediction of pulmonary complications after transthoracic oesophagectomy. Br J Surg 81:860–862, 1994.
4. Collard JM, Lengele B, Otte JB, et al: En bloc and standard esophagectomy by thoracoscopy. Ann Thorac Surg 56:675–679, 1993.
5. Gossot D, Cattan P, Fritsch S, et al: Can the morbidity of oesophagectomy be reduced by the thoracoscopic approach? Surg Endosc 9:1113–1115, 1995.

COMMENTARY

Manson Fok

This is a well-detailed technical paper describing the fine aspects of the procedure, and, again, we are impressed by how meticulously the extended dissection is carried out by our Japanese colleagues, even under the restricted access of thoracoscopy. There will always be a limitation to thoracoscopy in that the maneuverability of the dissecting instruments is hampered by the constraint of the thoracoports. Even with great care and good intentions, the dissection probably can never attain the same degree of en bloc radicality and oncologic clearance as an open resection. To carry out an extended dissection as described by the authors via thoracoscopy may prolong the duration of one-lung ventilation, that would nullify the prime objective of thoracoscopy, that is, to reduce perioperative pulmonary complication rates.

To date, there is no solid evidence in the form of a well-conducted prospective, randomized, controlled study with large patient numbers, to support that an ultraradical resection is superior to a conventional two-field resection. Even the oncologically unsound transhiatal resection has not been proven conclusively inferior in terms of long-term survival compared with transthoracic en bloc resection. In random patient groups, the 5-year survival rate after radical resection in major centers worldwide remains around 35% Thus, a thoracoscopic resection, although it may never attain the same radicality as an open resection, is still an oncologically sound resection, and, more importantly, a safe procedure, with the potential of decreasing operative morbidity and mortality when performed by experienced surgeons. It should, therefore, be considered in patients who have relative contraindications for open thoracotomy, and its merits should be fully studied in controlled trials.

For the majority of patients who have esophageal cancer, the tumor is often at an advanced stage by the time of presentation of symptoms, and prognosis is dismal. There is increasing evidence that adjuvant therapies, such as radiochemotherapy, rather than a more radical resection, provide the key for optimal local and systemic control of the disease. Therefore, a safe and sufficiently radical resection by thoracoscopy, together with adjuvant therapies as tolerated by the patient, is probably, at present, the optimal treatment of choice.

Chapter 35

Minimal Access Approach to Esophagectomy

Ninh T. Nguyen and James D. Luketich

The procedure of esophagectomy for treatment of patients who have either benign or malignant disease is surgically complex and challenging and can be associated with significant morbidity and mortality.[9] Conventional esophagectomy requires either laparotomy with transhiatal dissection or laparotomy combined with thoracotomy. Advances in surgical instrumentation and techniques now allow surgeons to perform complex procedures using a minimally invasive approach. These procedures include laparoscopic antireflux surgery, laparoscopic myotomy for achalasia, laparoscopic and thoracoscopic staging for esophageal cancer,[7, 13] video-assisted thorascopic (VAT) lobectomy,[6, 10] VAT Belsey fundoplication,[15, 19] VAT lung reduction surgery for emphysema,[5] and many others. In an effort to decrease the morbidity associated with esophageal resection, surgeons are beginning to facilitate esophagectomy by applying minimally invasive techniques to this procedure.

A number of authors have reported the use of video-assisted thoracoscopy or laparoscopy in performing esophagectomy.[3, 4, 8, 14, 17] Most reports have described a standard laparotomy with thoracoscopic mobilization of the esophagus used to complete the operation. Clear-cut advantages of thoracoscopic esophageal mobilization over thoracotomy or laparotomy with transhiatal dissection were not demonstrated in these studies. However, in one study, patients who underwent thoracoscopic esophagectomy had less postoperative pain and more complete recovery of vital capacity than did those who underwent open surgery.[1]

DePaula was the first to report a large series of 48 patients undergoing total laparoscopic transhiatal esophagectomy.[2] Two patients required conversion to open surgery, and two others required thoracoscopic assistance. In 1997, Swanstrom reported nine cases of laparoscopic total esophagectomy.[18] There were no conversions to laparotomy. One patient required a right thoracoscopy with intrathoracic anastomosis because of poor viability of the gastric tube.

In our institution, we have extensive experience in managing benign esophageal disorders using either laparoscopic or thoracoscopic techniques, or both. In addition, we routinely perform laparoscopic and thoracoscopic staging in patients who have esophageal carcinoma to establish eligibility for a neoadjuvant therapy protocol.[13] This experience has led us to apply these techniques to esophagectomy.[11]

Technique

Laparoscopic Transhiatal Esophagectomy

Our initial approach to minimally invasive esophagectomy was accomplished using a totally laparoscopic transhiatal technique. In this approach, the patient is placed in a supine position. The surgeon stands on the patient's right side and the assistant stands on the left. Five abdominal ports are placed (Fig. 35–1). The patient is placed in a steep reverse Trendelenburg position. The operative ports are similar to those we place when performing a laparoscopic Nissen fundoplication. The esophageal hiatus is exposed by retracting the left lobe of the liver upward using the Medi-flex (Velmed, Wexford, PA) self-retaining retractor system. The gastrohepatic ligament is divided, exposing the right crux of the diaphragm. The retroesophageal space is created, and the esophagus is mobilized circumferentially. The stomach is mobilized with division of the short gastric vessels using ultrasonic shears (Fig. 35–2). The gastrocolic omentum is divided, with preservation of the right gastroepiploic arcade. The stomach is retracted superiorly, and the left gastric vessels are identified and divided using the Endo-GIA stapler (U.S. Surgical Corporation, Norwalk, CT). Pyloroplasty closure is carried out with intracorporeal suturing using Endostitch (U.S. Surgical Corporation, Norwalk, CT). Gastroduodenoscopy with insufflation is used to confirm the completion of the pyloroplasty and the absence of leaks.

Periesophageal dissection is accomplished under laparoscopic visualization by retracting downward on the stomach and dividing the aortoesophageal branches. This dissection is carried up transhiatally into the mediastinum to the level of the left main stem bronchus. Periesophageal lymphadenectomy is performed en bloc with the esophagus. The esophagus, with a cuff of normal gastric cardia, is divided from the remaining stomach using (see Fig. 35–2) a 4.5-mm endoscopic stapler (Endo GIA-II, U.S. Surgical Corporation, Norwalk, CT). The gastric conduit is sutured to the esophageal specimen. A horizontal neck incision, 5 cm in length, is used to mobilize the cervical esophagus, and the specimen is removed through the neck incision after the attached gastric conduit is pulled up transhiatally to the cervical incision (Fig 35–3). An esophagogastric anastomosis is performed using a 25-mm EEA stapler (U.S. Surgical Corporation, Norwalk, CT) through a small gastrotomy. A nasogastric tube is directed through the anastomosis and placed down into the distal stomach. A loop of proximal jejunum is approximated to the anterior abdominal wall. The Seldinger technique is used to place a needle catheter feeding tube into the efferent limb of the jejunum for possible postoperative enteral feedings. Catheter position is checked by an insufflation of 10 ml of air.

Thoracoscopic and Laparoscopic Esophagectomy

In this approach, thoracoscopic mobilization of the esophagus is the initial procedure, followed by laparoscopic gastric mobilization with cervical anastomosis as described

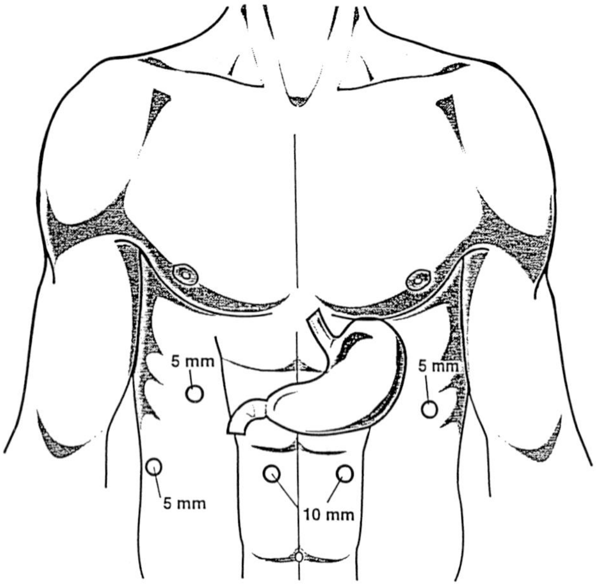

Figure 35–1. Abdominal trocars positioned for laparoscopic transhiatal esophagectomy.

previously. The patient is intubated with a double-lumen tube for single-lung ventilation and positioned in the left lateral decubitus position. Four thoracic trocars are introduced (Fig. 35–4). In the past, we used four 10-mm ports, but currently we use one 10-mm port and three 5-mm ports. The camera port is placed at the seventh intercostal space at the midaxillary line. A 5-mm port for the ultrasonic shears is placed at the eighth or ninth intercostal space, 2 cm behind the posterior axillary line. One 5-mm port is placed behind the tip of the scapula and one for retracting instruments is placed at the fourth intercostal space at the anterior axillary line. A 0-Surgitek Endostitch (U.S. Surgical Corporation, Norwalk, CT) suture is placed on the central tendon area of the diaphragm and brought percutaneously out of the thorax to facilitate downward retraction of the diaphragm and promote exposure of the distal esophagus. The mediastinal pleura overlying the esophagus is divided, and the esophagus and periesophageal tissues are circumferentially mobilized en bloc. A Penrose drain is placed around the esophagus to facilitate retraction (Fig. 35–5). The azygos vein is mobilized and divided using the Endo-GIA stapler with a vascular cartridge (U.S. Surgical Corporation, Norwalk, CT). The esophagus is mobilized from the diaphragmatic reflection up to the thoracic inlet. Periesophageal lymph nodes are sampled intraoperatively or mobilized to remain attached to the resected specimen. A 28 French chest tube is inserted through the camera port for postoperative drainage. The patient is then turned to the supine position. Laparoscopic gastric mobilization with cervical anastomosis is accomplished as described in the laparoscopic transhiatal approach.

Laparoscopic Gastric Mobilization With Right Mini-Thoracotomy

This technique is performed in unusual cases in which the gastric conduit is unable to reach the neck, thus requiring an intrathoracic anastomosis. Laparoscopic gastric mobilization with pyloroplasty is accomplished as previously described. The patient is repositioned in the left lateral decubitus position, and a right muscle-sparing thoracotomy is performed at the sixth intercostal space. The thoracic esophagus is mobilized up to the level of the azygos vein. The distal esophagus and proximal gastric cardia are resected, and either a hand-sewn or stapled anastomosis is performed in the chest.

Results

Minimally invasive esophagectomy was performed on 35 patients (23 men and 12 women) at our institution between June 1996 and June 1998. Indications for esophagectomy included esophageal carcinoma (N = 21),

Figure 35–2. Gastric conduit created with an endoscopic stapler.

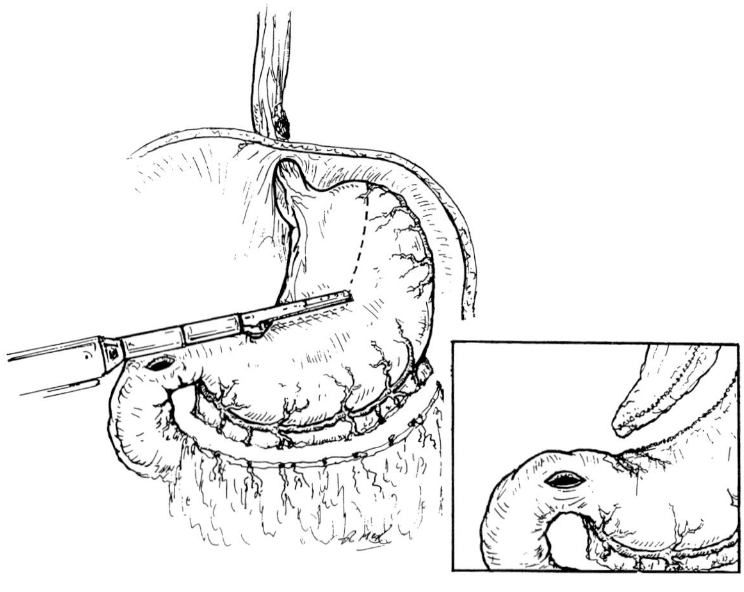

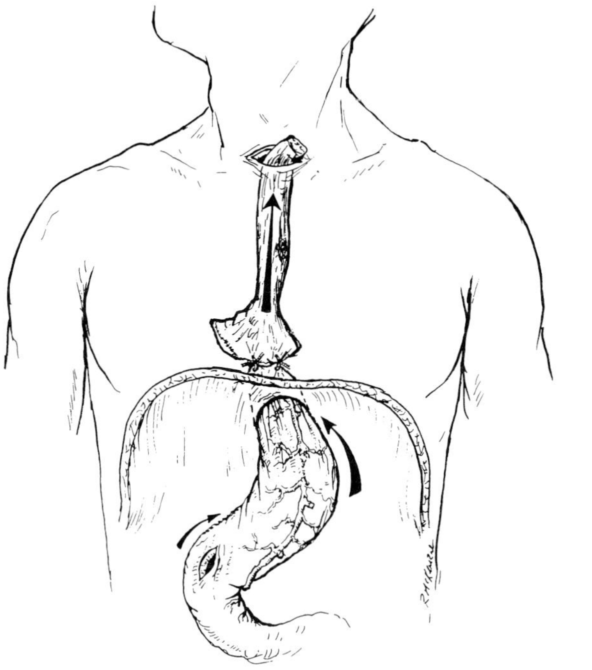

Figure 35–3. Transhiatal removal of an esophageal specimen with transhiatal pull-through of the gastric conduit.

locally advanced papillary thyroid carcinoma with esophageal involvement (N = 1), Barrett's esophagus with high-grade dysplasia (N = 7), benign tracheoesophageal fistula (N = 2), recalcitrant esophageal stricture (N = 2), and end-stage achalasia (N = 2). The mean age was 65.1 years with a range of 30 to 89 years. Twenty-one patients

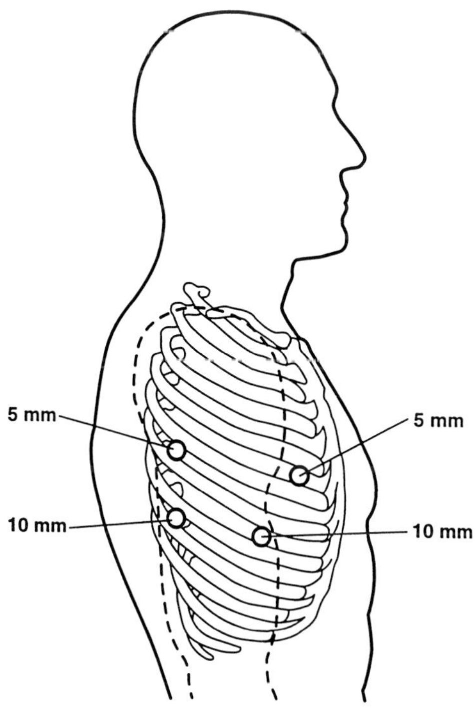

Figure 35–4. Thoracic trocar positioned on the right side of the chest for thoracoscopic and laparoscopic esophagectomy.

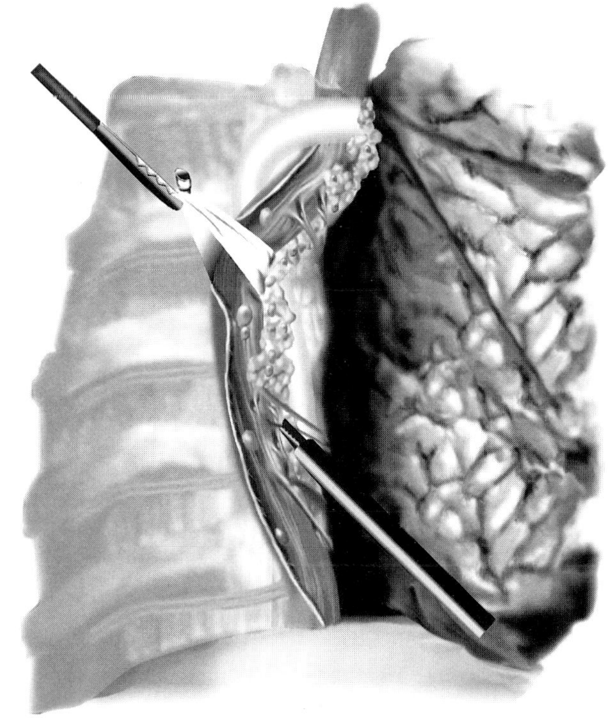

Figure 35–5. Thoracoscopic mobilization of the thoracic esophagus.

(60%) had undergone previous abdominal surgery, 12 had undergone previous esophageal surgery, 3 had hiatal hernia repair, 7 had undergone laparoscopic staging for esophageal cancer, and 2 had had laparoscopic Heller myotomy.

Our minimally invasive approach to esophagectomy included total laparoscopic transhiatal esophagectomy (N = 8), combined thoracoscopic and laparoscopic esophagectomy (N = 20), laparoscopic gastric mobilization with right muscle-sparing mini-thoracotomy (N = 6), and laparoscopic substernal gastric bypass (N = 1). Conversion to mini-laparotomy (5.7%) was necessary to achieve complete esophageal dissection in 1 patient and to facilitate gastric pullup in another. Pyloromyotomy was performed on 15 patients and pyloroplasty on 16 patients. A laparoscopic jejunostomy tube was placed in 20 patients. The mean operative time was 7.05 hours (range of 5.5 to 9.0 hours). The mean intensive care stay was 1.7 days (range of 0 to 7 days). The mean hospital stay was 9.3 days (range of 4 to 45 days). Minor complications included atrial fibrillation (N = 1), pleural effusion (N = 2), J-tube site infection (N = 2), hoarseness (N = 1), pneumonia (N = 1), and persistent air leaks (N = 1). Major complications included cervical anastomotic leak (N = 2), respiratory insufficiency (N = 2), myocardial infarction (N = 1), small bowel perforation (N = 1), and delayed gastric emptying requiring pyloroplasty (N = 3). There were no operative emergencies or deaths.

The final pathologic staging for patients who had esophageal malignancies included carcinoma in situ (N = 3), stage I (N = 3), stage IIa (N = 10), stage IIb (N = 2), stage III (N = 5), and stage IV (N = 1). All surgical margins were negative. The overall 30-day mortality was zero. Our median follow up was 7.5 months. One patient died at 4 months' follow-up as a result of progression of metastatic disease that was diagnosed at the time of operation.

Our Preferred Approach

We performed minimally invasive esophagectomy on 35 patients, and our initial results confirmed the feasibility and safety of this technique. This procedure continues to evolve, and, currently, our preferred approach is the combined laparoscopic and thoracoscopic technique.[12, 16] Such an approach facilitates more extensive lymph node dissection and improves our ability to easily mobilize the middle and proximal third of the esophagus. The azygos vein is routinely divided to promote dissection of the upper third of the esophagus. Laparoscopy is performed following thoracoscopy. Laparoscopy begins with placement of a jejunostomy catheter followed by gastric mobilization and pyloroplasty. The distal esophageal mobilization is performed just before creation of the gastric conduit, which limits carbon dioxide leaks during pneumoperitoneum. The esophageal specimen is retrieved through the neck incision, and a cervical anastomosis is created as is done in the open procedure. In this technique, all basic components of esophageal resection, except the cervical gastroesophageal anastomosis, were performed with a minimally invasive technique. In our last 20 consecutive cases, there were no conversions to open procedure and no additional access incisions.

Our initial approach was the laparoscopic transhiatal technique. In this operation, the patient is placed supine and the laparoscopy is performed with 5 abdominal ports. The advantages of this technique are that thoracoscopy with single-lung ventilation is not required, and there is no need to reposition the patient. The limitations we encountered with this approach include the small working space through the esophageal hiatus and level of difficulty involved in dissecting the middle and upper third of the esophagus, given the length of our available instruments and poor visualization.

Minimally invasive esophagectomy is a technically demanding operation, requiring advanced laparoscopic and thoracoscopic surgical skills. This procedure is promising but requires a steep learning curve. Appropriate instruments, including ultrasonic shears, an endoscopic stapler, and a liver retractor, necessary for performance of this procedure. Our experience, similar to that of DePaula and Swanstrom, confirms that esophagectomy can be performed safely by a totally laparoscopic or thoracoscopic approach.[2, 11, 12, 16, 18] Prospective trials with longer follow-up will be required to confirm any advantages of minimally invasive esophagectomy over conventional approaches. However, in comparing our patients who have undergone minimally invasive esophagectomy with those who have had an open procedure, it is our opinion that there is less pain and more rapid recovery following minimally invasive esophagectomy.

References

1. Akaishi T, Kaneda I, Higuchi N, et al: Thoracoscopic en bloc total esophagectomy with vertical mediastinal lymphadenectomy. J Thorac Cardiovasic Surg 112:1533–1541, 1996.
2. DePaula AL, Hashiba K, Ferreira EAB, et al: Transhiatal approach for esophagectomy. *In* Toouli J, Gossot D, Hunter JG (eds): Endosurgery. New York, Churchill Livingstone, 1996, pp. 293–299.
3. Dexter SPL, Martin IG, McMahon MJ: Radical thoracoscopic esophagectomy for cancer. Surg Endosc 10:147–151, 1996.
4. Jagot P, Sauvanet A, Berthoux L, Belghiti J: Laparoscopic mobilization of the stomach for esophageal replacement. Br J Surg 83:540–542, 1996.
5. Keenan RJ, Landreneau RJ, Sciurba FC, et al: Unilateral thoracoscopic surgical approach for diffuse emphysema. J Thorac Cardiovasc Surg 111:308–315, 1996.
6. Kirby TJ, Mack MJ, Landreneau RJ, et al: Lobectomy video-assisted thoracic surgery versus muscle-sparing thoracotomy. J Thorac Cardiovasc Surg 109:997–1002, 1995.
7. Krasna MJ, Reed CE, Jaklitsch MT, et al: Thoracoscopic staging of esophageal cancer: A prospective, multi-institutional trial. Ann Thorac Surg 60:1337–1340, 1995.
8. Law S, Fok M, Chu KM, et al: Thoracoscopic esophagectomy for esophageal cancer. Surgery 122:8–14, 1997.
9. Lee RB, Miller JI: Esophagectomy for cancer. Surg Clin North Am 77:1169–1196, 1997.
10. Luketich JD, Kassis ES, Landreneau RJ, et al: A comparison of total video thoracoscopic lobectomy and standard thoracotomy for early stage non-small cell lung cancer (NSCLC) (Abstract). Lung Cancer 18:98, 1997.
11. Luketich JD, Nguyen NT, Schauer P: Laparoscopic transhiatal esophagectomy for Barret's esophagus with high grade dysplasia, JSLS 1998;75–77
12. Luketich JD, Nguyen NT, Weigel TL, et al: The role of laparoscopy and video assisted thoracoscopy in esophagectomy (Abstract). Surg Endosc 12:554 1998.
13. Luketich JD, Schauer P, Landreneau R, et al: Minimally invasive surgical staging is superior to endoscopic ultrasound in detecting lymph node metastases in esophageal cancer. J Thorac Cardiovasc Surg 114:817–823, 1997.
14. McAnena OJ, Rogers J, Williams NS: Right thoracoscopically assisted esophagectomy for cancer. Br J Surg 821:236–238, 1994.
15. Nguyen NT, Schauer PR, Hutson W, et al: Preliminary results of thoracoscopic Belsey-Mark IV antireflux procedure. Surg Laparosc Endosc 8:185–188, 1998.
16. Nguyen NT, Schauer PR, Luketich JD: Combined laparoscopic and thoracoscopic approach to esophagectomy. J Am Coll Surg 188:328–332, 1999.
17. Robertson GM, Lloyd DM, Wicks AC, et al: No obvious advantages for thoracoscopic two-stage esophagectomy. Br J Surg 83:675–678, 1996.
18. Swanstrom LL, Hansen P: Laparoscopic total esophagectomy. Arch Surg 132:943–949, 1997.
19. Yang HK, Del Guercio LRM, Steichen FM: Thoracoscopic Belsey-Mark IV fundoplication. Surg Rounds 277–291, 1995.

Section V

Miscellaneous Thoracoscopic Procedures

Chapter 36

Anesthetic Considerations for Pediatric Thoracoscopic Procedures

Catherine P. Krucylak

The miniaturization of endoscopic instruments, advances in optics, and advances in anesthetic procedures have allowed thoracoscopy to be an effective and safe alternative to thoracotomy for a variety of diagnostic and therapeutic indications in infants and children. This technique allows direct examination of the entire hemithorax and its contents through a small opening without formal thoracotomy.[1, 2] Advances in technology have allowed the projection of the endoscopic image onto a television screen, which allows visualization of the procedure by the entire operating team. The ability to see what the surgeon is doing is of benefit to the anesthesiologist, who may now see when the surgeon is manipulating tissues that cause hemodynamic changes in the patient.[3]

Thoracoscopy offers advantages in the pediatric population because it avoids the large incision of a thoracotomy and, therefore, decreases the chance of scoliosis, breast deformity, winged scapula, and shoulder weakness.[4–6] The length of hospitalization postoperatively may be decreased, postoperative pain and disability are decreased,[7] and cosmetic appearance may be improved.[8] Depending on the procedure, adhesions may be minimal, which is necessary should definitive therapy include transplantation or reoperation. The pediatric patient is able to resume normal activity more quickly. In addition to the size of the surgical instruments, thoracoscopy may be limited by the hospital's ability to provide this procedure and by the patient's ability to tolerate one-lung ventilation.

Thoracoscopy can aid in the diagnosis and treatment of several common and uncommon pediatric problems. The severity of the condition of the patient, the size of the patient, and the equipment available to the anesthesiologist dictate the choice of anesthetic technique and perioperative care.

Pediatric patients who have pleural, pulmonary parenchymal, and intrathoracic chest wall processes; subdiaphragmatic lesions; mediastinal lesions;[9] and several minor congenital cardiac lesions may be able to benefit from video-assisted thoracoscopic surgical (VATS) techniques. Thoracoscopy has even become the technique of choice for persistent, recurrent pneumothorax and to drain an empyema resistant to thoracostomy tube drainage.[10] As the pediatric surgeon becomes more proficient with thoracoscopic techniques and develops new instruments or new ways to use existing ones, the anesthesiologist may face increasing challenges in providing safe, effective anesthetic for the patient that will allow the surgeon to work as quickly and effectively as possible. This chapter reviews anesthetic issues in the pediatric patient with specific attention to concerns of ventilatory management and positioning as they relate to performance of thoracoscopically assisted surgery.

Anesthesia for Minimal Access General Thoracic Surgery

The age of the pediatric patient determines important anesthetic concerns. The full-term newborn presenting for thoracoscopic surgery[11] may revert to fetal circulation in the presence of increased pulmonary vascular resistance caused by hypoxemia, hypothermia, hypervolemia, acidosis, stress, vasoactive drugs, decreases in systemic vascular resistance, or a combination of these conditions.[12] The ratio of surface area to weight in infants is approximately two times greater than that in adults; therefore, precautions to prevent heat loss intraoperatively should be an important part of the anesthetic plan. In addition, hypothermia less than 35°C (95°F) is a relative contraindication to extubation.[13] There is less surface area exposed to environmental air during a thoracoscopic surgical procedure than there would be during a thoracotomy, but the younger the child, the more care must be given to preventing heat loss. The operating room may be warmed, and overhead heating lamps or a warm air blanket device generally work well. In addition, intravenous fluids may be run through a warming device.

The chronically ill child often has parenteral fluids administered to supplement or replace enteral intake. It is important that such hyperalimentation or supplemental glucose not be interrupted without regular intraoperative measurement of the patient's glucose or electrolyte concentrations, or both. The stressed newborn may exhibit hypoglycemia, and glucose determinations should be obtained intraoperatively to ensure normoglycemia. Maintenance fluid administration for the infant and child may be calculated on the basis of the patient's weight: 4 ml/kg per hour for the first 10 kg of body weight, with an additional 2 ml/kg per hour for the second 10 kg of body weight and an additional 1 ml/kg per hour for every kg after 20 kg.

The anatomy of the pediatric airway differs significantly from that of the adult. The structures are obviously smaller and in closer approximation to one another. One can easily obstruct the airway when holding a mask on a child's face by placing a finger too firmly in the submandibular midline region, which causes occlusion of the airway by the relatively stiffer, longer epiglottis. The head is large in proportion to the rest of the body, therefore, a roll or blanket is usually required under the shoulders to avoid flexion of the head on the neck, and a doughnut-shaped pillow is needed to stabilize the head. The tongue is relatively larger and the mouth is relatively smaller, which allows less room for maneuvering airway equipment. Other differences exist that make the tracheal intubation of an otherwise healthy infant or small child more challenging. The larynx of the newborn is more cephalad, lying at about the level of C2–C3 compared with C5 in the adult.[14] The trachea of a newborn is only about 4 cm long from larynx to carina, and because head extension can move the tracheal tube cephalad by 1 cm, great care must be taken to place the tip of the tracheal tube 1.5 to 2 cm beyond the vocal cords[15] to avoid inadvertent tracheal extubation or bronchial cannulation.

Chest wall structure and composition impair the mechanics of breathing during the first year of life.[16] The highly compliant chest wall can also move paradoxically inward with inspiration, and it is not until the child is approximately 4 years old that the dynamic compliance of the chest wall decreases to equal that of the lungs.[17] It has been shown that after a thoracotomy, an infant or small child experiences fatigue or respiratory failure more easily than does an adult and that pain limits tidal volume when intercostal muscles damaged by thoracotomy attempt to stabilize the chest wall.[16] It has yet to be determined if the incisions for the thoracoscopic surgery produce as significant a disability in infants and young children.

In addition to pleurodesis for recurrent pneumothorax or effusions and drainage of an empyema,[18–20] thoracoscopy has been beneficial for diagnosis and intervention in a variety of childhood diseases.[21] Biopsies of lesions of the chest wall,[22] pleura,[2] pulmonary parenchyma,[1, 2, 23] mediastinum,[2] and subdiaphragmatic liver[9] can be obtained for staging or diagnosis in children who have metastatic or primary tumors. Thoracoscopy is a useful tool in second-look procedures[24] for suspicious or recurrent lesions and provides a unique opportunity to examine the entire hemithorax and obtain adequate biopsy specimens.[2] However, it is thought that pulmonary biopsies for diffuse interstitial lung disease in children, especially those younger than 8 years of age, should be performed by minithoracotomy and not thoracoscopy.[21] A dorsal sympathectomy via a thoracoscope is deemed to be the operative procedure of choice for palmar hyperhidrosis.[25] Thoracoscopy has also aided the approach to the dorsal spine for spinal fusion.[21] Intrathoracic cysts[26, 27] and sequestrated lung tissue[28] have been excised using thoracoscopy. Minimally invasive thoracoscopic decortication has been successful in a number of patients.[29] There has also been a report of a successful repair of a foramen of Bochdalek hernia in a teenaged patient, which was accomplished with a minimally invasive thoracoscopic technique.[30] Thymectomies, diaphragm plications, and aortopexy have all been accomplished successfully in pediatric patients by use of a minimally invasive technique.[31] Thoracoscopic lung biopsy has been reported in a 5-week-old (34-week gestation) infant weighing 2.1 kg.[23] A 1-day-old newborn had a bronchogenic cyst that was diagnosed prenatally and was unroofed thoracoscopically without complication other than recurrence and subsequent excision thoracoscopically when the patient was 1 year old.[11] The span of pediatric patients who have diseases that can benefit from general thoracoscopic surgical techniques is so broad that one cannot hope to manage all general minimally invasive thoracic surgery with one anesthetic plan.

Preoperative Evaluation

Anesthetic care begins with an assessment of the condition of the pediatric patient. Some disease processes allow the patient to be admitted the same day, whereas other patients may be critically ill with severe respiratory disability. A detailed history and carefully focused physical examination should act as a guide for further evaluation. A patient who has reactive airway disease or cystic fibrosis may benefit from optimization of medical therapy preoperatively. In addition to a thorough examination, the results of pulmonary function tests and a pulse oximetry reading in the preoperative area can help guide postoperative ventilatory management. The patient's level of respiratory comfort may be assessed by the level of current or stated activity and, during resting respiration, by the use of accessory muscles as well as grunting and nasal flaring. The estimation of pulmonary reserve may influence the type of anesthetic induction, the use of single- or double-lung ventilation intraoperatively, and the timing of withdrawal of ventilatory support postoperatively. When a biopsy or resection of a mediastinal mass is planned, the patient should be assessed for level of respiratory comfort while lying in the position he or she will assume intraoperatively. Chest roentgenography, and possibly computed tomography, should be used to evaluate the degree of the disease process in the chest. If the patient presents with a tumor or mass, it is critical to evaluate potential compression or invasion of the airway or vascular structures because on induction of anesthesia, a decrease in muscle tone may result in complete obstruction of ventilation or cardiovascular compromise.[32] Echocardiography may provide valuable information when performed with the patient in the recumbent position that will be assumed intraoperatively. In addition, physical examination may reveal symptoms, including dyspnea, wheezing, cough, orthopnea, congestion of the head and neck, that are indicative of increased risk of respiratory or cardiovascular compromise during sedation and general anesthesia.

Infants and children who receive chemotherapeutic medications may have significant respiratory or cardiovascular side effects associated with their treatments which can impact on their intraoperative and postoperative course. Radiation therapy to the head and neck may impair the degree of mouth opening and interfere with the ability to establish an artificial airway intraoperatively. A thorough assessment of the pediatric airway is extremely important. Attention should be focused on congenital or acquired features that could make the airway potentially difficult to secure intraoperatively. Previous reconstructive facial surgery should be noted, as should intraoperative or postoperative airway management problems. The teeth should be examined and every effort made to determine which are loose, if any. The potential for aspirating a dislodged tooth is real. The patient who has severe gastroesophageal reflux or the patient who presents for emergent surgery is at increased risk of aspiration, and appropriate precautions should be taken. Fasting parameters should be individualized for patients with intra-abdominal or intrathoracic masses of systemic disease that may delay gastric emptying. Otherwise healthy patients should follow preoperative fasting guidelines for children established at the operating institution (usually between 2 and 3 hours for clear liquids and 6 and 8 hours for milk and solids).[33]

The length of illness and preoperative medical condition should dictate the extent of laboratory evaluation. In the otherwise healthy patient, an evaluation of the hematocrit and type- and cross-matching for ensuring blood availability intraoperatively should suffice. In the healthy patient who has no intravenous access, these samples may be drawn after induction of anesthesia.

The choice of sedating a patient preoperatively should be made on an individual basis in consultation with the parents or guardian or the patient, if age-appropriate. A decrease in preoperative anxiety may lessen the trauma of separation from parents for a toddler. In patients who have emphysematous lungs or blebs, screaming preoperatively may put them at increased risk for spontaneous pneumothorax. In patients who have congenital cardiac lesions with right-to-left shunting, increased agitation may increase the amount of shunting because of an increase in pulmonary vascular resistance. The child who has a potentially difficult airway may find it more difficult to exchange air while screaming, with a resultant decrease in arterial oxygen saturation. Midazolam orally, intravenously,[34] or intranasally[35] is an effective premedication for the pediatric patient. An antisialagogue may be added to decrease secretions and therefore improve conditions during laryngoscopy or bronchoscopy. The premature patient or the infant less than 6 months of age may benefit from the vagolytic effects of an anticholinergic agent on induction of anesthesia. Ketamine orally or transmucosally has been suggested as an alternative premedication for patients with limited pulmonary reserve.[16]

Anesthetic Technique

The choice of anesthetic depends on the extent of the anticipated minimal access procedure, compliance of the patient, and experience of the anesthesiologist.

During a VATS procedure, the surgeon introduces a series of ports between the patient's ribs and produces an ipsilateral pneumothorax.[3] A camera is introduced through one port, allowing visualization of the entire thoracic cavity and placement of subsequent trocars for dissection or intervention. When performing thoracoscopy in pediatric patients, the surgeon and the anesthesiologist must work closely together, maintaining a sufficient pneumothorax to permit completion of the more complicated procedures.[10]

Use of a regional technique and local anesthetic techniques with sedation have been adequate for peripheral examination or resection. However, evaluation of mediastinal masses involves retraction of the visceral pleura, which causes discomfort and becomes difficult to obliterate with intravenous sedation. A stellate ganglion block can be added to anesthetize the visceral pleura.[2, 10] Cooperation for a local or regional technique is not usually possible when dealing with small children. Spontaneous respiration in all age groups (as young as 8 months) has been advocated to maintain a sufficient pneumothorax as well as adequate oxygenation.[2] In that report, all patients younger than 3 years of age received a general anesthetic and tracheal tube, whereas older children received sedation with intercostal nerve blocks to provide adequate parietal and pleural anesthesia as well as a stellate ganglion block to inhibit the visceral pleural cough reflex. Sedation and intercostal nerve blockade of four interspaces with 0.25% bupivacaine with epinephrine added provided adequate anesthesia for mediastinal biopsies and pleurodesis in five older children and young adults.[36] It has been speculated that thoracic epidurals can provide adequate anesthesia for peripheral procedures,[37] but there has been no report of their use for thoracoscopy in pediatric patients. Intravenous ketamine and 1% lidocaine locally to anesthetize the chest wall have been used for pulmonary biopsy in immunosuppressed children.[4] A regional technique with sedation (ketamine, midazolam, or propofol) may also be useful when an anterior mediastinal mass may compress the trachea and cause airway obstruction with induction of a general anesthetic.[36] If a regional technique is chosen, it is imperative that the sedation be easily reversible and that emergent intubation be easily and safely accomplished. Coagulopathies are contraindications for regional techniques, and there are limits to dosing local anesthetics because of the risk of toxicity on absorption.

General anesthetic in the pediatric population has been found to lessen the anxiety and discomfort experienced by pediatric patients during thoracoscopy and to allow placement of multiple instruments for more extensive manipulation than would be possible using local or regional anesthesia.[31]

Use of routine monitors for otherwise healthy pediatric patients should suffice. Such monitors include a four- or five-lead electrocardiograph, pulse oximeter, noninvasive blood pressure monitor, capnograph, esophageal stethoscope for auscultation, temperature monitor, and vapor analysis. Direct blood pressure measurement is indicated if circulatory instability, respiratory difficulty, or prolonged postoperative ventilatory support is anticipated.[16] Peripheral intravenous access must be similar to that placed for a thoracotomy because conversion to thoracotomy is occasionally necessary[11, 18] and intraoperative bleeding can occur.[7, 10, 38] If adequate peripheral access cannot be obtained, a central catheter may be placed. It should be placed at the side of the surgical procedure to prevent the possibility of bilateral pneumothoraces.[39]

In the pediatric patient who has an intravenous line, the choice of induction agent for general anesthetic can be governed by the cardiovascular and respiratory stability of the patient preoperatively. The infant or small child generally accepts inhalation induction with less protest than would be made to an injection unless there is an intravenous line already in place. Anesthesia can thus be induced with the patient spontaneously breathing nitrous oxide in oxygen through a mask as the concentrations of halothane or sevoflurane are progressively increased. At this time, the patient may be allowed to continue to breathe spontaneously through a mask, or a tracheal tube may be placed when the anesthetic is deep enough, but spontaneous ventilation is maintained. If there is no contraindication to intermittent positive pressure ventilation (emphysematous lung tissue or bullous lesions), a neuromuscular blocking agent may be given to facilitate tracheal intubation. Once the trachea is intubated, whether ventilation is spontaneous[1, 40] or controlled is determined by the ability to maintain adequate oxygenation during surgical intervention.[10] Both lungs may electively be ventilated intraoperatively,[19] but ventilation can also be separated, and one-lung ventilation may be necessary to complete the thoracoscopic procedure successfully. General anesthesia and two-lung ventilation may be employed for patients who cannot tolerate the collapse of one lung from a pulmonary standpoint and for procedures not requiring lung collapse for the desired exposure. It is preferred that the patient breathe spontaneously, because pulmonary expansion with positive pressure ventilation may not allow adequate exposure.[36]

Various techniques that can now be used to separate ventilation of the lungs have been developed in the past for bronchial blocking when secretions were troublesome, or when spillover from an abscess or cyst was feared during a thoracotomy and sealing of diseased areas to protect healthy lung tissue was indicated.[9] One-lung ventilation allows the surgeon to manipulate a deflated lung on the operative side. Retracting an inflated lung on the operative side is a challenge and provides a somewhat less acceptable operative field. After separation of ventilation is achieved, the operative lung is allowed to deflate by equilibration of the chest cavity with atmospheric pressure. Occasionally, the operative lung does not deflate passively[9, 39] and insufflation of air or carbon dioxide improves the surgeon's view. The intrathoracic 4 to 8 cm of water pressure does not usually cause hemodynamic compromise.[39] There has been a report of an air embolism during the insufflation of air for creation of a pneumothorax.[41] This was manifested by transient hypotension that resolved spontaneously. Care must be taken when insufflating gas to avoid creating an embolism into the pulmonary vessels or liver, which may manifest as cardiovascular collapse at the time of creation of the pneumothorax.[7]

One-lung ventilation may be achieved in several ways in the pediatric population. In older, larger children and young adults, a double-lumen tracheal tube [42] and a UNIVENT tube with a bronchial blocker built into the wall of the tube provide the most effective and efficient separation of ventilation. The smallest double-lumen tracheal tube available is a 26 French which is comparable in outer diameter with a 5.5-mm internal diameter (ID) tracheal tube.[39] This size may be suitable for children who are at least 8 years of age. The smallest UNIVENT tube with a bronchial blocker within the wall of the tube is a 6-mm ID tube, which is equivalent in outer diameter to a 7.5-mm ID tracheal tube and may be suitable in children who are at least 12 years of age. An advantage of the double-lumen or the UNIVENT tube is that either allows change from one-lung ventilation to two-lung ventilation without repositioning the tracheal tube. Separation of ventilation and one-lung ventilation may be achieved in smaller children and in infants with selective endobronchial intubation or blockade of a bronchus with a catheter, or a combination of both.[43]

In addition to achieving one-lung ventilation for surgery, selective intubation or blockade of a bronchus allows positive pressure ventilation for patients with emphysematous and bullous disease[44] and for patients with a distal tracheoesophageal fistula[45] and can help prevent infective material from a hydatid cyst,[46] abcess,[43] bronchiectasis, or hemorrhage from soiling the healthy lung during surgical manipulation.

Successful selective bronchial intubation has been described in neonates and infants.[44, 45, 47] A routine tracheal tube that is 0.5 to 1.0 mm smaller in size than is appropriate for the patient's trachea should be used.[44, 48] The correct length for endobronchial tube placement can be estimated from the lateral radiograph by measuring the distance from the mouth to the carina with the addition of 1 cm for projection into the bronchus. The right bronchus can usually be readily intubated in most infants and children by blindly advancing the tracheal tube and then confirming the position by auscultation, fiberoptic bronchoscopy, or radiography.[45, 46] In one report, selective right bronchial intubation was followed by a higher frequency of upper lobe collapse (50%). There was no upper lobe collapse after selective left bronchial intubation.[46] An easy modification of a tracheal tube has been described that enlarges the bevel at the distal end to avoid obstruction of the right upper lobe.[49, 50] In infants, children, and adults, the angle subtended by the right main bronchus favors inadvertent intubation of that bronchus[51]; however, that can be altered by the position of the bevel of the tracheal tube.[52] In one study, 10 patients acted as their own control group and in all the study patients, a left beveled tracheal tube entered the right main bronchus and a right beveled tracheal tube entered the left main bronchus.[52]

The most successful technique (92%) for blind left bronchial intubation involved turning the head to the contralateral side and rotating the tube 180 degrees.[53] Alternatively, a gum elastic bougie in patients who are at least 1 year of age[48] or a fiberoptic bronchoscope[45, 49, 54] may be used to pass the tracheal tube selectively into the appropriate bronchus.

Selective endobronchial blocking has been accomplished successfully with various catheters in infants and children. The Fogarty arterial embolectomy catheter has been the most widely reported,[9, 55, 56] but it has the disadvantage of not having a central lumen. Once the balloon is inflated to occlude the bronchus, a central lumen would allow easier deflation of the operative lung (not relying on absorption atelectasis), insufflation of oxygen to or maintenance of continuous positive airway pressure (CPAP) in the operative lung or suctioning of secretions from that lung. A 3 French Fogarty catheter should occlude the bronchus in an infant weighing less than 10 kg. A 4 French Fogarty catheter should adequately block the bronchus in a patient weighing up to 15 kg and a 5 to 8 French Fogarty catheter may be used for patients weighing more than15 kg.[16, 55]

The Fogarty catheter may be passed blindly after induction of general anesthesia. The tip should be curved slightly so that removal of the stylet does not dislodge the catheter.[50] The position of the catheter should be confirmed by auscultation, fluoroscopy,[9] or fiberoptic bronchoscopy, or with the rigid ventilating bronchoscope and telescope[43] because once the tracheal tube is placed, it is difficult to adjust the position of the Fogarty catheter. A simple, elegant blind technique for passing and positioning a bronchial blocker while maintaining continuous control of the airway during most of the procedure has been described.[55] The patient is preoxygenated and a tracheal tube is placed and connected to the ventilator. This tube is advanced into the appropriate main bronchus, and its position is confirmed by auscultation. A catheter is passed through the tracheal tube an appropriate distance, and the tracheal tube is withdrawn. Inflation of the catheter balloon during mask ventilation can confirm position, and the appropriate-sized tracheal tube is then placed. The catheter should be securely taped to the tracheal tube. The Fogarty arterial embolectomy catheter has a high-pressure, low-volume balloon and can cause damage to the bronchus if not properly inflated.[16] Bronchial rupture has been reported with its use.[57] A 5 French Fogarty catheter, inadvertently inflated with 4 cc of air caused a membranous tear in the right bronchus of a 4-year-old patient, which had to be surgically repaired.

A Swan-Ganz catheter may be used to occlude a bronchus selectively. Its placement with the aid or fiberoptic bronchoscopy has been described in a series of patients.[58] A Foley catheter with its distal tip amputated was passed over a guide wire to occlude the appropriate bronchus in another report.[59] In this description, the guide wire was passed through a tracheal tube that was blindly placed in the bronchus of the operative lung. Position was again confirmed with the fiberoptic bronchoscope. The pediatric fiberoptic bronchoscope usually fits through a 4.5-mm ID or larger tracheal tube. The ultrathin fiberoptic bronchoscopes can usually fit through a 3-mm ID or larger tracheal tube. Generally, 1 mm must be added to the outer diameter of the fiberscope to determine the smallest size tracheal tube that will accommodate it.

Simultaneous independent lung ventilation has been described with the pediatric double-lumen tube manufactured by Portex.[60] It consists of two separate tubes of different lengths attached side-by-side. Also there has been speculation that the manufacturer of UNIVENT tubes plans to release pediatric tubes in 3.5 mm and 4.0 mm ID sizes.[61]

With one-lung anesthesia, the risks of arterial hypoxemia and hypercapnia are a substantial consideration. One-lung ventilation creates a right-to-left transpulmonary shunt through the deflated operative lung. This shunt is not present during two-lung ventilation.[62] Hypoxic pulmonary vasoconstriction acts to decrease blood flow to the atelectatic (operative) lung. Also, the lateral decubitus position allows gravity to decrease the blood flow to the atelectatic (nondependent) lung. Surgical retraction compression of vessels should also help limit blood flow through the nonventilated lung. The occurrence of hypoxemia and hypercapnia caused by atelectasis and hypoventilation of the nonoperative (dependent) lung during spontaneous ventilation is often improved by controlled ventilation. Mild hypercarbia (Pa_{CO_2} = 55 mm Hg) has been shown to be unusual, but well tolerated, even in small pediatric patients.[39]

The location of the lesion and the nature of the procedure determine the patient's position.[9] For lesions in the apex of the lung or superior hemithorax, the patient is placed in the reverse Trendelenburg position. The Trendelenburg position is preferred for basilar masses. For lesions in the mediastinum, the patient may be rotated in an anterior or posterior direction. An axillary roll should be used under the dependent axilla and the extremities and head should be well padded. The patient should be prepared and drapes should be applied in a manner similar to that used for a thoracotomy because the surgeon should have the ability to convert the procedure to a thoracotomy quickly and easily.

After positioning the patient, the position of the bronchial blocker or bronchial tube, or both, must be confirmed. Anesthesia may be maintained with isoflurane, halothane, and oxygen or with intravenous agents such as fentanyl, ketamine, or propofol and neuromuscular blockade. Nitrous oxide is usually avoided to limit the distention of pockets of intrathoracic air. Isoflurane and halothane impair hypoxic pulmonary vasoconstriction and therefore cause intrapulmonary shunting to slightly different degrees, but that difference is clinically indistinguishable once CPAP of the operative lung and positive end expiratory pressure (PEEP) of the nonoperative lung are established.

In the presence of adequate one-lung ventilation (tidal volume is decreased by 20% and respiratory rate increased by 20%[13] from two-lung ventilation) and 100% oxygen, hypoxemia can be caused by a malpositioned tracheal or bronchial tube or bronchial blocker, inadequate ventilation of the dependent lung, or a severe ventilation/perfusion mismatch. CPAP to the operative (nondependent) lung acts to compress the pulmonary vasculature and thereby increase pulmonary vascular resistance and decrease blood flow.[3] If this fails to improve oxygenation, selective PEEP to the nonoperative (dependent) lung returns the lung to functional residual capacity, decreases the mechanical compression of pulmonary vessels, and recruits more alveoli for gas exchange.[62] An apparatus incorporating the Mapleson D Circuit can be assembled to provide PEEP to the ventilated (dependent) lung. It is possible to add too much PEEP and worsen arterial hypoxemia. Optimal oxygenation is achieved by a balance between CPAP and PEEP, and this balance may vary throughout the course of surgery.[3] Re-expansion and ventilation of the operative lung may become necessary. In one series, a significant number of patients did not tolerate one-lung ventilation or the lateral decubitus position.[23] If necessary, the tracheal tube can be withdrawn from the bronchus or the bronchial blocker balloon deflated to resume two-lung ventilation. Preoperative discussion with the surgeon should allow this to be a well-coordinated plan.

At the conclusion of surgery, the bronchial tube is repositioned within the trachea and the bronchial blocker is deflated. Two-lung ventilation is reinstituted and the pneumothorax is evacuated. The decision to leave a thoracostomy tube in place is determined by the presence or absence of an air leak in the reinflated lung. If continued drainage is required postoperatively, the thoracostomy tube can be inserted through the thoracoscopy incision, which allows adequate drainage. Thoracostomy tubes should be left in place in ventilator-dependent children.[63] An air leak may develop even through the stapled lung because of the high airway pressure.

After reversal of neuromuscular blockade and return of adequate spontaneous ventilation, most patients are easily extubated in the operating room and moved to the postanesthesia care unit for observation. They can then be admitted to the intensive care unit or ward for the duration of their hospitalization. Patients who have significant respiratory disability preoperatively or pulmonary hypertension[39] should be weaned from mechanical ventilation in the postoperative period. The breathing pattern of premature patients should be carefully observed for significant periodic breathing, the presence of which is a contraindication for removal of the breathing tube.[13]

Anesthesia for Minimal Access Cardiac Surgery

In the pediatric patient who has congenital heart disease, VATS is an option, but the anesthetic course can be complicated by the presence of shunt lesions, prematurity, and the potential need to maintain one-lung ventilation.[8] Although ligation of a patent ductus arteriosus (PDA) via a thoracotomy is a highly successful procedure, concerns over postthoracotomy syndrome[4, 5] and postoperative pain, as well as recent interest in endoscopic surgical techniques, have given rise to VATS for PDA,[64, 65] vascular rings,[66, 67] and ostium secundum fossa ovalis–type atrial septal defects.[68] Other successfully completed thoracoscopic cardiovascular procedures in pediatric patients include ligation of a large venous collateral to the left atrium in a 12-year-old patient who had Fontan physiology, and placement of an epicardial pacemaker for complete heart block in a newborn.[67] Thoracoscopically aided diaphragm plication is ideal in the patient who has phrenic nerve injury and diaphragm paresis. Chest wall trauma is avoided and recovery is maximized by minimizing pain and mechanical dysfunction.[66]

Minimal access surgery should not be performed in patients whose PDA is calcified, is larger than the descending aorta, or contains an occlusive device placed during cardiac catheterization. Likewise, thoracoscopic takedown of a vascular ring should not be attempted if the ring is composed entirely of vascular structures or if there is an aortic diverticulum compressing the airway.[67] A relative contraindication to thoracoscopy in these cases is a previous thoracotomy with pleural adhesions.[64] The minimally traumatic nature of thoracoscopy may justify surgery in the asymptomatic patient who has known vascular rings to prevent the long-term complication of airway dysfunction that usually occurs in patients who have repair after onset of symptoms.[66]

Preoperative Evaluation and Anesthetic Concerns

The same preoperative and anesthesia issues that are relevant in noncardiac surgery are also relevant in cardiac surgery. The population is young and small, consisting mostly of neonates, infants, and toddlers.[25] In addition, the patients who present for surgical interruption of a PDA are most likely to be premature.[67] In addition to the increased risk of transitional circulation, the premature patient is more likely to have hyaline membrane disease.[13] The potential for the development of retinopathy of prematurity must be considered in choosing an appropriate concentration of inspired oxygen.[69] In addition, heat loss is a major concern, and every effort must be taken to prevent a drop in patient temperature. Premature patients are likely to be mechanically ventilated and in congestive heart failure. The extent of their preoperative evaluation should be governed by the presence of other major systemic or cardiovascular diseases.

The presence of concurrent congenital cardiac lesions is not limited to the premature patient, and the possibility of intracardiac or extracardiac shunting because of complex congenital heart disease must be thoroughly evaluated. What effect lung manipulation, intraoperative ventilation, or hypoxic pulmonary vasoconstriction has on shunt hemodynamics has not been well documented. However, an increase in pulmonary vascular resistance will likely result in an increased right-to-left shunt[25] or reverse a left-to-right shunt, worsening arterial hypoxemia. In the patient who has existing diminished right ventricular function, an increase in pulmonary vascular resistance may lead to right ventricular failure. The anesthetic technique is chosen according to preoperative status, airway size, and anatomy. There should be blood available for transfusion before the placement of the trocars for the procedure. Antibiotics may be given prophylactically to decrease the risk of bacterial endocarditis.

Induction of anesthesia can be inhalational or intravenous for the otherwise healthy ambulatory patient. For the sick neonate or older child, an intravenous induction with fentanyl and pancuronium may be chosen. All patients undergoing minimal access surgery received a general anesthetic with neuromuscular blockade and a tracheal tube and were mechanically ventilated intraoperatively. Maintenance of anesthesia may be with low-dose fentanyl and isoflurane, halothane, or sevoflurane in oxygen and air. For intraoperative monitoring, in addition to the standard monitors (as discussed previously), pre- and postductal pulse oximetry should be used. If there are signs or symptoms of congestive heart failure, it is prudent to measure the blood pressure directly with an arterial line. The use of intraoperative real-time transesophageal echocardiography (TEE) with color flow mapping has been useful in patients weighing more than 3 kg to assess the efficacy of thoracoscopic PDA interruption as the clips are applied.[67, 70] TEE monitoring during ligation of the PDA may help improve the surgical result. Reintervention and complications associated with residual ductal flow may be avoided. Late recurrence of ductal flow may occur and may not be associated with intraoperative success.[4] Usually, preparations should be made for volume infusion and thoracotomy just before clip closure of the PDA.[67] If TEE was not used intraoperatively color flow Doppler echocardiography can be used before extubation to assess completeness of closure.[6, 64]

The institution and maintenance of one-lung ventilation can offer an easier field for the surgeon and can shorten the operating time.[55] If only the trachea was intubated, only one lung was effectively ventilated. A special fan-shaped retractor was used to retract the upper lobe of the left lung to provide sufficient exposure to allow unhindered manipulations. Premature patients weighing as little as 600 g have had successful thoracoscopic PDA interruption.[25] One-lung ventilation has been described for thoracoscopic PDA ligation in children as young as 1 month of age weighing 2.9 kg.[49] There is a report of thoracoscopic clippings of the PDA in three premature infants performed while the infants rested in their warmers in the intensive care unit.[65]

In the operating room, the patient for thoracoscopic PDA closure should be prepared in the standard posterolateral position as indicated for a thoracotomy. After completion of the procedure and substantiation by echocardiography that the ductal flow is interrupted, the tracheal tube is repositioned in the trachea if necessary and the lungs are re-expanded. Neuromuscular blockade may be reversed, and after return of spontaneous ventilation, the patient's trachea may be extubated. The patient may be sent to the intensive care unit or a ward for observation after leaving the postanesthesia care unit. If the patient was mechanically ventilated preoperatively or exhibited symptoms of congestive heart failure, pulmonary hypertension, or airway compromise, he or she should be weaned off mechanical ventilation postoperatively in the intensive care unit.

Pain Management

After thoracoscopy, most patients require only parenteral narcotics for adequate pain control or intravenous narcotics for the first 24 hours.[71] There is not much written about postoperative pain management after a thoracoscopic procedure.

Complications

Recurrent laryngeal nerve injury has been reported as an early complication of thoracoscopic PDA interruption.[5, 64, 67] Risk factors included a very small patient and extensive dissection. Early in their experience, one group also reported recurrence of ductal flow in five patients.[67] There have been two reports of conversion to thoracotomy for bleeding[67, 72] and one chylothorax[73] in patients undergoing minimal access cardiac surgery. Almost every group has reported a minimal number of conversions to thoracotomy to complete the surgical procedure. A TEE probe can cause bronchial obstruction in a child.[74, 75]

The ability to recognize the need to abandon thoracoscopy for better exposure and control is crucial to the successful use and outcome of thoracoscopic surgery.[63] Conversion to thoracotomy was the single largest complication reported, with indications varying by group and patient population. Postoperative recurrent or persistent pneumothorax that resolved spontaneously or required drainage with a thoracostomy tube was a relatively infrequent complication, even though this was the second most commonly reported complication. Intercostal artery injury during thoracostomy tube insertion[11] and bleeding postoperatively was reported in three patients,[10] and resulted in the need to transfuse the patients postoperatively. Conversion to a thoracotomy occurred in one patient because of an elevated carbon dioxide tension greater than 100 mm Hg.[24] There was one death as a result of respiratory insufficiency in a patient who had a diffuse interstitial process and in whom a bronchopleural fistula developed postoperatively after biopsy with a cup forceps.[10] An air embolism occurred on insufflation of air for trocar placement, which resulted in transient hypotension, but this was self-limited.[41] Treatment included initially evacuating the pneumothorax. It was thought that such a complication could have been avoided by recognizing that contralateral main bronchus intubation with lung collapse results in significant elevation of the ipsilateral hemithorax until the pneumothorax is established. The authors of the article now insert the needle into a higher interspace to avoid the hemidiaphragm. As previously mentioned, there was a perforation of a bronchus secondary to inadvertent overinflation of a Fogarty catheter balloon for bronchial occlusion.[57]

Potential complications that have not been reported in the pediatric population include cardiac fibrillation secondary to the use of a monopolar cautery near the myocardium.[9] A tension pneumothorax may be created as carbon dioxide or air is insufflated into the chest.[7]

References

1. Janik JS, Nagaraj HS, Groff DB: Thoracoscopic evaluation of intrathoracic lesions in children. J Thorac Cardiovasc Surg 83:408–413, 1982.
2. Ryckman FC, Rodgers BM: Thoracoscopy for intrathoracic neoplasia in children. J Pediatr Surg 17:521–524, 1982.
3. Mihalka J, Burrows FA, Burke RP, Javorski JJ: One-lung ventilation during video-assisted thoracoscopic ligation of a thoracic duct in a 3 year old child. J Cardiothorac Vasc Anesth 8:559–562, 1994.
4. Lavoie J, Javorski JJ, Donahue K, et al: Detection of residual flow by transesophageal echocardiography during video-assisted thoracoscopic patent ductus arteriosus interruption. Anesth Analg 80:1071–1075, 1995.
5. Laborde F, Noirhomme P, Karam J, et al: A new video-assisted thoracoscopic surgical technique for interruption of patent ductus arteriosus in infants and children. J Thorac Cardiovasc Surg 105:278–280, 1993.
6. Le Bret E, Folliguet TA, Laborde F: Videothoracoscopic surgical interruption of patent ductus arteriosus. Ann Thorac Surg 64:1492–1494, 1997.
7. Schropp KP: Thoracoscopy. Pediatr Ann 22:686–696, 1993.
8. Lobe TE: New developments: Pediatric surgery. Curr Probl Pediatr 23:348–357, 1993.
9. Cay DL, Csenderits LE, Lines V, et al: Selective bronchial blocking in children. Anaesth Intensive Care 3:127–130, 1975.
10. Rodgers BM: Pediatric thoracoscopy: Where have we come and what have we learned? Ann Thorac Surg 56:704–707, 1993.
11. Schier F, Waldschmidt J: Thoracoscopy in children. J Pediatr Surg 31:1640–1643, 1996.
12. Heymann MA: Postnatal regulation of the pulmonary circulation: A role for lipid mediators? Am Rev Respir Dis 136:222–224, 1987.
13. Benumof JL: Anesthesia for pediatric thoracic surgery. *In* Benumof JL (ed): Anesthesia for Thoracic Surgery. Philadelphia, WB Saunders, 1995, pp 657–695.
14. Westhorpe RN: The position of the larynx in children and its relationship to the ease of intubation. Anaesth Intensive Care 15:384–388, 1987.

15. Roopchand R, Roopnarinesingh S, Ramsevak S: Instability of the tracheal tube in neonates: A postmortem study. Anesthesia 44:107–109, 1989.
16. McDowall RH: Anesthesia for the pediatric patient. Chest Surg Clin North Am 7:831–868, 1997.
17. Motoyama EK: Pulmonary mechanics during early postnatal years. Pediatr Res 11:220, 1977.
18. Stovroff M, Teague G, Heiss KF, et al: Thoracoscopy in the management of pediatric empyema. J Pediatr Surg 30:1211–1215, 1998.
19. Davidoff AM, Hebra A, Kerr J, Stafford PW: Thoracoscopic management of empyema in children. J Laparoendosc Surg 6:S-51–S-54, 1996.
20. Kern JA, Rodgers BM: Thoracoscopy in the management of empyema in children. J Pediatr Surg 28:1128–1132, 1993.
21. de Campos JRM, Filho LOA, Werebe EC, et al: Thoracoscopy in children and adolescents. Chest 111:494–497, 1997.
22. Rodgers BM, Talbert JL: Thoracoscopy for diagnosis of intrathoracic lesions in children. J Pediatr Surg 11:703–708, 1976.
23. Rothenberg SS, Wagner JS, Chang JHT, Fan LL: The safety and efficacy of thoracoscopic lung biopsy for diagnosis and treatment in infants and children. J Pediatr Surg 31:100–104, 1996.
24. Holcomb GW III, Tomita SS, Haase GM, et al: Minimally invasive surgery in children with cancer. Cancer 76:121–128, 1995.
25. Lavoie J, Burrows FA, Hansen DD: Video-assisted thoracoscopic surgery for the treatment of congenital cardiac defects in the pediatric population. Anesth Analg 82:563–567, 1996.
26. Yim APC: Thoracoscopic resection of an esophageal cyst in a 4 year old girl. Chest 110:545–546, 1996.
27. Yim APC: Video-assisted thoracoscopic resection of type I cystic adenomatoid malformation in a 3 month old girl. Surg Endosc 9:1292–1294, 1995.
28. Watine O, Mensier E, Delecluse P, Ribet M: Pulmonary sequestration treated by video-assisted thoracoscopic resection. Eur J Cardiothorac Surg 8:155–156, 1994.
29. Rothenberg SS, Chang JHT: Thoracoscopic decortication in infants and children. Surg Endosc 11:93–94, 1997.
30. Silen ML, Canvasser DA, Kurkchubasche AG, et al: Video-assisted thoracic surgical repair of a Foramen of Bochdalek hernia. Ann Thorac Surg 60:448–450, 1995.
31. Lobe TE: Pediatric thoracoscopy. Semin Thorac Cardiovasc Surg 5:298–302, 1993.
32. Keon TP: Death on induction of anesthesia for cervical node biopsy. Anesthesiology 55:471–472, 1981.
33. Schreiner MS, Triebwasser A, Keon TP: Ingestion of liquids compared with preoperative fasting in pediatric outpatients. Anesthesiology 72:593–597, 1990.
34. Weldon BC, Watcha MF, White PF: Oral midazolam in children: Effect of time and adjunctive therapy. Anesth Analg 75:51–55, 1992.
35. Wilton NCT, Leigh J, Rosen DR, Pandit UA: Preanesthetic sedation of preschool children using intranasal midazolam. Anesthesiology 69:972–975, 1988.
36. McGahren ED, Kern JA, Rodgers BM: Anesthetic techniques for pediatric thoracoscopy. Ann Thorac Surg 60:927–930, 1995.
37. Tobias JD: Anesthetic implications of thoracoscopy in the pediatric patient. Anesthesiol Rev 21:133–138, 1994.
38. Rodgers BM, Moazam F, Talbert JL: Thoracoscopy in children. Ann Surg 189:176–180, 1979.
39. Rowe R, Andropoulus, D, Heard AM, et al: Anesthetic management of pediatric patients undergoing thoracoscopy. J Cardiothorac Vasc Anesth 8:563–566, 1994.
40. Graham DD, McGahren ED, Tribble CG, et al: Use of video-assisted thoracic surgery in the treatment of chylothorax. Ann Thorac Surg 57:1507–1512, 1994.
41. Rogers DA, Philippe PG, Lobe TE, et al: Thoracoscopy in children: An initial experience with an evolving technique. J Laparoendosc Surg 2:7–14, 1992.
42. Benumof JL: Separation of the two lungs (double-lumen tube and bronchial blocker intubation). *In* Benumof JL (ed): Anesthesia for Thoracic Surgery. Philadelphia, WB Saunders, 1995, pp 330–389.
43. Rao CC, Krishna G, Grosfeld JL, Weber TR: One-lung pediatric anesthesia. Anesth Analg 60:450–452, 1981.
44. Cullum AR, English ICW, Branthwaite MA: Endobronchial intubation in infancy. Anaesthesia 28:66–70, 1973.
45. Baraka A, Akel S, Haroun S, Yazigi A: One-lung ventilation of the newborn with tracheoesophageal fistula. Anesth Analg 67:189–191, 1988.
46. Baraka A, Slim M, Dajani A, Lakkis S: One-lung ventilation of children during surgical excision of hydatid cysts of the lung. Br J Anaesth 54:523–528, 1982.
47. Mathew OP, Thach BT: Selective bronchial obstruction for treatment of bullous interstitial emphysema. J Pediatr 96:475–477, 1980.
48. McLellan I: Endobronchial intubation in children. Anaesthesia 29:757–758, 1974.
49. Tan PPC, Chu JJ, Ho ACY, et al: A modified endotracheal tube for infants and small children undergoing video-assisted thoracoscopic surgery. Anesth Analg 86:1212–1213, 1998.
50. Hogg CE, Lorhan PH: Pediatric bronchial blocking. Anesthesiology 33:560–561, 1970.
51. Kubota Y, Toyoda Y, Nagata N, et al: Tracheo-bronchial angles in infants and children. Anesthesiology 64:374–376, 1986.
52. Baraka A, Akel S, Muallem M, et al: Bronchial intubation in children: Does the tube bevel determine the side of intubation? Anesthesiology 67:869–870, 1987.
53. Kubota H, Kubota Y, Toyoda Y, et al: Selective blind endobronchial intubation in children and adults. Anesthesiology 67:587–589, 1987.
54. Watson CB, Bowe EA, Burk W: One-lung ventilation for pediatric thoracic surgery: A new use for the fiberoptic bronchoscope. Anesthesiology 56:314–315, 1982.
55. Vakamudi M, Shenoy V, Haldar J, et al: A new technique for one-lung ventilation during video-assisted thoracoscopic surgical interruption of patent ductus arteriosus in children. J Thorac Cardiovasc Surg 110:273–274, 1995.
56. Vale R: Selective bronchial blocking in a small child. Br J Anaesth 41:453–454, 1969.
57. Borchardt RA, LaQuaglia MP, McDowall RH, Wilson RS: Bronchial injury during lung isolation in a pediatric patient. Anesth Analg 87:324–325, 1998.
58. Dalens B, Labbe A, Haberer JP: Selective endobronchial blocking vs. selective intubation. Anesthesiology 57:555–556, 1982.
59. Hammer GB, Manos SJ, Smith BM, et al: Single-lung ventilation in pediatric patients. Anesthesiology 84:1503–1506, 1996.
60. Marraro G: Simultaneous independent lung ventilation in pediatric patients. Crit Care Clin 8:131–145, 1992.
61. Turner MWH, Buchanan CCR, Brown SW: Paediatric one lung ventilation in the prone position. Paediatr Anaesth 7:427–429, 1997.
62. Benumof JL: Conventional and differential lung management of one-lung ventilation. *In* Benumof JL (ed): Anesthesia for Thoracic Surgery. Philadelphia, WB Saunders, 1995, pp 406–431.
63. Chen MK, Schropp KP, Lobe TE: Complications of minimal-access surgery in children. J Pediatr Surg 31:1161–1165, 1996.
64. Laborde F, Folliguet T, Batisse A, et al: Video-assisted thoracoscopic surgical interruption: The technique of choice for patent ductus arteriosus: Routine experience in 230 pediatric cases. J Thorac Cardiovasc Surg 110:1681–1685, 1995.
65. Forster R: Thoracoscopic clipping of patent ductus arteriosus in premature infants. Ann Thorac Surg 56:1418–1420, 1993.
66. Burke RP: Minimally invasive techniques for congenital heart surgery. Semin Thorac Cardiovasc Surg 9:337–344, 1997.
67. Burke RP, Wernovsky G, van der Velde M, et al: Video-assisted thoracoscopic surgery for congenital heart disease. J Thorac Cardiovasc Surg 109:499–508, 1995.

68. Chang CH, Lin PJ, Chu JJ, et al: Video-assisted cardiac surgery in closure of atrial septal defect. Ann Thorac Surg 62:697–701, 1996.
69. Phelps DL: Retinopathy of prematurity. N Engl J Med 326: 1078–1080, 1992.
70. Lavoie J, Burrows FA, Gentles TL, et al: Transesophageal echocardiography detects residual ductal flow during video-assisted thoracoscopic patent ductus arteriosus interruption. Can J Anaesth 41:310–313, 1993.
71. Blucher D, Lobe TE: Minimal access surgery in children: The state of the art. Int Surg 79:317–321, 1994.
72. Rothenberg SS, Chang JHT, Toews WH, Washington RL: Thoracoscopic closure of patent ductus arteriosus: A less traumatic and more cost-effective technique. J Pediatr Surg 30:1057–1060, 1995.
73. Burke RP, Rosenfeld HM, Wernovsky G, Jonas RA: Video-assisted thoracoscopic vascular ring division in infants and children. J Am Coll Cardiol 25:943–947, 1995.
74. Gilbert TB, Panico FG, McGill WA, et al: Bronchial obstruction by transesophageal echocardiography probe in a pediatric cardiac patient. Anesth Analg 74:156–158, 1992.
75. Zestos MM, Chehade M, Mossad E: A transesophageal echocardiography probe causes airway obstruction in an older child. J Cardiothorac Vasc Anesth 12:65–66, 1998.

COMMENTARY

Anthony P. C. Yim

The two main technical challenges in video-assisted thoracoscopic surgery for the pediatric population are (1) the ability to maintain selective one-lung ventilation and (2) instrumentation. The first point has been elegantly addressed by Dr. Catherine Krucylak in this chapter.

In our practice, we use main stem intubation with a single-lumen tube guided by a 1.8-mm outer diameter ultrafine flexible bronchoscope (LFP, Olympus) for toddlers or large infants. Right main stem intubation is often more difficult because of its short length. Right upper lobe ventilation can be easily compromised if care is not taken to ascertain the exact position of the tube. Carbon dioxide insufflation can be a useful adjunct to achieve lung collapse, but close monitoring of intrathoracic pressure is mandatory. As detailed in this chapter, the commercially available endotracheal tube with a bronchial blocker is rarely applicable to children younger than 12 years of age because of its size. For neonates (our youngest patient was a 22-day-old neonate), selective ventilation is difficult to achieve; nonetheless, simple procedures, such as pleural biopsy or drainage, can be satisfactorily performed using endotracheal intubation and lowered tidal volume or intermittent apnea. Close collaboration between the surgeon and the anesthesiologist is crucial to achieve optimal results.

Chapter 37

Pediatric Minimal Access Cardiothoracic Surgery

Evan R. Kokoska, Patrick A. Dillon, and Mark L. Silen

History and Evolution of Thoracoscopy

Hans Christian Jacobaeus is credited with the first major clinical contribution to laparoscopy in 1910 (see Chapter 1).[1] During this early experience, he explored the pleural, pericardial, and peritoneal cavities using a cystoscope, a procedure he termed *laparothorakoskapie.* His initial interest was in establishing the diagnosis of diseases such as cirrhosis, malignancy, syphilis, and tuberculosis (TB). After 1913, however, he focused his attention on thoracoscopy because "the most interesting use of the endoscope is for the examination of the pleural cavity," and it is a "simple method that can be performed without inconvenience."[2]

Jacobaeus subsequently expanded the indications for thoracoscopy, using the new technique for therapeutic and diagnostic purposes. He described a large series of patients in whom he used the thoracoscope to lyse pulmonary adhesions, allowing for complete lung collapse as a treatment for TB. This technique was generally successful, as many patients became "sputum-free,"[3] and it was widely adopted in both Europe and North America.[2, 3] The majority of patients treated by Jacobaeus were adults.

The major laparoscopic innovations during the 1950s involved advances in illumination and optics. Before this time, light was provided to the cavity of interest by either introducing lamps or reflecting light from external sources. In 1952, cold light was developed by Fourestier and colleagues; it consisted of a quartz rod that transmitted light from the proximal to the distal end of the laparoscope.[4] Subsequently a rod lens system was designed that significantly improved laparoscopic resolution. In 1981, charged coupling devices (CCDs), or "chips," allowed for the production of significantly smaller and lighter cameras. This advance also allowed for video technology in 1990, which ushered in the current era of video-assisted thoracic surgery (VATS). Recent innovations include endoscopic stapling devices, disposable trocars, safer electrocautery and lasers, and intracorporeal suturing devices. These advances in instrumentation have made thoracoscopy possible in both children and adults.

Improvements in anesthesia, antibiotics, critical care, and sterile technique from 1950 to 1980 resulted in decreased surgical mortality and made more complex surgical procedures possible. Interestingly, larger incisions became more frequent, and enthusiasm in North America for both laparoscopy and thoracoscopy waned. One critical driving force remained, however: demand from the consumer for safe, outpatient, or minimally invasive procedures at a reasonable cost. This remains a powerful force today.

Thoracoscopy in children was first described by Klimkovich and colleagues in 1971.[5] These pioneers conducted 45 thoracoscopic investigations in 43 children. The reported procedures consisted of both thoracic examination and adhesiolysis for mediastinal and lung tumors, pneumothorax, and empyema. In this series of patients, a diagnosis was established in 2 children, changed in 3, and confirmed in 30 others.

In North America, Rodgers was the earliest advocate of thoracoscopy for children. In 1976, he reported the first case series, which described the use of thoracoscopy for diagnostic biopsy in nine children with interstitial lung disease.[6] Before this, the standard technique for lung biopsy entailed pulmonary needle aspiration. This technique frequently obtained inadequate samples for diagnosis and was associated with significant morbidity and mortality. Using a combination of intravenous and local anesthesia, Rodgers performed thoracoscopy while the child was breathing spontaneously. There were no reported deaths and only three minor complications (bleeding and pneumothorax).[6] By 1979, his experience with pediatric thoracoscopy had increased to 27 biopsies in 24 immunosuppressed children.[7] This experience preceded by nearly a decade the first description of laparoscopic cholecystectomy.[8]

Within 3 years, the indications for thoracoscopic biopsy expanded to include intrathoracic tumors, mediastinal masses, and various pleural diseases. The overall diagnostic accuracy with 150 thoracoscopic procedures in children was 92%.[9] The indications and techniques for thoracoscopy in infants and children are somewhat different from those in adults and continue to evolve as expertise with endoscopic techniques is gained and advances in surgical equipment are made.

Pediatric Airway Anatomy and Management

Several anatomic differences distinguish the pediatric upper airway from that of the adult. It is important that these differences be appreciated as procedures are considered and undertaken. Laryngeal visualization may be compromised in children younger than 2 years of age owing to the relatively large size of the tongue with respect to the mandible. The larynx may also be difficult to visualize in newborns and infants because of its relatively cephalic and anterior position at the level of the C3 or C4 vertebral body. The adult larynx is typically at the level of C4 to C5. In addition, the floppy infant epiglottis may interfere with cord visualization and make endotracheal intubation difficult. These particular difficulties are infrequent in older children. The length of the trachea changes with age, being only 4 to 5 cm in infants[10] and up to 10 to 12 cm in adults.[11] Unintentional and intentional unilateral endobronchial intubation is thus easier in younger patients owing to the shorter tracheal length. As in adults, the right bronchus is more likely to be intubated than the left.[12]

Selection of the appropriate size and type of endotracheal tube is of considerable importance. The narrowest portion of the pediatric airway is at the level of the cricoid ring. To prevent mucosal ischemia, uncuffed endotracheal tubes are recommended for children younger than 10 years of age. The choice of optimal endotracheal tube size is influenced by factors in favor of larger tubes (e.g., easier suctioning, decreased resistance to flow) but ultimately by the need to avoid injury or damage to the airway (e.g., acquired subglottic stenosis). Several means of estimating the appropriate size of endotracheal tube for use in children have been described. Some are based on the height of the patient, others on the size of the fifth digit or on an age-based formula.[13–15] Regardless of the technique used to estimate size, the incidence of pressure-induced injury at the level of the cricoid ring is minimized if an adequate air leak is present around the tube. This can be assumed to be the case if a clinical leak is present at between 10 and 30 cm H_2O pressure. The size of the tube may need to be altered if intentional bronchial intubation or bronchial blockers are used (see later).

Intraoperative Monitoring

The anesthesiologist, along with the rest of the operating room team, must be prepared for formal thoracotomy in the event VATS is abandoned. Monitoring of these patients should be the same as for those subjected to a planned thoracotomy and should include pulse oximetry, end tidal CO_2, blood pressure, electrocardiogram, urine output, and core body temperature at a minimum. The decision not to use an indwelling arterial catheter or central venous catheter should be made on sound clinical grounds rather than because a less invasive operative technique requires less invasive monitoring. When these cannulae are used, central venous pressure, arterial blood pressure, and arterial blood gases should be monitored. Intraoperative fiberoptic bronchoscopy may be necessary for monitoring the appropriate position of either a double-lumen endotracheal tube or a bronchial blocker.

Two-Lung Ventilation

Many VATS procedures in children can be accomplished without one-lung ventilation. Pediatric surgeons discovered this because double-lumen endotracheal tubes generally cannot be used in patients who weigh less than 30 kg, and maintaining bronchial blockers in place can be difficult. Lung biopsy and the diagnosis and treatment of many pleural diseases do not necessarily require one-lung ventilation. In fact, in patients in whom spontaneous respirations are maintained, the pneumothorax obtained on the nondependent side may allow many VATS procedures to be accomplished quite easily. Our experience has been that CO_2 insufflation is rarely needed.

There are physiologic sequelae of general anesthesia, the lateral decubitus position, and unilateral pneumothorax that are relevant even in a two-lung ventilation technique.[16] Changes in pulmonary compliance are common from general anesthesia alone. Regional functional abnormalities of ventilation and perfusion occur independently as a result of the lateral decubitus position, and some of these abnormalities may persist into the postoperative period, making the dependent lung more susceptible to atelectasis.[17] Certainly, atelectasis is a common problem in the nondependent lung, which is compressed (mechanical compression or CO_2 insufflation) during the procedure. Right-to-left shunting of blood at the level of the lung may result in significant hypoxemia, although adequate concentrations of inhaled oxygen usually diminish or obviate this problem.

One-Lung Ventilation

One-lung ventilation may be necessary, or desired, for certain VATS procedures. These techniques may also be useful in patients undergoing standard thoracotomy.[18] The lateral decubitus position may be hazardous if infected material is allowed to flow into the unaffected dependent lung, and the first reported use of an intraoperative endobronchial blocker in a pediatric patient was in this clinical setting in 1969.[19] Subsequent reports confirmed the utility of endobronchial blockers during pulmonary resection in children.[20, 21] The method was later popularized with the adjunct of bronchoscopic positioning of the catheter tip by Ginsberg, and we have used his technique in children with great success.[22] The Fogarty embolectomy catheter is passed through the vocal cords, followed by passage of the endotracheal tube immediately adjacent to it. A flexible bronchoscope is passed through the endotracheal tube, and the tip of the Fogarty catheter is positioned in the main bronchus of the lung that is not to be ventilated. Sufficient air is introduced into the balloon to accomplish occlusion of the bronchus. After the endotracheal tube and Fogarty catheter are secured, the patient is put in the lateral decubitus position, and unilateral main stem bronchial blockade is demonstrated by auscultation. Repeat bronchoscopy may be necessary in the lateral decubitus position to replace the Fogarty catheter balloon if it becomes dislodged during positioning. Intraoperative fluoroscopy may also be useful to document correct positioning of the catheter. The use of a Swan-Ganz catheter, rather than a Fogarty catheter, has been advocated by some because it allows delivery of oxygen to the involved lung tissue through the distal port. This may minimize the degree of hypoxemia encountered intraoperatively. In addition, a commercially available endotracheal tube with a high-volume, low-pressure endobronchial blocker channel built into the wall has been developed and used clinically.[23] Unilateral bronchial blockers have been used clinically in the treatment of pulmonary interstitial emphysema and other forms of acquired (barotrauma) lung diseases in premature and newborn infants.[24]

There are two techniques other than placement of a bronchial blocker that can be used to accomplish one-lung ventilation in children. Double-lumen cuffed endotracheal tubes have a long and rich history in general thoracic surgery.[25, 26] It is generally held, however, that a body weight of at least 30 to 35 kg is necessary for the patient's airway to accommodate the smallest double-lumen device (28 French).[27] This size limitation essentially precludes the use of these devices for patients younger than approximately 8 years of age.

The second alternative is intentional intubation of a main stem bronchus with an endotracheal tube. In general, a single-lumen endotracheal tube, one half French smaller than a tube that would be appropriate for tracheal intubation, is used. Right main stem bronchus intubation can usually be accomplished blindly.[12, 27–29] Left main stem bronchus intubation usually requires the use of either fiberoptic bronchoscopy[30] or fluoroscopy[27] to ensure appropriate placement. Techniques have been described for increasing the likelihood of successful blind intubation of the left main stem bronchus,[29] but we prefer to ensure appropriate placement of an endobronchial tube with fiberoptic bronchoscopy.

Physiology of One-Lung Ventilation

Although general anesthesia alone causes changes in pulmonary compliance, and the lateral decubitus position may produce regional functional abnormalities of ventilation and perfusion, the pathophysiology of one-lung ventilation is much more dramatic. Any pulmonary blood flow to the nonventilated lung becomes right-to-left shunt flow. This shunt flow is in addition to any shunt flow occurring in the dependent (ventilated) lung due to the effects of anesthesia and/or positioning. The combination of these two intrapulmonary shunts during one-lung ventilation results in a much larger alveolar-arterial oxygen tension difference and lower $Pa{O_2}$ than during two-lung ventilation.

Reduction in the amount of pulmonary blood to the nonventilated lung during one-lung ventilation (decreased shunt fraction) occurs as a result of (1) simple gravitational forces due to the lateral decubitus position, (2) mechanical interference with blood flow (retraction), and (3) hypoxic pulmonary vasoconstriction. This latter mechanism can decrease blood flow to a hypoxic segment of lung by as much as 50%. Typically, the dependent lung in the lateral decubitus position during two-lung ventilation receives approximately 60% of pulmonary blood flow. Institution of one-lung ventilation causes a 50% decrease in the blood flow to the nonventilated lung due to hypoxic pulmonary vasoconstriction. The result is that the dependent lung receives 80% of pulmonary blood flow and the atelectatic lung receives only 20%.[31] This protective mechanism is critical in minimizing hypoxemia during one-lung ventilation. Certain measures can be undertaken during one-lung ventilation to optimize arterial $P{O_2}$. Maintaining two-lung ventilation as long as possible is a simple and effective maneuver. Once one-lung ventilation is begun, the inspired oxygen concentration should be maintained at 100%. Upper lung insufflation with oxygen at 10 cm H_2O pressure (if technically feasible) and application of 10 cm H_2O positive end expiratory pressure (PEEP) to the dependent lung are effective in maximizing arterial $P{O_2}$.[32] Upper lung insufflation with oxygen is not practical in pediatric patients who are being managed with unilateral bronchial intubation. In addition, unless a Swan-Ganz catheter is used as a bronchial blocker, oxygen cannot be used to insufflate the upper lung.

General Thoracoscopy Considerations

The development of smaller trocars, telescopes, and instrumentation has made pediatric thoracoscopy feasible. Thoracoscope size is limited by the size of the chest cavity, and we recommend the following: 3.75- to 4-mm trocar-telescope for patients younger than 2 years, 5 mm for those age 2 to 8 years, and 10 mm for those older than 8 years[33] (Fig. 37–1). If CO_2 insufflation is required to induce pneumothorax, a valved trocar is necessary. Otherwise, an unvalved port, such as the Thoracoport (Auto Suture Company, Division of U.S. Surgical Corp., Norwalk, CT), or a small stab wound can be used. The Thoracoport has external threads that enable it to maintain good position during manipulation. Although a 0-degree telescope is usually adequate, a 30-degree lens may be advantageous when an angled view is necessary, for example, during examination of the posterior mediastinum.[34] Thoracoscopic instruments are similar to those used for any open procedure. Most basic equipment will pass through a 5-mm port and include scissors, curved dissectors, retractors, various grasping instruments with ratcheted handles, and an atraumatic lung clamp. Unfortunately, the currently available fan retractors

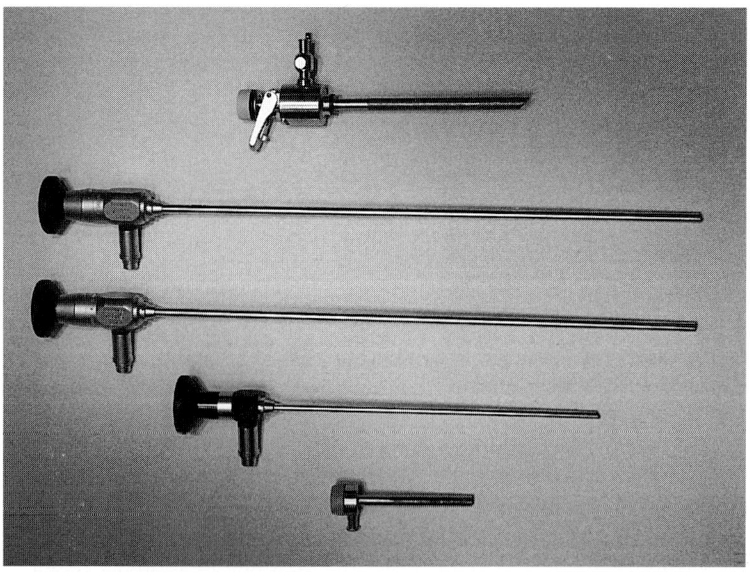

Figure 37–1. Trocar-telescopes for use in pediatric patients.

can be introduced only through a 10-mm port and are difficult but not impossible to use within small chest cavities. The EndoGIA device (U.S. Surgical Corp., Norwalk, CT) places two parallel sets of three rows of staples and divides the tissue in between, leaving an air- and watertight seal. A 12-mm trocar is required for EndoGIA use, and the device must be inserted at least 5 cm into the thoracic cavity for the anvil to open and function properly. For this reason, use of the EndoGIA is generally not possible in children younger than 4 to 5 years of age. For smaller children, Endo-loops (Ethicon Endosurgery, Inc., Cincinnati, OH) can be useful for lung biopsy. This instrument, which can be passed through a 5-mm trocar, places a ligature at the base of a snared piece of tissue before excision. An automated tissue morcellator may be useful for removing larger specimens. The resected tissue is placed in a bag, the neck of the bag is delivered through the trocar site, and a morcellator is used to break up the tissue into smaller pieces for easier removal. Use of this technique does not appear to significantly affect pathologic review.[35]

The recent development of safer laser equipment has had a significant impact on thoracoscopic surgery. One advantage of lasers is the ability to both cut and coagulate without changing instrumentation. In addition, the Nd:YAG laser seals lung parenchyma, thereby decreasing postoperative air leaks. Unlike electrocautery devices, lasers are not associated with cardiac fibrillation when working near the heart and pericardium.[36]

Preoperative imaging, utilizing modalities such as ultrasonography (US), computed tomography (CT), or magnetic resonance imaging (MRI), is required for planning optimal trocar placement, especially in infants and children with small chest cavities. With proper positioning, gravity maximizes visualization of the area of interest by displacing peripheral tissues, potentially allowing one to use fewer trocars. Patient positioning is dependent on the procedure and the anatomic location of the lesion. Either soft rolls or a beanbag can be used to secure the child in position on the table. For lateral decubitus positioning, the lower leg is flexed at the knee and hip and the upper leg is straight, with a pillow in between. The dependent arm is flexed at the elbow, with the superior arm either placed in the "praying position" with pillow support or extended on a padded Mayo stand. An axillary roll should be used to minimize the risk of brachial plexus injury. Overhead heaters and heating blankets are employed to maintain body temperature. The entire chest is prepared and draped to allow for trocar repositioning, chest tube drain-age sites, or open thoracotomy should this become necessary for either exposure or hemostasis. The operating surgeon is generally stationed on the side of the patient opposite the side of the lesion or area of interest (Fig. 37–2).

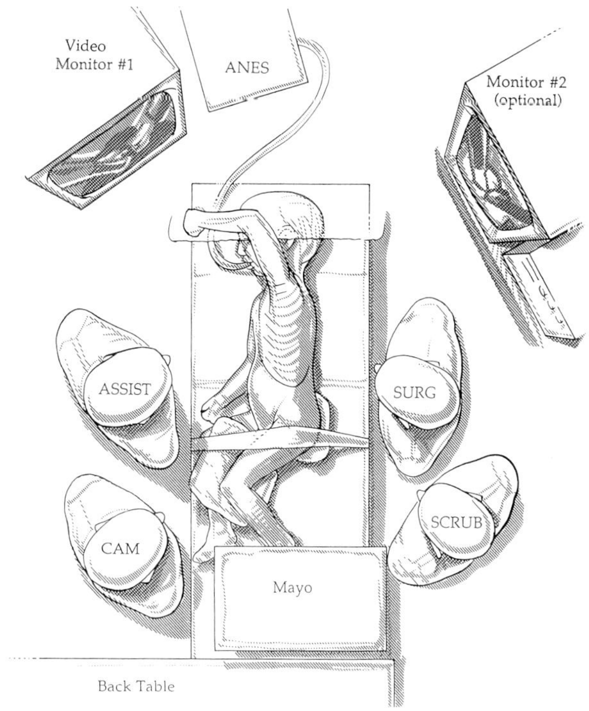

Figure 37–2. Placement of personnel for thoracoscopy for biopsy of an anterior mediastinal mass. The surgeon (SURG) stands at the back of the patient, on the side opposite the pathology. The scrub nurse (SCRUB) stands next to the surgeon and assists with retraction, and the camera operating assistant (CAM) stands across from the scrub nurse. Two monitors are used so that all personnel can look directly at a monitor. (From Rodgers BM: Thoracoscopic procedures in children. Semin Pediatr Surg 2:182–189, 1993, with permission.)

The initial trocar is usually placed in the midaxillary line, either inferiorly for apical lesions or superiorly for basilar lesions. Although some surgeons employ a Veres needle,[36] we prefer an open approach. A small transverse incision is made in the middle of the intercostal space, the underlying subcutaneous tissue and intercostal muscle are bluntly dissected, and the pleura is entered with a clamp. Tunneling of trocar sites, as is done during chest tube placement, is discouraged, as this limits telescope and instrument mobility.[33] Care must be taken during trocar insertion following complete lung collapse, because the diaphragm can rise as high as the third intercostal space.[35] The telescope is passed through the trocar, the entire pleural cavity is inspected, and additional trocars are placed, as needed, under direct thoracoscopic guidance. When one-lung anesthesia is deemed necessary but is incomplete, low-flow, low-pressure CO_2 insufflation (1 L/min; 2 to 4 mm Hg) may be utilized to facilitate total collapse of the lung.[37] Before closure, some recommend placing a small epidural catheter into the paravertebral region and infusing 0.25% bupivacaine with epinephrine (0.75 ml/kg) every 3 to 4 hours for postoperative analgesia.[33] For simple biopsies (pleural, mediastinal, or pulmonary) or when the visceral pleura is not violated, several authors aspirate the thorax with a small suction catheter and close without chest tube placement.[33, 35] Alternatively, a chest tube may be removed several hours after the procedure, allowing for earlier patient mobilization. For larger procedures, or following treatment of empyema, chest tubes can be placed through the original trocar sites. The fascia and skin are closed with absorbable suture and dressed with Steri-Strips. A postoperative chest radiograph should always be obtained to verify complete lung expansion.

Mediastinal Lesions

Thoracoscopy can be of great utility in evaluating mediastinal lesions in children. Biopsy and/or resection of mediastinal lesions is possible with proper localization, positioning, and thoracoscopic expertise. Mediastinal adenopathy may result from conditions such as lymphoma; fungal, viral, or mycobacterial infection; or granulomatous disease (e.g., sarcoidosis). Diagnosis can be confirmed in most of these patients by thoracoscopic lymph node biopsy when other less invasive methods (e.g., serology, bone marrow biopsy) have failed.

Several types of anterior mediastinal tumors are common in children, including germ cell neoplasms (teratomas) and dermoid cysts. These tumors require resection, because delay may result in necrosis, secondary infection, rupture, or malignant degeneration. Although anterior mediastinal tumors have traditionally been approached with median sternotomy or lateral thoracotomy, some of these lesions can currently be safely evaluated and/or treated with VATS.

VATS may be used for the evaluation of thymoma and as a means of thymic resection for the treatment of myasthenia gravis. Initial therapy for infants and children diagnosed with myasthenia gravis involves anti-acetylcholinesterase medication. Additional treatment includes a course of corticosteroids and occasionally plasmapheresis. For patients who have a transient or refractory response, a complete thymectomy is recommended. In rare cases in which a thymoma is associated with myasthenia gravis, thymectomy is also recommended.[38–41] One operative technique involves a combined thoracoscopic and transcervical approach. Initial dissection is accomplished in the neck and may require division of venous branches of the thymus to the innominate vein. A specially designed retractor (Cooper Thymectomy Retractor, Pilling-Weck Inc., Research Triangle Park, NC) is used to facilitate dissection in the anterior mediastinum. The mobilized thymus gland can then be placed within the mediastinum, the neck incision closed, and the remainder of the dissection accomplished with VATS. If thoracoscopy alone is employed for resection, one must verify complete removal of thymic tissue in the neck.[39] VATS may also be helpful for completion thymectomy in patients with refractory myasthenia gravis who have already undergone resection. This technique has the potential advantage of avoiding previously dissected tissue planes, thus facilitating the search for residual thymic tissue.[38] Bronchogenic and foregut duplication cysts are uncommon pediatric conditions that can be evaluated and potentially treated with a thoracoscopic approach.[39, 42–44] In addition, resection and/or biopsy of posterior mediastinal masses, such as neuroblastoma and ganglioneuroma, can be achieved with VATS.[45, 46] With these and all other uses of VATS, compromise of patient safety or inadequate treatment of the disease must result in conversion to a standard open operation.

Patient positioning for exploration of anterior or posterior mediastinal masses is either supine or prone, with the operative side slightly elevated (Figs. 37–3 and 37–4). The initial trocar should be placed near the midaxillary line in the fifth or sixth intercostal space. Before biopsy or excision, mediastinal masses may be aspirated with a long needle to ensure that the lesion is not of vascular origin.[33] Furthermore, aspirating a cystic lesion decreases its size and may facilitate excision. A puncture biopsy can be performed through either a 10-mm thoracoscope with a 5-mm biopsy channel or a 5-mm thoracoscope and a separate 5-mm trocar for placement of the biopsy instruments (such as Endo-loops). The latter technique is preferred in younger children. Alternatively, biopsies can be accomplished with partial resection.

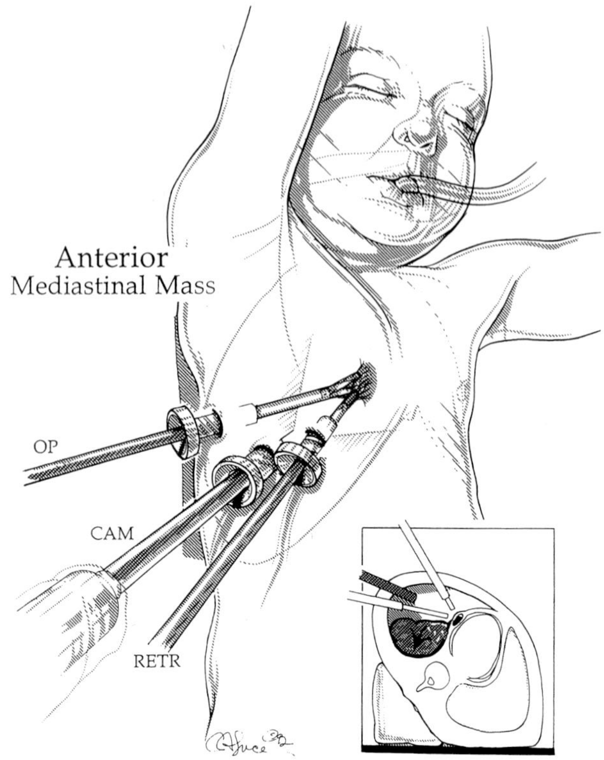

Figure 37–3. Orientation of patient and instruments for approach to an anterior mediastinal mass in a child. (*Inset*) The patient is placed in a 45-degree lateral decubitus position, allowing the lung to fall posteriorly. The telescope-camera port (CAM) is placed in the anterior axillary line, and the operating instruments (OP) are passed through a cannula placed posteriorly. Retracting instruments (RETR) are passed through an anteriorly placed port. (From Rodgers BM: Thoracoscopic procedures in children. Semin Pediatr Surg 2:182–189, 1993, with permission.)

For the majority of mediastinal lesions in children, other than lymph node diseases and neuroblastoma, complete excision is usually attempted. The pleura is opened and the lesion dissected from the surrounding structures using either hook cautery or scissors. A laser (KTP and/or Nd:YAG) can also be utilized when excising tissue.[35] When a cystic lesion is attached to a major structure (such as the esophagus or trachea), a partial cystectomy can be performed, and the remaining tissue can be destroyed with either laser coagulation or electrocautery.[33] Invasion of neoplastic tissue into surrounding structures, such as the phrenic nerve, is an indication for conversion to an open operation so that more definitive dissection and treatment can be undertaken.

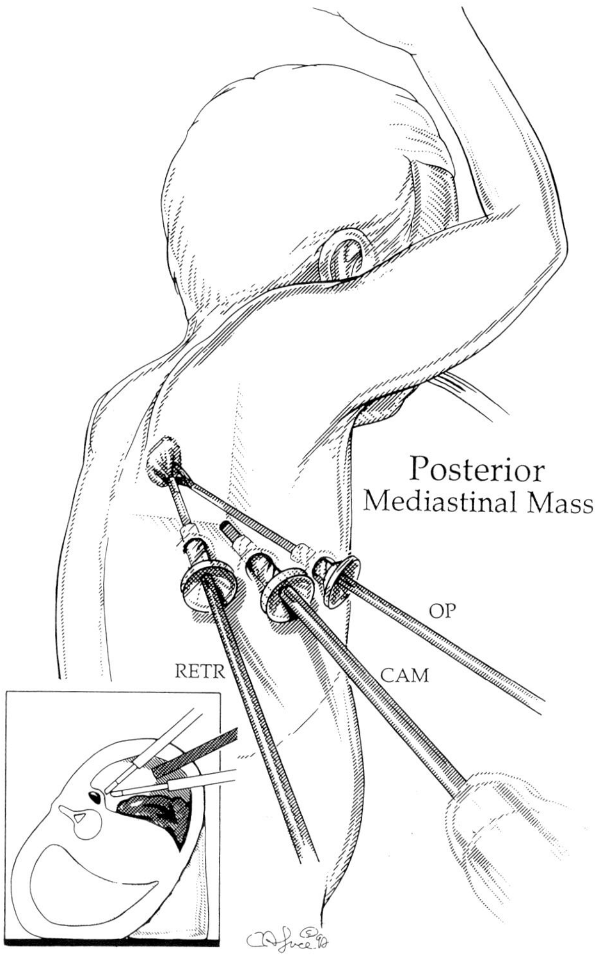

Figure 37–4. Orientation of patient and instruments for approach to a posterior mediastinal mass in a child. (*Inset*) The patient is placed in an exaggerated lateral decubitus position, allowing the lung to fall forward. The telescope-camera port (CAM) is placed in the posterior axillary line, with the operating instruments (OP) passed through a cannula placed anteriorly. The retracting instruments (RETR) are passed through a posteriorly placed port. (From Rodgers BM: Thoracoscopic procedures in children. Semin Pediatr Surg 2:182–189, 1993, with permission.)

Lung Biopsy

In children with suspected pneumonia or other primary pulmonary disease unresponsive to conventional antibiotics or other indicated therapies, thoracoscopic lung biopsy may be helpful. Other indications for pulmonary biopsy include lung masses that are suspicious for primary malignancy or metastasis. The full lateral decubitus position allows access to all surfaces of the lung. Some surgeons recommend one-lung anesthesia, and others prefer the child to be breathing spontaneously. The advantage of the latter is that areas of inflammation and atelectasis can be easily differentiated from uninvolved pulmonary parenchyma. A telescope is placed at the midaxillary line in the fourth or fifth intercostal space. An operating trocar is subsequently established anteriorly or posteriorly, depending on the site of greatest lung involvement, at the same intercostal space. An additional trocar may be necessary for lung retractor placement (Fig. 37–5).

For pediatric patients with primary or metastatic lung tumors, the utility of VATS continues to evolve and to be defined. Wedge resection or biopsy of the suspected lesion almost always provides adequate tissue for diagnosis.[47] At times, metastatic lesions are difficult to visualize owing to their small size, and localization may be improved with the use of intraoperative endoscopic US. Another useful technique for localizing lesions before VATS biopsy is CT-guided localization.[37] A small amount of the patient's blood is injected into the pulmonary parenchyma near the lesion, allowing for visualization of the area of diseased lung during thoracoscopy. In small children, biopsy can be performed with wedge resection and electrocautery. Alternatively, a cut biopsy forceps, an Endo-loop, or a vascular stapler can be employed.[35] The EndoGIA significantly facilitates lung biopsy in larger children. Chest tubes are not essential but may be placed if the pleural defect is large or if an air leak is present. Parenchymal lesions diagnosed ra-

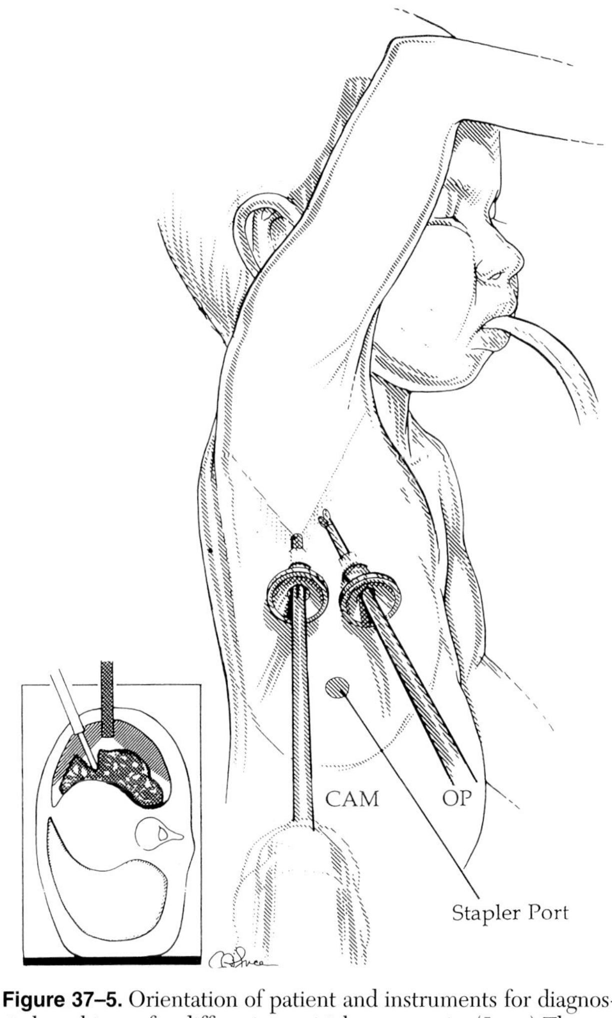

Figure 37–5. Orientation of patient and instruments for diagnostic lung biopsy for diffuse interstitial pneumonia. (*Inset*) The patient is placed in a full lateral decubitus position. The telescope-camera cannula (CAM) is placed in the region of the midaxillary line. The biopsy port (OP) is placed just anterior or posterior to this position in the same intercostal space. The cannula port for the EndoGIA stapler is indicated, well inferior to the others. (From Rodgers BM: Thoracoscopic procedures in children. Semin Pediatr Surg 2:182–189, 1993, with permission.)

diologically that cannot be visualized because of location or size may require an open procedure, which allows for manual palpation of the lung.[48]

Empyema

The increased use of thoracoscopy and its relatively low morbidity has resulted in its application in various pleural diseases. Among these, the treatment of empyema is the most common. Traditionally, a loculated empyema has been treated with selective thoracostomy tube placement and subsequent drainage. However, if the empyema remains undrained or if the patient does not clinically improve, open debridement and drainage, with or without rib resection, has been the standard operative therapy. Aggressive and early thoracoscopic debridement and irrigation with empyema drainage may avoid the need for subsequent open thoracotomy, and numerous studies have suggested that this practice may decrease hospital stay and minimize long-term morbidity.[33, 49–53] When treating patients with presumed empyema, it is usually helpful to localize the largest pleural collections with US or CT before surgery. A telescope is introduced into the largest cavity at the beginning of the debridement. Alternatively, initial access to the pleural cavity can be obtained through previous chest tube tracts.[49] The cavity is bluntly enlarged with the tip of the telescope, followed by placement of an additional trocar. The entire pleural cavity should be visualized and pleural fluid and fibrinous tissue collected for culture and sensitivity testing. Various grasping instruments are employed to break up adhesions and strip the "peel" from the pleural surface. The cavities are copiously irrigated with normal saline, and one or more chest tubes are placed. We prefer to delay chest tube removal until drainage is minimal.

Pneumothorax

VATS has also begun to play a major role in the treatment of spontaneous pneumothorax. In young patients, pneumothorax usually results from the spontaneous rupture of single or multiple blebs. These blebs are usually located at the apex of the upper lobe, and their rupture and the subsequent pneumothorax are initially treated conservatively with tube thoracostomy. Traditional thoracotomy with resection of the bleb and apical pleurodesis has generally been reserved for patients with persistent air leaks (greater than 1 week in duration) or for those patients with recurrence of pneumothorax. The lower morbidity associated with VATS appears to have influenced the recommended "waiting period," decreasing it to as little as 2 or 3 days.[39] Pleurodesis and bleb resection for persistent or recurrent pneumothorax can be easily achieved with VATS. The best technique for VATS pleurodesis is still actively debated. Mechanical abrasion can be achieved by attaching a portion of rough material (e.g., gauze or mesh) to the tip of a 5-mm biopsy forceps. Chemical pleurodesis has been performed by instilling talc under pressure (using either a bulb or an insufflator) through a 5-mm trocar. Talc pleurodesis should be avoided in patients who may eventually undergo lung transplantation (e.g., cystic fibrosis patients), because the resultant pleural sclerosis makes subsequent lung resection difficult.[39]

Chylothorax

Chylothorax can present during infancy and childhood. The primary causes of chylothorax in this population include idiopathic chylothorax of infancy, injury to the lymphatic channels following cardiac surgery or trauma, malignancy, congenital heart disease, or pulmonary lymphangiectasis. Chylothorax usually results in respiratory insufficiency and manifests as a pleural effusion on chest radiographs. The initial treatment of chylothorax is drainage by thoracocentesis or tube thoracostomy. This approach, when combined with a medium-chain triglyceride diet and/or elimination of enteral nutrition and initiation of total parenteral nutrition, results in resolution of chylothorax in over 80% of patients. If nonoperative therapy does not eliminate the lymphatic drainage, evaluation of the chest to identify the point of leakage may be accomplished using thoracoscopy. Surgical therapy may include ligation of the thoracic duct or pleurodesis. Covering the area with fibrin glue has also been attempted, and thoracoscopic placement of a pleuroperitoneal shunt has been highly effective in 85% to 95% of these patients.[54] The timing of surgical intervention remains controversial. A conservative approach has been to recommend 14 to 21 days of nonoperative therapy before considering surgical intervention. However, if less invasive techniques are employed, a shorter observation period, especially in children with right heart failure or central venous thrombosis, may be warranted.

Cerebrospinal Fluid Shunts

Thoracoscopic techniques can provide access to the thorax for management of children with cerebrospinal fluid shunts. For patients who require decompression into the pleural cavity, thoracoscopy can provide excellent visualization and minimize morbidity. With the patient in a prone position, a 5-mm incision is made overlying the sixth rib. The pleural space is then entered and a 5-mm cannula inserted. After visualization is established with a telescope, a site for insertion of the shunt can be identified, and it can be placed using the Seldinger technique. At the conclusion of shunt placement, the cannula site can be closed around a catheter that is removed with positive pressure ventilation. This approach, which eliminates the need for even a mini-thoracotomy, should decrease postoperative discomfort.[55]

Patent Ductus Arteriosus and Vascular Ring

Equipment miniaturization has made closure of patent ductus arteriosus (PDA) possible (see Chapter 75). There appear to be few age or size limitations to interruption of PDA with VATS. The thoracoscope (3.75 or 4 mm) is placed anterior to the midaxilla at the fourth or fifth intercostal space, and a working trocar is placed anteriorly. The left upper lobe is retracted inferomedially to expose the pleura covering the ductus. The PDA is identified and dissected free from the surrounding pleura and aorta. To achieve good exposure, it is important to dissect both proximal and distal margins of the ductus as well as both lateral aspects. Dissecting the pericardium on the pulmonary side may decrease the likelihood of recurrent laryngeal nerve injury. The PDA is occluded with two 8-mm titanium clips near and parallel to the aorta.[56] The clips should completely encircle the ductus, and success can be confirmed using transesophageal echocardiography. If flow is not interrupted, additional vascular clips are applied in the manner described earlier. The lung is expanded with positive pressure, and the pleural cavity is aspirated with a suction catheter. Chest tube placement may be unnecessary. Contraindications specific to VATS PDA interruption include a ductus diameter larger than the descending aorta; a ductus larger than the clip to be used (0.8 mm); the presence of pulmonary adhesions, which may make VATS excessively difficult; and calcification in the vessel wall.[56, 57] Complications of this technique include residual patency of the duct, recurrent laryngeal nerve injury, hemorrhage, chylothorax, and residual pneumothorax.[56–58] Recurrent laryngeal nerve injury is infrequent, because the operative field is magnified and thus better visualized using VATS.[59] In a series of over 300 patients undergoing VATS PDA interruption, the residual patency rate was 1.8% (0% in the final 200 patients).[56] A 12% residual patency rate at 2 months following surgery was reported by another group.[57] Although the experience with VATS PDA interruption is preliminary, the incidence of residual patency, as assessed by echocardiography, compares favorably with that reported for the transcatheter embolization device (38% at 1 year)[57, 60] and for open surgical ligation (23% at 4 months).[57, 61]

The use of VATS for division of a vascular ring has also been described.[57] These patients typically have symptoms consistent with varying degrees of esophageal and/or tracheal obstruction. The evaluation includes a standard chest radiograph and barium swallow. If these studies and the clinical picture are suggestive of a vascular ring, an MRI scan should be obtained. The surgical approach is similar to the one described for PDA interruption. The vascular ring is identified using the origin of the left subclavian artery for orientation. The ring elements are dissected from the underlying esophagus and divided between surgical clips. Additional fibrous bands that may encircle the esophagus can be divided with electrocautery. In a series of eight patients with vascular ring, two required open thoracotomy to divide the vascular structures. In one case, VATS was converted to an open procedure to control bleeding, and one patient developed a chylothorax. Preoperative symptoms were relieved in 88% of the patients.[57]

Anterior Spinal Exposure

Thoracoscopic anterior spinal release is in evolution but is easily performed in appropriately selected larger children. One-lung anesthesia is usually required, and 10-mm trocars are necessary for insertion of the current orthopedic instrumentation. Initial entry into the pleural cavity is made at the anterior axillary line superior to the spinal deformity. The ribs are counted by palpation from the inside of the chest for orientation, and an intervertebral disk space is marked with a K-wire for intraoperative radiographic confirmation. Two or more additional trocars are placed. In patients requiring exposure of T12–L3, the diaphragm may need to be divided and mobilized. An incision is made with electrocautery in the pleura overlying the most proximal deformed vertebral body anterior to the sympathetic chain and continued along all the vertebral bodies to be released. Segmental vessels at the appropriate levels are divided with ligature clips. The posterior pleura is dissected free from the vertebral bodies and their respective inner spaces. Anterior spinal release is then performed in conjunction with a pediatric spine surgeon. This involves release of the anterior longitudinal ligament and removal of the anterolateral portions of the annulus fibrosus at each affected disk level. The respective nucleus pulposus is then removed. If anterior fusion is deemed necessary, it is preferable to use bone chips from a portion of resected rib or iliac bone. The trocars are removed, and hemostasis is verified. A single chest tube is placed through one of the trocar sites. If posterior instrumentation is deemed necessary, the double-lumen endotracheal tube is exchanged for a single-lumen tube, and the patient is placed in a prone position.

ACKNOWLEDGMENTS

The authors wish to thank Debbie Sheil for her invaluable assistance in preparing this manuscript. The authors also wish to thank Dmitry Elentuck for translating the article by Klimkovich and colleagues[5] from Russian to English.

References

1. Jacobaeus HC: Ueber die Moglichkeit die Zystoskopie bei Untersuchung seroser Hohlungen anzuwenden. Muenchener Medizinische Wochenschrift 57:2090–2092, 1910.
2. Jacobaeus HC: The practical importance of thoracoscopy in surgery of the chest. Surg Gynecol Obstet 34:289–297, 1922.
3. Jacobaeus HC: The cauterization of adhesions in pneumothorax treatment of tuberculosis. Surg Gynecol Obstet 32:493–500, 1921.
4. Fourestier M, Gladu A, Vulmiere J: Perfectionnements a l'endoscopie medicale. Realisation bronchoscopique. Presse Med 60:1292–1294, 1952.
5. Klimkovich IG, Geldt VG, Okulov AB, et al: [Thoracoscopy in children]. Khirurgiia 47:19–24, 1971.
6. Rodgers BM, Talbert JL: Thoracoscopy for diagnosis of intrathoracic lesions in children. J Pediatr Surg 11:703–708, 1976.
7. Rodgers BM, Moazam F, Talbert JL: Thoracoscopy: Early diagnosis of interstitial pneumonitis in the immunologically suppressed child. Chest 75:126–130, 1979.
8. Dubois F, Berthelot G, Levard H: [Cholecystectomy by celioscopy]. Presse Med 18:980–982, 1989.
9. Ryckman FC, Rodgers BM: Thoracoscopy for intrathoracic neoplasia in children. J Pediatr Surg 17:521–524, 1982.
10. Yaster M: Anesthesia for surgical emergencies in newborns. *In* Rogers MC, Tinker JH, Covino BG, Longnecker DE (eds): Principles and Practice of Anesthesiology. St. Louis, Mosby–Year Book, 1993, pp 2137–2156.
11. Wolfe WG: Disorders of the lungs, pleura, and chest wall. I. Anatomy. *In* Sabiston DC Jr (ed): Textbook of Surgery. Philadelphia, WB Saunders, 1991, pp 1673–1682.
12. Kubota Y, Toyoda Y, Nagata N, et al: Tracheo-bronchial angles in infants and children. Anesthesiology 64:374–376, 1986.

13. van den Berg AA, Mphanza T: Choice of tracheal tube size for children: Finger size or age-related formula? Anaesthesia 52: 701–703, 1997.
14. King BR, Baker MD, Braitman LE, et al: Endotracheal tube selection in children: A comparison of four methods. Ann Emerg Med 22:530–534, 1993.
15. Shima T, Andoh K, Akama M, Hashimoto Y: The correct endotracheal tube size for infants and children. Masui 41:190–193, 1992.
16. Rehder K, Sessler AD, Marsh HM: General anesthesia and the lung. Am Rev Respir Dis 112:541–563, 1975.
17. Wulff KE, Aulin I: The regional lung function in the lateral decubitus position during anesthesia and operation. Acta Anaesthesiol Scand 16:195–205, 1972.
18. Wood RE, Campbell D, Razzuk MA, et al: Surgical advantages of selective unilateral ventilation. Ann Thorac Surg 14:173–180, 1972.
19. Vale R: Selective bronchial blocking in a small child: Case report. Br J Anaesth 41:453–454, 1969.
20. Hogg CE, Lorhan PH: Pediatric bronchial blocking. Anesthesiology 33:560–562, 1970.
21. Cay DL, Csenderits LE, Lines V, et al: Selective bronchial blocking in children. Anesth Intens Care 3:127–130, 1975.
22. Ginsberg RJ: New technique for one-lung anesthesia using an endobronchial blocker. J Thorac Cardiovasc Surg 82:542–546, 1981.
23. Karwande SV: A new tube for single lung ventilation. Chest 92:761–763, 1987.
24. Brooks JG, Bustamante SA, Koops BL, et al: Selective bronchial intubation for the treatment of severe localized pulmonary interstitial emphysema in newborn infants. J Pediatr 91:648–652, 1977.
25. Carlens E: A new flexible double lumen catheter for bronchospirometry. J Thorac Cardiovasc Surg 18:742–746, 1949.
26. Robertshaw FL: Low resistance double-lumen endobronchial tubes. Br J Anaesth 34:576–579, 1962.
27. Tobias JD: Anesthesia for thoracic surgery in children. Chest Surg Clin N Am 3:357–373, 1993.
28. Rowe R, Andropoulos D, Heard M, et al: Anesthetic management of pediatric patients undergoing thoracoscopy. J Cardiothorac Vasc Anesth 8:563–566, 1994.
29. Kubota H, Kubota Y, Toyoda Y, et al: Selective blind endobronchial intubation in children and adults. Anesthesiology 67:587–589, 1987.
30. Lee AC, Wu CL, Feins RH, Ward DS: The use of fiberoptic endoscopy in anesthesia. Chest Surg Clin N Am 6:329–347, 1996.
31. Banoub M, Nugent M: Thoracic anesthesia. *In* Rogers MC, Tinker JH, Covino BG, Longnecker DE (eds): Principles and Practice of Anesthesiology. St. Louis, Mosby-Year Book, 1993, pp 1719–1930.
32. Capan LM, Turndorf H, Patel C, et al: Optimization of arterial oxygenation during one-lung anesthesia. Anesth Analg 59:847–851, 1980.
33. Rodgers BM: Thoracoscopic procedures in children. Semin Pediatr Surg 2:182–189, 1993.
34. Bullard KM, Adzick NS: Pediatric thoracoscopy: A new vista. Pediatr Pulmonol 22:129–135, 1996.
35. Lobe TE: Pediatric thoracoscopy. Semin Thorac Cardiovasc Surg 5:298–302, 1993.
36. Rogers DA, Philippe PG, Lobe TE, et al: Thoracoscopy in children: An initial experience with an evolving technique. J Laparoendosc Surg 2:7–14, 1992.
37. Rothenberg SS: Thoracoscopy in infants and children. Semin Pediatr Surg 3:277–282, 1994.
38. Mineo TC, Pompeo E, Ambrogi V, et al: Video-assisted completion thymectomy in refractory myasthenia gravis. J Thorac Cardiovasc Surg 115:252–254, 1998.
39. Kaiser LR: Video-assisted thoracic surgery: Current state of the art. Ann Surg 220:720–734, 1994.
40. Sugarbaker DJ: Thoracoscopy in the management of anterior mediastinal masses. Ann Thorac Surg 56:653–656, 1993.
41. Kaiser LR: Thymoma: The use of minimally invasive resection techniques. Chest Surg Clin N Am 4:185–194, 1994.
42. Dillon PW, Cilley RE, Krummel TM: Video-assisted thoracoscopic excision of intrathoracic masses in children: Report of two cases. Surg Laparosc Endosc 3:433–436, 1993.
43. Ribet ME, Copin MC, Gosselin B: Bronchogenic cysts of the mediastinum. J Thorac Cardiovasc Surg 109:1003–1010, 1995.
44. Acuff TE, Mack MJ, Ryan WH, et al: Thoracoscopic excision of bronchogenic cysts. Ann Thorac Surg 55:200, 1993.
45. Naunheim KS: Video thoracoscopy for masses of the posterior mediastinum. Ann Thorac Surg 56:657–658, 1993.
46. Canvasser DA, Naunheim KS: Thoracoscopic management of posterior mediastinal tumors. Chest Surg Clin N Am 6:53–67, 1996.
47. Holcomb GW 3rd, Tomita SS, Haase GM, et al: Minimally invasive surgery in children with cancer. Cancer 76:121–128, 1995.
48. Rau B, Hunerbein M, Below C, Schlag PM: Video-assisted thoracic surgery: Staging and management of thoracic tumors. Surg Endosc 12:133–136, 1998.
49. Silen ML, Weber TR: Thoracoscopic debridement of loculated empyema thoracis in children. Ann Thorac Surg 59:1166–1168, 1995.
50. Chan W, Keyser-Gauvin E, Davis GM, et al: Empyema thoracis in children: A 26-year review of the Montreal Children's Hospital experience. J Pediatr Surg 32:870–872, 1997.
51. Stovroff M, Teague G, Heiss KF, et al: Thoracoscopy in the management of pediatric empyema. J Pediatr Surg 30:1211–1215, 1995.
52. Silen ML, Naunheim KS: Thoracoscopic approach to the management of empyema thoracis: Indications and results. Chest Surg Clin N Am 6:491–499, 1996.
53. Campbell PW 3rd: New developments in pediatric pneumonia and empyema. Curr Opin Pediatr 7:278–282, 1995.
54. Rodgers BM, McGahren ED III: Mediastinum and pleura. *In* Oldham KT, Colombani PM, Foglia RP (eds): Surgery of Infants and Children: Scientific Principles and Practice. Philadelphia, Lippincott-Raven Publishers, 1997, pp 915–933.
55. Holcomb GW 3rd, Smith HP: Laparoscopic and thoracoscopic assistance with CSF shunts in children. J Pediatr Surg 30: 1642–1643, 1995.
56. Laborde F, Folliguet TA, Etienne PY, et al: Video-thoracoscopic surgical interruption of patent ductus arteriosus: Routine experience in 332 pediatric cases. Eur J Cardiothorac Surg 11: 1052–1055, 1997.
57. Burke RP, Wernovsky G, van der Velde M, et al: Video-assisted thoracoscopic surgery for congenital heart disease. J Thorac Cardiovasc Surg 109:499–507, 1995.
58. Lupoglazoff JM, Laborde F, Magnier S, Casasoprana A: [Closure of patent ductus arteriosus by video-thoracoscopy in 45 children]. Arch Mal Coeur Vaiss 88:705–710, 1995.
59. Laborde F, Noirhomme P, Karam J, et al: A new video-assisted thoracoscopic surgical technique for interruption of patent ductus arteriosus in infants and children. J Thorac Cardiovasc Surg 105:278–280, 1993.
60. Hosking MC, Benson LN, Musewe N, et al: Transcatheter occlusion of the persistently patent ductus arteriosus: Forty-month follow-up and prevalence of residual shunting. Circulation 84: 2313–2317, 1991.
61. Sorensen KE, Kristensen B, Hansen OK: Frequency of occurrence of residual ductal flow after surgical ligation by color-flow mapping. Am J Cardiol 67:653–654, 1991.

COMMENTARY

Hock-Lim Tan

Thoracotomy in children is very safe today. Children, unlike adults, recover quickly, and because most chest diseases in children are benign, the surgical outcome of thoracotomy is almost always excellent. It is therefore difficult to justify *thoracoscopic* surgery when excellent results are already achieved by conventional treatment. The fact that thoracoscopic surgery can be performed is not seen as an indication, particularly when it often incurs higher costs, produces results that are not clearly superior, and is associated with significantly increased operating time. Videoscopic surgery, for those arguing against it, is often labeled "tedioscopic" surgery!

Why bother with video-assisted thoracic surgery (VATS)? The answer lies not in the immediate postoperative results but in the long-term morbidity. Checuti and associates[1] reported chest wall deformities in 33% (77/232) of patients who had undergone thoracotomy for esophageal atresia. These deformities were found in the group of patients who did *not* have associated vertebral abnormalities. In their group of 77 patients who developed chest wall deformities, 47 had anterior chest wall deformities alone, 18 had scoliosis, and 12 had a combination of both. Westfelt and associate[2] similarly reported 20 cases of scoliosis developing in 61 patients following thoracotomy for various conditions in childhood. Additionally, Van Biezen and associates[3] reported a 22% incidence (35/160) of scoliosis developing in children after thoracotomy for repair of aortic coarctation. An observation was made by the last group that the high-risk period for developing scoliosis began *3 years after* the procedure, and was not related to age or sex.

It is, therefore, clear that thoracotomy is not without long-term morbidity, and the development of VATS, as it is commonly known, apart from reducing the invasiveness to the child, may, by avoiding an open thoracotomy, result in significant reduction of chest wall deformities and scoliosis in the growing child over time.

Whatever the reason, VATS is here to stay. From the surgeon's viewpoint, it may be tedious, because it requires relearning many skills. However, for parents and children there are clear advantages to be gained from VATS. Its results do not need to be superior. The procedure just needs to be *safe* and to offer comparable results.

Safety is the paramount consideration. A thoracoscopist who is called on to perform an occasional procedure in a child should be aware that special problems exist with children. Most children requiring VATS already have a compromised respiratory system and can ill afford further compromise occasioned by the use of inappropriate anesthetic techniques.

This chapter addresses these issues, focusing on the anesthetic consideration and highlighting the differences between children and adults. It alerts the anesthetist, who may not be familiar with anesthesia in small children, to the risks of iatrogenic subglottic stenosis resulting from inappropriate endotracheal intubation. It also addresses the difficulty of single-lung ventilation, selective bronchial intubation, or both, in young children, and offers practical suggestions on selective bronchial occlusion. Although the authors state that thoracoscopic procedures are possible under spontaneous ventilation, in my opinion, there is very little margin for error. It is *essential* for all pediatric patients to be intubated, paralyzed, and ventilated so that the anesthetist has full control of the situation at all times.

Although the authors state that the thoracic cavity is not insufflated for thoracoscopy, it must be stated that this is an accepted alternative method of deflating the lung, and it is a practice I use, if necessary. I have found insufflation combined with blunt dissection particularly useful in decortication to break down loculi.

The section on thoracoscopic techniques broadly covers the types of procedures possible today. It also highlights some of the important technical difficulties of operating in a small space, such as the difficulty of deploying an Endo-GIA, and offers the practical alternative of using an Endoloop to snare a piece of lung for biopsy. One must, however, not forget that it is possible—and quite easy—to grab the lung, under thoracoscopic guidance, to perform an extracorporeal biopsy either through the trocar site or via a 1- to 2-cm mini-thoracotomy.

Laborde has described patent ductus arteriosus (PDA) ligation in a separate chapter, and it is similarly addressed in this chapter as well. This serves to highlight that this will be a very important clinical application, because information published to date shows that the results are at least as good as those obtained with conventional open surgery with reference to residual patency rate and incidence of recurrent laryngeal nerve damage. I would not be surprised if thoracoscopic PDA ligation replaces conventional thoracotomy almost entirely in the new millennium.

As in the case of PDA, there are several other relatively common conditions, such as tuberculosis and diaphragmatic hernia repair, that are not addressed in this chapter, but they occupy full chapters in their own right. The reader should, therefore refer, to these chapters for further details. Achalasia is also covered in a separate chapter.

Congenital abnormalities, such as cystic adenomatoid malformation and congenital lobar emphysema, are still currently managed by conventional thoracotomy. Although I have not had personal experience dealing with these conditions using minimally invasive methods, Dr. Yim has reported thoracoscopic resection of a cystic adenomatoid malformation.[4]

One other point I wish to make is that it is not always necessary to perform all procedures using endoscopy alone. One must not forget that an endoscopically assisted operation, such as the combination of VATS with a mini-thoracotomy, which allows the surgeon to insert one or two fingers for digital palpation, is a very useful technique.

There is no doubt that minimally invasive thoracoscopic surgery will become an important tool in the management of many pediatric conditions, because it will reduce the need for thoracotomy in many benign and malignant conditions in children such as infective empyema, and in the management of mediastinal tumors.

One can sense from reading this chapter that there is a rapidly expanding role for VATS in pediatrics. Most childhood diseases in the chest are completely curable with relatively simple procedures, such as decortication, excision, or ligation. If VATS can replace open thoracotomy for these disorders, its place in the armamentarium of the thoracic surgeon is assured. The authors have achieved the objective of demonstrating the broad spectrum of diseases that are now treatable via VATS, and have also comprehensively addressed the very crucial issue of safety.

References

1. Chetcuti P, Myers NA, Phelan PD, et al: Chest wall deformity in patients with repaired esophageal atresia. J Pediatr Surg 24:244–247, 1989.
2. Westfelt JN, Nordwall A: Thoracotomy and scoliosis. Spine 9:1124, 1125, 1991.
3. Van Biezen FC, Bakx PA, De Villeneuve VH, et al: Scoliosis in children after thoracotomy for aortic coarctation. J Bone Joint Surg Am 75:514–518, 1993.
4. Yim APC: Video-assisted thoracoscopic resection of type 1 cystic adenomatoid malformation in a 3 month old girl. Surg Endosc 9:1292–1294, 1995.

Chapter 38

The Diaphragm

Simon R. Knight and C. Peter Clarke

Anatomy

The diaphragm is a muscular structure consisting of two dome-shaped hemidiaphragms separating the abdominal and thoracic cavities. Each consists of radial muscles originating posteriorly from the costal margins and arcuate ligaments, which insert into a central area of tenderness. The nerve supply is from the third, fourth, and fifth cervical roots on each side via the phrenic nerves running down alongside the pericardium, with some minor lateral supply from the adjacent intercostal nerves. Posteriorly, the muscle is augmented by the right and left crurae. The right crura wraps around the esophageal hiatus and has a role in maintaining the integrity of the cardiac sphincter. The diaphragm is penetrated by the inferior vena cava, the aorta, and the esophagus (Fig. 38–1*A,B*). The blood supply is obtained directly from the aorta posteriorly, from the intercostal vessels, laterally and from the inferior mammary artery and the superior epigastric arteries anteriorly. The veins mainly run on the inferior surface to the inferior vena cava, but there may be some connection with the hepatic veins.

Intra-abdominal pressure is generally greater than intrathoracic pressure, and the normal position of the diaphragm is bowed upward, allowing the liver and spleen to have the protection of the rib cage (Fig. 38–2). The muscle fibers flatten the diaphragm during inspiration, increasing the size of the thoracic cavity, and relax during expiration, allowing intra-abdominal pressure to push the diaphragm upward.

The upper surface of each hemidiaphragm can be inspected by thoracoscopy from above, except that part immediately below the pericardial sac. The whole of the undersurface of the diaphragm can be inspected by laparoscopy, although complete inspection of the right hemidiaphragm is achieved only after mobilization of the liver.

Embryology

The diaphragm originates anteriorly from the septum transversum, laterally from paired lateral portions of the pleuroperitoneal folds, and posteriorly from a rather complexly shaped medial dorsal portion (Fig. 38–3). Muscle fibers migrate from the third, fourth, and fifth cervical myotomes, carrying their innervation with them. Delays in the fusion of the various parts can lead to congenital defects in the diaphragm, which are often associated with anomalies of the heart and lungs.

Technique of Video-Assisted Thoracic Surgery (VATS) on the Diaphragm

Anesthesia is administered via a double-lumen endotracheal tube that allows collapse of the lung. The patient is in the full lateral position, with the arm drawn upward to pull the scapula upward and forward, and the operating table is broken to reduce the prominence of the hip. Because it is easier for the operator to work in a forward direction, the arc placement of ports should be focused downward as shown in Figure 38–4. The telescope is at the apex of the arc toward the assistant, and three of four 5-mm ports are placed to allow passage of suturing instruments. For most purposes, a straight telescope is used, but a 30-degree telescope is useful in the posterior recesses of the diaphragm. If a small incision is required for larger instruments or staplers, it should be in the most anterior position, where the intercostal space is widest. Most of the more complicated procedures of the diaphragm require the operator to have facility in using endosurgical suturing techniques.[19]

Congenital Hernias

Congenital diaphragmatic hernia can occur anteriorly (Morgagni) between the digitations to the sternum and costal cartilage, and posteriorly (Bochdalek). Large posterior hernias caused by failure of maturation in the pleuroperitoneal canal are usually found on the left side and are associated with agenesis of the left lung; these hernias constitute a neonatal emergency. Smaller posterior hernias may present in adult life and can be confirmed and repaired by VATS techniques.[15] Morgagni hernias present with pain and breathlessness in later life and are best repaired from below.

Hiatal Hernias

Hernias through the esophageal hiatus are paraesophageal when part of the stomach finds its way into the chest alongside the esophagus with no dislocation of the cardiac sphincter or sliding hernias if the cardiac sphincter between the stomach and the esophagus slips up into the thorax (Fig. 38–5). Whereas paraesophageal hernias may be congenital, sliding hiatal hernias are usually acquired. Symptoms are caused by acid reflux associated with an incompetent sphincter mechanism.

A technique for repair of paraesophageal hernia, which uses a VATS approach has been outlined.[6] Uncomplicated

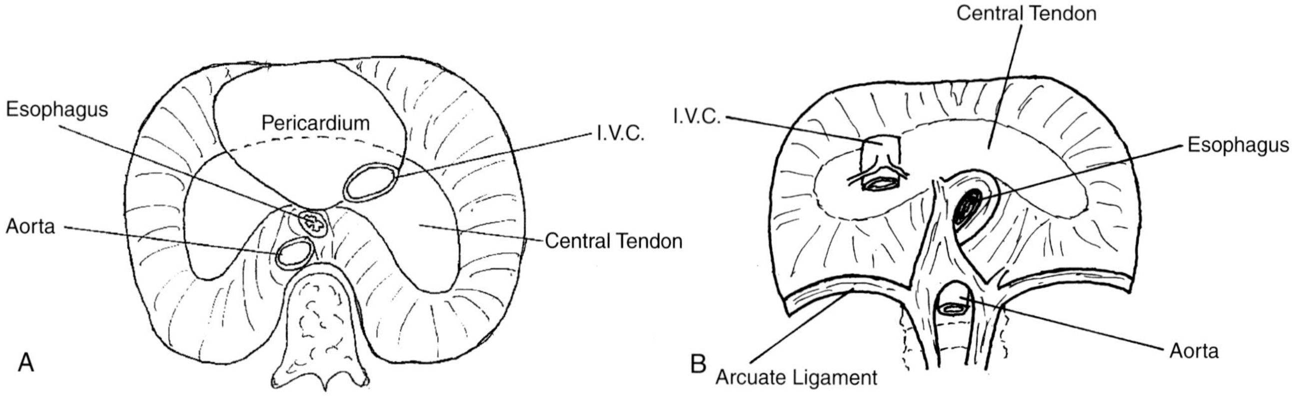

Figure 38–1. *A*, Shows the superior surface of the diaphragm; *B*, shows the inferior surface of the diaphragm. I.V.C. = inferior vena cava.

sliding hiatal hernias are most commonly dealt with by laparoscopic techniques,[2] but a technique for thoracoscopic fundoplication has been described,[13] which may be an advantage in obese patients or in those who have had previous abdominal surgery. A successful thoracoscopic repair following failed fundoplication for reflux in three children was reported by Sartotelli and associates.[14] The rationale for all these repairs is to reposition the esophagogastric junction below the diaphragm, reconstituting its angle and tightening the hiatus.

Eventration of the Diaphragm

Eventration of the diaphragm is a rare condition that may follow paralysis of the phrenic nerve or that may be caused by failure of muscular tissue to extend into the pleuroperitoneal membrane during development. The diaphragm moves paradoxically, or only a little, during respiratory effort, with secondarily impaired respiratory function and atelectasis of the basal segments of the lower lobe on the affected side, which is most commonly the left. Paralysis of the phrenic nerve, particularly if bilateral, can lead to acute respiratory failure in children, but diaphragmatic eventration usually presents in adults who have dyspnea or chronic cough, and needs to be differentiated from an old rupture or hernia of the diaphragm. Repair consists of plication of the diaphragm, with flattening and strengthening, which increases the vital capacity and prevents paradoxical movement. We favor a thoracoscopic approach (Figs. 38–6 and 38–7) using a suture plication technique, which has yielded good results in three patients.[5]

Several parallel 0 polypropelene sutures are placed in a drawstring manner and adjusted under vision until the desired flattening of the diaphragm is achieved. All three patients were dyspneic on exertion before surgery, and all could perform normal activities without dyspnea after repair. To date the period of follow-up is 24 months. Although measured improvement in pulmonary function tests has been modest (Fig. 38–8), the improvements in

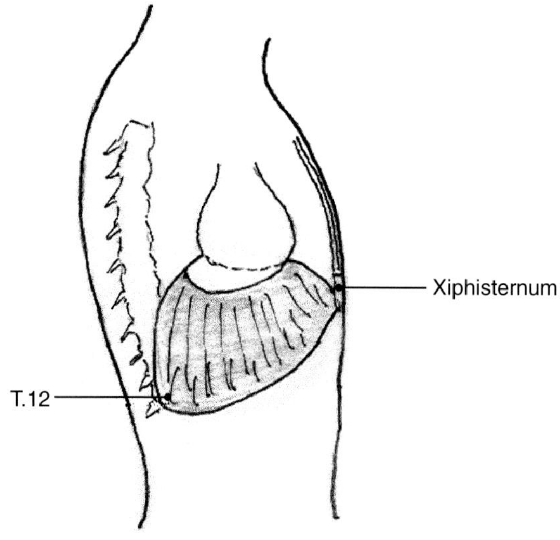

Figure 38–2. Lateral view of the diaphragm.

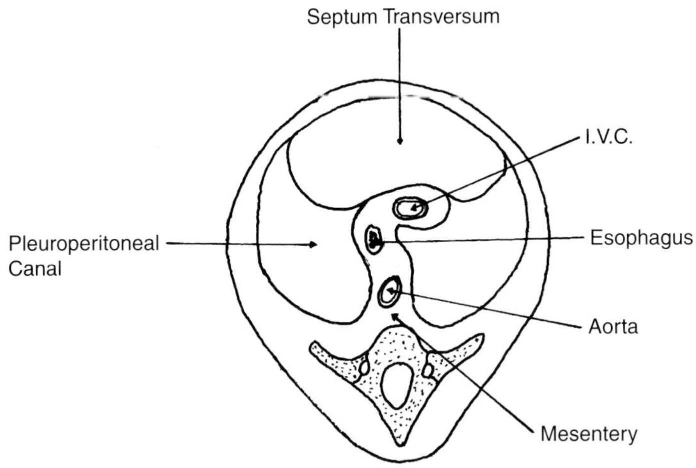

Figure 38–3. Shows embryology of the diaphragm.

ventilation perfusion studies show markedly increased function in the lower lobe, which explains the excellent clinical results in these patients (Figs. 38–9 and 38–10). Others have used a double-suture technique[10] or a similar multiple-suture technique.[17]

Permanent phrenic nerve paralysis, which is indistinguishable from eventration of the diaphragm, can be managed in a similar fashion.[4]

Trauma to the Diaphragm

Video-assisted thoracoscopy (VAT) is a valuable tool in the evaluation and management of thoracic trauma, a topic that is detailed more fully in another chapter (see Chapter 39). Injuries and ruptures of the diaphragm can be detected thoracoscopically, either acutely after injury,[8] or later, if a previously missed diaphragmatic injury is suspected.[7] In the acute situation, the safest course is to proceed to laparotomy or laparoscopy in view of the likelihood of associated intra-abdominal injuries. Blunt injuries of the diaphragm are generally caused by compression of the abdomen, and, in particular, there may be associated duodenal injuries. Penetrating injuries of the diaphragm may be associated with direct damage to the intestines or liver.

Ruptures of the diaphragm detected later do not pose the same problem as associated intra-abdominal injuries that are already manifest. Figure 38–11 shows a rupture of the diaphragm discovered 7 days after the

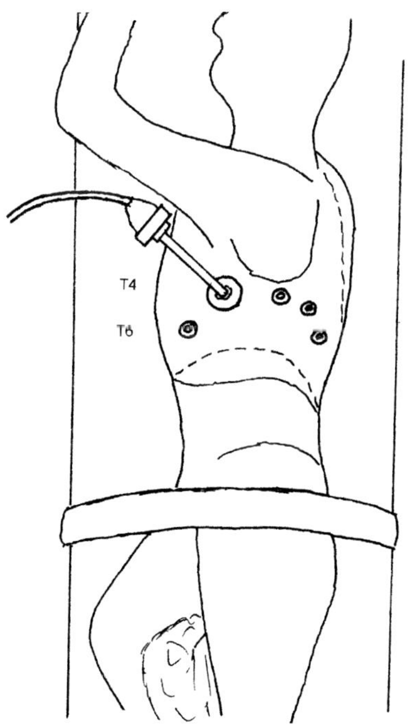

Figure 38–4. Shows placement of ports.

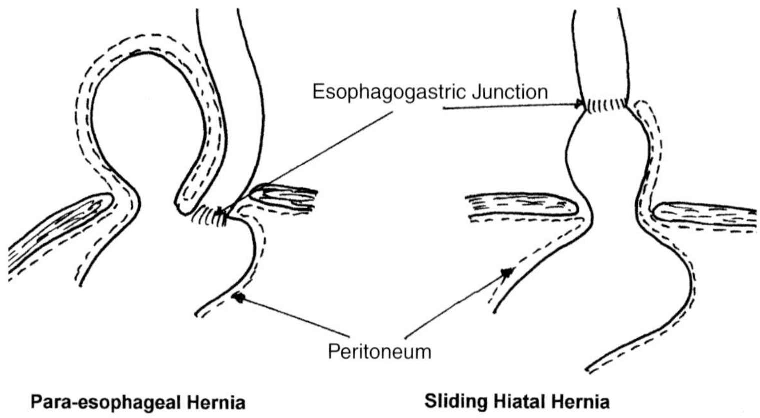

Figure 38–5. Shows types of hiatal hernia.

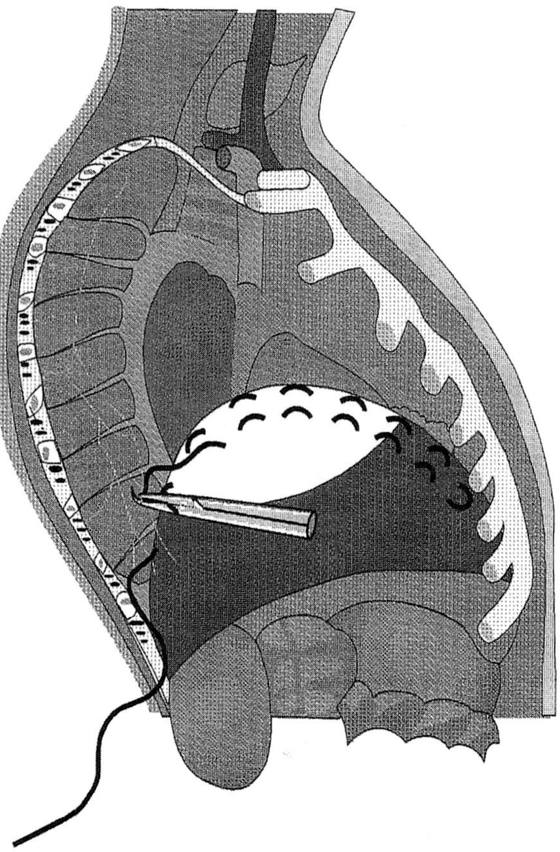

Figure 38–6. Thoracoscopic repair of eventration of the diaphragm: Placement of suture.

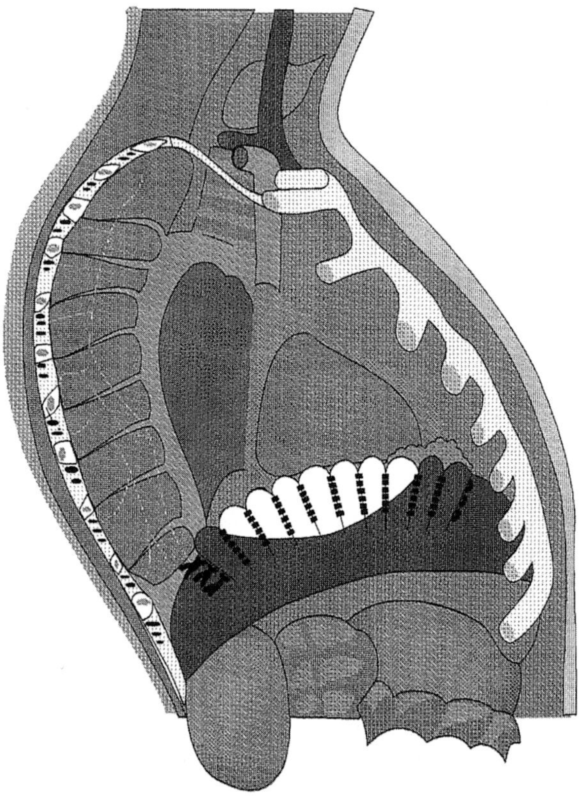

Figure 38–7. Thoracoscopic repair of eventration of the diaphragm: Sutures have been tightened.

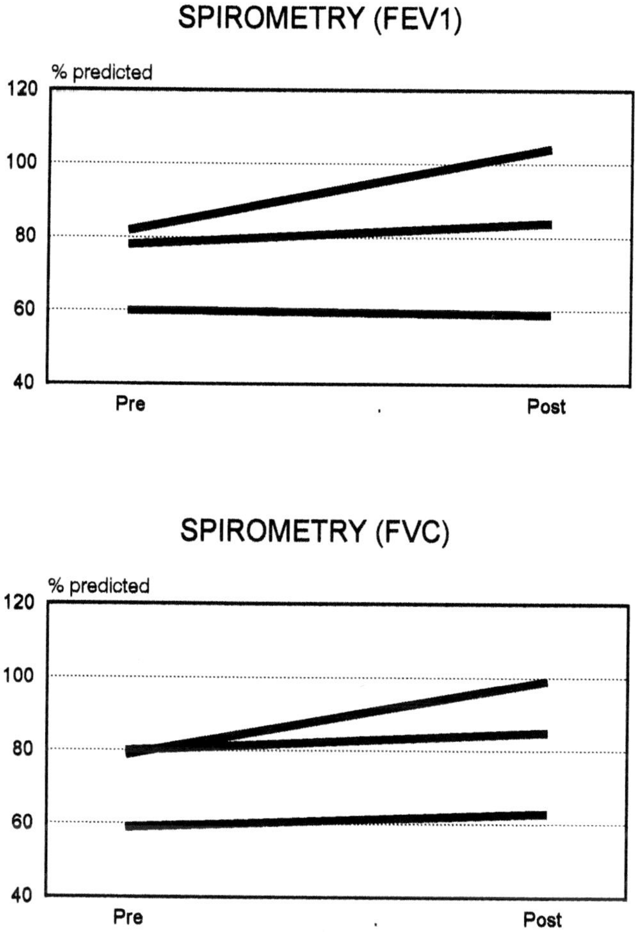

Figure 38–8. Changes in spirometry in patients having repair of eventration of the diaphragm.

acute injury. This was repaired thoracoscopically by direct sutures. We have performed VAT inspection in five patients who were suspected of having ruptured diaphragms sometime after the acute injury. Four ruptures were confirmed, of which two were repaired by VAT techniques and two by open thoracotomy. One patient proved to have an eventration of the diaphragm and not a rupture. Nel and Warren[12] were able to show in a prospective trial involving 55 patients who had knife wounds of the chest, a projected negative laparotomy rate of 63%. Laparotomy was avoided by thoracoscopic evaluation of the diaphragm, which detected only six actual diaphragmatic injuries. Minimal access techniques for the evaluation of thoracic trauma and, in particular, evaluation of integrity of the diaphragm,[11] have also been found useful in children.[1, 14]

Tumors of the Diaphragm

Primary tumors of the diaphragm are rare, and benign neoplasms are found more frequently than malignant ones.[16] Secondary tumors as part of general pleural seeding are more common and usually present as a pleural effusion. The most common benign tumors are fibromas and similar tumors of mesenchymal origin, but neurogenic tumors also occur.[9] The most common malignant tumors are correspondingly, fibrosarcoma and neurogenic sarcoma. Video thoracoscopy is useful for diagnosis, but treatment generally consists of wide excision and reconstitution of the diaphragm with prosthetic material, necessitating an open technique.

The diaphragm is also generally involved in the primary pleural tumor—malignant mesothelioma—which usually occurs many years after asbestos exposure. As is the case with other pleural tumors, the first manifestation is often a pleural effusion; however, a definitive diagnosis is hard to make based on aspiration cytology alone, and, generally, a thoracoscopic biopsy is required for histologic confirmation.

Miscellaneous Conditions

Catamenial pneumothorax is a rare condition caused by thoracic endometriosis, which usually involves the diaphragm. It can be detected and treated by VAT by fulgu-

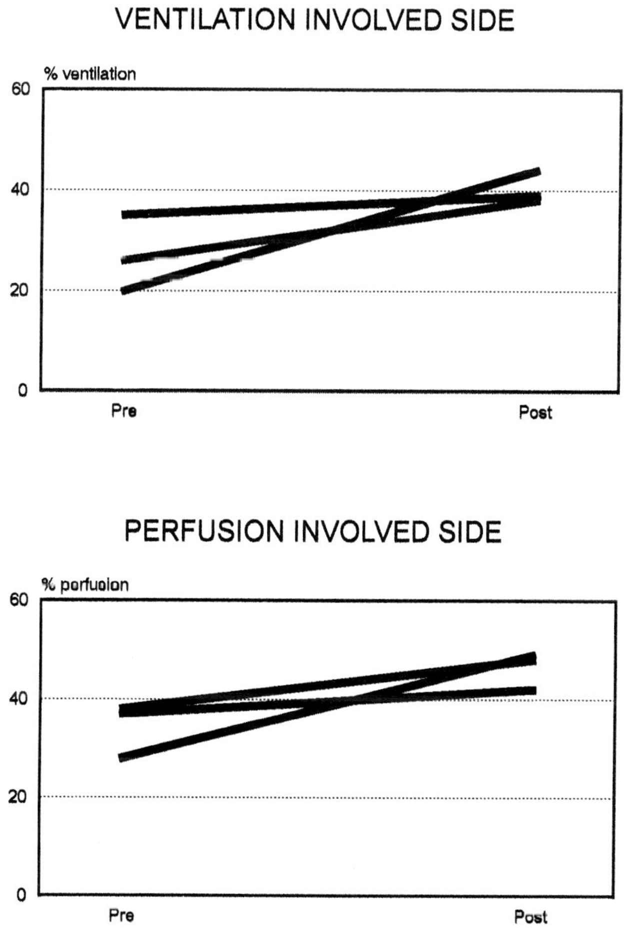

Figure 38–9. Changes in inhalation and perfusion in patients having repair of eventration of the diaphragm.

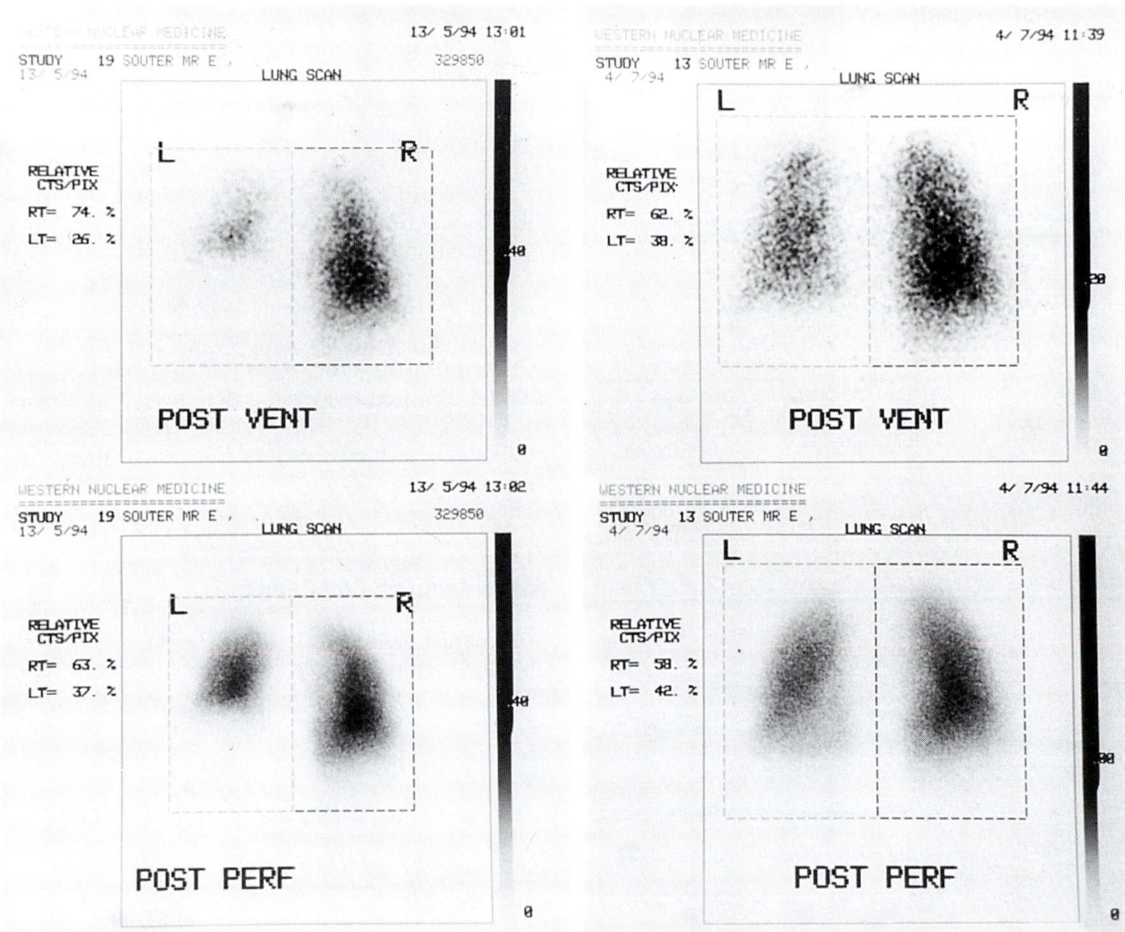

Figure 38–10. V/Q scan in one patient before and after repair of eventration of the diaphragm.

rating the ectopic endometrial tissue and performing pleurodesis.[10, 18]

Another condition that can be treated effectively by VAT techniques is an effusion that occurs during peritoneal dialysis because of small flaws in the diaphragm. These can be detected and closed, or pleurodesis can be performed,[3] which allows the patient to continue use of peritoneal dialysis.

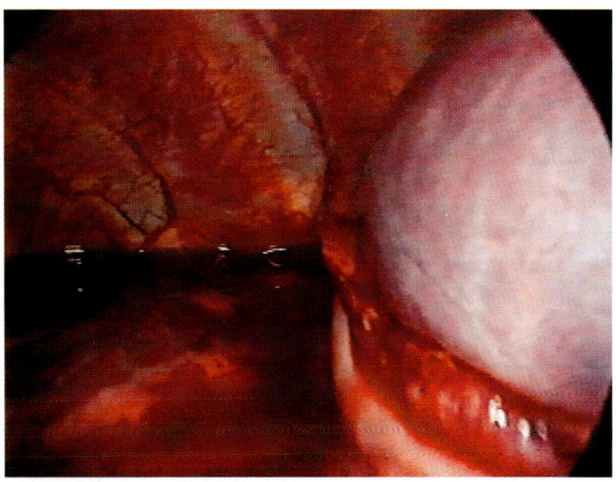

Figure 38–11. Thoracoscopic view of the diaphragm 7 days after injury, showing a linear rupture of the hemidiaphragm.

Summary

The diaphragm is inspected easily by VATS techniques, and this is useful in cases of trauma. If an acute injury is detected, a laparotomy or laparoscopy is required, because there is a likelihood of associated intra-abdominal injury; however, tears detected after the acute phase can be managed from above.

Repair of eventration of the diaphragm by VATS is the procedure of choice. Most congenital and hiatal hernias are best managed from below, but recurrent hernias may require revision from a thoracic approach.

All primary and secondary tumors of the diaphragm can be biopsied by a VATS approach, but most major resections require an open approach.

References

1. Chen MK, Schropp KP, Lobe TE: The use of minimal access surgery in pediatric trauma: A preliminary report. J Laparoendosc Surg 5:295–301, 1995.
2. Cuschieri A: Laparoscopic antireflux surgery and repair of hiatal hernia. World J Surg 17:40–43, 1993.
3. Di Bisceglie M, Paladini P, Voltolini L, et al: Videothoracoscopic

obliteration of pleuroperitoneal fistula in continuous peritoneal dialysis. Ann Thorac Surg 62:1509–1510, 1996.
4. Gharagozloo F, McReynolds SD, Snyder L: Thoracoscopic plication of the diaphragm. Surg Endosc 9:1204–1206, 1995.
5. Knight SR, Clarke CP: VATS plication of diaphragmatic eventration. Ann Thorac Cardiovasc Surg 4:240–243, 1998.
6. Hurley JP, McCarthy JF, Wood AE: Thoracoscopic assisted paraoesophageal hernia repair. Scand J Thorac Cardiovasc Surg 28:94–96, 1994.
7. Koehler RH, Smith RS: Thoracoscopic repair of missed diaphragmatic injury in penetrating trauma: Case report. J Trauma 36:424–427, 1994.
8. Lang-Lazdunski L, Mouroux J, Pons F, et al: Role of video thoracoscopy in chest trauma. Ann Thorac Surg 63:327–333, 1997.
9. McClenathan JH, Okada F: Primary neurilemoma of the diaphragm. Ann Thorac Surg 48:126–128, 1989.
10. Mouroux J, Padovani B, Poirier NC, et al: Technique for the repair of diaphragmatic eventration. Ann Thorac Surg 62: 905–907, 1996.
11. Namias N. McKenney M, Sosa JL, et al: Laparoscopic repair of a gunshot wound to the diaphragm. A case report. J Laparoendosc Surg 5:59–61, 1995.
12. Nel JH, Warren BL: Thoracoscopic evaluation of the diaphragm in patients with knife wounds of the left lower chest. Br J Surg 81:713–714, 1994.
13. Salo JA, Kivilvoto, T, Heikkila L, et al: Thoracoscopic fundoplication. Ann Chir Gynaecol 82:199–201, 1993.
14. Sartotelli KH, Rothenberg SS, Karrer FM, et al: Thoracoscopic repair of hiatal hernia following fundoplication: A new approach to an old problem. J Laparoendosc Surg 6 (suppl 1):591–593, 1996.
15. Sato Y, Ishikawa S, Onizuka M, et al: Thoracoscopic repair of diaphragmatic hernia. Thorac Cardiovasc Surg 44:54–55, 1996.
16. Sbokos CG, Salama FD, Powell V, et al: Primary fibrosarcoma of the diaphragm. Br J Dis Chest 71(1):49–52, 1977.
17. Suzumura Y, Terada Y, Sonobe M, et al: A case of unilateral diaphragmatic eventration treated by plication with thoracoscopic surgery. Chest 112:530–532, 1997.
18. Van Schil PE, Vercauteren SR, Vermiere PA, et al: Catamenial pneumothorax caused by thoracic endometriosis. Ann Thorac Surg 62:585–586, 1996.
19. Yamashita J, Iwasaki A, Kawahara K, et al: Thoracoscopic approach to the diagnosis and treatment of diaphragmatic disorders. Surg Laparosc Endosc 6:485–488, 1966.

COMMENTARY

Stephen R. Hazelrigg

The total reported experience of video-assisted thoracic surgery (VATS) in the treatment of diaphragmatic problems is not extensive, and, as such, makes any firm conclusions with regard to the role of VATS difficult. Although VATS may be used for repair of eventrations, this probably should be considered a moderate technical challenge to be reserved for those who have significant thoracoscopic experience. The potential for deep suture injury to abdominal organs and for sutures coming loose after intracorporeal knots exists, and the number of cases treated is still too small to advocate VATS as the gold standard. As noted, the majority of antireflux and hernia procedures are best performed from the abdomen.

In a patient who has stable trauma, thoracoscopy does seem to have a role in identifying, confirming, or repairing traumatic diaphragmatic tears. Similarly, diagnostic biopsy of the diaphragm for lesions is quick and easily performed by means of VATS. In diaphragmatic problems, VATS clearly has a role that will continue to be refined with time and experience.

Chapter 39

Chest Trauma

Ganga Prabhakar and Geoffrey M. Graeber

Thoracoscopy and video-assisted thoracic surgery (VATS) have come to play a definitive role in the diagnosis and management of thoracic trauma. The use of video-assisted surgery in managing traumatic chest injuries requires careful clinical decision-making, because the patient can be hemodynamically unstable and must meet specific criteria before VATS is used in diagnosis, treatment, or both. Our knowledge of VATS and how it may be employed in evaluation and treatment of trauma patients has expanded since previous reviews.[16, 17]

Trauma is the leading cause of death in children and adults up to 44 years of age, and it kills more Americans aged 1 to 34 than all other diseases combined.[19] As many as one fourth of all trauma deaths are a direct consequence of chest injury, and two thirds of these occur after the patient reaches the hospital.[19] Most thoracic injuries can be treated by close observation, volume replacement, respiratory care, serial chest radiographs, and tube thoracostomy. A small number have unstable hemodynamics and require treatment in the emergency room or thoracotomy in the operating room. Up to 21% of patients who have penetrating trauma of the thorax may require surgical intervention.[39]

This chapter discusses the role of VATS in treating patients who have limited, continuing, intrapleural hemorrhage and retained hemothoraces. It also examines the place of thoracoscopy and VATS in early empyema. The improved contribution of VATS in evaluating and treating acute diaphragmatic injuries is presented. The limitations of thoracoscopy in the treatment of pericardial, cardiac, and mediastinal injuries are evaluated. Finally, the technical aspects of performing VATS in trauma are reviewed.

History

The endoscopic examination of the thoracic cavity in a dog was first performed in Dresden, Germany, by Kelling in 1901. The human application was evaluated by Jacobaeus of Stockholm in 1903 and published in 1910.[25] He studied patients who had pulmonary tuberculosis and suggested the use of galvanocautery to lyse adhesions—Jacobaeus' operation. The thoracoscopic diagnosis and treatment of traumatic injury were undertaken in May 1943 by Braco in Brazil.[4] In 1946, he presented 5 patients who had penetrating wounds of the thorax, which were treated successfully by thoracoscopic evacuation of blood with reinfusion. Almost 30 years later, two additional reports were described in 1974 and 1975.[41, 42] The technique had an exponential rise in application after it was described by Jackson and Ferreira in 1976 for the diagnosis of diaphragmatic injuries.[24] In a larger study performed in 1981, in which rigid thoracoscopic evaluation was used, Jones and associates found that moderate continuing hemorrhage could be evacuated and treated in most patients by use of local anesthesia.[26] In 33 of 36 patients evaluated by this group, local anesthesia was appropriate; only 3 patients required general endotracheal anesthesia via double-lumen tube. A standard rigid thoracoscope, introduced through sites where chest tubes had been placed in the emergency department and withdrawn in the operating suite, was sufficient to evaluate and treat persistent hemorrhage. The use of a flexible fiberoptic bronchoscope, employed as a thoracoscope, has also been reported to control continuing intrapleural hemorrhage, remove clots, and re-expand the lung. For a complete review of the history of thoracoscopic surgery, the reader is advised to refer to Chapter 1.[8]

Contraindications to VATS in Trauma Patients

Before exploring the indications for using VATS in the evaluation of patients with chest trauma, the absolute contraindications for VATS in trauma patients must be understood. The proper use of VATS in these patients requires the best judgment of a mature surgeon, because miscalculation can be followed by the patient's demise. Thus, VATS has a limited, but clearly defined, role in the diagnosis and treatment of specific chest injuries. Inappropriate patient selection can lead to a desperate situation that will most likely result in the patient's death (Table 39–1). Obviously, if the patient is hemodynamically unstable, any VATS procedure is contraindicated. No patient who has systolic arterial pressure lower than 90 mm Hg is a candidate for a VATS procedure. Suspected injuries to the heart or great vessels caused by penetrating trauma also preclude a VATS procedure, because immediate catastrophic hemorrhage could occur at any time. These patients are best evaluated and treated by using standard incisions.

If the treating surgeon also has any reason to suspect a blunt injury to the vital structures, a VATS procedure should be abandoned in favor of an open approach. A widened mediastinum on standard radiographic examinations can also suggest a dangerous injury to the heart or great vessels. Such findings dictate that the patient should be explored through an open approach, because the risk of catastrophic hemorrhage is high. Similarly, suspected injuries to the trachea or a major bronchus require repair through an open approach, because endoscopic techniques at the present time are inadequate to repair a major tracheobronchial injury. Substantial hemorrhage also suggests significant injury to the heart or great vessels. Usually, a thoracotomy should be performed if the blood loss is greater than 500 ml/hour through a tube thoracostomy and if bleeding persists for more than 2 hours. The immediate loss of 1500 ml of blood on initial tube thoracostomy drainage usually heralds an injury to the heart or

Table 39–1. Contraindication to Thoracoscopic Surgery in Thoracic Trauma

Hemodynamic instability
- Signs of hypovolemic shock
- Cardiac arrhythmia

Suspected injuries to the heart or great vessels
- Widened mediastinum
- Blunt trauma with suspected cardiac contusion or other injury to the heart

Suspicion of major injuries to the trachea or bronchus

Substantial hemorrhage
- Bleeding of more than 500 ml per hour
- Initial drainage by tube thoracostomy of 1500 ml of pleural blood and clots

Inability to tolerate one-lung ventilation
- Previous injury or surgery
- Severe pulmonary contusion
- Intercurrent lung disease
- Bilateral lung injury

Other emergency conditions requiring major operative procedures to stabilize the patient
- Celiotomy
- Craniotomy

great vessels sufficient to warrant immediate open exploration. Similarly, any given patient who is unable to tolerate the collapse of one lung because of previous pleural disease, previous injury, surgical procedures, or concurrent pulmonary disease cannot undergo VATS.

If the patient is suffering from major life-threatening injury to other organs, this condition must be addressed first. A condition requiring a celiotomy or a craniotomy must be addressed and the patient stabilized before any VATS procedure can be considered. Realistically, VATS should be used only in a stable patient who can tolerate the procedure to achieve limited diagnostic and therapeutic goals.

Technical Considerations

The patient must be placed on the operating table so that a full thoracotomy may be performed if it should be necessary. Appliances that should be placed on the table to stabilize the patient include supports, a bean bag, straps, and tapes. The patient is fully secured to the table in a way that the table may be fully rotated as needed if a thoracotomy should be necessary. Preparation of the patient and draping should be wide enough to prepare for a potential full thoracotomy or any incision needed to correct major hemorrhage in the lungs, heart, or great vessels.

Careful preparation for appropriate anesthesia is mandatory for VATS procedures in treating trauma patients. The patient should have a double-lumen endotracheal tube in place, even though this can add significantly to the anesthetic time. Some trauma patients may decompensate their respiratory or cardiac status on single-lung ventilation. This can occur because of pulmonary contusion or hemothorax of the contralateral side. Proper monitoring should be instituted to maintain the patient and to plan for the eventuality of a major thoracic exploration. Electrocardiograph leads must be placed on the patient so that all possible leads may be evaluated. Continuous pulse oximetry is mandatory. An arterial line should be inserted to give an arterial wave form and provide access for blood gases should they be needed. A Foley catheter should be placed to monitor urine output.

Intravenous access is very important, because hemorrhage can be substantial. It is recommended that several large-bore lines be established for blood replacement. Transfusion requirements may be substantial if a particularly serious injury to the heart or major vessels is encountered. Usually, blood should be available, because major hemorrhage can ensue. If the hemorrhage occurs without proper preparation, universal donor blood may be needed for immediate transfusion to save the patient's life. A central line access site should be established as well. The placement of a large introducer in the internal jugular vein usually provides adequate access should it be needed. This port provides a site for blood replacement if hemorrhage occurs. It also offers access for placement of a Swan-Ganz catheter if it becomes necessary to monitor the cardiac performance of the patient closely. Separate intravenous lines should be maintained for cardiotropic drugs, vasoactive agents, and antibiotics. There should be constant vigilance for a possible contralateral pneumothorax, which may have gone unrecognized at the initial trauma evaluation.

Several other pieces of equipment are required in the preparation of a VATS procedure. There should be at least one, preferably two, electrocautery and suction units available. A bipolar unit can also be very helpful in cauterizing intrathoracic bleeding. Several different types of suction tips should be present: the standard Yankauer, the Poole (sump), and the endoscopic suction tip. Large volumes of warm saline irrigation may be required to evacuate the hemothorax before the source of bleeding is identified. Upon completion of the procedure, the port sites can be used for the newly inserted chest tubes.

Evaluation and Treatment of Persistent Intrathoracic Hemorrhage

Patients who have persistent hemorrhage after trauma may be selected for VATS evaluation and treatment if specific criteria are met (Table 39–2). The patients must be hemodynamically stable; those who are not should be taken to the operating room immediately for open correction through an incision appropriate for the injury.[16, 17, 26] If a patient experiences continued moderate hemorrhage (200 to 500 ml/hr) through tube thoracostomies that have re-expanded the lung, VATS evaluation and treatment are appropriate.

Between February 1992 and February 1993, Smith and associates conducted a prospective trial of videothoracoscopy at an urban trauma center to evaluate the efficacy of this modality in evaluating and treating patients who had thoracic injuries.[43] Of these patients they evaluated (22 had penetrating injuries, 2 had blunt injuries), 5 were taken to surgery for persistent hemorrhage from intercostal arterial injury (more than 1500 ml of blood loss in a 24-hour period). The use of diathermy achieved hemostasis in 3 patients without the use of thoracotomy.

Table 39–2. Indications for Thoracoscopy in Thoracic Trauma

Persistent hemorrhage	Moderate in nature Stable patient
Retained hemothorax	Evacuation of the clot Re-expansion of the lung
Empyema	Early intervention Evacuation of the pleural space Drainage Re-expansion of the lung Culture
Diaphragmatic injuries	Diagnosis Treatment
Chylothorax	
Removal of foreign bodies	Proper instrumentation Care to avoid major hemorrhage
Evaluation of heart and great vessels	Questionable diagnostic role Therapy requires open procedures for safety
Treatment of persistent air leak	Identity of cause Correct source

Retained Hemothorax After Thoracic Trauma

A logical extension of VATS for control of continued hemorrhage is the drainage of retained hemothoraces and residual pleural clot. For a detailed review of this indication, see the chapter on empyema and hemothorax.[2] Continued retention of liquid, clotted blood, or both in the thorax results in fibrothorax and entrapment of the lung secondary to failed resolution and resorption of the blood and clot.[11, 16] Of 9000 patients presenting to Ben Taub General Hospital in Houston, Texas, 3000 (33%) presented with hemothorax.[35] Of these patients, 2600 (85%) underwent drainage procedures; 85 patients (3.3%) required operative evacuation. In one retrospective review at an urban trauma center, Coselli and associates found that retained hemothoraces after tube thoracostomy placement occurred in fewer than 4% of 4766 patients who presented with traumatic hemothorax or hemopneumothorax.[11] Although this uncommon complication may be innocuous, it may result in a trapped lung, decreased pulmonary capabilities, prolonged time on a ventilator, and increased length of hospital stay, with a concomitant increase in hospital costs.

Several reports have focused on the use of VATS rather than standard thoracotomy for evacuating retained blood and clot from the traumatized pleural space. Smith and associates found that 9 of the 24 chest trauma patients they studied prospectively had clotted hemothoraces that would have required thoracotomies for evacuation.[43] In 8 of the 9 patients who had clotted hemothoraces, videothoracoscopy was used successfully to evacuate the clot and restore normal respiratory dynamics.[43] A time factor is related to success in evacuating the retained blood and clot as has been shown by Macini and associates.[32] They demonstrated that retained hemothoraces are more easily removed the sooner they are addressed. Ideally, clots and old blood should be removed within the first 24 hours after recognition. The longer the retained blood and clot remain in the pleural space, the more dense the resolving fibrosis becomes, making complete removal more difficult and time consuming.

Heniford and associates at the University of Louisville School of Medicine reviewed 25 patients who had retained thoracic collections after trauma.[22] These patients underwent 26 different thoracoscopic procedures for evacuation of retained blood in the pleural cavity. In 19 patients, thoracoscopic evacuation was successful. In 4 patients, thoracoscopy had to be abandoned, and an open thoracotomy had to be conducted to evacuate the clot successfully and re-expand the lung. In an additional 2 patients, subsequent procedures were required to achieve successful drainage of the retained collections. In their review, the authors found that the failure of thoracoscopy was directly proportional to the time lapse between the injury and the surgical procedure to remove the clot and re-expand the lung. Failure of thoracoscopy could also be correlated with the type of collection present in the chest but not with the mechanism of injury. It was found that when thoracoscopy was conducted within 7 days of admission, there were no patients who had any evidence of empyema at surgery. These authors concluded that videothoracoscopy is an accurate, safe, and reliable operative procedure used to achieve successful removal of retained thoracic collections after trauma. They indicated that their results reflected good postoperative results in 90% of the patients in whom the procedure was successfully conducted. The early evacuation of retained blood and fluid from the pleural space resulted in a reduced hospital stay and a concomitant decrease in possible complications. The authors believed that their results were good enough to suggest that videothoracoscopy should be the initial treatment for removal of retained thoracic collections in trauma patients, and that this modality should be used much earlier and more frequently in such patients to shorten hospital stay and decrease hospital costs.

In a paper on the role of videothoracoscopy in chest trauma, 12 patients evaluated at four French medical centers had an average of 1200 ml of fluid (range 500 to 2600 ml) in their thoracic cavities.[29] These authors noted that evacuation of the hemothorax was much more easily conducted if fewer than 10 days had transpired between the time the patient suffered the wound and the video-assisted thoracic exploration. In all but one of the patients, videothoracoscopy was successful in removing the clots around the lung. The sole patient of the 12 who required thoracotomy was operated on 31 days after a stab wound in the left chest. The adhesions were so dense and the blood clots so organized that surgeons had to open the chest to evacuate the maturing fibrothorax and re-expand the lung.

In a published randomized trial of retained hemothorax, one group was assigned to receive a second-tube thoracostomy and the other was to undergo VATS.[34] The group assigned to VATS had a smaller quantity of drainage over a shorter time, a shorter hospital stay, and lower costs. Ten of the 24 patients in the group of the second-tube thoracostomy required VATS or thoracotomy.

Evaluation and Treatment of Empyema

If bacterial contamination complicates a retained intrathoracic collection, empyema thoracis ensues. In series that have evaluated the role of thoracoscopy in diagnosing and treating conditions associated with chest trauma, empyema has occurred relatively infrequently. In fact, only 1 of the 42 patients evaluated and treated in a series reported in 1997 presented with post-traumatic empyema.[29] In most series of patients treated for chest injuries, post-traumatic empyema occurs in 2 to 10% of all cases of thoracic trauma.[13] In many instances that could lead to post-traumatic empyema, early evacuation of infected foreign material, with complete re-expansion of the lung, is the mainstay of therapy.[3, 13] Initial efforts to evacuate the contaminated blood clot and serum usually include multiple tube thoracostomies.[3] Chest tubes can have detrimental effects and can be the route through which bacteria infect the residual clot inside the pleural space.[12, 20] Moreover, prolonged emplacement of chest tubes may be correlated with the development of empyema.[12] Aggressive early thoracoscopic evacuation of the hemothorax may prevent empyema.[43] The incidence of empyema is reported to be less than 1% if the hemothorax occupies less than 35% of the thoracic cavity.[45] There was no incidence of empyema in a group of 105 patients who underwent complete evacuation of hematoma.[45] Some authors have suggested early guided percutaneous drainage,[7] but this has not been widely accepted because of the difficulty of evacuating the infected pleural cavity completely.

Chapter 8 provides more detailed information on the role of VATS in empyema.[2] The largest number of patients in a given series treated by VATS for empyema thoracis appears to be the 76 reported by Landreneau and associates in 1995.[28] Eight of these patients were treated successfully by videothoracoscopy for empyemas arising in retained intrathoracic hematomas caused by chest trauma. O'Brien and associates reported 8 cases of empyema thoracis following penetrating chest injury; these were treated successfully by thoracoscopy.[38] Two patients required subsequent thoracoscopic procedures to release trapped lung and control persistent air leaks. VATS has been reported to be successful in 54% of chronic emphyemas of all causes; whether the same result can be obtained with empyemas of traumatic etiology remains to be seen.[37] Striffeler and associates published their VATS experience with 67 patients who had a preoperative diagnosis of stage II empyema[1] from all causes.[46] Nineteen (28%) patients required conversion to an open procedure because advanced disease was found. Trauma was the cause of empyema in 7% of patients in whom VATS was successfully employed. No preoperative investigation, including computed tomography (CT) scan, was useful in differentiating the patients in whom VATS was likely to be successful. Empyema recurred in 2 (4%) patients who required further surgery.

The Diagnosis and Management of Diaphragmatic Injuries

One of the more perplexing problems of thoracic trauma is the diagnosis of diaphragmatic injuries. It is particularly difficult in the immediate postinjury state. According to some sources, approximately 30% of all diaphragmatic injuries are missed, even when chest radiography, CT, and diagnostic peritoneal lavage are appropriately employed.[14, 30] In an attempt to improve diagnostic acumen, some authors have recommended the use of videolaparoscopy for diagnosis of diaphragmatic injury.[9] Despite some favorable reports, laparoscopy may be inadequate in diagnosing all diaphragmatic injuries, and may even be potentially dangerous, because the air insufflation required for laparoscopy may cause tension pneumothorax by entering the chest through a diaphragmatic defect.[23] Thoracoscopy, on the other hand, does not require air insufflation, yet it gives an excellent view of the diaphragm. For these reasons, some authors advocate the regular use of VATS to assess the diaphragm and determine whether diaphragmatic injury has occurred.[26, 27, 47] The treating surgeon has to realize that injury to intra-abdominal viscera frequently accompanies diaphragmatic injury. Any attempt to correct a diaphragmatic injury without proper preparation for, and correction of, injury to intraperitoneal viscera can leave the patient with a serious, untreated intra-abdominal injury. Such an injury can lead to critical complications.

The chronicled experience of thoracoscopy in evaluating diaphragmatic injuries has been increasing for several years. Over a 6-month period, Uribe and associates evaluated 28 patients who had penetrating thoracoabdominal trauma.[47] Their prospective evaluation by thoracoscopy was conducted in a major trauma center in patients who were hemodynamically stable and who had no indication for immediate celiotomy. All the patients demonstrated sufficient findings of thoracic injury on chest radiography and physical examination to justify surgical exploration. Of 28 patients, 24 suffered stab wounds and 4 had gunshot wounds. The authors were able to identify diaphragmatic injury by thoracoscopy in 9 (32%) patients. All patients who had diaphragmatic injuries underwent celiotomy for confirmation of the injury and appropriate repair. Of the nine (89%) patients undergoing celiotomy, 8 were found to have significant injuries to intra-abdominal viscera, which required direct repair. The authors judged that thoracoscopy was a good diagnostic methodology that was safe in diagnosing diaphragmatic injury; however, their experience underlines the fact that intra-abdominal repair for injuries suffered by intraperitoneal organs is significant and requires direct surgical attention.

Nel and Warren assessed the role of thoracoscopy in evaluating the status of the diaphragm in 55 patients who suffered penetrating knife wounds to the left lower chest.[37] This prospective study showed that those who had positive thoracoscopic findings needed to proceed to laparotomy and that those who had an uninvolved diaphragm could be observed. Twenty-two patients underwent laparotomy and 32 were observed; 1 patient had inconclusive findings at thoracoscopy. Thoracoscopy was 100% sensitive, 90% specific, and 94% accurate in assessing the diaphragm for the presence of diaphragmatic injury. The authors reported that if they had conducted the mandatory celiotomy for supposed diaphragmatic injuries, there would have been a 63% negativity rate. They deemed thoracoscopy as particularly effective, because their actual negative rate was only 6%. Therefore, they concluded that thoracoscopy was a safe and reliable method for evaluating the diaphragm in left lower thoracic stab wounds.

Spann and associates conducted a prospective study on stable patients to evaluate the accuracy of VATS compared with that of exploratory celiotomy in assessing diaphragmatic and thoracoabdominal injuries.[44] Patients underwent both VATS and subsequent celiotomy under the same general anaesthetic. The intraoperative thoracoscopic findings were not presented to the abdominal surgeons who conducted the celiotomies. During the enrollment period of 12 months, 26 patients were entered into the study. Diaphragmatic injuries were identified in 8 (31%) patients. All eight injuries in these patients were identified by VATS. Six of the 8 (75%) patients who had diaphragmatic injuries sustained associated injury to intrathoracic or intra-abdominal organs. The authors found that there was no mortality and no procedural morbidity associated with VATS. More importantly, they found that there were no injuries missed by VATS in patients who underwent surgery. The authors believed their findings supported the position that VATS was a safe, expeditious, and accurate method of evaluating the diaphragm in injured patients. They concluded that VATS was at least comparable in accuracy with exploratory celiotomy and that use of VATS technique could reduce the incidence of negative celiotomies.

In a prospective study conducted in France by Lang-Lazdunski and associates, 14 patients whom they evaluated by VATS had diaphragmatic injuries.[29] In 7 of the 14 patients, VATS showed that the diaphragm had no perceptible injury. These patients were, therefore, not explored either through a thoracic or abdominal incision but were observed. In all instances, VATS yielded a correct evaluation of the status of diaphragmatic injuries. Four patients were identified as having major diaphragmatic injuries and were converted to open thoracotomy. Two additional patients were diagnosed as having diaphragmatic injuries of a lesser nature and underwent minithoracotomy (consisting of a 5-cm incision) to repair the diaphragm. One patient had a small diaphragmatic injury identified, which was able to be closed by endoscopic suture repair techniques. The experience of these surgeons reflects their personal bias for performing a major open procedure to repair any type of substantial diaphragmatic injury and assess both intrathoracic and intra-abdominal organ trauma.

The Management of Chylothorax

Chylothorax is a relatively rare but treatable condition, which may be attributed to trauma. The reader is referred to Chapter 9 for a more detailed discussion of chylothorax.[15] Extensive experience of VATS at the University of Virginia was reported by Graham and associates.[18] In their series performed between 1987 and 1993, 12 VATS procedures were used to treat 10 patients for chylothorax. The patients ranged in age from 7 months to 82 years, and the reasons for surgery included two iatrogenic conditions, two congenital conditions, two caval thromboses, two cases of amyloid disease, one case of blunt trauma, and one metastatic carcinoid tumor. In 8 patients, talc pleurodesis alone was used to resolve the chylothorax. Talc pleurodesis was performed in 1 patient in association with clipping of the thoracic duct and application of fibrin glue. The final patient in the series required clipping of a pleural defect with application of fibrin glue. In 2 of the patients, a video-assisted operation was used in conjunction with pleuroperitoneal shunting. In all cases, the effusion resolved after the patients had been treated by VATS with no subsequent intervention. The authors concluded that VATS offered an effective means of treating chylothorax regardless of its cause, because access could be gained to the thoracic duct and pleural space without performance of major thoracotomy.

In their experience, Lang-Lazdunski and associated encountered 1 patient who had post-traumatic chylothorax.[29] They approached the chylothorax via a more direct procedure. Once the injury to the thoracic duct was recognized, a small thoracotomy was performed with video assistance, and the open end of the thoracic duct was clipped. No pleurodesis was performed.

Complete discussions of chylothorax and the anatomy of the thoracic duct was available.[31] Several successful surgical techniques other than the thoracoscopic procedures have been described for correcting injuries to the thoracic duct and treating chylothorax.[10] These should be consulted for a more thorough discussion of the thoracic duct, its anatomy, and the problems of its repair.

Management of Retained Foreign Bodies

The most extensive reported experience of VATS in removing symptomatic foreign bodies from the thorax comes from France. Lang-Lazdunski and associates treated 4 patients in their series collected from the experience of four hospitals.[29] One patient had painful metal shrapnel embedded in the lingula, which was removed by VATS resection. Another had a Kirschner wire removed from the right pleural space after it migrated from a scapular repair into the chest and caused a hemothorax. Two patients had bullets removed from the chest by use of VATS. These authors cautioned, however, that VATS assessment of possible cardiac and great vessel injuries can be dangerous, because catastrophic hemorrhage or serious arrhythmias can ensue. In 1 patient who had a bullet removed, lethal cardiac arrhythmias claimed the patient's life approximately 36 hours after the projectile had been successfully removed. Bartek and colleagues reported using VATS to remove glass fragments from the chest of a patient.[5] Had the fragments not been removed thoracoscopically, the patient would have required a thoracotomy. The mere presence of a missile in or around the heart or the great vessels is not a mandate for removal.[33] The long-term follow-up results do not indicate that erosion into the vital structures is common.[6]

Evaluation of the Heart, Pericardium, and Great Vessels

The incident cited previously of fatal arrhythmia after removal of a bullet is a good warning concerning use of VATS in evaluating potential injuries to the heart, great vessels, and pericardium.[29] VATS procedures should not be used in treating injuries to these structures; only open techniques should be used. The potential for life-threatening hemorrhage is real in treating injuries to these structures. VATS techniques are usually inadequate for controlling such a hemorrhage and would prove totally inadequate to achieve a successful repair.

Some authors have proposed using VATS for exploring the heart, great vessels, and pericardium when a negative evaluation is anticipated (i.e., if the chance of finding an injury is small, even though its potential presence has been entertained). Hermansson and associates reported their success in using VATS to diagnose pleuropericardial rupture secondary to blunt trauma.[21] Fortunately, no injury to the heart had occurred. Thoracoscopic placement of a pericardial window has been described for apparently stable patients who have suffered penetrating trauma.[36] Exploration of the pleural and pericardial spaces by laparoscopic techniques has been described, but it is potentially dangerous on two counts.[40] The patient may suffer tension pneumothorax or tension pneumopericardium with disastrous cardiovascular results. Serious, uncontrollable hemorrhage could ensue secondary to a clot being dislodged over a major injury. Hence, such approaches are mentioned only to discourage their use.

Management of Persistent Air Leak

Lang-Lazdunski and associates treated 5 patients for persistent pneumothorax and air leaks in their series of 42 trauma patients treated by VATS.[29] VATS was particularly effective in treating direct lung injuries and in ensuring that chest tubes were placed properly. In the 5 patients the surgeons treated, the mean period of persistent air leak was 11 days. In 1 patient who had an air leak persisting for 7 days despite tube thoracostomy, CT scan revealed a large rib fragment lacerating the underlying pulmonary parenchyma. The patient had an uneventful postoperative course after the fragment was removed by VATS. The remaining hematoma was evacuated, and the lung was fully re-expanded. The second and third patients required positive pressure ventilation for serious multiple traumas. A pneumothorax developed in both patients and persisted despite tube thoracostomies. One patient had ruptured apical blebs, which were successfully stapled. The other had a pulmonary contusion and a poorly compliant lung. Both had successful VATS pleural abrasions. A fourth patient suffered a large left-sided hemopneumothorax secondary to a stab wound. VATS was employed and a large pulmonary laceration was identified due to a persistent air leak. VATS stapling techniques were used to control the air leak successfully. The last patient had suffered a thoracic stab wound and had a persistent pneumothorax despite tube thoracostomy. A VATS procedure revealed that the tube was extrapleural, and a small pulmonary parenchymal laceration was identified. The patient experienced an uneventful recovery after two properly placed tubes were secured in the pleural space by VATS guidance and visualization.

Summary

The use of VATS in trauma has to be tempered by mature judgment. Stabilization of patients who have trauma, along with a complete and thorough assessment, comes first and foremost. VATS should not be used in the unstable patient, and should be used cautiously in the presence of bilateral lung injury. VATS, however, has become a significant aid in assessing and managing slow, continuing hemorrhage, retained hemothorax, empyema, and diaphragmatic and thoracic duct injuries. The role of minimally invasive thoracic surgery in heart and great vessel injury is limited. The next few years will see a greater expansion in the application of VATS for trauma along with a more widespread use of this resurgent technology.

References

1. Andrews NC, Parker EF, Shaw RP, et al: Management of nontuberculous empyema. Am Rev Respir Dis 85:935–936, 1962.
2. Angelillo-Mackinlay T: Hemothorax and empyema. *In* Yim AP, Hazelrigg SH, Izzat MB, et al (eds): Minimal Access Cardiothoracic Surgery. Philadelphia; WB Saunders, 1999.
3. Aram KV, Grover FL, Richardson JD, et al: Post traumatic empyema. Ann Thorac Surg 23:254–258, 1997.
4. Braco JMC: Thoracoscopy as a method of exploration in penetrating injuries of the thorax. Dis Chest 12:330–335, 1946.
5. Bartek JP, Grasch A, Hazelrigg SR: Thoracoscopic retrieval of foreign bodies after penetrating chest trauma. Ann Thorac Surg 63:1783–1785, 1997.
6. Bland EF, Beebe GW: Missiles in the heart: A twenty year follow-up report of World War II cases. N Engl J Med 274:1039–1046, 1966.
7. Block EFJ, Kinton OC, Windsor J, et al: Guided percutaneous drainage for post-traumatic empyema thoracis. Surgery 117: 282–287, 1995.
8. Braimbridge M: History. *In* Yim AP, Hazelrigg SH, Izzat MB, et al (eds): Minimal Access Cardiothoracic Surgery. Philadelphia; WB Saunders, 1999.
9. Chen JC, Wilson SE: Diaphragmatic injuries: Recognition and management in sixty-two patients. Ann Surg 57:810–815, 1991.
10. Cevese PG, Vecchioni R, Cordiano C, et al: Surgical techniques for operating on the thoracic duct. Surg Gynecol Obstet 140:958–962, 1975.
11. Coselli JS, Mattox KL, Beall AC: Reevaluation of early evacuation of clotted hemothorax. Am J Surg 148:786–790, 1984.
12. Eddy AC, Luna GK, Copass M: Empyema thoracis in patients undergoing emergent closed tube thoracostomy for thoracic trauma. Am J Surg 157:494–497, 1989.
13. Fallon WF, Jr: Post traumatic empyema. J Am Coll Surg 179:483–492, 1994.
14. Feliciano DV, Cruse PA, Mattox KL, et al: Delayed diagnosis of injuries to the diaphragm after penetrating wounds. J Trauma 28:1135–1144, 1989.
15. Ferguson MK: Chylothorax. *In* Yim AP, Hazelrigg SH, Izzat MB, et al (eds): Minimal Access Cardiothoracic Surgery. Philadelphia, WB Saunders, 1999.
16. Graeber GM, Jones DR: The role of thoracoscopy in thoracic trauma. Ann Thorac Surg 56:646–648, 1993.
17. Graeber GM: Thoracic Trauma. *In* Daniels TA, Kizer LJ (eds): Thoracoscopic Surgery. Boston, Little, Brown, and Co. 1993, pp 221–233.
18. Graham DD, McGahren ED, Tribble CG, et al: Use of video-assisted thoracic surgery in the treatment of chylothorax. Ann Thorac Surg 57:1507–1511, 1994.

19. Gregory GJ, Carrico CJ: Trauma: Management of the acutely injured patient. *In* Sabiston DC, Lyerly HK (eds): Surgery: The Biological Basis of Modern Surgical Practice. Philadelphia, WB Saunders, 1997, pp 296–339.
20. Helling TS, Gyles NR, Eisenstein CH, et al: Complications following blunt and penetrating injuries in 216 victims of chest trauma requiring tube thoracostomy. J Trauma 29:1367–1370, 1989.
21. Hermansson U, Konstantinov I, Traffs S: Lung injury with pleuropericardial rupture successfully treated by video-assisted thoracoscopy; Case report. J Trauma 40:1024–1025, 1996.
22. Heniford BT, Carillo EH, Spain DA, et al: The role of thoracoscopy in the management of retained thoracic collections after trauma. Ann Thorac Surg 63:940–943, 1997.
23. Ivatury RR, Sungn RJ, Weksler B, et al: Laparoscopy in the evaluation of the intrathoracic abdomen after penetrating injury. J Trauma 33:101–109, 1992.
24. Jackson AM, Ferreira AA: Thoracoscopy as an aid to the diagnosis of diaphragmatic injury in penetrating wounds of the left lower chest. Injury 7:213–217, 1976.
25. Jacobaeus HC: Possibility of the use of cystoscope for investigating serious cavities. Munch Med Wochenschr 57:2090, 1910.
26. Jones JW, Kitahama A, Webb WR, et al: Emergency thoracoscopy: A logical approach to chest trauma management. J Trauma 21:280–284, 1981.
27. Kern JA, Tribble CG, Spotnitz WD, et al: Thoracoscopy in the subacute management of patients with thoracoabdominal trauma. Chest 104:942–945, 1993.
28. Landreneau RJ, Keenan RJ, Hazelrigg SR, et al: Thoracoscopy for empyema and hemothorax. Chest 109:18–24, 1995.
29. Lang-Lazdunski L, Mouroux J, Pons F, et al: The role of videothoracoscopy in the chest trauma. Ann Thorac Surg 63:327–333, 1997.
30. Madden MR, Paul DE, Finkelstein JL, et al: Occult diaphragmatic injury from stab wounds to the lower chest and abdomen. J Trauma 29:292–298, 1989.
31. Malthaner RA, McKneally MR: Anatomy of the thoracic duct and chylothorax. *In* Pearson FG, Deslauriers J, Ginsberg RJ, et al (eds): Thoracic Surgery. New York, Churchill-Livingstone 1995, pp 1069–1081.
32. Macini M, Smith LM, Nein A, et al: Evacuation of clotted blood in hemothorax using thoracoscopy: Case reports. J Trauma 34:144–147, 1993.
33. Mattox KL: Indications for thoracotomy: Deciding to operate. Surg Clin North Am 69:47–58, 1989.
34. Meyer DM, Jessen ME, Wait MA, et al: Early evacuation of traumatic retained hemothoraces using thoracoscopy: A prospective, randomized trial. Ann Thorac Surg 64:1396–1401, 1997.
35. Milfeld DJ, Mattox KL, Beall Jr AC: Early evacuation of clotted hemothorax. Am J Surg 136:686–692, 1978.
36. Morales CH, Salinas CM, Henao CA, et al: Thoracoscopic pericardial window and penetrating cardiac trauma. J Trauma 42:273–275, 1997.
37. Nel JM, Warren BL: Thoracoscopic evaluation of the diaphragm in patients with knife wounds of the left lower chest. Br J Surg 81:713–714, 1994.
38. O'Brien J, Cohen M, Solit R, et al: Thoracoscopic drainage and decortication as definitive treatment for empyema thoracis following penetrating chest injury. J Trauma 36:536–540, 1994.
39. Oparah SS, Mandal AK: Operative management of penetrating wounds of the chest in civilian practice. J Thorac Cardiovasc Surg 77:162–168, 1979.
40. Porter JM: Diagnostic laparoscopy and laparoscopic transdiaphragmatic pericardial window in a patient with an epigastric stab wound: Case report. J Laparoendosc Surg 6:51–54, 1996.
41. Senno A, Moallem S, Quijano ER, et al: Thoracoscopy with the fiberoptic bronchoscope. J Thorac Cardiovasc Surg 67:606–611, 1974.
42. Senno A, Moallem S, Quijano ER, et al: Fiberoptic thoracoscopy. NY State J Med 75:51–56, 1975.
43. Smith RS, Fry WR, Tsoi EKM, et al: Preliminary report on videothoracoscopy in the evaluation and treatment of thoracic injury. Am J Surg 166:690–695, 1993.
44. Spann JC, Nwariaku FE, Wait M: Evaluation of video-assisted thoracoscopic surgery in the diagnosis of diaphragmatic injuries. Am J Surg 170:628–631, 1995.
45. Stein A, Achnier G: Penetrating stab wounds of the chest. S Afr Med J 39:63–67, 1965.
46. Striffeler H, Gugger M, Hof VM, et al: Video-assisted thoracoscopic surgery for fibrinopurulent empyema in 67 patients. Ann Thorac Surg 65:319–323, 1998.
47. Uribe RA, Pachon CE, Frame SB, et al: A prospective evaluation of thoracoscopy for the diagnosis of penetrating thoracoabdominal trauma. J Trauma 37:650–654, 1994.

COMMENTARY

Stephen R. Hazelrigg

The role of video-assisted thoracic surgery (VATS) in thoracic trauma has been a slowly evolving area because of the fact that it is only applicable in a small percentage of trauma patients. As noted in the chapter, VATS is recommended only in hemodynamically stable patients, and these procedures have been used most frequently in diagnosing diaphragmatic injuries, treating retained hemothoraces and continuous low level bleeding, and for resolving late complications such as empyema.

Diaphragmatic lacerations are often difficult to diagnose in penetrating trauma. It has been estimated that the diagnosis is missed in 20% of cases and a significant number of patients eventually develop hernias with strangulated bowel. For this reason,using VATS to diagnose potential injuries when the penetrating trauma is in proximity to the diaphragm seems prudent.

Retained hemothoraces that reveal more than one third of the hemithorax on radiograph should be drained, and VATS is an ideal way to accomplish this. The prospective study by Meyer and associates supports this use of VATS. The number of retained hemothoraces that require VATS should be less than 5%. Undrained hemothoraces do increase the risk of fibrothorax and empyema, and VATS successfully drains the hemothorax in virtually all cases operated upon within a week of the trauma.

VATS is an effective tool for managing empyemas in the fibropurulent phase but is rarely helpful in the fibrous phase; hence, one needs to operate upon these within 3 weeks to have a significant chance of success in avoiding thoracotomy.

Persistent chest tube bleeding in a hemodynamically stable patient who has trauma has been successfully managed in more than 90% of cases with VATS alone. Endoscopic clips, staples, cautery, or suture may be required, and an intercostal vessel is the most common source of the bleeding.

Overall, the use of VATS in a hemodynamically stable patient avoids thoracotomy and enhances diagnostic capability. Sensible use of VATS in trauma enhances the thoracic surgeon's options in managing these patients.

Chapter 40

Spinal Deformities

Alvin H. Crawford and Randall K. Wolf

The conventional approaches to the spine have been posterolateral, costotransverse, and anterior. To reach the anterior spine, anterior thoracotomy has traditionally been used. Problems associated with thoracotomy include a long incision, rib resection, significant ribspreading, tissue desiccation, alteration of pulmonary and shoulder girdle function, as well as significant pain, associated morbidity, and poor cosmesis. The field of video-assisted thoracoscopy (VAT) presents the spinal surgeon an endoscopic option for approaching the anterior vertebral column.

VAT offers the potential of decreasing surgical morbidity associated with traditional open procedures. It is a new technique as opposed to a new operation, and the goals and objectives are the same as those for thoracotomy. Surgical instruments, guided by an endoscope are able to gain access to the chest, without breaking ribs, through an approximately 1-inch long incision (portal) rather than through the 8- to 10-inch long incision required by thoracotomy. The endoscope can be linked to a video camera and inserted through portals that also allow use of other instruments. Camera optics provide magnification. This technique has been reported extensively in both medical and lay press.[8, 11, 19]

Thoracoscopy has been employed in treating lung lesions for more than 80 years.[4] The development of laparoscopic cholecystectomy has awakened a new interest in this technique and led to the development of many new therapeutic and diagnostic applications of video-assisted thoracic surgery (VATS). Most recently, the technology has been used in spinal surgery. Mack[7] and Regan[15] initiated clinical trials at the Texas Back Institute in the early 1990s. At about the same time, Eismont conducted animal studies[18] and Blackman[1] conducted animal, cadaveric, and clinical studies. Others have reported clinical[3, 6, 10, 12] and biomechanical[20] experiences with the technique. This technology was presented at the Scoliosis Research Society meeting in Dublin, Ireland, in 1993,[15] and also at the National Association of Spinal Surgeons in San Diego, California, in the same year.[17] As a result, a published summary of the procedure appeared in *USA Today* in December 1993.[19] Regan presented a comprehensive multi-authored atlas and accompanying video atlas of endoscopic spine surgery.[16]

The introduction of video technology with multichip cameras has significantly enhanced the capability of identifying structures in the chest through very small incisions or portals. The use of this technology has also been instrumental in allowing spinal surgeons to perform resection of the annulus fibrosis, the intervertebral disk, single or multiple ribs, and the vertebral end plate. Bone graft from the iliac crest or adjacent ribs can be placed into the intervertebral disk space through four or five portals as opposed to a 9- to 12-inch incision, thus enhancing the cosmetic effect of the scoliosis surgery.

In December 1993, at Children's Hospital Medical Center in Cincinnati, we began performing video-assisted thoracic surgery (VATS) for anterior release of severe spinal deformities in children and adolescents. We believed that the potential benefits of this procedure would include minimal invasiveness, better visualization and magnification, diminished postoperative pain and ventilatory compromise, reduced blood loss, decreased hospitalization, reduced health-care costs, improved wound care, and earlier return to prehospital activities, with minimal shoulder dysfunction. Reduced infection risks to patients and operating room personnel were also anticipated because of the decrease in operative time and exposure.

Indications in Children and Adolescents

We believed that VATS should be performed on patients who would usually require anterior spinal release surgery.[2] Indications included the following:

1. Rigid idiopathic scoliosis deformities at or above 75 degrees in magnitude with correction to less than 50 degrees on side-bending radiographs
2. Prevention of crankshaft phenomenon in the skeletally immature child who has more than a 50-degree curvature
3. Kyphotic deformities greater than 70 degrees
4. Neuromuscular deformities accompanied by at-risk pulmonary status
5. Progressive spinal deformity and metabolic disease
6. Severe rib hump deformity not corrected by spinal instrumentation
7. Neurofibromatosis with intrathoracic tumors in addition to a significant spinal deformity
8. Pseudarthrosis following anterior intervertebral fusion
9. Anterior hemiepiphysiodesis for congenital scoliosis
10. Incision and excision biopsy

We have now extended our indications to include all the procedures to the thoracic spine that were previously approached by thoracotomy.[9]

Contraindications

Relative contraindications to the VATS approach include:

1. Inability to tolerate single-lung ventilation
2. Severe or acute respiratory insufficiency
3. High airway pressures with positive pressure ventilation
4. Pleural symphysis
5. Empyema
6. Previous thoracotomy

Many spinal deformities occur in children who have congenital cardiothoracic problems requiring thoracotomy in the neonatal period and early childhood. There are, on occasion, significant adhesions following these procedures. We have now performed VATS in patients following previous thoracotomy, although resection of adhesions is time consuming and there is a higher risk of infection.

Training

VATS is an extremely demanding procedure that requires experience. Techniques for obtaining experience with this procedure include the use of animate laboratories, models, cadaveric laboratories, proctoring, hybrid procedures (endoscopic and open), and visitation to active centers for observation or teleconference surgeries with interactive discussions. Study groups to aid in instrument design and upgrading are also necessary. We have found the goat and the sheep to be the best animate models for thoracoscopy; however, the porcine model (which appears to be readily available and less expensive) is equally effective. Ultimately, credentialing will be necessary before one can operate on patients.

Team Coordination

The ability to perform VATS for spinal deformity revolves around a team of surgeons (access surgeon and spinal surgeon), anesthesiologists, nurses, and surgical technicians who complement each other in carrying out this task. Video monitoring and taping of the procedure is recommended. The bony thorax, unlike the abdomen, provides its own fixed space once the lung is collapsed, so insufflation (used in laparoscopy to create a space) is unnecessary and potentially dangerous. The anesthesiologist must be capable of using a flexible bronchoscope and selectively deflating one lung. This can be done best with the use of a double-lumen tube, although bronchial blockers may be necessary in small children. The access surgeon, who may be either a general, thoracic, or spinal surgeon, is responsible for handling the thoracoscope and providing visualization and illumination of the endothoracic anatomy. The spinal surgeon performs the procedure. The particular operating room setup is a variable (Fig. 40–1).

Some surgeons prefer to work on the same side of the table, usually facing the patient, who is in the lateral decubitus position. Others prefer to work opposite each other, viewing the intrathoracic contents by placing monitors directly across from them and usually looking over the associate's shoulder. One must realize that the monitor seen from the posterior position is a mirror image of that seen from the anterior position. Some surgeons have commented anecdotally about turning one of the monitors upside down, but we have no personal experience of this (Fig. 40–2).

Hand-eye coordination and knowledge of intrathoracic anatomy are paramount. The endoscopic hardware includes various angled thoracoscopes capable of magnifying up to 15 times, as well as specialized thoracospinal instruments (e.g., rongeurs, curets, periosteal elevators, electrocautery, harmonic scalpel, and suction irrigation devices) (Fig. 40–3).

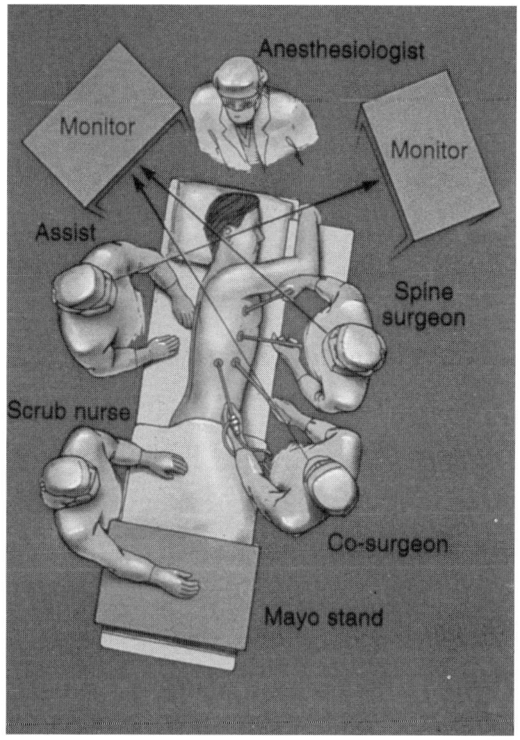

Figure 40–1. Conventional setup for video-assisted thoracoscopic spinal surgery. Note the anesthesiologist is at the head of the table and the monitors are positioned over the shoulders of the assisting surgeon and the spinal surgeon. The scrub nurse is at the area of the pelvis and the patient is prepped and draped so that he or she is in the left lateral decubitus position with the right side up. (From Crawford AH: Video-assisted thoracoscopy. Spine: State of the Art Reviews II: 341–359. Philadelphia, Hanley & Belfus, 1997, with permission.)

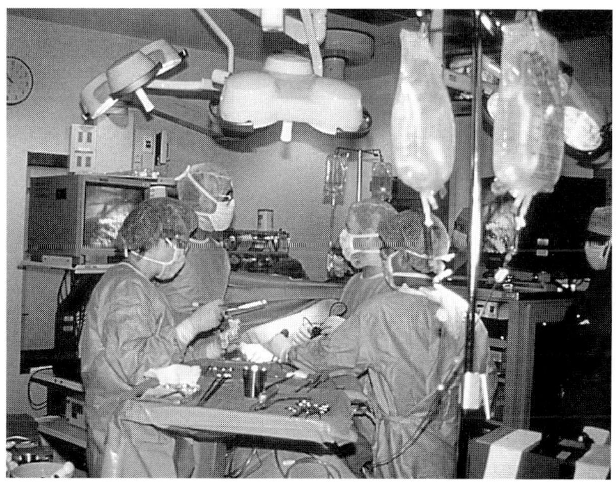

Figure 40–2. The conventional setup as used at Cincinnati Children's Hospital. This view looks from the foot of the table directly toward the head of the table. One of the monitors can be seen on the left just behind the surgeon and scrub nurse. (From Crawford AH: Video-assisted thoracoscopy. Spine: State of the Art Reviews II: 341–359. Philadelphia, Hanley & Belfus, 1997, with permission.)

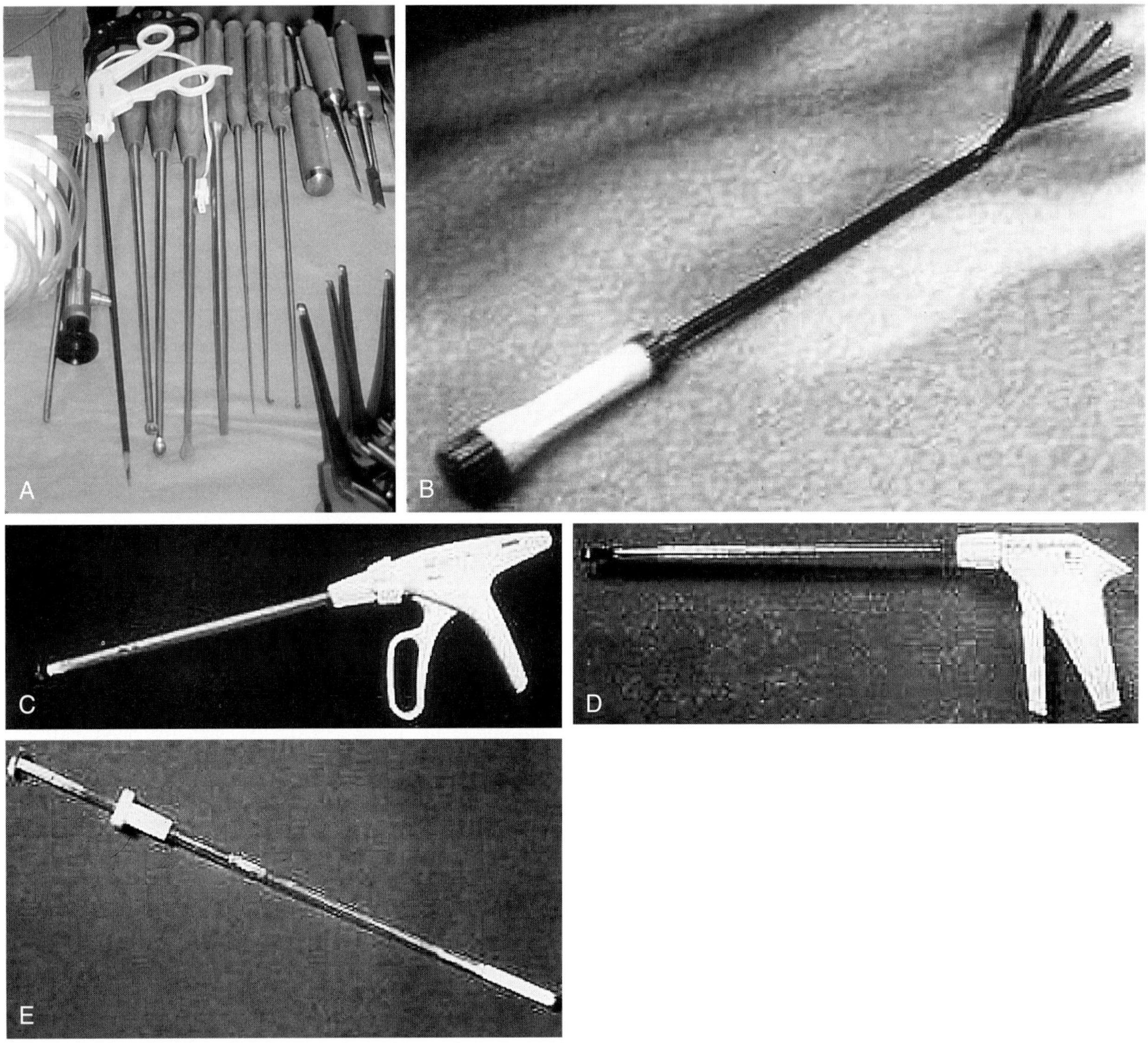

Figure 40–3. *A,* The endoscopic instruments are longer than the conventional instruments, which are shown in the top right corner. The endoscopic instruments are just to the left. There are thin- and wide-shanked instruments. The wide-shanked instrument is used mostly in laparoscopic surgery. Abdominal laparoscopic surgery requires continuous insufflation to displace the viscera. The wide shank of the instrument allows a tight seal at the portal interface. Insufflation is not required in the thoracic cavity. (From Crawford AH: Video-assisted thoracoscopy. Spine: State of the Art Reviews II: 341–359. Philadelphia, Hanley & Belfus, 1997, with permission.) *B,* A number of disposable and reusable retractors are available, but the Endo Tract II (Auto Suture Co., Division of U.S. Surgical Corp.) fan retractor has been the most useful for retracting the atelectatic lung. The articulating arm is especially helpful in gently depressing the diaphragm for exposure to the lower dorsal spine. (From Regan JJ, McAfee PC, Mack MJ: Atlas of Endoscopic Spine Surgery. St. Louis, Quality Medical Publishing, 1995, with permission.) *C,* Clip appliers are used for hemostasis and blood vessel ligation before division, which commonly occurs during sectioning of the segmental vein and artery. The position of the segmental vessels in the trough of the vertebral body may restrict the use of end-clipping devices. (From Regan JJ, McAfee PC, Mack MJ: Atlas of Endoscopic spine surgery. St. Louis, Quality Medical Publishing, 1995, with permission.) *D,* A right-angled grasper can be used to elevate the vessel for ligation with an endoscopic vascular clip applier. The ideal clip applier is yet to be manufactured for endoscopic spine surgery. (From Regan JJ, McAfee PC, Mack MJ: Atlas of Endoscopic Spine Surgery. St. Louis, Quality Medical Publishing, 1995, with permission.) *E,* Epidural venous and bone bleeding are common in thoracoscopic spinal procedures. Hemostasis can be maintained with endoscopically applied Endo-Avitene followed by application of a cottonoid or sponge. (From Regan JJ, McAfee PC, Mack MJ: Atlas of Endoscopic Spine Surgery. St. Louis, Quality Medical Publishing, 1995, with permission.)

Operative Technique

General anesthesia is administered via a double-lumen endothracheal tube or bronchial blocker, and the patient is turned to the lateral decubitus position. The anesthesiologist should observe deflation of the lung before draping is carried out, and 10 minutes are allowed to achieve complete resorption atelectasis. Routine intraoperative monitoring for thoracic procedures (i.e., arterial pressure line, pulse oximeter, and end-tidal carbon dioxide measurement) is initiated. Because the majority of thoracic spinal deformities appear on the right side, the patient is usually placed in the left lateral decubitus position with a kidney rest support (Fig. 40–4).

Although not sterilely draped, the arm is hyperflexed at the shoulder to allow the placement of portals high into the axilla. The Mayo stand is situated so that electrocautery, suction, and light source are fully accessible from both sides of the table. The topographic anatomy, specifically the scapular borders, the 12th rib, and the iliac crest, are identified and outlined with a water marker. Usually four to five portals are necessary. The first portal is most frequently placed at or about the T6 or T7 interspace in the posterior axillary line. Entry at this level usually avoids the diaphragm (Fig. 40–5).

The reverse L-shaped configuration of portals is most popular. We prefer to make the incision through the dermis with a scalpel followed by electrocautery through the subcutaneous tissue and intercostal muscles and into the chest cavity. The incision is made over the top of the rib to avoid the intercostal vessels. The index finger can be used to sweep the space, thus ensuring that the lung is down and preventing injury. There tends to be less bleeding when the electrocautery is used to dissect the intercostal muscles surrounding the portal into the chest cavity. This procedure is safe and can be observed through the scope. More important is the coagulation of the vessels. Nothing is worse than experiencing a steady drip around the visual port, requiring removal of the scope and continuous wiping. A 15-mm trocar is used, through which a 10-mm, 30-degree, angled rigid telescope is placed. The 30-degree scope allows direct vision into the intervertebral disk spaces, without either impeding the surgical instrumentation or obscuring the operative field. The end of the scope is kept in warm saline solution or in a scope warmer until it is used. This prevents fogging when the chest is entered. The thoracoscope is introduced and the lung is observed as it deflates. The reverse L-shaped configuration for portal sites is most popular. The instruments can be switched from portal to portal as the need arises (Fig. 40–6).

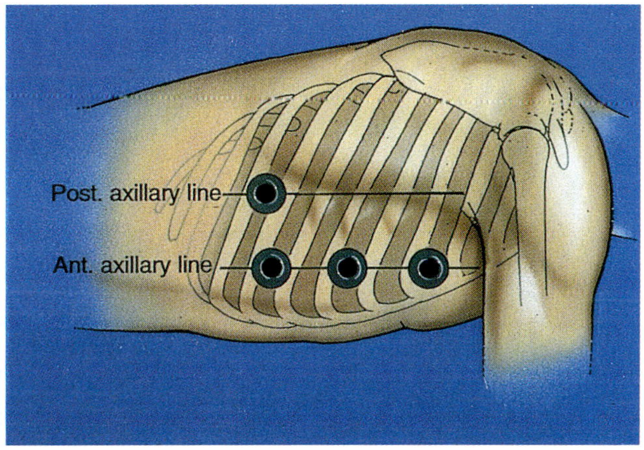

Figure 40–5. The first portal for an anterior thoracoscopic release of the spine is created along the posterior axillary line at T6 or T7 intercostal spaces. Subsequent portals are created along the anterior axillary line. (From Regan JJ, McAfee PC, Mack MJ: Atlas of Endoscopic Spine Surgery. St. Louis, Quality Medical Publishing, 1995, with permission.)

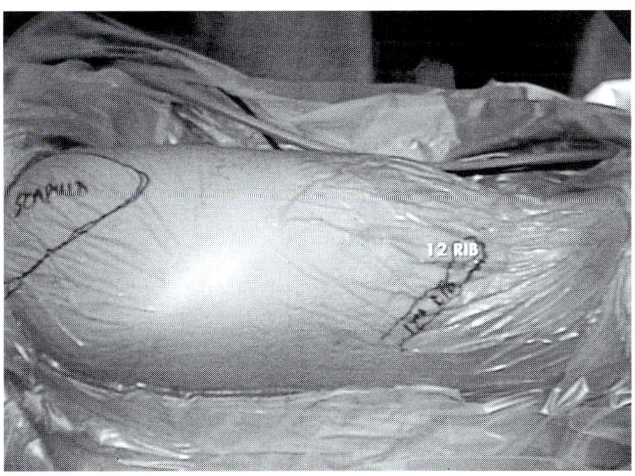

Figure 40–4. The patient is in the lateral decubitus position with the scapula on the left and the 12th rib on the right. The arm is flexed to allow greater access to the superior axilla, but prepped and draped out of the field. (From Crawford AH: Video-assisted thoracoscopy. Spine: State of the Art Reviews II: 341–359. Philadelphia, Hanley & Belfus, 1997, with permission.)

A panoramic assessment and evaluation of the intrathoracic space should be carried out in an effort to determine the anatomy as well as possible sites for other portals that would allow a more direct working approach to the intervertebral disks. The portals should be as far apart as possible (Fig. 40–7).

Rotating the patient anteriorly and using the Trendelenburg position for the lower thoracic spine or the reverse Trendelenburg position for the upper thoracic spine usually causes the lung to fall away from the operative field when it is completely collapsed, obviating the need for retraction instruments.[7] The superior thoracic spine is well visualized without retraction once the lung is completely deflated. Retraction of the diaphragm is necessary below T9 to T10. Several lung retractors are commercially available. Most involve a spreading mechanism that can be activated inside the chest cavity. The spreading can be destructive to the lung and great vessels. To avoid pleural injury, the lung retractor should be visualized in the open and closed positions following its insertion. By percussing the chest and visualizing the percussions from within, the direction and route the instruments would travel to the spine can be extrapolated. The primary and other working portal sites are selected by this method. We use rigid as well as flexible ports for positioning and inserting instruments.

Insufflation in the thoracic cavity is not necessary be-

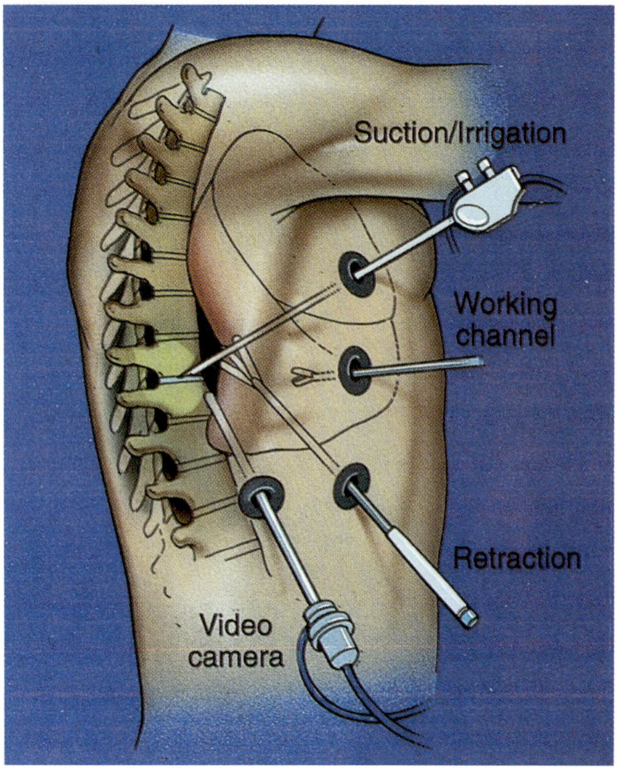

Figure 40–6. Multiple portals along the lateral chest wall provide access for a thoracoscope and instrumentation. (From Regan JJ, McAfee PC, Mack MJ: Atlas of Endoscopic Spine Surgery. St. Louis, Quality Medical Publishing, 1995, with permission.)

cause of the rigidity of the chest wall and the ability to collapse the ipsilateral lung, so open trocars are used. A variety of disposable trocars are available (Fig. 40–8).

A rigid thoracoport is important for preventing damage to the thoracoscope as the surgeon attempts to navigate the resistant rib cage fulcrum. We have found that flexible

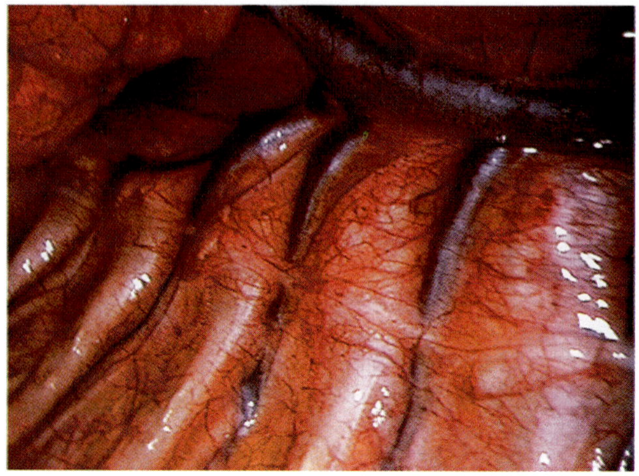

Figure 40–7. View of the upper portion of the thoracic spine, where the superior intercostal veins enter into the azygos vein. Note the mounds and valleys along the vertebral column. The mounds are the intervertebral disks and the valleys are the vertebral bodies. The segmental vessels cross the spine over the vertebral bodies (valleys) and continue as the intercostals. Also note the sympathetic chain crossing horizontally just above the head of the ribs in the foreground of this view. (From Crawford AH: Video-assisted thoracoscopy. Spine: State of the Art Reviews II: 341–359. Philadelphia, Hanley & Belfus, 1997, with permission.)

ports cause less intercostal neuralgia. We can occasionally place more than one instrument (e.g., suction, rongeur, grasper, and Cherry dissector) through a flexible thoracoport. The camera and viewing field are rotated 90 degrees from the standard VATS position, because the spinal surgeon is most comfortable viewing and approaching the spine via horizontal projection.

Once the spinal anatomy has been identified, it is important to select the levels to perform annulotomy and diskectomy. The ribs are counted by palpation with a blunt grasping instrument. The superior intercostal vein usually

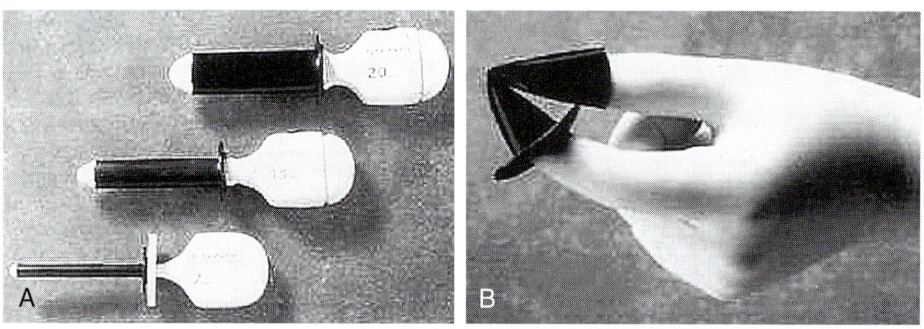

Figure 40–8. *A*, Another available disposable trocar is the Flexipath (Ethicon Endo-Surgery, Cincinnati, Ohio). (From Regan JJ, McAfee PC, Mack MJ: Atlas of Endoscopic Spine Surgery. St. Louis, Quality Medical Publishing, 1995, with permission.) *B*, The advantage of these trocars is that they are flexible and conform to the intercostal space, thereby minimizing intraoperative pressure on the intercostal nerve. They also allow passage of rigid orthopedic instruments. The disadvantage of the flexible device is that delicate manipulations may be more difficult to perform because of dragging or purchase of the instruments by the compressed trocar. To decrease operative expenses, consideration should also be given to the variety of nondisposable trocars that are available. (From Regan JJ, McAfee PC, Mack MJ: Atlas of Endoscopic Spine Surgery. St. Louis, Quality Medical Publishing, 1995, with permission.)

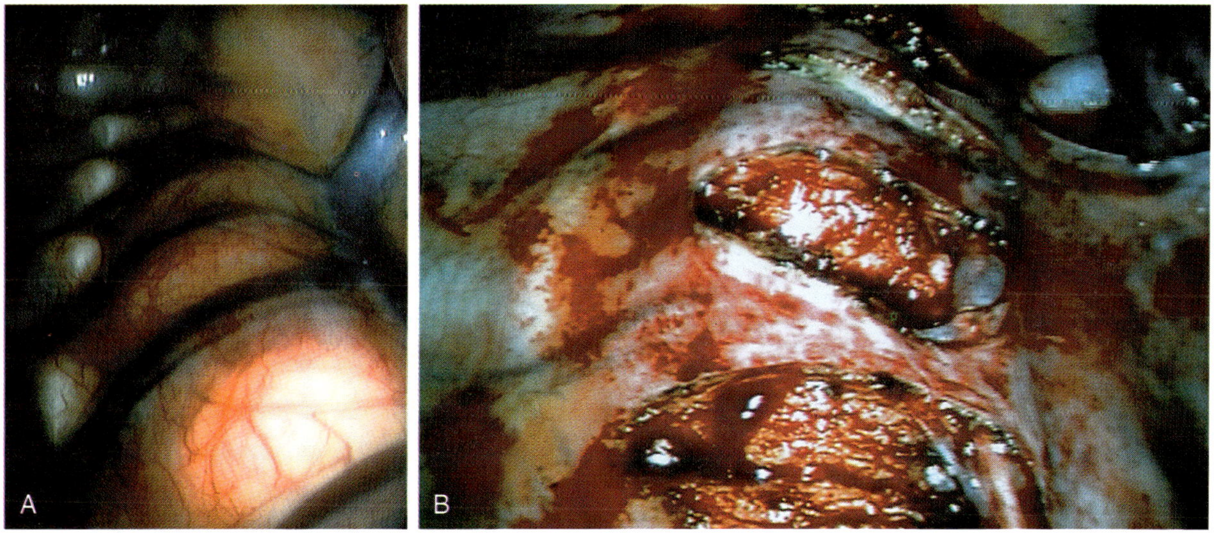

Figure 40–9. A panoramic view of the vertebral column of a child who has significant angular deformity and dysplasia. *A*, Note the abnormality of the rib heads. The azygos system can be seen in the foreground next to the deflated lung in the top right-hand corner of this illustration. *B*, This child underwent annulotomy and disk excision with preservation of the segmental vessels. (From Crawford AH: Video-assisted thoracoscopy. Spine: State of the Art Reviews II: 341–359. Philadelphia, Hanley & Belfus, 1997, with permission.)

empties into the azygos circulation at or about the T3 or T4 interspace. If there is a question of the specific level, a spinal needle is inserted into an intervertebral disk and a radiograph is taken. The vertebral column is approached through the parietal pleura. We prefer to use a harmonic scalpel for opening the parietal pleura in a longitudinal fashion over the vertebral column along the length of the operative field, in a fashion very similar to what is done when a transthoracic thoracotomy is performed. The intervertebral disk is identified by the mounds observed on the spinal column and the vertebral bodies by the valleys. The segmental vessels are noted to nest in the valleys directly overlying the bodies. Multilevel anterior diskectomies are necessary for correcting severe spinal deformity. This anterior release of the spinal curvature usually requires diskectomy at six to eight levels.

Controversy has arisen as to whether the segmental vessels should be transligated to allow better exposure or whether they should be preserved. We advise the surgeon perform the procedure he or she finds most comfortable or to use the same procedure as would be done for a thoracotomy, that is, preservation or ligation of the segmental vessels (Fig. 40–9).

A recent report from the Minnesota Spine Center of 6000 cross-ligations of the segmental vessels in 1197 cases failed to present a neuropathic consequence.[21] Transligation of the segmental vessels appears to be fairly safe. We use the harmonic scalpel to incise the pleura and ligate the segmental vessels. We have also used monopolar and bipolar electrocautery to approach the vertebral bodies through the parietal pleura. A small Robinson catheter is placed over an extended tip electrocautery Bovie, leaving 3 to 4 mm of cutting surface to use as a scalpel (Fig. 40–10).

Endoscissors or a pleural dissector can be used to incise the pleura as well. The segmental vessels are coagulated with a bipolar electrocautery or harmonic scalpel, incised, and allowed to retract with the pleura. The pleura is elevated and retracted with thoracoscopic periosteal elevators and blunt dissectors. Any vessels that appear to be at risk for bleeding are coagulated when encountered. We prefer use of the harmonic scalpel or bipolar coagulation of vessels; however, suture ligature or endoscopic clips may be employed (Fig. 40–11).

Once the pleura has been completely dissected the surgeon may proceed directly to excision of the annulus at the level of the intervertebral disk. The spinal surgeon should use a technique that he or she finds comfortable. The procedure should be performed in an orderly and sequential fashion; every effort should be made to avoid fencing the instruments by manipulating only one instrument at a time. A transverse cut is made across the vertebral body,

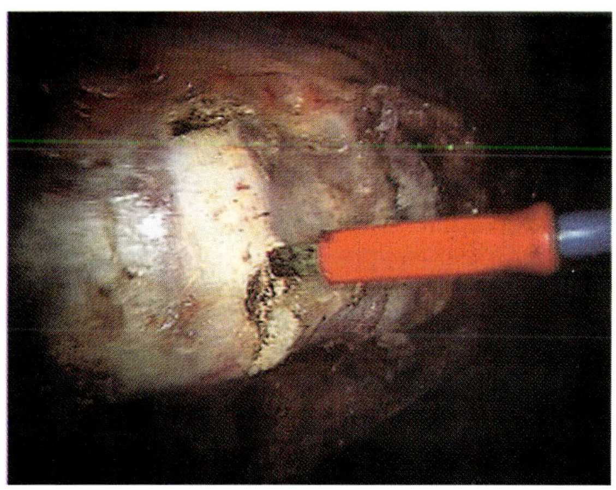

Figure 40–10. A Robinson catheter has been placed over an extended Bovie cautery, as seen in this illustration. The parietal pleura has been retracted and an annulotomy is being carried out. Note the deflated lung in the foreground of the photograph.

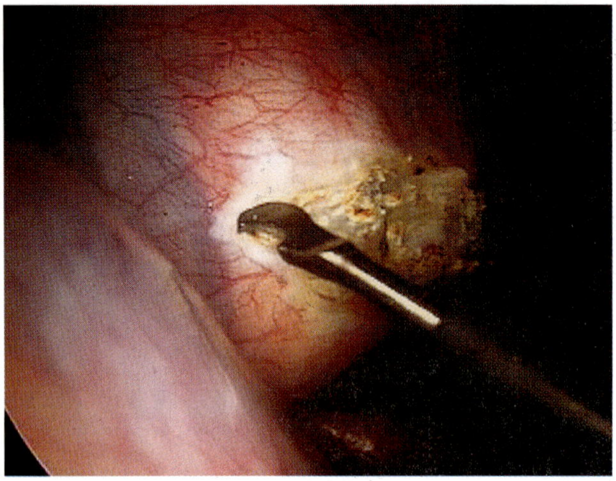

Figure 40–11. This device is an UltraCision harmonic scalpel (Ethicon Endosurgery, Inc., Cincinnati, OH). The use of this scalpel greatly decreases thermal burns, char, and desiccation, as noted with a monopolar Bovie catheter. The hemostasis is excellent, and, as a result, we have recently used this primarily for pleural and subperiosteal dissection, as well as control of segmental vessels.

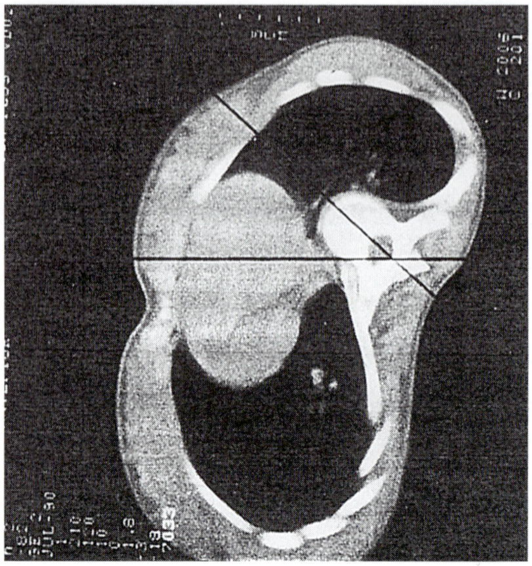

Figure 40–12. The computed tomographic cut through the midthorax illustrates the rotation of the thoracic spine secondary to scoliosis. The distance from the chest wall to the deformed spine is always less on the convexity, and, occasionally, this allows conventional length instrumentation (rongeurs, curets, and elevators) to be used instead of special endoscopic instruments. (From Crawford AH: Video-assisted thoracoscopy. Spine: State of the Art Reviews II: 341–359. Philadelphia, Hanley & Belfus, 1997, with permission.)

anterior to the rib heads, and parallel to the disk that is both rostral and caudal to it. An elevator is then used for lifting the periosteum toward the vertebral end plate and isolating the disk. A transverse cut is made across the annulus fibrosis and continued down to the level of the nucleus pulposus. Rongeurs, curets, and periosteal elevators are then used as necessary to ensure complete removal of the disk material and the end plates. In the case of severe deformities, the spine may be rotated toward the chest wall and moved close enough for the use of conventional length instruments (Fig. 40–12).

The length of the rongeurs' jaws should be measured to the hinge so that the depth of penetration toward the posterior longitudinal ligament can be determined. In a young child, it is often possible to elevate the vertebral end-plate apophysis and completely excise the intervertebral contents back to the posterior longitudinal ligament (Fig. 40–13).

With experience, the surgeon improves the ability to excise the annulus and disk space contents in an approximately 250-degree arc, or almost from pedicle to pedicle. Particular attention is directed to the release of the annulus on the concave side. Caudally, we have approached the L2 disk through thoracoscopy, and we consider it less than safe to attempt to extend below this limit. We are comfortable excising the T2 to T3 interspace in the rostral direction.

Following excision of the annulus and removal of the disk space contents down to the end plate in mature patients and cancellous bone in the skeletally immature, a small piece of Gelfoam or Surgicel is inserted. The spinal column segment should be stressed by rotating the periosteal elevator in the disk space, exercising moderate force following each release to see if mobility has been achieved. The complete anterior release should improve the mobility and correction of the spine substantially. Some surgeons believe this complete release down to cancellous bone is enough to enhance fusion, and they do not insert a bone graft. We now harvest bone by removing a rib and performing a fusion. Rib harvesting can also achieve an internal costoplasty. Others have taken bits of iliac crest bone, portions of ribs or allografts, and more recently metallic cages, and placed them into the disk space. Following completion of the procedure, efforts are made to remove all disk fragments and debris from the thoracic cavity; the pleura can either be sutured or allowed to remain open. In our procedures, we no longer attempt pleural closure. All efforts are made to control bleeding. A chest tube is then placed through the posterior and most inferior portal. The thoracoscope is used to observe the chest tube as it is placed alongside the vertebral column, lest it seek its way into one of the intervertebral spaces. The chest tube is then connected to the water seal, and the anesthesiologist inflates the lung to determine whether there is an air leak. A careful inspection should be made to check for any evidence of cloudiness in the fluid irrigant, and it should be ascertained that no injury to the thoracic duct has occurred. Marcaine is injected into each port, followed by deep layer and subcuticular closure. The patient is usually reintubated and turned to the prone position for a posterior spinal fusion (Fig. 40–14).

During the procedure, the greater splanchnic nervous sympathetic chain is usually transected at one of several levels; this does not cause permanent residual problems. However, the parents and the pediatric patient should be made aware that there is a possibility of a hot and cold "sympathetic release" phenomenon on the contralateral-ipsilateral lower extremity following this kind of surgery. This phenomenon is very similar to what is experienced after a transthoracic thoracotomy is performed.

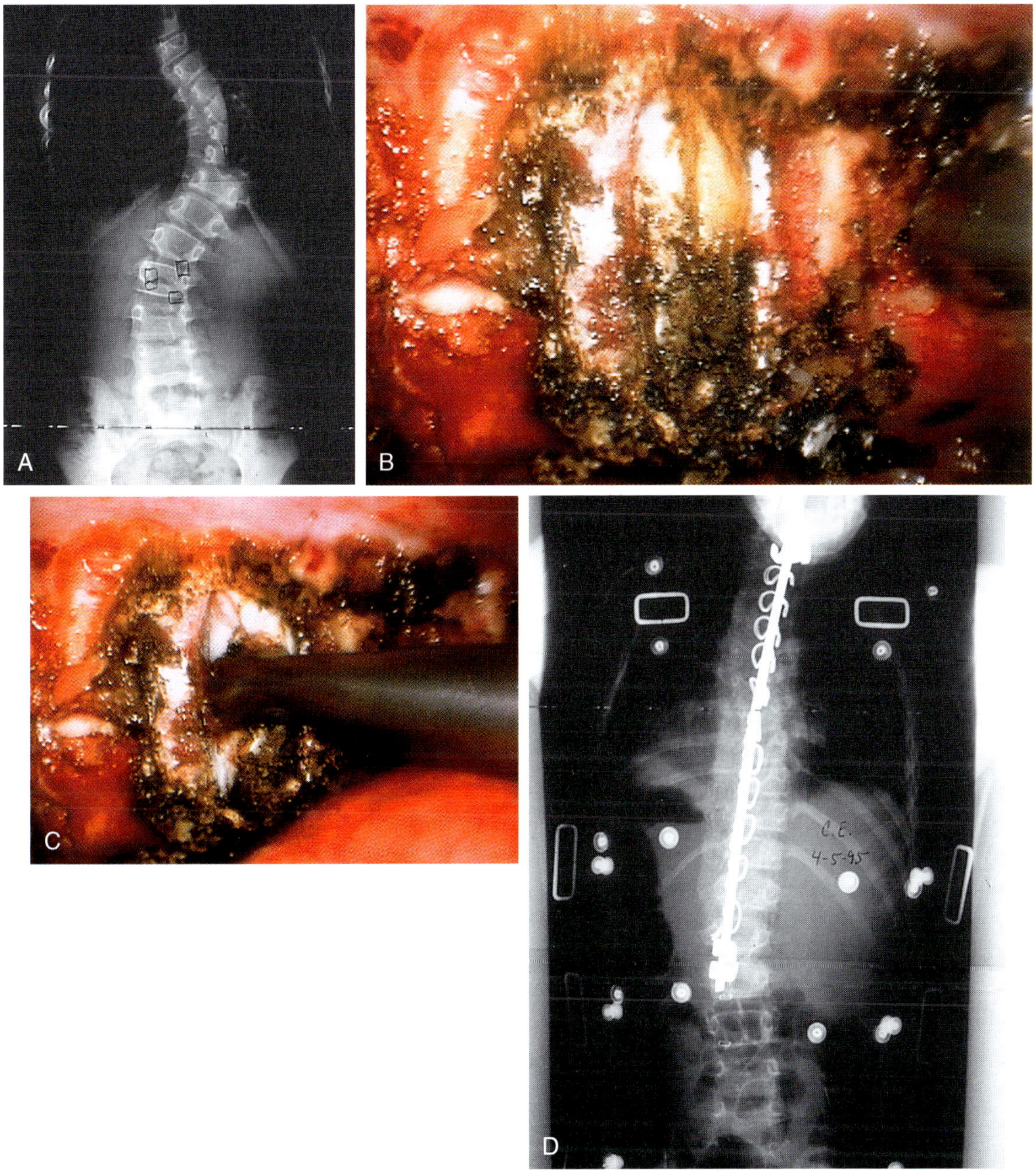

Figure 40–13. This 9-year-old child presented with a severe spinal deformity and surgery was recommended. *A,* Preoperative standing posteroanterior (PA) radiograph illustrating a double primary thoracic curvature. *B,* Thoracoscopic view: The intercostal vessels were sacrificed in this child. Note in the mid-foreground, the vertebral end plates are exposed as well as the annulus fibrosis. A periosteal elevator is seen on the right. *C,* The periosteal elevator, which was placed in between the cartilaginous end-plate apophysis and the vertebral body, lifted the cartilaginous apophysis from the vertebral body. The entire annulus-apophysis complex was then excised with a rongeur. *D,* Postoperative PA radiograph showing correction achieved with a clawed sublaminar wiring construct. (From Crawford AH: Video-assisted thoracoscopy. Spine: State of the Art Reviews II: 341–359. Philadelphia, Hanley & Belfus, 1997, with permission.)

We have performed VATS thoracoplasty[10] (i.e., convex rib resections through the thoracoscope) in an effort to decrease the rib hump. If costoplasty is carried out, fragments of rib can be placed in the intervertebral disk spaces to enhance fusion. After completion of the thoracoscopic release or fusion, or both, the child in most cases is turned to the supine position and reintubated. After moving the child to a prone position, a posterior spinal fusion with instrumentation is then carried out. Some centers have reported performing VATS in the prone position with simultaneous anterior release and posterior exposure to decrease reintubation and turnover time. In very severe cases, an anterior release and intervertebral fusion may be preferred, with the patient placed in either halo-femoral or

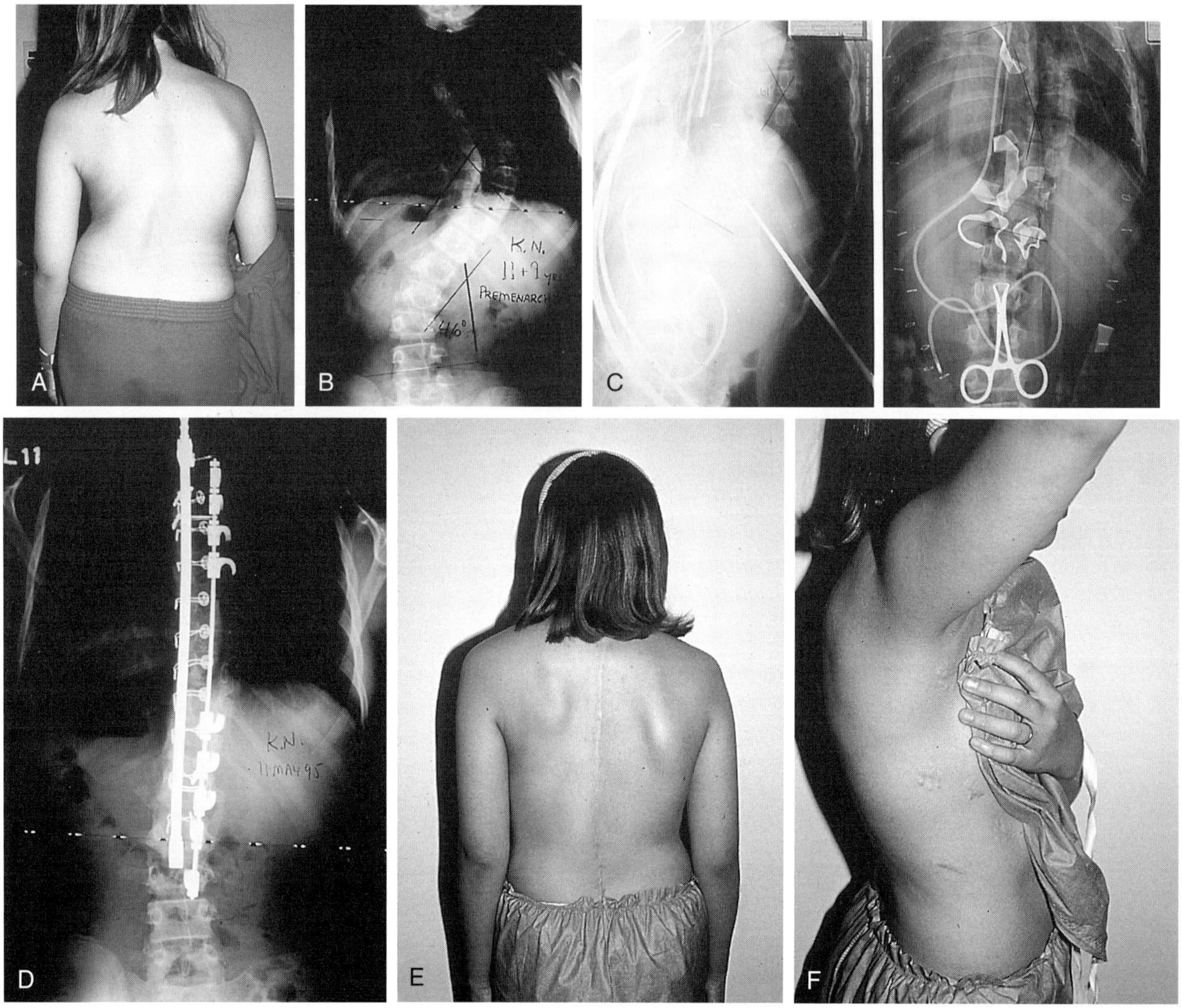

Figure 40–14. This 11-year-old child presented with a severe spinal deformity and underwent anterior release followed by posterior interspinous segmental instrumentation. The initial curvature of 80 degrees had been decreased to 30 degrees at the time of instrumentation. The final correction was down to 7 degrees. *A,* Standing clinical photograph showing severe right chest deformity and truncal shift to the right. *B,* Standing posteroanterior (PA) radiograph before video-assisted thoracic surgery (VATS), showing right dorsal deformity of 80 degrees. *C,* Intraoperative radiographs following VATS, showing on the left a curvature of 61 degrees and a marker (towel clip) in the right radiograph following posterior soft tissue exposure showing a curvature of 30 degrees. *D,* Standing postoperative radiograph following VATS anterior release and posterior spinal fusion with segmental instrumentation. The curvature has been corrected and truncal balance restored. *E,* Posterior clinical photograph of the same child 1 year after surgery. There has been tremendous clinical improvement. *F,* Note the portal incisions in the axilla. The scar from thoracotomy would be 12 to 15 inches long. (From Crawford AH: Video-assisted thoracoscopy. Spine: State of the Art Reviews II: 341–359. Philadelphia, Hanley & Belfus, 1997, with permission.)

halo-wheelchair traction in an effort to further decrease the severity of the deformity. These types of patients usually undergo posterior spinal fusion within the next 7 to 10 days.

Piccetti[14] and Blackman[1] have performed corrective and stabilizing instrumentation via VATS.

Possible Complications

Bleeding. Remain calm and keep in mind that the field is magnified 15 times. The scrub person should have a radiopaque sponge with a heavy suture attached and loaded on a sponge stick. This device should be available at all times to allow the surgeon to exert pressure on the source of bleeding. It is important that a suture tie is secured to the radiopaque sponge for easy retrieval, and the sponge stick fits through one of the portals. Apply direct pressure and clear the field for visualization. An endoscopic monopolar electrosurgical device with an extension tip is usually sufficient for achieving hemostasis; however, endoscopic bipolar forceps, an argon Bovie coagulator, or both may be needed. Endoscopic clip appliers and a variety of hemostatic agents (e.g., absorbable gelatin sponges, topical thrombin, collagen hemostat) should also be readily available. The scrub person should ensure that instrumentation for performing an open thoracotomy incision is set up on the sterile back table. This arrangement avoids delay and confusion in the event of an emergency.

Lung Tissue Trauma. Although the lung is deflated and retracted away from the spine, damage to delicate lung tissue can occur at any time. Prolonged air leak is the most prevalent complication of thoracoscopy.[5] The scrub person should ensure that an endoscopic suture ligature or stapling device is ready for sealing air leaks.

Dural Tear. A dural tear can be recognized by the leakage of clear cerebrospinal fluid (CSF) from the disk space. Hemostatic agents (e.g., absorbable gelatin sponges, topical thrombin, collagen hemostat) will often seal small CSF leaks. A neurosurgical consultation should be obtained if the dural tear continues to leak CSF.

Lymphatic Injury. The presence of cloudy fluid in the endothoracic space after irrigation and suctioning may indicate a lymphatic injury. A lymphatic injury is closed with an endoscopic clip applier and small surgical stainless steel clips or an endoscopic argon Bovie coagulator device.

Spinal Cord Injury. If somatosensory evoked potential (SSEP) monitoring reveals a spinal cord compromise, the anesthesia care provider immediately administers corticosteroids, and the surgeon changes the position of the endoscopic instruments.

Sympathectomy. Trans-section of the sympathetic nerve causes little or no morbidity; however, the surgeon informs the patient and his or her family members of the possibility of temperature and skin color changes below the level of injury.

The entire anterior release and intervertebral fusion requires approximately 2 to 4 hours to complete. Throughout the intraoperative period, the circulating nurse remains in close contact with the patient's family members by giving them frequent updates on the patient's condition. At the completion of surgery, the anesthesia care provider extubates the patient. Before surgical team members transport the patient to the intensive care unit (ICU), the circulating nurse gives a detailed report to the ICU nurse to assist him or her in planning patient care activities.[13]

Although thoracoscopy offers a safe approach to the release of the anterior thoracic spine via a minimal incision, there are some risks involved. Possible complications from VATS procedures are the same as those that may occur with open thoracotomy procedures. We consider the procedure to be minimal from the standpoint of the incision, but we do not necessarily consider this surgery to be minimally invasive. Conversion to an open thoracotomy does not represent failure.

Other uses of this technique have included anterior hemiephiphyseal ablation and strut (rib) graft fusion for pseudarthrosis and severe kyphosis (Fig. 40–15), as well as incision of intercostal nerve neurofibroma (Fig. 40–16).

Benefits

The benefits of the technique appear to be slightly reduced surgical time, less tissue damage, improved cosmesis, decreased blood loss, reduced postoperative pain, improved postoperative respiratory functions, and shorter stays in the ICU and the hospital. There is a reduced potential for infection, as well as decreased rehabilitation of the shoulder. The small incisions used in the VATS approach preclude the need for rib retraction and result in reduced postoperative pain and improved respiratory function. Surgeons aspirate residual fluid directly from the patient's pleural cavity and completely inflate the lung at the completion of VATS procedures. Subsequently, the amount of chest tube drainage is less, and the chest tube can usually be discontinued 24 hours after surgery. Early removal of the chest tube improves the patient's mobility

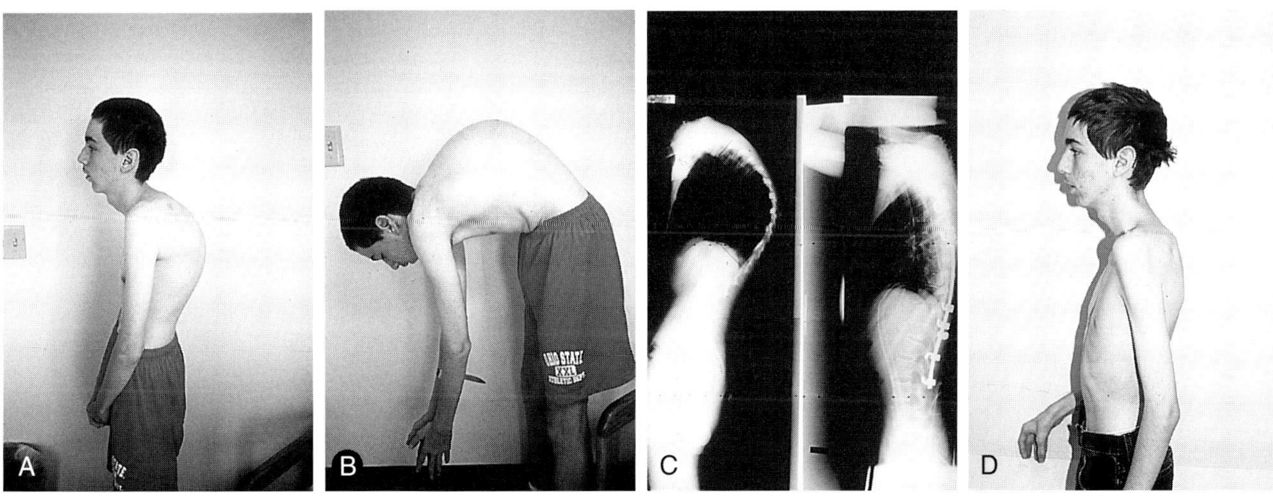

Figure 40–15. This 16-year-old boy presented with a 98-degree kyphosis. He underwent video-assisted thoracic surgery anterior release and rib grafting of the intervertebral disk. His clinical and radiographic correction was excellent. *A*, Standing lateral photograph showing significant adolescent kyphosis. Note protrusion of chin and hyperlordosis of cervical spine. *B*, Bending lateral photograph showing exaggeration of thoracic kyphosis. *C*, Preoperative radiograph and postoperative lateral radiograph showing excellent correction. *D*, Clinical lateral photograph 6 months after surgery showing correction. (From Crawford AH: Video-assisted thoracoscopy. Spine: State of the Art Reviews II: 341–359. Philadelphia, Hanley & Belfus, 1997, with permission.)

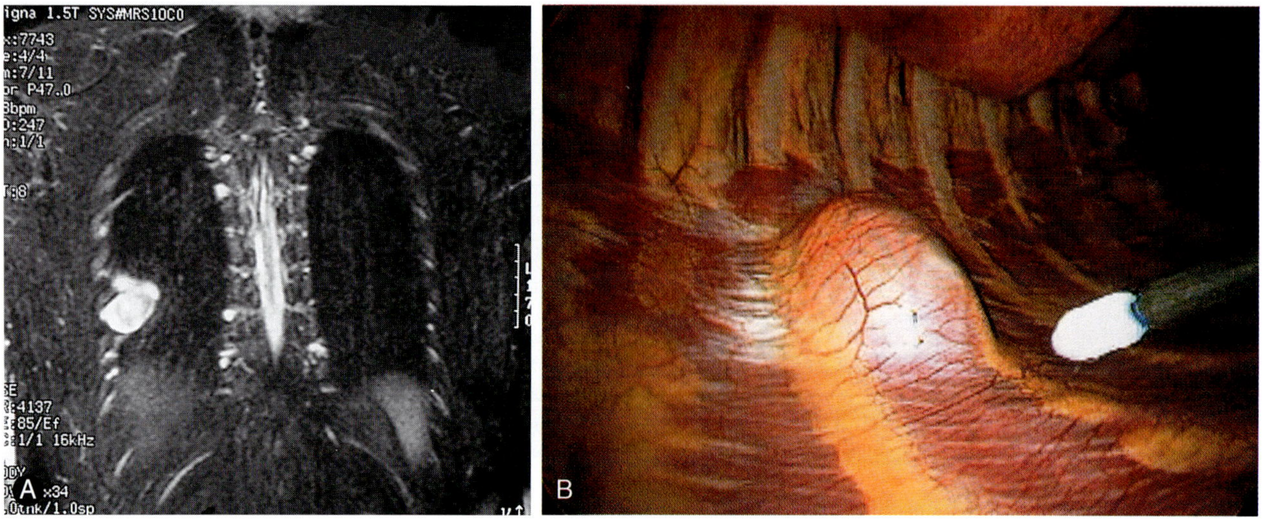

Figure 40–16. This 16-year-old child with type I neurofibromatosis was noted on magnetic resonance imaging to have a neurofibroma of an intercostal nerve. The lesion was removed by video-assisted thoracic surgery (VATS). *A,* MRI scan showing an intrathoracic mass on an intercostal nerve. *B,* Thoracoscopic view of lesion. (From Crawford AH: Video-assisted thoracoscopy. Spine: State of the Art Reviews II: 341–359. Philadelphia, Hanley & Belfus, 1997, with permission.)

and hastens convalescence. Using the VATS approach to anterior thoracic release in scoliosis surgery, we have shortened the average postoperative ICU stay from several days to 24 hours, and we have minimized body image distortions by creating smaller surgical incisions. These benefits should result in an overall decreased cost for the procedure, despite the fact that the procedure is somewhat costly, in fact more so than the conventional open technique, because of the amount of technology required. However, this is a startup fee and should decrease with the number of procedures performed. Unquestionably, using VATS, the same procedures can be performed with thoracotomy. They yield the same technical results, less morbidity, and a faster return to a normal functional lifestyle.

Disadvantages of Endoscopic Transthoracic Techniques

The learning curve for VATS is fairly steep. We recommend animate or cadavaric training before performing the procedure on humans. The specialized elongated instruments require 3-D perception. There is minimal tactile feedback, and assessing spatial depth can be difficult. The surgical team has to feel comfortable and qualified to treat unexpected bleeding complications with thoracoscopic instrumentation or be prepared to perform a thoracotomy. The anesthesiologist must be qualified in the management of single-lung ventilation and capable of troubleshooting. It is very disconcerting to have the lung expand unexpectedly during the procedure.

Limitations

The limitations of the procedure at this time include the inability of routinely inserting corrective implants for spinal deformities into the thoracic cage. If corrective implants could be introduced and activated within the four to five portals usually required for anterior release, thus alleviating the posterior midline scar, the procedure could truly be cosmetic. This limitation is currently being addressed. Another problem that needs to be resolved is the time required to remove the disk and end plate fragments. Currently the rongeur, curet, or other instrument has to be removed and reinserted with each bite. A mechanized device for removal of disk fragments would speed up the procedure.

The Future

We believe that the future potential of VATS in the management of spinal deformities is unlimited. For example, suturing techniques can be developed to offer closure of the parietal pleura over the excised intervertebral disk space. Autologous or homologous bone can be routinely placed into the disk space to obtain fusion and ensure a more stable spine once posterior instrumentation and fusion have been carried out. Voice-activated robotic instrument holders may replace the access, or visualization, surgeon. An advantage could be that they listen but do not talk back!

The ultimate success of the technique lies in the development of corrective instrumentation that could be applied through the portals. We think that the emerging technology of implant and instrumentation devices will ultimately give us the ability to perform corrective and stabilizing instrumentation by VATS. The future also includes the ability to use a heads-up display, which would relieve the surgeon and his or her associate from having to view monitors. Special glasses would allow the display to be part of the surgeons' direct optics. At some centers, 3-D video assistance has been used, and some surgeons are very comfortable with it. Robotics is not used as frequently in thoracic spinal surgery as in laparoscopy, but it could have the potential of improving visualization with lung retraction capabilities in the chest.

The procedure also allows for the possibility of navigational direction of transthoracic anatomy, such as the futuristic concept of interoperative magnetic resonance imaging (MRI), with the images coming up on the screen in real time. With this technologic capability, a probe could be passed into the thorax to demonstrate the distance to the target site. Video-assisted thoracoscopy and telesurgery are excellent tools for teaching, in that telepresence and telecommunication can be achieved through the videoscope and then transmitted via telephone technology to local conference centers as well as abroad. Unlimited capabilities are possible with this new technology.

References

1. Blackman R: Multiple level anterior thoracic discectomy using an endoscopic exposure. Exhibit #5, Dublin, Ireland. September 18–23, 1993.
2. Crawford AH, Wolf RK, Wall EJ, et al: Pediatric spinal deformity. *In* Regan JJ McAfee PC, Mack MJ (eds): Atlas of Endoscopic Spine Surgery. St. Louis, Quality Medical Publishing, 1995.
3. Crawford AH: Video-assisted thoracoscopy. Spine: State of the Art Reviews II. Philadelphia, Hanley & Belfus, 1997.
4. Jacobaeus HC: Possibility of the use of cystoscope for the investigation of the serous cavities. Munchen Med Wochenschr 57:3090–3092, 1910.
5. Kaser LR, Barvaria JE: Complications of thoracoscopy. Ann Thorac Surg 56:796–798, 1993.
6. Mack MJ, Regan JJ, Bobechko WP, et al: Application of thoracoscopy for diseases of the spine. Ann Thorac Surg 56:736–738, 1993.
7. Mack MJ, Regan JJ, McFee PC, et al: Video-assisted thoracic surgery for the anterior approach to the thoracic spine. Ann Thorac Surg 59:1102–1106, 1995.
8. Medical science. New York Times. September 19, 1991.
9. Mehlman CT, Crawford AH: Video-assisted thoracoscopic surgery: Pediatric orthopaedic applications. *In* Zdeblick T (ed): Anterior Approaches in Spine Surgery. St. Louis, Quality Medical Publishing, 1997.
10. Mehlman CT, Crawford AH, Wolf RK: Video-assisted thoracoscopic surgery (VATS): Endoscopic thoracoplasty technique. Spine 22:2178–2182, 1997.
11. Nash, JM: The kindest cut of all. Time. March 23, 1992.
12. Newton PO, Wenger DR, Mubarak SJ, et al: Anterior release and fusion in pediatric spinal deformity: A comparison of early outcome and cost of thoracoscopic and open thoracotomy approaches. Spine 22:1398–1406, 1997.
13. Nymberg SM, Crawford AH: Video-assisted thoracoscopic releases of scoliotic anterior spines. AORN J 63:561–575, 1996.
14. Picetti G III, Blackman RG, O'Neal K, Luque E: Anterior endoscopic correction and fusion of scoliosis. Orthopaedics 20: 1285–1287, 1998.
15. Regan JJ, Mack MJ, Picetti GD III: A comparison of VAT to open thoracotomy in thoracic spinal surgery. Scoliosis Research Society, Dublin, Ireland. September 18–23, 1993.
16. Regan JJ: Equipment and instrumentation for endoscopic spine surgery. *In* Regan JJ, McAfee PC, Mack MJ (eds): Atlas of Endoscopic Spine Surgery. St. Louis, Quality Medical Publishing, 1995.
17. Regan JJ: Video-Assisted Thoracoscopic Surgery. National Association of Spinal Surgeons. Annual Meeting, San Diego, CA, 1993.
18. Riley LH, Lebwohl NH, Eismont FJ: Thoracoscopic corpectomy: Description of a new technique and its outcome in a canine model. Paper #69. Scoliosis Research Society, Dublin, Ireland. September 18–23, 1993.
19. Snider M: TV-aided back surgery—video-assisted thoracoscopy. USA Today, December 1993; Life section.
20. Wall EJ, Bylski-Austrow DI, Shelton FS, et al: Endoscopic discectomy increases thoracic spine flexibility as effectively as open discectomy: A mechanical study in a porcine model. Spine 23:9–16, 1998.
21. Winter RB, Lonstein JE, Denis F, et al: The risk of paraplegia secondary to segmental vessel ligation: An analysis of 1197 consecutive anterior operations. Orthop Trans 19:616, 1995–1996.

COMMENTARY

George D. Picetti III and Kelly C. O'Neal

Minimal access techniques have significantly altered the practice of spinal surgery. The authors eloquently state the rationale behind thoracoscopic diskectomy, anterior release, and fusion of the thoracic and thoracolumbar spine in deformity surgery. They justifiably emphasize the importance of radical diskectomy, decortication, and fusion and document the feasibility of achieving these goals using an endoscopic technique. The aims are not only to mobilize the spine but also to obtain correction and solid arthrodesis.

At the Northern California Kaiser Permanente Spine Center, we have performed more than 150 endoscopic procedures for spinal deformity. In 35 procedures, not only release, but correction, instrumentation, and fusion were achieved by a strictly endoscopic technique.

Initially, all cases included participation by a thoracic surgeon. Of late, we enlist a thoracic surgeon only when instrumentation is planned, but not for endoscopic anterior release, hemivertebrectomy, hemiepiphysiodesis, and so forth.

Operating room setup costs are minimal because thoracic surgeons are already using the video equipment and access instrumentation that are needed. All the equipment we currently use is nondisposable, including our ports.

There is a significant learning curve for these procedures. With experience, most cases are handled more quickly and effectively than by conventional open techniques. Our most recent endoscopic scoliosis cases with release, instrumentation, and fusion of six to eight levels were performed in less than 4 hours.

Chapter 41

Thoracoscopic First Rib Resection for Thoracic Outlet Syndrome

Randall K. Wolf, Alvin H. Crawford, and Beverly Hahn

Resection of the first rib is performed for surgical treatment of thoracic outlet syndrome (TOS). TOS refers to compression of the subclavian vessels or the brachial plexus, or both, by the first rib and adjacent structures at the superior aperture of the chest.[5] Sir James Paget in 1875 in London and von Schroetter in 1884 in Vienna reported thrombosis of the subclavian vein caused by TOS. This vascular form of TOS is known as Paget–von Schroetter syndrome. However, the most common symptoms are neurologic and are related to compression of the brachial plexus in the distribution of the ulnar nerve.

The anatomy, clinical presentation, and evaluation of the patient with TOS have been extensively reviewed by Urschel and associates,[5, 10, 11] and the reader is referred to Urschel's textbook chapters for clear, concise, and exhaustive information concerning the history, anatomy, presentation, testing, and accepted management of TOS, which is beyond the scope of this presentation. This chapter presents a thoracoscopic surgical technique for excision of the first rib for treatment of TOS.

Anatomy

First, we focus on the forces that can cause compression on the thoracic outlet and the anatomy as seen from inside the thorax. The subclavian vessels and brachial plexus drape over the first rib as they transverse the cervicoaxillary canal and exit to the upper extremity. Compression of the contents in this canal can be caused by the muscles, ligaments, or bony structures that compose the borders. This includes the scalenus anticus and medius muscles, the subclavius muscle, the costocoracoid ligament, the cervical rib, the first rib, and anomalies of the first rib or clavicle.

On thoracoscopic examination, the first rib can be easily identified in the "roof" of the thorax. The first rib is a wide, flat rib that forms a C in the apex of the chest cavity. It can be "palpated" indirectly using an endoscopic kittner and can be clearly visualized. Care should be taken to note the relationship of the internal mammary artery anteriorly and the sympathetic chain posteriorly to the borders of the first rib. On the left, the subclavian artery is also easily visualized on thoracoscopic examination (Fig. 41–1).

Clinical Presentation

The spectrum of thoracic outlet compression symptoms ranges from mild to disabling,[13] and the specific symptoms can be divided by the structure that is most compressed, be it artery, vein, or nerve. The cause can be congenital, traumatic, or acquired. Brachial plexus compression accounts for the majority of cases that are evaluated surgically, and presenting symptoms may include pain, paresthesias, and motor weakness, usually in the distribution of the ulnar nerve. Subclavian artery compression can present as arm claudication, pulselessness, or arterial thrombosis. Subclavian vein compression may present with acute pain and edema of the arm secondary to venous thrombosis or, more chronically, as Paget–von Schroetter syndrome.

The most effective single procedure is probably resection of the first thoracic rib. The most successful approach reported is the transaxillary approach, initially described by Atkins,[2] reported by Roos,[9] and popularized by Urschel. By completely resecting the first rib, Urschel reported 85% good results in properly selected patients.[10]

The diagnostic evaluation should include a history, physical examination, chest radiograph, cervical spine films, electromyogram, and ulnar nerve conduction velocities. Arterial and venous compression in TOS requires contrast studies. A complete cardiologic workup is necessary in selected patients, as is complete neurologic workup in some patients. Once other disease processes have been eliminated and appropriate medical therapy has been ineffective or deemed not appropriate, surgical therapy may be entertained.

Procedure

The room setup is depicted in Figure 41–2. Both surgeons position themselves on the anterior side of the patient, who is placed in the lateral position after induction of general anesthesia with a double-lumen tube (Figs. 41–3 and 41–4). Three 10-mm thoracic ports are used for the operation: the two highest ports, in the anterior third and lateral fifth intercostal spaces, are for the working instruments, and a lower port on the lateral wall in the sixth intercostal space is used for a rigid 30-degree scope (Figs. 41–5 and 41–6). The thoracoscopic approach to first rib resection has been reported by Ohtsuka and colleagues.[6] Endoscopic instruments, including endoscopic elevators, curettes, and rongeurs (Sofamor Danek, Nashville, TN), were altered from the regular orthopedic tools by extension and modification to pass through 10-mm endoscopic ports.[8] An endoscopic drill (Midas Rex, Pneumatic Tools Inc., TX) capable of pulverizing bone through ports with a coarse ball tip revolving at high speed was also initially used. The harmonic scalpel (Ethicon Endosurgery, Inc., Cincinnati, OH), which operates with ultrasonic energy,

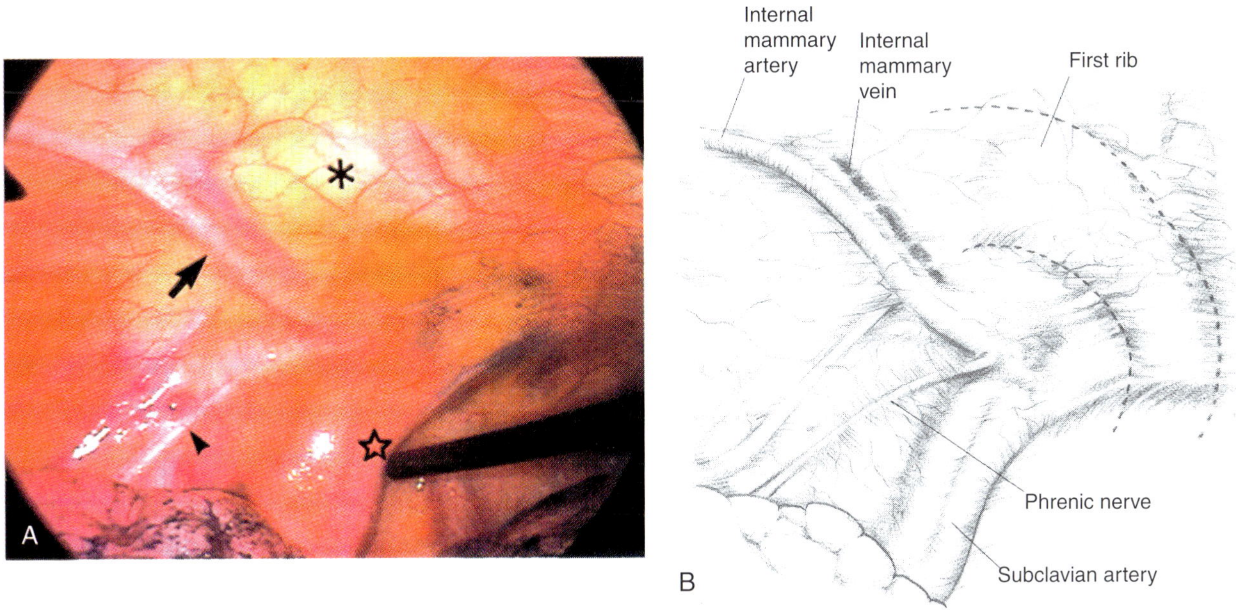

Figure 41–1. The anatomy of the thoracic outlet as seen through the thoracoscope and accompanying artist's rendition.

producing less smoke and lower heat than regular electrocautery, was routinely used to facilitate endoscopic dissection of the first rib.[1]

Initially, the parietal pleura as well as intercostal muscles are sharply dissected from the costal edge of the first rib using the harmonic scalpel (Figs. 41–7 and 41–8). The subclavian vein, artery, and brachial plexus, lying from anterior to posterior and draped over of the first rib, are bluntly freed using an endoscopic Cobb elevator and endoscopic curettes. Next, cautious dissection with a spinous process elevator frees the ribs circumferentially. An endoscopic drill is then used to divide the rib. The vessels and nerve are protected from the revolving drill by placing an endoscopic elevator behind the rib. The powdered tissue is evacuated by suction. Currently, the drill has been replaced by an endoscopic rib cutter (Fig. 41–9). The endoscopic rib cutter is employed to divide the first rib both anteriorly and posteriorly in its midportion. The divided rib is then removed through one of the port incisions. Endoscopic orthopedic rongeurs are then used to trim the resected ends of the rib back to the transverse process posteriorly and anteriorly to the manubrium (Fig. 41–10). Final assessment should include palpation of the transverse process posteriorly, as well as the costochondral junction anteriorly. This allows complete excision of the first rib, a technical point emphasized by Urschel.

A few technical aspects of the thoracoscopic first rib resection are worth emphasizing. Care must be taken in developing the plane of dissection, and it is recommended to dissect anterior to the vein initially. After transection of the rib, any additional muscle attachments, such as the scalenus anticus or medius, can be divided under direct vision. The rib can be delivered easily through one of the port sites after removing the port. During this dissection, the mammary artery anteriorly and the sympathetic chain posteriorly are clearly observed and preserved. Port sites are best placed at some distance from the target to allow adequate manipulation of the instruments in a comfortable arc. After complete thoracoscopic first rib excision, the contents of the neurovascular bundle drape gently across the apex of the pleural cavity. The extent of rib resection and its immediate effect on the structures of the thoracic outlet are clearly visualized.

Results

In six cases performed by Wolf and associates, the first rib was removed by this technique to decompress the subclavian vessels and brachial plexus lying on the first rib. In the first patient, who presented with right subclavian vein thrombosis, the symptoms on the right side resolved completely after the procedure. Symptoms subsequently developed in his left arm, and the same procedure was performed on the left side. The duration of the initial operation was 110 minutes. However, the operation times were reduced with experience to 100 minutes for second case and 75 minutes for third case. Blood loss was minimal in each case, and the hospital stays were 3, 2, and 1 day in the first, second, and third cases, respectively. A year after surgery, the patient who had Paget-Schroetter syndrome is still asymptomatic. More recently, in the last three patients the endoscopic rib cutter has been used to transect the first rib. The rib cutter appears to add safety to the division maneuver and is relatively easy to use compared with the drill. Fischel (personal communication) has completed six cases of first rib resection, with histories including trauma, sudden onset of numbness, long-standing pain, and weakness secondary to an overhead lifting job. Conservative treatments had failed in all these patients. All had good improvement with relief of pain and numbness. Only one reported some tingling in the fifth finger on postoperative day 10.

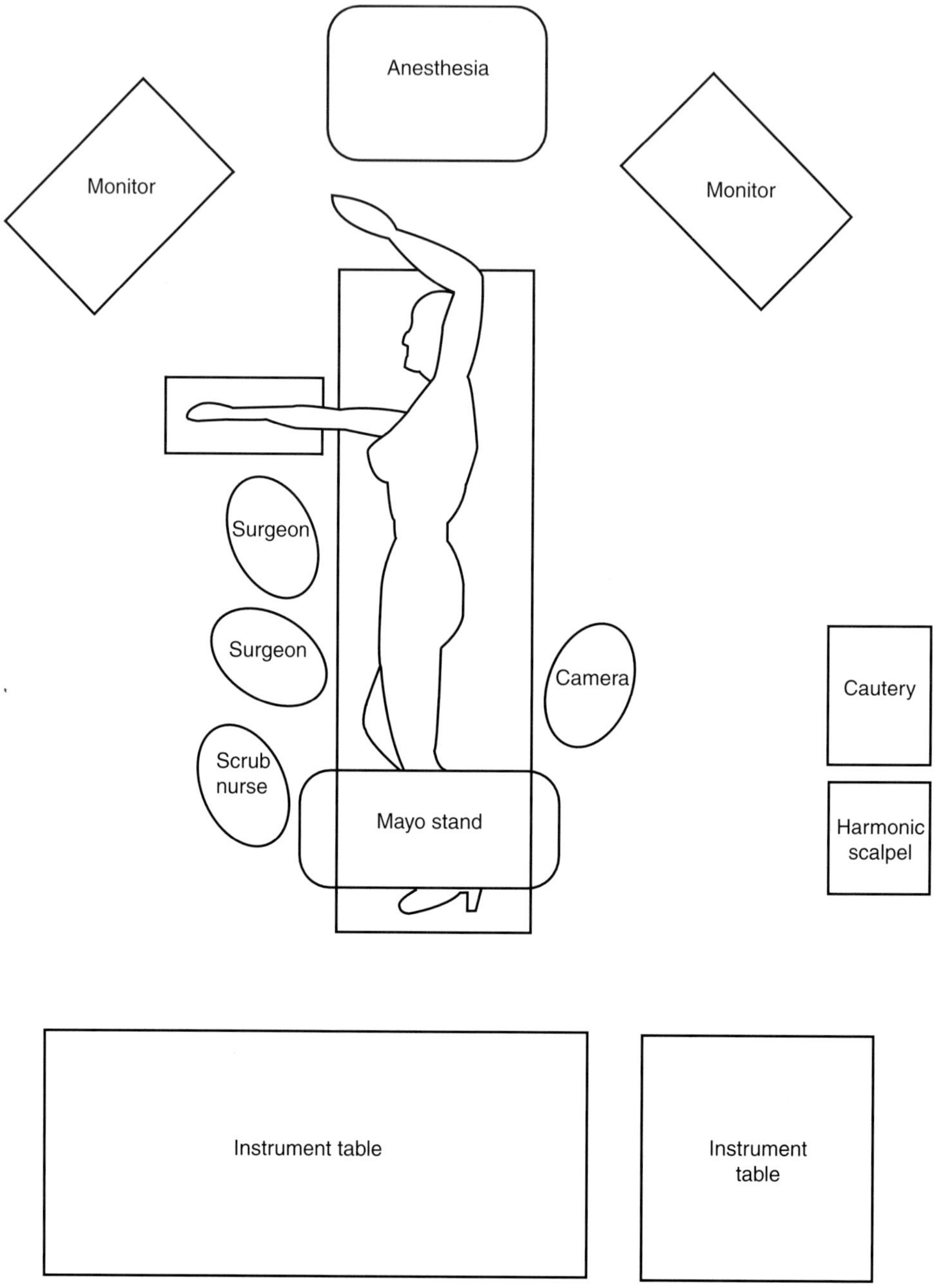

Figure 41–2. Room setup for thoracoscopic first rib resection.

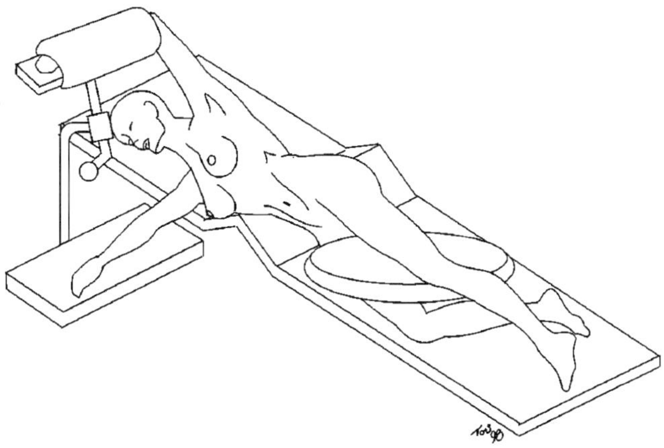

Figure 41–3. Patient positioned for left thoracoscopic first rib resection (port 1).

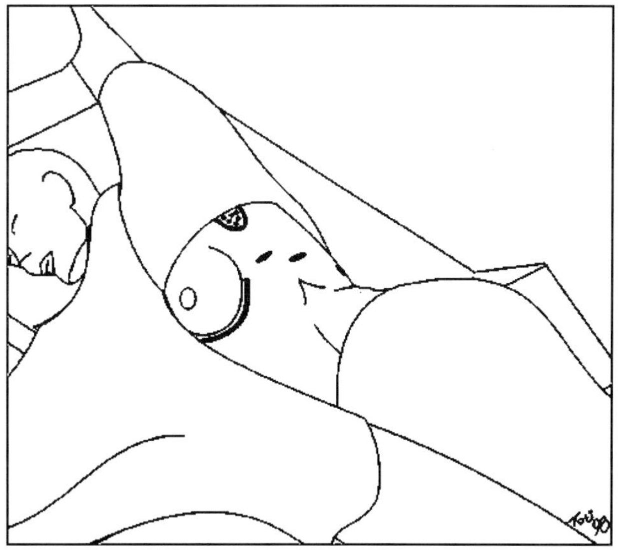

Figure 41–5. Topical anatomy for thoracoscopic first rib resection.

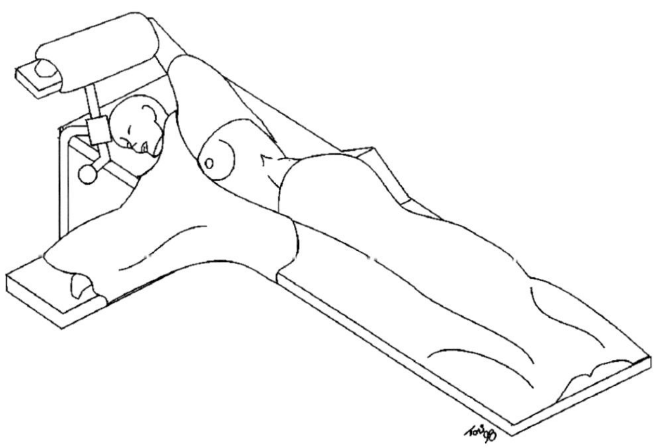

Figure 41–4. Patient draped for left thoracoscopic first rib resection (port 2).

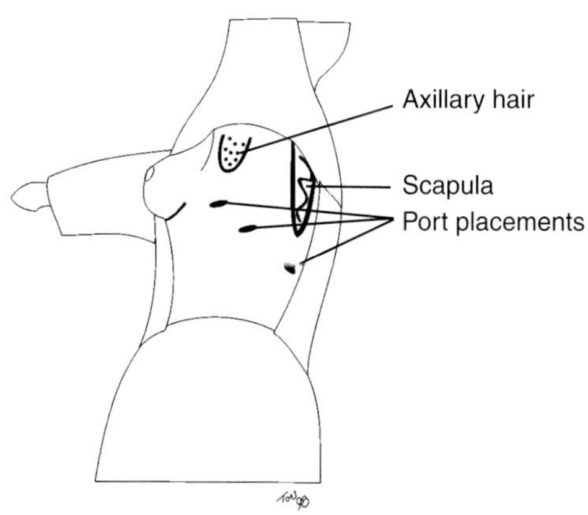

Figure 41–6. Ports for thoracoscopic first rib resection.

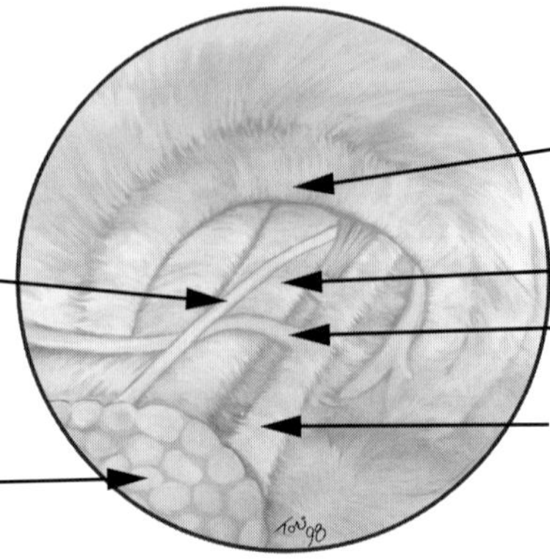

Figure 41–7. Thoracoscopic view of the left first rib.

Comments

Surgical treatment for neurologic TOS has a long history going back to the last century, but it is still controversial.[3, 4, 7] Patients who have neurologic or vascular symptoms can be treated successfully by resecting the first rib, usually through a transaxillary approach. The transaxillary resection of the first rib has been detailed by Urschel.[5, 10, 11] Advantages of this open technique are that it can be accomplished without major muscle division, without brachial plexus retraction, and with an acceptable cosmetic result. The disadvantages of the open transaxillary approach include limited visualization of the important structures and possibility of injury to the intercostobrachialis cutaneous nerve.

This chapter has described an alternative approach for resection of the first rib using new tools developed for endoscopic orthopedic surgery. The endoscopic drill and, more recently, a thoracoscopic rib cutter allow thoracoscopic division of the first rib through ports, and the harmonic scalpel facilitates thoracoscopic dissection and exposure of the first rib, providing smokeless views.

Excellent visualization of the thoracic outlet is the main advantage of the thoracoscopic approach. It is dramatic to observe the contents of the thoracic outlet drape gently across the superior thorax after the first rib has been successfully excised thoracoscopically. Complete excision of the first rib is possible using this thoracoscopic technique (Fig 41–11). Urschel stated that thoracoscopy expedites the transaxillary approach and helps teach the procedure.[12] With the totally thoracoscopic approach, the pleu-

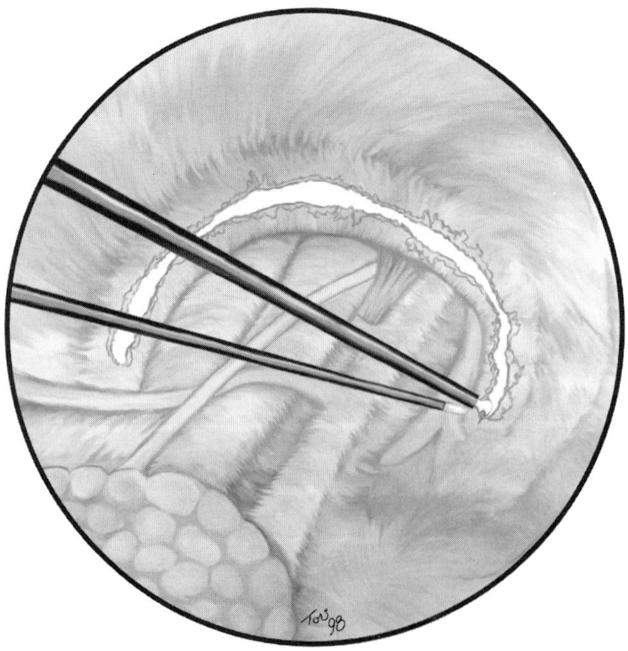

Figure 41–8. Initial dissection of the pleura overlying the first rib as performed with the harmonic scalpel.

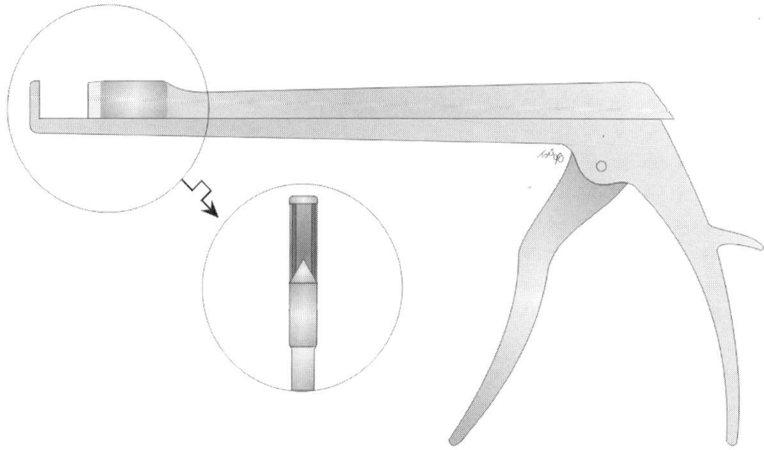

Figure 41–9. Thoracoscopic rib cutter (Sofamor Danek, Nashville, TN).

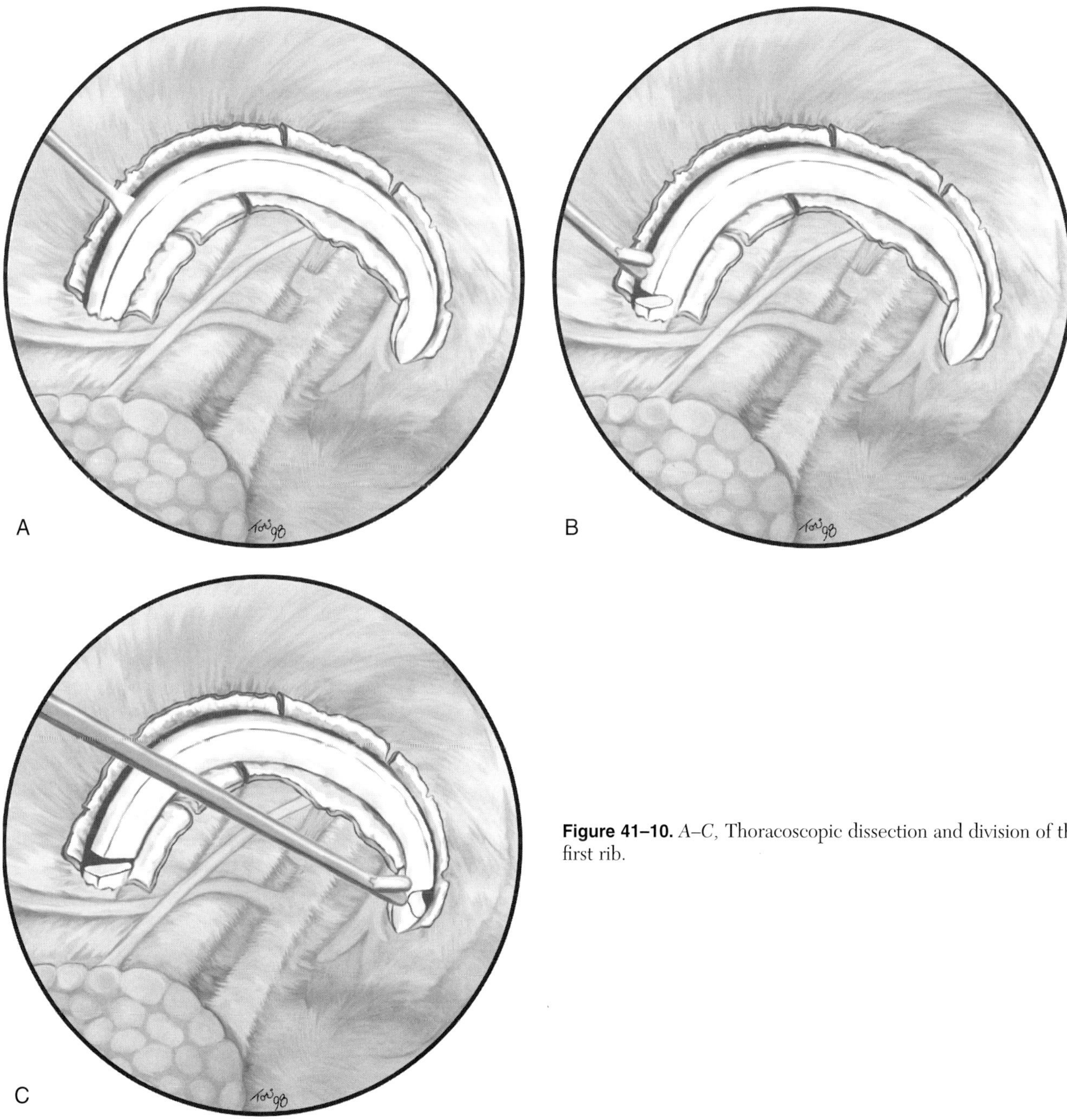

Figure 41–10. *A–C,* Thoracoscopic dissection and division of the first rib.

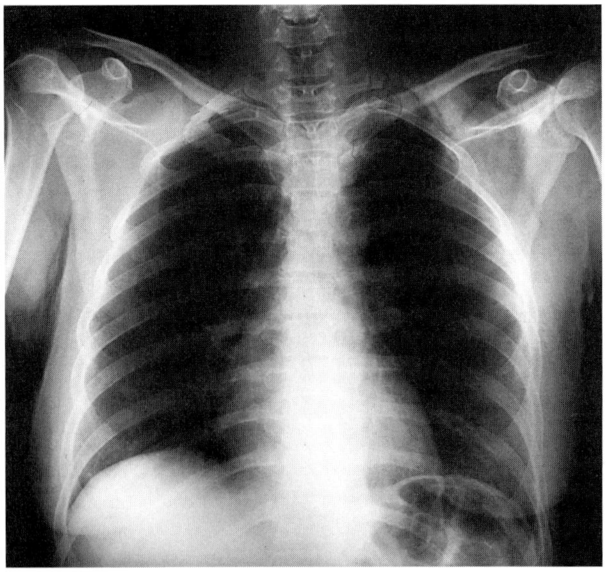

Figure 41–11. Postoperative chest posteroanterior radiograph demonstrating complete excision of the left first rib in a 45-year-old female with neurologic symptoms in the left arm. Symptoms completely resolved immediately after operation.

ral side of the first rib is visualized in its entirety, and the anatomic relationship of the first rib to the adjacent structures is clearly identified.

Thoracoscopic first rib resection is feasible and reproducible using new instruments. With future instrument and technical processes, this approach is expected to become a minimally invasive alternative for resection of the first rib.

References

1. Amaral JF: The experimental development of an ultrasonically activated scalpel for laparoscopic use. Surg Laparosc Endosc 4:92–99, 1994.
2. Atkins HJB: Sympathectomy by the axillary approach. Cancer 1:538, 1954.
3. Lindgren KA, Oksala I: Long-term outcome of surgery for thoracic outlet syndrome. Am J Surg 169:358–360, 1995.
4. MacKinnon SE: Thoracic outlet syndrome. Ann Thorac Surg 58:287–289, 1994.
5. MacKinnon SE, Patterson GA, Urschel HC: Thoracic outlet syndromes *In* Pearson FG, et al (eds): Thoracic Surgery, Churchill Livingstone, 1995.
6. Ohtsuka T, Wolf RK, Dunsker SB: Port-access first rib resection with new instrument: A report of two cases. J Surg Endosc (in press).
7. Poole GV, Thomae KR: Thoracic outlet syndrome reconsidered. Am Surg 62:287–291, 1996.
8. Regan JJ: Equipment and instrumentation for endoscopic spine surgery. *In* Regan JJ, McAfee PC, Mack MJ (eds): Atlas of Endoscopic Spine Surgery. St. Louis, Quality Medical Publishing, 1995.
9. Roos DB: Transaxillary approach for first rib resection to relieve thoracic outlet syndrome. Ann Surg 163:354–358, 1996.
10. Urschel HC: Thoracic outlet syndrome, *In* Shields TW, et al: General Thoracic Surgery. Philadelphia, Lea & Febiger, 1989.
11. Urschel HC: Thoracic outlet syndrome. *In* Sabiston DC, Spencer FC: Surgery of the Chest. Philadelphia, WB Saunders, 1990.
12. Urschel HC: The transaxillary approach for treatment of thoracic outlet syndromes. Semin Thorac Cardiovasc Surg 8:214–220, 1996.
13. Wilson SE, et al: Thoracic outlet disorders. *In* Veith FJ, Hobson RW, Williams RA, et al (eds): Vascular Surgery, Principles and Practice. New York, McGraw-Hill, 1993.

COMMENTARY

Stephen R. Hazelrigg

This represents an interesting application of video-assisted thoracoscopic surgery, which appears to have some distinct advantages. The transaxillary approach is certainly a good cosmetic procedure, but its greatest drawback is the lack of visualization, especially for anyone but the operating surgeon. VATS allows better appreciation of the anatomic relationships and the capability of easier teaching. The newly developed instruments, that is, bone cutters, have enabled this procedure to be performed totally thoracoscopically. The only caution revolves around the possible vascular injuries that could potentially occur and that need to be addressed. The less than ideal exposure for vascular injuries would also apply to the transaxillary route.

This procedure has been performed infrequently thoracoscopically and requires more experience before we can confidently recommend its routine use. Because of its potential problems, it should probably be considered as an advanced procedure to be performed only after a significant thoracoscopic experience has been gained.

Chapter 42

Hydatid Cysts of the Lung

Basem Shabb and Firass Abiad

Hydatid disease has been known since the time of Hippocrates[1] and is still endemic in many countries. The lung is the second most commonly involved organ, after the liver. Although there have been recent advances in the areas of diagnosis and medical therapy of the disease, surgery remains the mainstay of therapy. The most commonly performed surgical procedure is open thoracotomy with chemical sterilization followed by cystotomy and capitonnage. The thoracoscopic approach to hydatid disease has been applied with minimal morbidity.[2,3] It has proved to be a safe procedure with the advantage of less postoperative pain, shortened hospital stay, and reduced costs. The long-term results are comparable to the open technique.

Incidence and Pathology

Hydatid disease in humans is most often caused by the parasite *Echinococcus granulosus,* which produces the common macrocystic disease. *E. multilocularis* is a rare form that leads to an aggressive type of infiltrating disease in humans. *E. granulosus* is most commonly found in areas where sheep and cattle constitute important industries, such as the Middle East, South America, and eastern Europe. *E. multilocularis* is noted in Japan and parts of central Europe.

The annual incidence of cystic echinicoccosis can range from less than 1 to 220 per 100,000 inhabitants in various endemic areas, but the incidence seems to be declining with better hygiene.[4] The mortality rate (2 to 4%) from cystic echinococcosis may increase considerably if medical treatment and care are inadequate.

Echinococcal infection is a parasitic disease that humans share with other vertebrates. The worm spends its life cycle in two hosts, an intermediate host and a definitive host. The definitive hosts include dog, wolf, fox, and jackal. Humans are an intermediate host and are infected by intimate handling of the final host, usually an infected dog. The worm resides in the intestine of the primary host and excretes its eggs in the stools. The intermediate host, usually sheep or cow, ingests the eggs and the ingested embryo penetrates the small bowel wall and travels via the portal circulation to the liver. In the liver, the embryo develops into the disease-producing larval form.[5] Most of the larvae develop into hydatid cysts of the liver, but some occasionally pass through and into the lungs or any other organ.

The liver (60 to 70%) and the lung (20 to 30%) are the most frequently involved organs. Humans usually generate an active cellular reaction against the cyst, forming a fibrous layer around it known as the pericyst. The cyst wall itself is known as the endocyst and is usually easily separated from the pericyst. The endocyst consists of a laminated acellular membrane and a single cell layer composed of germinated epithelium. These cells are responsible for reproduction by producing protoscolices, which float in the cyst fluid. If spilled into the peritoneal or pleural cavity by rupture or surgery, the protoscolices may develop into new cysts.

Diagnosis

The hydatid cyst can lay dormant for many years before giving rise to symptoms. In a small number of cases, the first presentation might be cyst rupture into the bronchial tree, with the patient expectorating the laminated membranes. Spontaneous cure has been noted if the endocyst was completely expectorated. The majority of patients, however, have symptoms and signs due to compression of the surrounding structures or complications of the cyst such as rupture or infection. Patients usually present with cough with or without hemoptysis. Fever may be present and usually is a sign of infection. The cyst may rupture into the pleura, giving rise to pneumohydrothorax and dyspnea. The cyst can also be an accidental finding on a chest radiograph that is requested for other reasons. In endemic areas, the diagnosis should be considered in patients who have a solitary pulmonary nodule. The diagnosis can usually be made by a radiograph that shows well-defined solitary or multiple cysts (Fig. 42–1). Calcifications may be present and are usually associated with the death of the organism. In such cases, especially if the serologic titers are negative or low, the cyst should be treated conservatively because the likelihood of complications is minimal. Specific radiologic signs are present infrequently. An air leak between the pericyst and the endocyst may give rise to a "crescent" sign.[6] The "water lily" sign is seen in ruptured cysts with the collapsed membrane in the cavity. Computed tomography is especially helpful in demonstrating water density in a homogeneous cyst (Fig. 42–2). It can show loculations and daughter cysts and delineate other organ involvement when such is suspected.[7,8] Ultrasonography of the abdomen is part of the preoperative work up to detect any simultaneous liver cysts.

The diagnosis of hydatid cyst is further ascertained by using serologic testing. Tests such as the indirect hemagglutination assay are based on detection of antiechinococcal antibody, immunoglobulin G (IgG), or immunoglobulin M (IgM) in the patient's serum. These tests are highly sensitive and specific at the time of illness and are useful in the follow-up of patients for detection of recurrence.[9] The Casoni intradermal test that was used in the past has become obsolete because it is both inaccurate and potentially dangerous.

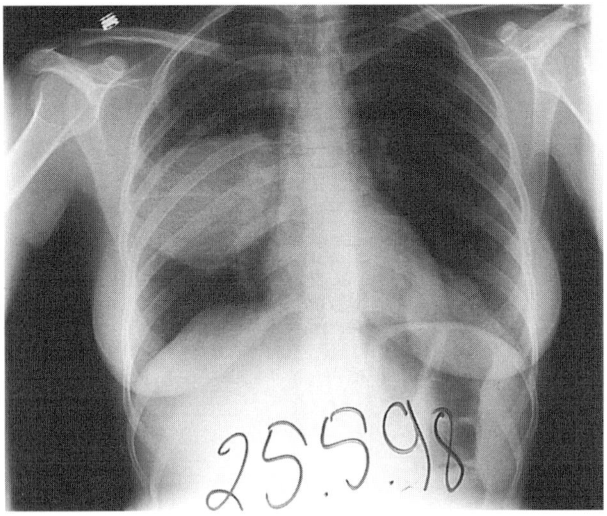

Figure 42–1. Hydatid cyst filling the right middle lobe.

Medical Therapy

Although surgery remains the mainstay of therapy for hydatid disease of the lung, medical therapy has become an integral part in the treatment of hydatid disease.[10] Benzimidazole drugs, such as mebendazole and albendazole, are active against the organism. Both have been used extensively, although its higher rate of gastrointestinal absorption favors albendazole. Studies have not yet shown that medical therapy can replace surgery. Drugs are effective in 30 to 40% of patients. Furthermore, they should be taken for long periods and have significant gastrointestinal, neurologic, hematologic, and hepatic toxicity.[11] They can, however, be used as the primary mode of therapy for small cysts or disseminated disease. There is also some evidence that medical therapy can play an important adjuvant role to surgery by preventing the dissemination of the protoscolices at the time of operation and thus reducing the recurrence rate of the disease.[12]

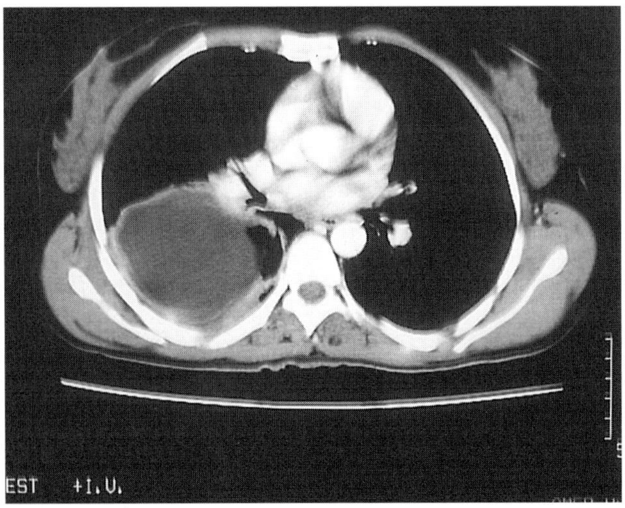

Figure 42–2. Computed tomography of the lung in a patient with a ruptured hydatid cyst. The cyst shows homogeneous water density except for a rim of air density—an appearance consistent with rupture.

Surgical Therapy

Surgery for pulmonary hydatid disease has evolved over the last four decades. The type of surgery for pulmonary hydatidosis depends on the extent of pulmonary disease and the present complications. The surgical options are many. Strict scolicidal asepsis and the complete evacuation of the endocyst remain the basic principles of management. Anatomic resections were performed frequently in the past but now are rarely indicated except in patients in whom a cyst occupies more than 50% of a lobe or if chronic suppuration has resulted in the destruction of the lobe. Other surgeons advocate Barrette's method of delivering the cyst intact, which ensures strict scolicidal asepsis.[13] However, accidental rupture can be catastrophic. In addition, the unsuspected presence of multiple daughter cysts can complicate the intact delivery technique. Many surgeons therefore prefer to resort to a technique of chemical sterilization before performing a cystostomy and evacuation of the cyst contents.[14–16] The standard approach consists of a posterolateral thoracotomy. Spillage of the cyst fluid harboring living protoscolices can be catastrophic. The result can be anaphylaxis and shock or dissemination of the disease. Therefore, the operative field is protected with pads soaked with a scolicidal agent. Several scolicidal agents have been proposed.[17] Formaldehyde was originally used but was then abandoned because of its systemic toxicity. Other agents are hydrogen peroxide and hypertonic saline. At the American University of Beirut Medical Center, we have used 0.5% cetrimide (cetyltrimethylammonium bromide), which is safe, more potent, and effective against daughter cysts. The cyst is chemically sterilized, a cystostomy is performed, and the cyst contents are evacuated. It is vitally important to evacuate all the laminated membrane because recurrence of the cysts and suppurative complications have been associated with residual membrane. Bronchial openings are sutured. Two main techniques have been advocated to minimize suppurative and bronchopleural complications resulting from the residual cavity after evacuation. The residual cavity is either imbricated (capitonnage) or marsupialized. In bilateral cysts, a two-stage thoracotomy is the option preferred by many surgeons. If simultaneous liver hydatid cysts are present, a transdiaphragmatic route to evacuate the liver cysts is preferred if possible.

Video-Assisted Thoracoscopic Surgery for Pulmonary Hydatidosis

Video-assisted thoracoscopic surgery aims to perform the same operation as open surgery but in a less invasive manner. The basic principles of hydatid surgery—strict scolicidal asepsis and complete evacuation of the cyst—are adhered to. The preferred operation is the standard cystostomy and evacuation followed by partial imbrication.

Cyst rupture or infection with resultant empyema are not considered contraindications to performing the operation thoracoscopically, although they render it more difficult.

Operative Technique

All patients undergo video-assisted thoracoscopy under general anesthesia. A double-lumen intubation is used. The patient is placed in the lateral position. A 10-mm 0-degree scope is introduced through a chest tube incision away from the cyst. Thin adhesions may be noted in patients with intact cysts, whereas dense adhesions are often seen with ruptured and secondarily infected cysts. The cyst is usually seen as a relatively tense mass surfacing from the lung parenchyma. Two or three accessory ports are necessary, all inserted under direct vision (Fig. 42–3). One port is used to stabilize the pericyst and another is used to aspirate the cyst using high-power suction. The pleural cavity is routinely irrigated with 0.5% cetrimide. The cyst is carefully mobilized away from the chest wall. The dissection should be performed with care not to rupture the cyst. A long 19-gauge needle is introduced into the cavity under negative pressure transmitted from an aspirated 60-ml syringe connected to a three-way stopcock (Fig. 42–4). Cetrimide, 0.5% is then injected into the cavity. The amount injected is less than that aspirated. After 5 minutes, the 0.5% cetrimide is aspirated and the pericyst is opened with electrocautery at its uppermost portion to prevent spillage (Fig. 42–5). High-power suction is then introduced into the cavity, aspirating the germinal membrane and the contents of the cavity (Fig. 42–6). The telescope is then introduced into the cavity itself to check for daughter cysts and ensure complete evacuation of the cavity (Fig. 42–7), which is irrigated several times with 0.5% cetrimide. The pericyst is partially imbricated with several rows of endoscopic staples (Fig. 42–8). The lung is inflated and the staple line is checked for air leaks and is reinforced if necessary with additional staples. No attempt is made to resect the pericyst. A single chest tube is left in one of the anterior ports. The chest tube is usually removed in 3 to 4 days.

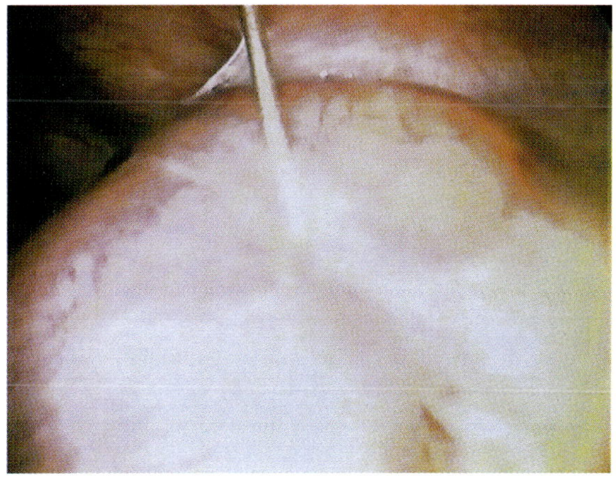

Figure 42–4. The needle is inserted into the cyst cavity.

Results

From March 1993 to December 1997, eight patients with one or more hydatid cysts of the lung underwent video-assisted thoracoscopic treatment. The ages ranged from 19 to 62 years with a mean of 31 years. There were four males and four females. The indirect hemagglutination assay was positive in four patients, negative in two patients, and was not performed in two patients. Of a total of 11 cysts, 6 were ruptured and 5 were intact. The intact cysts were larger than the ruptured cysts. The largest cyst measured 16 cm in diameter, and the smallest was 3 cm. All patients underwent radiologic evaluation with chest radiography and computed tomography.

All patients underwent the operation using the technique described previously. There was no mortality. All chest tubes were removed within 4 days. Excluding one patient who remained hospitalized for removal of a liver hydatid cyst, the average hospital stay was 5.6 days. Two patients had fever secondary to pneumonitis for which they received intravenous antibiotics. Both recovered uneventfully. The procedure had to be converted to an open thoracotomy in one patient because the pericyst

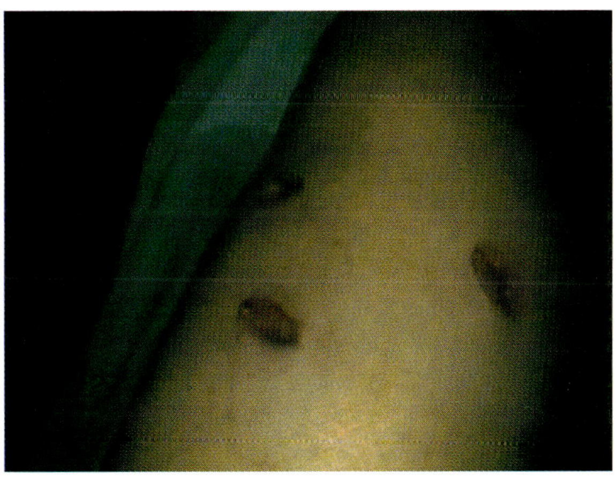

Figure 42–3. Three trocars are usually needed. Their position depends on the location of the cyst.

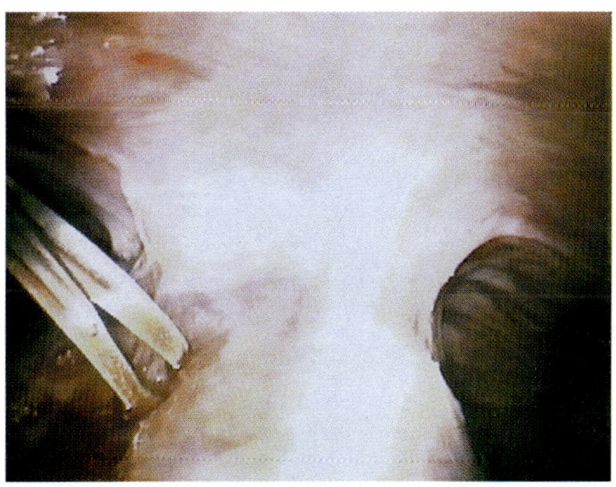

Figure 42–5. Cystotomy is performed using electrocautery and scissors.

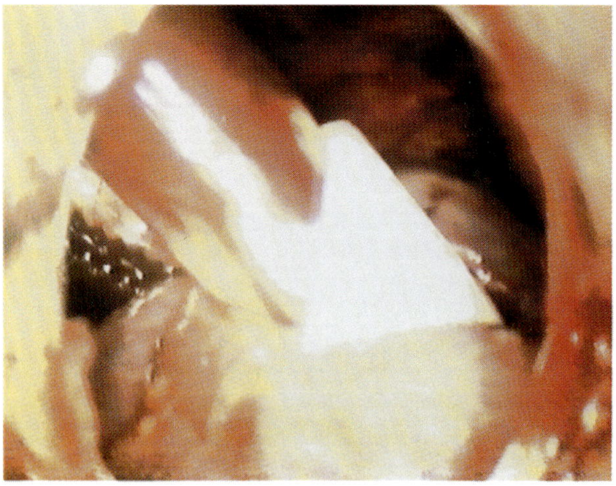

Figure 42–6. Laminated membranes are suctioned out using high-power suction.

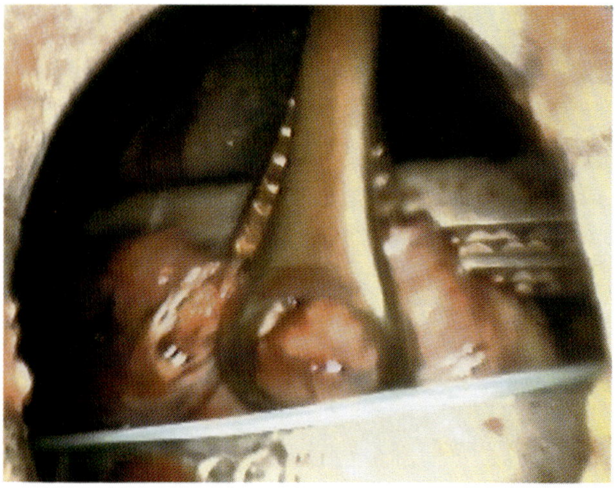

Figure 42–8. Closure and partial imbrication of the residual cavity using endoscopic stapler.

failed to close with the endoscopic stapler. A small posterolateral thoracotomy was employed to imbricate the pericyst.

The patients were followed up for 12 to 42 months. One patient with a small ruptured cyst was lost to follow-up. No recurrences were noted. All residual cavities resolved with no sequelae, with the larger cavities requiring up to 4 months to heal (Fig. 42–9). No secondary procedures were performed.

Complications

The most feared intraoperative complication is cyst rupture with resultant spillage of the cyst fluid into the pleural cavity.[18] This may result in anaphylactic shock. If the cyst has not been chemically sterilized, dissemination of the disease can occur.

In the perioperative period, the common complications are air leaks, pneumonitis, and secondary infection of the residual cavity. Suturing of all bronchial openings prevents major air leaks, whereas minor ones close within a short time. Pneumonitis is a more frequent occurrence when other scolicidal agents, such as formalin, are used. Secondary infection of the cavity is not common and is seen more often with ruptured or infected cysts. In these cases, the cysts should be completely evacuated and all debris removed. If chronic infection has destroyed most of the lobe, a lobectomy is the preferred procedure.

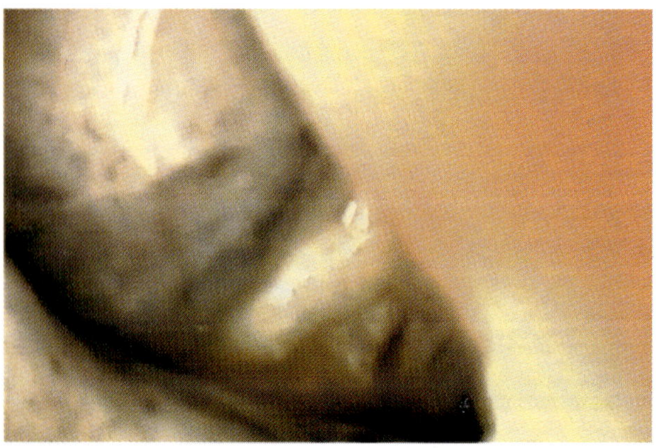

Figure 42–7. View from within the cyst, showing the fibrotic outer layer with no residual laminated membrane.

The major late complication of hydatid disease of the lung is recurrence. The recurrence rate in multiple series has ranged from 2 to 10%. Factors associated with recurrence are spillage at the time of operation and incomplete evacuation of the cyst, thus leaving residual germinal membrane behind. Although some surgeons claim that certain procedures such as anatomic resections and delivering the cyst intact are associated with lower rates of recurrence, there have not been any well-performed studies to prove this. Furthermore, the results of the less invasive operation—cystotomy and evacuation—have shown a comparable recurrence rate when the previously mentioned surgical principles are adhered to. When used as an adjunct to surgery, medical therapy may also have an important role in decreasing the recurrence rate.

Conclusion

Video-assisted thoracoscopy has gained acceptance as an alternative to open thoracotomy in many conditions because of the increased pain and morbidity associated with an open thoracotomy. In addition, video-assisted techniques offer better visualization and magnification. Thoracoscopic treatment of pulmonary hydatid disease using strict scolicidal asepsis can be applied thoracoscopically. No residual cavity problems were noted in either infected or intact cysts when meticulous evacuation of debris and airtight closure of the pericyst was employed. In addition, thoracoscopy is associated with minimal morbidity and a short hospitalization.

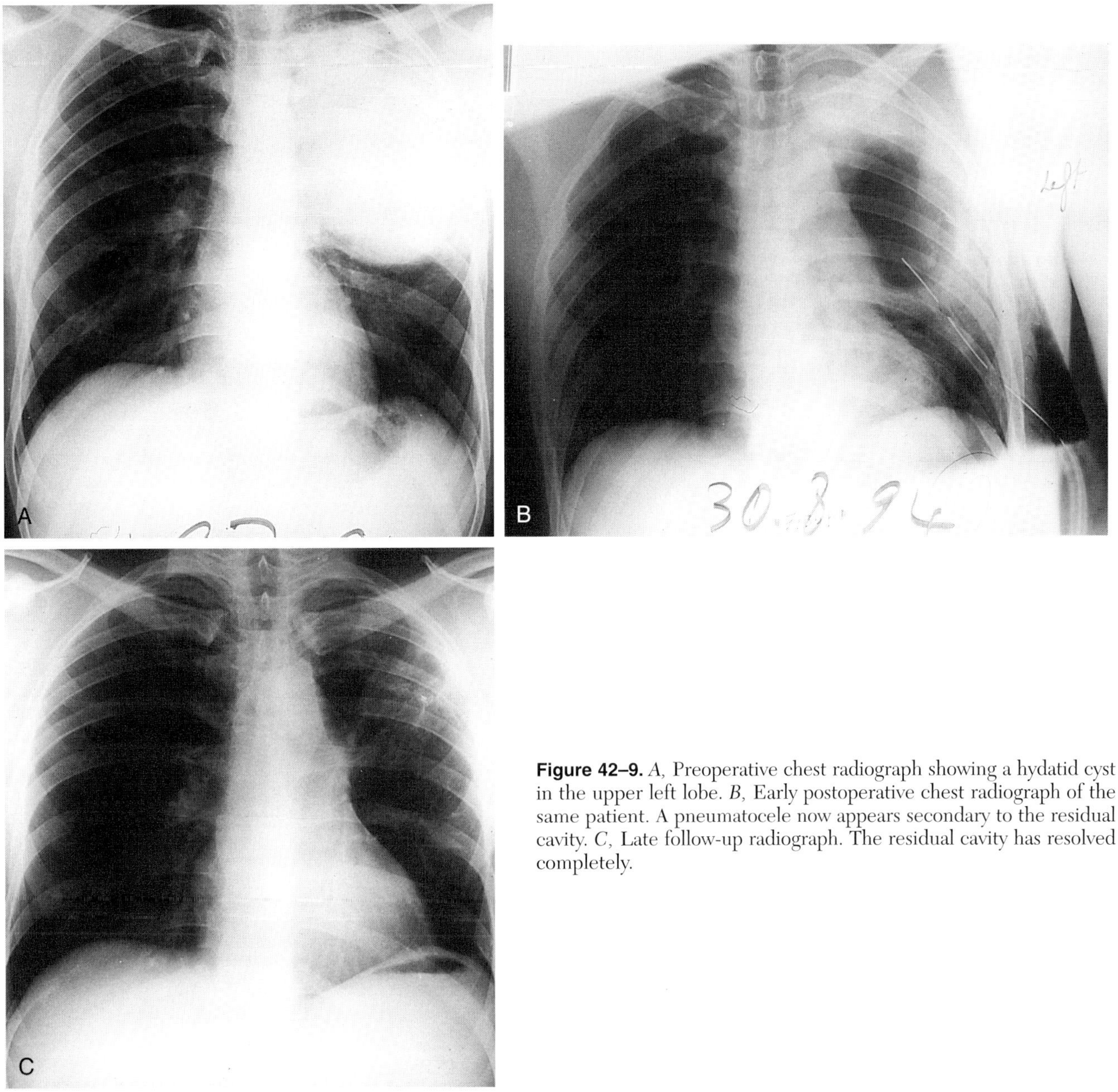

Figure 42–9. *A*, Preoperative chest radiograph showing a hydatid cyst in the upper left lobe. *B*, Early postoperative chest radiograph of the same patient. A pneumatocele now appears secondary to the residual cavity. *C*, Late follow-up radiograph. The residual cavity has resolved completely.

References

1. Hippocrates. Aphorisms VII: 55.
2. Shabb B, Taha AM, Khoury GH: Thoracoscopic treatment of two patients with infected hydatid cyst. Med J Infect Parasit Dis X(4):236–237, 1995.
3. Paterson H, Blyth D: Thoracoscopic evacuation of dead hydatid cysts. J Thorac Cardiovasc 111:1280–1281, 1996.
4. World Health Organization Informed Working Group on Echinococcosis: Guidelines for treatment of cystic and alveolar echinococcosis in humans. Bull World Health Org 74:231–242, 1996.
5. McGree PB, Nelson GS: Larval cestode infections. *In* Strickland GT (ed): Hunter's Tropical Medicine, 6th ed. Philadelphia, WB Saunders, 1984, p 771.
6. Tuncel E: Pulmonary air meniscus sign. Respiration 46:139–144, 1984.
7. Grabbe E, Kern P, Heller M: Human echinococcosis: Diagnostic value of computed tomography. Tropenmed Parasitol 32: 35–38, 1981.
8. Beggs I: The radiology of hydatid disease. AJR Am J Roentgenol 145:639–648, 1985.
9. Chemtai AK, Bowry TR, Ahmad Z: Evaluation of five immunodiagnostic techniques in echinococcosis patients. Bull World Health Org 59:767, 1981.
10. Mawhorter S, Temeck B, Chang R, et al: Nonsurgical therapy for pulmonary hydatid disease. Chest 112:1432–1436, 1997.
11. Teggi A, Lastilla MG, De Rosa F: Therapy of human hydatid disease with mebendazole and albendazole. Antimicrob Agents Chemother 37:1679–1684, 1993.
12. Morris DL, Chinnery JB, Hardcastle JD: Can albendazole reduce the risk of implantation of spilled protoscoleces? An animal study. Trans R Soc Trop Med Hyg 80:481–484, 1986.
13. Barret NR: Surgical treatment of hydatid cysts of the lung. Thorax 2:21–57, 1947.
14. Qian Z: Thoracic hydatid cysts: A report of 842 cases treated over a thirty year period. Ann Thorac Surg 46:342–346, 1988.
15. Dogan R, Yuksel M, Cetin G, et al: Surgical treatment of hydatid

cysts of the lung: Report on 1055 patients. Thorax 44:192–199, 1989.
16. Burgos L, Baquerizo A, Munoz W, et al: Experience in the surgical treatment of 331 patients with pulmonary hydatidosis. J Thorac Cardiovasc Surg 102:427–430,1991.
17. Meymeriam E, George MS, Luttermoser W, et al: Laboratory evaluation of chemical scolicides as adjuncts to hydatid surgery. Ann Surg 158:221–226, 1963.
18. Scgiller CF: Complications of *Echinococcus* cyst rupture: A study of 30 cases. JAMA 19:220–222,1966.

COMMENTARY

Anthony P. C. Yim

Echinococcosis or hydatid disease, although uncommon in Western countries, continues to be a major health problem in regions like the Middle East and Australasia. The disease can involve virtually any organ system, and a high index of suspicion is needed for diagnosis. The disease can involve the lung, the heart, or the thoracic spine. As the authors of this chapter point out, the surgical approach of extruding intact hydatid cysts as originally advocated by Barrett is risky and has fallen out of favor. The thoracoscopic approach described in this chapter, with instillation of scolicide followed by suction removal of all the cyst contents including the germinal membrane, is a viable alternative to the open technique for peripheral cysts in experienced hands. However, the inability to use bimanual palpation in video-assisted thoracoscopic surgery makes it more likely that smaller and more deeply placed cysts will be missed. Centrally located cysts may require anatomic resection for removal. Another treatment modality that deserves more attention is the percutaneous approach for instillation and aspiration under imaging guidance. It could be used as an adjuvant therapy to surgery for recurrent or missed pulmonary cysts when prior operation renders future surgical intervention difficult or hazardous.

Chapter 43

Complications and Pitfalls in Video-Assisted Thoracic Surgery

William S. Walker

Video-assisted thoracic surgery (VATS) has evolved over the past 8 years to encompass a wide range of minor and major surgical procedures. Inevitably, there have been and will continue to be instances in which complications have arisen or have clearly had the potential to do so. The immediate relevance of these events is to the safety and well-being of the patient, which is naturally of paramount importance. Quite apart from these considerations, however, adverse outcomes arouse scrutiny from patients, relatives, support groups, health care purchasers, and the legal profession. Thus, a potentially superior new procedure may acquire an undeservedly bad reputation when performed incorrectly or without due care. This entirely avoidable outcome can impair development, adversely affect the general uptake of a procedure, and place those who continue to use it (even with excellent results) in an invidious and exposed position.

Remarkably few serious intraoperative events have been reported in the literature on VATS procedures, perhaps because these events, together with the "near misses" we have all experienced, are often the subject of conversation rather than a journal article. It is the purpose of this chapter to review the existing published experience of VATS procedures within the context of the associated reported complications and problems and to consider aspects and technical issues that may be known to or understood by those with a detailed experience of VATS but may not yet be well reported. There is clearly little point to each surgeon rediscovering the same problems and solutions; thus, it is to be hoped that the overview of current knowledge presented in this chapter may be of help by highlighting potential pitfalls and the strategies that have been found to be of value in dealing with different areas of difficulty or concern.

Legal Considerations

Any complication may form the basis of litigation; therefore, it is of particular importance that the surgeon undertaking VATS procedures is conversant with the potential complications and pitfalls in this field, especially as applied to the procedures of relevance to his or her practice. Case law in Great Britain[1] has, for example, established the position of the medical practitioner as someone who "exercising and professing to have that special skill . . . exercises the ordinary skill of an ordinary competent man exercising that particular art." This clearly translates into the assumption that a surgeon practising VATS procedures (and therefore implicitly claiming special skill in that field) must exhibit an appropriate level of competence, including the ability to anticipate and manage complications. Whereas the specifics of case or codified law vary from region to region, there seems little reason to assume that significant deviation from this principle will occur. The obvious comparators for most VATS cases are the reported outcomes with established open thoracic procedures. These have benefited from a learning curve often extending over nearly 50 years. Ironically, these cases have almost always escaped any form of systematic appraisal prior to general adoption. It is also the case that a sizable group of general thoracic surgeons continue to regard VATS as excessively employed, and a majority have significant reservations regarding its use in certain areas.[38] Consequently, justifying deviation from established practice toward a VATS approach may require detailed records with adequate documentation of training, current experience, meticulous operative procedure, and advance planning.

Sources and Types of Actual and Potential Complication

Complications and pitfalls occurring in association with VATS procedures may occur in or stem from all three perioperative phases (Table 43–1).

The Preoperative Phase

Preoperative assessment affords the opportunity to select optimal candidates for VATS and, by recognizing potential pitfalls, avoid complications. In this context, it is important to recognize that psychological factors may be of considerable importance in determining the incidence of perceived complications.

Addressing Patient Expectation

There has been a trend for patients to self-select for minimal-access procedures on the basis of Internet reports, newspaper articles, and hearsay. This can create a significant reality gap between what the patient has been led (or has led himself or herself) to believe and the actual outcomes that may reasonably be anticipated. It is important to stress to the patient during preoperative counseling that, in general terms, a VATS procedure is a less traumatic approach to performing the same operative procedure used for a standard open operation. It may therefore involve all the complications known to relate to open surgery and, additionally, intraoperative complications specific to the particular VATS procedure. Although VATS is expected to be less painful, it is *not* free from pain. Simi-

Table 43–1. Classification of Complications Occurring in Association with VATS Procedures

Preoperative
Patient selection
Patient expectation
Operative
Equipment
Anesthesia
Operator skill issues
Complications common to open surgery
Specific complications related to VATS itself
Postoperative
Complications common to open surgery
Specific complications related to VATS itself
Failure to achieve therapeutic goals

larly, extirpative surgery involving the loss of functioning lung will still result in degradation in respiratory function. This is the time to discuss with the patient the possibility of conversion to open thoracotomy if the intraoperative events or findings determine that this is the safest course of action. This outcome must be presented for what it is—a continuation of intelligent surgical practice into the operative phase—rather than ignored and then later defended in a retrospective attempt to excuse an apparent failure of technique.

Preoperative Assessment

Elderly patients and those with reduced pulmonary function normally constitute increased-risk groups for thoracic surgical procedures. These patients appear to experience better outcomes with a VATS approach[13, 25] than with open thoracotomy. Therefore, they may be particularly appropriate candidates for a VATS approach, but that does not mean that the risks of operation should be underplayed.

Grossly overweight patients are unlikely to make good VATS subjects. Port lengths are generally insufficient to allow satisfactory entry into the chest, and manipulation of instruments and adequate ventilatory control may be difficult to achieve. Anticoagulant and nonsteroidal anti-inflammatory medications are relative contraindications, as they may result in excessive intraoperative oozing, which can render endoscopic surgery hazardous by obscuring the operator's view.

The surgeon should question whether a VATS procedure really is the least invasive form of surgery for the patient or whether some other even less invasive procedure might achieve the same result more simply. Limited parietal injury—the chief benefit of a VATS approach—can be less important than minimizing the internal operative procedure. For example, a subxyphoid pericardial window is a much better choice for an end-stage malignant pericardial effusion than a VATS pericardial window. Also, some patients, such as those in intensive care on ventilation undergoing lung biopsy for severe lung changes, may be unlikely to tolerate single-lung ventilation, in which case a VATS approach would at best be difficult and potentially could be hazardous.

Anticipated Intrathoracic Pathology

Intrathoracic adhesions are a relative contraindication to VATS. They increase operative time and result in damaged lung. More importantly, they obscure vision both directly and via increased blood loss, which then increases the risk of an intraoperative complication. Moderate adhesions are manageable and may be tackled by an experienced VATS surgeon after assessing the intrathoracic appearances at preliminary videoendoscopy, but patients with obvious dense adhesions on the initial chest film should not be scheduled for a VATS procedure.

In general, a VATS approach to definitive therapy, as opposed to biopsy or palliative care issues, is relevant in earlier disease stages. It is important, therefore, to conform to established selection criteria. Deviation from this policy will significantly increase the risk and attendant liability of complications, as the surgeon will then be attempting to manage disease that lies outside the correct limit of a VATS approach.

Consideration should be given to the location of pulmonary nodules. Is it truly realistic to anticipate a successful thoracoscopic excision, or could the lesion lie too deep for this to be a safe maneuver? Careful scrutiny of the preoperative computed tomography (CT) images may help clarify this issue. Nodules located far from the pleural surface are unlikely to be suitable choices for a VATS approach.[14] Small lesions (< 1 cm) may be difficult to locate, but identification might be facilitated by the use of CT-guided hook wire or dye markers.[39, 50]

Operative Factors

Equipment

Imaging. VATS surgery currently exists in two main forms: true endoscopic surgery, in which the operative view is obtained entirely using a videothoracoscope and is displayed on a video screen, and hybrid approaches, in which the surgeon may also operate partly under direct vision through a small wound, guided by light from the videothoracoscope. It is not within the scope of this chapter to consider the relative merits of these two approaches. However, regardless of the preferred technique, a high-grade camera and light source combination is clearly a prerequisite.

Videoendoscopic equipment is generally reliable, but failure during surgery requires obligatory conversion to an open procedure and may be exceptionally dangerous if it occurs during a crucial operative maneuver, such as dissection or clamping a major vessel. Simple anticipation and training will resolve the risk of complications as distinct from inconvenience resulting from equipment failure. Most equipment problems are "finger" problems—wrong or bad connections or inappropriate setup. The surgeon should know how the equipment connects together and works, and a member of the surgical team should be encouraged to take a special interest in the equipment. Few situations are more frustrating to a surgeon during surgery than knowing which button to press but being in the position of trying to explain this while scrubbed to someone with no technical knowledge and no awareness of (and usually no interest in) the principles of videoendoscopic surgical equipment. A dedicated, or at least consistent, unit for thoracic surgical use will help to ensure that the equipment is understood and correctly adjusted during the operative procedure. Simple but useful measures include ensuring that a supply of spare light-source bulbs are available and that backup camera and light source units are within the surgical suite, if possible.

It should be a cardinal principle for the surgeon to check over the equipment before the procedure, just as the anesthesiologist checks the anesthetic machine, and a pilot an aircraft's systems. This is a surgical responsibility and an opportunity to avoid a serious complication.

Surgical Endostaplers. VATS procedures, particularly pulmonary resections, require extensive use of endoscopic staplers. These can be a significant source of complications. We and others[10, 62] have experienced failure of vascular stapling devices (Fig. 43–1), and we would now recommend that a vascular clamp be placed centrally on a pulmonary vein (Fig.43–2) or main artery prior to division. Once the stapler has been fired, the central closure line can be inspected (Fig. 43–3) and confirmed to be satisfactory before the clamp is released. This method provides continuous vascular control. Despite these observations, endoscopic staplers are exceptionally reliable, and failure is most often a complication caused by incorrect handling of the device by the surgical team. Specifically, the cartridge must be verified to be correctly loaded, the correct staple leg length must be chosen for the tissue to be divided (Table 43–2), tissue must not encroach on the hinge mechanism, and loose staples must be carefully removed. Excess staples can be a nuisance, as they may fall off the cartridge after firing and litter the chest cavity, potentially interfering with the stapler mechanism. It is helpful to coat the jaws of the stapler with a water-soluble lubricating jelly, as this will retain surplus staples on the fired cartridge so that they do not contaminate the operative field. The stapler is then rinsed in water before reloading in preparation for the next firing.

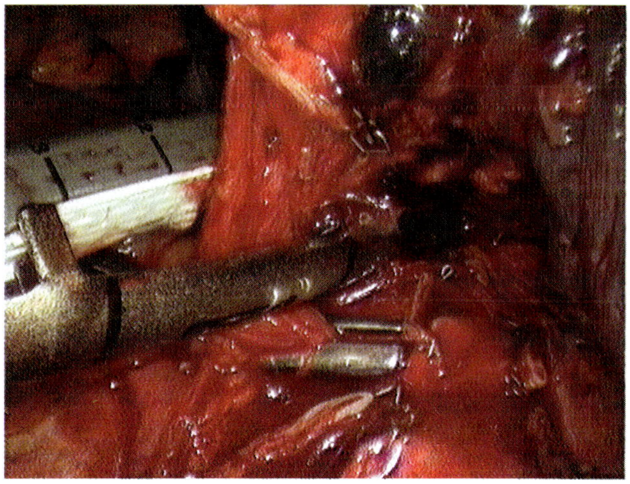

Figure 43–2. Left lower lobectomy with use of centrally placed vascular clamp to control the lower left pulmonary vein before division by an endostapler.

Electrocautery. Cautery is of great value in VATS procedures, but use of monopolar cautery presents potential risks, predominantly from unintentional injury to intrathoracic tissues. Mechanisms include lack of appreciation of the extent of current flow—as with potential spinal cord injury during cautery ablation of the sympathetic chain; inadvertent burn complications due to insulation breaks in instruments; and arcing caused by capacitive coupling problems. This last issue[56] is perhaps least appreciated and relates to the use of electrically insulated cannulae. Conductive metal cannulae allow charge accumulated on instruments (notably the endoscope) to dissipate through the patient's body and consequently obviate the risk of spontaneous discharge burns. If extensive use of cautery,

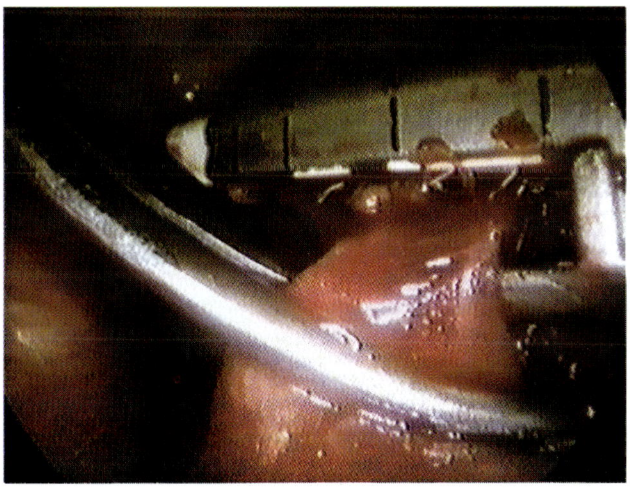

Figure 43–1. Failure of Endo GIA vascular stapler on left upper pulmonary vein. Note distorted staples and torn bleeding vein. This device could not be made to release initially.

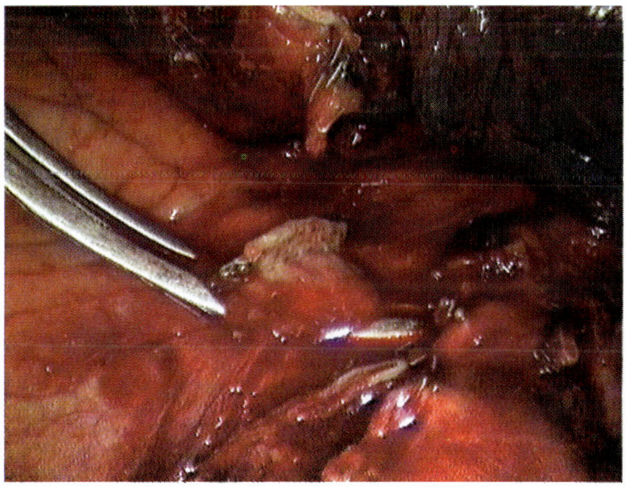

Figure 43–3. Appearance after firing stapler. The closure line is entirely satisfactory; therefore, the clamp may be released with confidence.

Table 43–2. Endoscopic Stapler Sizes and Useage

Cartridge Color	Stapler Leg Length	Typical Thoracic Tissue
Gray	2 mm	Small pulmonary arteries
White	2.5 mm	Large pulmonary arteries Pulmonary veins Azygos vein
Blue	3.5 mm	Peripheral lung parenchyma Segmental bronchi Esophageal wall
Green	4.8 mm	Main bronchus and lobar bronchi Central pulmonary parenchyma Stomach

either monopolar or bipolar, is required, it may be helpful to utilize a carbon dioxide (CO_2) through flow system, which reduces combustion risks by eliminating oxygen from the thoracic cavity and also improves the view by clearing smoke.

In any situation where cautery is used near the heart, it is sensible to apply remote defibrillation pads to the patient prior to surgery so that ventricular fibrillation can be easily corrected. The most obvious procedures in which this might apply are formation of a pericardial window and endoscopic dissection of the internal mammary artery.

Anesthesia

Anesthetic considerations regarding VATS procedures have been discussed in detail elsewhere (see Chapters 3, 4, and 36) and will only be considered here insofar as anaesthetic events have the capacity to induce surgical complications.

Intrapleural CO_2 insufflation may be used to create space in the ipsilateral hemithorax when a single endotracheal tube is employed or to aid pulmonary collapse when a double-lumen tube is used. Although CO_2 insufflation appears to be safe in clinical practice,[59] experimental evidence[23, 28] suggests that it has the potential for serious detrimental effects, including mediastinal distortion, elevated central venous pressure, and decreased cardiac output. Intrapleural pressure should not exceed 10 mm Hg (probably less in children), and the flow rate should be restricted to a maximum of 2 L/min to prevent rapid mediastinal movement.

A misplaced double-lumen tube almost always results in air trapping and hyperexpansion of the ipsilateral lung, which makes thoracoscopic surgery impossible. Auscultation and observation are unreliable indicators of satisfactory tube position,[53] which is often disturbed when the patient is turned into the lateral decubitus position. Either the anesthesiologist or the surgeon should perform a fiberoptic bronchoscopy to check and, if necessary, adjust the tube position once the patient has been finally positioned. If a tube moves during surgery, it is often possible to reposition it under bronchoscopic guidance,[4] but if this cannot be rapidly achieved, this situation should be taken as an indication for conversion to an open procedure.

A collapsed lung may cause worrisome hypoxia because of right-to-left intrapulmonary shunting. This problem is particularly noticable in the initial phase of pulmonary collapse before hypoxic pulmonary vasoconstriction has occurred. Continuous positive airway pressure is an often-advocated anesthetic solution to this problem,[6, 24] but it may create potentially dangerous operating conditions for a VATS procedure, as the lung will often re-expand to a troublesome degree. In our experience, either intermittent insufflation of the operative lung with oxygen or delivery of continuous oxygen to the lung is a useful alternative strategy that will result in much less pulmonary expansion. Contralateral pneumothorax has occurred only once in our experience of approximately 900 major VATS procedures. This rare event presents an unmanageable situation in which the mediastinum is pushed toward the surgeon while hypoxia prevents adequate deflation of the operative lung, so that conversion to open thoracotomy is mandatory.

Operator Skill Issues

Selection of Operative Approach. The operative approaches relevant to most procedures have now been well described by various authors. There are several fundamental concepts,[31] however, that are generally applicable. The principle of triangulation should be adhered to for lesser procedures at least (see Chapter 5). Small patients have small interspaces; therefore, postoperative pain may be improved by the use of a 5-mm videothoracoscope rather than a 10-mm one and by the insertion of larger instruments through the wider anterior interspaces. Regardless of patient size, excessive leverage must be avoided at port sites to reduce the risk of intercostal nerve injury.

Assessing Operability. Many problems occur in VATS procedures when the surgeon does not continue the process of assessment of operability into the operative phase. Conversion to an open procedure should be an elective maneuver—not the response to an operation that has gone seriously wrong. On initial appraisal at videothoracoscopy, the surgeon should determine whether the assumptions made during preoperative assessment are correct. Successful wedge excision of a pulmonary nodule, for example, presupposes that it can be reliably located. Physical palpation by fingertip or the use of a pledget mounted on a Robert's forceps provides the best form of identification, but ultrasonic or tactile sensor probes[44, 51] may be helpful. Smaller lesions will have required preliminary hook wire or dye marker localization, in which case the success of the localization process will have to be judged carefully (see Chapter 15). It remains the case that unless absolute localization can be achieved and confirmed if necessary by frozen section, conversion to open thoracotomy must occur. Finally, it must be determined whether the nodule is located too deep within the lung substance for safe wedge excision.

The surgeon must consider whether a VATS operative procedure will meet the established requirements of surgery for malignant disease with regard to adequacy of local tissue clearance and lymph node management. Will a VATS approach lead to an excessively prolonged procedure (and hence increase the risk of postoperative pulmonary complications), when an open approach would be much quicker? Even when it seems obvious that an open approach will be necessary, however, VATS assessment offers the opportunity to detect the presence of hitherto unsuspected causes of irresectability in malignant cases and thereby avoid an unnecessary open thoracotomy.[3, 46]

Patients with inflammatory lung disease should undergo particularly careful scrutiny before surgery. Highly vascular adhesions and lymph nodes with large feeding vessels may be present. We have had only one life-threatening intraoperative hemorrhage occurring during more than 160 VATS major pulmonary resections.[57] This occurred during attempts to clear densely adherent inflammatory nodes from the pulmonary artery within the fissure with a consequent 2.3-L hemorrhage. This patient went on to make an entirely uneventful postoperative recovery, but we would now regard the presence of inflammatory nodes adherent to the sheath of the pulmonary artery as an absolute indication for conversion to an open procedure.

Surgical Ability. The skills required in VATS are different from but additive to existing skills required for open thoracic surgery. Specifically, the surgeon must develop sufficient hand-to-eye coordination to allow surgery to proceed safely on the basis of a monitor display. Three-dimensional awareness (i.e., the intuitive reconstruction of a three-dimensional concept of the operative field based on a synthesis of the two-dimensional view presented on the monitor and the surgeon's own memory of the detailed topographic anatomy of the relevant region) is an essential prerequisite for advanced VATS procedures such as dissection within the pulmonary hilum.

Whereas simple operations such as lung biopsy or wedge resection and pneumothorax surgery may be less taxing than complex procedures, it must be said that some individuals are not sufficiently adept at endoscopic surgery to allow them to undertake more major procedures. Where this limitation applies, it is incumbent on the surgeon to recognize this reality and always operate within his or her own capabilities. Equally, even the most dextrous surgeon would be foolhardy and open to justifiable criticism if he or she were to embark on a program of major VATS procedures without appropriate guidance and training. Adequate training in VATS surgery is clearly essential, as is theability to retrieve untoward situations by rapid recourse to open thoracotomy with appropriate surgical intervention. Therefore, the general recommendation must be that the surgeon and team are experienced in general thoracic (and, where appropriate, cardiac) surgery,[54] trained in VATS techniques, and educated regarding the specifics of the procedure to be performed. Conversely, skill level should certainly not be used as a reason for selecting an operative procedure. For example, wedge resection of a peripheral pulmonary cancer may be a straightforward and tempting VATS procedure in elderly or unfit patients,[52] but there is ample evidence from conventional surgery[19, 58] to demonstrate that it should not be performed simply to achieve a VATS approach when lobectomy would otherwise have been the selected procedure.

Operative Technique. The significance of postoperative air leakage following VATS surgery has been apparent since the initial review of the VATS study group data.[22] Prolonged air leakage reduces the value of a VATS approach by impeding early discharge and exposing the patient to drain-related pain. Gentle handling of lung parenchyma is essential to minimize pulmonary tears, and staple lines must be scrutinized carefully. Various additive measures including pericardial[9] and polytetrafluoroethylene (PTFE)[55] buttress strips may be of value in shortening the period of leakage. Experience with PTFE is limited, but Hazelrigg and associates[20] reported a 2.6-day reduction in air leakage with the use of pericardial buttresses in a prospective randomized study of lung volume reduction surgery—a measure that paid for itself by reducing patient stay by 2.8 days. There is now some suspicion that pericardial buttresses may be associated with the formation of severe and dense adhesions, which can make reoperative procedures both difficult and dangerous. This could be viewed as a late complication of this technique and may have implications regarding patient selection. Light activated polymerizing tissue sealant has proved highly effective at sealing lung tears and fissure lines in preliminary studies,[36] may allow much earlier discharge after any procedure involving lung stapling, and has the advantage of being reabsorbable.

Bronchus closure with endostaplers is generally very reliable, but the stump must be carefully scrutinized and reinforced with sutures if the staple line appears suspect in any area. Utilizing this policy, we have experienced only one bronchopleural fistula early in our experience (0.66%) of 150 VATS lobectomies.[57] During the initial experience of VATS lobectomy, concern over the use of 3.5-mm staplers to divide lobar bronchi led Kirkby and associates[29] to recommend that separate division of the major segmental group bronchi was preferable on the basis that a more reliable bronchial closure was achieved. Further development of endostapler design has provided devices with 4.8-mm staples; thus, this recommendation is no longer relevant.

Malignant tissues must be handled with caution during VATS procedures. Rough handling may increase the risk of tearing through cancerous tissues, with consequent contamination of the operative field, and instruments which then have the potential to disseminate malignant cells into the port sites. A plastic delivery bag must be used for all malignant specimens other than simple bite biopsies. These should be taken using a biopsy forceps inserted through a physical port tube, which will protect the soft tissues of the chest wall. Implantation of malignant cells in VATS port sites has been well described in a paper by Downey and associates on behalf of the VATS Study Group,[17] in a more general review by Collard and Reymond,[8] and in further recent case reports.[48, 60] Although these accounts—which total 26 reported events—present a serious complication, they require interpretation. Half the patients with port site implants in the aforementioned reports underwent surgery for intrathoracic metastatic disease (eight cases) or for biopsy of mesothelioma (five cases). An increased risk of wound implantation might, therefore, have been anticipated in these cases regardless of the surgical approach adopted. Also, the denominator is unknown but probably runs into thousands, making the true incidence of this problem low overall. One recent estimate calculated the risk taken over all cases to be 0.08%,[35] which is similar to an incidence of 0.13% determined in a recent questionnaire survey of 21 surgical groups undertaking a total of 1530 VATS lobectomy cases.[40]

Safety and Conversion

Overall, operative safety reported in mixed series of VATS procedures appears generally high. Jancovici and associates,[26] presenting a review of 937 cases from the French Thorax Group, described a 12.4% conversion rate with 0% intraoperative mortality and 0.5% inpatient mortality. Comparable reports describe the results obtained with mixed groups from other European,[43] North American,[13] and Asian centers.[64] Conversion to open thoracotomy may occur because of technical difficulties or because an open operation is considered more appropriate. Rates of 2 to 15% appear average, but the threshold for conversion will vary between centers, depending on attitudes toward primary malignant disease. Allen and associates,[2] reporting the Mayo Clinic experience, for example, described a consistent and unusually high 25% conversion rate for a mixed series of moderate-complexity cases.

Operative complication rates for the most complex VATS operations appear similar to those for general experience. Mackinlay[40] specifically sought conversion data for his survey of 1530 VATS lobectomy cases and found an average rate of 11% (range, 1 to 30%). Fifty-one (3.3%) intraoperative accidents occurred because of either surgical maneuvers or instrument failure, but only 17 (1.1%) of these required immediate conversion. None were fatal. One intraoperative death did occur (0.06%), but this reflected a primary cardiac event. Peracchia and associates[45] reviewed 107 thoracoscopic esophagectomies collected from the literature. Conversion was required in 12 (11.2%), with no intraoperative deaths.

Planning for disaster management should, in the author's opinion, be to the fore in every VATS program. In large part, disaster can be avoided by good training, careful surgery, and the application of some elementary safety principles, but major bleeding can occur, and when it does, immediate action is required. Appropriate strategies must be in place to manage such an event, including positioning and draping the patient so that rapid conversion to a major thoracotomy is feasible and ensuring that the necessary equipment and trays are available. All major VATS cases should benefit from arterial pressure monitoring, a large-caliber intravenous line, and blood readily available within the operating theater area. The instinctive reaction to hemorrhage is to control bleeding with a vascular clamp. This is a dangerous policy, as the operative view is usually lost within seconds, making it difficult to apply a clamp effectively and safely within that time frame. A safer alternative would be to use those few seconds of vision to insert a swab mounted on a stick through the utility incision, so that an assistant can control blood loss by pressing on the bleeding point while the surgeon opens the chest.

The Postoperative Phase

Postoperative events following VATS procedures may be considered under three broad headings: procedure efficacy compared with conventional surgery, complications common to open surgery, and cost and resource issues.

Efficacy

Although a detailed comparative review of the relative merits of VATS and open approaches is beyond the scope of this chapter, it is fair to observe that a failed or substandard outcome resulting from a VATS procedure would be a very significant complication of that approach. However, a substantial body of literature is now available testifying to equivalent outcomes between open and VATS approaches for a range of procedures, including early-stage empyema,[41] pneumothorax,[6, 27, 61] lung volume reduction,[30] wedge excision of nodules,[5] metastasectomy,[16] and management of benign esophageal disease.[42] Major pulmonary resection would appear to be safe and to have equivalent survival results for stage I lung cancer.[34, 40, 47, 57, 65] In others, notably the excision of malignant mediastinal masses and esophagectomy,[45] considerable scepticism persists and is reflected in modest procedure uptake.

Postoperative Complications

There are no complications manifesting in the postoperative period that are unique to VATS procedures. Air leakage and port site implantation have been considered previously. Wound infection can occur but is no more or less likely than with open surgery. There is cause for concern, however, regarding the validity of sterilization for complex reusable instruments and flexible endoscopes, particularly for instruments that are not autoclaved.[18] Little data currently are available in this respect, but viral infection may be a future consideration.

Pain is a significant complication of open thoracic surgery[12] that is consistently reported to be reduced by a VATS approach, although relatively few authors have provided documentary evidence to support this assertion.[27, 32, 34, 57, 63]

Dieter and Kuzycz,[15] in their recent review of complications and contraindications of thoracoscopy, raise the specter of associated cardiovascular complications with a VATS approach but report that they have not experienced significant problems in this regard and do not cite references to support these assertions. In our own experience, such problems have been minimal. Of a series comprising 895 major operative intrathoracic procedures (as opposed to biopsy procedures) as of December 1997, we have experienced only two 30-day deaths from pulmonary embolism—both were patients with a history of recurrent emboli—and a supraventricular tachyarrhythmia incidence of 2.5%. Clinically significant myocardial infarction has not occurred. Therefore, we would not consider that cardiovascular problems were a feature of either the intraoperative or postoperative phase in VATS surgery.

Cost and Resource Issues

Whether or not cost represents a complication is debatable, but in the context of current economic restrictions in health care provision, it is certainly a complicating factor. There can be little doubt that a VATS procedure is generally more expensive with regard to surgical disposable costs, but many authors comment on reduced patient stay, which provides a significant cost offset. There are serious difficulties in comparing cost-related issues between different countries, as the overall cost and cost share calculations vary significantly. The available evidence, however, would support the view that when all aspects of patient cost are summated, lung biopsy,[7] pneumothorax surgery,[11, 49] pulmonary wedge excision,[21] lung volume reduction,[20, 37] and major lung resection[33] are (or can be) either cost-effective or cost-neutral procedures.

Summary

To summarize,

- Many complications related to a VATS approach may be anticipated and are therefore potentially avoidable.
- Careful patient selection and counseling are essential.
- The surgeon should ensure that equipment functions correctly prior to commencing surgery and that his or her own level of competence and skill is appropriate to the intended procedure. Planned measures must be in place to allow rapid and safe conversion to open thoracotomy in the event of an intraoperative disaster.
- Careful operative technique is essential, and particular care is required in the handling of malignant tissue. The operative situation should be the subject of continued appraisal to assess whether a procedure is progressing as planned or whether an unsatisfactory or potentially dangerous situation may be developing.
- Review of the literature demonstrates that VATS procedures are associated with an excellent intraoperative safety record, postoperative complication rates equal to or less than conventional surgery, and equivalent functional results.

References

1. Allen MS, Deschamps C, Jones DM, et al: Video-assisted thoracic surgical procedures: The Mayo experience. Mayo Clinic Proceedings 71:351–359, 1996.
2. Asamura H, Nakayama H, Kondo H, et al: Thoracoscopic evaluation of histologically/cytologically proven or suspected lung cancer: A VATS exploration. Lung Cancer 16:183–190, 1997.
3. Benumof J, Partridge B, Salvatierra C, et al: Margin of safety in positioning modern double-lumen endotracheal tubes. Anaesthesiology 67:729–738, 1987.
4. Bernard A: Resection of pulmonary nodules using video-assisted thoracic surgery. Ann Thor Surg 61: 202–205, 1996.
5. Bolam v. Friern Hospital management committee. All England Reports, 1957, 2, p 118.
6. Caplan L, Turndorf H, Patel C, et al: Optimization of arterial oxygenation during one lung anaesthesia. Anesthes Analges 59:847–851, 1980.
7. Carnochan FM, Walker WS, Cameron EWJ: Efficacy of video assisted thoracoscopic lung biopsy: An historical comparison with open lung biopsy. Thorax 49:361–363, 1994.
8. Collard JM, Reymond MA: Video-assisted thoracic surgery (VATS) for cancer. Int Surg 81:343–346, 1996.
9. Cooper JD: Technique to reduce air leaks after resection of emphysematous lung. Ann Thorac Surg 57:1038–1039, 1994.
10. Craig SR, Walker WS: Potential complications of vascular stapling in thoracoscopic surgery. Ann Thorac Surg 59:736–738, 1995.
11. Crisci R, Coloni GF: Video-assisted thoracoscopic surgery versus thoracotomy for recurrent spontaneous pneumothorax. Eur J Cardiothorac Surg 10:556–560, 1996.
12. Dajczman E, Gordon A, Kreisman H, et al: Long term post-thoracotomy pain. Chest 99:270–274, 1991.
13. De Camp MM Jr, Jaklitsch MT, Mentzer SJ, et al: The safety and versatility of video-thoracoscopy: A prospective analysis of 895 consecutive cases. J Am Coll Surg 181:113–120, 1995.
14. Demy TL, Wagner-Mann CC, James MA, et al: Feasibility of mathematical models to predict success in video-assisted thoracic surgery lung nodule excision. Am J Surg 174:20–23, 1997.
15. Dieter RA, Kuzycz GB: Complications and contraindications of thoracoscopy. Int Surg 82:232–239, 1997.
16. Dowling RD, Landreneau RJ, Miller DL: Video-assisted thoracoscopic surgery for resection of lung metastases. Chest 113(suppl a):2S–5S, 1998.
17. Downey RJ, McCormack P, LoCicero J III: Dissemination of malignancies following video-assisted thoracic surgery: A report of 21 cases. J Thorac Cardiovasc Surg, 111:954–960, 1996.
18. Ducel G, Henry A: Prevention of the risk of infection in endoscopy. The price to pay. Eur J Coelio Surg 1:61–67, 1997.
19. Ginsberg R, Rubinstein L: A randomized trial of lobectomy versus limited resection in patients with T1N0 non–small cell lung cancer (Abstract 304). Lung Cancer 7(suppl): 83, 1991.
20. Hazelrigg SR, Boley TM, Naunheim KS, et al: Effect of bovine pericardial strips on air leak after stapled pulmonary resection. Ann Thorac Surg 63:1573–1575, 1997.
21. Hazelrigg SR, Nunchuck SK, Landreneau RJ, et al: Cost analysis for thoracoscopy: Thoracoscopic wedge resection. Ann Thor Surg 56:633–653, 1993.
22. Hazelrigg SR, Nunchuck SK, LoCicero LJ III: Video-assisted thoracic surgery study group data. Ann Thorac Surg 56: 1039–1044, 1993.
23. Hill RC, Jones DR, Vance RA, et al: Selective lung ventilation during thoracoscopy: Effects of insufflation on hemodynamics. Ann Thorac Surg 61:945–948, 1996.
24. Horswell JL: Anesthetic techniques for thoracoscopy. Ann Thorac Surg 56:624–629, 1993.
25. Jaklitsch MT, De Camp MM Jr, Liptay MJ, et al: Video-assisted thoracic surgery in the elderly—a review of 307 cases. Chest 110:751–758, 1996.
26. Jancovici R, Lang-Lazdunski L, Pons F, et al: Complications of video-assisted thoracic surgery: A five-year experience. Ann Thorac Surg 61:533–537, 1996.
27. Jiminez-Merchan R, Garcia-Diaz F, Arenas-Linares C, et al: Comparative retrospective study of surgical treatment of spontaneous pneumothorax. Thoracotomy vs. thoracoscopy. Surg Endosc 11:919–922, 1997.
28. Jones DR, Graeber GM, Tanguilig GS, et al: Effects of insufflation on hemodynamics during thoracoscopic procedures. Ann Thorac Surg 55:1379–1382, 1993.

29. Kirkby TJ, Mack MJ, Landreneau RJ, et al: Initial experience with video-assisted thoracoscopic lobectomy. Ann Thorac Surg 56:1248–1253, 1993.
30. Kotloff RM, Tino G, Bavaria JE, et al: Bilateral lung volume reduction surgery for advanced emphysema: A comparison of median sternotomy and thoracoscopic approaches. Chest 110:1399–1406, 1996.
31. Landreneau RJ, Mack MJ, Hazelrigg SR, et al: Video-assisted thoracic surgery: Basic technical concepts and intercostal approach strategies. Ann Thorac Surg 54:800–807, 1992.
32. Landreneau RJ, Mack MJ, Hazelrigg SR, et al: Prevalence of chronic pain after pulmonary resection by thoracotomy or video-assisted thoracic surgery. J Thorac Cardiovasc Surg 107:1079–1086, 1994.
33. Lewis RJ, Caccavale RJ, Sisler GE, et al: Is video-assisted thoracic surgery cost effective? N J Med 93:35–41, 1996.
34. Lewis RJ, Caccavale RJ, Sisler GE, et al: One hundred video-assisted thoracic surgical simultaneously stapled lobectomies without rib spreading. Ann Thorac Surg 63:1415–1422, 1997.
35. Lewis RJ, Caccavale RJ, Sisler GE, et al: Does VATS favor seeding of carcinoma of the lung more than a conventional operation? Int Surg 82:127–130, 1997.
36. Maccharini P: Data presented at 12th EACTS meeting, Copenhagan, Denmark, September 1997.
37. Mack MJ: Cost-effective and surgically effective lung volume reduction surgery (Editorial). Chest 111:268, 1997.
38. Mack MJ, Scruggs GR, Kelly KM, et al: Video-assisted thoracic surgery: Has technology found its place? Ann Thorac Surg 64:211–215, 1997.
39. Mack MJ, Shennib H, Landreneau RJ, et al: Techniques for localization of pulmonary nodules for thoracoscopic resection. J Thorac Cardiovasc Surg 106:550–553, 1993.
40. Mackinlay TA: VATS lobectomy: An international survey. Presented at the IVth International Symposium on Thoracoscopy and Video Assisted Thoracic Surgery, Sao-Paulo, May 1997.
41. Mackinlay TA, Lyons GA, Chimondeguy DJ, et al: VATS debridement versus thoracotomy in the treatment of loculated postpneumonia empyema. Ann Thorac Surg 61:1626–1630, 1996.
42. McBride PJ, Hinder RA, Filipi C, et al: Surgical treatment of spastic conditions of the esophagus. Int Surg 82:113–118, 1997.
43. McCarthy JF, Hurley JP, Wood AE: The diverse potential of thoracoscopic assisted surgery. Int Surg 82:29–31, 1997.
44. Ohtsuka T, Furuse A, Kohno T, et al: New tactile sensor techniques for localization of pulmonary nodules. Int Surg 82:12–14, 1997.
45. Peracchia A, Rosati R, Fumagalli U, et al: Thoracoscopic dissection of the esophagus for cancer. Int Surg 82:1–4, 1997.
46. Roviaro G, Varoli F, Rebuffat C, et al: Videothoracoscopic staging and treatment of lung cancer. Ann Thorac Surg 59:971–974, 1995.
47. Roviaro G, Varoli F, Rebuffat C, et al: Videothoracoscopic operative staging for lung cancer. Int Surg 81:252–254, 1996.
48. Sartorelli KH, Partrick D, Meagher DP Jr: Port-site recurrence after thoracoscopic resection of pulmonary metastasis owing to osteogenic sarcoma. J Pediatr Surg 31:1443–1444, 1996.
49. Schramel FMNH, Sutedja TG, Braber JCE, et al: Cost-effectiveness of video-assisted thoracoscopic surgery versus conservative treatment for first time or recurrent spontaneous pneumothorax. Eur Resp J 9:1821–1825, 1996.
50. Shaw RM, Spirn PW, Salazar AM, et al: Localization of peripheral pulmonary nodules for thoracoscopic excision: Value of CT-guided wire placement. Am J Roentgenol 161:279–283, 1993.
51. Shennib H, Bret P: Intraoperative transthoracic ultrasonographic localization of occult lung lesions. Ann Thorac Surg 55:767–769, 1993.
52. Shennib HA, Landeneau R, Mulder DS, et al: Video-assisted thoracoscopic resection of T1 lung cancer high-risk patients. Ann Surg 218:555–558, 1993.
53. Smith G, Hirsch N, Ehrenwerth J: Placement of double lumen endobronchial tubes. Correlation between clinical impression and bronchoscopic findings. Br J Anaesthes 58:1317–1320, 1986.
54. Statement of the AATS/STS joint committee on thoracoscopy and video assisted thoracic surgery. J Thorac Cardiovasc Surg 104:1, 1992.
55. Vaughn CC, Wolner E, Dahan M, et al: Prevention of air leaks after pulmonary wedge resection. Ann Thorac Surg 63:864–866, 1997.
56. Voyles CR, Tucker RD: Education and engineering solutions for potential problems with laparoscopic monopolar electrosurgery. Am J Surgery 164:57–62, 1992.
57. Walker WS: VATS lobectomy—The Edinburgh Experience. Semin Thorac Cardiovasc Surg 10:291–299, 1998.
58. Warren WH, Penfield Faber L: Segmentectomy versus lobectomy in patients with stage 1 pulmonary carcinoma. J Thorac Cardiovasc Surg 107:1087–1094, 1994.
59. Wolfer R, Krasna M, Hasnain JU, et al: Hemodynamnic effects of carbon dioxide insufflation during thoracoscopy. Ann Thorac Surg 58:404–408, 1994.
60. Yim APC: Port site recurrence following video-assisted thoracoscopic surgery. Surg Endosc 9:1133–1135, 1995.
61. Yim AP: Video-assisted thoracoscopic management of primary pneumothorax. Ann Acad Med Singapore 25:668–672, 1996.
62. Yim APC, Ho JKS: Malfunctioning of vascular staple cutter during thoracoscopic lobectomy. J Thorac Cardiovasc Surg 109: 1252, 1995.
63. Yim AP, Ko KM, Chau WS, et al: Video-assisted thoracoscopic anatomic lung resections. The initial Hong Kong experience. Chest 109:13–17, 1996.
64. Yim APC, Liu H-P: Complications and failures of video-assisted thoracic surgery: Experience from two centres in Asia. Ann Thorac Surg 61:538–541, 1996.
65. Yim APC, Liu H-P: Thoracoscopic major lung resection—Indications, technique and early results: Experience from two centers in Asia. Surg Laparosc Endosc 7:241–244, 1997.

Chapter 44

Cost-Containment Strategies

Hui-Ping Liu

Over the past few years, video-assisted endoscopic surgery has become popular in a number of specialties, including biliary, gynecologic, arthroscopic, plastic, and spinal surgery. Endoscopic surgery of the chest has also generated enthusiasm during the past 5 years.[1–26] Video-assisted thoracic surgery (VATS) is being performed with increasing frequency, and the applicable instrumentation and video equipment have evolved at a rapid pace. Each year, newly developed procedures are performed in increasing numbers and for a growing variety of indications. Surgical equipment suppliers and innovative surgeons have designed and developed instruments such as endoscissors, endostaplers, endoretractors, and other endoscopic equipment to be used through refined thoracic trocars. Although there are obvious benefits of smaller incisions and shorter hospital stays, the benefit of lower health care costs has rarely been addressed. Much of this equipment can be quite expensive and, if used injudiciously, can raise operative costs. This chapter is based on 5 years of VATS experience and outlines basic strategies and surgical skills that can enhance the cost-effectiveness of VATS.

Surgical Techniques

The surgical techniques necessary to perform cost-effective diagnostic and therapeutic procedures can be divided into three categories: common basic skills, endoscopic technique, and video-assisted technique using an extended manipulating incision. All these techniques are based on traditional surgical principles. They allow one to perform standard procedures with minimal invasion of the chest cavity and are based on the surgical techniques of dissection, suturing, hemostasis, and tissue approximation that are familiar to us in the open setting.

Common Basic Skills

Adhesiolysis

Fibrinous adhesions can often be easily separated with light pressure using a conventional ring forceps (Fig. 44–1). More extensive pleural adhesions require careful dissection and control of bleeders using electrocautery. One should dissect only the adhesions necessary for visualization and performance of the procedure.

Hemostasis

A standard electrocautery with a malleable extender (Fig. 44–2) works as well as any coagulator or argon beam device. It can be as effective as the endoscopic surgical hook for dissection and hemostasis and does not require the purchase of additional expensive equipment.

Dissection

Careful, stepwise dissection is the key. Whenever possible, two hands should be used—one to lift, and the other to dissect the tissue. The blunt tip of a conventional wall suction tube (Fig. 44–3) is an excellent instrument and allows the dissection to be accomplished safely and quickly. Standard electrocautery is usually used to cut tissue and to achieve hemostasis during dissection.

Tumor or Lymph Node Biopsy

VATS is a highly productive and safe method of obtaining biopsy specimens. Before starting the biopsy, electrocautery is used to penetrate the capsule of the mass. A cup biopsy forceps is applied directly on the lesion to obtain an accurate tissue sample. Frequently, several bites of tissue are obtained for histologic confirmation. All the bleeders are controlled with diathermy.

Suction and Evacuation

Conventional instruments such as a long-handled clamp and a large-bore Silastic suction tube (Fig. 44–4) can be used to break down a blood clot or empyema cavity. The fibrous pleural "peel" can be decorticated and removed by changing the position of the instruments through different incisions. Changing the position of the scope also improves visual orientation and allows better access to certain areas for further debridement.

Endo-loop Ligation

A homemade loop of polydioxanone suture (PDS II, Ethicon) with a pretied knot (Fig. 44–5) is an excellent cost-effective technique for bulla ablation in a patient with spontaneous pneumothorax. At least two to three such loops are used to ligate each bulla (Fig. 44–6).

Wedge Resection and Suturing

To avoid excessive use of expensive endoscopic stapling devices, wedge resection of lung parenchyma can be accomplished using a conventional suturing method as in open thoracotomy (Fig. 44–7). Flexing the operating table or using a small Tuffier retractor may facilitate the wedge resection and suturing of the lung parenchyma. If desired, a homemade loop can be used to ligate the final bridge of tissue (Fig. 44–8), which is then divided with scissors. Using an Endo-loop is especially helpful if the angle for applying staples or sutures is awkward, and it may be less costly than using additional staples.

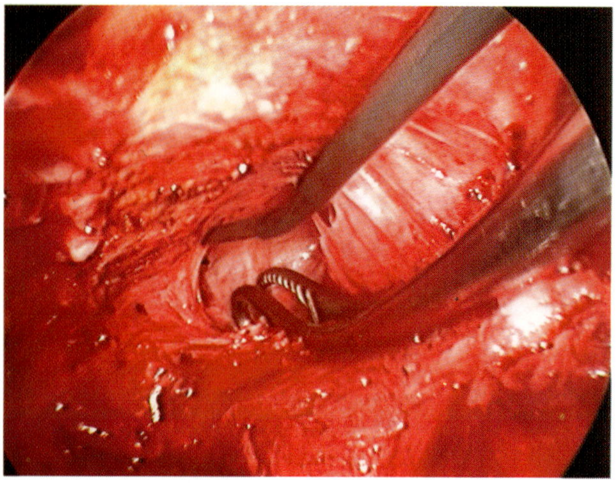

Figure 44–1. Adhesiolysis using conventional ring forceps and electrocautery.

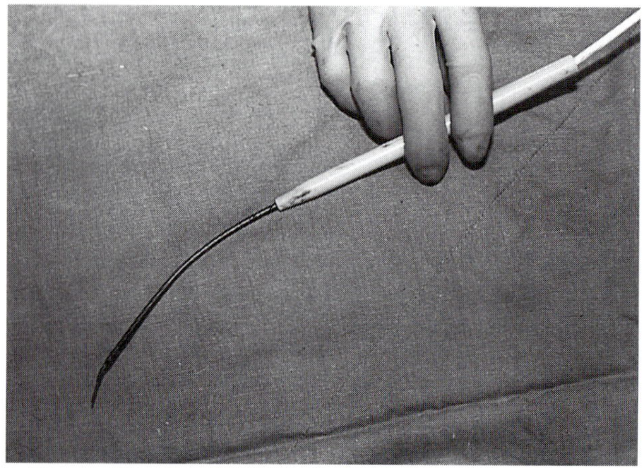

Figure 44–2. Standard electrocautery with malleable extender.

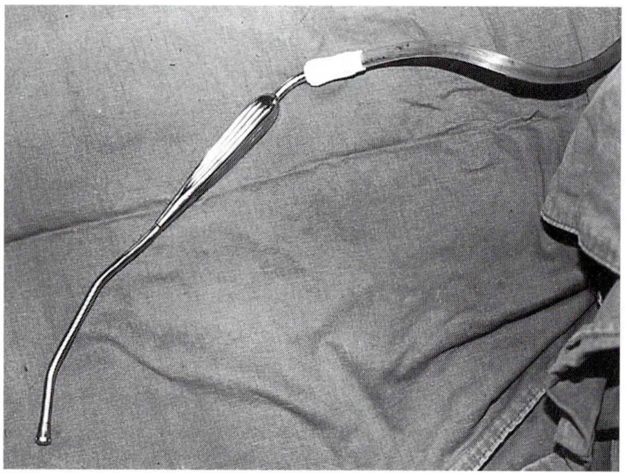

Figure 44–3. Blunt tip of conventional wall suction tube.

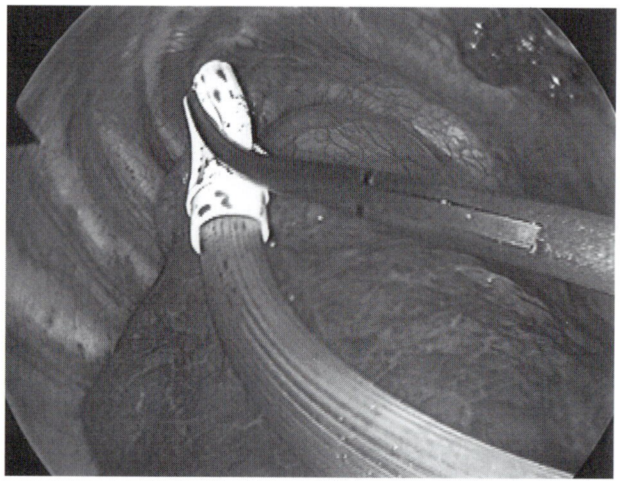

Figure 44–4. Large-bore Silastic suction tube grasped by long-handled clamp.

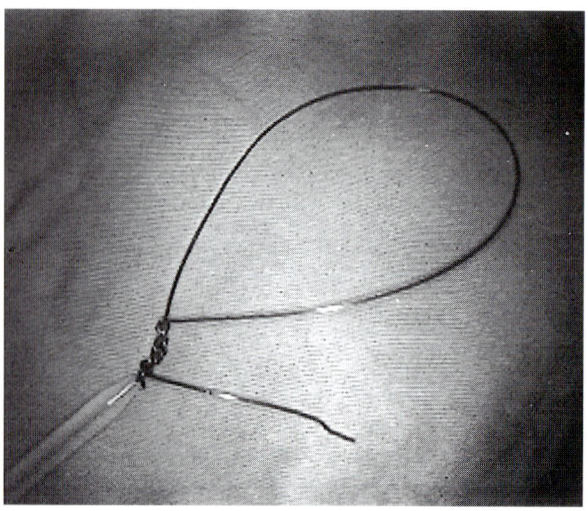

Figure 44–5. Homemade loop with pretied knot.

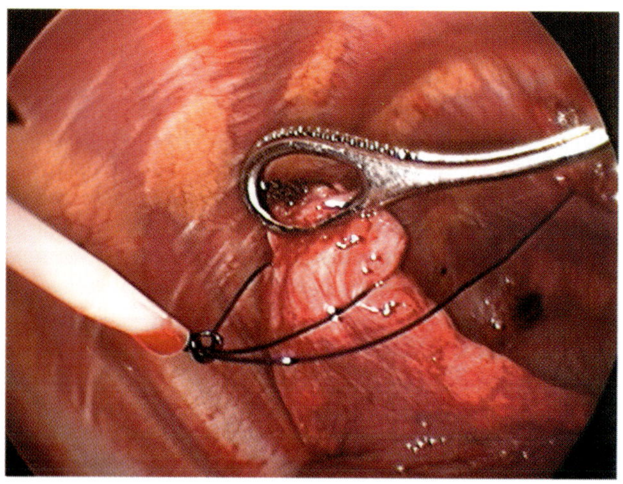

Figure 44–6. Bulla ligation using homemade loop.

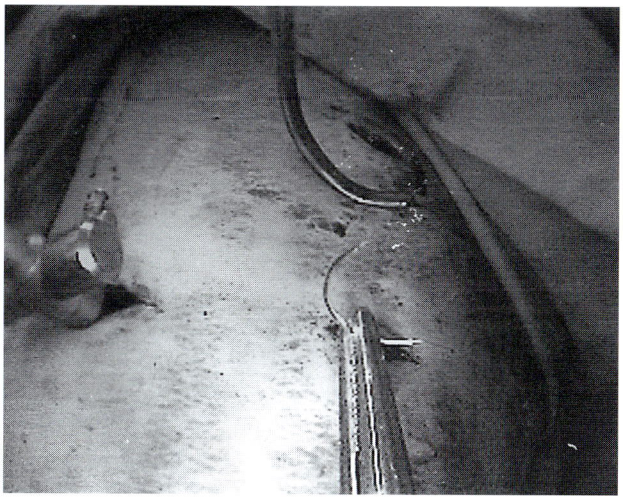

Figure 44–7. Endoscopic suturing in a conventional way.

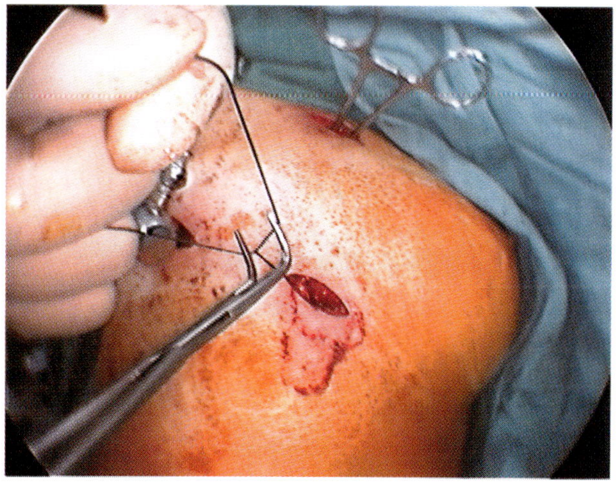

Figure 44–9. Externally tied knot cinched down using conventional right-angled hemostat.

Vessel Ligation

The extended manipulating incision accommodates a conventional right-angled hemostat and aids in identifying and dissecting the pulmonary vessels. Blunt dissection using a "pusher" or the tip of a wall suction tube aids in the exposure of the interlobar vessels. After the vessel has been cleared circumferentially, it is encircled with 2–0 or 3–0 silk sutures. Either the suture is tied directly through the extended manipulating incision or the externally tied knot is cinched down inside the thoracic cavity using a right-angled hemostat (Fig. 44–9) or homemade knot pusher. The vessel is then divided as in open thoracotomy.

Intraoperative Bleeding

During VATS, rapid access to control active bleeding is usually restricted. Careful dissection and control of blood vessels before dividing them are mandatory. To control bleeding quickly, a conventional vascular clamp should always be available at the beginning of the surgical procedure. Once an active bleeder is encountered, the clamp should be applied immediately to control the hemorrhage until the chest can be opened. Small bleeders are usually controlled using standard electrocautery.

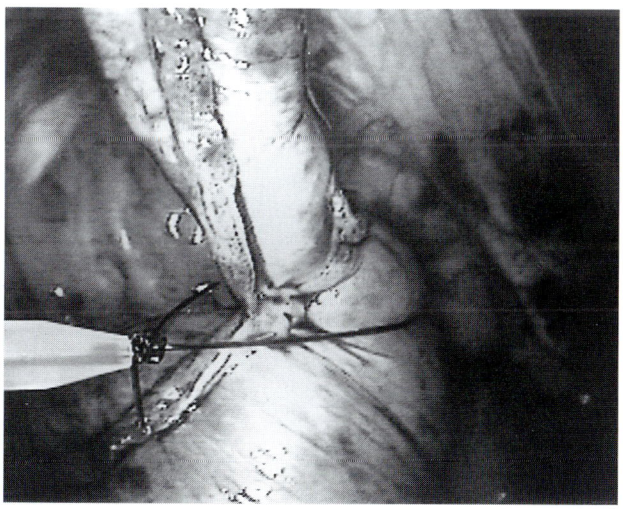

Figure 44–8. Homemade loop used to ligate the final bridge of stapled tissue.

Bronchial Closure

Traditional 3.5- or 4.5-mm staples are usually used to close the bronchus. They may also be used to staple vessels or lung parenchyma through the extended manipulating incision to expedite the procedure.

Endoscopic Technique

The first point of entry (1 to 2 cm) allows initial inspection of the chest cavity. After the pathology is determined, the initial point of entry is used to assist in selecting all subsequent entry points. Depending on the location of the lesion, additional incisions are located to form a working pyramid.[16] Three incisions (two additional, positioned opposite each other) are normally required and are triangulated so that the incision for the scope is the farthest from the target. This allows for a broad field of vision. No disposable trocars or Thoracoports are used. The presence of trocar ports makes it difficult to use conventional instruments. The telescope is the only device that requires placement through a reusable trocar. All procedures can be performed using conventional thoracic surgical instruments directly through incisions (Fig. 44–10). The entire thoracic procedure is accomplished by visualization of projected images on the video monitor. Procedures such as bulla ablation, wedge resection of a small lung nodule, tumor biopsy, mediastinal tumor removal (<5 cm), evacuation of blood clot or purulent debris, and creation of pericardial window can all be accomplished entirely with the aforementioned endoscopic technique.

Video-Assisted Technique Using an Extended Manipulating Incision

The extended manipulating incision is best created directly over or close to the underlying pathology (usually 4 to 6 cm in length). It allows the surgeon to use one or more

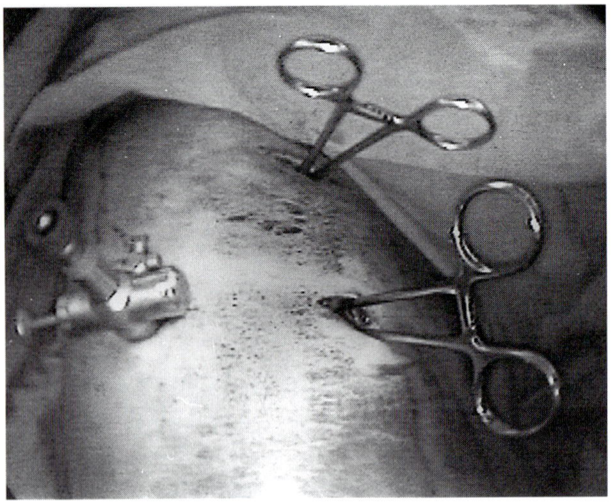

Figure 44–10. Conventional instruments pass directly through incisions.

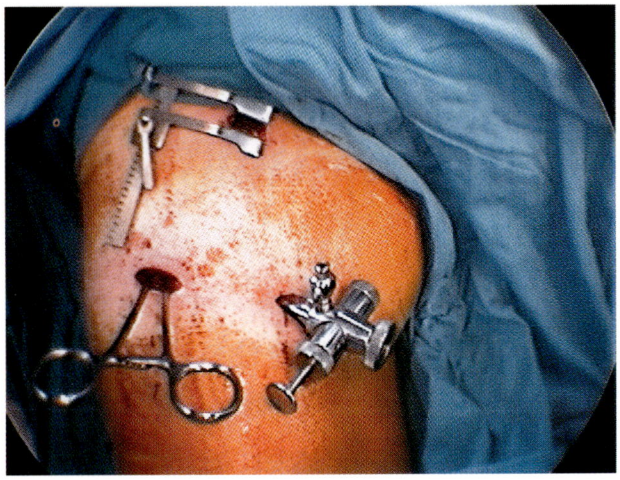

Figure 44–12. Small retractor facilitates direct visualization to expedite the procedure.

conventional instruments through this extended wound (Fig. 44–11). The incision is made to accommodate standard instruments such as a conventional stapling device, aortic cross-clamp, ring forceps, right-angled hemostat, standard needle holders, and forceps, which can be passed into it for manipulation and eventually for specimen retrieval. Certain intrathoracic procedures may require the use of a small Tuffier retractor, which facilitates direct visualization to expedite the procedure (Fig. 44–12). However, flexing the operating table usually opens up the intercostal spaces, making use of the retractor unnecessary. This is done when performing lobectomy and pneumonectomy as well as esophagectomy. Conventional wedge resection of a lung nodule without an EndoGIA endostapler can be accomplished in this manner, combined with endoscopic suturing technique.

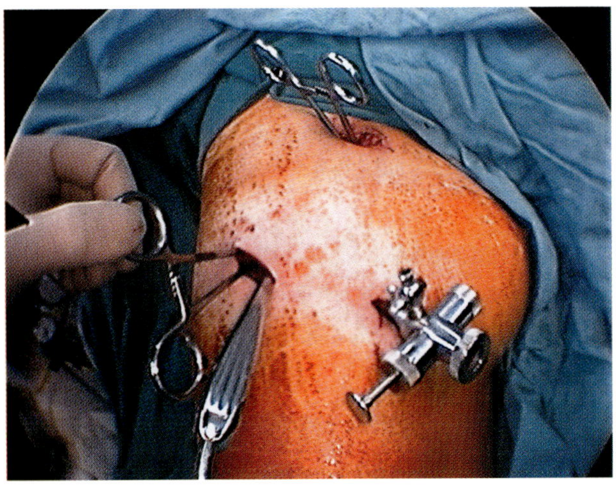

Figure 44–11. One or more instruments pass through extended manipulation incision.

Discussion

VATS is now well established and provides excellent results with low mortality and morbidity. In the past, most of these chest lesions were resected through open thoracotomy; today, the majority of patients can be operated on in a minimally invasive manner.[14] The advantages are less postoperative pain, faster recuperation, and shorter hospital stay. Although VATS permits a less invasive approach to the treatment of diseases of the chest, the surgical skills needed to ensure patient safety may be difficult to obtain in developing countries. Cost containment, though desirable in the West, is a high priority in developing countries.[8, 24] The high cost of consumables has deterred many hospitals from widely applying VATS technique. To complement the advances in VATS, cost-containment strategies have been designed to minimize health care budgets in many Asian countries.[8, 11, 26]

The procedures and techniques described here do not differ greatly from those reported in the literature[14]; however, the complication rate in the series reported by Yim and Liu[26] is similar to or less than that in other reported series, without the use of expensive and disposable endoscopic equipment. One patient had a dislodged Endo-loop ligature after a forceful sneeze 2 days postoperatively.[13, 27] This occurred in one of the first three patients in which we used Endo-loop (chromic catgut) for bulla ligation.[13] After that, we changed to a homemade loop of PDS II for bulla ligation without any subsequent complications. It is our impression that thoracoscopic Endo-loop ligation of the visceral pleura and the base of the bulla is as good as if not better than stapler resection for the prevention of air leaks.[27] Homemade Endo-loop ligation is more cost-effective than other techniques that use thoracoscopy in treating patients with primary spontaneous pneumothorax.[14, 15]

Our conversion rate to open surgery is quite low.[8, 26] The reason for this might be that we use conventional thoracic instruments and operative strategy, as in open surgery.

New surgical approaches will undoubtedly bring their

own complications. Some of these are immediately obvious, but others may become apparent only as more procedures are performed. Our complication rates are comparable to those reported by Kaiser and Bavaria.[28] Persistent air leak, which is the most common nonfatal complication, usually occurs in patients with pneumothorax, often because of diffuse bullous emphysematous changes in the lung parenchyma. The cost-containing technique of loop ligation and suturing[21, 27] is as effective as other techniques and provides similar results.

When active hemorrhage occurs, extension of the wound for control of bleeders is usually indicated. Long conventional clamps (Satinsky or curved vascular clamps) seem to be the best devices to control active bleeders through the extended manipulating incision before the chest is opened. In a comparison of endoscopic and conventional thoracic instruments, we found that there was a significant difference in manipulation, especially during bleeding. Rapid access is usually restricted through a thoracic trocar. Surgeons should take advantage of every opportunity to use familiar, already available instruments to perform simple and safe procedures. There is little doubt that at the present time, with the exception of stapling devices, no disposable instrumentation is better than standard long cardiothoracic instruments. With the combined use of conventional instruments, dissecting, grasping, suturing, and other means of vessel control will become much easier and thus expedite the procedure. Because an airtight system is unnecessary in performing VATS, we strongly recommend the use of conventional instruments without trocars. Those who rely excessively on disposable endoscopic instruments will find themselves in trouble when facing complications such as active hemorrhage. By incorporating conventional instruments, VATS can be performed in a fashion similar to that for open thoracotomy but with more natural hand manipulation.

Formal thoracic surgery requires long and painful incisions, often to perform relatively simple procedures. With the development of VATS, these incisions can be avoided without compromising the treatment goals set for the patient. This is especially noteworthy in the management of small peripheral lung nodules. One may use an endostapling device to simply wedge-resect the nodule. However, this device alone costs over $400, which may be one-and-a-half times the average annual per capita income in some developing countries.[24] In our experience, patients with lung nodules (who are not willing or cannot afford to pay for the expensive endostapling device) can undergo wedge resection through an extended manipulating incision and standard suturing technique with or without using rib-spreading video-assisted exposure. Some might argue that the benefits in terms of shorter hospital stays counterbalance the high cost of the equipment. However, this may not always be true. In Asia, there is frequently a longer hospital stay for thoracic surgery patients because of cheaper hospital charges compared with those in the West. There is also a common perception among many Asian patients that they need to stay in the hospital for as long as those who undergo open thoracic procedures.[24] The cost of the hospital stay is only a small fraction of total expenditures for endoscopic procedures. Thus the decreased costs of the hospital stay in most developing countries will not counterbalance the high cost of the consumables. Only stringent use of endoscopic equipment, trocars, and especially endostapling devices will keep the operative costs to a minimum. This is of paramount importance in achieving a cost-effective VATS procedure.

Analyses of the total costs for endoscopic surgery clearly show that the increased expenditure for equipment is not offset by the saving from decreased hospital stay and shorter recovery period.[29] VATS is significantly more costly than the equivalent open procedure if disposable instruments and staplers are used injudiciously. VATS occasionally offers greater technical challenges and thus takes longer to perform than comparable open procedures. In these circumstances, operating room charges are increased; this is in addition to the costs of purchasing the necessary video equipment. But if surgeons use conventional instruments through extended manipulating incisions, the operating time should decrease. Also, as surgeons become more experienced and learn which VATS procedures offer the most significant benefits, a more selective approach will decrease operative time and eventually result in cost savings.

The future of VATS is exciting, and the field is experiencing ongoing change. Conventional wisdom holds that as VATS techniques become more prevalent and sophisticated, many related questions will be raised. Presently, the usefulness of VATS in the treatment of pulmonary disease is not fully defined, and the debate over VATS continues to unfold. It is of paramount importance for each thoracic surgeon who performs VATS to be committed to establishing a cost-effective procedure. The enthusiasm for its use in certain situations must be tempered so as not to compromise a treatment objective that could be achieved definitively by another approach. Although patients sometimes request the use of a minimally invasive approach, VATS must be utilized in appropriate settings and in appropriate medical situations. This is a tool that all thoracic surgeons should have in their surgical armamentariums, but they should make an effort to curtail the use of costly technology and endoscopic equipment as much as possible. VATS costs will decrease with proper patient selection and attention to the aforementioned surgical techniques.

If a procedure can be performed effectively in a conventional way and can yield an equivalent minimally invasive result, there is no reason to encourage the use of costly new technology and endoscopic equipment in performing VATS. In our enthusiasm to endorse the development and application of new technology and equipment, we must reflect on both patient outcomes and economic impact.

References

1. Akashi A, Ohashi, Yoden Y, et al: Thoracoscopic surgery combined with a supraclavicular approach for removing superior mediastinal tumor. Surg Endosc 11:74–76, 1997.
2. Hazelrigg SR, Nunchuck SK, LoCicero J: Video assisted thoracic surgery group data. Ann Thorac Surg 56:1039–1044, 1993.
3. Hurtgen M, Linder A, Friedel G, et al: Video-assisted thoraco-

scopic pleurodesis: A survey conducted by the German Society for Thoracic Surgery. Thorac Cardiovasc Surg 44:199–203, 1996.
4. Keller CA, Ruppel G, Hibbert A, et al: Thoracoscopic lung volume reduction surgery reduces dyspnea and improves exercise capacity in patients with emphysema. Am J Respir Crit Care Med 156:60–67, 1997.
5. Landreneau RJ, Mark MJ, Hazelrigg SR, et al: Video-assisted thoracic surgery: Basic technical concepts and intercostal approach strategies. Ann Thorac Surg 54:800–807, 1992.
6. Landreneau RJ, Keenan RJ, Hazelrigg SR, et al: Thoracoscopy for empyema and hemothorax. Chest 109:18–24, 1996.
7. Liu HP, Lin PJ, Chang JP, Chang CH: Video-assisted thoracic surgery: Manipulation without trocar in 112 consecutive procedures. Chest 104:1452–1454, 1993.
8. Liu HP, Chang CH, Lin PJ, et al: Video-assisted thoracic surgery: The Chang Gung experience. J Thorac Cardiovasc Surg 108:834–840, 1994.
9. Liu HP, Chang CH, Lin PJ, et al: Thoracoscopic management of effusive pericardial disease: Indications and technique. Ann Thorac Surg 58:1695–1697, 1994.
10. Liu HP, Chang CH, Lin PJ, Chang JP: Video-assisted endoscopic esophagectomies with stapled intrathoracic esophagogastric anastomosis. World J Surg 19:745–747, 1995.
11. Liu HP, Chang CH, Lin PJ, et al: Thoracoscopic-assisted lobectomy: Preliminary experience and results. Chest 107:853–855, 1995.
12. Liu HP, Lin PJ, Hsieh MJ, et al: Application of thoracoscopy for lung metastases. Chest 107:266–268, 1995.
13. Liu HP, Lin PJ, Hsieh MJ, et al: Thoracoscopic surgery as a routine procedure for spontaneous pneumothorax: Results from 82 patients. Chest 107:559–562, 1995.
14. Mack MJ, Hazelrigg SR, Landreneau RJ, et al: The first international symposium on thoracoscopic surgery. Ann Thorac Surg 56:609–804, 1993.
15. Naunheim KS, Mack MJ, Hazelrigg SR, et al: Safety and efficacy of video-assisted thoracic surgical techniques for the treatment of spontaneous pneumothorax. J Thorac Cardiovasc Surg 109:1252, 1995.
16. Roviaro GC, Rebuffat C, Varoli F, et al: Major thoracoscopic operations: Pulmonary resection and mediastinal mass excision. Int Surg 81:354–358, 1996.
17. Walker WS, Craig SR: Video-assisted thoracoscopic pulmonary surgery: Current status and potential evolution. Eur J Cardiothorac Surg 10:161–167, 1996.
18. Yim APC: Minimizing chest wall trauma in video assisted thoracic surgery. J Thorac Cardiovasc Surg 109:1255–1256, 1995.
19. Yim APC, Low JM, Ng SK, et al: Video-assisted thoracoscopic surgery in the paediatric population. J Paediatr Child Health 31:192–196, 1995.
20. Yim APC, Ho JKS: 100 consecutive cases of video assisted thoracoscopic surgery for primary spontaneous pneumothorax. Surg Endosc 9:332–336, 1995.
21. Yim APC: Video assisted thoracoscopic suturing of apical bullae—an alternative to staple resection in the management of primary spontaneous pneumothorax. Surg Endosc 9:1013–1016, 1995.
22. Yim APC, Kay R, Ho JK: Video assisted thoracoscopic thymectomy for myasthenia gravis. Chest 108:1440–1443, 1995.
23. Yim APC, Lee TWE: Homemade knot pusher for extracorporeal ties. Aust N Z J Surg 65:510–511, 1995.
24. Yim APC: Cost containing strategies in video-assisted thoracoscopic surgery: An Asian perspective. Surg Endosc 10:1198–200, 1996.
25. Yim APC, Ko KM, Chau WS, et al: Video assisted thoracoscopic anatomical lung resections: The initial Hong Kong experience. Chest 109:13–17, 1996.
26. Yim APC, Liu HP: Complications and failures of video-assisted thoracic surgery experience from two centers in Asia. Ann Thorac Surg 61:538–541, 1996.
27. Liu HP, Chang CH, Lin PJ, et al: Thoracoscopic loop ligation of parenchymal blebs and bullae: Is it effective and safe? J Thorac Cardiovasc Surg 113:50–54, 1997.
28. Kaiser LR, Bavaria JE: Complications of thoracoscopy. Ann Thorac Surg 56:796–798, 1993.
29. Miller JI Jr: Thoracoscopic surgery. *In* Kaiser LR (ed): Economics of Thoracoscopic Surgery. Boston, Little, Brown, 1993, pp 255–259.

COMMENTARY

Anthony P. C. Yim

Within a short time, VATS has become the preferred approach in the management of a variety of thoracic conditions. We, like others, have witnessed an increase in case referrals which probably reflects increased acceptance by both patients and their referring physicians for earlier surgical intervention. This, however, could place extra demands on health care, mainly because of the high cost of the equipment. The argument in the West that the cost of the equipment is counterbalanced by the shorter hospital stay cannot be applied to developing countries, where hospital costs are only a fraction of those in the United States. Also, there is little pressure in these countries from insurance companies for early discharge from the hospital.

Cost containment, though important in the West, is an essential priority in developing countries if VATS is not to be limited to the privileged few who can afford it. Careful patient selection is by far the most important strategy for reducing costs. For example, a peripheral lung nodule located on a flat surface of a lobe is better approached using minithoracotomy and standard suturing technique with video assistance rather than trying to resect it using purely endoscopic techniques. This chapter by Dr. Liu gives many useful suggestions as to how VATS could be made more cost-effective.

VATS is still in evolution. Technology and techniques will continue to improve, but cost containment is an important issue that we cannot afford to ignore.

Chapter 45

Endoscopic Fetal Surgery

Jun Wu, Jan A. Deprest, Edward Gratacos, Hirotoshi Yamamoto, and Toni E. Lerut

Most prenatally diagnosed malformations are best managed after birth. However, a few congenital anomalies may result in fetal death in utero or cause permanent sequelae and therefore may benefit from correction before birth.[1] There is an international consensus on the criteria and indications for fetal surgery endorsed by the International Fetal Medicine and Surgery Society (Table 45–1).[2, 3] This list may expand as prenatal diagnosis, pathophysiologic insight, instruments, and surgical techniques are improved.[4] However, fetal surgery through hysterotomy still poses significant risks and side effects to both the mother and the fetus. The main problem remaining is the high incidence of preterm labor directly related to the large uterine incision required for fetal exposure.[5]

The current expansion of video-endoscopic surgery, combined with years of experience in clinical fetoscopy and experimental fetal surgery, forms the basis of the concept of endoscopic fetal surgery.[6] Given the "keyhole" access, making it possible to keep the fetus in its natural environment and ultimately inducing less maternal trauma, endoscopic fetal surgery is an attractive, minimally invasive alternative to open procedures.[7–9] Meanwhile, its feasibility has been supported by experimental and clinical data, which will be reviewed in this chapter.

Animal Model

In order to study the feasibility of endoscopic surgery in utero, our team[10] and others[11] developed an experimental model in the pregnant ewe (Fig. 45–1). Intra-amniotic access to the fetus should be atraumatic and leakproof and should avoid separation or rupture of the chorionic and amniotic membranes, which are strong triggers of premature uterine contractions[12, 13] and may eventually cause amniotic band syndrome.[14] Therefore, we designed a short and atraumatic cannula with a balloon tip.[15] The balloon allows secure fixation of the cannula inside the amniotic cavity, whereas the soft, flexible tip reduces the risk of direct fetal injury. Endoscopes were initially 2- to 4-mm rod lens telescopes, but today small 0.5- to 2-mm fiber endoscopes with a resolution of up to 50,000 pixels are available. The fetus can be monitored through endoscopically placed pulse oximetry and temperature probes.[7, 10]

To minimize maternal invasiveness further, a percutaneous technique for direct endoscopic access to the sheep uterus has been reported.[16, 17] Under ultrasonographic guidance, a 20-gauge spinal needle is advanced through the maternal abdomen and uterus and directly into the amniotic cavity. Trocars are then inserted percutaneously into the amniotic cavity using ultrasonographic and fetoscopic guidance.

Endoscopic surgery needs a working space, which in laparoscopy is most commonly provided by carbon dioxide insufflation. Using this technique for uterine distention, we observed fetal acidosis due to absorption of carbon dioxide.[18] However, later experiments by Saiki and colleagues[19] demonstrated that this may be reduced by maternal hyperventilation. We preferred to distend the amniotic cavity by amnioinfusion with Hartmann's solution. The solution, warmed to 38°C, enabled us to maintain a stable fetal temperature throughout a 180-minute procedure,[10] with no evidence of a shift of fluid to the maternal compartment.[20] Hence, two of the major problems of open fetal surgery, hypothermia and dehydration, can be avoided by this approach. Fetal retinal injury caused by bright light exposure has been excluded by animal experiments.[21, 22]

Rather than using unipolar electrosurgery and electrolyte-poor fluids such as glycine,[23] we use a bipolar cutting probe. The asymmetry of the electrodes (a needle tip and a broad-based ring) allows sufficient energy to be generated at the tip of the instrument to allow electrical cutting. Alternatively, a laser fiber can be used.[58, 59]

Experimental Endoscopic Fetal Surgery

Successful treatment of unborn patients relies on a better understanding of the pathophysiology of the disease and the technical feasibility of prenatal interventions. To achieve these, animal experiments are the first step. The feasibility of fetal endoscopic surgery was first tested in San Francisco on a cleft lip model.[24] In our institution, a surgical trial was performed in fetal lambs by creating a lower urinary tract obstruction in early and late second trimester.[7] This procedure included dissection and ligation of delicate structures such as the urachus within the umbilical cord and the penile and abdominal urethra. Fetal survival rates were higher than historic controls that had undergone a similar open procedure.[25] Using a semirigid fiberoptic and a flexible 3-mm endoscope, we performed tracheoscopy and foregut endoscopy in the fetal lamb model without significant mucosal or other trauma.[15] This technique could become a valuable research tool for the study of fetal gastrointestinal and pulmonary physiologic factors in vivo. Similar endoscopic techniques have been used to place a transabdominal stent in the ovine fetal bladder in an attempt to salvage renal function in urinary tract obstruction.[8] Another procedure repaired a myelomeningocele defect in utero,[26] demonstrating that complex surgical procedures can be performed through an endoscopic approach. The neurologic deficit associated with open spina bifida is apparently not directly caused by the primary defect but may be due to chronic mechanical and chemical trauma because the unprotected neural tissue is exposed to the intrauterine environment. This theory is

Table 45–1. Criteria for Fetal Surgery

Accurate diagnosis and staging possible, with exclusion of associated anomalies
Natural history of the disease is documented and prognosis established
Currently, postnatal therapy is either ineffective or too late.
In utero surgery has been proved feasible in animal models, reversing deleterious effect of the condition
Interventions are performed in specialized multidisciplinary fetal treatment centers within strict protocols, after education of the mother and full consent of the couple

strongly supported by both animal experiments and early observations in human gestation.[27–30] Therefore, prenatal correction of myelomeningocele seems reasonable.[30]

The limiting factor for open fetal surgery is uterine irritability. To test the hypothesis that endoscopic access to the uterine cavity is associated with less uterine activity than by hysterotomy, we studied the effect of endoscopic uterine access on the postoperative myometrial activity in five rhesus monkeys during midtrimester pregnancy (90 to 108 gestational days; term, 165 to 175 days). The electrical myometrial recordings on the first postoperative day showed that endoscopic cannulation induces no significant premature contraction in the nonhuman primate.[31]

Congenital diaphragmatic hernia has become the focus of current research. Because of the poor outcome of in utero complete anatomic repair, an alternative approach is needed. An interesting option is tracheal occlusion to accelerate lung growth. The pulmonary expansion gradually reduces the fetal viscera into the abdominal cavity,

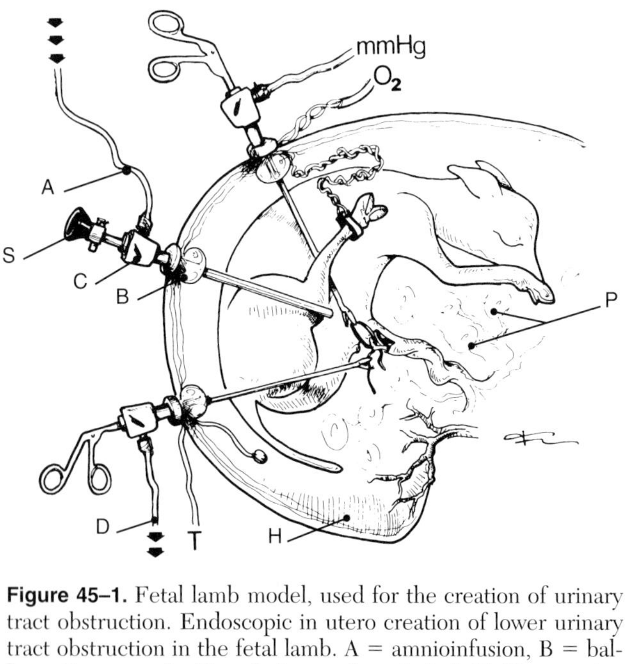

Figure 45–1. Fetal lamb model, used for the creation of urinary tract obstruction. Endoscopic in utero creation of lower urinary tract obstruction in the fetal lamb. A = amnioinfusion, B = balloon, C = cannula, D = drainage of amniotic fluid, H = uterine horn, mm Hg = pressure transducer, O_2 = pulse oximetry, S = telescope, T = temperature probe, P = placental cotyledons. (From Deprest JA, Luks F, Peers K, et al: Intrauterine endoscopic creation of urinary tract obstruction in the fetal lamb: A model for fetal surgery. Am J Obstet Gynecol 172:1422–1426, 1995, with permission.)

and pulmonary growth may avoid the most critical neonatal problems associated with pulmonary hypoplasia. Formal hernia repair is then delayed until the neonate's condition is sufficiently stable.[32, 33] Many investigators are now exploring this new approach, including the fetoscopic modification of such a procedure. We have been investigating the tracheoscopic placement of a detachable balloon, serving as an endotracheal "plug" (Fig. 45–2). The tracheal obstruction results in reactive pulmonary hyperplasia as demonstrated by morphometry and DNA analysis.[34] Others have used clips or endotracheal stents.[35, 36] However, some concern has been raised about the quality of these lungs, as accelerated growth appears to be associated with a progressive decrease of the type II pneumocytes and a concomitant decrease in surfactant secretion.[34, 37–39] We have demonstrated that temporary occlusion of the trachea may counteract this problem.[40] We suggest using an endotracheal balloon, which would, at least in theory, allow in utero reversal of tracheal occlusion by simple ultrasonographically guided puncture.

Operative fetoscopy also opens new perspectives in fetal gene therapy, particularly in directing it to individual fetal organs. Most research is focused on pulmonary diseases, such as cystic fibrosis and surfactant protein B deficiency. Current topics are how to deliver the transgene selectively to the lung tissue and how to achieve effective transfection. When the vectors are delivered by intra-amniotic injection,[41–43] all organs in contact with the amniotic fluid may become transfected. Moreover, the gene expression to lung tissue is limited because of dilution and inhibition of vector by amniotic fluid. We (unpublished data) and other groups[44] are testing the potential benefit of endoscopic techniques. Through fetal tracheoscopy, an endotracheal balloon is used to occlude the fetal trachea after vector administration. Preliminary data show that fetal lung is successfully targeted with a significant level of gene transfer, and there is no significant transfection to other fetal organs or to the mother.

Another new application is video-fetoscopy–assisted fetal tissue engineering. Treatment of several congenital anomalies is frequently hindered by the lack of enough tissue for surgical reconstruction in the neonatal period. Video-fetoscopy has been used to harvest fetal tissue, which is then processed through tissue engineering techniques in vitro while the pregnancy is continuing. At delivery, the newborn can benefit from having autologous, expanded tissue promptly available for surgical reconstruction at birth. This concept has been experimented with for bladder augmentation and skin replacement.[45, 46]

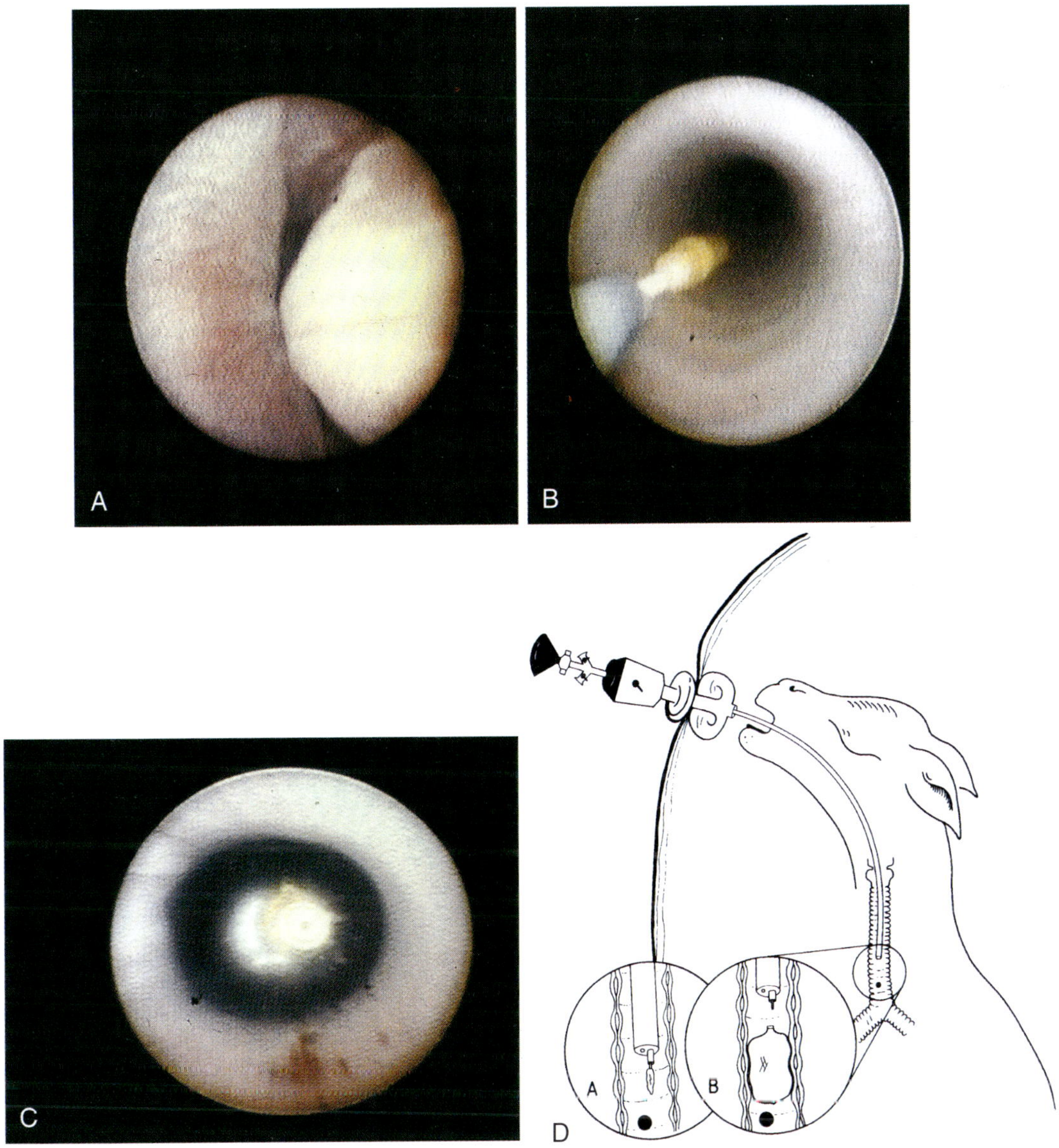

Figure 45–2. Fetal tracheoscopic placement of an endoluminal detachable balloon plug in a lamb model. *A*, view of the fetal vocal cords. *B*, View of the trachea with the catheter in its lumen. *C*, View at the time of maximal balloon inflation. *D*, Schematic view of the technique. (From Evrard VA, Flageole H, Deprest JA: Intrauterine tracheal obstruction, as treatment for congenital diaphragmatic hernia decreases amniotic fluid sodium and chloride concentrations in the fetal lamb. Ann Surg 226:753–758, 1997, with permission.)

Clinical Applications of Endoscopic Fetal Surgery

Clinical experience with endoscopic fetal surgery is still limited. Some fetal conditions discussed in the following sections do not meet the criteria listed in Table 45–1. At present, most reported experience deals with operative fetoscopy on the placenta and cord.

Operative Fetoscopy on the Placenta and Cord and Fetofetal Transfusion Syndromes in Monochorionic Twins

Fetofetal transfusion syndrome (FFTS) may affect 4 to 35% of monochorionic twins (Fig. 45–3). When occurring before 28 weeks' gestation, FFTS is associated with more than 80% fetal or perinatal loss, and, therefore, an attempt to improve its prognosis seems justified.[68] For years, the standard of therapy has been drainage of amniotic fluid, aiming to prevent the polyhydramnios-related complications. This therapy results in a mean fetal survival of 60%, but the rate of neurologic sequelae in survivors has been consistently reported to be about 20%.[47] Fetoscopic neodymium:yttrium-aluminum-garnet (Nd:YAG) laser coagulation of anastomosing vessels has been proposed as a "causal" therapy for severe FFTS before 28 weeks' gestation, as the vascular territory of both fetuses is being divided by this procedure (Fig. 45–4).[48–50] To date, more than 220 cases of FFTS treated with this procedure have been reported (Fig. 45–5). Fetal survival after this procedure was 54.5%, with a risk of neurologic injury in survivors about 5%. Particularly lower neurological morbidity compares favorably with drainage of amniotic fluid,[51] although there is no randomized trial supporting this statement.

A second potential application in monochorionic twins is cord obliteration in cases of feto-fetal transfusion with one nonviable twin. This has resulted in cases of FFTS with one fetus affected with a nonviable condition, or a monochorionic pregnancy with an acardiac fetus. In the case of such a parasitic fetus, the mortality of the cotwin may be up to 50%, mainly from high-output cardiac failure in the normal twin or as a consequence of polyhydramnios and prematurity.[52] Therapy consists of the arrest of the transfusion process by cord obliteration, which can be achieved by ultrasonographically guided cord embolization, cord coagulation, or cord ligation (Fig. 45–6).[53] Sonoendoscopic cord ligation (Fig. 45–7) is probably the most frequently performed procedure and results in immediate, complete, and permanent arterial and venous interruption of flow.[54] Twenty-three cases of cord ligation have been published so far.[67] In two cases, hemorrhage or lack of workspace did not allow adequate visualization, and cord ligation could not be performed. For the 21 successful ligations, the survival rate was 66% (n = 14). Once again, preterm labor was not a clinically significant problem, but a 47% rate of preterm premature rupture of membranes (PPROM) was observed.[57] It has been suggested that the use of two or more access ports and increased operating time are cofactors associated with PPROM, but this remains to be proven.

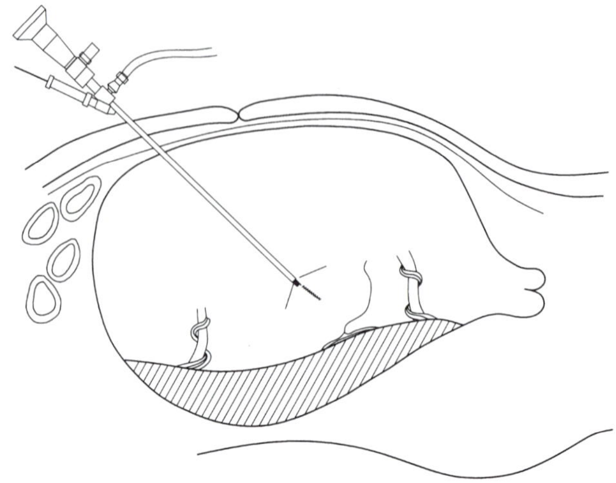

Figure 45–4. Percutaneous Nd:YAG laser coagulation in a case of posterior placenta. The fetoscope and laser fiber incline in optimal conditions toward the intertwin membrane and chorionic vessels. (From Deprest JA, Van Schoubroeck D, Van Ballaer P, et al: Alternative access for fetoscopic Nd:YAG laser in TSS with anterior placenta. Ultrasound Obstet Gynecol 347–352, 1998, with permission.)

Sacrococcygeal Teratoma

Sacrococcygeal teratoma (SCT) is the most common prenatally diagnosed tumor; it is usually treated after birth. In some cases, SCT is associated with high fetal mortality caused by high-output fetal cardiac failure resulting from the vascular steal in arteriovenous shunts within the tumor. In 1996, Hecher and Hackeloer[55] treated a fetus with SCT at 20 weeks, aiming to reduce the blood flow and tumor growth. Using a 0.4-mm ND:YAG laser fiber, the blood vessels under the surface of the tumor were coagulated fetoscopically. The cystic parts of the tumor were punctured to reduce its volume. The procedure was repeated at 26 weeks. At 37 weeks, a girl weighing 3500 g was delivered by elective cesarean section and underwent surgical treatment the same day. The patient was healthy and developing normally at 8 months of age. This represents a different approach to the previously suggested open fetal surgical approach, in which the tumor is removed in toto.[56]

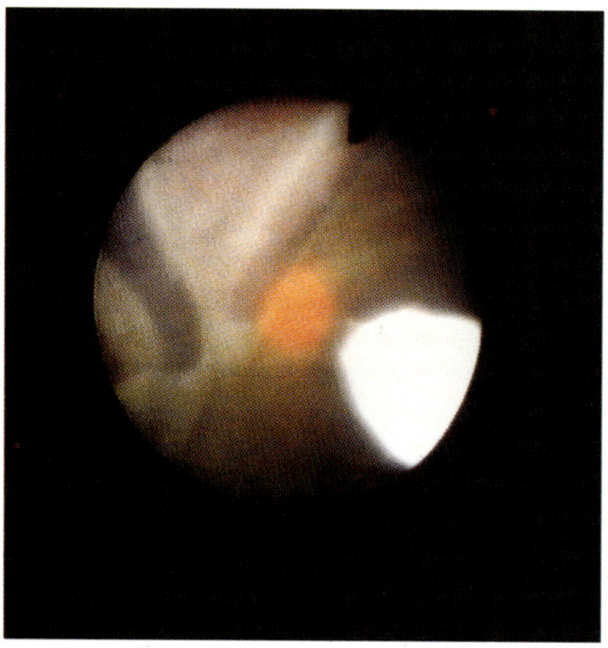

Figure 45–3. Superficial chorionic plate vessels crossing the intertwin membrane. A 400-μm Nd:YAG laser fiber is used to coagulate vessels. (From Deprest JA, Lerut T, Vandenberghe K: Endoscopic fetal surgery: A new perspective in fetal surgery. Prenat Diagn 17:1247–1260, 1997, with permission.)

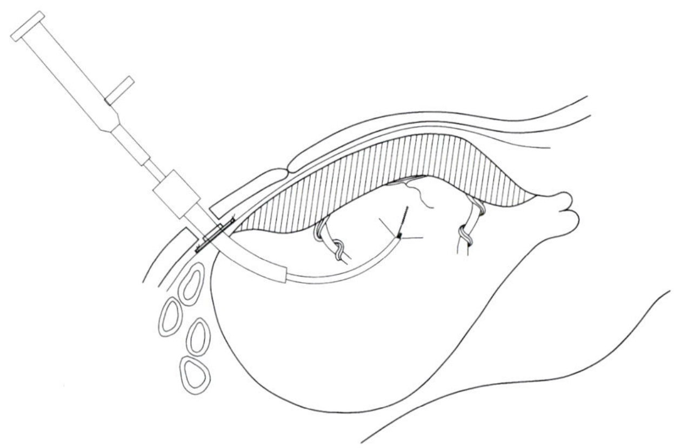

Figure 45–5. Extraplacental approach through minilaparotomy for Nd:YAG laser coagulation. Bowels have been retracted, and a trocar has been introduced. The cannula has been fixed with a molnar disc and the bent fetoscope inserted, allowing full visualization of the intertwin membrane and the intertwin vessels. (From Deprest JA, Van Schoubroeck D, Van Ballaer P, et al: Alternative access for fetoscopic Nd:YAG laser in TTS with anterior placenta. Ultrasound Obstet Gynecol 347–352, 1998, with permission.)

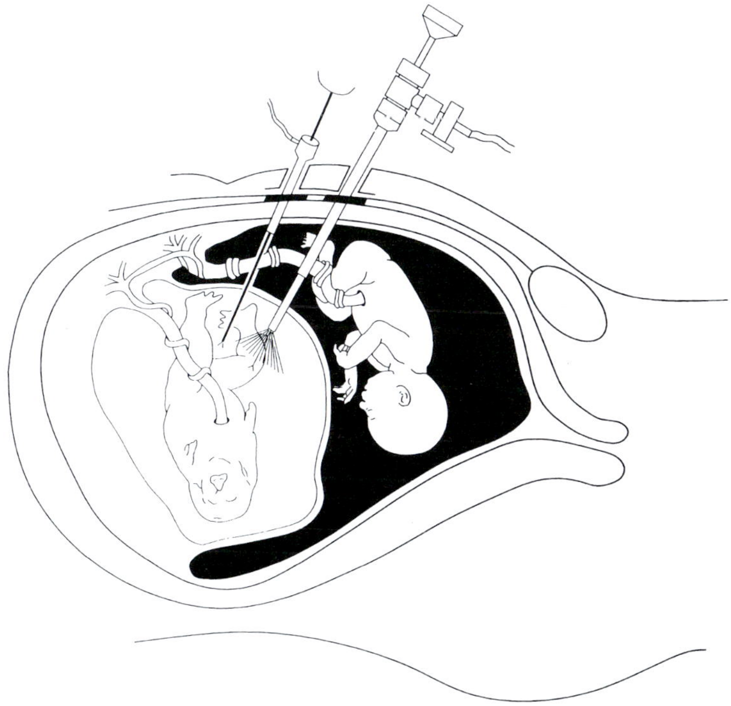

Figure 45–6. Technique of two-port fetoscopic cord ligation. The amniotic sac of the acardiac, lying under the placenta, has been opened. Instruments are inserted into that sac to do the actual procedure. Ports are attached to the fascia with a retention disk. Amnioinfusion goes in by the scope, and drainage is performed through the ports. (From Deprest JA, Evrard V, Van Ballaer P, et al: Experiences with fetoscopic cord ligation. Eur J Obstet Gynaecol Reprod Biol 81:157–164, 1998, with permission.)

Congenital Diaphragmatic Hernia

Successful clipping of the trachea was reported in 6 cases of congenital diaphragmatic hernia. Four of six patients survived and, once again, the fetoscopic modification of the procedure seemed to reduce the need for tocolytic agents used in the same procedure performed by hysterotomy.[57]

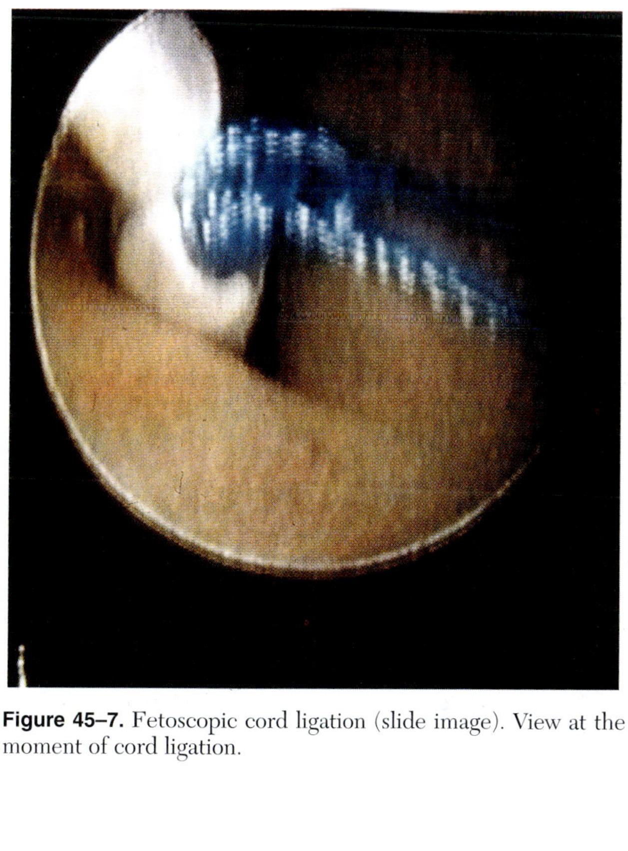

Figure 45–7. Fetoscopic cord ligation (slide image). View at the moment of cord ligation.

Lower Urinary Tract Obstruction

The sequence of lower urinary tract obstruction is hydroureteronephrosis, renal dysplasia, and pulmonary hypoplasia. In highly selected cases, urinary diversion can prevent further renal damage and allow normal pulmonary development. The first endoscopic vesicostomy was performed in 1992 by MacMahon and colleagues.[58] At 17.5 weeks' gestation they created a functional vesicostomy using a 3-mm endoscope and Nd:YAG laser fiber, but it closed by 33 weeks' gestation. The baby was born with a prune belly but had normal renal function. Quintero and colleagues[59, 60] have suggested that in utero fetal cystoscopy be performed to diagnose and assess the causes of lower urinary tract obstruction. These authors passed a thin endoscope through the lumen of a needle to observe the fetal bladder and urethral and ureteric orifices. They also placed shunts under fetoscopic guidance and ablated posterior urethral valves in a 24-week-old fetus, restoring urethral patency, but the fetus later died. The potential for fetal cystoscopy is currently being evaluated.[59, 61]

Myelomeningocele

In utero fetoscopic covering of myelomeningocele by gluing a maternal split-thickness skin graft at 23 weeks' gestation was carried out in four cases.[62] Two fetuses were born at 28 and 35 weeks' gestation, respectively, and are currently nearly 1 and 3 years old. They both suffer from mild motor and somatosensory deficits. A third fetus died of prematurity and sequelae of chorioamnionitis. The fourth fetus died intraoperatively from placental abruption. Although the indications for this procedure are under debate, this report once again illustrates the feasibility of performing complex operations through fetal endoscopy.

Amniotic Band Syndrome

Amniotic band syndrome is a sporadic condition that occurs in approximately 1 in 1200 to 1 in 15,000 live births. Without treatment, it may result in amputations, constriction, and other deformities in the fetus. Experimental work in sheep showed that fetoscopic release of the constriction can restore anatomy and function of the limb.[63] Two cases were successfully treated using endoscopic fetal surgery at 22 and 23 weeks' gestation, respectively.[64] Adequate blood flow distal to the obstruction and limb function were preserved. The extremities that were saved have a significantly improved function.

Conclusion

Endoscopic fetal surgery is a new approach to fetal therapy. For successful treatment of unborn patients, the development of animal models, instruments, and expertise has been and still is necessary. The clinical application should be considered only in centers that have a multidisciplinary team with a formal research protocol. The experience in each individual center is small, and this substantially limits the availability of evidence-based conclusions. A collaboration between centers is essential for monitoring outcomes, complications, or side effects. Now, a collaborative project (The Eurofoetus Project) has been granted by the European Commission. Its aims are (1) the achievement of technical developments meeting the requirements of intrauterine endoscopic surgery; (2) overcoming the current limitations, such as PPROM associated with invasive uterine procedures; (3) the design and implementation of a computer- and internet-based system for an international registry recording all available experience in endoscopic fetal surgery. This initiative can be accessed, joined, or consulted via the internet (http://www.eurofoetus.org). The group will establish an international registry on fetoscopic procedures. The incorporation of new participants reporting their experiences is encouraged. An open multicenter randomized trial to establish the place of the most commonly performed fetoscopic procedure (Nd:YAG laser for TTS) is being launched.

References

1. Harrison MR: Fetal surgery. Am J Obstet Gynecol 174:1255–1264, 1996.
2. Harrison MR, Golbus MS, Filly RA: The Unborn Patient. Philadelphia, WB Saunders, 1991, pp 8–13.
3. Adzick NS, Harrison MR: Fetal surgical therapy. Lancet 343: 897–902, 1994.
4. Deprest JA, Lerut T, Vandenberghe K: Operative fetoscopy: New perspective in fetal therapy? Prenat Diag 17:1247–1260, 1997.
5. Flake AW, Harrison MR: Fetal surgery. Annu Rev Med 46:67–78, 1995.
6. Luks FI, Deprest JA: Endoscopic fetal surgery: A new alternative? (Editorial) Eur J Obstet Gynecol Reprod Biol 52:1–3, 1993.
7. Deprest JA, Luks F, Peers K, et al: Intrauterine endoscopic creation of urinary tract obstruction in the fetal lamb: A model for fetal surgery. Am J Obstet Gynecol 172:1422–1426, 1995.
8. Estes JM, MacGillivray T, Hedrick M, et al: Fetoscopic surgery for the treatment of congenital anomalies. J Pediatr Surg 27: 950–954, 1992.
9. VanderWall KJ, Skarsgard E, Filly R, et al: Fetendo-clip: A fetal endoscopic tracheal clip procedure in a human fetus. J Pediatr Surg 32:970–972, 1997.
10. Luks FI, Deprest J, Vandenberghe K, et al: A model for fetal surgery through intrauterine endoscopy. J Pediatr Surg 29:1007–1009, 1994.
11. Estes JM, Szabo B, Harrison MR: Techniques for in utero endoscopic surgery. A new approach for fetal intervention. Surg Endosc 6:215–218, 1992.
12. Harrison MR, Anderson GD, Rosen M, et al: Fetal surgery in the primate I: Anesthetic, surgical and tocolytic management to maximize fetal-maternal survival. J Pediatr Surg 17:115–122, 1982.
13. Graf JL, Bealer J, Gibbs D, et al: Chorioamniotic membrane separation: A potentially lethal finding. Fetal Diagn Ther 12: 81–84, 1997.
14. Deprest J, Evrard V, Van Schoubroeck D, Vandenberghe K: Fetoscopic cord ligation. Lancet 348:890–891, 1996.
15. Luks FI, Deprest JA, Vandenberghe K, et al: Fetoscopy-guided fetal endoscopy in a sheep model. J Am Coll Surg 178:609–612, 1994.
16. Kohl T, Szabo B, Suda M, et al: Percutaneous fetal access and uterine closure for fetoscopic surgery. Lessons learned from 16 consecutive procedures in pregnant sheep. Surg Endosc 11: 819–824, 1997.
17. VanderWall KJ, Bruch S, Meuli M, et al: Fetal endoscopic ('Fetendo') tracheal clip. J Pediatr Surg 31:1101–1103, 1996.
18. Luks FI, Deprest JA, Marcus M: Carbon dioxide pneumoamnios causes acidosis in fetal lamb. Fetal Diagn Ther 9:105–109, 1994.
19. Saiki Y, Litwin D, Bigras JL, et al: Reducing the deleterious effect of intrauterine CO_2 during fetoscopic surgery. J Surg Res 69:51–54, 1997.
20. Evrard VA, Verbeke EA, Peers K, et al: Amnioinfusion with Hartmann's solution: A safe distention medium for endoscopic fetal surgery in the ovine model. Fetal Diagn Ther 12:188–192, 1997.
21. Quintero RA, Crossland WJ, Cotton DB: Effect of endoscopic white light on the developing visual pathway: A histologic, histochemical, and behavioral study. Am J Obstet Gynecol 171: 1142–1148, 1994.
22. Deprest JA, Luks FI, Peers KH, et al: Intro-uterine exposure to videoendoscopic light in the fetal lamb. Am J Obstet Gynecol 172:427, 1995.
23. Ford WD, Cool J, Byard M, Allanson M: Glycine as a potential window for minimal access fetal surgery. Fetal Diagn Ther 12:145–148, 1997.
24. Estes JM, Whitby D, Lorenz H, et al: Endoscopic creation and repair of fetal cleft lip. Plast Reconstr Surg 90:743–746, 1992.
25. Bussi A, Ares L, Wieckowski J, et al: Creation of experimental urethral obstruction in utero: Evaluation of fetal renal function. Eur J Pediatr Surg 3:161–165, 1993.
26. Copeland MI, Bruner J, Richards W, et al: A model for in utero endoscopic treatment of myelomeningocele. Neurosurgery 33: 542–544, 1993.
27. Meuli M, Meult-Simmen C, Yingling C, et al: In utero repair of experimental myelomeningocele saves neurological function at birth. J Pediatr Surg 31:397–402, 1996.
28. Meuli M, Meult-Simmen C, Hutchins G, et al: In utero surgery rescues neurological function at birth in sheep with spina bifida. Nat Med 1:342–347, 1995.
29. Meult-Simmen C, Meuli M, Hutchins G, et al: Fetal reconstructive surgery: Experimental use of the latissimus dorsi flap to correct myelomeningocele in utero. Plast Reconstr Surg 96: 1007–1117, 1995.
30. Meuli M, Meult-Simmen C, Hutchins G, et al. The spinal cord lesion in human fetuses with myelomeningocele: Implications for fetal surgery. J Pediatr Surg 32:448–452, 1997.

31. van der Wildt B, Luks F, Steegers E, et al: Absence of electrical uterine activity after endoscopic access for fetal surgery in the rhesus monkey (Letter). Eur J Obstet Gynecol Reprod Biol 58:213–214, 1995.
32. DiFiore JW, Fauza DO, Slavin R, et al: Experimental fetal tracheal ligation reverses the structural and physiologic effect of pulmonary hypoplasia in congenital diaphragmatic hernia. J Pediatr Surg 29:248–257, 1994.
33. DiFiore JW, Fauza D, Slavin R, Wilson JM: Experimental fetal tracheal ligation and congenital diaphragmatic hernia: A pulmonary vascular morphometric analysis. J Pediatr Surg 30: 917–923, 1995.
34. Flageole H, Evrard V, Vandenberghe K, et al: Tracheoscopic endotracheal occlusion in the ovine model: Technique and pulmonary effects. J Pediatr Surg 32:1328–1331, 1997.
35. Skarsgard ED, Meuli M, VanderWall K, et al: Fetal endoscopic tracheal occlusion ('Fetendo-PLUG') for congenital diaphragmatic hernia. J Pediatr Surg 31:1335, 1996.
36. Luks FI, Gilchrist B, Jackson B, et al: Endoscopic tracheal obstruction with an expanding device in a fetal lamb model: Preliminary considerations. Fetal Diagn Ther 11:67–71, 1996.
37. O'Toole SJ, Karamanoukian H, Irish M, et al: Tracheal ligation: The dark side of in utero congenital diaphragmatic hernia treatment. J Pediatr Surg 32:407, 1997.
38. Piedboeuf B, Laberge J, Ghitulescu G, et al: Deleterious effect of tracheal obstruction on type II pneumocytes in fetal sheep (Abstract). Pediatr 41:473–479, 1997.
39. Douar AM, Themis M, Coutelle C: Fetal somatic gene therapy (Abstract). Mol Hum Reprod 41:633–641, 1996.
40. Flageole H, Evrard VA, Piedboeuf B, et al: The plug-unplug sequence: An important step to achieve type II pneumocyte maturation in the fetal lamb model. J Pediatr Surg 33:299–303, 1998.
41. McCray PB, Armstrong K, Zabner J, et al: Adenoviral-mediated gene transfer to pulmonary epithelia in vitro and in vivo (Abstract). J Clin Invest 95:2620–2632, 1995.
42. Sekhon HS, Larson J: In utero gene transfer into the pulmonary epithelium (Abstract). Nat Med 1:1201–1203, 1995.
43. Douar AM, Adebakin S, Themis M, et al: Foetal gene delivery in mice by intra-amniotic administration of rotroviral producer cells and adenovirus (Abstract). Gene Ther 4:883–890, 1997.
44. Sylvester KG, Yang EY, Cass DL, et al: Fetoscopic gene therapy for congenital lung disease (Abstract). J Pediatr Surg 32:964–969, 1997.
45. Fauza DO, Fishman SJ, Mehegan K, Atala A: Videofetoscopically assisted fetal tissue engineering: Bladder augmentation (Abstract). J Pediatr Surg 33:7–12, 1998.
46. Fauza DO, Fishman SJ, Mehegan K, Atala A: Videofetoscopically assisted fetal tissue engineering: Skin replacement (Abstract). J Pediatr Surg 33:357–361, 1998.
47. Ville Y: Monochorionic twin pregnancies: "Les liaisons dangereuses" (Abstract). Ultrasound Obstet Gynecol 10:82–85,1997.
48. De Lia JE, Cruikshank DP, Keye WR: Fetoscopic neodymium: YAG laser occlusion of placental vessels in severe twin-twin transfusion syndrome (Abstract). Obstet Gynecol 75:1046–1053, 1990.
49. Ville Y, Hyett J, Hecher K, Nicolaides K: Preliminary experience with endoscopic laser surgery for severe twin-twin transfusion syndrome (Abstract). N Engl J Med 332:224–227, 1995.
50. Deprest JA, Van Schoubroeck D, Van Ballaer PP, et al: Alternative technique for Nd:YAG laser coagulation in twin-to-twin transfusion syndrome with anterior placenta. Ultrasound Obstet Gynecol 11:347–352, 1998.
51. Ville Y, Van Pebergh P, Gagnon A, et al: Surgical treatment of twin-to-twin transfusion syndrome: Coagulation of anastomoses with a Nd:YAG laser under endosonographic control. Forty four cases (Abstract). J Gynecol Obstet Biol Reprod Paris 26: 175–181, 1997.
52. Moore TR, Gale S, Bernischke K: Perinatal outcome of forty-nine pregnancies complicated by acardiac twinning (Abstract). Am J Obstet Gynecol 163:907–912, 1990.
53. Ville Y, Hyett JA, Vandenbussche F, Nicolaides KH: Endoscopic laser coagulation of umbilical cord vessels in twin reversed arterial perfusion sequence (Abstract). Ultrasound Obstet Gynecol; 4:396–398, 1994.
54. Quintero RA, Romero R, Reich H, et al: In utero percutaneous umbilical cord ligation in the management of complicated monochorionic multiple gestations. Ultrasound Obstet Gynecol 8:16–22, 1996.
55. Hecher K, Hackeloer BJ: Intrauterine endoscopic laser surgery for fetal sacrococcygeal teratoma (Letter). Lancet 347:470, 1996.
56. Langer JC, Harrison MR, Schmidt KG, et al: Fetal hydrops and death from sacrococcygeal teratoma: Rationale for fetal surgery (Abstract). Am J Obstet Gynecol 1989;160:1145–1150, 1989.
57. Mychaliska G, Graf J, Filly R, et al: Endoscopic fetal tracheal occlusion for treatment of CDH: Technical innovations and clinical outcomes (Abstract). Presented at the 16th annual meeting of the International Fetal Medicine and Surgery Society, June 1–5, 1997, Alyeska Resort, Alaska, USA.
58. MacMahon RA, Renou PMM, Shekelton PA, Paterson PJ: In utero cystostomy (Abstract). Lancet 340:234, 1992.
59. Quintero RA, Johnson M, Romero R, et al: In-utero percutaneous cystoscopy in the management of fetal lower obstructive uropathy. Lancet 346:537–540, 1995.
60. Quintero RA, Hume R, Smith C, et al: Percutaneous fetal cystoscopy and endoscopic fulguration of posterior urethral valves (Abstract). Am J Obstet Gynecol 172:206, 1995.
61. Johnson MP, Quintero R, Freedman AU, et al: Development of a fetal cystoscopy program (Abstract). Presented at the 16th Annual Meeting of the International Fetal Medicine and Surgery Society, June 1–5, Alyeska Resort, Alaska, 1997.
62. Bruner JP, Richards WO, Tulipan NB, et al: Endoscopic coverage of fetal myelomeningocele in utero. Am J Obstet Gynecol 180:153–158, 1999.
63. Crombleholme TM, Dirkes K, Whitney T, et al: Amniotic band syndrome in fetal lambs. I: Fetoscopic release and morphometric outcome. J Pediatr Surg 30:974, 1995.
64. Quintero RA, Morales WJ, Phillips J, et al: In utero lysis of amniotic bands (Abstract). Ultrasound Obstet Gynecol 19:316–320, 1997.
65. Evrard V, Flageole H, Deprest JA, et al: Intrauterine tracheal obstruction, as treatment for congenital diaphragmatic hernia, decreases amniotic fluid sodium and chloride concentrations in the fetal lamb. Ann Surg 226:753–758, 1997.
66. Deprest JA, Lerut T, Vandenberghe K: Endoscopic fetal surgery: A new perspective in fetal surgery? Prenatal Diagnosis 17:1247–1260, 1997.
67. Deprest JA, Evrard V, Van Ballaer P, et al: Experience with fetoscopic cord ligation. Eur J Obstet Gynecol Reprod Biol 81: 157–164, 1998.
68. Gonsoulin W, Moise K, Kirshon B, et al: Outcome of twin-twin transfusion diagnosed before 28 weeks of gestation. Obstet Gynecol 75:214–216, 1990.

COMMENTARY

W. D. Andrew Ford

This chapter reflects the ingenuity involved in the rapid development of a completely new dimension in surgery. Until the 1970s, there was no scope for fetal interventions because there was no way of detecting the vast majority of fetal abnormalities. No sooner had destructive anomalies become visible on antenatal ultrasonography, however, there was increasing pressure to change the course of those lesions that might lead to the death of the fetus or to irreparable damage that would permanently diminish the quality of life. Lesions that were unlikely to lead to the death of the fetus or newborn or to permanent damage, have not been potential candidates for surgery and are not likely to be until such time as the major problems with the preterm labor seen after fetal intervention have been overcome.

Initial attempts at fetal surgery mimicked procedures that would otherwise have been performed after birth. This was especially true for fetuses with congenital diaphragmatic hernia. These interventions led to a procedure-related fetal loss rate as high, or higher, than the natural history of the lesion. The procedures required an extensive hysterotomy, which often led to immediate preterm labor or intrauterine fetal death from the shutdown of the fetoplacental circulation. Furthermore, they required toxic tocolysis for the mother in an attempt to limit preterm labor. Conversely, the placement of urinary tract shunt catheters into fetuses with obstructed urinary tracts produced low fetal mortality from the procedure itself, with reduced rates of preterm labor. These procedures were carried out through small trochars with the aid of ultrasonographic guidance.

This work led to the belief that if fetal interventions could be carried out through small access sites in the uterus, employing procedures that reduced fetal stress, preterm delivery rates would be reduced and there would be better survival from the procedure itself. Therefore, miniaturized approaches to the fetus and the surgery have been developed as fast as possible but are still in the early phase of development in a limited number of centers worldwide. Nevertheless, when they have been developed to the point that they can be carried out simply, by many centers, fetal intervention for anatomic abnormalities will become an accepted method of salvaging the fetus and improving survival and the quality of that survival after birth. We are on the threshold of those developments now, with exciting prospects on the horizon after a decade of disappointments.

Apart from fetoscopy, there are other minimally invasive procedures that have been carried out to improve the outcome of the fetus with a lethal abnormality. The size of hysterotomies has been reduced to the point that maternal-fetal risks have decreased. This has been partly successful, at least in Philadelphia, where congenital diaphragmatic hernia has now been treated successfully with a small hysterotomy that exposes the fetal neck. A clip is then applied to the trachea. One advantage of using the hysterotomy is that the procedure is faster than placing multiple ports. In addition, it is less operator-dependent than fetoscopy, as surgeons can learn the techniques operating directly on a child rather than operating fetoscopically in a liquid through the mother. Therefore, the search for procedures that use minimal invasion of the uterus to correct major defects, be it fetoscopic or through a minihysterotomy, are becoming a priority. For example, correction of spina bifida in utero has been carried out fetoscopically, but a small hysterotomy is apparently just as effective.

The procedures described use an actual image of the fetus. This may not, however, be necessary. There are other potential interventions that are less invasive in which the imaging is indirect. For example, when there is a space-occupying lesion causing the eventual demise of the fetus, ablation of part of that lesion may allow the fetus to survive in good condition until birth. Indirect visualization of the fetus with ultrasonography allows the placement of probes that can then be used to obliterate such a tumor. In this way, the placement of a thermocoagulating probe has been used to partly destroy a sacrococcygeal teratoma and its feeding blood vessels in a situation in which the fetus was in high-output cardiac failure and likely to die. The rare case of a pulmonary cystic adenomatoid malformation that does not regress in utero and causes fetal cardiac failure because of the diminished venous return may be amenable to similar treatment. In this instance, simple injections of sclerosants into the pulmonary lesion would not work because they could make the tumor swell, thereby worsening the situation.

Congenital diaphragmatic hernia may also be treatable in a similar indirect manner if a tracheal blocking agent could be injected into the trachea of the fetus while imaging with ultrasonography, rather than the fetoscopic visualization of the neck, mobilizing the trachea, or endoscopic visualization of the inside of the trachea itself after placing a flexible scope through the fetus' mouth. The procedure could become much simpler but would rely on ultrasonographic machines of high resolution or the use of computed tomography.

Lesions that can be treated with fetoscopic imaging of the fetus exist and will continue to grow in number. The future, in fact, looks much more promising for fetal interventions and surgery than has the past and present, and we are looking forward to an era of growth rather than one of setbacks, which has happened in the past. Fetoscopy will play a major role in that growth.

Section VI

Endoscopy and Imaging

Chapter 46

Interventional Bronchoscopy

Peter Ferson, Rodney J. Landreneau, Robert J. Keenan, James D. Luketich, and Tracey L. Weigel

The application of endoscopic methods to evaluate and treat disorders of the airways is an essential skill for practicing thoracic surgeons. The unusual location of the trachea, originating at the larynx in an almost subcutaneous position and ending in the posterior mediastinum behind the great vessels, makes surgical exposure through standard incisions difficult. Thus, endoscopic management of problems involving the trachea and main airways may offer the most direct approach. As with most facets of surgical practice, endoscopic technology is constantly changing. Thoracic surgeons must therefore be aware not only of the historical development of techniques[1] but also of currently available methods and instrumentation, so that they can select the appropriate equipment and use it effectively.

Development

Bozzini is credited with the first report of examining various body orifices with light transmitted through a hollow tube. Using a wax candle and a mirror as a light source, he performed vaginal and rectal examinations, and in 1806 he used his device to inspect the pharynx and possibly the upper esophagus.[2–4]

Kussmaul recruited a sword swallower as a subject and in 1868 successfully visualized the esophagus and stomach using a lighted tube designed by Desormeaux for urethroscopy.[3, 5] This took place in the city of Freiburg, where 30 years later, in 1897, Gustave Killian performed the first examination of the trachea and bronchi by inserting an esophagoscope through the larynx to visualize the subglottic airway. Like Kussmaul, Killian enlisted the services of a paid volunteer for his early efforts. That same year, he reported the first clinical application: the removal of a foreign body from the bronchus.[6]

During the first half of the 20th century, refinement in technique and equipment for bronchoscopy centered on the use of rigid instruments. The major participant in this development was Chevalier Jackson, whose clinics in Pittsburgh and Philadelphia became world-recognized centers of bronchoesophagology. His published descriptions of methods have become classics for students of upper airway disorders.[7]

The development of flexible viewing instruments resulted in great changes in the methods of investigating the upper aerodigestive system. Hirschowitz and coworkers described the use of a flexible gastroscope at a meeting in 1957,[8] and Ikeda and coworkers in 1968 reported on the use of a flexible bronchofiberscope.[9] The use of flexible scopes for evaluating and treating disorders of the pharynx, larynx, tracheobronchial tree, esophagus, and stomach is now standard procedure. When compared with their rigid counterparts, flexible scopes offer greater patient acceptability, fewer anesthetic requirements, better visibility, and increased versatility. There remain, however, specific indications for the use of rigid instruments both alone and in conjunction with flexible devices.

Bronchoscopes

Flexible Bronchoscopes

The flexible endoscope consists of a plastic-covered tube containing several compartments. Two bundles of optical fibers are present—one to carry light to the distal end, and the other to carry the visual image back to the control end. Newer instruments may eliminate the viewing fiberoptic bundle by placing a camera chip directly on the end of the scope and transmitting the image along electrical circuits through the scope to a video monitor. Most bronchoscopes contain an empty channel for suctioning, irrigating, and introducing instruments.

The length of fiberscopes is related to their application, with shorter instruments for nasopharyngeal use. Diameter sizes range from 2.2 to 6.4 mm. The smaller-diameter endoscopes tend to have greater flexibility at the expense of lower-quality optics and smaller or absent working channels. With larger diameters one finds better optics as well as increased size and number of working channels. A suction channel of 2.6-mm diameter is almost the same size as a rigid suction tube that could be inserted through a rigid bronchoscope (Fig. 46–1). Flexible bronchoscopes with two working channels (Olympus Corp., Strongsville, OH) permit simultaneous suctioning and instrumentation.

When selecting a bronchoscope, one must consider factors related to each patient, such as the need to visualize very distal airways, the need for suctioning, and the degree of airway obstruction that will be produced by the endoscope (with or without an endotracheal tube in place). The potential hazard with using larger-diameter flexible bron-

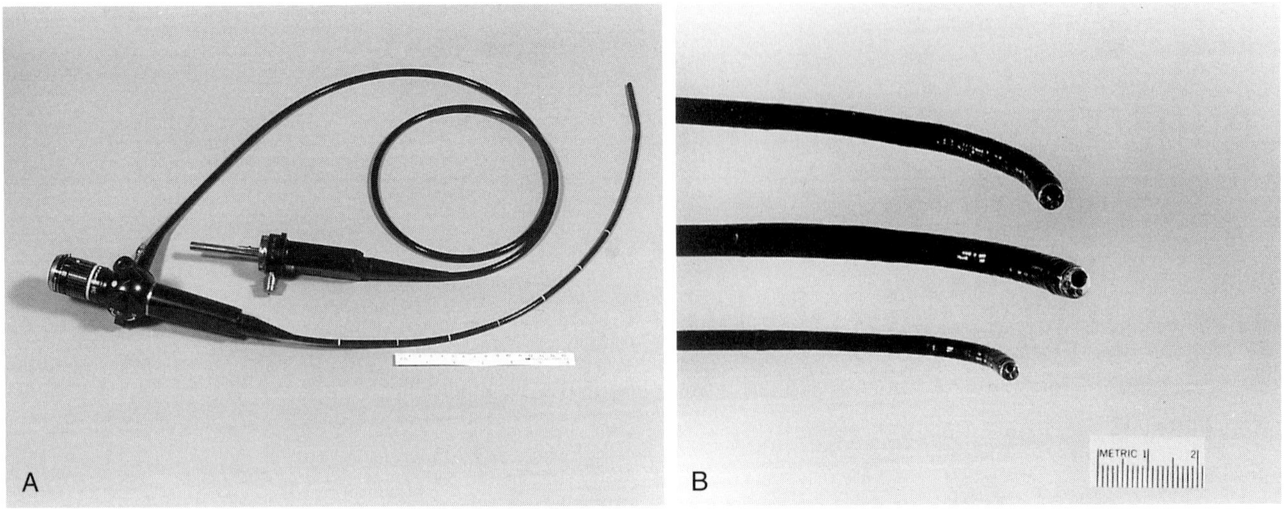

Figure 46–1. *A*, A standard adult-size flexible fiberoptic bronchoscope. *B*, The distal ends of flexible bronchoscopes with varying diameters. The size of the light bundle and the suction channel is also variable.

choscopes is that larger scopes produce greater airway compromise when inserted.

There are several options for image visualization with flexible instruments. An individual operator may view directly into the vision port of the flexible bronchoscope. A beam-splitting teaching attachment allows direct vision by the operator while an assistant watches through a side arm. If a video camera is attached to the viewing port, the image can be projected on a monitor for group viewing, and the image can be recorded for later demonstration (Fig. 46–2). A still camera can also be attached to the viewing port for documentation purposes. If video display is used, the operator can perform the procedure while watching on the video screen. This method can be disorienting to inexperienced observers, particularly when performing bronchoscopy, in which the anterior-posterior and lateral relationships are more apparent than with esophagoscopy. It is easier to maintain orientation with a beam splitter that allows the operator to view directly into the scope, but this may detract from the intensity of illumination.

Rigid Bronchoscopes

As with flexible scopes, rigid bronchoscopes are available in an array of lengths and diameters (Fig. 46–3). The bronchoscopes are hollow tubes with a light mechanism that delivers either a distally positioned light source or a proximally diverted light beam. The distal end is beveled to allow careful insertion between the vocal cords. Side perforations along the distal portion of the bronchoscope tube permit ventilation into the trachea when the bronchoscope is advanced down one main stem bronchus. The external end has a variety of attachments, depending on the manufacturer. A securely fitting window plug is present to allow

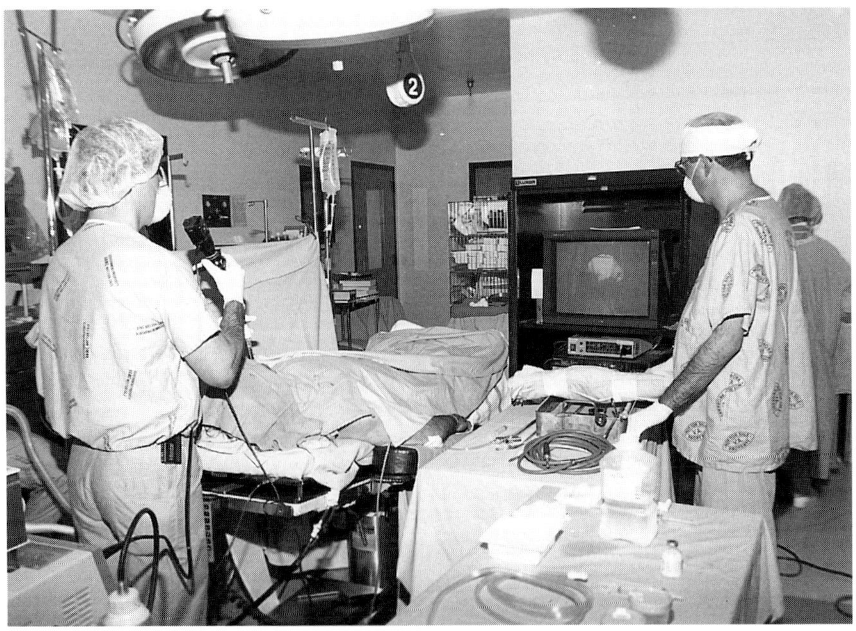

Figure 46–2. The image from a flexible bronchoscope can be projected onto a video monitor. (From Myers EN [ed]: Operative Otolaryngology: Head and Neck Surgery. Philadelphia, WB Saunders, 1997, with permission.)

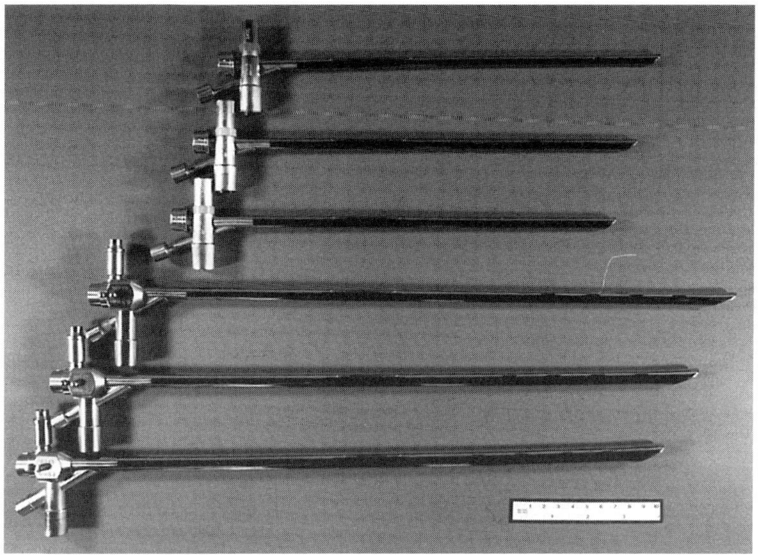

Figure 46–3. An array of rigid bronchoscopes. The inner diameters range from 4 to 8.5 mm and the lengths are 30 and 43 cm. (From Myers EN [ed]: Operative Otolaryngology: Head and Neck Surgery. Philadelphia, WB Saunders, 1997, with permission.)

the system to be closed for conventional ventilation. Most bronchoscopes have an inlet for connecting a jet ventilator to permit working with an open system (Fig. 46–4). Rigid suction tubes, with or without cautery capability, should be matched to the length of the bronchoscope, as should biopsy forceps and foreign body forceps.

Vision may be directly through the tube, or a magnified image of endobronchial anatomy may be obtained by utilizing a telescopic attachment (either forward or angled viewing). As with flexible bronchoscopes, viewing may be directly through the telescope, or a video camera may be attached to its external eyepiece to project the image. Still cameras may also be attached for documentation (Fig. 46–5).

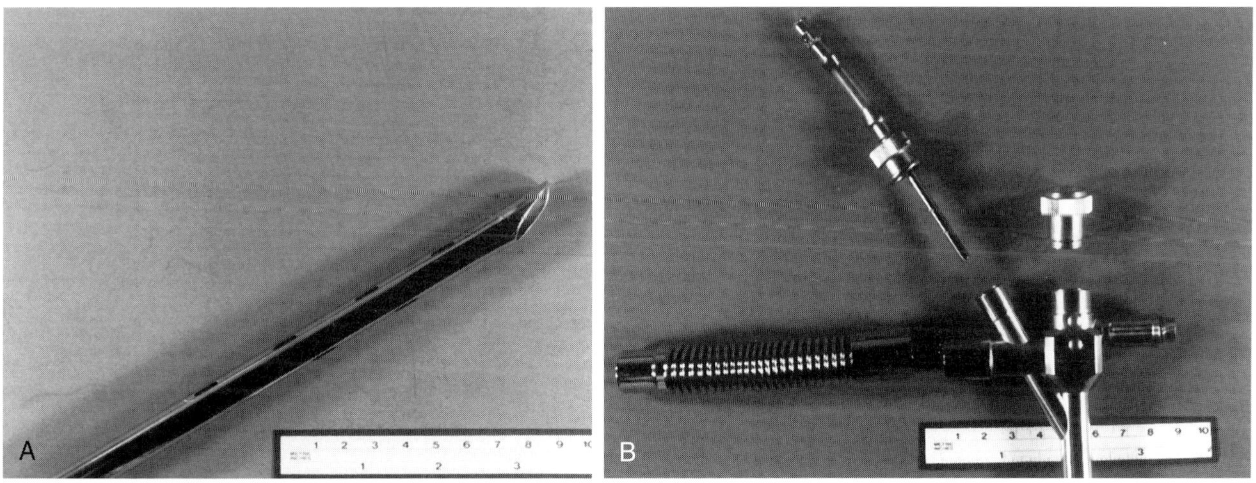

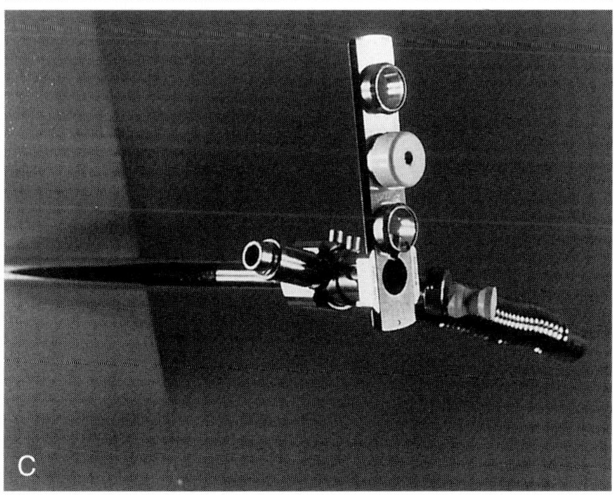

Figure 46–4. *A*, The distal end of the rigid bronchoscope is angled to enable atraumatic insertion between the vocal cords. This also enhances passage through strictures. The multiple side holes distribute the ventilation throughout the trachea and main bronchi, particularly when the bronchoscope is inserted into a distal bronchus. *B*, The proximal end of the rigid bronchoscope has connections for the anesthesia circuit for conventional positive pressure ventilation, a jet ventilation port, a sealed window plug, and the fiberoptic light carrier. *C*, A multiple-port window plug facilitates opening of the bronchoscope for insertion of a suction tube, working instruments, or a telescope without concern for misplacement of the window plug. (From Myers EN [ed]: Operative Otolaryngology: Head and Neck Surgery. Philadelphia, WB Saunders, 1997, with permission.)

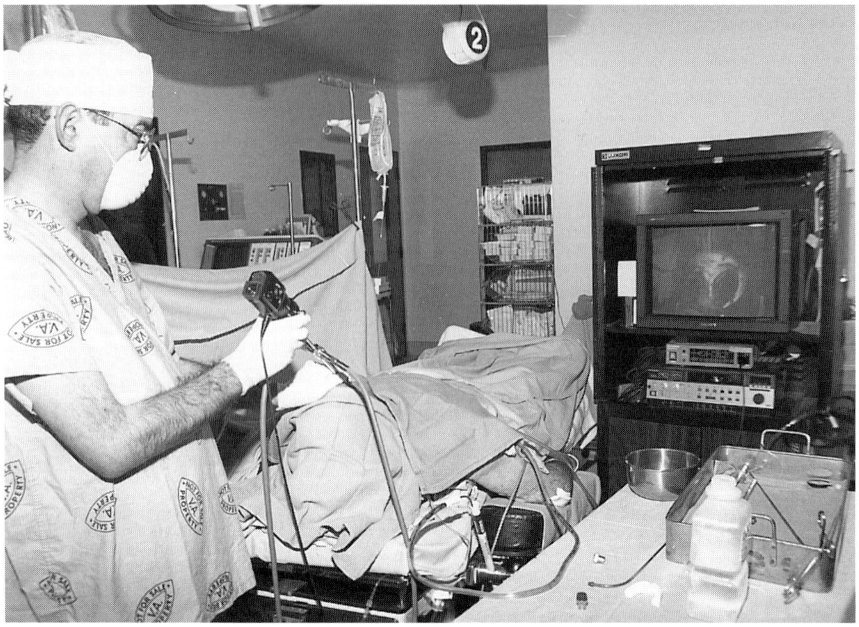

Figure 46–5. Video display of the endobronchial findings is accomplished by inserting a telescope through the rigid bronchoscope and connecting a video camera to the telescope.

Bronchoscopy Technique

The decision to perform rigid or flexible bronchoscopy does not have to be an exclusionary choice. The two methods can be combined to use the advantages of each. Whereas a rigid bronchoscope gives better airway control and allows insertion of larger suctioning and grasping instruments, a flexible bronchoscope permits more direct viewing (in spite of the use of telescopes through the rigid bronchoscope) and provides more mobility in the distal bronchi. Complex procedures involving difficult biopsies, lasering of tumors or strictures, and retrieval of foreign bodies may be enhanced by combining rigid and flexible bronchoscopy. When a large rigid bronchoscope is used, a flexible bronchoscope with a second light source can be advanced through the rigid instrument to take advantage of the flexible instrument's mobility in the distal airways.

Flexible Bronchoscopy

Local anesthesia is used for most routine flexible bronchoscopic examinations. Sedation with 1 to 2 mg of midazolam and 50 to 100 μg of fentanyl given intravenously immediately before initiation of the local anesthesia is usually sufficient. Continuous pulse oximetry and electrocardiogram monitoring are utilized, along with noninvasive blood pressure monitoring.

Application of topical anesthetic can be performed in a variety of ways. We prefer to spray the posterior pharynx with 10% lidocaine and to apply 2% lidocaine jelly to the nasal passage. A long right-angle spring-loaded forceps facilitates the direct application of small pieces of cotton soaked in 4% lidocaine into the pyriform sinuses (Fig. 46–6). An alternative method for achieving local anesthesia is to administer 4% lidocaine aerosol 10 minutes before the procedure. An additional 2 to 3 ml of 1% lidocaine is then directed through the bronchoscope into the larynx and upper trachea. Further applications of 2 to 3 ml of 1% lidocaine can be directed through the bronchoscope as needed to accomplish adequate distal airway anesthesia.

A few patients will not tolerate local anesthesia because of severe anxiety or an excessive gag reflex. General anesthesia may also be needed to control the airway in patients who have had laryngeal surgery or primary laryngeal deformities or when the patient must be totally immobilized and unresponsive for careful examination or manipulation of the airway. With general anesthesia, the flexible bronchoscope can be passed through a ventilation adapter (Portex Inc., Wilmington, MA) and the procedure performed through the endotracheal tube (Fig. 46–7). Care must be taken in the selection of a bronchoscope and endotracheal tube so that there is sufficient airway to ventilate the patient yet a large enough bronchoscope to perform the planned procedure. Inexperienced personnel sometimes place too large a bronchoscope into an endotracheal tube without adequate lubrication. When the anesthesiologist complains of an inability to ventilate, it may be discovered that the bronchoscope is stuck in the endotracheal tube. This scenario can usually be remedied by instilling saline solution through the endotracheal tube alongside the bronchoscope. If this does not loosen the bronchoscope, the endotracheal tube can be removed with the bronchoscope and the patient re-intubated.

Rigid Bronchoscopy

Although rigid bronchoscopy can be performed successfully with local anesthesia, general anesthesia is almost always used. For severe abnormalities of the pharynx and upper trachea, spontaneous ventilation adds a measure of security, particularly until the trachea can be intubated with the bronchoscope. For most routine examinations, however, insertion of the bronchoscope and examination or manipulation of the airways are easier and safer with the patient paralyzed. Anesthetic induction proceeds in a fashion similar to that for routine endotracheal intubation,

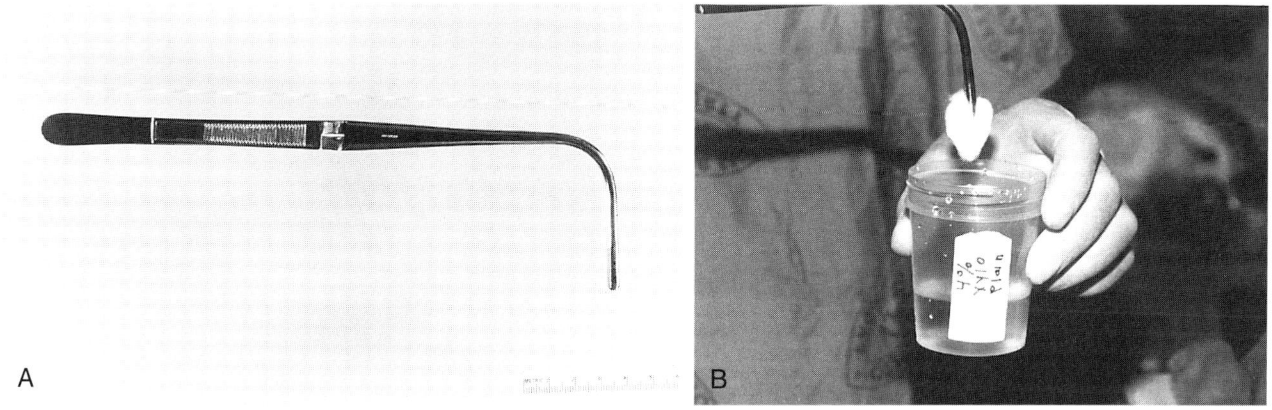

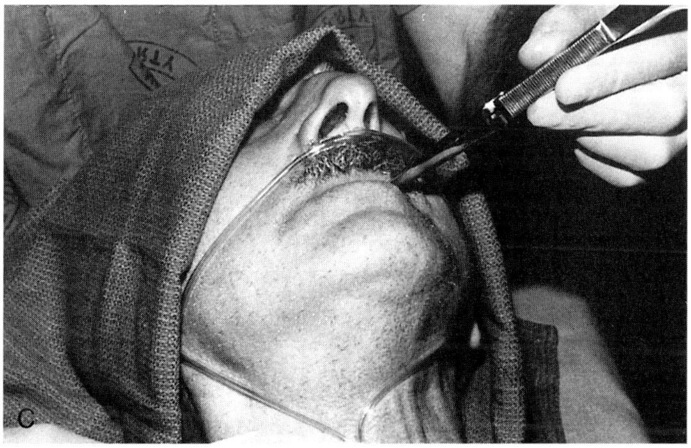

Figure 46–6. *A–C,* A spring-loaded right-angled forceps is used to hold a small piece of cotton soaked in 4% lidocaine against the pyriform sinus.

with the patient ventilated via a mask until total relaxation is achieved. The bronchoscope is then inserted instead of an endotracheal tube, and ventilation is performed through the bronchoscope.

The most difficult part of rigid bronchoscopy is proper visualization of the larynx and passage of the bronchoscope. Several guidelines facilitate this maneuver. First, there is a common tendency to hyperextend the neck, often by elevating the shoulders and dropping the head. For the initial part of the procedure, it is better to have the neck in a more neutral position and the head slightly forward (the "sniffing" position). The second guideline pertains to the actual exposure of the larynx. This can be accomplished by visualizing through the bronchoscope as it is directed posterior to the epiglottis and then used to elevate the epiglottis anteriorly, exposing the vocal cords (Fig. 46–8). Even for an experienced operator, this can sometimes be difficult owing to the small area exposed at any one time. It is usually easier to use a standard laryngoscope to elevate the epiglottis, exposing the larynx. While this exposure is maintained with the laryngoscope held in the left hand, the bronchoscope can be guided to the larynx with the right hand. At this point, the laryngoscope is removed and the left hand is placed on the teeth or upper jaw to protect these structures and to serve as a fulcrum point for the bronchoscope (Fig. 46–9). This latter method was well described by Jackson and Jackson in their detailed description of bronchoscopic techniques.[7]

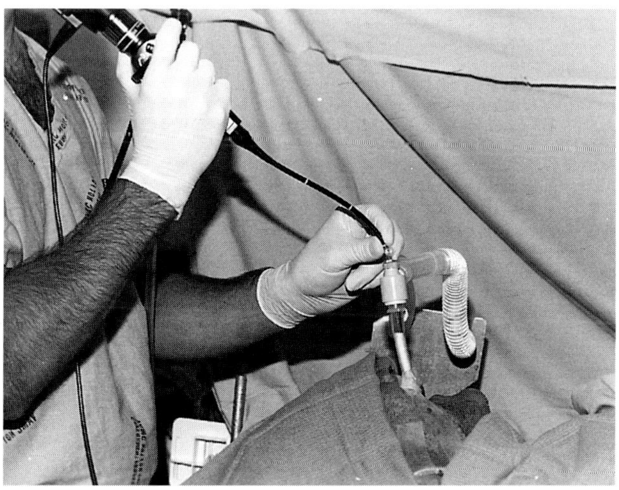

Figure 46–7. The right-angled adapter with a perforated membrane permits flexible bronchoscopy through an endotracheal tube while positive pressure ventilation is continued.

Once the bronchoscope has been inserted into the trachea, ventilation is initiated. This can be accomplished by spontaneous breathing if the patient is not paralyzed. Standard positive pressure ventilation may be used if the system is closed with either a window plug or a rubber diaphragm through which a telescope is inserted. Even with such closure, a large retrograde air leak through the larynx is usually present, and high gas flow from the anesthesia machine will need to be maintained. Alternatively, high-frequency jet ventilation can be used. This permits an open system and eases the insertion and use of instruments and telescopes. Occasionally, a separate catheter

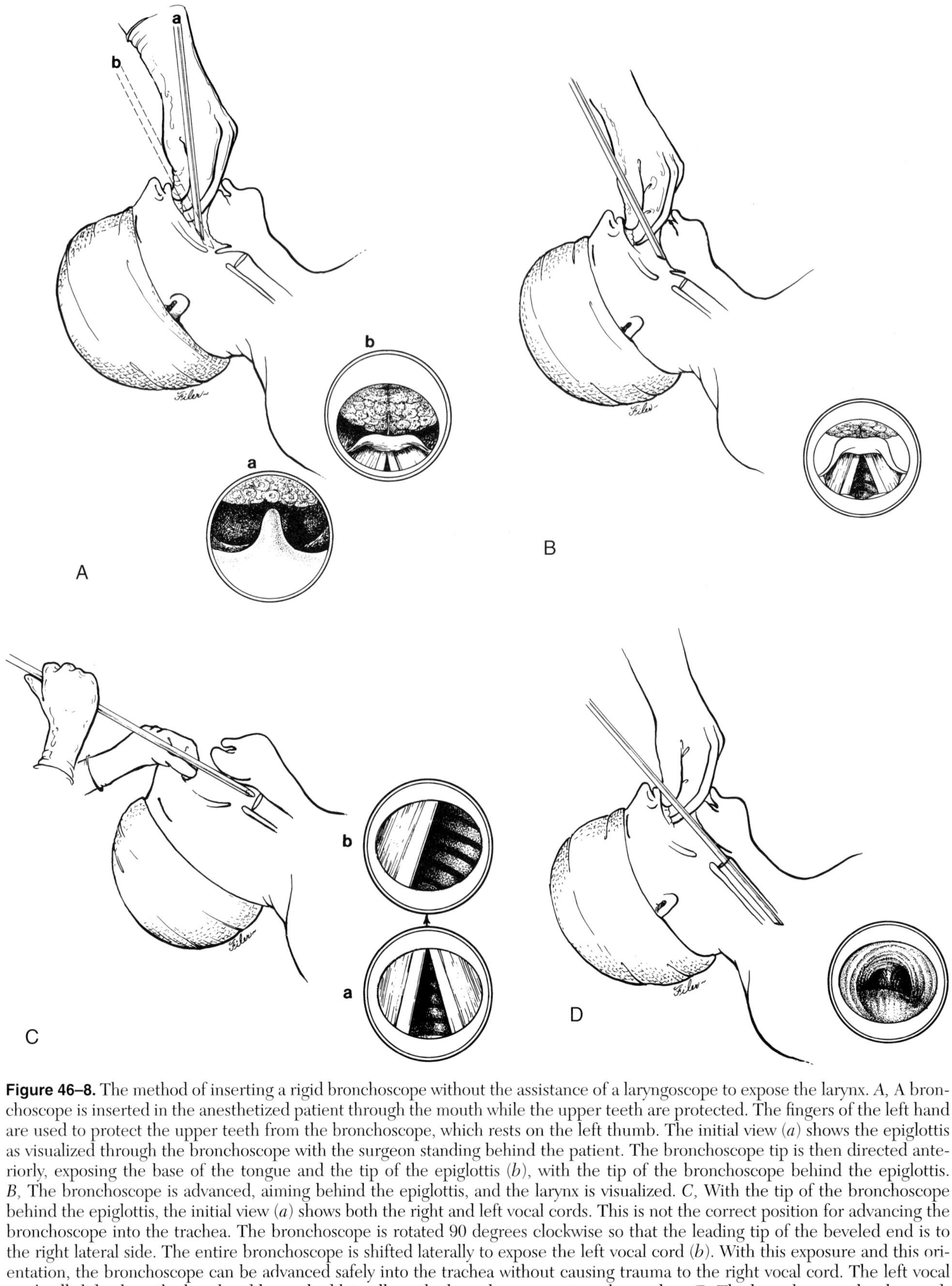

Figure 46–8. The method of inserting a rigid bronchoscope without the assistance of a laryngoscope to expose the larynx. *A,* A bronchoscope is inserted in the anesthetized patient through the mouth while the upper teeth are protected. The fingers of the left hand are used to protect the upper teeth from the bronchoscope, which rests on the left thumb. The initial view (*a*) shows the epiglottis as visualized through the bronchoscope with the surgeon standing behind the patient. The bronchoscope tip is then directed anteriorly, exposing the base of the tongue and the tip of the epiglottis (*b*), with the tip of the bronchoscope behind the epiglottis. *B,* The bronchoscope is advanced, aiming behind the epiglottis, and the larynx is visualized. *C,* With the tip of the bronchoscope behind the epiglottis, the initial view (*a*) shows both the right and left vocal cords. This is not the correct position for advancing the bronchoscope into the trachea. The bronchoscope is rotated 90 degrees clockwise so that the leading tip of the beveled end is to the right lateral side. The entire bronchoscope is shifted laterally to expose the left vocal cord (*b*). With this exposure and this orientation, the bronchoscope can be advanced safely into the trachea without causing trauma to the right vocal cord. The left vocal cord will slide along the bevel and be pushed laterally as the bronchoscope enters the trachea. *D,* The bronchoscope has been advanced past the larynx into the trachea for distal tracheal examination. It is important at this point that the upper hand be placed in a firm position to protect the teeth and upper jaw from pressure from the bronchoscope. The bronchoscope should rest on the left thumb and not against the teeth. This is similar to an open bridge cue-stick position when shooting billiards. (From Myers EN [ed]: Operative Otolaryngology: Head and Neck Surgery. Philadelphia, WB Saunders, 1997, with permission.)

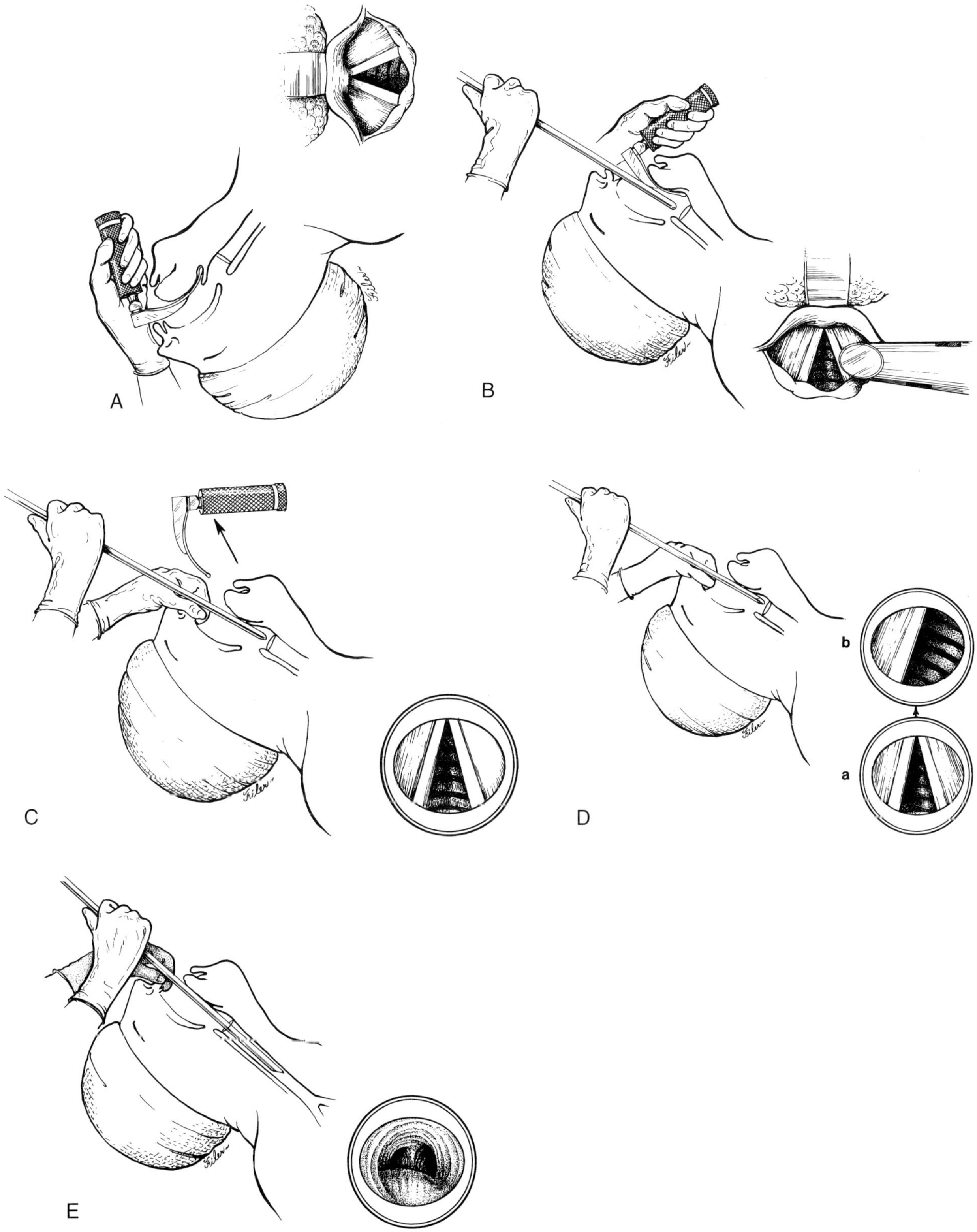

Figure 46–9. The method of exposing the larynx assisted by a laryngoscope for introduction of a rigid bronchoscope. *A,* The larynx is exposed directly using the laryngoscope to elevate the tongue and epiglottis. *B,* While the larynx is visualized through the laryngoscope held in the left hand, the bronchoscope is inserted behind the epiglottis with the right hand. *C,* The operator's view is now directed down the shaft of the bronchoscope. The laryngoscope is removed, and the left hand is placed on the upper teeth to support the bronchoscope. *D, E,* The technique from this point is the same as that outlined in Figure 46-8. (From Myers EN [ed]: Operative Otolaryngology: Head and Neck Surgery. Philadelphia, WB Saunders, 1997, with permission.)

placed through the larynx beside the bronchoscope can be used for jet ventilation (Fig. 46–10).

When a telescope is inserted, care must be exercised to avoid advancing it beyond the bronchoscope, particularly with side-viewing telescopes. The telescope can be blindly advanced into the bronchus and traumatize the airway. A video camera can be attached to the telescope for projection of the image, and still photography can be performed with a camera attached to the telescope.

Applications

Pulmonary Masses

Evaluation of undiagnosed pulmonary masses involves a variety of standard diagnostic procedures, including chest roentgenograms and computed tomography scans, sputum analysis, percutaneous needle biopsy, and bronchoscopy. Although rigid bronchoscopy permits visualization of the main bronchi for inspection and biopsy, a flexible bronchoscope can demonstrate the segmental and subsegmental bronchi more clearly. With flexible bronchoscopes, biopsy specimens of more distally located tumors and those in the upper lobes can be easily obtained. Fluoroscopic guidance assists in the biopsy of masses that cannot be visualized endobronchially (Fig. 46–11).

In addition to obtaining a tissue diagnosis, bronchoscopic evaluation in patients who are candidates for surgical resection helps in planning a resection strategy with respect to the endobronchial extent of a tumor. Edema and extrinsic compression suggesting peribronchial infiltration by the malignant process can signal the need for more extensive resection than otherwise planned.

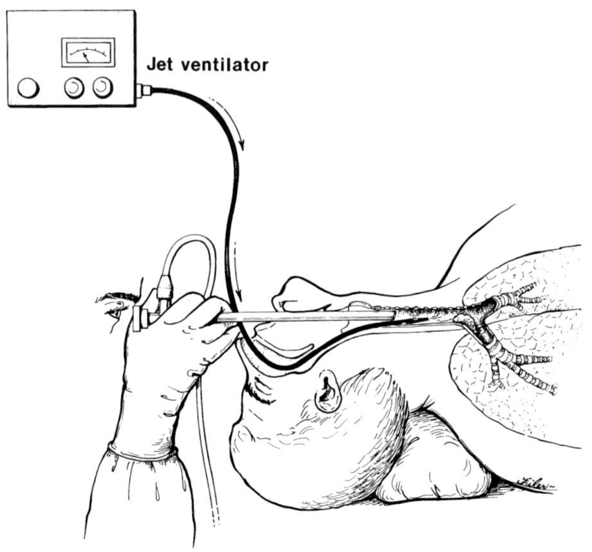

Figure 46–10. A flexible nasotracheal suction catheter can be used for jet ventilation. When a complex bronchoscopic procedure requires removal and reinsertion of the bronchoscope, this method allows for continued ventilation when the bronchoscope has been removed. (From Myers EN [ed]: Operative Otolaryngology: Head and Neck Surgery. Philadelphia, WB Saunders, 1997, with permission.)

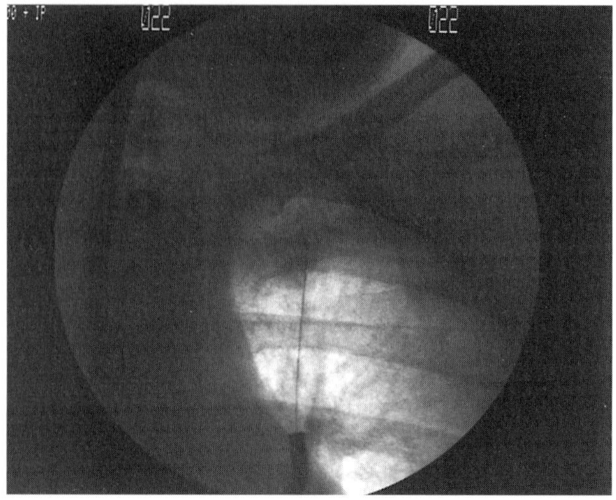

Figure 46–11. Fluoroscopic guidance is used to obtain a specimen from a peripheral lung mass. The mass could not be seen through the bronchoscope.

Pulmonary Infiltrates

Diffuse pulmonary infiltrates may be associated with either chronic progressive respiratory insufficiency or acute respiratory failure and sepsis. For patients with chronic respiratory insufficiency, bronchoscopy can obtain transbronchial biopsy specimens of the lung parenchyma. In certain disorders, such as sarcoid, this method has been shown to have a high positive diagnostic yield.[10]

A patient with acute respiratory insufficiency and pulmonary infiltrates is often immunosuppressed from malignancy or chemotherapy or following transplantation. Infection is the most common cause of the respiratory failure, although infiltrating neoplastic processes may also be present. Flexible bronchoscopy is beneficial for obtaining culture specimens by direct endobronchial aspiration, bronchoalveolar lavage, and transbronchial biopsy.[4]

The diagnostic yield of flexible bronchoscopy in both acute and chronic pulmonary infiltrates is not as great as that of open lung biopsy, but bronchoscopy is clearly a less invasive first step that should be considered.[11]

Hemoptysis

Flexible bronchoscopy is an important diagnostic method in the evaluation of patients with hemoptysis. A threefold purpose is served by bronchoscopic evaluation. First, the source of the hemoptysis can be localized. An endobronchial source of active bleeding may be identified. If no lesions are seen, it is often possible to identify the bronchial segmental orifice from which the bleeding is originating. Second, a tissue diagnosis can be obtained if an endobronchial lesion is present. Third, direct therapeutic intervention, such as laser coagulation of a bleeding lesion, can be undertaken to control the bleeding.

When massive hemoptysis occurs, rigid bronchoscopy is frequently necessary to control the airway and provide more extensive endobronchial suction capabilities. In such instances, a flexible bronchoscope can be inserted through the rigid bronchoscope to completely evaluate the distal airways.

Obstructing Lesions

Airway obstruction can occur from endobronchial tumors, from benign strictures, or from functional abnormalities such as malacia. Although some of these lesions are amenable to primary resection, endobronchial evaluation is essential. Frequently the abnormalities are not surgically correctable, and bronchoscopic therapy is undertaken.

The use of flexible bronchoscopy in the evaluation of strictures of the major airways must be undertaken with great caution. Unlike the rigid bronchoscope, which allows ventilation through its central lumen, the flexible bronchoscope essentially obstructs whatever portion of the lumen it occupies. If the flexible bronchoscope is inserted into a narrowed airway, it may obstruct distal ventilation. This is particularly true in the trachea, where tumor or benign stricture may be severely narrowing the airway. The remaining lumen may be easily obstructed if the flexible bronchoscope is advanced into a narrow portion. Subsequent edema from the instrumentation may further compromise the airway. Rigid bronchoscopy is therefore essential for thorough evaluation of lesions causing proximal airway obstruction. The ability to pass the bronchoscope beyond the obstruction, thus establishing distal ventilation, adds security that is not possible with a flexible bronchoscope. Once the initial evaluation is completed, appropriate therapeutic intervention can be initiated through the rigid instrument.

Careful use of a flexible bronchoscope permits evaluation of the larynx and trachea proximal to an obstructing lesion. Flexible bronchoscopy is also essential in evaluating functional strictures such as malacic segments, where the changing nature of the obstruction with voluntary forced inspiration and expiration must be demonstrated.

The application of flexible bronchoscopy in the treatment of tracheal or proximal bronchial strictures is similarly limited. When an obstructing malignancy is present, ablation with an Nd:YAG laser, passed through a flexible bronchoscope, is possible. The Nd:YAG laser is preferred over the carbon dioxide laser because of its greater depth of tissue penetration and because the laser beam can be delivered through a flexible fiber introduced through the working channel of a flexible bronchoscope. Although the carbon dioxide laser is also effective, it must be delivered through a rigid system with straight optics. Use of the laser is best performed with the patient under general anesthesia, and care must be taken to avoid igniting the endotracheal tube. Laser ablation of large obstructing tumors can be tedious and time consuming. Progress with the laser is slow, and it is almost impossible to use effectively when any bleeding occurs. For these reasons, we use the Nd:YAG laser initially to cauterize the surface of the lesion and then insert a rigid bronchoscope to debride the tumor with biopsy forceps. Further laser application can be performed through a flexible bronchoscope introduced through the rigid instrument. Any significant bleeding is much easier to control with an insulated suction or cautery. Occasionally, troublesome bleeding can occur. When this happens, the presence of the rigid bronchoscope permits a tamponade of hemostatic gauze to be transiently inserted into the offending area, and then the other main stem bronchus can be separately ventilated. When the stenosis is secondary to an unresectable neoplasm, endobronchial ablation may also be followed by placement of an intraluminal stent and catheters for brachytherapy, when appropriate.

Photodynamic ablation is a newer method for dealing with unresectable malignant lesions of the airways. An intravenous photosensitizer is injected (Photofrin II, Sanofi Winthrop Pharmaceuticals, New York, NY), and 24 to 48 hours later, bronchoscopy is performed and a laser fiber is introduced to expose the involved area to light with a wavelength of 630 nm. Selective destruction of the neoplasm results, and follow-up endoscopic debridement can be performed 48 hours after the treatment. Our early experience with the use of photodynamic therapy for endobronchial lesions has been favorable. We have used this modality in 16 patients with obstructing or bleeding tracheobronchial tumors. Symptomatic relief was achieved in 13 (81%) of these patients. In all the patients who received photodynamic therapy for hemoptysis, the bleeding was controlled and no further bleeding occurred. It remains to be seen, however, whether this method has any benefit over established methods such as endobronchial laser, external beam radiotherapy, or endobronchial brachytherapy.

Management of unresectable benign strictures typically involves dilatation of the involved airway. Dilatation is best performed using rigid bronchoscopic techniques. This can be accomplished by passing dilators directly through the open end of the bronchoscope, with the use of dilating balloon catheters through the bronchoscope, or by passing serially larger rigid bronchoscopes through the stricture. Although laser excision of a stricture can be accomplished with the rigid bronchoscope alone, we prefer to manage this problem with a combined fiberoptic and rigid bronchoscope approach. The laser fiber can be guided by a flexible bronchoscope that has been inserted through a rigid bronchoscope. This method combines the airway access of a rigid bronchoscope with the distal flexibility of the fiberoptic system. After the stenotic segment has been dilated or excised, an internal stent is usually placed if formal open surgical resection of the airway lesion is not possible.

Stent Placement

Tracheal and bronchial stents are either Silastic tubes or expandable wire devices (Fig. 46–12). Following dilatation or laser excision of benign or malignant strictures, placement of intraluminal stents is effective in avoiding recurrence of obstruction.[2] Straight stents may be placed to support local segments of the trachea or main stem bronchi, or inverted Y stents may be positioned at the carina. When combined with a tracheostomy for upper tracheal stenosis, a T-shaped stent is quite functional.[12]

The results following placement of Silastic airway stents, in appropriately selected patients, have been gratifying. Sonett and coworkers[2] reported a series of 57 patients with a variety of benign, malignant, and post-

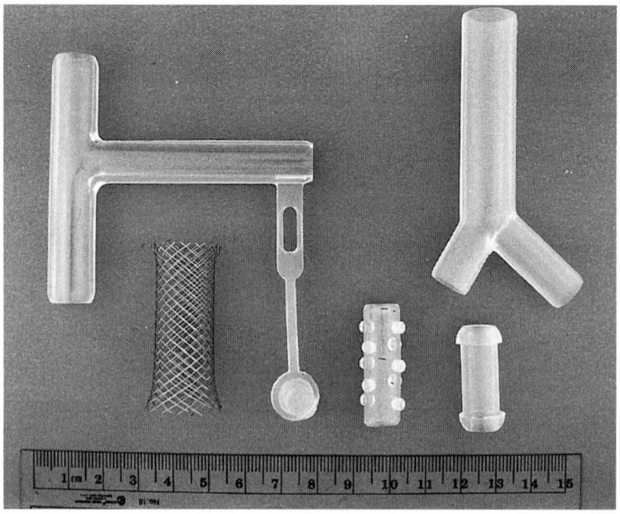

Figure 46–12. Tracheal and bronchial stents. *Top row,* T-tube tracheal stent; tracheobronchial Y stent (Hood Laboratories, Pembroke, MA). *Bottom row,* Expandable wire tracheal stent (Schneider Inc., Minneapolis, MN); bronchial stent with multiple fixation points (Bryan Corp., Woburn, MA); bronchial stent with flanged ends (Hood Laboratories).

transplantation airway obstruction who were managed with Silastic stents. Symptomatic relief was obtained in 8 of 10 patients (80%) with benign strictures and in 20 of 23 patients (87%) with malignant disease. There were no procedure-related deaths.[7, 13, 14]

Dumon[13] reported in 1990 on the insertion of 118 silicone stents in 66 patients. This series was expanded by Colt and Dumon[15] in 1995 and included the placement of 502 silicone stents in 286 patients. Of note was the limited mean follow-up period of 3.3 months for patients with malignant obstuction.

Yim and coworkers[14] placed silicone stents in 30 patients. Twenty-seven of these patients had malignant airway obstruction—10 from primary bronchial cancer, 4 from endobronchial metastasis, and 13 from esophageal cancer. They noted very short survival times—2 months for patients with carcinoma of the bronchus and 3 months for those with carcinoma of the esophagus. This short-term survival accentuates the need for quick, effective palliation and the avoidance of repetitive debriding procedures. In that regard, Yim and colleagues noted that use of silicone stents avoided the possibility of recurrent obstruction due to tissue ingrowth, as can occur with mesh stents.[14]

Experience with expandable wire stents has not been as extensive as that with Silastic stents. Expandable wire stents offer relatively easy insertion because they can be placed through a flexible bronchoscope with fluoroscopic guidance. Unlike Silastic stents, wire stents can be modified after insertion to conform to bronchial openings. For instance, a right main stem bronchial stent inserted into the bronchus intermedius would obstruct the right upper lobe orifice. With an expandable wire stent, however, the portion of the wire mesh covering the right upper lobe can be excised using a laser through the flexible bronchoscope (Fig. 46–13). Expandable wire stents are difficult to remove or reposition and have problems with tissue ingrowth.[16] Wire stents covered with an impermeable membrane are available (Schneider Corporation, Plymouth, MA) and may solve the problem of tissue ingrowth, but experience with these devices is limited. Our use of covered wire stents in patients with esophageal cancer has raised concern about migration of the stent.

Silastic stent insertion can be challenging and requires considerable experience with use of a rigid bronchoscope. Straight stents of the double-ended flange type (Hood Laboratories, Pembroke, MA) are best inserted over a small rigid bronchoscope, as shown in Figure 46–14. Stents with multiple fixation points (Bryan Corporation, Woburn, MA) are best inserted through a large bronchoscope in collapsed fashion and re-expanded after insertion. When a Silastic stent fails to properly expand, it buckles or kinks in the airway. This can usually be corrected by dilating the stent and the surrounding stricture with either a vascular angioplasty balloon catheter (for smaller-diameter stents) or an esophageal or pyloric dilating balloon catheter (for tracheal stents) (Fig. 46–15). Similar balloon dilatation may be used with wire stents that fail to fully expand, but care must be used to avoid overdistention of wire stents.

Inverted Y stents are particularly difficult to insert. Figure 46–16 demonstrates the method of such insertion. Whereas the stent must be placed with a rigid bronchoscope, the adequacy of stent positioning is best evaluated with a small-diameter flexible bronchoscope that can be passed through the stent without dislodging it.

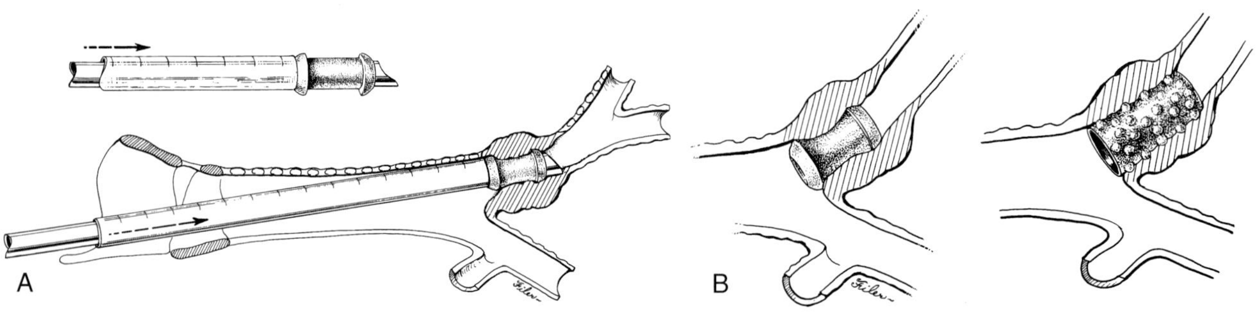

Figure 46–13. *A,* A wire stent has been placed in the distal left main stem bronchus. The stent can be seen to cover the orifice of the left upper lobe. *B,* A portion of the stent has been removed by using an Nd:YAG laser. The upper lobe is now unobstucted. (Reprinted with permission from the Society of Thoracic Surgeons. From Sonnett JR, Keenan RJ, Ferson PF, et al: Endobronchial management of benign, malignant and lung transplant airway stenoses. Ann Thorac Surg 59:1417–1422, 1995.)

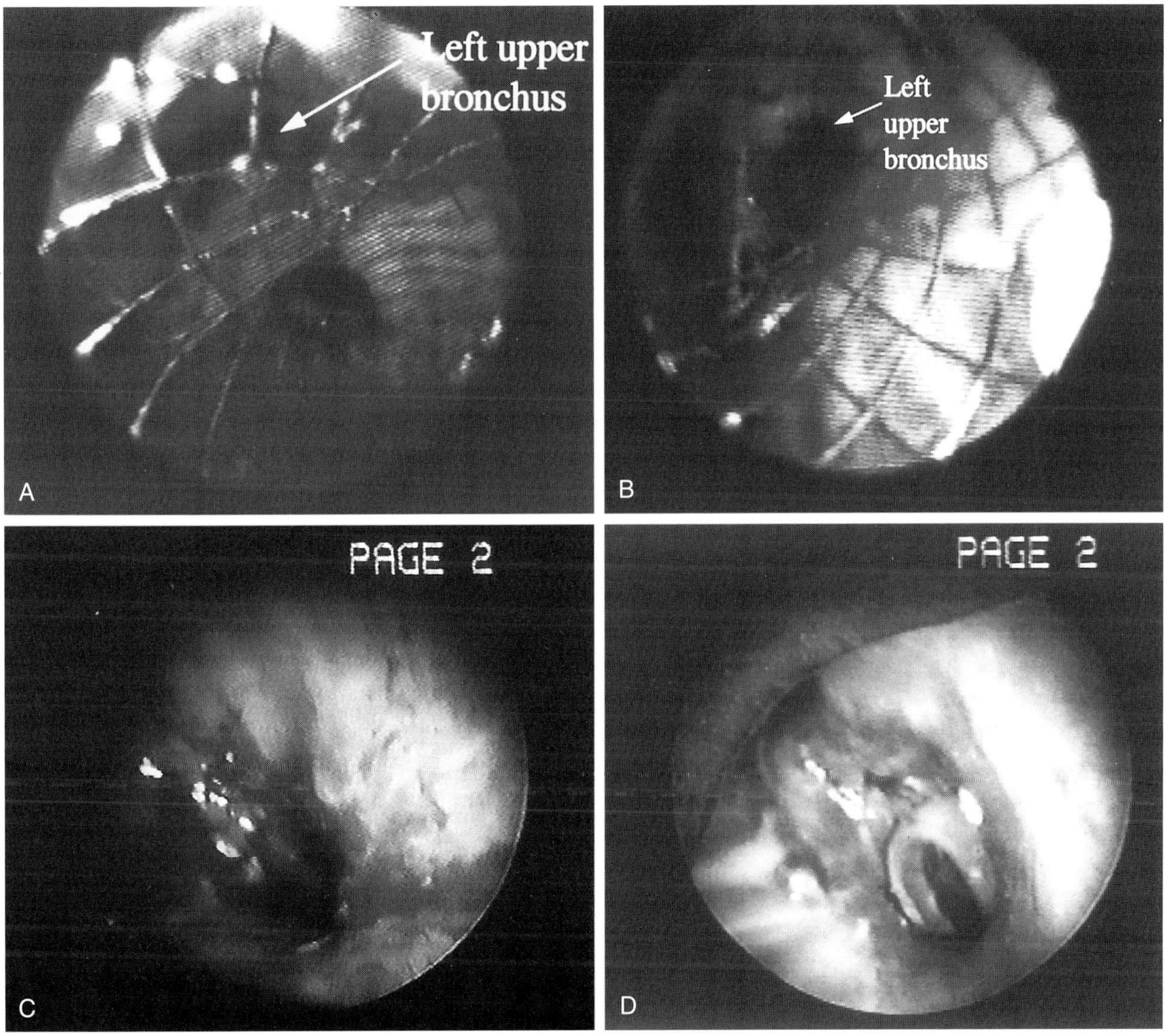

Figure 46–14. *A*, Placement of a Silastic bronchial stent. The stent is placed outside a small rigid bronchoscope and dislodged at the site of stricture by a chest tube that was previously placed on the bronchoscope. *B*, Silastic stents are secured in place either by flanges at each end or by multiple small projections that grasp the surrounding tissue. These latter stents must be placed through the channel of a larger bronchoscope (they cannot be placed as shown in *A*). *C*, Bronchoscopic view of an obstructing tumor in the right main stem bronchus. *D*, A Silastic stent (Hood Laboratories, Pembroke, MA) has been placed in the right bronchus. As in most cases of proximal right main stem obstructing tumors, the right upper lobe was obliterated; thus the stent extends to the bronchus intermedius. (Reprinted with permission from the Society of Thoracic Surgeons. From Sonnett JR, Keenan RJ, Ferson PF, et al: Endobronchial management of benign, malignant and lung transplant airway stenoses. Ann Thorac Surg 59:1417–1422, 1995.)

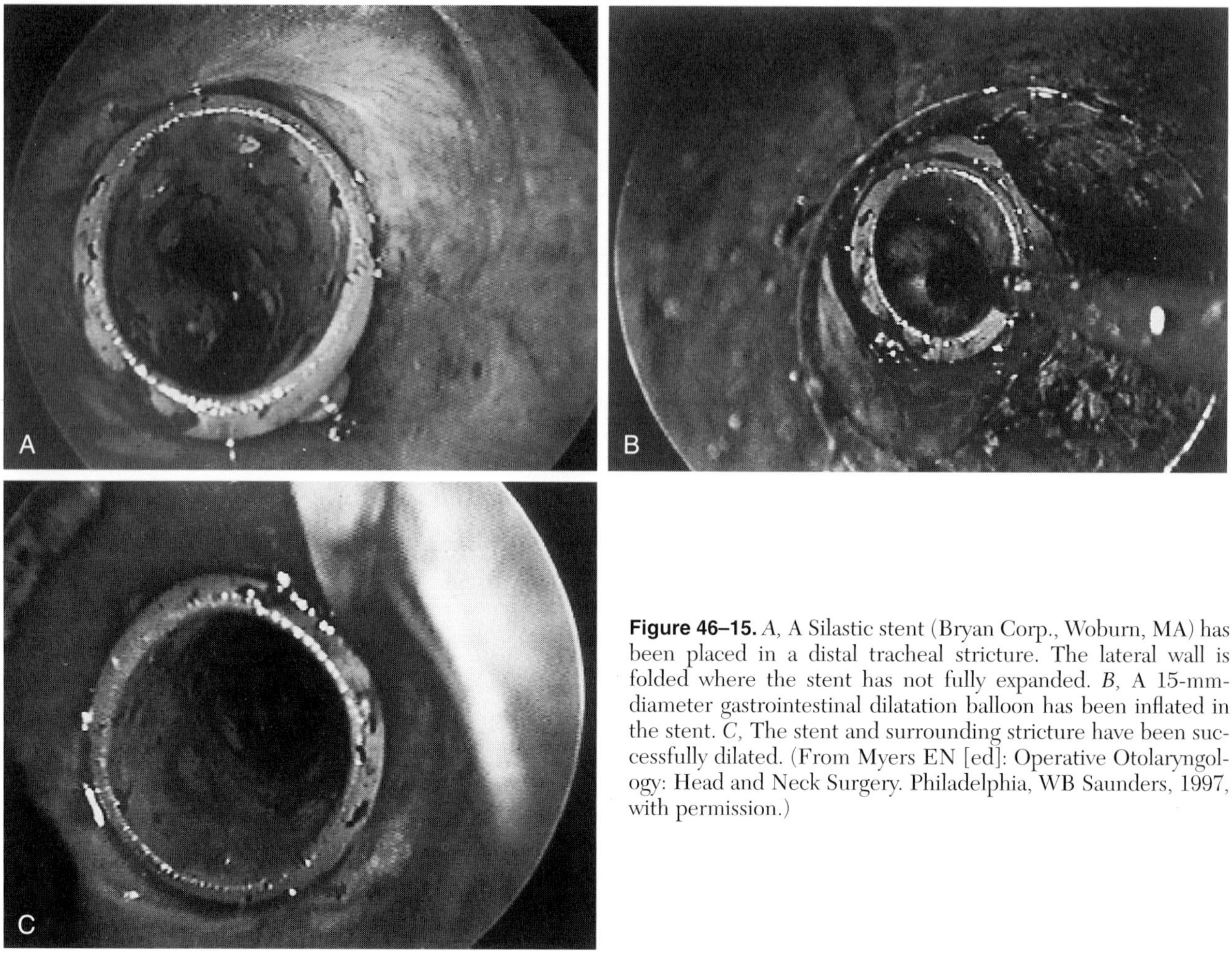

Figure 46–15. *A*, A Silastic stent (Bryan Corp., Woburn, MA) has been placed in a distal tracheal stricture. The lateral wall is folded where the stent has not fully expanded. *B*, A 15-mm-diameter gastrointestinal dilatation balloon has been inflated in the stent. *C*, The stent and surrounding stricture have been successfully dilated. (From Myers EN [ed]: Operative Otolaryngology: Head and Neck Surgery. Philadelphia, WB Saunders, 1997, with permission.)

Foreign Bodies

Foreign body retrieval from the trachea and bronchi has traditionally called for rigid bronchoscopy. With newer grasping devices that can be advanced through a flexible bronchoscope, the need for rigid bronchoscopy is no longer absolute. The key to bronchoscopic removal of foreign bodies is the availability of proper instrumentation. Standard bronchoscope biopsy forceps are almost always inadequate for securely grasping and retrieving foreign bodies from the airway. An array of flexible instruments with umbrella-type expanding and collapsing tined ends, wire basket extraction catheters, and balloon embolectomy catheters can be used to dislodge and remove peanuts, teeth, aspirated food particles, or whatever might make its way into the trachea (Fig. 46–17). Again, fiberoptic methods can be combined with rigid bronchoscopic techniques to facilitate the procedure.

Foreign body extraction is best performed under general anesthesia to avoid the frustration of chasing a moving target while the patient breathes or coughs. With large objects such as teeth, it may be necessary to withdraw the endotracheal tube and the bronchoscope as a unit after the object is securely grasped and withdrawn against the end of the endotracheal tube (Fig. 46–18). There are times when rigid bronchoscopy will be necessary, such as for the removal of sharp objects or aspirated soft food. As with the flexible bronchoscope, special forceps are necessary for foreign body removal with the rigid bronchoscope (Fig. 46–19). Whenever foreign body extraction is attempted, rigid bronchoscopic equipment should be immediately available in case attempts at removal with the flexible bronchoscope are unsuccessful.

Pulmonary Hygiene

A frequent application of flexible bronchoscopy is for the aspiration of bronchial secretions that the patient is having difficulty clearing. For thoracic surgeons, this is most often a problem in the postoperative period when atelectasis has been unresponsive to incentive spirometry, coughing, chest physiotherapy, or nasotracheal suctioning. A bronchoscope with a fairly large suction channel is usually chosen to remove secretions from the obstructed airway. Results are best when this is performed early, before lobar atelectasis has been present for more than 24 hours. The larynx is relatively insensitive in the early postoperative period, and bronchoscopy requires less local anesthesia and less sedation than usual. Care must be taken, however, to

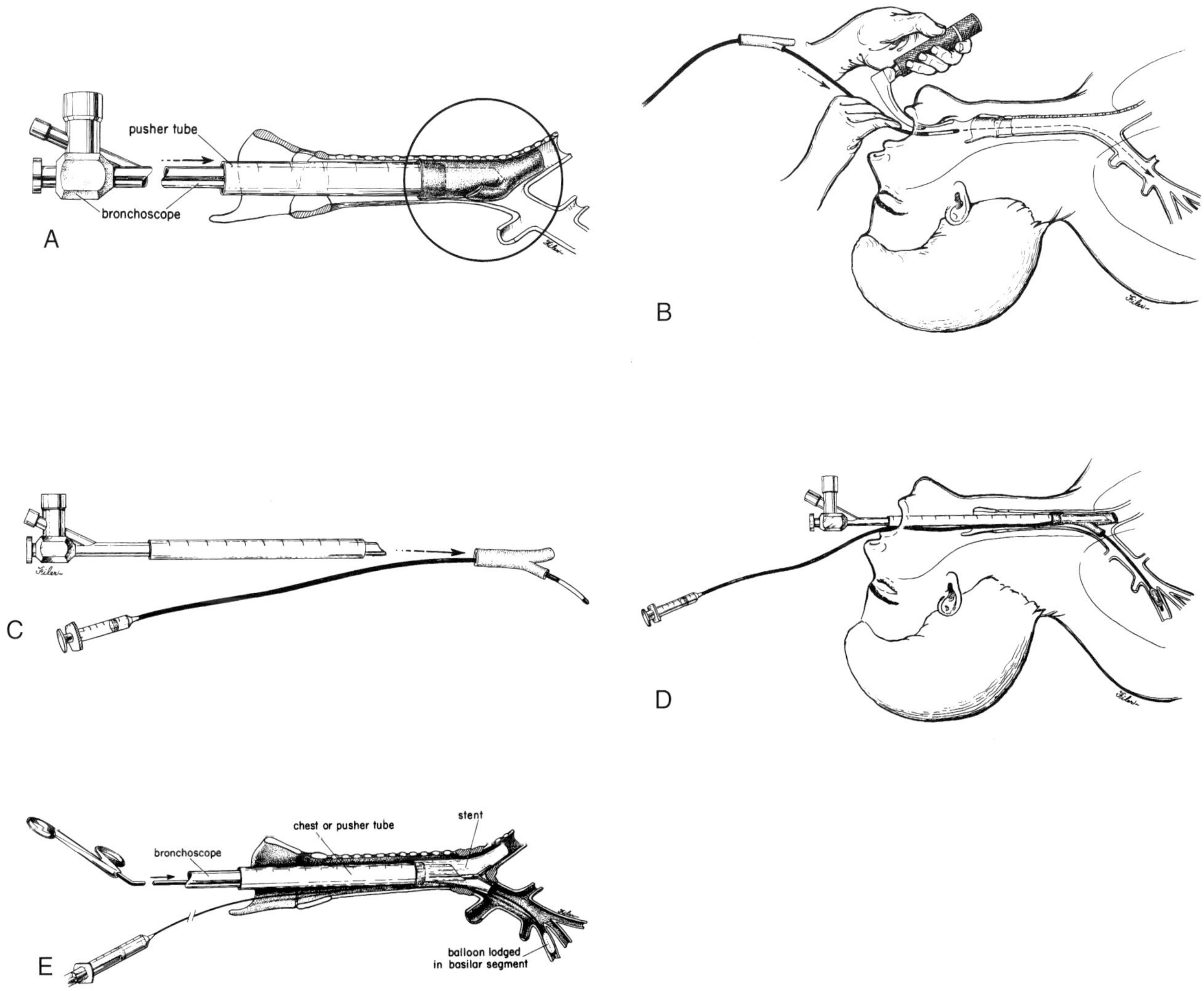

Figure 46–16. *A,* A Y stent may be placed at the tracheal bifurcation by inserting it over a rigid bronchoscope (a 6.5-mm Storz bronchoscope, 43 cm long). The bronchoscope extends down the left limb of the stent. After the bronchoscope has been directed into the left main stem bronchus, the stent is dislodged with a chest tube that has been trimmed to the appropriate length and previously placed on the bronchoscope above the stent. When the stent is dislodged from the bronchoscope, the right limb may fail to properly enter the right main stem bronchus. *B,* In order to direct the right limb of the stent into the right bronchus, a balloon embolectomy catheter (4 or 5 French) is first passed through the larynx and bronchoscopically guided into the distal right bronchus, where it is inflated to secure it in place. The catheter should have been passed through the right limb of the stent before this placement. *C,* A chest tube is placed on the bronchoscope, and then the exposed end of the bronchoscope is inserted through the stent and out the left limb. *D,* The entire assembly is passed through the larynx and guided to the carina, with the end of the bronchoscope in the left main stem bronchus. The chest tube is then used to push the stent off the bronchoscope as the bronchoscope is carefully withdrawn. *E,* When the bifurcation of the stent is visible, this should be firmly secured with an *open* alligator-type foreign body forceps. Pressure against the stent and the carina prevents the stent from migrating while the bronchoscope and chest tube are removed.

Illustration continued on following page

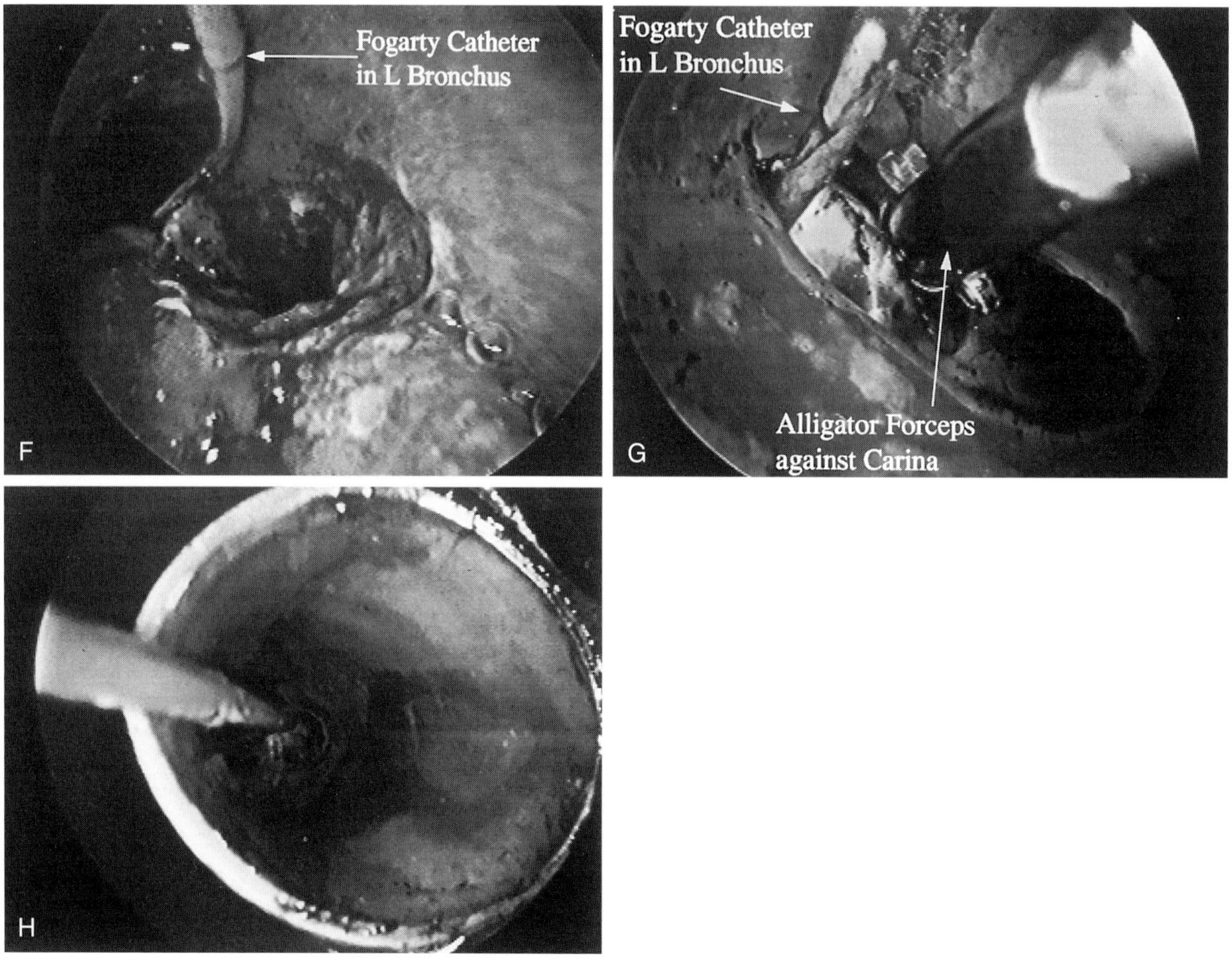

Figure 46–16. (*Continued*) *F,* Bronchoscopic view of the carina with invasive cancer that has been debrided. A Fogarty catheter has been placed down the left main stem bronchus. The right limb of the stent will be guided into the right bronchus over the rigid bronchoscope. In this patient, the right upper lobe is totally occluded, so the long bronchial limb of the stent will be placed on the right side extending into the bronchus intermedius. *G,* The stent has been discharged from the end of the rigid bronchoscope, and an open alligator forceps is used to hold the stent against the carina while the bronchoscope is withdrawn. *H,* The proximal end of the stent is now exposed after the bronchoscope has been withdrawn. Notice that the proximal lip of the stent is free within the lumen and is not tight against the wall of the trachea. If the end of the stent, either proximal or distal, has a tight fit with the airway wall, granulation and subsequent overgrowth will occur.

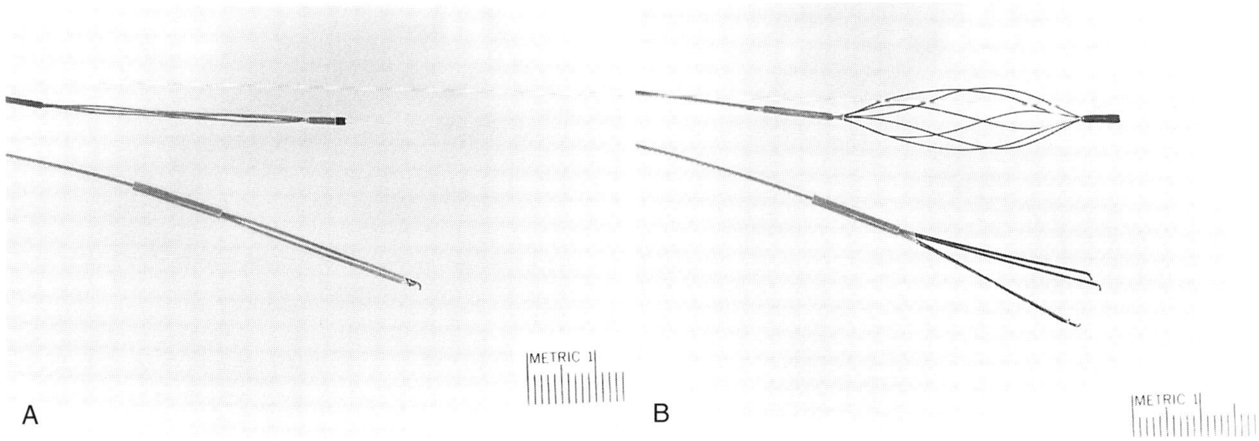

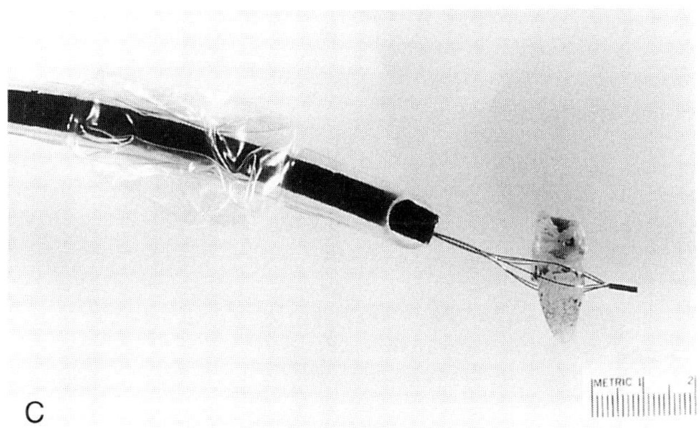

Figure 46–17. Multiple-pronged grasping forceps and basket devices can be used for foreign body removal through a flexible bronchoscope. *A,* The instruments are passed through the bronchoscope channel inside a sheath. *B, C,* When extended from the insertion sheath, they can engage the foreign body. (From Myers EN [ed]: Operative Otolaryngology: Head and Neck Surgery. Philadelphia, WB Saunders, 1997, with permission.)

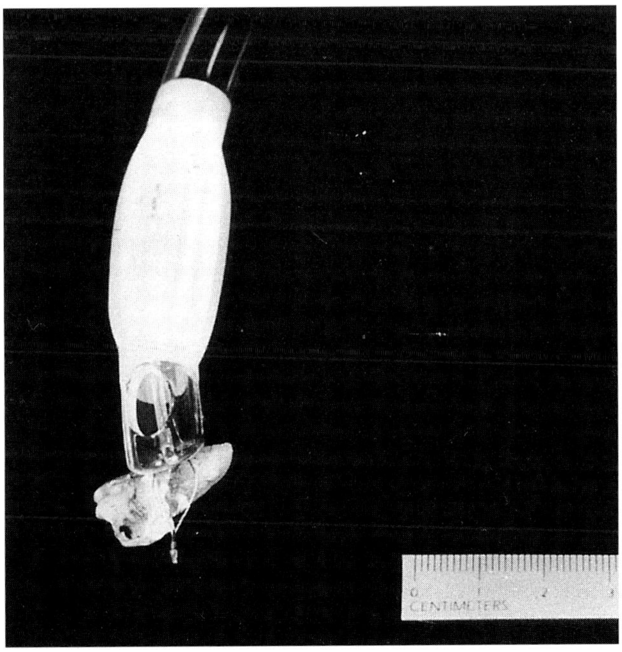

Figure 46–18. Many foreign bodies, once grasped, cannot be removed through the endotracheal tube. They should be withdrawn tightly against the end of the endotracheal tube, and then the tube, bronchoscope, and foreign body are removed as one unit.

carefully monitor patient oxygenation and vital signs during such a therapeutic bronchoscopic procedure.

Intubation Assistance

When visualization of laryngeal structures is difficult as a result of a small oral aperture or anterior displacement of the larynx, the flexible bronchoscope can serve as a guide for endotracheal intubation. The endotracheal tube is placed over the bronchoscope and then advanced into the trachea along the course of the bronchoscope, which has been visually guided into the trachea. This same technique is applicable for endotracheal intubation when previous laryngeal or pharyngeal surgery has obscured visibility. When confronted with a patient with edema and distortion of oropharyngeal structures secondary to maxillofacial trauma, intubation with a flexible bronchoscope can be useful, but one must always bear in mind that a tracheotomy may be necessary when trauma is severe.

In all circumstances in which endotracheal intubation guided by the flexible bronchoscope is considered, it must be remembered that this procedure is safest and easiest when the patient is breathing spontaneously. Muscle relaxants cause the pharyngeal structures to collapse on themselves, totally obscuring the laryngeal opening. This can make visualization with the flexible bronchoscope impossible. If, however, the patient is still breathing spontaneously, the active retraction of the pharyngeal muscles with respiration maintains an open passage to

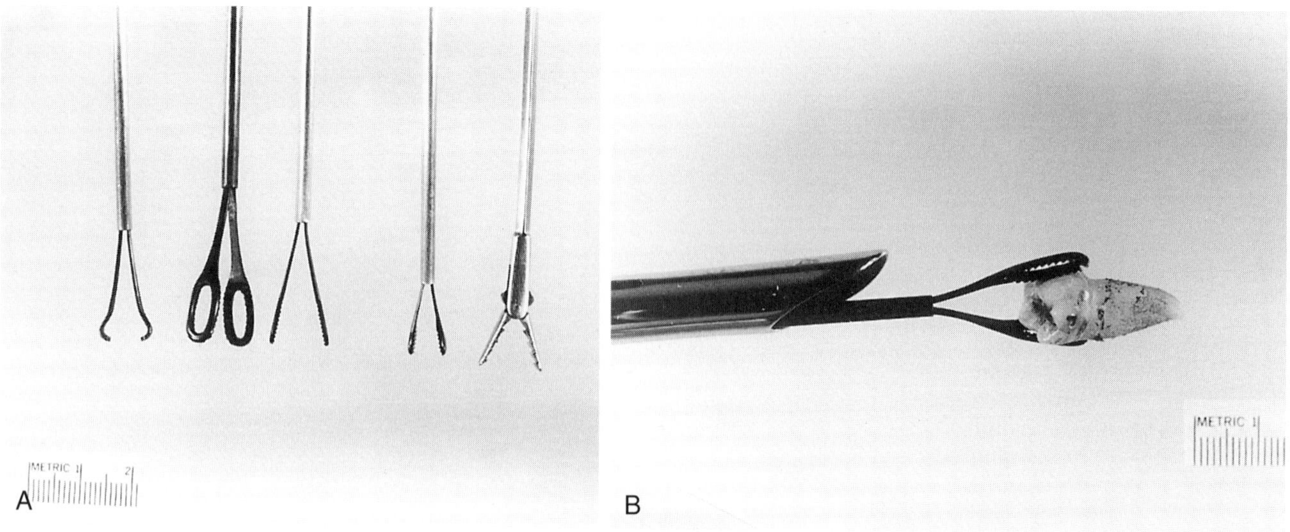

Figure 46–19. *A,* Foreign body forceps for use with a rigid bronchoscope. The jaws are individually designed for grasping different-shaped objects. *B,* Many foreign bodies, such as teeth, are too large to remove through the rigid bronchoscope. They should be secured against the opening of the bronchoscope, and then the bronchoscope and foreign body are removed in unison. The bronchoscope helps protect the larynx from injury by the foreign body during removal.

the larynx that can be followed with the bronchoscope. When the patient has already been paralyzed, use of a laryngoscope may provide enough retraction of pharyngeal structures to enable bronchoscopic visualization of the larynx, but this is not always true. If the larynx cannot be adequately visualized, and if ventilation cannot be maintained with a face mask, an urgent tracheotomy will be necessary.

Use of the flexible bronchoscope is also an important adjunctive maneuver for the proper positioning of a double-lumen endotracheal tube or a standard endotracheal tube with bronchial blocker attachment to accomplish independent unilateral pulmonary collapse during thoracic surgical procedures. For these purposes, a small-diameter bronchoscope must be used to traverse the smaller diameters of double-lumen endotracheal tubes.

Summary

The ability to endoscopically manage problems involving the trachea and proximal airways is an essential skill for thoracic surgeons. A wide variety of abnormalities may require such intervention, often in an urgent fashion. Thorough knowledge of established techniques and equipment is therefore necessary to allow the surgeon to act properly.

References

1. Berci G: History of endoscopy. *In* Berci G (ed): Endoscopy. New York, Appleton-Century-Crofts, 1976, pp xix–xxiii.
2. Sonett JR, Keenan RJ, Ferson PF, et al: Endobronchial management of benign, malignant and lung transplant airway stenoses. Ann Thorac Surg 59:1417–1422, 1995.
3. Stock CR: Esophagoscopy. Ear Nose Throat J 64:502–503, 1985.
4. Williams D: The role of fiberoptic bronchoscopy in the evaluation of immunocompromised hosts with diffuse pulmonary infiltrates. Am Rev Respir Dis 131:880–885, 1985.
5. Grant AK: A century of upper gastrointestinal tract endoscopy. Med J Aust 2:903–906, 1973.
6. Zollner F: Gustav Killian—father of bronchoscopy: Historical vignette. Arch Otolaryngol 82:656–659, 1965.
7. Jackson C, Jackson CL: Technique of bronchoscopy and laryngoscopy. *In* Bronchoesophagology. Philadelphia, WB Saunders, 1950, pp 40–67.
8. Hirschowitz BI, Curtiss LE, Peters CW, Pollard HM: Demonstration of a new gastroscope, the "fiberscope." Gastroenterology 35:50–53, 1958.
9. Ikeda S, Yanai N, Ishikawa S: Flexible bronchofiberscope. Keio J Med 17:1–16, 1968.
10. Fulkerson WJ: Current concepts in fiberoptic bronchoscopy. N Engl J Med 311:511—515, 1984.
11. Burt ME: Prospective evaluation of aspiration needle, cutting needle, transbronchial, and open lung biopsy in patients with pulmonary infiltrates. Ann Thorac Surg 32:2, 1981.
12. Cooper JD, Pearson FG, Patterson GA, et al: Use of silicone stents in the management of airway problems. Ann Thorac Surg 47:371–378, 1989.
13. Dumon JF: A dedicated tracheobronchial stent. Chest 97:328–332, 1990.
14. Yim AP, Abdulah VJ, Izzat MB: Which stent to use for tracheobronchial stenoses: Metallic or silicone? Ann Thorac Surg 62:844–887, 1996.
15. Colt HG, Dumon JF: Airway stents: Present and future. Clin Chest Med 16:465–478, 1995.
16. Rousseau H, Dahan M, Lauque D, et al: Self-expandable prostheses in the tracheobronchial tree. Radiology 188:199–203, 1993.

Chapter 47

Interventional Esophagoscopy

Angus C. W. Chan and S. C. Sydney Chung

The first esophagoscopy was credited to Aldolf Kussmaul (after whom a clinical sign of acidotic breathing was named), who in the early 19th century used a rigid hollow tube and light reflected from a spirit lamp to view the inside of the esophagus and stomach in professional sword swallowers. Clinically useful esophagoscopy using rigid open-lumen esophagoscopes (Haslinger or Chevalier Jackson types) required general anesthesia and muscle relaxation (Fig. 47–1). With the development of fiberoptic endoscopes, flexible endoscopy, which does not require general anesthesia, has largely replaced rigid esophagoscopy for both diagnostic and therapeutic purposes. The modern esophagoscope uses a charged coupling device (CCD) to transmit the image from the tip of the endoscope to a video monitor.

Besides allowing an accurate visual diagnosis and enabling tissue to be obtained for histologic diagnosis, esophagoscopy can be therapeutic for many conditions of the esophagus. Many ingenious accessories have been designed to be used in conjunction with the endoscope to achieve this aim. Interventional endoscopy is greatly facilitated by video-endoscopy, as both the operator (who controls the endoscope) and the assistant (who controls the accessories) can see what is going on (Fig. 47–2).

Removal of Foreign Bodies

Psychotic patients and prisoners may swallow objects of all descriptions. Children have a propensity for swallowing a variety of small items, particularly coins. The elderly, who may have reduced gingival sensation, may swallow dentures, toothpicks, and food boluses. In Asia, accidentally swallowed bones, particularly fish bones, are common causes of hospital attendance because of the custom of eating meat without first removing the bones.[1]

Most swallowed foreign bodies traverse the gastrointestinal tract uneventfully. Although perforation of various parts of the gut by sharp objects has been reported, once the foreign body has passed the gastroesophageal junction, retrieval is generally not indicated. An exception has to be made for disk batteries, which can become eroded and leak alkali, causing perforation. These batteries should be removed as soon as possible if they are still within reach of the endoscope.

Patients who have swallowed bones may complain of discomfort on swallowing, foreign body sensation in the throat, and blood-stained saliva. Identical symptoms may be reported after the bone has passed, causing a mucosal laceration (Fig. 47–3). Fever, pain and tenderness in the neck, widening of the prevertebral space, and air in the soft tissues of the neck on radiology are signs that perforation has already occurred. Sudden total dysphagia with the inability to swallow even saliva results from impaction of a food bolus on a pre-existing esophageal stricture.

Most fish bones are lodged in the valleculae or the pyriform fossae, but they may become impacted at any site in the esophagus. Sharp objects that perforate the esophagus at the region of the aortic arch may cause torrential hemorrhage from an aortoesophageal fistula, the result of an abscess caused by the bone eroding the aorta. This catastrophic event typically occurs several days after the bone is swallowed and is heralded by a smaller warning bleed.

For patients with a history of fish bone ingestion, the oropharynx and hypopharynx should be inspected with a direct laryngoscope, and bones lodged in these areas can be easily removed. Patients who complain of retrosternal pain should have flexible esophagoscopy.

A large variety of accessories are available for removing foreign bodies. Most foreign bodies can now be removed with a flexible gastroscope without the need for general anesthesia.[2] Ordinary biopsy forceps may suffice for small fish bones. Crocodile forceps have a firmer grip and are suitable for larger fish bones or pork bones. Coins are best grasped by the edge with rat-tooth forceps. Polypectomy loops and stone baskets may be useful for odd-shaped objects. It is generally easier to push food boluses into the stomach than to remove them. If an identical or similar object is available, a practice run of trying to catch it with the chosen accessory outside the patient may be helpful. Objects that cannot be safely extracted because of their size and shape can be pushed into the stomach and fragmented before piecemeal removal. Lasers can be used in these cases to break up hard objects such as dentures.[3]

Removal of a pointed object grasped by endoscopic forceps through the cricopharyngeus may be difficult and may cause laceration at the upper esophageal sphincter. There is also a risk of the foreign body being dropped into the trachea. For these reasons, use of an overtube to protect the cricopharyngeus and the airway is mandatory. The overtube is preloaded onto the endoscope and slid into place after the scope is passed into the esophagus (Fig. 47–4). Foreign bodies lodged in the upper esophagus may have to be pushed into the distal esophagus to allow passage of the overtube. After the foreign body is securely grasped, the endoscope, together with the foreign body, is withdrawn into the overtube. With the overtube as protection against the sharp foreign body, the whole ensemble is removed together.

After the foreign body is removed, a complete examination of the esophagus is necessary to assess the damage caused and to exclude a stricture distal to the site of impaction.

Dilatation of Strictures

Benign strictures from corrosive ingestion and reflux disease respond well to endoscopic dilatation. The stricture is

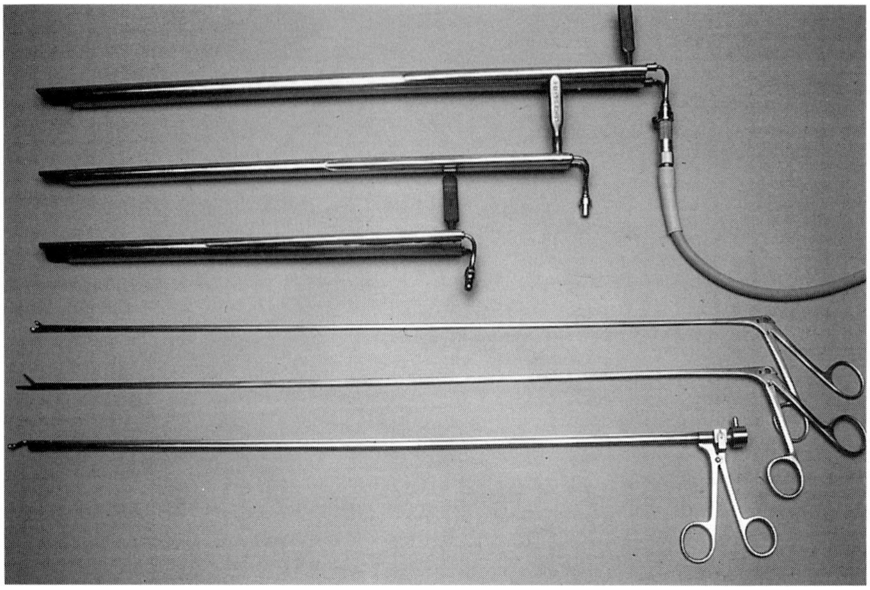

Figure 47–1. Negas rigid esophagoscopy set (Downs Manufacturer, England).

gradually dilated, usually on a weekly basis, until a diameter of 16 or 17 mm is achieved. For malignant strictures, dilatation gives only temporary relief. Dilatation alone provides poor palliation, but it is a useful adjunct in the management of malignant dysphagia, as it allows endoscopic access to a tight malignant stricture. Postirradiation strictures are fibrotic and fragile, but good results can be obtained by dilatation if precautions are taken.[4]

There are many types of dilators: Eder-Peustow metal olives, tapered dilators such as the Savary-Gillard or the American dilators, and balloon catheters (Figs. 47–5 and 47–6). The basic principle is the same: A guide wire is first passed under endoscopic (and fluoroscopic) guidance through the stricture; then the endoscope is removed, leaving the guide wire in place. Dilators of increasing size are then railroaded over the guide wire to dilate the stricture (Fig. 47–7).

Whether x-ray control is necessary for all cases of esophageal dilatation is often hotly debated. Our own view is that fluoroscopy should always be available. Endoscopic treatment for malignant esophageal obstruction is difficult, and perforation is a disaster: we need all the help we can get.

The first step in esophageal dilatation is passage of the guide wire. This is easy if the endoscope can be passed through the stricture; the guide wire is merely passed through the biopsy channel of the scope to lie along the greater curvature of the antrum. The scope is then removed slowly, with the endoscopist feeding the wire in during the process. The nurse-assistant should hold onto the guide wire once the scope leaves the mouth. If the scope can pass the stricture, it does not matter what kind of guide wire is used. The Savary-type stainless steel piano wire has the advantage of being stiff. Because of this, it

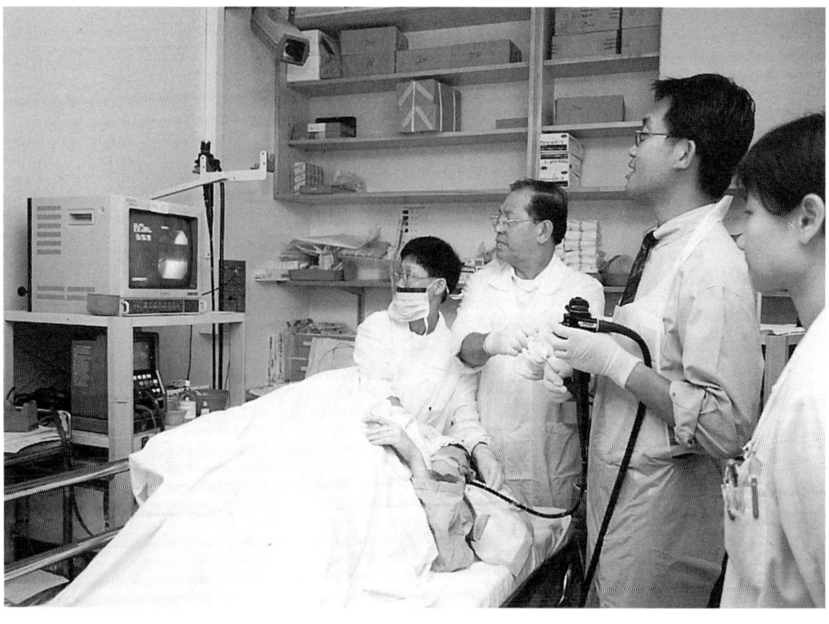

Figure 47–2. Video flexible endoscope with connected television system.

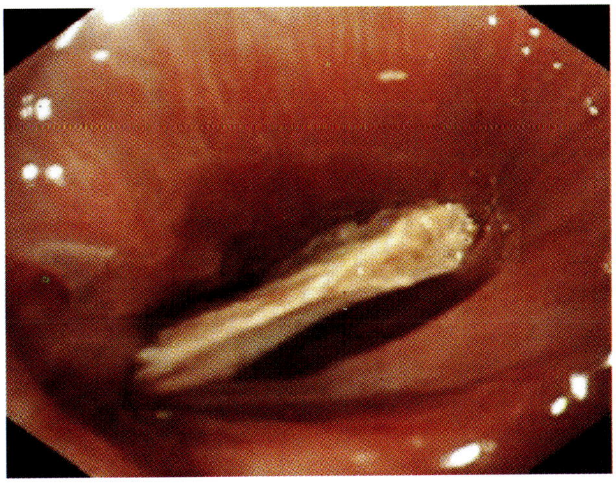

Figure 47–3. Duck bone lodged in the upper esophagus.

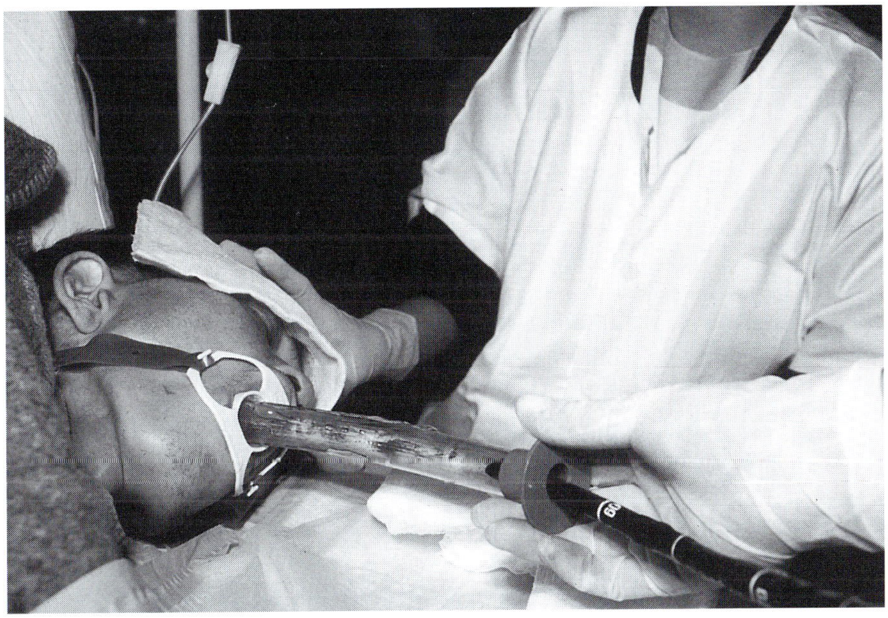

Figure 47–4. Overtube preloaded onto the endoscope and slid into the esophagus.

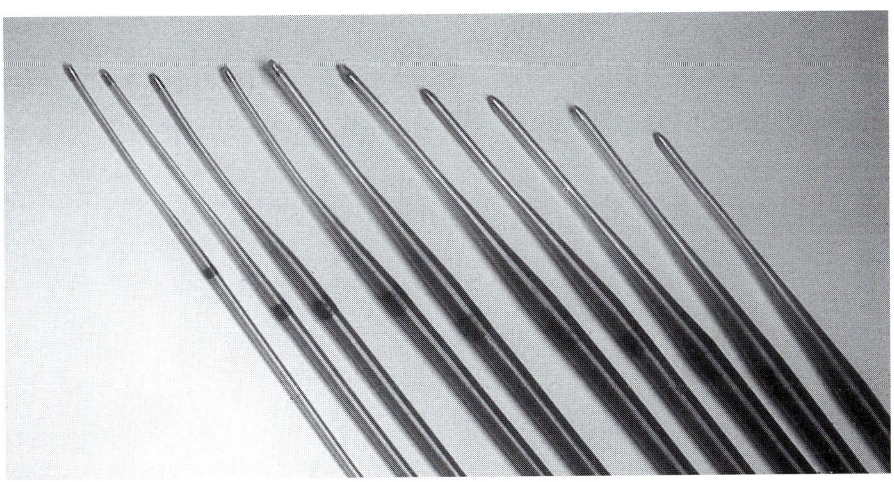

Figure 47–5. Savary-Gillard dilators.

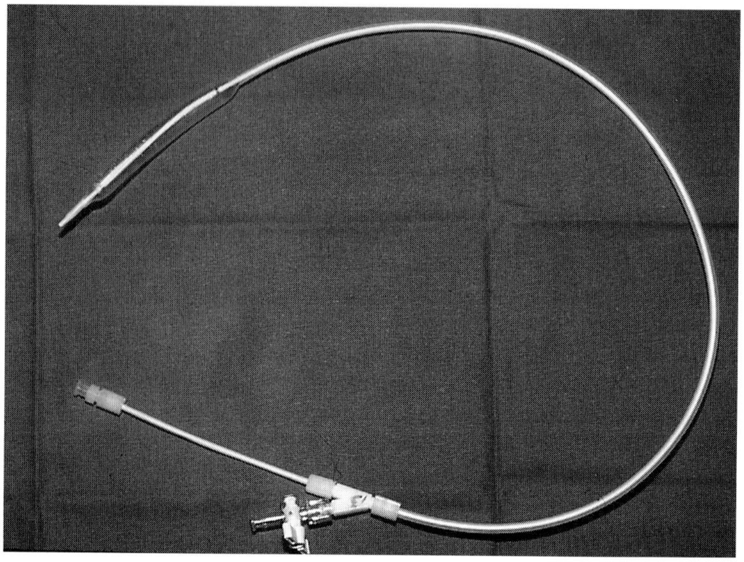

Figure 47–6. Esophageal balloon catheter.

keeps a straighter course through the throat, and it is easier to railroad dilators over the wire during dilator passage through the pharynx.

If the endoscope cannot pass the stricture, the guide wire must be passed under x-ray control. In effect, the tip of the guide wire acts as a lumen finder. In these cases, the Savary wire is not suitable, as the spring tip is too rigid. We prefer to use 0.035-in. Teflon-coated wires—the same ones used for endoscopic retrograde cholangiopancreatography (ERCP). These wires have a flexible tip and are much safer and easier to pass than the Savary wire. They should be used routinely if the endoscope cannot pass the tumor. As these wires are more flexible, a pulling-back action should be applied on the wire when passing dilators over them—otherwise, a loop can easily form at the back of the throat.

If a 0.035-in. wire does not pass, the following tricks may be useful:

- Use a wire with a longer flexible tip; it may bend back on itself and form a loop. The apex of the loop may be able to negotiate the stricture more easily.
- Use a wire with a J tip.
- Use a hydrophilic "slippery" wire.
- Inject some contrast using a metal-tipped ERCP catheter to outline the stricture (beware of aspiration). The guide wire can then be passed through the metal-tipped catheter. The slight bend in the catheter may help the wire negotiate the stricture. Using a catheter to guide the guide wire is most useful in very long strictures—which may need to be negotiated by steps.
- Use a balloon catheter to guide the guide wire. By inflating and deflating the balloon, the tip of the guide wire can be pointed in different directions.

After negotiating a difficult stricture, it may be wise to check that the guide wire is within the lumen of the gut be-

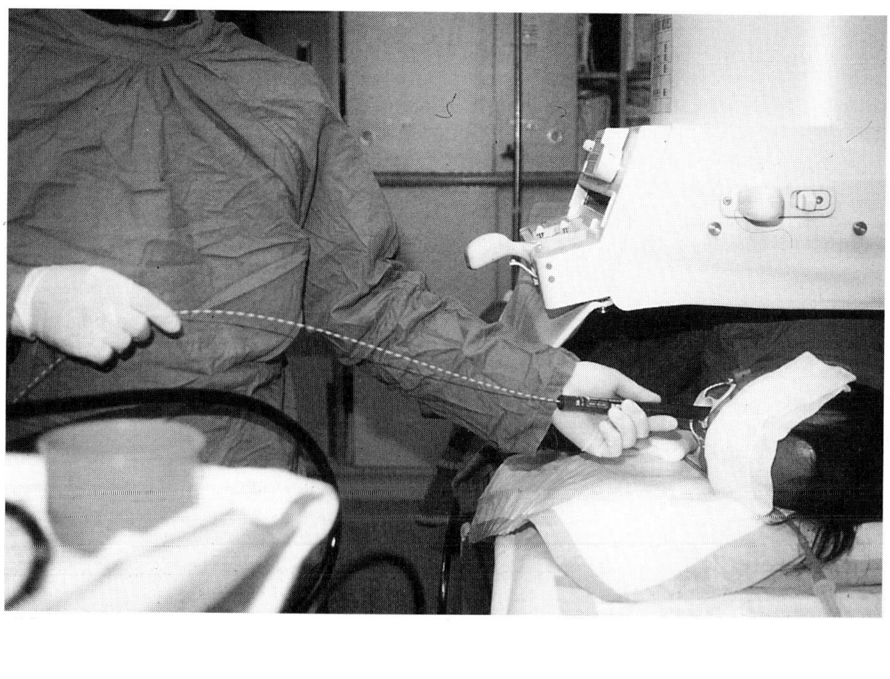

Figure 47–7. Slide the dilator with an extended left elbow while the right hand is holding the guide wire to provide countertraction.

fore dilatation. This can be done by railroading a metal-tipped ERCP catheter over the wire, removing the wire, and then injecting some contrast. If correct position is confirmed, the wire is replaced through the catheter, and dilatation can be performed with confidence.

For dilating malignant strictures, we use Savary-Gillard dilators almost exclusively. The house rules are:

1. Always use fluoroscopy.
2. If the scope cannot pass the tumor, always start with the smallest dilator.
3. If the scope can pass, start with a dilator the same size as the endoscope.
4. Never skip dilators.
5. The "rule of three" states that a maximum of three dilators of increasing size should be used after resistance is met. Although this is generally a good rule, it does not take into account how rigid the stricture is. A feel for the rigidity of the stricture and the amount of resistance encountered can be gained only by experience. Proceed with caution in postirradiation (and corrosive) strictures.
6. If in doubt whether to use one more dilator, don't. Bring the patient back another time.

Malignant Dysphagia

Malignant dysphagia may be due to either luminal obstruction (cancer of the esophagus or cardia) or extrinsic compression (cancer of the bronchus or mediastinal lymph nodes). Although patients should be given every opportunity to undergo resection for cure, in a large proportion of patients, surgery is inappropriate, either because the disease is too advanced or because the patient's general condition precludes a major operation. In these patients, endoscopy can rapidly restore the ability to swallow and help maintain a reasonable quality of life in the time remaining.[5]

In managing patients with malignant dysphagia, we must recognize what can be achieved: reboring a passage does not restore perfect swallowing. Indeed, the quality of swallowing after a palliative resection or even a surgical bypass is often superior to that achieved by endoscopy. Tumor growth will reobstruct the endoscopically rebored lumen, necessitating repeat treatment. Esophageal prostheses may be blocked by food bolus or tumor overgrowth. The less-than-perfect swallowing and the need for repeat treatment should be explained to the patient at the outset.

The choice of which endoscopic method to use is determined chiefly by the length and geometry of the tumor. Other factors that may influence the decision are (1) the patient's acceptance of the need for repeat procedures, (2) the performance status and life expectancy of the patient, and (3) economic factors, especially if expandable metal stents are considered.

Laser treatment is best for short segment strictures that are exophytic.[6] We prefer to start at the distal end of the tumor and work up, aiming to vaporize the tumor and restore a patent passageway (Fig. 47–8). The newer holmium laser is easier to use than the Nd:YAG, as coaxial gas cooling is not necessary and the laser can be fired with the tip of the fiber touching the tumor without destroying the fiber.

Alcohol injection[7, 8] is inexpensive and does not require special equipment. Absolute alcohol (0.5- to 1-ml aliquots) is injected into the protuberant part of the tumor. Resistance to the injection and blanching of the tissue indicate that the alcohol has entered the tissue. Typically 5 to 10 ml are injected per session. Tissue swelling occurs almost immediately and may cause worsening of the dysphagia immediately after the procedure. The tissue sloughs in 3 to 5 days. Because the tissue effect is delayed, it is difficult to gauge the depth of injury at the time of treatment. Esophageal perforation and tracheoesophageal fistula may occur if large volumes are injected. We recommend using smaller volumes and repeating the procedure twice weekly until adequate relief of dysphagia is obtained. Recurrent dysphagia from tumor regrowth occurs 4 to 6 weeks later and may be treated by repeat injection.

The BICAP probe[9] consists of a metal olive with six electrodes arranged in a circumferential array. When activated, it delivers a 1-cm-long circumferential electrical burn to the tissue in contact with it. The BICAP device is suitable for circumferential tumors and is especially useful for cancer of the cardia—where other forms of treatment are difficult because of angulation. Treatment with the

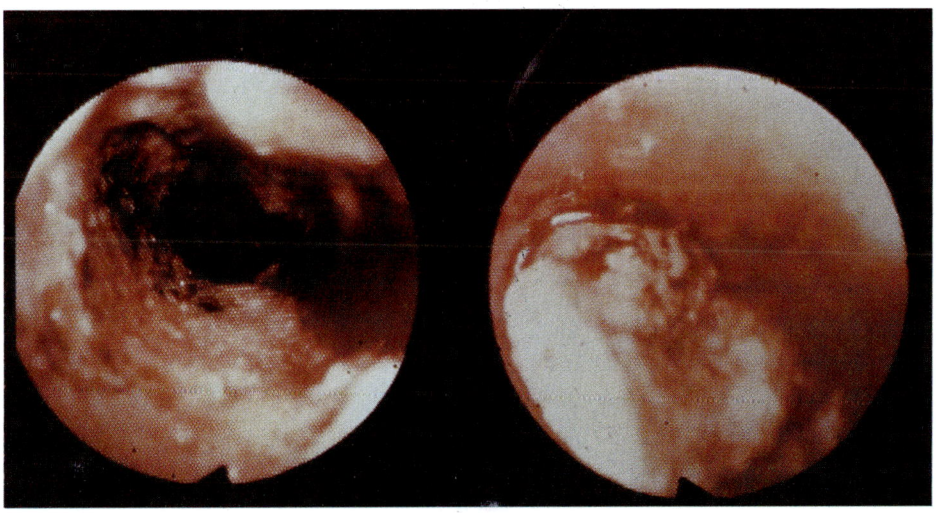

Figure 47–8. *Left,* Exophytic esophageal tumor. *Right,* Laser recanalization.

BICAP device is performed with radiologic and endoscopic control. The tumor is first dilated to a 15-mm diameter. As passage of the probe through the throat can be difficult, a Savary wire is necessary. If an ERCP wire is used for the dilatation, it should be exchanged for a stiffer wire. The BICAP probe is then passed over the wire. The endoscope is inserted to visually monitor the procedure. The BICAP probe is placed in contact with the tumor and activated. We use a setting of 7 with 2-second pulses, with 5 to 10 pulses for each 1-cm segment of tumor. After delivering the burn to one area, the probe is advanced 1 cm to treat the next segment.

Stent insertion[10] can be used for most tumors and is the only option available for a patient with a tracheoesophageal fistula (Fig. 47–9). In the past, insertion of a plastic stent could be a rather brutal procedure. The stricture was first dilated to 15 or 16 mm, and the prosthesis, mounted on an introducer, was rammed through the tumor. The procedure-related mortality was around 10%, largely due to perforation during dilatation and stent insertion.

To obtain satisfactory results, the stent should bridge the whole extent of the tumor. The length of the tumor should be carefully measured by the endoscope. The stent should be at least 3 cm longer than the tumor so that there is some margin for error and some room for the tumor to grow. Precise localization of the tumor on fluoroscopy is essential for accurate stent placement. A simple and reliable way to do so is to inject 0.2 to 0.5 ml of Lipiodol into the normal esophageal mucosa just proximal and distal to the tumor using a sclerotherapy needle.[11] In the past, we relied on metal markers taped to the skin, but these can fall off or change in relative position if the patient turns during the procedure.

The advent of self-expanding esophageal stents[12–14] has made stenting much easier and safer. There are a number of expandable metal stents on the market. They differ in design, material, and method of deployment. The radical force exerted and the resistance to kinking differ greatly. When choosing a particular stent for a particular patient, one should consider the elasticity of the tumor and whether the tumor is angulated. These stents are introduced in the collapsed state and expanded to the maximal diameter of around 20 mm after deployment. Prior dilatation is not mandatory unless the tumor is very tight. In any case, gentle dilatation to 12 mm is sufficient. The dreaded complication of esophageal perforation can be eliminated. Because the diameter of expandable stents is larger, the quality of swallowing is better. The first-generation stents have an open mesh design, and tumor ingrowth can cause recurrent obstruction. Newer designs have membrane covers to prevent tumor ingrowth[15] and are suitable for tracheoesophageal fistulae[16] (Fig. 47–10).

Self-expanding metal stents have revolutionized the palliative treatment of malignant dysphagia[17] (Fig. 47–11). Good-quality swallowing can now be achieved atraumatically and with little morbidity. These stents have become the treatment of choice for patients with inoperable esophageal and cardia cancers in most centers. Their one drawback is their high cost. If used in patients with reasonable life expectancies, however, these stents are cost-effective because readmissions and reinterventions can be avoided.

Variceal Bleeding

Injection sclerotherapy was once the treatment of choice for bleeding varices. Injection of sclerosants into (intravariceal injection) and around (paravariceal injection) varices can control active hemorrhage and reduce the chance of rebleeding by obliterating the varices. Because an irritant sub-

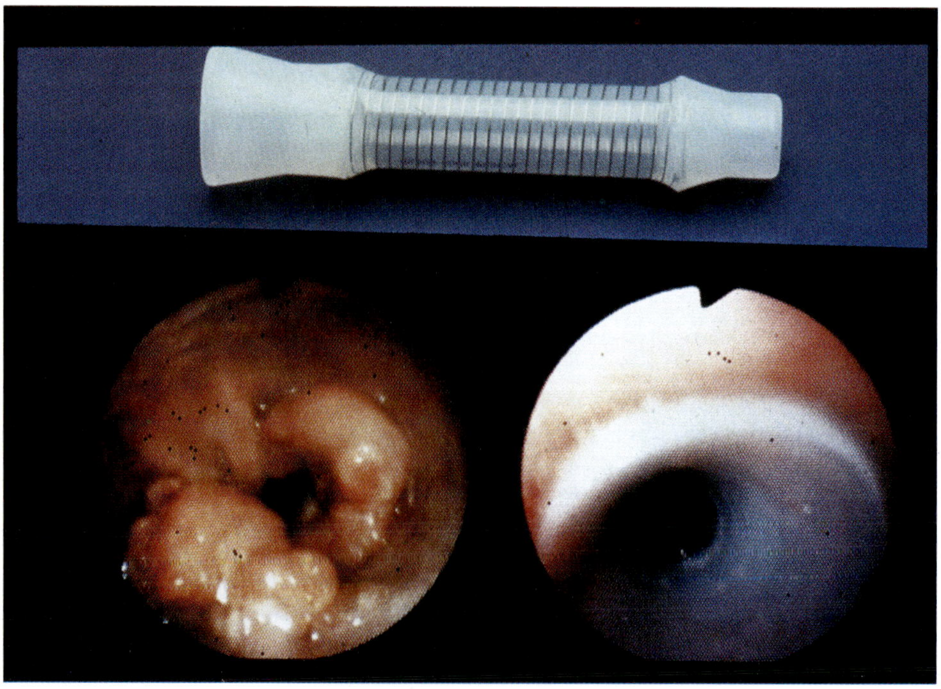

Figure 47–9. Esophageal tumor stented by a Wilson-Cook prosthesis.

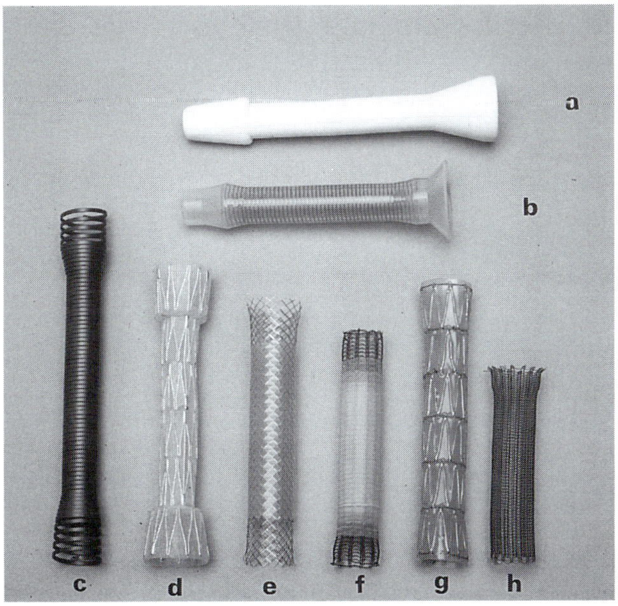

Figure 47–10. (a) Atkinson endo-prosthesis. (b) Wilson-Cook prosthesis reinforced with metal ring. (c–h) Self-expandable metal stents: (c) Esophagocoil, (d) Song stent, (e) Wallstent, (f) Ultraflex stent (covered), (g) Gianturco-Z stent, (h) Ultraflex stent (noncovered).

stance is injected, sclerotherapy is associated with complications such as ulceration and stricture formation.

Band ligation, using a principle similar to ligation of hemorrhoids, was introduced by Stiegmann and colleagues.[18] The ligation device comprises a "friction-fit" adaptor that fits onto the end of the endoscope, an inner cylinder preloaded with an elastic O ring, and a trip wire for pulling the inner cylinder into the adaptor to release the ring (Fig. 47–12). With the endoscope en face with the varix, suction is applied to suck the varix into the cup. When a "red-out" appears (signifying that the varix is fully sucked into the cup and is touching the lens of the endoscope), the trip wire is pulled to release the band (Fig. 47–13). Meta-analyses of randomized controlled trials have demonstrated that banding is superior to sclerotherapy and should now be used as first-line treatment of bleeding varices.[19]

The original banding device can apply only one band at a time, and the endoscope needs to be removed and the band reloaded for each firing. To facilitate repeated endoscope insertion, an overtube is used. Overtubes are uncomfortable and carry a risk of pharyngeal and esophageal laceration. There are now commercially available multiple-band ligators that can apply multiple bands with a single passage of the endoscope. They are quicker and easier to use but are more costly. Detachable mini-loops can also be used to ligate esophageal varices. They are slightly more cumbersome to use but can apply an unlimited number of bands without removing the endoscope.

Achalasia

The spastic lower esophageal sphincter in achalasia may be disrupted by pneumatic balloon dilatation. The balloon, ranging from 30 to 40 mm in diameter, may be either mounted on the shaft of the endoscope or, more commonly, railroaded over a guide wire. The balloon is slowly inflated to 260 to 300 mm Hg over 3 minutes. Blood staining of the balloon on removal signifies successful dilatation. Success in relieving dysphagia can be achieved in over 85% of cases.[20] There is a small risk of perforation. Pneumatic balloon dilatation is the treatment of choice for achalasia in most units.

A more novel way of treating achalasia is the direct injection of botulinum toxin (Botox) into the sphincter.[21]

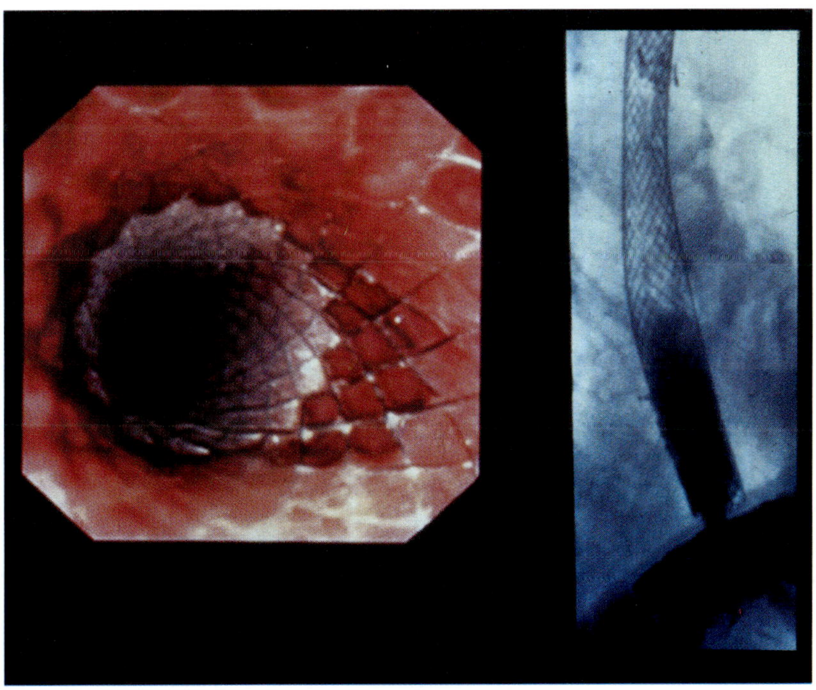

Figure 47–11. Endoscopic view of covered Wallstent after stenting, showing patency of the stent on contrast study.

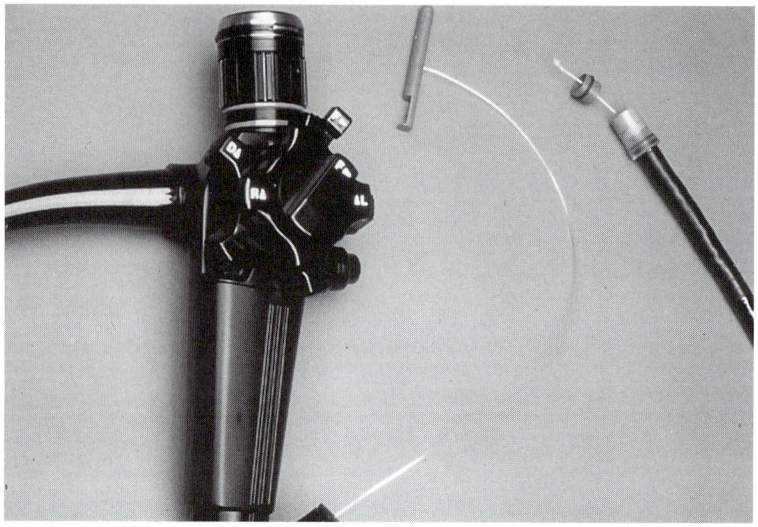

Figure 47–12. Esophageal variceal banding ligation device loaded onto the endoscope.

The toxin causes paralysis of the sphincter. The advantage of this method is that it is safe; there is no risk of perforation. However, the effect of botulinum toxin injection is not permanent, and recurrence is the rule after several months. For this reason, it cannot be recommended for routine use.

Endoscopic Incision of Pharyngeal Diverticulum

Endoscopic division of the septum between the esophagus and the diverticulum has been described as a treatment option for pharyngeal diverticulum. Dohlman and Mattsson[22] used a specially designed double-lipped laryngoscope that straddles the septum and divided the septum with electrocautery. The procedure was performed with the patient under general anesthesia. More recently, Ishioka and colleagues[23] and Mulder and colleagues[24] performed the incision using flexible endoscopes with the patient under local anesthesia. The procedure was advocated for symptomatic patients who are high surgical risks.

Endoscopic Mucosectomy for Mucosal Carcinoma

It is now possible to detect early cancer and dysplasia in the esophagus by spraying 1.5% Lugol's iodine onto the esophageal mucosa. The iodine stains the glycogen in the normal mucosa brown, whereas dysplastic and cancerous areas remain unstained.[25] For small lesions (<3 cm in diameter) confined to the mucosa without lymph node metastasis, mucosectomy is an alternative to surgical resection.

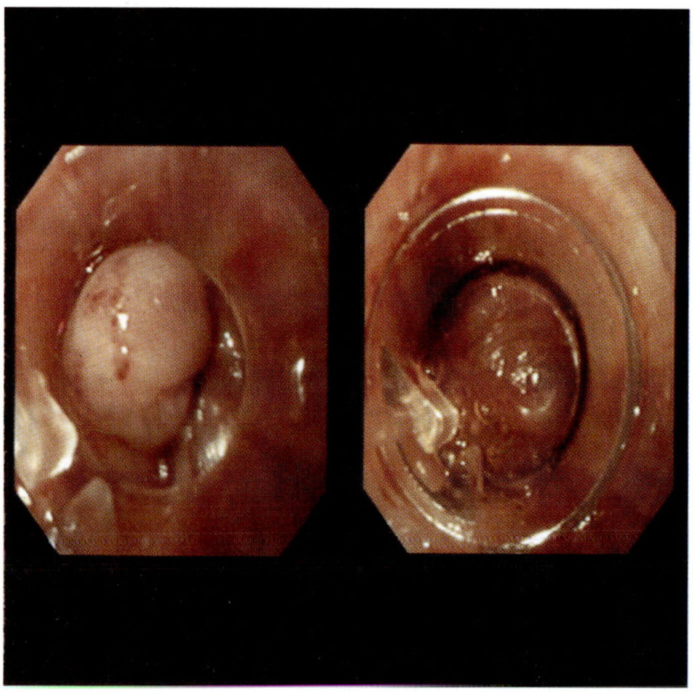

Figure 47–13. *A*, Esophageal varices ready for banding. *B*, Banded varices.

Accurate staging by endosonography is mandatory in choosing patients for mucosal resection. Saline is first injected submucosally to lift up the lesion. The affected area is then resected using a diathermy snare. This can be achieved by using a double-channel endoscope and using grasping forceps in one channel to lift up the lesion while the snare is passed in the second channel. A more elegant method is to use a suction cup attached to the tip of the endoscope.[26] The snare is prelooped onto the cup; suction is applied to suck the affected area into cup. The snare is then tightened around the affected area, and resection is performed by electrocautery.

References

1. Tong MC, Woo JK, Sham CL, Van Hasselt CA: Ingested foreign bodies—a contemporary management approach. J Laryngol Otol 109:965–970. 1995.
2. Chu KM, Choi HK, Tuen HH, et al: A prospective randomized trial comparing the use of the flexible gastroscope versus the bronchoscope in the management of foreign body ingestion. Gastrointest Endosc 47:23–27, 1998.
3. Lam YH, Ng EKW, Chung SCS, Li AKC: Laser-assisted removal of a foreign body impacted in the esophagus. Laser Surg Med 20:480–482, 1997.
4. Wax MK, Amirali A, Ulewicz DE, Lough R: Safety of esophagoscopy in the irradiated esophagus. Ann Otol Rhinol Laryngol 106:297–300, 1997.
5. Lambert R: Endoscopic treatment of esophago-gastric tumors. Endoscopy 26:28–35, 1994.
6. Fleischer D, Sivak MV: Endoscopic Nd:YAG laser therapy as palliation for esophagogastric cancer: Parameters affecting initial outcome. Gastroenterology 89:827–831, 1985.
7. Payne-James JJ, Spiller RC, Misiewicz JJ, Silk DBA: Use of ethanol-induced tumor necrosis to palliate dysphagia in patients with esophagogastric cancer. Gastrointest Endosc 36:43–46, 1990.
8. Chung SCS, Leong HT, Choi CYC, et al: Palliation of malignant esophageal obstruction by endoscopic alcohol injection. Endoscopy 26:275–277, 1994.
9. Fleischer D: A comparison of endoscopic laser therapy and BICAP tumor probe therapy for esophageal cancer. Am J Gastroenterol 82:608–612, 1987.
10. Bennett JR: Intubation of gastroesophageal malignancies: A survey of current practice in Britain, 1980. Gut 22:336–338, 1981.
11. Chan ACW, Leong HT, Chung SCS, Li AKC: Lipiodol as a reliable marker for stenting in malignant esophageal stricture. Gastrointest Endosc 40:520–521, 1994.
12. Grund KE, Storek D, Becker HD: Highly flexible self-expanding meshed metal stents for palliation of malignant esophagogastric obstruction. Endoscopy 27:486–494, 1995.
13. Knyrim K, Wagner HJ, Bethge N, et al: A controlled trial of an expandable metal stent for palliation of esophageal obstruction due to inoperable cancer. N Engl J Med 329:1345–1346, 1993.
14. De Palma GD, Matteo E, Romano G, et al: Plastic prosthesis versus expandable metal stents for palliation of inoperable esophageal thoracic carcinoma: A controlled prospective study. Gastrointest Endosc 43:478–482, 1996.
15. Song HY, Choi KC, Kwon HC, et al: Esophageal strictures: Treatment with a new design of modified Gianturco stent. Radiology 184:729–734, 1992.
16. Raijman I, Lynch P: Coated expandable esophageal stents in the treatment of digestive-respiratory fistulas. Am J Gastroenterol 92:2188–2191, 1997.
17. Segalin A, Bonavina L, Carazzone A, et al: Improving results of esophageal stenting: A study on 160 consecutive unselected patients. Endoscopy 29:701–709, 1997.
18. Stiegmann GV, Goff JS, Michaletz-Onody PA, et al: Endoscopic sclerotherapy as compared with endoscopic ligation for bleeding esophageal varices. N Engl J Med 326: 1527–1532, 1992.
19. Laine L, Cook D: Endoscopic ligation compared with sclerotherapy for treatment of esophageal variceal bleeding: A meta-analysis. Ann Intern Med 123:280–287, 1995.
20. Wehrmann T, Jacobi V, Jung M, et al: Pneumatic dilation in achalasia with a low-compliance balloon: Results of a 5-year prospective evaluation. Gastrointest Endosc 42:31–36, 1995.
21. Annese V, Basciani M, Perri F, et al: Controlled trial of botulinum toxin injection versus placebo and pneumatic dilation in achalasia. Gastroenterology 111:1418–1424, 1996.
22. Dohlman G, Mattsson O: The endoscopic operation for hypopharyngeal diverticula. Arch Otolaryngol 71:744–752, 1960.
23. Ishioka S, Sakai P, Maluf-Filho F, Melo JM: Endoscopic incision of Zenker's diverticula. Endoscopy 27:433–437, 1995.
24. Mulder CJJ, Hartog G, Robijn RJ, Thies JE: Flexible endoscopic treatment of Zenker's diverticulum: A new approach. Endoscopy 27:438–442, 1995.
25. Sugimachi K, Kitamura K, Baba K, et al: Endoscopic diagnosis of early carcinoma of the esophagus using Lugol's solution. Gastrointest Endosc 38:657–661, 1992.
26. Inoue H, Noguchi O, Saito N, et al: Endoscopic mucosectomy for early cancer using a pre-looped plastic cap. Gastrointest Endosc 40:263–264, 1994.

Chapter 48

Interventional Radiology in the Chest

Joseph B. Zwischenberger, Eric vanSonnenberg, Scott K. Alpard, and Brian W. Goodacre

Because of the precision of imaging and the technical developments in needle placement and catheterization, interventional radiology has assumed an important role in the diagnosis and treatment of thoracic disorders. These radiologic techniques provide many benefits: They aid the pulmonologist and thoracic surgeon diagnostically, they may benefit the thoracic surgeon as a temporizing maneuver, and they may obviate surgery in selected cases. A host of procedures are available to diagnose and treat thoracic disorders: guided diagnostic and therapeutic thoracentesis; drainage of empyemas or noninfected pleural collections; drainage of lung and mediastinal abscesses; pericardial drainage; transthoracic biopsy of pulmonary, mediastinal, pleural, and hilar lesions; pleural sclerosis; treatment of pneumothoraces; esophageal and tracheobronchial stenting; removal of pleural foreign bodies; and brachytherapy. This chapter highlights the indications, techniques, and results of interventional radiologic procedures for various thoracic disorders.

Choice of Imaging Guidance

The choice of imaging to detect thoracic fluid collections and guide drainage depends on the availability of the modalities, the imaging characteristics and location of the collection, and the comfort and expertise of the operator. Ultrasound (US) is portable, does not expose the patient and operator to radiation, and is relatively inexpensive.[1] Computed tomography (CT) is the preferred modality for those collections that are inaccessible to US, are obscured on US because of overlying lung, or are inadequately displayed by US. Fluoroscopy is used for tube exchanges and to determine cavity communication and loculations (by injecting contrast into the cavity). Some operators prefer to mark the overlying skin site in US or CT and then transfer the patient to the fluoroscopy suite to complete catheter insertion. In most cases, we perform the entire procedure in either US or CT and reserve fluoroscopy for postprocedure catheter injections when necessary.

Ultrasound and CT provide an assessment of adequacy of drainage immediately after the procedure. A "postdrainage" set of images should be obtained on the completion of the initial procedure; these images reveal whether the entire collection has been drained and whether an additional catheter (or catheters) needs to be inserted.

Magnetic resonance imaging (MRI) currently has no role in the percutaneous drainage of thoracic collections. Whether "drainability" can be assessed by the superior resolution of MRI with respect to internal contents (compared with CT or US) has not been determined. The capability of MRI guidance exists with nonferromagnetic needles now available. At present, MRI guidance is more theoretical than practical.

Diagnosis and Treatment of Thoracic Fluid Collections: *Diagnostic Thoracentesis*

Diagnostic thoracentesis has emerged as a common procedure. Standard ward "taps" have been replaced in many situations by US-guided thoracentesis. Indications for sonographic guidance are (1) failed ward "taps"; (2) a very small amount of pleural fluid; (3) compromised respiratory status, such that the development of iatrogenic pneumothorax would be extremely deleterious to the patient; (4) cases in which the patient is respirator dependent; and (5) known loculations. Diagnostic US-guided "taps" can be done in the radiology department, on the ward, or in the intensive care unit.

Evaluation of aspirated pleural fluid should include pH level; determination of the presence and concentration of white blood cells and bacteria; and measurement of glucose, protein, and lactic dehydrogenase (LDH). Exudative material is diagnosed by a pH less than 7.1, low glucose, the presence of white blood cells, and elevated protein and LDH. The presence of bacteria on Gram's stain or culture provides a diagnosis of infection. "Sterile" collections may be seen in patients on antibiotics; however, these collections require drainage if clinical evidence of infection exists.

Needle aspiration may be adequate to drain noninfected pleural effusions. A helpful maneuver for large serous or malignant collections is to insert a small sheath or catheter (5 to 7 F) to facilitate fluid removal. For large effusions, insertion of a multi-sidehole pigtail catheter connected to water-sealed drainage at −20 cm H_2O suction usually proves adequate.

Percutaneous Thoracic Biopsy

Fluoroscopic, CT, or sonographic guidance may be used for percutaneous biopsy. Fluoroscopy is chosen whenever possible because of its ease and relatively low cost. If a lesion is visible in two 90-degree planes, fluoroscopic guidance is adequate. In general, lesions larger than 1.5 to 2.0 cm are amenable to fluoroscopic biopsy; lesions measuring 0.5 to 1.5 cm are appropriate for CT guidance. CT is particularly advantageous for lesions not seen in two planes on conventional radiography. US may be used for pleural lesions or pulmonary lesions that abut the pleura. Sonography has the advantage that neither the patient nor the operator is exposed to radiation. CT and usually US permit accurate and unequivocal documentation of needle position in the lesion.

The main drawback to CT guidance is time required to place a needle stepwise into the lesion with intermittent scanning, which can be impossible for small lesions when the patient is unable to reproducibly suspend respiration. With the advent of "fluoro-CT," rapid scanning and reconstruction time allow CT images to be displaced at six "frames" per second. The needle can then be advanced as the localizing scans are obtained, conferring a benefit of traditional fluoroscopic or sonographic guidance to CT biopsy. CT is the most expensive guidance system but gives the greatest opportunity to achieve a diagnosis.

Diagnosis by transthoracic biopsy is achieved in 70 to 90% of cases (90% for malignancy). An assortment of benign conditions, including histoplasmosis, coccidioidomycosis, tuberculosis, nocardiosis, aspergillosis, mucormycosis, hamartoma, and bacterial and opportunistic infections, may be diagnosed. The typical assortment of bronchogenic, metastatic, and less common pulmonary tumors (carcinoid, lymphoma) all may be diagnosed by percutaneous biopsy.

Pneumothorax occurs in 10 to 60% of patients undergoing percutaneous biopsy. A chest tube is inserted in 5 to 25% of patients. Patients with underlying lung disease (emphysema, chronic bronchitis) are at increased risk for development of large pneumothoraces. Pulmonary hemorrhage, hemothorax, and pain are less frequent complications.

Percutaneous Biopsy of Mediastinal and Hilar Lesions

When fluoroscopy was the sole guidance method, mediastinal and hilar lesions were considered hazardous for transthoracic biopsy by most authors. Presently, CT permits precise localization of major vessels, allowing safe biopsy in many if not most cases of mediastinal and hilar lesions. With current high-resolution CT, biopsy specimens of most hilar and mediastinal lesions larger than 1 cm may be obtained under CT guidance (Fig. 48–1*A*, *B*).

A frequently used system for biopsy is the coaxial technique, in which an outer needle slides over an inner localizing needle. After removal of the inner guiding needle, multiple biopsy passes are obtained coaxially through the outer cannula by 21- or 22-gauge needles. Biopsy specimens may be obtained from mediastinal lesions in the pretracheal, aorticopulmonary window, and subcarinal regions and from pericardial and diaphragmatic nodes. Specimens from lesions in the anterior, middle, and posterior mediastinum may be obtained as well.

Major complications of these biopsies are uncommon but include bleeding, pneumothorax, and pericarditis. Pericardial tamponade has been reported but fortunately is rare. Mediastinal and hilar biopsies permit staging of pulmonary malignancy and may preclude unnecessary thoracotomy if a diagnosis of incurability is made on the basis of the biopsy findings.

Therapeutic Thoracentesis

Small (5 to 9 French) catheters may be inserted under US guidance alongside the localizing guided needle. These catheters permit therapeutic thoracentesis for evacuation of serous or noninfected fluid. US is the guidance procedure of choice for most thoracenteses; CT is reserved for loculated collections or otherwise complicated collections, particularly in obese patients. With noninfected collections, catheters usually remain in place for a short time; with malignant effusions, catheters frequently are left in place for a longer period, and sclerosing agents may be infused.

Drainage of Infected Collections

Empyema

Undrained pus in the chest may be a source of systemic sepsis or the inciting cause of the multiple sequelae of the systemic inflammatory response syndrome (SIRS) and therefore requires urgent drainage. The major indication for catheter drainage is localized purulence or persistent infection despite an initial thoracostomy tube. Ongoing sepsis usually occurs because of suboptimal positioning

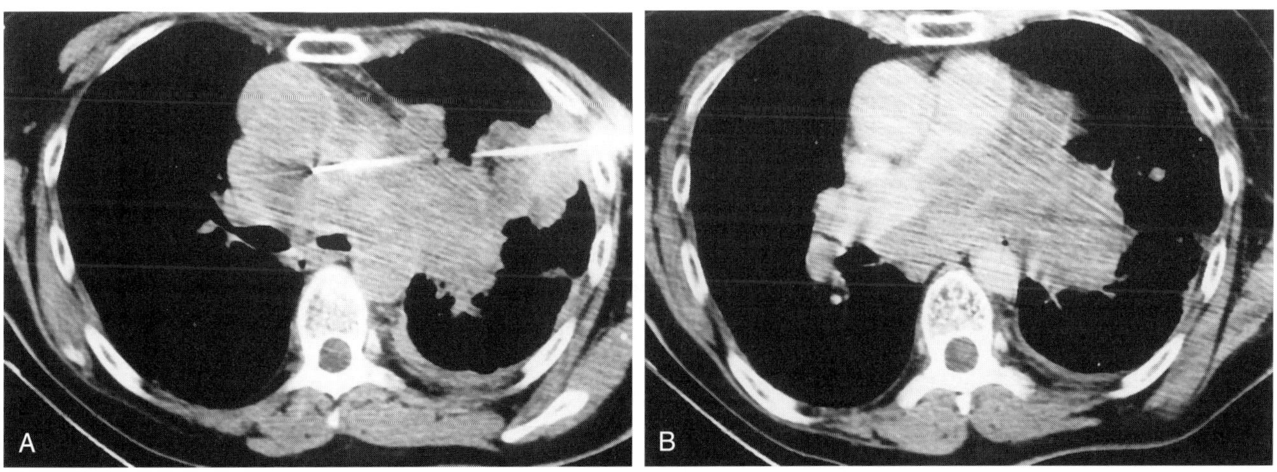

Figure 48–1. *A*, Mediastinal biopsy via a left approach through postobstructive pneumonia. *B*, A biopsy deep into the mediastinum is performed for staging; the results were positive for bronchogenic carcinoma, precluding operation.

of a thoracotomy tube that leaves undrained pus (Fig. 48–2*A–C*) or because of additional infected fluid loculations.

Antibiotic therapy accompanies drainage of all infected thoracic collections. Drained fluid should be cultured for aerobic and anaerobic bacteria, atypical mycobacteria, and fungus. A thoracic surgeon/interventional radiologist team is essential to help decide whether percutaneous drainage or operation would be more effective and appropriate in a given situation.

The success rate for drainage of the various thoracic collections ranges from 80 to 95% and depends on the complexity of the collection, the underlying status of the patient, and the technical adequacy of catheter(s) placement.[2–7] Stage II empyema (organizing fibropurulent) collections result in less successful tube drainage. Complications are avoided by meticulous imaging and image planning. Guiding principles of percutaneous drainage are essential and should include inserting catheters over the top of ribs rather than beneath the ribs (where the intercostal vessels course) and avoiding injury to the internal mammary arteries and deep mediastinal structures The use of intravenous contrast media to highlight mediastinal and hilar vessels is essential in many cases.

If diagnostic aspiration reveals infection by Gram's stain or by culture, percutaneous drainage is indicated. For large or free-flowing empyemas, US is used as the guidance system. For loculated and less accessible collections, CT is the modality of choice. Radiologically guided catheters may be placed de novo or after a large-bore thoracostomy tube has proved ineffective. The latter occurs when these tubes migrate into the major fissure or are remote from the empyema.

Technique and Materials

Thoracic drainage may be accomplished either by trocar or Seldinger technique. With either method, using US or CT guidance, the collection is localized, and a fine 22-gauge needle localizer initially is inserted. This fine needle serves as a marker, allows aspiration of a small amount of fluid to determine the contents of the collection, and serves as a guide for catheter insertion. If the initial placement is not optimally situated, additional needles are placed until a repetitive optimal route of catheter insertion is obtained.

When using the trocar method, we prefer the "tandem trocar technique with a protective guidewire."[8] With this method, after appropriate localization with the fine needle, trocar puncture is made. The stylette is removed, and approximately 1 ml is aspirated to confirm that the tip of the catheter is within the collection. A floppy-tip guidewire is then inserted through both the cannula and catheter and is coiled in the collection. The catheter then slides over both its internal metal cannula and the guide wire, thereby facilitating smooth entry into the collection. The cannula

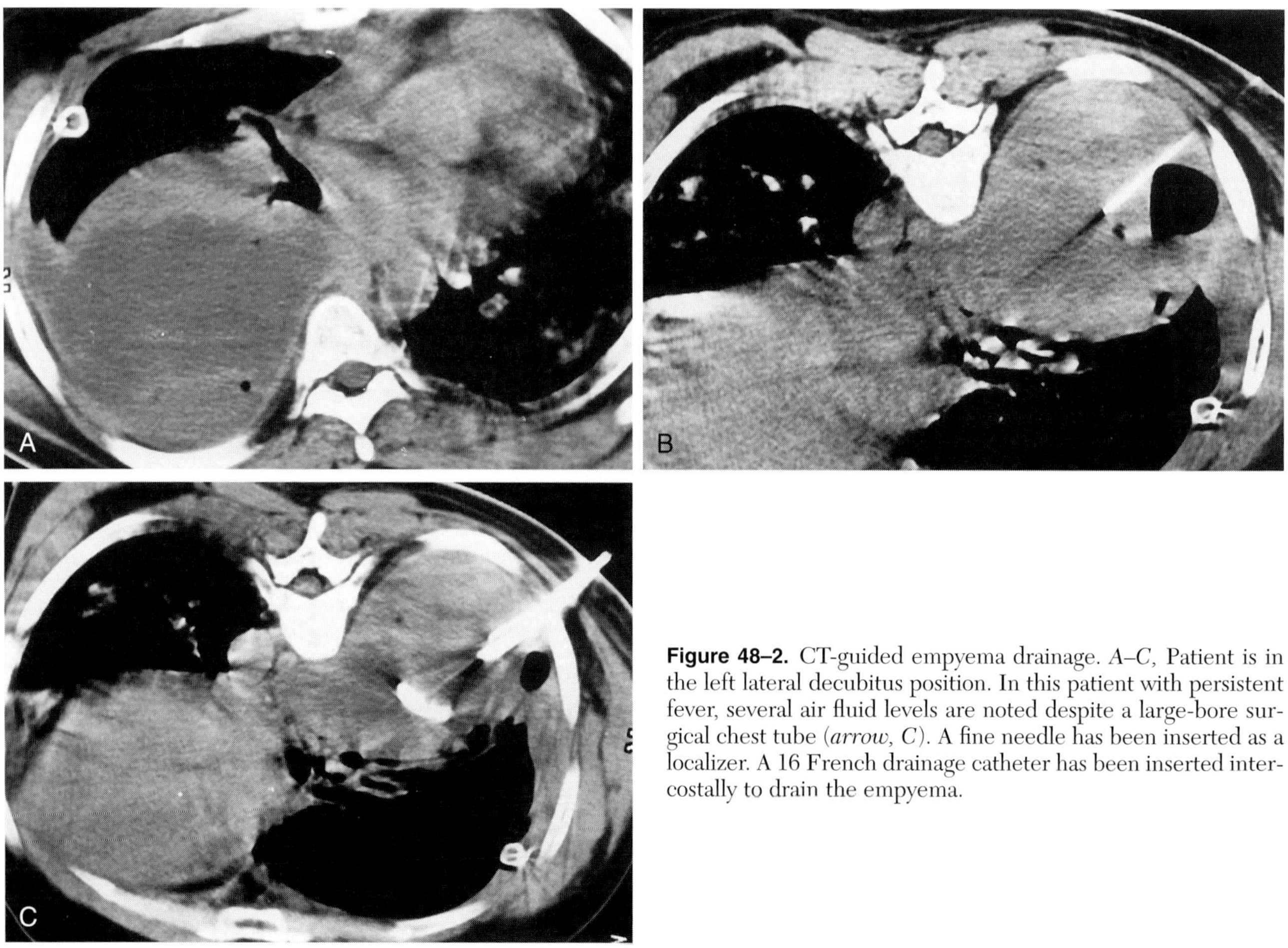

Figure 48–2. CT-guided empyema drainage. *A–C,* Patient is in the left lateral decubitus position. In this patient with persistent fever, several air fluid levels are noted despite a large-bore surgical chest tube (*arrow, C*). A fine needle has been inserted as a localizer. A 16 French drainage catheter has been inserted intercostally to drain the empyema.

and guide wire are removed, the catheter is locked, and the fluid is aspirated. Alternatively, the Seldinger technique may be used. Either a coaxial system with a small needle can be used, or a larger needle with a 0.035-in. or 0.038-in. guide wire may be preferred.

Once the catheter is situated within the collection, the contents are aspirated as completely as possible. If more than one discrete collection has been localized, each collection deserves its own catheter. Once the abscess or collection is evacuated, a postdrainage set of images should be obtained. The radiologist can then determine whether a second catheter is necessary.

Catheter size varies in the chest from small 5 F catheters to 30 F catheters. Generally, single-lumen catheters are preferred in the chest to avoid the introduction of air into the pleural space or parenchyma. The choice of catheters depends on the viscosity of the collection. For serous or parapneumonic effusions, 7 F to 9 F catheters are sufficient, although even smaller catheters may be used successfully. For thicker collections, such as most empyemas, hematomas, and organizing collections, 12 F to 30 F drains are utilized. Pleural drainage may be augmented by the instillation of urokinase. After a vial with 250,000 units of urokinase is mixed with 20 to 50 ml of saline, the mixture is delivered into the collection and left in place for 15 to 30 minutes. Saline irrigation of the collection immediately afterward helps to evacuate the lysed material. Catheters are routinely attached to three-chamber collection devices at approximately −20 cm of H_2O of suction. Gently saline irrigation is performed on the ward to augment drainage and to maintain catheter patency. Complications occur in 5 to 10% of patients undergoing catheter drainage of empyemas. Dislodgement of the catheter is the most frequent problem. Bleeding is rare.

Sclerotherapy

Sclerotherapy of the pleural cavity is frequently used to treat symptomatic malignant effusions. Investigations are currently underway to determine superiority of bedside talc/saline sclerotherapy versus talc insufflation during video-assisted thoracic surgery (VATS). For bedside sclerotherapy, a 7 F pigtail catheter usually is sufficient. The effusion is drained "dry," then 5 to 10 ml of lidocaine or bupivacaine HCl (Marcaine) is instilled in the chest while the patient is rolled to ensure coating of the entire parietal pleura (Trendelenburg, roll 360°, then reverse Trendelenburg, roll 360°). Five grams of sterile talc are instilled in 100 ml of saline as the patient is again rolled to coat the parietal pleura. The patient should be sedated with intravenous or intramuscular narcotics for pain control prior to talc sclerotherapy. The pigtail catheter or chest tube is then placed on the chamber suction until the drainage is less than 100 ml over 12 hours.

Brachytherapy

Brachytherapy, the placement of interstitial or intracavitary radioactive sources into a desired target to facilitate the safe delivery of high-radiation doses to tumors, with selective sparing of normal surrounding tissue,[9] is performed for recurrent or refractory tumor that abuts or is in the pleural space. Brachytherapy has been explored as an alternative treatment modality to manage selected tumors arising in or metastasizing to the chest. A fine needle for localization is inserted into the recurrent tumor. This is followed by placement of a large (16-gauge) needle into the lesion. Several needles may be necessary. Radiation pellets are loaded into the large needles for local therapy. Tumor shrinkage has occurred in some patients. Care must be taken in placing these large needles; the potential for bleeding or pneumothorax exists and theoretically is greater than with fine needles. To date, brachytherapy may improve local outcome and, possibly, survival in selected situations and should be considered as a viable treatment option in planning a multimodality approach. The treatment is well tolerated, with few reported complications. Future directions for the use of brachytherapy include video-assisted thoracoscopy for the placement of radioactive sources in an unresectable tumor in the lung or chest wall; percutaneous brachytherapy for superficial lesions of the chest wall[9]; and radiolabeled monoclonal antibodies for direct targeting of tumor cell antigens.[11]

Drainage of Pneumothorax

The most common indication for radiologic drainage of pleural air is the development of a postbiopsy pneumothorax; spontaneous pneumothorax and post–central venous access catheter placement are other indications. Multi-sidehole catheter insertion can be performed either with CT or fluoroscopic (or, rarely, US) guidance. Evacuation of the pneumothorax is performed for patient comfort and safety or to continue a percutaneous biopsy if an intervening pneumothorax makes accurate localization of the lesion difficult. Ironically, planned introduction of a pneumothorax is becoming an important maneuver for the interventional radiologist to allow needle access to mediastinal, subcarinal, or aortopulmonary window nodes. A controlled amount of intrapleural air is inserted (i.e., a "controlled" pneumothorax) to push the lung parenchyma away from the incoming biopsy needle and prevent puncture of and injury to underlying lung parenchyma.

A recent application of radiologically guided drainage of pneumothorax is in patients with severe pulmonary disease who develop loculated pneumothoraces. Compromised ventilatory status in these patients suggests that evacuating dead space and improving the volume of ventilated lung may be of benefit. The common situation is in a patient with adult respiratory distress syndrome (ARDS) who develops multiple loculated spontaneous pneumothoraces. Multi-sidehole small catheters (7 F to 10 F) usually suffice for drainage in these situations.[11]

By convention, catheters are inserted in the second intercostal space in the midclavicular line. However, when a biopsy is being done with the patient in the prone position, the catheter may be inserted in the axillary line or even somewhat posterior to obviate turning the patient (twice) and using valuable CT time. Initially, the pneumothorax should be evacuated by syringe suction. If the air leak is large or persistent, the catheter can be connected to three-chamber suction and the patient observed. If an airleak persists for more than 2 hours, the patient should be admitted for observation. Often a one-way flap valve (Heimlich valve) is all that is necessary to effect reexpansion and seal a small air leak.

Lung Abscess

Antibiotics and postural drainage are the mainstays of medical therapy for lung abscesses. Bronchoscopy can be of value to loosen secretions or to remove an obstructing foreign body that may have caused the abscess. For lung abscesses that drain poorly, are refractory to standard medical therapy, are large (>6 to 8 cm in diameter), or occur in patients on ventilator assistance, or when expeditious evacuation of pus is necessary because of the clinical status of the patient, the next therapeutic step traditionally has been surgery.

Percutaneous drainage offers an alternative that is more aggressive than medical therapy alone but less invasive than standard surgical drainage and will be successful in 80 to 90% of cases. Imaging guidance provides information that allows safe access for drainage. Radiologically guided drainage of lung abscess is most often performed with CT guidance.[5, 12, 13] The tandem trocar or Seldinger technique may be used for catheter insertion. An important guideline is that the lung abscess should be accessed at a point where the abscess is juxtaposed to the pleura or where there is adjacent inflammation between the abscess and the pleura. Traversing normal lung en route into a lung abscess is not preferred because of the potential risk of inducing a bronchopleural fistula and empyema. If there is no other route to the abscess than through normal lung, this principle must be violated; in most cases, there are no negative sequelae.

Another important principle of lung abscess drainage is that the affected side should not be placed in a nondependent position; this avoids spillage of infected contents from the lung abscess into the unaffected contralateral lung.

Once the catheter is in place, the abscess is evacuated as completely as possible and the cavity is gently irrigated with saline. Following drainage, patients will often expectorate purulent material that aids in evacuation of pus from the abscess cavity. Postdrainage films demonstrate whether the abscess has been entirely evacuated. Most lung abscesses are unilocular, but if necessary, a second catheter can be inserted to drain a second collection.

Improvement after drainage of lung abscess may be dramatic; usually the catheter can be removed within 5 to 7 days. Occasionally, drainage is more protracted. Ward irrigation of the catheter is performed with saline.

Infected cystic pulmonary collections are formes frustes of lung abscesses and may include infected pneumatoceles, necrotic tumors, and sequestrations. Like lung abscesses, these collections may require drainage and are amenable to percutaneous radiologic therapy. The technique of percutaneous drainage is similar to that described for lung abscess. Drainage of cavities with fungus balls may be augmented by direct instillation of antifungal agents.[14]

Mediastinal Collections

Mediastinal abscesses are among the most challenging infections to treat. These collections are not always well defined; access may be difficult, and the patient is often severely ill. A less invasive approach than surgery is often sought for the aforementioned reasons, and therefore percutaneous drainage may be indicated. CT is used almost exclusively to guide drainage of mediastinal abscesses because of their deep location, long access paths, and the intimate relation between the collection and adjacent mediastinal vessels.[15] An important principle in mediastinal abscess drainage is to avoid the internal mammary arteries. Injury to the internal mammary artery by incoming needles or catheters can result in significant bleeding. For deep mediastinal abscesses, advantage may be taken of pleural effusion or pneumothoraces to provide a nontranspulmonary approach for mediastinal abscess drainage. Should an empyema result, this also can be treated percutaneously.

The most common mediastinal abscess requiring percutaneous drainage is postoperative and follows esophageal surgery. Infected duplication cyst, lymphocele, mediastinal pancreatic pseudocyst, and hematoma are additional types of mediastinal collections that may require drainage. Unusual infections such as histoplasmosis may produce mediastinal abscesses, and infected tumors may require drainage. Multiple catheters may be needed to drain these complex collections.

Postoperative pericardial effusions that become secondarily infected may require percutaneous drainage. Ultrasound is the modality of choice for imaging guidance. Successful percutaneous drainage can obviate the need for reoperation in many cases.

Anterior Mediastinal Lesions: Trans-sternal or Parasternal Biopsy with Computed Tomography Guidance

Diagnostic biopsy of anterior mediastinal lesions can be performed endoscopically (via the bronchi), surgically (by using mediastinoscopy or thoracoscopy), or percutaneously. The percutaneous approach is effective, minimally invasive, can be an outpatient procedure, and is less expensive than surgery. Pneumothorax, however, is a potential risk when biopsy specimens are taken from anterior mediastinal lesions behind the sternum. Pneumothorax occurs if the biopsy needle traverses the visceral pleura and the lung at two separate locations on its path to the lesion. Recently, we have employed two new techniques to access mediastinal and aortopulmonary window lesions. The first, "iatrogenic controlled pneumothorax," allows the lung to fall away from the mediastinal parietal pleura to avoid lung puncture. The second is the use of saline injections to increase the soft tissue mediastinal space to allow a safe extrapulmonary access for biopsy (Fig. 48–3*A–C*).

Trans-sternal biopsy, another consideration to access anterior mediastinal lesions, is a two-step procedure; first the sternum is punctured to gain access to the lesion, then a biopsy needle is inserted coaxially to obtain the specimen. This method avoids puncture of the lung during access to anterior mediastinal lesions.

All interventions are performed under conscious sedation with intravenous midazolam. With CT guidance, the site of entry of the trans-sternal needle is marked on the skin. The skin area is prepared and draped, and 1% lidocaine is injected into the soft tissues below the entry site on the skin and to the periosteum of the outer layer of

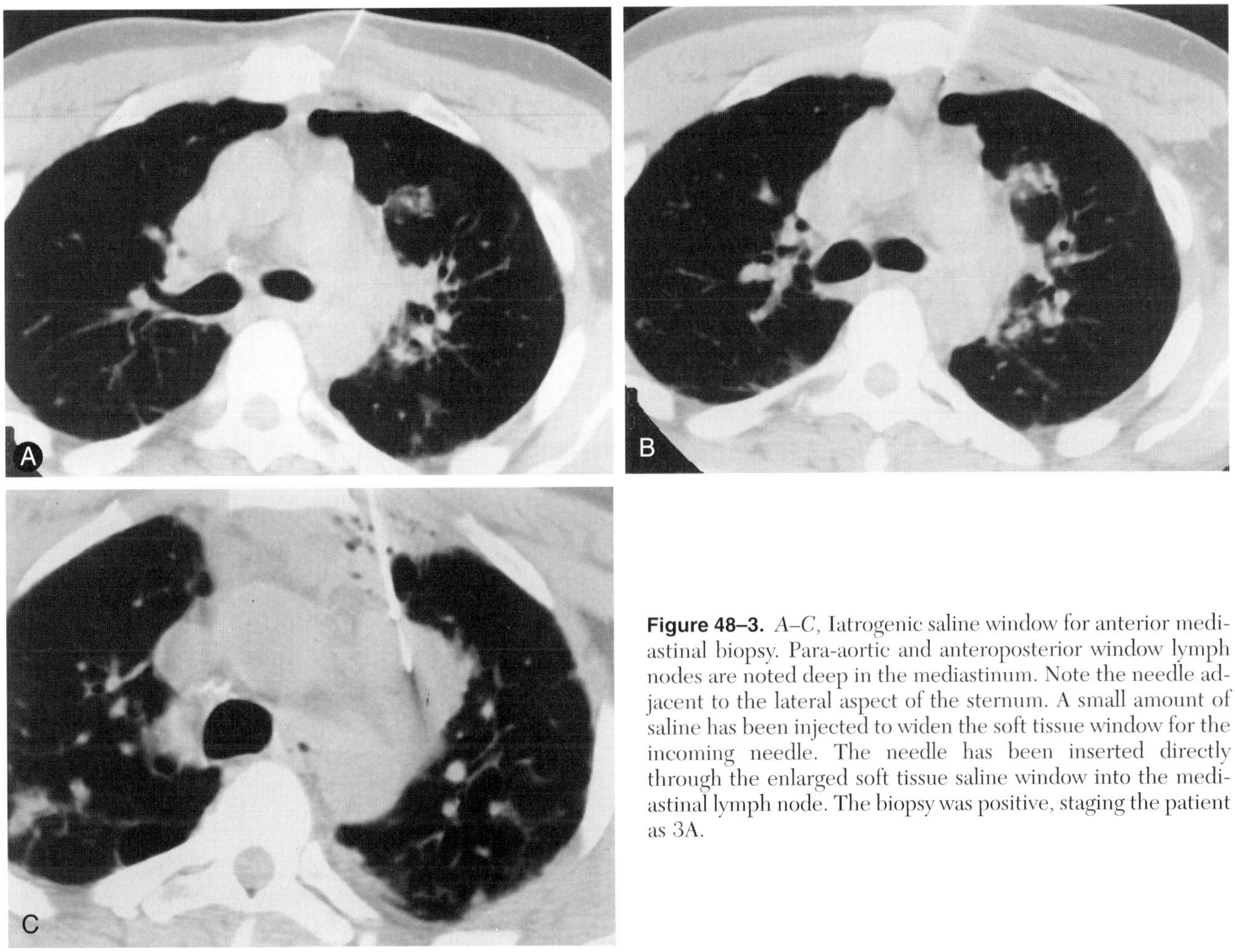

Figure 48–3. *A–C,* Iatrogenic saline window for anterior mediastinal biopsy. Para-aortic and anteroposterior window lymph nodes are noted deep in the mediastinum. Note the needle adjacent to the lateral aspect of the sternum. A small amount of saline has been injected to widen the soft tissue window for the incoming needle. The needle has been inserted directly through the enlarged soft tissue saline window into the mediastinal lymph node. The biopsy was positive, staging the patient as 3A.

the sternum. The alignment of the trans-sternal needle with the mass is reassessed with CT. The posterior cortex of the sternum is infiltrated with 1% lidocaine and traversed in the same fashion as the outer layer. CT confirms optimal alignment of the trans-sternal needle with the mass (see Fig. 48–1). The distance between the tip of the trans-sternal needle and the lesion is measured. Specimens are obtained with the previously described needles in a coaxial fashion. Tissue samples are examined immediately by a cytopathologist in the CT suite. Following the procedure, a CT scan through the midportion of the chest is performed to assess for pneumothorax. Trans-sternal needle insertion produces minimal discomfort and is well tolerated by patients. The patients are observed in the radiology department for 2 hours before being discharged to their homes or sent back to a hospital room for chest tube management.

Percutaneous routes for biopsy of anterior mediastinal masses vary with the location of the lesion. Sonographic guidance is beneficial when a suprasternal route is used, as the needle can be controlled in real time.[19–21] CT or MRI may be used in selected large lesions.[18–20] When the lesion extends laterally to the sternal border,[22] a direct extrapleural approach can be used.

The diagnostic accuracy of percutaneous biopsy ranges from 74.5 to 90.3%.[22, 23] The sensitivity of percutaneous biopsy of mediastinal lesions is high for metastatic disease and germ cell tumors and increases for lymphoma if immunohistochemical cytologic methods are used.[24–27] Transbronchial biopsy provides diagnostic-quality specimens in only 23 to 32% of cases.[28–31]

Biopsy specimens of anterior mediastinal lesions can also be obtained surgically through mediastinoscopy or endoscopic thoracostomy. Cervical and transthoracic mediastinoscopy yields positive results in 74.5% of cases.[33] There is consensus that although no deaths were reported in a compiled series of 2259 patients who underwent mediastinoscopy, significant adverse consequences, including mortality, can occur if the procedure is performed by inexperienced operators.[33] Life-threatening complications such as hemorrhage, tracheobronchial injury, esophageal injury, recurrent nerve palsy, pneumothorax, wound infection, and hematoma may result from mediastinoscopy.[34]

No complications related to the trans-sternal route are reported[27] or have occurred in our series. A bone marrow biopsy of the sternum, however, has been associated with manubriosternal separation in a patient with malnutrition and osteoporosis.[35] Deaths related to injury of the right ventricle or major vessels from uncontrolled penetration by the sternal bone marrow needle have been described.[36, 37] Use of CT guidance for controlled needle placement and positioning of smaller needles increases the safety of the procedure. Pain that may be experienced by the patient while the needle traverses the sternum is prevented with both appropriate local anesthesia of the periosteum and finesse in needle insertion. Our experience with trans-sternal biopsy suggests this is a safe and well-tolerated alternative route for biopsies of anterior mediastinal lesions.

Management of Pulmonary Arteriovenous Malformation

Arteriovenous malformations of the lung are congenital abnormalities that have a direct connection between a pulmonary artery and pulmonary vein, such that the normal capillary bed is circumvented. These lesions are usually subpleural in location and frequently are multiple (58%) or bilateral (42%) and predominate in the lower lobes (55 to 84%).[38] First described in 1977,[39] the effectiveness and advantages of embolization over surgery have made the former treatment of choice for pulmonary arteriovenous malformations (PAVMs).[39–41]

Preliminary steps in evaluating patients with suspected PAVM are chest radiography and arterial blood gases (ABGs). Chest films occasionally demonstrate the lobular soft tissue mass, the feeding artery coursing the hilum, and the draining vein passing into the left atrium. Plain film findings are not reliably present; thus, a suggestive ABG with a negative chest x-ray should not deter further investigation. CT has a high sensitivity in diagnosing and localizing PAVMs.[42] CT typically shows a noncalcified nodule or serpiginous mass with feeding arteries and draining veins. Helical CT and three-dimensional techniques provide further identification and characterization.[43]

However, although CT is very sensitive this method cannot always determine location, size, and number of PAVMs.[44] Radionucleotide shunt studies using technetium-99m albumin demonstrate right-to-left shunting; however, anatomic detail of location, size, and number of PAVMs again cannot be determined. Pulmonary angiography is the gold standard for diagnosing PAVM. A simple malformation has a single feeding artery, an intervening aneurysm, and a single draining vein. Complex lesions possess several arteries and veins with an irregular, frequently septated, connecting nidus. Further experience by three-dimensional imaging should make this a front-line diagnostic study.

Indications for treatment of PAVM include alleviating symptoms and signs of the left-to-right shunt. The goal of therapy is to eliminate shunts in which the feeding artery is 3 mm or larger. Lesions of this size may increase the patient's risk for stroke. Smaller lesions may require therapy when numerous enough to result in significant hypoxemia. Conservative therapy is associated with an unacceptably high rate of complications (e.g., paradoxical embolus, right heart failure, systemic embolic abscess, hypoxemia with dyspnea and fatigue), with morbidity and mortality rates up to 33% and 29%, respectively.[38]

Preceding embolization, a bilateral diagnostic pulmonary angiogram is done to determine the number, location, and architecture of the lesions. A 7 F multipurpose catheter (Cordis, Miami, FL, or Cook, Inc., Bloomington, IN) or similar catheter is advanced into the pulmonary circulation. This catheter is capable of selecting most branches, especially in the lower and upper lobes.

The optimal site to occlude in a feeding artery is the narrowest segment distal to any significant supply to normal lung. There is frequently dilatation of the artery immediately before it enters the aneurysm. Coil emboli are currently the primary agents used for transcatheter occlusion of PAVMs. The proper coil diameter to use is approximately 20% larger than the expected true diameter of the vessel. If too small, the coil may potentially migrate through the PAVM. If too large, it will elongate and displace itself and the top of the catheter from the target vessel. The longer the coil, the more stainless steel there is to induce vessel thrombosis; however, the longer the coil, the greater the tendency to displace the catheter tip from the target vessel during deployment of the coil.[45] Use of shorter coils and a floppy guidewire to push the coil is also less likely to cause the catheter tip to recoil and dislodge from the target vessel. Delivering coils through an occlusion balloon catheter (Medi-Tech/Boston Scientific, Natick, MA) is helpful when embolizing high-flow malformations or lesions in which it is difficult to maintain stable catheter position. White and colleagues[46] favor detachable balloons over coils for occluding PAVMs, as immediate cross-sectional occlusion of the segmental artery is obtained in a position preserving the most normal branches. However, in specific anatomic situations (oversized arteries and for occlusion of an aneurysm of a PAVM), coils have advantages over balloons.[46] Following embolization, a control angiogram is performed to confirm occlusion of the PAVM and to look for any residual feeding arteries or previously undetected malformations.

Major clinical complications of embolotherapy are rare.[40, 41, 47] As the geometry of pulmonary arteries changes with respiratory excursions, catheters tend to become wedged, and air can be introduced. The most common symptoms caused by air embolization are angina and bradycardia, which occur when air enters the right coronary artery, the ostium of which is anterior and nondependent in the supine patient. Paradoxical migration of embolization devices occurs in fewer than 1% of procedures and has been associated with no adverse sequela. Phlebotomy should be done at the start of the procedure in patients with elevated hematocrits to minimize thrombotic complications. After embolization, patients are instructed to use an incentive spirometer for several days to prevent atelectasis. Pleuritic chest pain with occasional fever occurs in more than 20% of patients. This is probably due to pulmonary infarction. Acetaminophen or nonsteroidal anti-inflammatory or other agents can be prescribed to control this self-limited problem.

Occlusion of nearly all significant lesions can be achieved, although several catheterizations may be necessary.[40, 41] Dyspnea and fatigue improve, and patients are protected against macroscopic paradoxical emboli. Complex lesions and diffuse involvement of a region of the lung present the greatest challenges. Several therapeutic sessions may be necessary to occlude the numerous channels present in these lesions. The diffuse variety may also necessitate sacrifice of substantial amounts of normal lung tissue. Persistence or recurrence of a malformation occurs in fewer than 10% of cases and is usually caused by a nonembolized artery or, rarely, by recanalization.

After therapy, patients should have repeat chest radiographs, ABGs, and clinical assessment at one day, one month, and then every 3 to 5 years to look for new, persistent, and/or recurrent malformations. Slow growth of PAVMs also has been documented.[48] It is likely that helical CT scanning will play an important role in follow-up, possible replacing ABGs.[42] Persistence of the aneurysm or nidus without significant reduction in size probably indicates continued perfusion.

Management of Hemoptysis

Successful control of hemoptysis remains a challenge. Bronchial artery embolization (BAE) is an effective vascular procedure, which, when successful, results in immediate cessation of bleeding.[49, 50] Long-term benefits vary, depending on the disease and underlying patient condition. BAE is indicated whenever hemoptysis cannot be controlled by conservative or surgical management. Hemoptysis exceeding the amount of 300 ml per day is considered life threatening and is initially treated best by embolization.[51] Embolization should be the first choice for treatment for episodes of mild hemoptysis occurring over weeks or months. In recent years, the indications for embolization have increased and include cases in which the patient has mild bleeding and diffuse lung disease that requires respiratory therapy (such as in cystic fibrosis). This aggressive approach to management is a reflection of the development of safer techniques using digital subtraction angiography and nonionic contrast agents, and the techniques are unlikely to cause neurotoxic damage to the spinal cord.[50] The frequent occurrence of a common bronchial trunk giving origin to a right and left bronchial artery in more than 45% of patients was noted.[50]

The search for bleeding often begins with bronchoscopy to identify the side of bleeding.[51] In a large number of patients, the findings of the chest x-ray or computed axial tomography scan, along with the patient's subjective localization of bleeding point, are sufficient to obviate a bronchoscopic examination. Occasionally, patients with massive hemoptysis require immediate angiography and embolization without previous assessment. The search for the bleeding site begins by performing a bronchial arteriogram. If an abnormality is identified, immediate embolization is performed. However, if the bronchial arteriogram is normal or does not yield a significant abnormality, the angiographic search is continued, pursuant to the changes seen on the chest radiograph or by bronchoscopic location of the bleeding site. The branches of subclavian and axillary arteries, most notable the internal mammary artery, are the most common feeding vessels in the region of upper lobes. The intercostal vessels commonly feed the abnormal lung parenchyma.[52] Occasionally, in the basal segments of the inferior phrenic artery branches, there may be a main supply source. A vessel from the neck and lateral chest wall may become a source for blood flow to the lesion.[53, 54] The most common angiographic feature in hemoptysis is the enlargement of the systemic vessel supplying the abnormal site; these may be associated with systemic-to-pulmonary artery shunting.

It is important to embolize distal branches and preserve the proximal trunk of the vessel. This has a twofold purpose: (1) the important mediastinal and spinal cord branches remain patent; and (2) access to the area of bleeding is available if a second intervention is required. Particles ranging in size from 0.5 to 2.0 mm in diameter are preferred. Occlusive therapy is usually begun by using the smallest particles; as flow to the area of interest gradually decreases, larger particles are used to achieve better occlusion.[54] Gelfoam (Upjohn, Kalamazoo, MI) is the most commonly used agent.[55] However, if the patient rebleeds from the same source, the use of a permanent occlusive material such as Ivalon (Ivalon, San Diego, CA) is more appropriate. A polymerizing liquid material such as Cyanoacrilate (B Braum, Melsung, Germany) should be reserved for special cases when other materials fail.

Whenever therapeutic embolization is performed, the catheter should be advanced distal to the origin of the mediastinal and spinal cord branches. These small vessels may not be visible on the initial arteriogram, but during embolization, the distal branches gradually occlude and the hemodynamic changes redistribute the blood flow, revealing more proximal branches. The occlusive material is pushed through the catheter. This prevents reflux and undesirable embolization of nontarget vessels.

A pseudoaneurysm of the pulmonary artery branches should be embolized with coils or detachable balloons. Detachable balloons are preferable to coils, particularly in patients with hyperdynamic flow, as they can be chosen to suit both the anatomy and size of the vessel to be embolized.

In 64 patients with hemoptysis from tuberculosis,[50] overall immediate control of bleeding by BAE was achieved in 49 of 64 patients (76.6%). The percentage of immediate control for massive hemoptysis may be as high as 82.8%.[50] Long-term control of massive hemoptysis reaches 87%,[50] using all treatment modalities including embolization with chemotherapy and surgery when possible. Recurrent hemoptysis yields a lower rate of control for both immediate (68.9%) and long-term (76%) results.[50] Rebleeding occurs in approximately 21% of patients, usually nonmassive, allowing for nonemergency re-embolization or clinical follow-up. Patients with chronic diffuse disease such as interstitial sarcoidosis, cystic fibrosis, bilateral diffuse tuberculosis, aspergillosis, and bleeding bronchial carcinoma tend to have poorer results in bleeding control because of the progressive course of the disease and gradual deterioration of the patient's condition.[56] However, BAE still controls acute hemoptysis in most of these patients.

Following successful embolization procedures, patients may complain of retrosternal pain and dysphagia. These symptoms are related to tissue ischemia in the distribution of the embolized vessel; the pain often subsides within a short time. Although more serious complications occasionally have been reported (e.g., bronchoesophageal fistula, necrotic changes in the bronchial wall, and esophageal and spinal cord injury), current techniques are quite safe.[50] A careful approach should be used whenever the subclavian artery branches are embolized. Also, occlusive therapy of any intercostal artery should be done gradually, with frequent test angiograms,[52] to greatly reduce the possibility of neurotoxic damage or retrograde dislodgement of embolic particles by distant embolization.

Conclusions

Interventional radiologic techniques offer many options and benefits in the care of patients with thoracic disorders. Imaging-guided catheter techniques provide unsurpassed precision and accuracy in performance of these procedures. CT-guided needle biopsy has an important place in the diagnostic approach to parenchymal as well as mediastinal tumors. Transcatheter arterial embolization has made a significant contribution to the management of the patient with massive hemoptysis and is the procedure of choice for treatment of pulmonary arteriovenous malformations. Percutaneous catheter drainage of intrathoracic collections has developed as a natural extension of similar interventional radiologic procedures in the abdomen. The advent of CT and sonography, which allow detection and characterization of pleural and parenchymal collections, combined with advances in drainage catheter design and interventional techniques, has made image-guided management of intrathoracic collections a safe and effective alternative to traditional surgical therapy.

References

1. McGahan JP: Aspiration and drainage procedures in the intensive care unit: Percutaneous sonographic guidance. Radiology 154:531–532, 1985.
2. Mueller PR, vanSonnenberg E: Interventional radiology in the chest and abdomen. N Engl J Med 322:1364–1374, 1990.
3. Westcott JL: Percutaneous catheter drainage of pleural effusion and empyema. AJR 144:1189–1193, 1985.
4. Silverman SG, Mueller PR, Saini S, et al: Thoracic empyema: Management with image-guided catheter drainage. Radiology 169:5–9, 1988.
5. O'Moore PV, Mueller PR, Simeone JF, et al: Sonographic guidance in diagnostic and therapeutic interventions in the pleural space. AJR 149:1–5, 1987.
6. van Sonnenberg E, Nakamoto S, Mueller PR, et al: CT- and ultrasound-guided catheter drainage of empyemas after chest-tube failure. Radiology 151:349–353, 1984.
7. Stavas J, vanSonnenberg E, Casola G, Wittich GR: Percutaneous drainage of infected and noninfected thoracic fluid collections. J Thorac Imaging 2:80–87, 1987.
8. vanSonnenberg E, Polansky AD, Wittich GR, et al: Guidewire protection for trocar puncture of fluid collections. AJR 145: 831–832, 1985.
9. Raben A, Mychalczak B: Brachytherapy for non-small cell lung cancer and selected neoplasms of the chest. Chest 112:2765–2865, 1997.
10. Sanchez R, vanSonnenberg E, D'Agostino H, et al: Percutaneous tissue ablation by radiofrequency thermal energy as a prelim to tumour ablation. Min Invas Therap 2:299–305, 1993.
11. Hilaris BS: Lung brachytherapy: An overview and current indications. Chest Surg Clin North Am 4:45–53, 1994.
12. Chon KS, vanSonnenberg E, D'Agostino HB, et al: CT-guided percutaneous catheter drainage of loculated thoracic air collections in patients with severe pulmonary compromise. Presented at the 79th Scientific Assembly and Annual Meeting of the Radiological Society of North America, Chicago, IL, November 28th through December 3rd, 1993.
13. vanSonnenberg E, D'Agostino H, Casola G, et al: Lung abscess: CT-guided drainage. Radiology 178:347–351, 1991.
14. Al-Salem AH, Ali EA: Computed tomography–guided percutaneous needle aspiration of lung abscesses in neonates and children. Pediatr Surg Int 12:417–419, 1997.
15. Rumbak M, Kohler G, Eastrige C, et al: Topical treatment of life-threatening haemoptysis from aspergillomas. Thorax 51:253–255, 1996.
16. vanSonnenberg E, Casola G, D'Agostino HB, et al: Interventional radiology in the chest. Chest 102:608–612, 1992.
17. Werneck K, Vassallo P, Peters PE, vonBassewitz DB: Mediastinal tumors: Biopsy under US guidance. Radiology 172:473–476, 1989.
18. Ikezoe J, Morimoto S, Arisawa J, et al: Percutaneous biopsy of thoracic lesions: Value of sonography for needle guidance. AJR 154:1181–1185, 1990.
19. Saltiel AA, Matalon TAS, Turner DA: MR-guided needle biopsy of mediastinal mass. J Intervent Radiol 5:165–166, 1990.
20. Gardner D, vanSonnenberg E, D'Agostino HB, et al: CT-guided transthoracic needle biopsy. Cardiovas Intervent Radiol 14:17–23, 1991.
21. Cameron DC: Modified "Tores" biopsy needle use in CT-guided mediastinal and paraspinal biopsy. Australas Radiol 33:101–104, 1989.
22. Glassberg RM, Sussman SK, Glickstein MF: CT anatomy of the internal mammary vessels: Importance in planning percutaneous transthoracic procedures. AJR 155:397–400, 1990.
23. vanSonnenberg E, Casola G, Ho M, et al: Difficult thoracic lesions: CT-guided biopsy experience in 150 cases. Radiology 167:457–461, 1988.
24. de Gregorio Ariza MA, Alfonso Aguiran ER, Villavieja Atance JL, et al: Transthoracic aspiration biopsy of pulmonary and mediastinal lesions. Eur J Radiol 12:98–103, 1991.
25. Herman SJ, Holub RV, Weisbrod GL, Chamberlain DW: Anterior mediastinal masses: Utility of transthoracic needle biopsy. Radiology 180:167–170, 1991.
26. Weisbrod GL: Percutaneous fine-needle aspiration biopsy of the mediastinum. Clin Chest Med 8:27–41, 1987.
27. Swanson DC, Wittich GR: CT-guided transsternal biopsy of a mediastinal mass. J Intervent Radiol 5:163–164, 1990.
28. Westcott JL: Percutaneous transthoracic needle biopsy. Radiology 169:593–601, 1988.
29. Harrow EM, Oldenburg FA, Lingenfelter MS, Smith AM: Transbronchial needle aspiration in clinical practice: A five-year experience. Chest 96:1269–1272, 1989.
30. Gay PC, Brutinel WM: Transbronchial needle aspiration in the practice of bronchoscopy. Mayo Clinic Proc 64:158–162, 1989.
31. Mehta AC, Kavuru MS, Meeker DP, et al: Transbronchial needle aspiration for histology specimens. Chest 96:1228–1232, 1989.
32. Wagner ED, Ramzy I, Greenberg SD, Gonzalez JM: Transbronchial fine-needle aspiration. Reliability and limitations. Am J Clin Pathol 92:36–41, 1989.
33. Pattison CW, Westaby, S, Wetter A, Townsend ER: Mediastinoscopy in the investigation of primary mediastinal lymphadenopathy. Scand J Thorac Cardiovasc Surg 23:177–179, 1989.
34. Ginsberg RJ: Evaluation of the mediastinum by invasive techniques. Surg Clin North Am 67:1025–1035, 1987.
35. Eastlund DT: Sternal-manubrial separation as a complication of marrow aspiration in a patient with protein-calorie malnutrition and osteoporosis. Acta Haematol 83:42–44, 1990.
36. Bakir F: Fatal sternal puncture: Report of a case. Dis Chest 44:435–439, 1963.
37. Pascali VL, Lazzaro P, Fiori A: Is a sternal bone marrow biopsy still a hazardous technique? Report of three further fatal cases. Am J Forensic Med Pathol 8:42–44, 1987
38. Burke CM, Safai C, Nelson DP, Raffin TA: Pulmonary arteriove-

nous malformations: A critical update. Am Rev Resp Dis 134: 334–339, 1986.
39. Porstmann W: Therapeutic embolization of arteriovenous pulmonary fistula by catheter technique. *In* Kelop O (ed). Current Concepts in Pediatric Radiology. Berlin, Springer, 1997, pp 23–31.
40. White RI Jr, Lynch-Nyhan A, Terry P, et al: Pulmonary arteriovenous malformations: Techniques and long-term outcome of embolotherapy. Radiology 169:663–669, 1988.
41. Chilvers ER, Whyte MKB, Jackson JE, et al: Effect of percutaneous transcatheter embolization on pulmonary function, right-to-left shunt, and arterial oxygenation in patients with pulmonary arteriovenous malformations. Am Rev Respir Dis 142:420–425, 1990.
42. Remy J, Remy-Jardin M, Wattine L, Deffontaines C: Pulmonary arteriovenous malformations: Evaluation with CT of the chest before and after treatment. Radiology 182:809–816, 1992.
43 Remy J, Remy-Jardin M, Giraud F, Wattine L: Angioarchitecture of pulmonary arteriovenous malformations: Clinical utility of three-dimensional helical CT. Radiology 191:657–664, 1994.
44. Barzilai B, Waggoner AD, Spessert C, et al: Two-dimensional contrast echocardiography in the detection and follow-up of congenital pulmonary arteriovenous malformations. Am J Cardiol 68:1507–1510, 1991.
45. Chuang VP, Wallace S, Gianturco C, et al: Complications of coil embolization: Prevention and management. Am J Roentgenol 137:809–813, 1981.
46 White RI Jr, Pollak JS, Wirth JA: Pulmonary arteriovenous malformations: Diagnosis and transcatheter embolotherapy. J Vasc Intervent Rad 7:787–804, 1996.
47. Remy-Jardin M, Wattine L, Remy J: Transcatheter occlusion of pulmonary arterial circulation and collateral supply: Failures, incidents, and complications. Radiology 18:699–705, 1991.
48. Teragaki M, Akioka K, Yasuda M, et al: Case report hereditary hemorrhagic telangiectasia with growing pulmonary arteriovenous fistulas followed for 24 years. Am J Med Sci 295:545–547, 1988.
49. Remy J, Arnaud A, Fardou H, et al: Treatment of hemoptysis by embolization of bronchial arteries. Radiology 122:33–37, 1977.
50. Uflacker R, Kaemmerer A, Picon P, et al: Bronchial artery embolization in the management of hemoptysis: Technical aspects and long-term results. Radiology 157:637–644, 1985.
51. Uflacker R, Kaemmerer A, Neves C, et al: Management of massive hemoptysis by bronchial artery embolization. Radiology 146:627–634, 1983.
52. Vujic I, Pile R, Parker E, et al: Control of massive hemoptysis by embolization of intercostal arteries. Radiology 137:617–621, 1980.
53. Jardin M, Remy J: Control of hemoptysis: Systemic angiography and anastomoses of the internal mammary artery. Radiology 168:377–383, 1988.
54. Cohen AM, Doershuk CF, Stern RC: Bronchial artery embolization to control hemoptysis cystic fibrosis. Radiology 175:401–405, 1990.
55. Matsumoto AH, Sohocki PV, Barth CH: Technical note: Superselective Gelfoam embolotherapy using a highly visible small caliber catheter. Cardiovasc Intervent Radiol 11:303–306, 1988.
56. Hayakawa K, Tanaka F, Torizuka T, et al: Bronchial artery embolization for hemoptysis: Immediate and long-term results. Cardiovasc Intervent Radiol 15:154–159, 1992.

COMMENTARY

Stephen R. Hazelrigg

This chapter nicely reviews a variety of techniques now used routinely by invasive radiologists. In many cases, they may complement the effort of the thoracic surgeon, and a team approach generally yields the best results for the patient. Indications in several areas remain controversial. The percutaneous needle biopsy (PNB) of lung nodules has proven safe, but in many places is overused. A definitive benign diagnosis is obtained by PNB in less than 20% of cases, and in most patients a diagnosis of malignancy leads to a thoracic surgical procedure. Hence, PNB avoids a surgical procedure in only a small percentage of cases and is often an unneccessary step that may cause some degree of morbidity (i.e., pneumothorax). We prefer to reserve PNB for nonsurgical candidates, for diagnosis of metastases, or for patients in whom there is a high suspicion of a nonsurgical diagnosis.

The role of mediastinal node biopsy is still evolving. In most patients, a diagnosis can be obtained by transbronchial biopsy. The radiologic needle biopsy must be weighed against other options, such as cervical mediastinoscopy and thoracoscopic techniques.

The use of catheter drainage for empyema has proven valuable during the fibropurulent phase, in which there are multiple loculations. This procedure is performed after chest tube drainage has been attempted. How this compares with thoracoscopic video-assisted thoracic surgery (VATS) debridement and drainage is not known, but for good-risk patients we have opted for VATS drainage and have used radiologically guided drains for subsequent loculations.

Overall, this chapter provides a valuable assessment of the role of the radiology service in thoracic surgery. Knowing the options for treatment will allow us to make better informed decisions in managing the problems of our patients.

Section VII

Cardiac Surgery

Chapter 49

Pioneering Minimally Invasive Coronary Surgery: A Historical Perspective

Evgenii V. Kolesov

The modern features of minimally invasive coronary artery surgery did not appear all at once. Bricks of the building were tempered from time to time in different and often far distant kilns.

Precursors

A typical textbook from the early 20th century, *Lehrbuch der Chirurgie,* edited by Wullstein and Wilms,[96] contains only a short chapter describing heart wounds. However, in that same year (1910) Alexis Carrel[20] published a description of the first experimental coronary artery grafting procedure. He created a shunt between the descending aorta and the left coronary artery using a free carotid artery graft. At a time when even pneumothorax was considered a very serious problem, Carrel's efforts must have looked like the visions of a far-sighted genius. Despite Carrel's efforts, full-fledged experimental studies obviously directed to the clinical use of coronary artery bypass grafting did not appear until the middle of the century.

Early Experiments

Starting in the 1940s, Murray[74–76] developed a number of direct suture anastomoses of systemic arteries, including the internal mammary artery, to the coronary artery, as well as procedures involving free arterial grafting. Studies from 1956 to 1965 aimed not just to solve the immediate suturing problems but also to protect against jeopardizing the coronary circulation.[1, 8, 9, 15, 28, 29, 31, 63, 71, 73, 83, 88, 90] These studies first used blood perfusion or autoperfusion to prevent cardiac fibrillation, then moved on to cardiopulmonary bypass and cardioplegia to achieve a motionless arterial target for the suturing process.

The idea of rapid revascularization of the coronary artery, thereby preventing serious disturbances in the function of the heart, represented another step toward minimally invasive coronary artery bypass grafts. Rapid anastomoses were first created with nonsuture instruments (e.g., tubes, cannulas, rings).[7, 9, 21, 24, 27] A pioneer of experimental surgery, V. P. Demikhov in Moscow, successfully performed a left internal mammary artery–to–left anterior descending coronary artery anastomosis by means of a cannula on the beating heart of a dog in 1953.[23]

Meanwhile, other groups attempted to accelerate suturing techniques with automatic suturing instruments. This work was conducted mainly in Russia.[4, 79, 80] In 1965, Amosova and Sinyakin[3] used a circular vessel-suturing apparatus (VCA-4 or ASC-4, the Russian abbreviation) in experimental studies in dogs, but not clinically. At the same time, Kahn and colleagues[32] experimented with Russian and American vascular staplers for coronary anastomoses in calves, with promising results. Further work was delayed until recent renewed efforts by Tulleken and colleagues,[91] Werker and Kon,[94] Nataf and colleagues,[77, 78] and others.

Origins of Contemporary Minimally Invasive Coronary Artery Bypass Grafts

The following is a reminiscence of W. Longmire, one of the pioneers of coronary surgery in the 1950s[68, 93]: "At the time we were doing the coronary thromboendarterectomy procedure, I think we also performed a couple of the earliest internal mammary artery to coronary anastomoses. We were forced into it when the coronary artery that we were endarterectomizing disintegrated, and in desperation, we anastomosed the internal mammary artery to the distal end of the right coronary artery and later decided that it was a good operation."

In 1961, Goetz and colleagues[27] described their experiments with nonsutured internal mammary artery anastomoses. In the addendum to their paper, they reported a clinical case of joining the right internal mammary artery to the right coronary artery on the beating heart by means of a tantalum ring. In a personal communication to Olearchyk,[79] Goetz reported that it took 17 minutes to establish the ring connection and that catheterization 2 weeks after surgery confirmed the patency of the anastomosis. The patient was put on anticoagulants and remained symptom free for more than 1 year. He later developed a fatal inferior myocardial infarction; there was no autopsy. Further trials were not performed. In 1973, Garrett and colleagues reported a case of saphenous vein graft performed on a beating heart 9 years earlier in

1964.[26] These various attempts, however, did not encourage less invasive surgery at the time.

The only group whose work steadily reflected the concepts on minimally invasive coronary surgery was the clinic in St. Petersburg (then Leningrad), where substantial creative research was directed by Professor Vasilii I. Kolesov. Olearchyk[80] described many activities of this pioneer and recognized him as "the founder of coronary revascularization." Kolesov (Fig. 49–1) became involved in the treatment of ischemic heart disease in the mid-1950s. He first used the Fieschi operation (i.e., ligation of both internal mammary arteries in the hope of increasing collateral flow to the mediastinal and coronary arteries).[40, 43] Next he used the Vineberg procedure (i.e., tunneling of bleeding internal mammary arteries into the left ventricle wall).[43, 65, 95] Finally, Kolesov introduced direct suturing anastomoses between internal mammary arteries and coronary arteries.[41, 45, 47, 48] He performed the first such procedure in February 1964, and until May 1967, Kolesov's clinic was the only site where coronary revascularization was systematically performed.[80] The key principle that governed this group was characterized by Kolesov in the monograph *Surgery of the Coronary Arteries* (1977): "Our scientific opinions are based on our own clinical experience, accumulation of facts and its thorough analysis."[51]

Kolesov's clinic experimented with various coronary bypass techniques (Table 49–1): mammary-coronary anastomoses in combination with tunneling of the mammary artery (1965),[43] use of the gastroepiploic artery for Vineberg procedures (1966),[46] retrograde (1968)[61] and bilateral internal mammary anastomoses (1969),[80] and the use of abdominal arteries for grafting on an experimental basis.[64] He also pioneered the use of internal mammary artery–coronary artery anastomoses for treatment of acute myocardial infarction and preinfarction conditions.[54, 60]

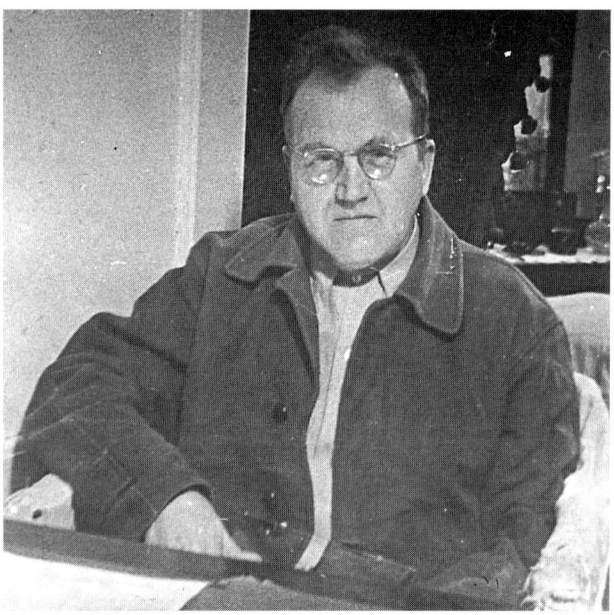

Figure 49–1. Professor Vasilii I. Kolesov in the mid-1950s when he started working in the field of coronary revascularization.

Kolesov's group gradually dispersed after Kolesov retired in 1976, and he died in 1992. Because his key works are published in Russian and are not easily accessible, it seems fitting to cite his concepts in this chapter.

Kolesov's Milestones

Kolesov was probably the first investigator to realize that coronary intervention in a clinical setting could be less dangerous than an analogous experimental procedure. In his 1966 monograph he wrote, "Artificial perfusion of coronary arteries, while extremely important in animal studies, is not always necessary in clinical practice."[43] This insight motivated Kolesov to begin clinical experiments on "beating heart" coronary artery bypass grafts.[40–45, 47–49, 55]

Basic Techniques. Kolesov compared suture and nonsuture techniques and concluded that "connecting cannulas are too crude to create anastomosis in vessels with a diameter of 1 to 1.5 mm."[51] Also, "Our experimental and clinical experience showed that anastomosis with sutures has advantages, and this is our method of choice."[43]

The Conduit. Because of Kolesov's extensive experience with the internal mammary artery in various revascularization procedures (e.g., the Fieschi and Vineberg operations),[40, 43, 46] he held to this preference, even when studies elsewhere used free vein grafts.[25] He had a chance to meet with Dr. Rene Favaloro (Fig. 49–2), but in general, he was devoted to arterial grafting,[49, 58, 64] and he wrote a chapter titled "Free Transplantation of Autologous Arteries in Aorto-Coronary Bypass" in his 1977 monograph.[51]

Indications. To Kolesov, surgical treatment of ischemic heart disease was always palliative; he believed that it was impossible to cure the entire arterial wall or to halt the progression of atherosclerosis. Kolesov wrote, "The chase for surgical repair of all involved coronary arteries is barely reasonable."[51] Thus, Kolesov insisted that the surgeon must treat life-threatening lesions and restore circulation to the most damaged segments of the coronary arteries.[50, 52, 53, 56, 62] He believed that complete occlusions or subocclusions were absolute indications for coronary intervention.[50, 51, 59] He also believed that major anatomic damage must be ameliorated, even in the face of fair clinical function. He advised that lesser stenoses be assessed, for instance, by using simple needle punctures to study endovascular pressures.[48] Today, sophisticated pressure and flow wire probes are used for the same purpose,[81] and some recent studies have challenged compulsory complete revascularization.[10, 92]

Coronary Angiography. Kolesov's first patients (cited in 1966–1967) underwent surgery without coronary angiography.[43, 48] This probably had a lasting influence on Kolesov. He neither overestimated nor underestimated the value of this technique. He wrote, "Concerning the severity of pathological alterations of the vessel wall itself,

Table 49–1. Beating Heart Coronary Artery Bypass Grafts at the Clinic Directed by V. I. Kolesov (1964–1975)

Date	Procedure	Stapler	Access	CPB
IMA-CORONARY ANASTOMOSIS				
Chronic Ischemic Heart Disease				
Feb. 25, 1964	IMA-coronary (branch of circumflex artery) suture end-to-end anastomosis	No	Thoracotomy	No
Jan. 26, 1965	IMA-LAD suture end-to-side anastomosis with tunneling IMA into myocardium	No	Thoracotomy	No
Mar. 22, 1967	First stapler-facilitated IMA-LAD anastomosis	ASC-4	Thoracotomy	No
Dec. 11, 1968	Retrograde IMA-LAD anastomosis	ASC-4	Sternotomy	No
June 10, 1969	Double IMA anastomosis	ASC-4	Thoracotomy	No
Mar. 5, 1970	Double IMA-LAD anastomosis: from left IMA ante- and retrograde	ASC-4	Thoracotomy	No
Jan. 21, 1971	First vacuum stapler–facilitated IMA-LAD anastomosis	ASC-v	Thoracotomy	No
Acute Ischemic Heart Disease				
Feb. 5, 1968	IMA-LAD suture end-to-end anastomosis	No	Thoracotomy	No
May 17, 1968	IMA-LAD suture end-to-side anastomosis	No	Thoracotomy	No
May 21, 1968	IMA-LAD anastomosis	ASC-4	Thoracotomy	No
Feb. 11, 1972	AMI with clinical death IMA-LAD anastomosis	ASC-v	Sternotomy	No
Jan. 28, 1975	AMI with pulmonary edema; IMA-LAD anastomosis bypass	ASC-v	Sternotomy	13 min
AORTOCORONARY BYPASS WITH VEIN OR FREE AFTERIAL GRAFTS				
June 16, 1971	Aorta-RCA bypass with autoartery superficial femoral artery (substituted with transplant of great saphenous vein); suture connection end-to-end	No	Sternotomy	Yes, with iliac artery blood return
Jan. 19, 1972	Aorta-RCA autovein bypass	ASC-4	Sternotomy	Yes
	+			
	IMA-LAD suture end-to-side anastomosis	No		No
Feb. 22, 1972	Aorta-RCA autovein bypass	ASC-4	Sternotomy	Yes
	+			
	IMA-LAD anastomosis	ASC-v		Yes
Mar. 1, 1973	Aorta-RCA autovein bypass	ASC-v	Sternotomy	No

CPB = cardiopulmonary bypass; IMA = internal mammary artery; LAD = left anterior descending artery; AMI = acute myocardial infarction; RCA = right coronary artery

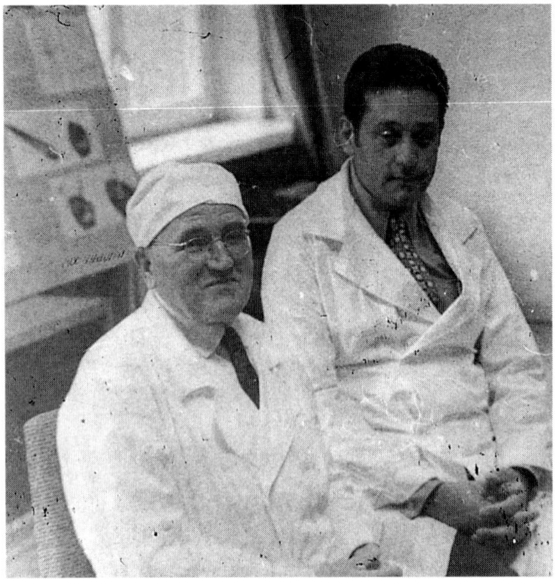

Figure 49–2. Several distinguished surgeons visited the clinic of Professor V. I. Kolesov after the 10th International Cardiovascular Congress, which took place in Moscow in August 1971. Among them was Dr. Rene Favaloro (*right*).

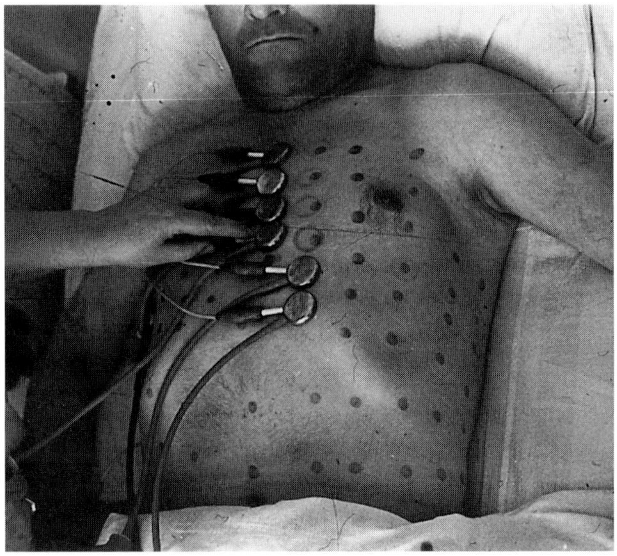

Figure 49–3. Mosaic electrocardiotopography (MECTG). Monopolar potentials were registered from more than 100 points from anterior and back surfaces of the thorax, as well as from the upper abdominal wall.

coronary angiography gives only approximate impressions. The experience of surgical interventions on coronary arteries tells that vascular walls in reality are much more damaged than would be assumed from angiographic pictures. . . . Angiography, in spite of its importance, could not be the only method of patient study or the only criterion in determining indications for surgical treatment of ischemic heart disease."[51] Kolesov's group used intraoperative epicardial ultrasonography to better localize stenoses within the coronary arteries[35, 51] and experimented with remote thermography of the heart surface as well.[36] In modern clinical practice, such complementary studies are well accepted.[82]

Noninvasive Diagnosis. The following remark by Kolesov is typical: "In the majority of publications about clinical use of mammary-coronary artery anastomosis, data from ECG studies and other non-invasive methods are scarcely mentioned. However, we pay serious attention to those methods. They can be safely repeated many times and studied comparatively."[51] Among the noninvasive methods used by Kolesov was mosaic electrocardiotopography (MECTG)[66, 95] (Fig. 49–3). This method involves registering monopolar electrocardiogram (ECG) tracings from more than 100 points around the thorax and upper abdominal wall (see Fig. 49–3). Such "electrical portraits of the heart"[2, 33, 66, 95] were correlated with angiographic patterns. Later, MECTG was connected with a bicycle system for stress testing.

The Clamping Test and Ischemic Preconditioning. Some investigative surgeons in the group claimed that the heart would be more stable after brief clamping of the coronary artery. Although this was not recognized as a preconditioning maneuver, it was used routinely as a test (Fig. 49–4). Kolesov, however, stressed its important clinical application: "To perform coronary grafting without cardiopulmonary bypass is possible if patients have significant localized narrowing of the coronary arteries and if the clamping test and ECG control are used during the operation, with registration of electrical potentials from the epicardium itself."[51]

Epicardial ECG. Epicardial ECG (EpiECG) is derived from studies of MECTG and surface potentials of the heart (Fig. 49–5) and is more sensitive than conventional

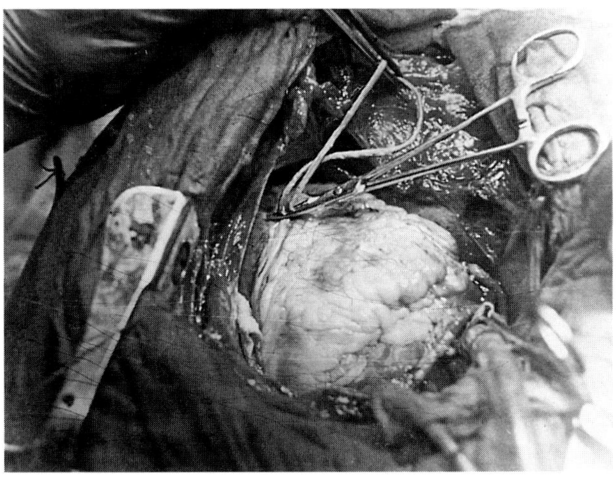

Figure 49–4. The clamping test. The coronary artery with surrounding tissues is compressed with a soft rubber tourniquet for 6 to 8 minutes. The heart activity, arterial pressure, and electrocardiogram tracings are controlled during and after the test. *Right,* an autovein stapler-facilitated aortocoronary shunt has already been performed. Also shown is a right atrium cannula for partial cardiopulmonary bypass (operation performed January 19, 1972, Table 49–1).

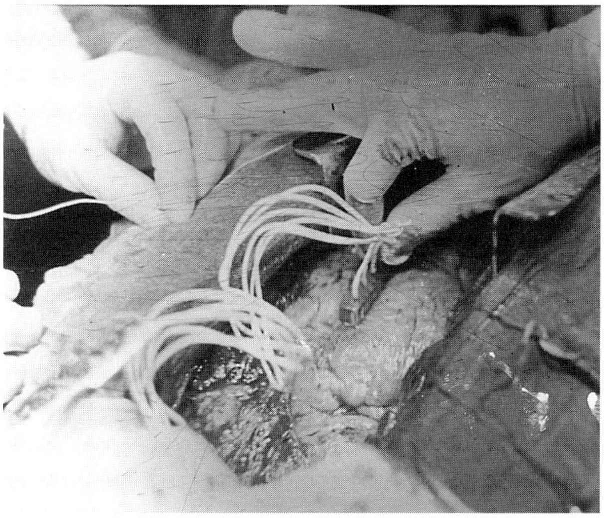

Figure 49–5. Studies of epicardial electrocardiogram during coronary revascularization operation with a 6-pin electrode.

ECG. It also better reflects the conditions of the region affected by revascularization.[39, 51] In this procedure, surface wire electrodes are used for monitoring throughout the surgical procedure and the early postoperative period (Fig. 49–6). The electrodes are treated and extracted like temporary pacemaker wires. This method has proved to be highly effective and quite simple.

Cardiopulmonary Bypass. Despite the widespread use of cardiopulmonary bypass, Kolesov preferred to avoid or at least simplify it. "For seriously ill persons, cardiopulmonary bypass is a heavy burden and it must be avoided as often as possible. For this reason the vast majority of our patients were operated upon without cardiopulmonary bypass."[51] However, Kolesov was not dogmatic (see Table 49–1). For emergency operations and for right coronary grafting, he used partial cardiopulmonary bypass through a standard sternotomy (Fig. 49–7; see Fig. 49–4). If cardiopulmonary bypass was necessary when a thoracotomy approach was used, a single large cannula was inserted through the right ventricle conus or pulmonary artery. Arterial return was established preferably through the external iliac artery, but sometimes through the femoral artery.

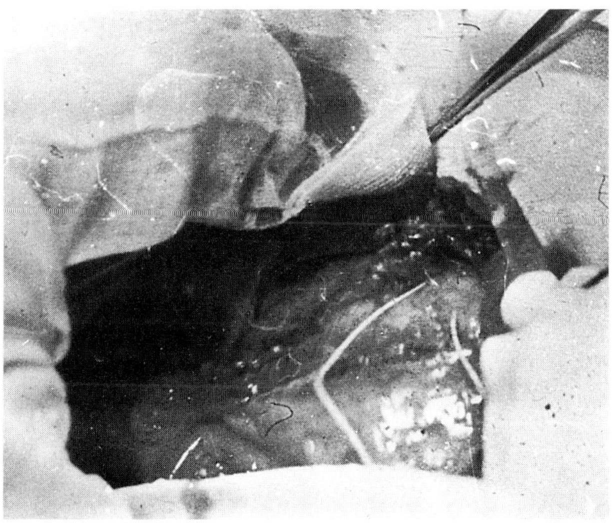

Figure 49–6. Wire epicardial electrodes were used for control of the situation in the region of revascularization during the clamping test and the coronary bypass procedure and in the early postoperative period.

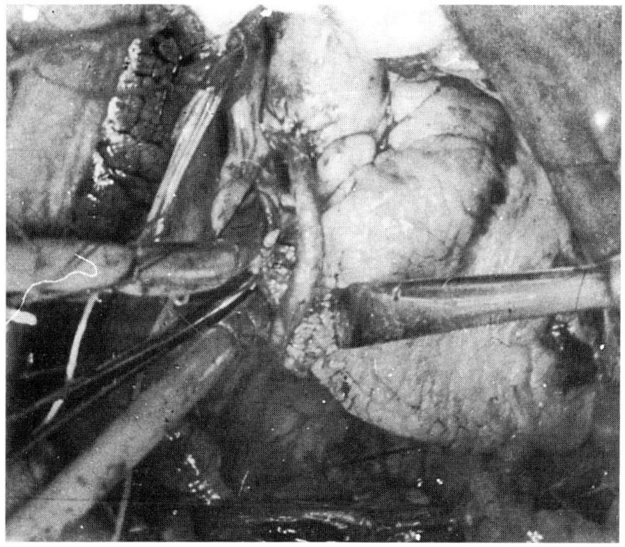

Figure 49–7. Autoarterial aortocoronary shunting with partial cardiopulmonary bypass. Oxygenated blood return was established through the right iliac artery (operation performed June 16, 1971, Table 49–1).

The Beating Heart and Stabilization. Kolesov's first cases were often performed with end-to-end suture techniques, with the arteries lifted off the heart for stabilization. In end-to-side anastomoses, a simple hand-and-loop stabilization was applied. In these early days, it would have been difficult to imagine that the doctrine of stabilization would reach the enormous scale of today's clinical practice.[14, 18, 30, 86] Because Kolesov often used interrupted sutures, a faulty stitch could easily be removed and replaced. The group later turned to mechanical suturing devices.[57]

Staplers. After 2 years of animal research, V. I. Kolesov and E. V. Kolesov began using the ASC-4 stapler clinically in 1967 (Fig. 49–8; see Table 49–1). Although this device could produce a functioning anastomosis in about 2 to 3 minutes, the method had serious drawbacks. It required prolonged training, and arteries had to be completely everted. This maneuver was too crude for sclerotic arteries; hence I proposed to use suction to maintain the ends of the arteries in an everted position. Although this idea was initially met with great skepticism, we were able to maintain the arteries everted up to 90 degrees. Several models of suction staplers were produced and patented, starting in 1970[34, 37, 38] (Fig. 49–9). In clinical practice,

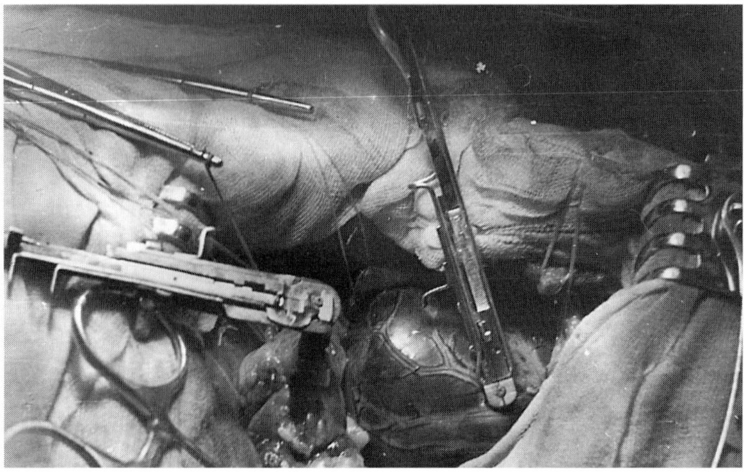

Figure 49–8. In this experiment, a completely everted arterial end is held with mechanical pincers in an ASC-4 stapler (*left*). A similar result was achieved with a vacuum stapler (*right*) on a shorter portion of coronary artery that was gently and "automatically" held over a flat head of the stapler. The latter is simpler and more solid.

these staplers were used to produce end-to-end anastomoses for occluded or suboccluded (about 90% stenosis) coronary arteries (Figs. 49–10 and 49–11).

The Era of Minimally Invasive Coronary Artery Bypass Grafts

In the last two decades, minimally invasive procedures have burst into all domains of general and thoracic surgery, including interventional cardiology and cardiovascular surgery. Trapp and Bisarya[89] and Ankeney[5] in 1975 and several later groups[6, 67, 72] surveyed ways of avoiding cardiopulmonary bypass. Wide clinical application of off-pump coronary grafting was pioneered in South America by Benetti and colleagues[11, 12] and Buffolo and colleagues[16] and spread widely. This evolved into minimally invasive direct coronary grafting with the efforts of investigators such as Subramanian,[86] Robinson and colleagues,[84] Calafiore and colleagues,[17–19] Jansen,[30] and Yim and Liu.[97] Introduction of video assistance by Mack[69, 70] and Nataf[78] and their colleagues greatly reduced the invasiveness of the procedure and developed it further. Recently, robotics have emerged as means to expand these techniques,[22, 85] and complete thoracoscopic coronary surgery is on the threshold.

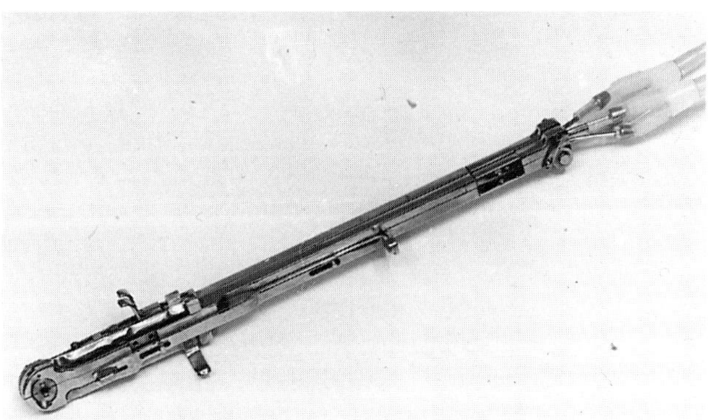

Figure 49–9. A late-model vacuum stapler with four independent suction lines and the ability to grip the artery end and lock the machine with one hand.

Epilogue

The development of coronary artery surgery covers practically the entire 20th century, with the intervals between breakthroughs becoming progressively shorter. However, one can see a distressing gap between origination and general acceptance of ideas regarding less invasive coronary surgery. Information was widely available in international journals, but the preoccupation with vein bypass grafting and obligatory cardiopulmonary bypass was too strong, and the alternatives were overlooked for many years. At last, the value of prior experiences has been recognized, and the field is progressing based on previously overshadowed principles.

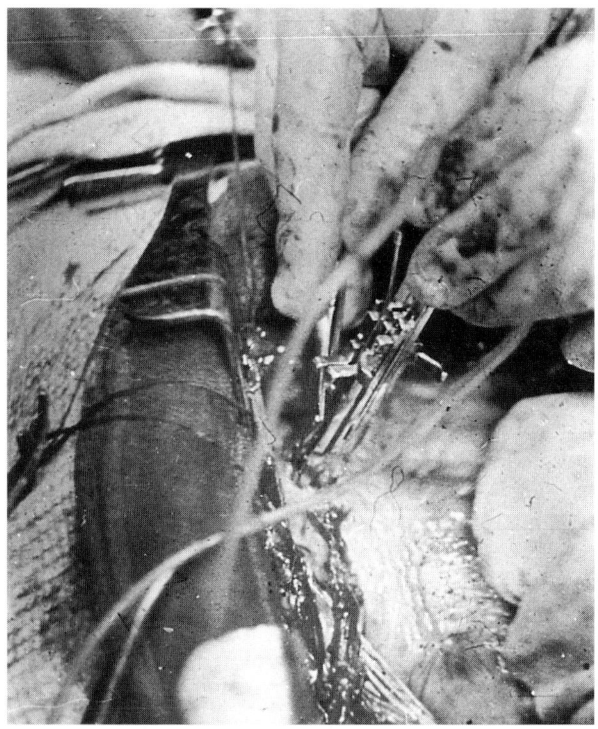

Figure 49–10. Mammary artery to coronary artery (left anterior descending artery [LAD]) anastomosis with vacuum stapler (seen between suction tubes of the instrument).

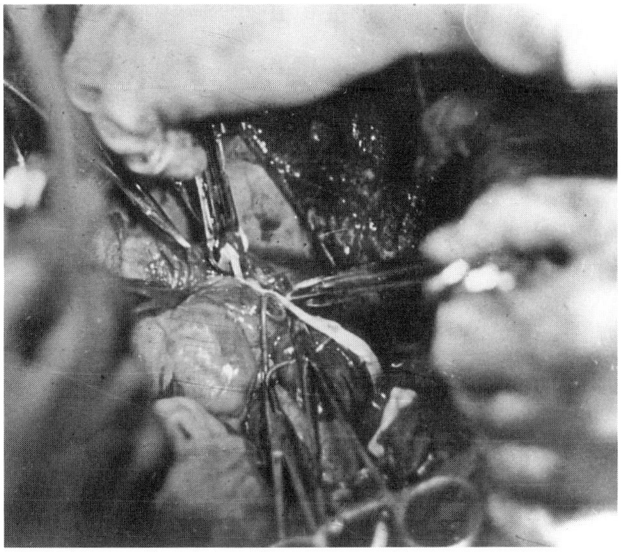

Figure 49–11. The stapler connection of the autovein graft (seen as a white strip) to the right coronary artery.

References

1. Absolon KB, Aust JB, Varco RL, Lillehei CW: Surgical treatment of occlusive coronary artery disease by endarterectomy or anastomotic replacement. Surg Gynecol Obstet 103:180–185, 1956.
2. Amirov RZ: Electrocardiotopography [Russian]. Moscow, Meditsina Publishers, 1965.
3. Amosova VV, Sinyakin SI: Mechanical suture for the mammary coronary vascular anastomosis [Russian]. *In* The Studies in Cardiology. Gor'ky, Gor'ky Medical Institute Publishing, 1965, pp 247–254.
4. Androsov PI: Mechanical Suturing in Vascular Surgery [Russian]. Moscow, Medgiz Publishers, 1960.
5. Ankeney JL: To use or not to use the pump oxygenator in coronary bypass operations. Ann Thorac Surg 19:108–109, 1975.
6. Archer R, Ott DA, Patiravincini R, et al: Coronary revascularization without cardiopulmonary bypass. Tex Heart Inst J 11:52–57, 1984.
7. Arnulf G: Original documents on the use of internal mammary artery for myocardial revascularization. *In* Fournial G, Glock T, Roux D, Dalous PH (eds): Internal Thoracic Artery for Myocardial Revascularization. Toulouse, Paul Sabatier University Publishing, 1990, pp 19–23.
8. Baker NH, Grindlay JH: Technique of experimental systemic to coronary artery anastomosis. Staff Meeting Mayo Clin 34:497, 1959.
9. Ballinger WF, Padula RT, Fishman NH, Camishion RC: Operations upon coronary arteries: Evaluation of absorbable intra luminal gelatin tubes, sutures and tissue adhesive. J Thorac Cardiovasc Surg 48:790, 1964.
10. BARI (bypass angioplasty revascularization investigation) Investigators: Comparison of coronary bypass with angioplasty in patients with multivessel disease. N Engl J Med 335:217–225, 1996.
11. Benetti FJ, Ballester C, Sani G, et al: Video assisted coronary bypass surgery. J Card Surg 10:620–625, 1995.
12. Benetti FJ, Naselli G, Wood M, Geffner L: Direct myocardial revascularization without extracorporeal circulation: Experience in 700 patients. Chest 100:312–316, 1991.
13. Bonatti J, Hangler H: Meta analysis of results in minimally invasive coronary artery bypass grafting. Cor Europaeum 6: 150–158, 1997.
14. Borst C, Santamore WP, Smedira NG, Bredee JJ: Minimally invasive coronary artery bypass grafting: On the beating heart and via limited access. Ann Thorac Surg 63(suppl 6):S1–5, 1997.
15. Botham RG, Joung WP: An experimental study of systemic coronary anastomosis. Surg Gynecol Obstet 108:361–365, 1959.
16. Buffolo E, Andrade JCS, Branco JNR, et al: Myocardial revascularization without extracorporeal circulation: Seven year experience in 593 cases. Eur J Cardiothorac Surg 4:504–508, 1990.
17. Calafiore AM, Di Giammarco G, Teodori G, et al: Left anterior descending coronary artery grafting via left anterior small thoracotomy without cardiopulmonary bypass. Ann Thorac Surg 61:1658–1665, 1996.
18. Calafiore AM: Technique and results pre and post stabilization era. Symposium Facts and Myths of Minimally Invasive Cardiac Surgery, New Orleans, January 24, 1998, p 20.
19. Calafiore AM, Teodori G, Di Giammarco G, et al: Minimally invasive coronary artery bypass grafting on a beating heart. Ann Thorac Surg 63(suppl 6):S72–S75, 1997.
20. Carrel A: On experimental surgery of the thoracic aorta and the heart. Ann Surg 52:83–95, 1910.
21. Carter EL, Roth EJ: Direct nonsuture coronary anastomosis in the dog. Ann Surg 148:212–218, 1958.
22. Damiano R: Will robotic assistance enable us to perform totally endoscopic CABG? Symposium Facts and Myths of Minimally Invasive Cardiac Surgery, New Orleans, January 24, 1998, p 26.
23. Demikhov VP: Experimental Transplantation of Vital Organs. New York, Consultant Bureau Publishing, 1962.
24. Dmitrieva EM: Thoracico-coronary arterial anastomosis [Russian]. *In* Lavrova TF (ed): Surgical Correction of Coronary Insufficiency. Voronezh, Voronezh University Publushing, 1974, pp 100–109.
25. Favaloro R: Surgical Treatment of Coronary Arteriosclerosis. Baltimore, Williams & Wilkins, 1970, pp 1–132.
26. Garrett HE, Dennis EW, DeBakey ME: Aortocoronary bypass with saphenous vein graft: Seven years follow up. JAMA 223: 792–794, 1973.
27. Goetz RH, Rohman M, Haller JD, et al: Internal mammary coronary artery anastomosis: A non-suture method employing tantalum rings. J Thorac Cardiovasc Surg 41:378–386, 1961.
28. Gottesman L: Direct surgical relief of coronary artery occlusion. Am J Cardiol 2:315–320, 1958.
29. Hall RI, Khouri EM, Gregg DE: Coronary-internal mammary anastomosis in dogs. Surgery 50:560, 1961.
30. Jansen EWL: Towards Minimally Invasive Coronary Artery Bypass Grafting. Utrecht, University of Utrecht Publishing, 1998.
31. Julian OC, Lopez-Belio M, Moorehead D, Lima A: Direct surgical procedures on the coronary arteries: Experimental studies. J Thorac Surg 34:654–660, 1957.
32. Kahn DR, Mallina RF, Wilson WS, Sloan H: The use of the American and Russian vascular staplers for coronary artery anastomosis in calves. J Thorac Cardiovasc Surg 50:699–705, 1965.
33. Kienle FL: The electrical heart portrait. *In* IV Congressus Cardiologicus Europeus. Prague, Prague University Publishing, 1964, p 171.
34. Kolesov EV: The usage of staplers for internal thoracic artery–coronary artery anastomoses. In Fournial G, Glock I, Roux D, Dalous Ph (eds): Internal Thoracic Artery for Myocardial Revascularization. Toulouse, Paul Sabatier University Publishing, 1990, pp 217–218.
35. Kolesov EV, Dvorjashin YE. Ultrasonic detection of the atherosclerotic coronary obstructions [Russian]. Vestn Khir 11:14–18, 1970.
36. Kolesov EV, Chernjaev YS, Krasnorogov B, Chernova CD: The usage of thermovision for intraoperative diagnostic stud-

ies in the reconstructive coronary heart surgery [Russian]. *In* Miroshnikov MM, Gvozdev MP (eds): Thermo-Vision in Medicine, Vol I. Leningrad, State Optical Institute Publishing, 1976, pp 197–203.
37. Kolesov EV, Gurevich IY: The method of evertion and fixation of the end of an artery with a help of vacuum [Russian]. Patent SU No. 269408. Published by SU Patent Institute, April 17, 1970, Bulletin No. 15.
38. Kolesov EV, Smirnov BA, Fedotov VM, Lipovsky IL: Instrument for establishing vascular anastomosis. US Patent No. 4,350,160, September 21, 1982.
39. Kolesov EV, Volodkovich NG, Tokarevich KK, et al: The usage of epicardial electrocardiography in surgery of coronary arteries [Russian]. Klin Med 7:73–77, 1975.
40. Kolesov VI: Results of surgical treatment of stenocardia and acute myocardial infarction [Russian]. Vestn Khir 2:87–95, 1963.
41. Kolesov VI: Straight operations on coronary arteries [Russian]. *In* Bakulev AN (ed): Surgical Treatment of Coronary Heart Disease. Moscow, Meditsina Publishers, 1965, pp 162–166.
42. Kolesov VI: Contemporary problems in surgical treatment of coronary disease of the heart: Pamphlet of main lecture [Russian]. Leningrad, Meditsina Publishers, 1965.
43. Kolesov VI (ed): Surgical Treatment of Coronary Disease of the Heart [Russian]. Leningrad, Meditsina Publishers, 1966.
44. Kolesov VI: Coronary-thoracic arterial anastomosis as a means of treating of coronary disease of the heart [Russian]. Klin Med 7:7–12, 1966.
45. Kolesov VI: An application of coronary-thoracic vascular anastomosis in coronary disease of the heart [Russian]. *In* Kolesov VI (ed): Surgical Treatment of Cardiovascular, Neoplastic and Endocrine Diseases. Leningrad, First Medical Institute of IP Pavlov, 1967, pp 48–54.
46. Kolesov VI: Implantation of systemic arteries into the myocardium as the means of treatment of stenocardia [Russian]. *In* Kolesov VI (ed): Surgical Treatment of Cardiovascular, Neoplastic and Endocrine Diseases. Leningrad, First Medical Institute of IP Pavlov, 1967, pp 54–58.
47. Kolesov VI: The first experience in the treatment of angina pectoris by establishment of coronary-systemic vascular anastomosis [Russian]. Kardiologiia 4:20–25, 1967.
48. Kolesov VI: Mammary artery–coronary artery anastomosis as method of treatment for angina pectoris. J Thorac Cardiovasc Surg 54:535–544, 1967.
49. Kolesov VI: Replacement of occluded vitally important arteries with free arterial autotransplantation [Russian]. *In* Chronic Ischemic Heart Disease. Vilnius, Vilnius University Publishing, 1971, pp 158–164.
50. Kolesov VI: Direct myocardial revascularization in ischemic heart disease (indications, technique, results) [Russian]. Klin Med 7:35–44, 1976.
51. Kolesov VI: Surgery of the Coronary Arteries [Russian]. Leningrad, Meditsina Publishers, 1977.
52. Kolesov VI: Basic trends in the development of coronary surgery [Russian]. Vestn Khir 8:3–7, 1978.
53. Kolesov VI: Remote results of mammary-coronary arterial anastomosis [Russian]. Vestn Khir 1:49–53, 1982.
54. Kolesov VI: From ligation of the internal mammary arteries to their employment for coronary anastomosing. *In* Fournial G, Glock I, Roux D, Dalous Ph (eds): Internal Thoracic Artery for Myocardial Revascularization. Toulouse, Paul Sabatier University Publishing, 1990, pp 25–27.
55. Kolesov VI, Kolesov EV: Treatment of angina pectoris by means of mammary-coronary anastomosis. Bul Soc Int Chir 28:366–371, 1969.
56. Kolesov VI, Kolesov EV: Twenty year results with internal thoracic artery–coronary artery anastomosis. J Thorac Cardiovasc Surg 101:360–361, 1991.
57. Kolesov VI, Kolesov EV, Gurevich IY, Leosko VA: Vasosuturing apparatuses in surgery of coronary arteries [Russian]. Med Tekh 6:24–28, 1970.
58. Kolesov VI, Kolesov EV, Tsareva AN, et al: Surgery of some vitally important small arteries [Russian]. Vestn Khir 7:54–61, 1971.
59. Kolesov VI, Kolesov EV, Tsareva AN, et al: Principles of myocardial revascularization in chronic and acute coronary insufficiency [Russian]. In All-Union Scientific Cardiologic Conference Devoted to 100th Jubilee of GF Lang. Moscow, All-Union Scientific Cardiologic Society Publishing, 1975, pp 27–28.
60. Kolesov VI, Kolesov EV, Volodkovich NG: Mammary artery coronary artery anastomosis as method of treatment for angina pectoris and myocardial infarction [Russian]. Khirurgiia 1:151–152, 1970.
61. Kolesov VI, Petukhov JA: Retrograde mammary-coronary arterial anastomosis and its place among other methods of myocardium revascularization [Russian]. Vestn Khir 2:7–13, 1976.
62. Kolesov VI, Pikaleva VY, Kolesov EV, Mamedov KH: Hemodynamic changes in patients with ischemic disease of the heart before and after construction of the mammary coronary arterial anastomosis [Russian]. Kardiologiia 6:78–82, 1973.
63. Kolesov VI, Potashov LV: Operations on the coronary arteries [Russian]. Exp Chir Anaesth 10:3–8, 1965.
64. Kolesov VI, Romankova MP, Volodkovich NG, Dulaev VK: Experimental study of the coronary-systemic arterial anastomosis for possible myocardium revascularization [Russian]. Vestn Khir 3:9–14, 1975.
65. Kolesov VI, Tokarevich KK, Tsaregorodtsev AA: The usage of Vineberg operation as a source of the myocardium additional blood supply [Russian]. *In* Bakulev AN (ed): Surgical Treatment of Coronary Heart Disease. Moscow, Meditsina Publishers, 1965, pp 185–188.
66. Kolesov VI, Tsareva AN, Kolesov EV, et al: Selection of the operations on the coronary arteries for treatment of ischemic heart disease [Russian]. Vestn Khir 9:3–8, 1972.
67. Laborde F, Abdelmeguid I, Piwnica A: Aortocoronary bypass without extracorporeal circulation: Why and when? Eur J Cardiothorac Surg 3:152–155, 1989.
68. Longmire WP, Cannon JA, Kattus AA: Direct-vision coronary endarterectomy for angina pectoris. N Engl J Med 259:993–999, 1958.
69. Mack M, Aronoff RJ, Acuff TE, et al: The present role of thoracoscopy in the diagnosis and treatment of diseases of the chest. Ann Thorac Surg 54:403–409, 1992.
70. Mack M, Acuff TE, Casimir-Ahn H, et al: Video-assisted coronary bypass grafting on the beating heart. Ann Thorac Surg 63(suppl 6):S100–S103, 1997.
71. Mamiya RT, Cooper T, Willman VI, et al: Distal relocation of the origin of the left coronary artery by subclavian–left coronary anastomosis. Surg Gynecol Obstet 113:599, 1961.
72. Moshkovitz Y, Luskv A, Mohr R: Coronary artery bypass without cardiopulmonary bypass: Analysis of short-term and mid-term outcome in 220 patients. J Thorac Cardiovasc Surg 110:979–987, 1995.
73. Moore TC, Riberi A: Maintenance of coronary circulation during systemic–to–coronary artery anastomosis. Surgery 43: 245, 1958.
74. Murray G: Heparin in surgical treatment of blood vessels. Arch Surg 40:307, 1940.
75. Murray G: Surgery of coronary heart disease. Angiology 4: 526, 1953.
76. Murray G, Porcheron R, Hilario J, Roschlau W: Anastomosis of a systemic artery to the coronary. Can Med Assoc J 71:594, 1954.
77. Nataf P, Kirsch W, Hill AC, et al: Nonpenetrating clips for coronary anastomosis. Ann Surg 63(suppl 6):S135–S137, 1997.

78. Nataf P, Lima L, Regan M, et al: Minimally invasive coronary surgery with thoracoscopic internal mammary dissection: Surgical technique. J Card Surg 11:288–292, 1996.
79. Olearchyk AS: Coronary revascularization: Past, present and future [Ukrainian]. J Ukr Med Assoc North Am 35:3–34, 1988.
80. Olearchyk AS: Vasilii I. Kolesov: A pioneer of coronary revascularization by internal mammary–coronary artery grafting. J Thorac Cardiovasc Surg 96:13–18, 1988.
81. Pfister AJ, Zaki MS, Garcia JM, et al: Coronary artery bypass without cardiopulmonary bypass. Ann Thorac Surg 54:1085–1092, 1992.
81a. Pijls NHJ, Willem Bech J, De Bruyne B, van Straten A: Clinical assessment of functional stenosis severity: Use of coronary pressure measurements for the decision to bypass a lesion. Ann Surg 63(suppl 6):S6–S11, 1997.
82. Pirolo JS, Fredi JL, Shuman TA, et al: Intracoronary ultrasound-guided CABG in patients with angiographically noncritical lesions. Ann Thorac Surg 64:375–379, 1997.
83. Pronin VI, Dobrova NB, Zingerman LS: Revascularization of the heart by means of straight reconstructive operations on the coronary arteries [Russian]. *In* Creation of Organ Anastomoses in Experiment and Clinic. Ryazan', Ryazan' Medical Institute Publishing, 1962, pp 97–101.
84. Robinson MC, Gross DR, Zeman W, Steje-Larsen E: Minimally invasive coronary artery bypass grafting: A new method using an anterior mediastinotomy. J Card Surg 10:529–536, 1995.
85. Shennib H: Telemanipulation enhances precision in minimally invasive cardiac surgery. Symposium Facts and Myths of Minimally Invasive Cardiac Surgery, New Orleans, January 24, 1998, p 25.
86. Subramanian VA: Less invasive arterial CABG on a beating heart. Ann Thorac Surg 63(suppl 6):S68–S71, 1997.
87. Subramanian VA, Sani G, Benetti FJ, Calafiore AM: Minimally invasive coronary artery bypass surgery: A multicenter report of preliminary experience. Circulation 92(suppl 1):645, 1995.
88. Thal A, Perry JF, Miller FA, Wangensteen OH: Direct suture anastomosis of the coronary arteries in the dog. Surgery 40: 1023–1029, 1956.
89. Trapp WG, Bisarya R: Placement of coronary artery bypass graft without pump oxygenator. Ann Thorac Surg 19:1–9, 1975.
90. Tsoy AA: Anastomosis of the internal mammary artery with the coronary artery and curettage of the latter in experiment [Russian]. *In* Bakulev AN (ed): Surgical Treatment of Coronary Heart Disease. Moscow, Meditsina Publishers, 1965, pp 171–174.
91. Tulleken CAF, Verdaasdonk RM, Mansvelt Beck HJ: Nonocclusive excimer laser–assisted end-to-side anastomosis. Ann Surg 63(suppl 6):S138–S142, 1997.
92. Van Brussel BL, Plokker HWM, Voors AA, et al: Different clinical outcome in coronary artery bypass with single and sequential vein grafts: A fifteen-year follow-up study. J Thorac Cardiovasc Surg 112:69–78, 1996.
93. Westaby S: Coronary surgery without cardiopulmonary bypass. Br Heart J 73:203–205, 1995.
94. Werker PMN, Kon M: Review of facilitated approaches to vascular anastomosis surgery. Ann Surg 63(suppl 6):S122–S127, 1997.
95. Volodkovich NG, Kolesov EV: The usage of mosaic electrocardiotopography for detection of localized myocardial damaged areas [Russian]. Kardiologiia 11:99–103, 1973.
96. Wullstein, Wilms (eds): Lehrbuch der Chirurgie, Zweite umgearbeitet Auflage, Erster Band. Jena, Verlag G. Fischer, 1910.
97. Yim AP, Liu HP: Complications and failures of video-assisted thoracic surgery: Experience from two centres in Asia. Ann Thorac Surg 61:538–541, 1996.

COMMENTARY

W. Gerald Rainer

In this chapter, Professor Kolesov has made a valuable contribution to the history of the development of surgery for myocardial revascularization. He recounts the role of his father, Vasilii Kolesov, who was a pioneer in the use of the internal mammary artery for myocardial revascularization and performed the first internal mammary–coronary anastomosis in humans. Evgenii Kolesov has also contributed to a more complete bibliography on this topic by including many articles in the European and Russian literature that are not usually acknowledged by current writers.

Although this chapter speaks to the issue of minimally invasive coronary surgery, much of Vasilii Kolesov's work and the work of other pioneers cannot accurately be called "minimally invasive." Certainly there were many attempts in the early days of coronary bypass surgery in both experimental animals and humans to omit the use of extracorporeal circulation, and this has had some return to acceptance. It is my opinion, however, that the place of minimally invasive coronary surgery has not yet been accurately defined and will be clarified only after careful study of the long-term results (5 to 10 years) regarding the patency of anastomoses performed on delicate vessels under less than ideal circumstances.

The contributors to this text are to be given credit for examining all aspects of coronary surgery (historical, experimental, and clinical) and attempting to put the role of minimally invasive coronary surgery into its present perspective and lay the groundwork for the definition of its role in the future.

Chapter 50

Patient Selection for Minimally Invasive Coronary Artery Bypass

Valavanur A. Subramanian

The surgical treatment of coronary artery disease is constantly undergoing alteration and refinement in order to meet the changing clinical challenges brought on by an aging population with recurrent disease, the competitive status of coronary stenting, and the need for cost containment in cardiac surgery. Because of this, clinical interest in less or minimally invasive coronary artery bypass surgery has grown.[1, 6–8] These procedures fall into two categories:

1. Beating heart surgery using local coronary occlusion without cardiopulmonary bypass either by (a) minimally invasive direct coronary artery bypass (MIDCAB) grafting with strategically placed minimal access incisions, that is, mini left and right thoracotomy (left internal mammary artery [LIMA] to left anterior descending artery [LAD] and right internal mammary artery [RIMA] to right coronary artery [RCA] grafts), mini-sternotomy for LAD-RCA grafting, subxiphoid incision (right gastroepiploic artery to distal RCA or posterior descending artery [PDA]), and mini left lateral thoracotomy (radial artery graft from descending aorta to marginal branches); or (b) coronary artery bypass graft (CABG) via midline sternotomy without cardiopulmonary bypass (off-pump CABG).
2. Port access bypass surgery via mini-thoracotomy with peripheral cannulation, cardiopulmonary bypass, endoluminal ascending aortic occlusion, and cardioplegic arrest.

The advantages of port access include no sternotomy and the ability to perform multivessel grafting with coronary anastomosis on a stopped heart in a bloodless field analogous to conventional CABG. However, the disadvantages include the requirement for cardiopulmonary bypass and its attendant significant complications, the potential for retrograde aortic dissection and atherosclerotic emboli from cannulation, a steeper learning curve, and the expense for necessary equipment.

The advantages of MIDCAB include no sternotomy, no cardiopulmonary bypass, and no manipulation of the aorta. The disadvantages of MIDCAB include limited application (single vessel, i.e., LAD, RCA, PDA) and a significant learning curve (internal mammary artery [IMA] harvest and anastomosis on a beating heart).

The advantages of off-pump full sternotomy CABG include elimination of cardiopulmonary bypass, potential for multivessel grafting, and, ideally, the avoidance of aortic manipulation by relying exclusively on arterial graft conduits. Disadvantages of this approach involve the difficulty of approaching the posterior vessels in a predictable manner.

The premise for adopting these less invasive approaches is that patient morbidity can be reduced without compromising the safety and efficacy of CABG. Despite encouraging early clinical results,[2–5, 10] CABG without cardiopulmonary bypass via midline sternotomy or mini-thoracotomy has raised concerns about technical limitations and the efficacy of anastomosis. Recently, the introduction of surgical instrumentation to facilitate IMA harvest via mini-thoracotomy and mechanical local immobilization and stabilization of the coronary artery during anastomosis in beating heart surgery has enabled the standardization of surgical techniques with predictable good results.[9]

The incidence of retrograde aortic dissection and migration of the endoaortic balloon in the port access technique has been reduced by modifications in catheter designs and the introduction of central cannulation techniques via mini-thoracotomy incision.

Owing to its evolutionary nature, no indications or contraindications for minimally invasive CABG can be generalized; this depends on the surgeon's experience and confidence in his or her technique, the acceptance of this procedure by the cardiologist and the patient, and the results obtained.

The initial impression was that the MIDCAB procedure would be applicable to only a small segment, roughly 5% of the total CABG population. In our center, the overall percentage of patients who underwent MIDCAB over the past $3\frac{1}{2}$ years has been 9.2%. Interestingly, within the last year, the percentage of patients undergoing MIDCAB in the isolated CABG population has risen to 19.2%. In addition, initially it was predicted that only single-vessel disease was applicable to the MIDCAB technique; however, over the last 2 years, double-vessel bypass grafting via mini-thoracotomy or a subxiphoid approach has been performed in 15% of MIDCAB procedures.

This chapter defines the indications and contraindications for MIDCAB and the intraoperative exclusions that necessitate converting a planned MIDCAB to a standard conventional coronary bypass surgery. Many of the preoperative contraindications for MIDCAB will probably change with innovations in MIDCAB techniques, including mechanical local coronary artery stabilizers, temporary intracoronary shunts, various enabling chest wall retractors for IMA harvest, and instruments for off-pump sternotomy CABG.

Contraindications and Exclusions

The contraindications and exclusions for MIDCAB surgery are mainly anatomic and strictly related to the difficulty of performing the anastomosis or finding the LAD.

In some patients, unfavorable conditions can be detected preoperatively; in the great majority, however, patients are excluded from the procedure intraoperatively.

A correct evaluation of the preoperative angiogram is the first step in determining the feasibility of the anastomosis. The anastomotic site is 2 to 4 cm below the second diagonal branch, and attention must be focused on this point. Different angiographic projections can show the internal size of the distal LAD, the quality of its walls, and LAD position relative to the epicardial surface. Perioperative contraindications to MIDCAB include a small-sized LAD (internal size <1.5 mm), a calcified LAD, and an intramyocardial LAD. The latter situation can be detected angiographically from the right anterior oblique projection when the vessel is clearly seen going downward and, after several centimeters, upward, or it can be suspected if the LAD goes straight toward the apex without any curve. Evaluation of the vessel's internal size or wall quality can be unclear if the LAD is occluded and poorly recannulated. All these situations can be evaluated before the operation.

Another perioperative contraindication is stenosis or occlusion of the left subclavian artery, although the LIMA can be reversed if the LAD is occluded and the territory is not wide, as I did in one case in which the LIMA was accidentally injured. However, I do not recommend this solution electively. Alternatively, coronary-coronary anastomosis from the large diagonal branch to the LAD with a free graft can be used if the diagonal branch is big and the LAD lesion is after the takeoff of the diagonal. Infrequently, the right gastroepiploic artery brought into the left chest via a small subxiphoid approach has been anastomosed to distal LAD.

Patient characteristics influencing access to the LAD and LIMA may be the basis for preoperative contraindications. Although entry via the fourth intercostal space is generally the optimal level, various patient-related factors can affect the ease of access. These include the degree of curvature of the chest wall (the more curved, the easier the IMA visualization and dissection), the length of the chest wall (the longer the chest, the more difficult the proximal IMA access), chronic lung disease (the downward and medial displacement of the heart requires a lower entry level for the correct site of grafting and longer IMA dissection), cardiomegaly and abnormal course of the coronary artery (buried or displaced), and obesity. In both routine and difficult cases, the use of video-assisted thoracoscopy with an endoscope and screen or headset imaging is increasing.

Intraoperatively, some patients can be excluded from the procedure and the thoracotomy reversed to a median sternotomy in several situations:

1. If the LAD position is substernal, the anastomosis is impossible to do.
2. If the LAD is not visible (in some patients, it is deep in the epicardial fat), the anastomosis can be dangerous. Each case has to be evaluated individually, as small fat emboli can accidentally be introduced into the coronary artery.
3. The quality of the wall can be layered (onion-skin like). This anatomy is accompanied by calcifications of the posterior and lateral walls and must be carefully evaluated, as the beating heart can cause tears that are impossible to repair.
4. A very lateral LAD is a potentially dangerous situation, as surgical exposure can be difficult and the quality of the anastomosis reduced.

The first step is to open the pericardium and check the position and quality of the vessel, which will confirm the feasibility of the procedure.

In summary, preoperative contraindications for MIDCAB include:

1. A small-sized coronary artery target site (coronary arteries <1.5 mm)
2. Diffusely calcified coronary arteries
3. Intramyocardial LAD
4. Stenosis or occlusion of left subclavian artery

Relative preoperative contraindications for MIDCAB are:

1. Obesity
2. Large, dense breast tissue
3. Pulmonary hypertension with laterally displaced right ventricle pushing the left ventricle posteriorly

Intraoperative exclusions for MIDCAB are:

1. LAD position substernal
2. LAD not visible
3. Laterally placed LAD
4. Extremely fatty heart
5. Very thin, onion-skin–like coronary artery wall (easily torn by a beating heart if the immobilization technique is not good)

The high rate of conversion to sternotomy (5 of 19 cases; 26%) in patients undergoing RIMA-RCA MIDCAB (because of diffuseness of the disease and difficulty immobilizing the mid-RCA), in combination with the low early patency rate of RIMA-RCA grafts (20% occlusion), leads me to believe that this operation should be performed only in rare instances when the RCA is of good caliber and quality in a thin patient with a short anteroposterior chest diameter.

For RCA grafting, I currently use the right gastroepiploic artery to the distal RCA or PDA by a subxiphoid approach. This technique is rapidly gaining popularity and has become effective by application of a new stabilizer platform (CardioThoracic Systems, Cupertino, CA) to the distal RCA as well as the PDA.

Anatomic Indications for MIDCAB

Ideal anatomic indications for LIMA–LAD by MIDCAB technique are:

1. LAD more than 2 mm beyond the first major diagonal branch
2. Thin tubular heart on chest radiograph
3. Thin chest wall with wide intercostal spaces
4. Reoperative coronary bypass graft with deteriorated saphenous vein graft (SVG)
5. Totally occluded LAD with good collaterals to the distal LAD
6. Noncalcified LAD
7. Left ventricular dysfunction

Clinical Indications for MIDCAB

1. Patients with high risk for cardiopulmonary bypass (renal failure, extreme chronic obstructive pulmonary disease, advanced age, advanced aortic atherosclerosis, calcified aorta, previous radiation to the mediastinum, documented severe cerebrovascular disease with previous history of stroke, primary hematologic disturbances, immunosuppressive state secondary to cancer and prior transplantation, diffuse peripheral vascular disease, insulin-dependent diabetes mellitus in combination with any of the other comorbid factors). Other considerations for avoidance of cardiopulmonary bypass may include religious or social preferences of the patient.
2. Reoperative CABG for prior failed SVG grafts to the LAD or RCA or for single-vessel CABG. This indication has become increasingly popular. In our center, 28% of our patients are reoperative candidates. Operation by a MIDCAB without cardiopulmonary bypass becomes a simple operation with few of the traditional complications associated with the conventional reoperative coronary bypass grafting (entry into the cardiac structures, atherosclerotic emboli, bleeding, and respiratory insufficiency).
3. Isolated single-vessel LAD, RCA, or obtuse marginal disease when percutaneous transluminal coronary angioplasty (PTCA) and stenting have been done previously and there is now restenosis.
4. Isolated single-vessel LAD, RCA, and obtuse marginal disease when PTCA is not advisable—proximal severe complex stenosis—or PTCA will not be successful or is not possible—occluded LAD.

LIMA–LAD grafts by MIDCAB as an adjunct in patients undergoing major noncardiac surgery (e.g., carotid endarterectomy, abdominal aneurysm resection [transabdominal or endoluminal grafting], and right hemicolectomy) have been performed in a few patients. This indication will become more frequent as the experience grows. Because of the excellent results with LIMA–LAD grafting in patients with poor left ventricular function, patients with ischemic cardiomyopathy and congestive heart failure are being referred for LIMA–LAD. The early results in 24 patients at our center have been gratifying. The striking difference between the standard results with conventional coronary bypass grafting in patients with congestive heart failure and ischemic cardiomyopathy and the results with LIMA–LAD MIDCAB may be due to the use of cardiopulmonary bypass and the global ischemia inherent in the conventional procedure. These patients tolerated the MIDCAB grafting well and were able to resume increased functional capacity in a short time. Elderly patients with bad left ventricular function and good target LADs who are not candidates for transplantation may be offered LIMA–LAD MIDCAB as an alternative to medical therapy.

There is also a trend in applying LIMA–LAD MIDCAB as therapy for culprit lesions in patients with multiple-vessel disease, questioning the necessity of complete revascularization in these patients. The information obtained by intracoronary Doppler wire analysis of the significance of coronary artery lesions may shed some light on the applicability of this approach in the future. The question of whether LIMA–LAD MIDCAB will be a primary strategy for LAD disease instead of catheter-based therapy will be answered by future comparative data on stenting and PTCA vs. LIMA–LAD MIDCAB.

Intramyocardial LAD is a special situation, but with the immobilization technique using the CTS stabilizer, the intramyocardial LAD can be dissected from its location and the anastomosis performed safely.

Surgical Indications in Double-Vessel Disease

An ideal case would be a patient who needs bypass grafting of the LAD, with an occluded RCA and a good distal RCA and PDA visible on angiogram. This patient would be an excellent candidate for bilateral arterial grafting, using the right gastroepiploic to the distal RCA or the PDA by a mini-subxiphoid access and LIMA–LAD by a left mini-thoracotomy approach. The performance of sequential LIMA–LAD–diagonal grafting is increasing, thus expanding double-vessel grafting. In addition, we are liberally using composite grafting in radial artery grafts from LIMA to the ramus intermedius as well as the first circumflex marginal branches.

Besides the mini right and left anterior thoracotomy and the subxiphoid approach, two new access approaches have emerged as important innovations in the MIDCAB field. High midlateral MIDCAB with the incision placed on either the third or fourth space above the nipple, starting from the midclavicular line and going toward the posterior axillary line in front of the scapula, gives an excellent exposure to the proximal LAD, the first diagonal branch, the ramus intermedius, and the first obtuse marginal branch just beyond the left atrial appendage. The CTS stabilizer is deployed in all these coronary artery target sites, and sequential LIMA grafting as well as composite grafting to these targets has been performed as a double bypass graft. This is an important access technique for the treatment of left main coronary artery disease. Further technical innovations that involve isolating the RIMA, either by a thoracoscopic approach on the right side or through a direct approach through the third-space incision to be used for the proximal LAD, will expand the indications for bilateral mammary artery grafting to the proximal LAD and the first obtuse marginal branch for left main coronary artery stenosis by this high midlateral MIDCAB access technique.

The lateral MIDCAB[10] access technique has been used increasingly for the second obtuse marginal branch and posterior lateral branch of the circumflex coronary artery, and especially in reoperative coronary bypass grafting. The approach can be through the bed of the seventh or sixth rib posteriorly beyond the tip of the scapular. The graft is placed into the descending thoracic aorta either by saphenous vein graft or by a radial artery conduit, and the anastomosis of the coronary artery is placed in retrograde fashion using either the conventional immobilization technique or the CTS stabilizer technique.

With the introduction of mechanical stabilizers (CTS retractor and Medtronic Octopus device [Minneapolis, MN]), off-pump CABG via a full midline sternotomy is being performed in multivessel grafting for LAD, diagonal RCA, and high ramus intermedius branches with considerable technical comfort and success. A relative contraindication is grafting of circumflex marginal branches in a large heart with bad left ventricular function. In addition, patients at high risk for sternotomy complications (chronic obstructive pulmonary disease, renal failure, obesity, severe diabetes, or immune deficiency) should probably not undergo this operation. For such patients, a MIDCAB and adjunct PTCA or stenting may be the best approach.

Future Indications for MIDCAB

MIDCAB surgery will be applied more frequently as the safety and efficacy of various techniques are established and scientifically validated. Current ongoing trials include POEM (patency, outcome, and economics of MIDCAB), MIST (mini-CABG vs. stent trial), and MORE (myocardial optimal revascularization trial). Hybrid MIDCAB with PTCA and stent will become increasingly frequent along with bilateral mammary grafting for left main coronary arterial stenosis by mini-thoracotomy. Laparoscopic dissection of the right gastroepiploic artery for distal LAD and PDA grafting by minimally invasive approaches will also increase. New paradigms for coronary artery bypass will use LIMA–LAD MIDCAB plus preventive cardiology by risk factor modification or stent of the circumflex artery or RCA.

Ambulatory MIDCAB procedures may become a reality, leading to totally noninvasive CABG on a beating heart with strategically placed ports using arterial grafts, port-introduced coronary artery stabilizers, and robotically assisted microsurgical anastomosis with ports. In the past, procedures for myocardial revascularization were performed by separate groups: interventional cardiologists and cardiac surgeons. In the future, different procedures will be performed by teams of operators with different backgrounds at one physical plant (comprehensive optimal revascularization center).

References

1. Acuff TE, Landreneau RJ, Griffith BP, Mack MJ: Minimally invasive coronary artery bypass grafting. Ann Thorac Surg 61:135 137, 1996.
2. Benetti FJ, Naselli G, Wood M, Gefner L: Direct myocardial revascularization without extracorporeal circulation. Chest 100: 312–316, 1991.
3. Buffolo E, de Andrade JCS, Branco JNR, et al: Coronary artery bypass grafting without cardiopulmonary bypass. Ann Thorac Surg 61:63–66, 1996.
4. Calafiore AM, DiGiammarco G, Teodori G, et al: Left anterior descending coronary artery grafting via left anterior small thoracotomy without cardiopulmonary bypass. Ann Thorac Surg 61:1658–1665, 1996.
5. Pfister AJ, Zaki MS, Garcia JM, et al: Coronary artery bypass without cardiopulmonary bypass. Ann Thorac Surg 54:108–192, 1992.
6. Robinson MC, Gross DR, Zeman W, Stedje-Larsen E: Minimally invasive coronary artery bypass grafting: A new method using an anterior mediastinotomy. J Card Surg 10:529–536, 1995.
7. Stevens JH, Burdon TA, Peters WS, et al: Port-access coronary artery bypass grafting: A proposed surgical method. J Thorac Cardiovasc Surg 111:567–573, 1996.
8. Subramanian VA: Clinical experience with minimally invasive reoperative coronary bypass surgery. Eur J Cardiothorac Surg 10:1058–1063, 1996.
9. Subramanian VA, McCabe JC, Geller CM: Minimally invasive direct coronary artery bypass grafting: Two-year clinical experience. Ann Thorac Surg 64:1648–1655, 1997.
10. Subramanian VA, Sani G, Benetti FJ, Calafiore AM: Minimally invasive coronary bypass surgery: A multi-center report of preliminary clinical experience. Circulation 92(suppl I):I1645, 1995.

COMMENTARY

Eugene K. W. Sim

Minimally invasive techniques are rapidly gaining acceptance as methods of coronary revascularization. Dr. Subramanian's excellent summary of indications for use of MIDCAB includes good pointers on the types of cases to avoid and how to determine this preoperatively.

Excellent results for MIDCAB and beating heart surgery have been reported by Subramanian and associates[1] and Jansen and colleagues,[2] but less than ideal outcomes have probably been under-reported. Routine angiography performed after MIDCAB showed disturbingly high rates of anastomotic and graft abnormalities, and routine use of intraoperative angiography has resulted in a significant number of graft revisions. Concerns about poor results have been voiced by Reardon and colleagues,[3] citing empiric examples of cases referred for heart transplant following MIDCAB. However, most surgeons agree that better results have been obtained in more recent series with the use of stabilizers.

Excellent results can be obtained from conventional coronary bypass surgery using cardiopulmonary bypass, with minimal morbidity and mortality in most patients. In considering the indications for MIDCAB or beating heart surgery, the physician's experience, the learning curve, and the institutional volume in determining which patients will benefit are important factors. Contraindications to MIDCAB include small vessels, diffusely diseased vessels, calcified vessels, and those with an intramyocardial course. These can be difficult to determine preoperatively, especially in vessels that are totally occluded, when the angiographic size and quality of the vessel may be extremely deceptive. Intramyocardial coronary arteries are not encountered often and are not always easy to predict preoperatively. Recently, Ohtsuka and colleagues[4] from Japan used ultrafast computed tomography to aid in preoperative planning for such patients. Although this appears to be an extremely expensive way of determining suitability for MIDCAB, the concept of image-guided surgery is yet to be fully explored.

References

1. Subramanian VA, McCabe JC, Geller CM: Minimally invasive direct coronary artery bypass grafting: two-year clinical experience. Ann Thorac Surg 64:1648–1655, 1997.
2. Jansen EWL, Borst C, Lahpor JR, et al: Coronary artery bypass grafting without cardiopulmonary bypass using the octopus method: Results in the first one hundred patients. J Thorac Cardiovasc Surg 116:60–67, 1998.
3. Reardon MJ, Espada R, Letsou GV, et al: Minimally invasive coronary artery surgery—a word of caution [Editorial]. J Thorac Cardiovasc Surg 114:419–420, 1997.
4. Ohtsuka T, Takamoto S, Endoh M, et al: Ultrafast computed tomography for minimally invasive coronary artery bypass grafting. J Thorac Cardiovasc Surg 116:173–174, 1998.

Chapter 51

Preoperative Assessment for Minimally Invasive Cardiac Surgery

Dan M. Meyer

Minimally invasive cardiac surgery has become a major area of clinical and industrial activity. Public awareness of this surgical option has played a major role in stimulating physician interest in this area as well. It is the responsibility of physicians to ensure that the important tenets of both coronary and valvular surgery are not compromised to adapt to these newfound pressures. This process begins with the preoperative assessment, which must follow the same strict criteria as required for the standard surgical approach.

Assessment

Assessment of patients for minimally invasive coronary surgery involves some of the same fundamental issues in conventional cardiac procedures. Whereas classic trials such as the Coronary Artery Surgery Study (CASS)[13] indicated that the combination of significant three-vessel coronary artery disease and decreased left ventricular systolic function necessitates surgical myocardial revascularization, current techniques do not follow these criteria.[12] At a minimum, there should be some evidence of unstable angina or reversible ischemia. Conversely, the indications for minimally invasive valvular surgery directly parallel those for conventional elective aortic and mitral valve repair or replacement.

With the rapid emergence of this technique, the indications have similarly evolved[3] (Table 51–1). Initially and conservatively, the minimally invasive approach focused on two groups of patients. The first group comprises those patients with unstable angina and isolated proximal/mid–left anterior descending coronary artery (LAD) and/or right coronary artery (RCA) disease who have failed attempts at angioplasty or stenting or who have complex lesions that are not amenable to percutaneous techniques. Patients with ostial lesions and complex or multiple lesions of the LAD fall into this category, as do those in whom the potential improved durability of the left internal thoracic artery (LITA) graft to the LAD is preferred over angioplasty.

The second major group of patients consists of those with associated conditions that put them at high risk from cardiopulmonary bypass (CPB). These patients have renal insufficiency or failure, chronic obstructive pulmonary disease, calcific aortic disease, diffuse cerebrovascular or peripheral vascular disease, or severe left ventricular dysfunction. Also, patients who require reoperation because of restenosis in the LAD distribution would be included in this group.[6] In a report by Arom and associates,[2] 72 patients undergoing minimally invasive coronary bypass procedures were categorized as either low (group A) or high (group B) risk. Those in group A were healthy, low-risk patients with disease of the LAD, RCA, or both. In contrast, group B patients had major contraindications to conventional CPB procedures. Results showed a 30-day mortality of 2% for group A and 6% for group B. The length of stay was 4 days for group A and 5.5 days for group B. Allen and associates[1] showed that patients subjected to minimally invasive techniques have decreased morbidity at reoperation, possibly from avoiding the detrimental physiologic and cerebral effects of CPB and not simply because of the smaller access incisions.

More recently, patients with circumflex artery, distal RCA–posterior descending coronary artery (PDA), and multivessel disease have been approached using minimally invasive techniques. More complex revascularizations in patients with multivessel disease include a combination of minimally invasive and angioplasty or stenting techniques or all-arterial revascularization with the use of the right gastroepiploic artery (RGEA), radial artery T graft, and right inferior epigastric artery (RIEA) as an extension off the LITA or RGEA.

Exclusion criteria for minimally invasive coronary surgery are almost nonexistent. Previous use of the ITA and subclavian artery stenosis or occlusion are contraindications. A history of radiation therapy to the chest wall would qualify as only a relative contraindication secondary to possible thermal injury to the ITA. Patients who require immediate surgery, such as those in cardiogenic shock, are not suitable for minimally invasive techniques because of the time necessary to mobilize the LITA and the longer time needed to perform the anastomosis. Early in the minimally invasive experience, the procedure was limited to vessels on the anterior surface of the heart, as they were accessible by either the right or the left ITA. With the assistance of the new myocardial stabilization platforms, vessels on the posterior aspect of heart are more accessible, and their involvement is no longer a contraindication.

As discussed later, patients with small LADs (internal diameter <1.5 mm) or calcified vessels are not typically advised to undergo this procedure, although these are not absolute contraindications (Table 51–2). An intramyocardial LAD, however, is likely the primary contraindication to the minimally invasive approach. A laterally positioned LAD requires more extensive dissection of the LITA or extension of the LITA with another arterial conduit, such as the RIEA. Aortic insufficiency is not a contraindication to minimally invasive revascularization using either a beating or arrested port access technique. In the former condition, no CPB is needed; in the latter situation, retrograde cardioplegia can be used, and the aortic root can be vented throughout the procedure.[10]

Table 51–1. Indications for Minimally Invasive Coronary Surgery

Isolated proximal/mid-LAD or RCA stenosis not amenable to PTCA (complex stenosis, total occlusion of LAD)
Patient/physician preference
Restenosis after PTCA/stenting
High risk from cardiopulmonary bypass because of comorbidity
Reoperation
In combination with angioplasty in patients with multivessel disease

LAD = left anterior descending artery; RCA = right coronary artery; PTCA = percutaneous transluminal coronary angioplasty.

With minimally invasive valve surgery, most contraindications are related to potential problems with access to the aortic or mitral valve. These problems would become apparent during the preoperative assessment, when a chest radiograph would demonstrate a rotated heart with the aorta positioned toward the midline. An extreme condition in which a minimally invasive procedure has not provided adequate exposure is pectus excavatum, in which the heart is located entirely in the left hemithorax. From a technical standpoint, a calcified or atheromatous ascending aorta on preoperative transesophageal echocardiography (TEE) would be a contraindication to a minimally invasive valvular or port access approach.

History

As there are few contraindications to this technique, issues discovered in the history are also uncommon. As discussed earlier, patients requiring emergency operation are not typically candiates for this procedure, because time is necessary to prepare the ITA for use. Patients with severe chronic obstructive pulmonary disease may not easily tolerate single-lung ventilation; therefore, mobilization of the internal mammary artery without isolation of the lung would be problematic but not contraindicated. For minimally invasive valvular surgery, the patients must exhibit the same symptoms as required for conventional valve surgery, be it syncope, angina, or congestive heart failure.

Physical Examination

On physical examination, body habitus is a key issue that affects the enthusiasm to perform any minimally invasive cardiac procedure. An excessive body habitus may preclude intervention. Specifically, obesity could be considered problematic, as the distance between the chest wall and heart might be too great. This may also be true to some extent in female patients. Peripheral vascular disease, a disease process that may favor the use of minimally invasive techniques because of these patients' associated comorbidity, also introduces limitations with respect to the use of femoral cannulation for either emergent placement on CPB or use of port access approaches. Moreover, these patients may have evidence of atheromatous disease of the ascending aorta on TEE.

Table 51–2. Contraindications to Minimally Invasive Coronary Surgery

Intramyocardial LAD
Diffusely calcified LAD (<1.5 mm)
Severe pulmonary hypertension with large left ventricle
Above factors may correlate with more common graft occlusion

LAD = left anterior descending artery.

Radiographic Evaluation

Radiographic evaluation is critical in predicting the feasibility of performing the planned procedure. A chest radiograph depicting the heart as rotated may indicate that the LAD will be out of sight to the operating surgeon, making access difficult. Instead, one may see only the diagonal branch and mistake this for the LAD.[5] This is especially true for patients with significant deposits of epicardial fat. In aortic valve surgery, a chest radiograph showing an aorta that is rotated toward the midline may similarly make surgical access difficult.

Pulmonary Function

The need for formal pulmonary function testing in the patient population undergoing minimal access cardiac surgery is fairly limited. Clearly, patient tolerance to single-lung ventilation is helpful, especially if a thoracoscopic approach to the LITA is to be used. However, recently available ITA retractors offer excellent visualization without the need for a double-lumen endotracheal tube. In minimally invasive valvular surgery, no specific pulmonary function testing is routinely recommended.

Cardiac Catheterization

The most important aspect of the preoperative assessment for minimal access coronary surgery is cardiac catheterization. Cardiac catheterization must demonstrate a hemodynamically significant lesion amenable to surgical revascularization techniques. Typically, isolated proximal or middle LAD or RCA stenosis is present. The quality of the vessel must also be amenable to bypass. Early guidelines stated that the distal LAD should be greater than 1.5 mm in diameter and not calcified (Table 51–3). However, as experience has grown, the size of the coronary artery has not been absolutely specified. The specific anatomic course of the vessel is also important information, and this must be defined with angiography. With the very limited exposure available to the operating surgeon, landmarks are less useful for deciding on the location of the vessel. Critical assessment of the catheterization is undertaken to ensure that the LAD and not the diagonal branch is the prominent epicardial vessel. Finally, and most importantly, an intramyocardial course of the LAD must be ruled in or out, as this will dictate whether a minimally invasive approach is a feasible option. An intramyocardial course is an

Table 51–3. Ideal Anatomic Conditions for Minimally Invasive Coronary Surgery

LAD >2 mm
Noncalcified LAD
Thin chest wall with wide intercostal spaces
Reoperative coronary artery bypass graft with deteriorated saphenous vein graft
Totally occluded LAD with good collaterals to distal LAD
Tubular heart on chest radiograph

LAD = left anterior descending artery.

absolute contraindication, as this would prohibit access to the vessel.

Other information that must be obtained from preoperative cardiac catheterization includes the position of any large septal perforators off the LAD. It is possible to injure these vessels if they are manipulated during isolation of the LAD segment at the site of the proposed anastomosis. Furthermore, these vessels could be difficult to control if the orifice of the septal branch is in the area of the proposed anastomosis, as back-bleeding could hamper visualization efforts. Additionally, careful examination of the left main coronary artery is important to ensure that this region is not involved. For patients requiring reoperation, a patent LITA would be favorable additional information.

Culprit Vessel Identification

The next issue revolves around the preoperative assessment of the significance of a stenotic coronary lesion. As increasing attention is given to revascularization efforts in patients with multivessel disease, parameters will be needed to guide the surgeon to the most hemodynamically significant lesion. Dobutamine stress echocardiography[11] and thallium scintigraphy[4] can detect regional wall motion abnormalities and areas of reversible ischemia. More specific information may be obtained from coronary Doppler studies, which have recently been applied to patients with multivessel disease. Pijls and associates[8] assessed a parameter that determined whether a particular stenosis was responsible for reversible myocardial ischemia. The myocardial fractional flow reserve (FFR_{myo}) index was obtained by simultaneous measurement of mean aortic pressure and trans-stenotic coronary pressure and indicated the influence of an epicardial coronary stenosis on maximal achievable blood flow in the supplied myocardial territory. If the FFR_{myo} was less than .75, revascularization was indicated; if the FFR_{myo} was greater than .75, revascularization was likely not necessary. The authors concluded that this index might impact clinical decision-making when assessing patients for minimally invasive cardiac surgery. Recent comparisons between the diagnostic accuracy of this technique in predicting inducible ischemia and that of more standard tools such as exercise testing, dobutamine stress echocardiography, and thallium scintigraphy have favored the use of FFR_{myo}.[9] Other invasive techniques to assess the significance of specific coronary stenosis include quantitative coronary arteriography and intracoronary ultrasonography, neither of which clearly defines a relationship between morphologic abnormalities and impairment of blood flow. A related technique, Doppler-derived coronary flow reserve, has not delivered consistent results.[7]

Conclusion

Preoperative assessment of patients undergoing minimally invasive cardiac surgery requires an understanding of the indications for the procedure as well as the caveats discussed earlier. Selecting patients with an appropriate body habitus is important in the initial assessment. Chest radiography may provide information about accessibility of coronary arteries or particular valves. Careful review of the cardiac catheterization is required to ascertain the exact course of the vessel and the location of associated septal branches. Most importantly, however, assessment of the catheterization is imperative to ensure against the presence of an intramyocardial vessel. Finally, newer studies may be used to help in selecting the specific coronary artery that requires revascularization. By combining these aspects of the preoperative assessment, minimal access cardiac surgery may prove to be a safe and beneficial option in a select group of cardiac patients.

References

1. Allen KB, Matheny RG, Robison RJ, et al: Minimally invasive versus conventional reoperative coronary artery bypass. Ann Thorac Surg 64:616–622, 1997.
2. Arom KV, Emery RW, Nicoloff DM, et al: Minimally invasive direct coronary artery bypass grafting: Experimental and clinical experiences. Ann Thorac Surg 63:S48–S52, 1997.
3. Calafiore AM, Angelini GD, Bergsland J, Salerno TA: Minimally invasive coronary artery bypass grafting. Ann Thorac Surg 62:1545–1548, 1996.
4. Dilsizian V, Rocco TP, Freedman NMT, et al: Enhanced detection of ischemic but viable myocardium by the reinjection of thallium after stress-redistribution imaging. N Engl J Med 323:141–146, 1990.
5. Machiraju VR: Correspondence. Ann Thorac Surg 64:294, 1997.
6. Mack MJ, Acuff TE, Casimir-Ahn H, et al: Video-assisted coronary bypass grafting on the beating heart. Ann Thorac Surg 63:S100–S103, 1997.
7. Ofili EO, Labovitz J, Kern MJ: Coronary flow velocity dynamics in normal and diseased arteries. Am J Cardiol 71:3D–9D, 1993.
8. Pijls NHJ, Bech GJW, De Bruyne B, van Straten A: Clinical assessment of functional stenosis severity: Use of coronary pressure measurements for the decision to bypass a lesion. Ann Thorac Surg 63:S6–S11, 1997.
9. Pijls NHJ, De Bruyne B, Peels K, et al: Measurement of fractional flow reserve to assess the functional severity of coronary artery stenoses. N Engl J Med 334:1703–1708, 1996.
10. Ribakove GH, Galloway AC, Grossi EA, et al: Port-access coronary artery bypass grafting. Semin Thorac Cardiovasc Surg 9:312–319, 1997.
11. Sawada SG, Segar DS, Ryan T, et al: Echocardiographic detection of coronary artery disease during dobutamine infusion. Circulation 83:1605–1614, 1991.
12. Subramanian VA: Less invasive arterial CABG on a beating heart. Ann Thorac Surg 63:S68–S71, 1997.
13. The Principal Investigators of CASS and their Associates: The National Heart, Lung, and Blood Institute Coronary Artery Surgery Study (CASS). Circulation 63(suppl I):I-1–I-39, 1981.

COMMENTARY

Kit V. Arom

Minimally invasive cardiac surgery presently revolves around the issues of *incision* and use of *cardiopulmonary bypass.* Minimally invasive cardiac surgery uses a small skin incision, approximately 10 to 12 cm long. The incision can be located at any appropriate area on the chest wall. The chest cavity or the mediastinal cavity is entered through the intercostal space, by a subxiphoid approach, by the removal or dislocation of the costal cartilage, or by partial sternotomy.

The question arises whether a port access approach using the heart-lung machine with a small incision at the appropriate chest wall site and a groin incision for arterial and venous cannulation is a less invasive approach. The answer at the present time is yes. Currently, all intracardiac surgery and some extracardiac surgery for both congenital and acquired disease, in which a limited incision is made and the heart-lung machine is used are considered to be minimally invasive.

This excellent chapter covers the global preoperative assessment, not only for minimally invasive coronary artery bypass surgery but also for minimally invasive valvular surgery and port access approaches. I totally agree with Dr. Meyer that the preoperative assessment must follow the same strict criteria required for the standard surgical approach. It should also involve some of the fundamental issues present in conventional cardiac surgical procedures.

There is no controversy concerning the indications for and assessment of valvular surgery that can be accomplished through a small skin incision. However, the various types of approaches, such as removal or dislocation of the costal cartilage with or without sacrificing the right internal mammary artery and the approach through the intercostal space and partial sternotomy, all of which are being done with or without groin cannulation, remain controversial in terms of which technique is safest and most cost-effective.

Indications and assessment for coronary artery bypass surgery are still controversial. The early indications for minimally invasive coronary artery bypass surgery for single- and double-vessel disease remain true today. However, this could change in the future as surgeons develop better techniques for complete revascularization on a beating heart in patients with three-vessel disease and poor left ventricular function. It is this subset of patients that can benefit the most in terms of good, immediate, and long-term clinical outcomes from this type of surgical revascularization. With improved outcomes, minimally invasive coronary bypass procedures will be more widely accepted.

What we are missing are long-term clinical results in patients who have more than one-vessel disease, such as disease of the proximal LAD and diagonal artery. Many of these patients may get only a LIMA-to-LAD graft via a limited incisional approach because experts believe that long-term outcomes are not compromised when the branch of the LAD is not bypassed. This conclusion has been drawn without any specific preoperative assessment or documented outcome results. Some investigators suggest that in a patient with significant proximal LAD and RCA disease, staged bilateral thoracotomy is the best approach, but again, this is without any preoperative assessment. In this particular circumstance, a partial sternotomy can be accomplished and two vessels can be bypassed in the same setting with less tissue injury and with obvious cost savings. The assessment of myocardial flow reserve is crucial in a patient with three-vessel disease undergoing revascularization via a limited access. If myocardial flow reserve studies suggest significant multivessel disease, the patient should be treated with either a hybrid type of procedure or conventional coronary artery bypass surgery.

I also agree with the author that for minimally invasive coronary artery bypass surgery we should focus on two groups of patients and analyze them according to their preoperative indications and assessment of comorbidity. These patients are not the same in terms of intraoperative risk and postoperative surgical outcomes.

Performing anastomosis on a beating heart via a limited access requires exceptional skill and attention to detail. Preoperative assessment begins with patient habitus selection, preoperative evaluation of cardiac position on chest x-ray, and coronary angiogram. The size of the target artery, location of the branch, and collateral circulation all play important roles in the success of minimally invasive coronary artery bypass surgery.

Chapter 52

Anesthetic Considerations for Minimally Invasive Cardiac Surgery

Peter E. Krucylak

Cardiac surgery as practiced until recently involved operations performed via sternotomy with the patient supported by the use of cardiopulmonary bypass (CPB). But the routine use of sternotomy and CPB in the performance of cardiac surgery has been questioned, particularly during coronary artery bypass graft (CABG) procedures. With the rapid introduction of minimally invasive (also referred to as minimal access) procedures, the anesthesiologist assumes a more interactive role during surgery.

The two major goals driving the development of minimally invasive cardiac surgery are the desire to avoid CPB and the desire to use smaller incisions.[1] The range of minimal access approaches has many anesthetic implications. Much of the monitoring that is used during conventional CABG involves direct observation of the heart. This is obviously not possible with smaller incisions, requiring the use of new technologies such as transesophageal echocardiography (TEE) to supplement hemodynamic monitors such as measurement of pulmonary pressures. Many of the anesthetic concerns depend on the type of surgical exposure and on whether CPB is used. This discussion includes traditional anesthetic methods that have been applied to this surgical population as well as new techniques of intraoperative management that have been developed to meet the specific needs of minimally invasive cardiac procedures.

Anesthesia for Cases Not Involving Cardiopulmonary Bypass

Minimally invasive direct coronary artery bypass (MIDCAB) is a procedure that involves a myocardial revascularization operation that avoids both median sternotomy and CPB.[2] The anastomosis of the bypass graft is done under direct vision without the aid of video-assisted methods. The myocardium is stabilized by pharmacologic or mechanical means to facilitate surgery.

Preoperative Assessment

The preoperative evaluation for patients undergoing MIDCAB is initially the same as for patients undergoing any form of myocardial revascularization. Attention is directed to the indices of left ventricular function as well as the patient's exercise tolerance. Patients are not necessarily excluded from undergoing a MIDCAB procedure owing to poor left ventricular function, because many of these patients may do better with a MIDCAB than with coronary revascularization using CPB. Akins and associates demonstrated that septal function is better preserved by performing coronary artery bypass without CPB.[3] The performance of coronary surgery without cross-clamping the aorta may also increase myocardial production of heat shock proteins that are cardioprotective.[4]

The extent of coronary lesions is scrutinized carefully. If the degree of stenosis is greater than 95%, vessel occlusion is usually well tolerated. If the degree of stenosis is less than 95%, vessel occlusion may cause hemodynamic decompensation and arrhythmia.[5] The presence of collateral vascularization is noted on inspection of data from cardiac catheterization. There are several types of data that support the preceding statements. First, during percutaneous transluminal coronary angioplasty, patients with coronary lesions causing less than 80% stenosis suffered an increased incidence of arrhythmias during coronary artery balloon occlusion.[6] Second, in cases of MIDCAB, areas of myocardial ischemia, characterized by regional wall motion abnormalities, typically occurred only with lesions causing less than 75% occlusion.[7] Last, the presence of high-grade coronary lesions may allow the formation of collateral vessels so that interruption of coronary flow is well tolerated.[8] Based on this type of data, Westaby and Benetti argue that MIDCAB should be done only if the coronary stenosis is greater than 75% or if there are collateral vessels to the area of myocardium at risk from vessel occlusion.[7] Discussion with the surgeon helps plan the order of coronary graft placement. In cases in which the left anterior descending artery and the right coronary artery are to be bypassed, it may be preferable to perform the anastomosis to the left anterior descending artery first in order that the patient may better tolerate subsequent manipulation to the heart.[9]

Patient Safety and Positioning

The patient is typically placed in a right lateral decubitus position (30 to 60 degrees from the horizontal plane) with the arm safely secured above the head.[10] This position affords access to the left hemithorax for harvest of the left internal mammary artery, as well as access to the groin for femoral vessel cannulation if CPB becomes necessary. External pacing and defibrillator pads (R2 Pads, Cardiotronics Systems, Draper, UT) are placed as appropriate.

A perfusionist and CPB machine are available on immediate notice for cases that need to be converted to conventional surgical methods using CPB. Early in the surgeon's learning curve, it may be advisable to place guide wires in the femoral artery and vein in case emergency CPB or placement of an intra-aortic balloon pump is necessary. A catheter in the femoral artery may also serve as a source for oxygenated blood when a coronary artery shunt is necessary.[11]

During CABG performed via sternotomy, epicardial pacing wires are often placed before chest closure. This method of pacing may not be available during MIDCAB, owing to limited exposure of the epicardial surface. Wasnick argues that atrioventricular pacing via a pulmonary artery catheter is necessary to manage these patients.[12] In his case series, as many as 35% of patients required transvenous pacing during MIDCAB.[13] Alternative means of backup pacing include the use of Zoll pads for external pacing or epicardial pacing wires, when available.

Monitoring

In the absence of firm outcome data, the choice of monitors during MIDCAB can take many forms. Pawlowski and associates advocate the use of minimal monitoring for minimally invasive cardiac surgery unless a specific indication exists for more intensive monitoring.[14] Their standard monitors include an arterial catheter, central venous pressure, and possibly TEE to help guide the administration of myocardial-depressant drugs. The decision to use a pulmonary artery catheter in addition to these monitors is often based on factors such as degree of left ventricular dysfunction or institutional preferences. In contrast to this simplistic view, more intensive monitoring may be required because the heart cannot be directly visualized.

Electrocardiography must be used with care during MIDCAB, because the V5 lead is often more lateral than usual and behaves more like a V6 lead. The use of automated ST-segment monitoring helps extend the utility of electrocardiogram (ECG) monitoring. Occlusion of the left anterior descending artery during MIDCAB can cause regional ischemia with ST-segment elevations.[15] Figure 52–1 shows ST-segment elevation that resolved immediately after reperfusion of the left anterior descending artery.

The relatively new technology of TEE helps identify areas of hypokinetic or akinetic myocardium at risk during a test clamp period and also helps document recovery from a period of regional ischemia. Although TEE has been used as a monitor for myocardial ischemia, there have been reports of TEE failing to diagnose intraoperative myocardial infarction.[16] The routine use of TEE in detecting regional wall motion abnormalities may lead to many false-positive diagnoses, as only 6% of such abnormalities are associated with cardiac morbidity.[17] The use of mechanical stabilizers on the surface of the heart may appear as areas of hypokinesis or akinesis on TEE. Inspection of the anterior surface of the heart using a gastric short-axis view of the heart by TEE before stabilizer application is necessary to get a true picture of anterior wall function.

The integrated use of TEE, ECG, and changes in pulmonary capillary wedge pressure (PCWP) is the most complete way to detect myocardial ischemia.[18] In addition to the modalities mentioned previously, myocardial ischemia can be detected by the elevation of PCWP or the new onset of V waves on the PCWP waveform.[19] This mode of myocardial ischemia detection is limited by the fact that the pulmonary artery catheter is not continuously in the wedge position. Table 52–1 lists equipment and drugs used during MIDCAB.

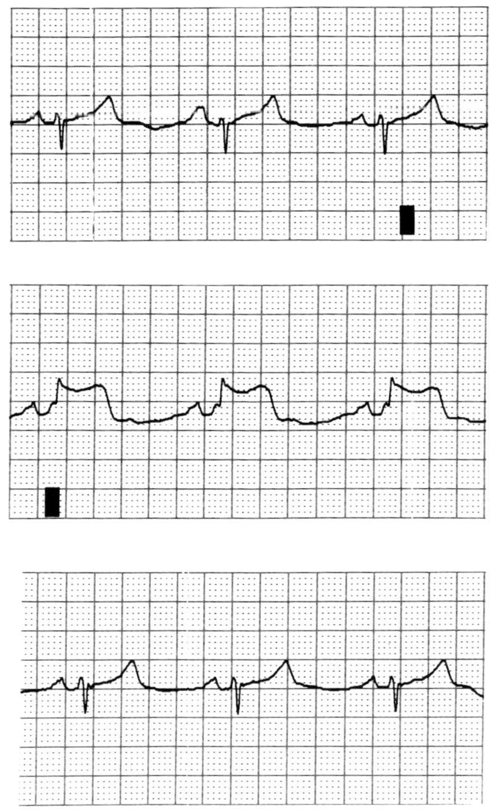

Figure 52–1. *Top,* Electrocardiogram trace (lead II) before left anterior descending artery occlusion. *Middle,* One minute following occlusion, showing ST-segment elevation. *Bottom,* One minute after reperfusion, showing normalization of the ST segments.

Induction of Anesthesia

One of the goals of minimal access techniques for coronary revascularization is the more efficient use of hospital resources, including the use of postoperative intensive care units. The induction and maintenance of general anesthe-

Table 52–1. Equipment and Drug Setup for Minimally Invasive Direct Coronary Artery Bypass

Equipment
Arterial catheter; Swan-Ganz catheter (optional)
External defibrillator pads (R2 Pads, Cardiotronics Systems, Draper, UT)
Double-lumen or UNIVENT tube
Pediatric fiberoptic bronchoscope
Transesophageal echocardiography
Cardiopulmonary bypass standby
Room temperature at 22°C; warming blanket
Drugs
Nitroglycerin (50 mg in 250 cc)
Esmolol (draw up 10 cc syringe; mix 2.5 g in 250 cc)
Phenylephrine (100 μg/kg)
Heparin (10,000 U drawn up in syringe)
Halothane vaporizer (optional)

sia for MIDCAB should ideally allow rapid weaning with minimum postoperative mechanical ventilation. Short-acting intravenous agents such as thiopental or propofol are ideal for rapid induction of anesthesia and rapid offset. The use of newer muscle relaxants such as rocuronium allows rapid offset as well as hemodynamic stability. Pancuronium is relatively contraindicated because of associated tachycardia from a vagolytic effect and its long duration of action.

The use of one-lung ventilation (OLV) may be helpful during harvest of the left internal mammary artery, particularly early in a surgeon's experience. In place of OLV, the use of smaller tidal volumes may provide adequate conditions for harvest. Special concerns such as hyperinflation or scarring of the left lung may prompt the use of OLV.[14] OLV may be provided by the use of double-lumen endotracheal tubes or UNIVENT tubes that incorporate a bronchial blocker.[20] If OLV is used, the left lung should be reinflated before closure to ensure that the graft is not kinked.[21]

Maintenance of Anesthesia

The main hemodynamic goal of anesthetic management during MIDCAB is to enhance myocardial oxygen delivery without creating an increase in oxygen demand. The specific goals of intraoperative management of patients undergoing MIDCAB include avoidance of tachycardia and induction of bradycardia when necessary, while maintaining adequate oxygen delivery. Maintenance of general anesthesia may be provided by inhaled agents such as isoflurane or by the use of total intravenous anesthesia. Total intravenous anesthesia with a propofol infusion is useful when the patient is transported to the cardiac catheterization laboratory or for sedation of patients who remain intubated after MIDCAB. Limiting the dose of narcotics or using ultrarapid agents such as remifentanil facilitates early extubation. Early extubation should be avoided in the setting of persistent myocardial ischemia, hypothermia, global myocardial dysfunction, and coexisting pulmonary disease.[14]

Management of Vessel Occlusion

Reported regional ischemic times range from 9 minutes[22] to 28 minutes.[23] The role of the anesthesiologist during this period is maintenance of acceptable hemodynamic parameters while enhancing the operating conditions. To maintain a quiet surgical field, it may be necessary to tolerate some degree of hypotension during construction of the anastomosis.[24]

Heparin must be given before snaring of the left anterior descending artery to prevent clot formation in the vessel. Heparin doses used in this population are usually 100 to 150 U/kg.[25] This dose must obviously be supplemented when the procedure is converted to a conventional CABG. The endpoint for heparin monitoring during a MIDCAB procedure is an activated clotting time (ACT) of at least 250 seconds.[26] Heparin may be neutralized at the conclusion of the procedure according to the surgeon's preference.[14]

Novel strategies of myocardial protection must be used during MIDCAB. Preconditioning can be induced pharmacologically with alpha-adrenergic, cholinergic, and adenosine receptor agonists and volatile anesthetic agents or with intermittent periods of ischemia before the main ischemic insult.[27]

Ischemic preconditioning has been reported to be beneficial in cases of inadequate protection with cardioplegia.[28] Periods of preconditioning as short as 3 minutes have been shown to be protective in humans undergoing conventional coronary bypass surgery.[29] Even with periods of ischemia as short as 5 minutes, the protective effects can last 1 to 2 hours.[30] Ischemic preconditioning has been reported to have multiple beneficial effects, including limiting infarct size in a rabbit model,[31] delaying cell death,[32] and reducing the incidence of reperfusion arrhythmias.[33] Preconditioning reduces troponin-T release in patients undergoing cardiac surgery.[34] The actual mechanism of action of ischemic preconditioning probably involves adenosine receptors.

Intracoronary adenosine has been used to precondition the myocardium before percutaneous transluminal coronary angioplasty of the left anterior descending artery with excellent results, specifically, fewer ST-segment changes of the intracardiac ECG.[35] There are theoretical concerns about infusing intracoronary adenosine into the right or circumflex coronary arteries because of the risk of conduction disturbances, specifically, atrioventricular block. Brief periods of myocardial ischemia result in the release of adenosine as a consequence of adenosine triphosphate (ATP) metabolism.[36] Although the exact molecular mechanism is unknown, it is apparent that the adenosine receptor activates protein kinase C, which in turn protects the myocardium by an unknown mechanism.[37] Adenosine may also act as a coronary and collateral vessel dilator, thus increasing oxygen supply in cases of regional ischemia.[38] There are practical reasons that limit the routine use of adenosine, such as systemic hypotension after parenteral infusion of the drug.[37] Despite this concern, adenosine has been used for preconditioning using a slow infusion of 12 mg over 20 minutes with few side effects.[39]

Volatile anesthetic agents, particularly halothane and isoflurane, have been shown to limit myocardial stunning,[40] decrease infarct size,[41] reduce reperfusion arrhythmias,[42] and improve postischemia left ventricular function.[43] There are several factors that make volatile anesthetic agents cardioprotective. Halothane limits myocardial contractility and thus myocardial oxygen consumption. Isoflurane is a coronary vasodilator and improves coronary blood flow.[38] Volatile anesthetics preserve myocardial ATP levels and improve ATP regeneration following reperfusion.[43] Volatile agents, particularly isoflurane, are well tolerated during MIDCAB and also enable a smooth and rapid extubation.

It is estimated that one third of patients will exhibit signs of ischemia during vessel occlusion.[44, 45] These patients may need volume or pharmacologic resuscitation, especially during revascularization of the right coronary artery.[20, 46] Ischemia and hemodynamic instability are more frequent during revascularization of the right coronary artery as compared with the left anterior descending artery.[46] This is probably related to the increased amount of surgical manipulation needed to accomplish the right coronary artery anastomosis.[46] The rapid institution of pacing may be necessary using either external pacing leads or an intravenous pacemaker. Often an epicardial pacing wire can be placed to provide the capability for ventricular pacing.

Rare cases may require the urgent or emergent institution of CPB. Placement of guide wires in the femoral artery and vein is a reasonable safety measure when rapid institution of CPB is necessary or for placement of an intra-aortic balloon pump.[47] This is particularly useful early in an institution's experience performing MIDCAB.

The placement of shunts across the occluded area of the bypassed vessel has been described as a means of avoiding regional ischemia. Early systems were complex and technically difficult to use.[48] More recent shunt systems have been specifically developed for MIDCAB procedures.[45] The ability to shunt across a region of ischemia is useful for restoring normal hemodynamic performance and for controlling arrhythmias.[11] Placement of shunts may be particularly useful in patients with low degrees of stenosis of the right coronary artery and thus little likelihood of collateral circulation.[49]

Myocardial stabilization is critical to the ability to perform MIDCAB. Early attempts to stabilize the heart included the liberal use of induced bradycardia. Table 52–2 lists the drugs that have been used during MIDCAB to induce bradycardia. Esmolol is a popular agent because of its ability to induce bradycardia and its anti-ischemic effects. Esmolol is typically titrated to a heart rate of 50 to 60 bpm, starting with 10- to 30-mg boluses. Metoprolol is an economical alternative to esmolol, requiring a dose of 0.5 to 1 mg every 5 minutes, titrated to a heart rate of 60 bpm. The use of high-dose esmolol may require mechanical circulatory support during surgery, such as use of the Sternotomy Hemopump (Johnson & Johnson Interventional Systems Company, Rancho Cordova, CA).[50] High doses of esmolol may also be used in patients supported on CPB to provide the advantage of a relatively quiet surgical field without the use of cardioplegia.[51] Esmolol helps control the heart rate, decreases myocardial consumption, stabilizes the surgical field, and has been demonstrated to attenuate regional ischemia during vessel occlusion during percutaneous transluminal coronary angioplasty.[52] Jacobsohn and associates reported that a dose of less than 150 μg/kg/min reliably produced a heart rate of 50 to 60 bpm.[53] The use of esmolol alone fails to produce a sufficient reduction in heart rate to continue with surgery in 40% of cases.[54]

Table 52–2. Drugs That Induce Bradycardia During Minimally Invasive Direct Coronary Artery Bypass

Drug	Dose	Comments
Esmolol[53]	50–150 μg/kg/min	Serum half-life = 9 min
Adenosine[57]	0.2–0.3 mg/kg	Causes 15–30 sec of asystole
Verapamil[55]	5-mg doses titrated to desired heart rate	May cause unacceptable hypotension
Diltiazem[58]	0.1 mg/kg/hr starting dose	May cause unacceptable hypotension
Neostigmine[58]	1–3-mg bolus	Will reverse muscle paralysis

A number of other agents have been used to induce bradycardia. Calcium channel blockers, particularly verapamil, have been used for this purpose.[55] The results of calcium channel blockers have been disappointing because of associated vasodilatation. Esmolol has been shown to be comparable to verapamil in terms of hemodynamic effects during CABG without the use of CPB, but esmolol demonstrates superior antiarrhythmic effects.[56]

Adenosine has been used to cause transient asystole during MIDCAB. The appropriate dose of adenosine is 0.2 to 0.3 mg/kg, which reliably causes atrioventricular node blockade for 15 to 30 seconds, with return of hemodynamic parameters within 40 to 60 seconds.[57] A bolus of adenosine can also be used for brief asystole when placing partial aortic clamps (C clamps). Persantine (5 mg) is given before occlusion of the target vessel to potentiate the effects of adenosine.[14] An average of nine doses of adenosine have been used per anastomosis, with return of normal arterial blood pressure occurring within 35 seconds.[39]

The last category of drugs that can induce bradycardia are anticholinesterases such as neostigmine. Neostigmine causes the accumulation of acetylcholine at muscarinic and nicotinic sites and is also a direct cholinergic agonist.[58] The chief advantage of neostigmine is the lack of negative inotropism, as seen with esmolol or calcium channel antagonists. Side effects of neostigmine include reversal of muscle relaxation and bronchospasm in patients with reactive airways.[58]

The use of pharmacologic stabilization often results in a decrease in the cardiac index of approximately 25%[59] and often offers inadequate surgical conditions.[60] Table 52–3 reports hemodynamic changes with the use of esmolol to decrease heart rate at our institution.

Other methods of myocardial stabilization include the use of mechanical stabilizers that attach to the surface of the heart. Two such mechanical devices have become widely available: the IMA Access Retractor system and the Octopus system. The simpler of the two systems is the IMA Access Retractor (CardioThoracic Systems [CTS], Cupertino, CA). This consists of a mechanical "foot" that is attached to the anterior wall of the heart, thus limiting the motion of that area of myocardium. Use of this system results in stable operating conditions and results in little impairment of cardiac output and coronary perfusion pressure.[61] Subramanian presented preliminary data that use of the CTS device may also increase graft patency rates from 92% to 96%.[62] While using the CTS device, the anterior wall of the left ventricle appears hypokinetic on TEE, which may alter interpretation of the echocardiogram when monitoring for regional areas of ischemia.

The Octopus stabilizer is a more complex suction device that attaches to the epicardial surface of the heart. The suction portion of the device is immobilized with two tentacles that attach to the operating table.[63] The Octopus allows manipulation of the heart, which may allow grafting of vessels other than the left anterior descending artery. Grundeman and associates examined the hemodynamic consequences of such cardiac displacement using a pig model.[64] During vertical displacement of the heart, the stroke volume and cardiac output decreased 44%. Some of

Table 52–3. Hemodynamics During Minimally Invasive Direct Coronary Artery Bypass With Pharmacologic Stabilization

	Supine	OLV	LAD Artery Clamped	LAD Artery Open
MAP (mm Hg)	94 ± 15.1	83.8 ± 16.1	77 ± 10.9	72.3 ± 5.1*
PCWP (mm Hg)	11.6 ± 0.55	12.2 ± 4.8	13.8 ± 3.4	13.2 ± 2.8
CI (L/min/m^2)	1.92 ± 0.55	2.36 ± 0.95	1.98 ± 0.8	1.98 ± 0.4
DO_2 (ml/min)	574.6 ± 63.0	810.3 ± 384.3	670.3 ± 305.2	642.3 ± 156.6
HR (min^{-1})	54 ± 5.8	57.5 ± 8.9	55 ± 7.6	57.3 ± 10.3
SVI (ml/m^2)	35.4 ± 7.8	40.3 ± 10.6	36.0 ± 13.7	35.3 ± 8.7
Esmolol (μg/kg/min)	11.7 ± 19.1	25.2 ± 28.5	100.8 ± 83.8*	41.7 ± 58.5

Results are reported as mean ± SD; n = 6.
OLV = one-lung ventilation; LAD = left anterior descending; MAP = mean arterial pressure; PCWP = pulmonary capillary wedge pressure; CI = cardiac index; DO_2 = oxygen delivery; HR = heart rate; SVI = stroke volume index.
*$P < .05$.

this decrease can be avoided by placing the pig in Trendelenburg's position, at the expense of increased ventricular preload and tachycardia. The Octopus device does not alter coronary blood flow, even during cardiac displacement.[65]

Comparison of pharmacologic vs. mechanical stabilization techniques shows clear advantages to the use of mechanical devices. A direct comparison by Jurmann and associates demonstrated that patients who had mechanical stabilization devices rather than pharmacologic stabilization had less of a decrease in ejection fraction and cardiac output while having no change in end-diastolic chamber dimensions.[66] The use of mechanical stabilization preserves cardiac function while significantly reducing the range of motion of the target vessel.[67] The use of these devices is strongly urged, given the superior limitation of myocardial motion as well as better preservation of hemodynamic parameters.

Intraoperative Complications

The most serious morbidity of MIDCAB is perioperative myocardial infarction. Even though the reported series to date are relatively small, it appears that the rate of myocardial infarction is approximately 1 to 3%.[59] It is uncertain whether myocardial infarctions are related to technical problems at the site of anastomosis, spasm of the internal mammary artery, or other unidentified factors. Many patients exhibit ST-segment elevation on surface ECG, but not all these patients have myocardial infarctions. Also unclear is the mortality associated with having a perioperative infarction during MIDCAB.

Episodes of hypotension and low cardiac output are also seen during MIDCAB; these appear to be necessary to allow revascularization while avoiding CPB. The episodes of hypotension tend to be brief and are associated with surgical manipulation of the heart or attempts at inducing bradycardia. Persistent hypotension after termination of these maneuvers is worrisome, as this may indicate a myocardial infarction. Reperfusion arrhythmias may be seen after release of vessel occlusion, particularly if the native vessel was not severely occluded. The use of a prophylactic dose of lidocaine helps prevent these arrhythmias.

Bleeding is often limited during MIDCAB and rarely requires transfusion unless the patient is already anemic. Hypothermia is a common event that may delay extubation for 3 to 4 hours.[68] A decline in the patient's temperature occurs because it is typical to prepare the patient for a conventional CABG, including preparation of the legs. Once the patient's legs have been prepped, a sterile sheet may be placed over the legs with a warming blanket placed over the sterile sheet. In the case of conversion to sternotomy and saphenous vein harvest, the warming blanket can be removed while maintaining sterility of the leg.

MIDCAB procedures are converted to conventional CABG in approximately 6 to 7% of cases.[69, 70] Reasons for the change in procedure include difficulty mobilizing or inability to locate the left anterior descending artery and hemodynamic instability.[71] Even though there is a change in surgical procedure, the anesthesiologist can still manage the patient with the goal of an early extubation, assuming that the remainder of the procedure is without incident.

Reperfusion Monitoring

The long-term graft patency results after MIDCAB are unknown. There is interest in determining the condition of the anastomosis soon after the procedure. Angiography is the "gold standard" by which the results of an anastomosis can be judged.[72] Angiography can be performed in the operating room, adding 15 minutes to the surgical time,[72] or after transport to the cardiac catheterization suite immediately after operation.[73] A propofol infusion can be used to maintain anesthesia if immediate transport to the catheterization laboratory is necessary.[74] Immediate postoperative angiography may lead to revision of one fifth of all grafts.[75]

Although angiography remains the gold standard for evaluation of a coronary artery anastomosis, its routine use is cumbersome. Other imaging technologies, such as thermography and myocardial contrast echocardiography, have been suggested for routine monitoring. The use of thermography does not provide a detailed view of the anastomosis, but despite this limitation, thermography may affect the management of up to 16% of coronary bypass operations.[76]

Myocardial contrast echocardiography (MCE) involves the use of sonicated albumin microspheres to enhance echocardiographic contrast. MCE has been shown to illustrate the distribution of an ultrasound contrast agent into the distribution of the left anterior descending artery after

MIDCAB but gives no information concerning the quality of the anastomosis site.[77] The use of MCE during conventional CABG may identify up to 16% of cases in which additional revascularization may be beneficial.[78] The use of MCE will increase as TEE becomes more readily available in cardiac surgical suites and as the technology for providing echocardiographic contrast becomes simplified.

Postoperative Analgesia

The amount of pain after MIDCAB has been poorly described. In keeping with the minimally invasive nature of MIDCAB, proponents argue that there is less pain involved than with a sternotomy. It is sometimes difficult to assess the cause of pain in the postoperative period. The possibility of myocardial ischemia or infarction should be entertained if there appears to be an excessive amount of pain.

A number of pain-control methods are available for use in this population. Intravenous opioids can be effective, particularly if used in conjunction with patient-controlled analgesia. Intercostal blocks are uniquely well suited and provide 6 hours of analgesia.[79] The use of parenteral nonsteroidal anti-inflammatory drugs such as ketorolac helps manage the pain from chest tubes. The early removal of chest tubes can also help patients feel more comfortable. Chaney advocates the use of epidural or intrathecal narcotics for analgesia following cardiac surgery performed via median sternotomy.[80] There is considerable resistance to this approach, however, given the risk of injury from epidural hematoma.

Anesthesia for Cases Involving Cardiopulmonary Bypass

Although in a recent survey, Shennib and associates reported that 81% of cardiac surgeons surveyed would rather eliminate CPB from heart surgery than eliminate a median sternotomy approach,[81] many surgeons now believe that median sternotomy is also responsible for a significant portion of postoperative morbidity. The port access approach aims to eliminate the need for median sternotomy while the use of CPB is maintained. The introduction of port access techniques has meant additional responsibilities for cardiac anesthesiologists involved in these cases.

Port Access Techniques

Heartport (Redwood City, CA) is a system that relies on percutaneously placed catheters to support a patient's circulation with CPB and allow the administration of cardioplegia to arrest the heart with the chest closed. Cannulas are placed percutaneously in the femoral artery and vein to provide systemic flow to the patient. The position of the femoral venous cannula in the right atrium and inferior vena cava can be confirmed by fluoroscopy or TEE. A percutaneous pulmonary artery vent cannula is placed by the anesthesiologist; the position of this cannula is also checked with fluoroscopy. This vent is used to decompress the left ventricle. The anesthesiologist then places an optional coronary sinus cannula via the internal jugular vein, guided by fluoroscopy and TEE.[82]

Figure 52–2 demonstrates the appearance of the coronary sinus by TEE; correct placement of the retrograde catheter is signaled by the obliteration of the channel on TEE. The coronary sinus catheter is routinely used during mitral valve procedures and is optional during other procedures. Last, an endoaortic catheter with an occlusion balloon is inserted with the tip in the ascending aorta. This catheter provides the means for delivering antegrade cardioplegia. This last catheter can be located by fluoroscopy but is readily visible by TEE, and the position can be rechecked intermittently during the operation. TEE is used for mitral valve surgery using the Heartport system to reassess the mitral valve before surgery, guide placement of the endoaortic balloon, measure aortic diameter before inflation of the endoaortic catheter, evaluate efficacy of deairing maneuvers, evaluate adequacy of the mitral valve surgery, and help guide weaning from CPB.[83]

Monitoring techniques are used during port access CPB cases to ensure adequate venous drainage, arterial flow, venting, and aortic occlusion. Troubleshooting a CPB system may be unfamiliar to many anesthesiologists. Venous return in this system is augmented by a centrifugal pump rather than relying solely on gravity drainage.[84] Conventional femoral venous cannulation without augmentation of venous return can support only 75 to 80% of a normal cardiac output.[85] An excessive pulmonary artery vent flow (5% of total bypass flow) indicates poor positioning of the venous cannula.[85] Potential migration of the endoaortic clamp may be detected by a variety of methods, including TEE of the aorta, transcranial Doppler of the right carotid artery, balloon pressure measurements, and comparison of the aortic root pressure and the systemic arterial pressure.[84] Use of low filling volume in the endoaortic clamp is associated with catheter migration.[86] Reliance on only retrograde cardioplegia may not reliably protect the right ventricular free wall, which may result in hemodynamic instability and atrioventricular conduction block.[87] Other concerns include the high cost of this largely disposable system and the increased operating times owing to the lengthy process of placing the percutaneous cannulas.

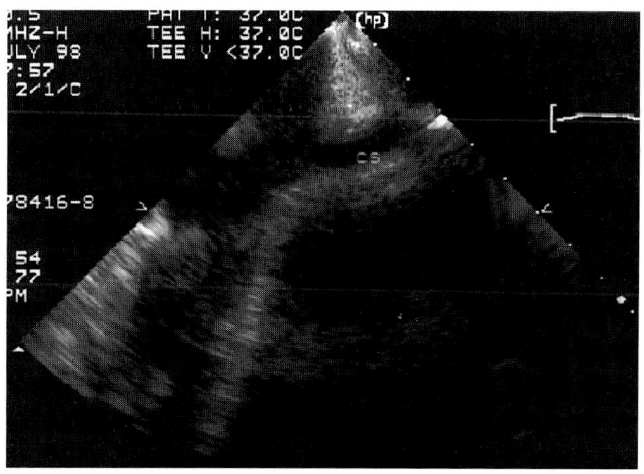

Figure 52–2. Coronary sinus appearance by transesophageal echocardiography. The coronary sinus (CS) is best visualized by retroflexion of the probe.

Traditional Cardiopulmonary Bypass via Smaller Incisions

Valvular surgery requires the use of CPB because of the intracardiac nature of the procedure. Cosgrove and Sabik described a technique for aortic valve replacement performed with a minimally invasive right parasternal approach.[88] Access to the heart for defibrillation and pacing is limited, but the technique relies on placing the arterial bypass cannula directly into the ascending aorta. TEE is used to assist in cardiac monitoring as well as in de-airing the heart before release of the aortic cross-clamp. A similar approach for mitral valve replacement has been described using a superior vena cava cannula in addition to a femoral venous cannula positioned in the inferior vena cava.[89] The ventricular pacing wire should be placed while the aortic clamp is still on, because it is easier to do with the heart decompressed.[90] Chitwood and associates described a minimal access procedure for mitral valve surgery that uses a specially designed transthoracic aortic cross-clamp.[91] These approaches use familiar techniques such as external aortic cross-clamps and surgically placed bypass cannulas. The anesthetic management of these patients has been described and differs little from established anesthetic techniques.[92]

References

1. Izzat MB, Yim APC: Minimally invasive cardiac surgery, a fleeting fancy or a lasting prospect? Int J Cardiol 59:223–225, 1997.
2. Calafiore AM, Angelini GD, Bergsland J, Salerno TA: Minimally invasive coronary artery bypass grafting. Ann Thorac Surg 62:1545–1548, 1996.
3. Akins CW, Boucher CA, Pohost GM: Prevention of interventricular septal function in patients having coronary artery bypass grafts without cardiopulmonary bypass. Am Heart J 107:304–309, 1984.
4. Perrault LP, Bel A, de Chaumarray T, et al: Beating heart coronary artery bypass surgery is associated with increased myocardial production of heat shock proteins (Abstracts). Circulation 94:I–170, 1996.
5. Westaby S: Coronary surgery without cardiopulmonary bypass. Br Heart J 73:203–205, 1995.
6. Airaksinen KEJ, Ikaheimo MJ, Huikuri HV: Stenosis severity and the occurrence of ventricular ectopic activity during acute coronary occlusion during balloon angioplasty. Am J Cardiol 76:346–349, 1995.
7. Westaby S, Benetti FJ: Less invasive coronary surgery: Consensus from the Oxford meeting. Ann Thorac Surg 62:924–931, 1996.
8. Borst C, Jansen EWL, Grundeman PF: Less invasive coronary artery bypass grafting: Without cardiopulmonary bypass and via reduced surgical access. Heart 77:302–303, 1997.
9. Vural KM, Tasdemir O, Karagoz HY, Bayazit K: Avoiding early or late failure in "off-pump" coronary artery bypass grafting. Ann Thorac Surg 62:945–946, 1996.
10. Benetti FJ, Ballester C, Sani G, et al: Video assisted coronary bypass surgery. J Card Surg 10:620–625, 1995.
11. Borges MF, Spohn PK, Coulson AS: Arrhythmia/ischemia management during minimally invasive cardiac operation. Ann Thorac Surg 64:843–844, 1997.
12. Wasnick JD: Minimally invasive direct coronary artery bypass procedure and pacing pulmonary artery catheter (Letter). J Cardiothorac Vasc Anesth 10:975, 1996.
13. Wasnick JD, Acuff T: Anesthesia and minimally invasive thoracoscopically assisted coronary artery bypass: A brief clinical report. J Cardiothorac Vasc Anesth 11:552–555, 1997.
14. Pawlowski J, Haering JM, Communale ME, et al: Minimally invasive anesthesia should accompany minimally invasive surgery. J Cardiothorac Vasc Anesth 11:536–537, 1997.
15. Schaff HV: New surgical techniques: Implications for the cardiac anesthesiologist: Mini-thoracotomy for coronary revascularization without cardiopulmonary bypass. J Cardiothorac Vasc Anesth 11(suppl 1):6–9, 1997.
16. Chung F, Seyone C, Rakowski H: Transesophageal echocardiogram may fail to diagnose perioperative myocardial infarction. Can J Anaesth 38:98–101, 1991.
17. Jopling MW: Pro: Automated electrocardiogram ST-segment monitoring should be used in the monitoring of cardiac surgical patients. J Cardiothorac Vasc Anesth 10:678–680, 1996.
18. Wickey GS, Larach DR, Keifer JC, et al: Combined interpretation of transesophageal echocardiography, electrocardiography, and pulmonary artery wedge waveform to detect myocardial ischemia. J Cardiothorac Anesth 4:102–104, 1990.
19. Kaplan JA, Wells PH: Early diagnosis of myocardial ischemia using the pulmonary artery catheter. Anesth Analg 60:789–793, 1981.
20. Benetti FJ: Experience with surgery on the beating heart. *In* Emery RW, Arom KV, Fonger JD, et al (eds): Techniques for Minimally Invasive Direct Coronary Artery Bypass (MIDCAB) Surgery. Philadelphia, Hanley & Belfus, 1997, pp 23–26.
21. Duncan S, Fonger JD: Operative MIDCAB nursing. *In* Emery RW, Arom KV, Fonger JD, et al (eds): Techniques for Minimally Invasive Direct Coronary Artery Bypass (MIDCAB) Surgery. Philadelphia, Hanley & Belfus, 1997, pp 119–125.
22. Boonstra PW, Grandjean JG, Mariani MA: Improved method for direct coronary grafting without CPB via anterolateral small thoracotomy. Ann Thorac Surg 63:567–569, 1997.
23. Stanbridge RL, Hadjinikolaou LK, Cohen AS, et al: Minimally invasive coronary revascularization through parasternal incisions without cardiopulmonary bypass. Ann Thorac Surg 63:S53–S56, 1997.
24. Wasnick JD, Hoffman WJ, Acuff T, Mack M: Anesthetic management of coronary artery bypass via minithoracotomy with video assistance. J Cardiothorac Vasc Anesth 9:731–733, 1995.
25. Benetti FJ, Mariani MA, Ballester C: Direct coronary surgery without cardiopulmonary bypass in acute myocardial infarction. J Cardiovasc Surg 37:391–395, 1996.
26. Grandjean JG, Mariani MA, Ebels T: Coronary reoperation via small laparotomy using right gastroepiploic artery without CPB. Ann Thorac Surg 61:1853–1855, 1996.
27. Mentzer RM, Lasley RD: Ischemic preconditioning. *In* Emery RW, Arom KV, Fonger JD, et al (eds): Techniques for Minimally Invasive Direct Coronary Artery Bypass (MIDCAB) Surgery. Philadelphia, Hanley & Belfus, 1997, pp 113–118.
28. Galinanes M, Argano V, Hearse DJ: Can ischemic preconditioning ensure optimal myocardial protection when delivery of cardioplegia is impaired? Circulation 92:II-389–II-394, 1995.
29. Yelton DM, Alkhulaifi AM, Pugsley WB: Preconditioning the human myocardium. Lancet 342:276–277, 1993.
30. Alkhulaifi AM, Jenkins DP, Pugsley WB, Treasure T: Ischaemic preconditioning and cardiac surgery. Eur J Cardiothorac Surg 10:792–798, 1996.
31. Cohen MV, Liu GS, Downey JM: Preconditioning causes improved wall motion as well as smaller infarcts after transient coronary occlusion in rabbits. Circulation 84:341–349, 1991.
32. Murry CE, Jennings RB, Reimer KA: Preconditioning with ischemia: A delay of lethal cell injury in ischemic myocardium. Circulation 74:1124–1136, 1986.
33. Shiki K, Hearse DJ: Preconditioning of ischemic myocardium: Reperfusion-induced arrhythmias. Am J Physiol 253: H1470–H1476, 1987.

34. Jenkins DP, Pugsley WB, Kemp M, et al: Ischaemic preconditioning reduces troponin-T release in patients undergoing cardiac surgery (Abstract). Heart 75:P71, 1996.
35. Leesar MA, Stoddard M, Ahmed M, et al: Preconditioning of human myocardium with adenosine during coronary angioplasty. Circulation 95:2500–2507, 1997.
36. Przyklenk K, Kloner RA: Ischemic preconditioning: Exploring the paradox. Prog Cardiovasc Dis 40:517–547, 1998.
37. Downey JM, Cohen MV, Ytrehus K, Liu Y: Cellular mechanisms in ischemic preconditioning: The role of adenosine and protein kinase C. Ann N Y Acad Sci 723:82–98, 1994.
38. Finegan BA: Myocardial protection: Is there anything better than ice? Can J Anaesth 45:R32–R36, 1998.
39. Robinson MC, Thielmeier KA, Hill BB: Transient ventricular asystole using adenosine during minimally invasive and open sternotomy coronary artery bypass grafting. Ann Thorac Surg 63:S30–S34, 1997.
40. Warltier DC, Al-Wathiqui MH, Kampine JP, Schmeling WT: Recovery of contractile function of stunned myocardium in chronically instrumented dogs is enhanced by halothane or isoflurane. Anesthesiology 69:552–565, 1988.
41. Davis RF, Sidi A: Effects of isoflurane on the extent of myocardial necrosis and on systemic hemodynamics, regional myocardial blood flow, and regional myocardial metabolism in dogs after coronary artery occlusion. Anesth Analg 69:575–586, 1989.
42. Buljubasic N, Marijic J, Stowe DF, et al: Halothane reduces dysrhythmias and improves contractile function after global hypoperfusion in isolated hearts. Anesth Analg 74:384–394, 1992.
43. Coetzee A, Moolman J: Halothane and the reperfusion injury in the intact animal model. Anesth Analg 76:734–744, 1993.
44. Elefteriades JA: Mini-CABG: A step forward or backward? The "pro" point of view. J Cardiothorac Vasc Anesth 11:661–668, 1997.
45. Rivetti LA, Gandria SMA: Initial experience using an intraluminal shunt during revascularization of the beating heart. Ann Thorac Surg 63:1742–1747, 1997.
46. Collard E, Ducart A, Buche M, et al: Perioperative cardiac events during coronary-artery surgery without cardiopulmonary bypass (Abstract). Anesth Analg 84:SCA97, 1997.
47. Arom KV, Emery RW, Nicoloff DM: Conversion to sternotomy. *In* Emery RW, Arom KV, Fonger JD, et al (eds): Techniques for Minimally Invasive Direct Coronary Artery Bypass (MIDCAB) Surgery. Philadelphia, Hanley & Belfus, 1997, pp 73–76.
48. Trapp WG, Bisarya R: Placement of coronary artery bypass graft without pump oxygenator. Ann Thorac Surg 19:1–9, 1975.
49. Lima LE, Nataf P, Gandjbakhch I, et al: Thoracoscopic IMA dissection and direct suture (La Pitie technique). *In* Emery RW, Arom KV, Fonger JD, et al (eds): Techniques for Minimally Invasive Direct Coronary Artery Bypass (MIDCAB) Surgery. Philadelphia, Hanley & Belfus, 1997, pp 55–62.
50. Abramson DC, Pivalizza EG, Gottschalk LI: Drug management for coronary revascularization without cardiac standstill: The use of high-dose esmolol. J Cardiothorac Vasc Anesth 9:184–188, 1995.
51. Grocott HP, Grichnik K: Partial cardiopulmonary bypass, high dose esmolol, and a left thoracotomy for reoperative coronary artery bypass graft surgery (Abstract). Anesth Analg 82:SCA129, 1996.
52. Labovitz AJ, Barth C, Castello R, et al: Attenuation of myocardial ischemia during coronary occlusion by ultrashort-acting beta adrenergic blockade. Am Heart J 121:1347–1352, 1991.
53. Jacobsohn E, Ferdinand F, Albertucci M, et al: Minimally invasive CABG: Anesthetic technique and outcome (Abstract). Anesth Analg 84:S91, 1997.
54. Robinson MC: Identification and management of coronary arteries: Immobilization and control. *In* Emery RW, Arom KV, Fonger JD, et al (eds): Techniques for Minimally Invasive Direct Coronary Artery Bypass (MIDCAB) Surgery. Philadelphia, Hanley & Belfus, 1997, pp 79–86.
55. Buffolo E, de Andrade JCS, Branco JNR, et al: Coronary artery bypass grafting without cardiopulmonary bypass. Ann Thorac Surg 61:63–66, 1996.
56. Rajek A, Podesser A, Kupilik N, et al: Effect of α-blockers versus calcium channel blockers in myocardial revascularization without cardio-pulmonary bypass in pigs (Abstract). Br J Anaesth 76:A.39, 1996.
57. Thielmeier KA, Robinson MC: Role of adenosine-induced ventricular asystole during minimally invasive CABG optimizing the surgical field (Abstract). Anesthesiology 85:A162, 1996.
58. Hesselvik JF, Ortega RA, Shemin RJ: The use of neostigmine to decrease the heart rate in a patient undergoing minimally invasive coronary artery bypass surgery. J Cardiothorac Vasc Anesth 11:883–884, 1997.
59. Benetti F, Mariani MA, Sani G, et al: Video-assisted minimally invasive coronary operations without cardiopulmonary bypass: A multicenter study. J Thorac Cardiovasc Surg 112:1478–1484, 1996.
60. Pagni S, Qaqish NK, Senior DG, Spence PA: Anastomotic complications in minimally invasive coronary bypass grafting. Ann Thorac Surg 63:S64–S67, 1997.
61. Boonstra PW, Grandjean JG, Mariani MA: Local immobilization of the left anterior descending artery for minimally invasive coronary bypass grafting. Ann Thorac Surg 63:S76–S78, 1997.
62. Subramanian VA: Less invasive arterial CABG on a beating heart. Ann Thorac Surg 63:S68–S71, 1997.
63. Borst C, Jansen EWL, Tulleken CA, et al: Coronary artery bypass grafting without cardiopulmonary bypass and without interruption of native coronary flow using a novel anastomosis site restraining device ("Octopus"). J Am Coll Cardiol 27:1356–1364, 1996.
64. Grundeman PF, Borst C, van Herwaarden JA, et al: Hemodynamic changes during displacement of the beating heart by the Utrecht Octopus method. Ann Thorac Surg 63:S88–S92, 1997.
65. Grundeman PF, Borst C, van Herwaarden JA, Verlaan CWJ: Ninety degrees anterior displacement of the beating porcine heart using the Octopus tissue stabilizer: Does it limit coronary flow? (Abstract). Circulation 96:I–681, 1997.
66. Jurmann MJ, Menon A, Guggenberger H, et al: Pharmacologic versus mechanical stabilization of the heart during minimally invasive coronary artery bypass: Effects on left ventricular geometry and hemodynamics (Abstract). Circulation 96:I-680, 1997.
67. Shennib H, Lee AGL, Akin J: Safe and effective method of stabilization for coronary artery bypass grafting on the beating heart. Ann Thorac Surg 63:988–992, 1997.
68. Juneja R, Mehta Y, Mishra Y, Trehan N: Minimally invasive coronary artery surgery: Anesthetic considerations. J Cardiothorac Vasc Anesth 11:123–124, 1997.
69. Landreneau RJ, Mack MJ, Magovern JA, et al: "Keyhole" coronary artery bypass surgery. Ann Surg 224:453–462, 1996.
70. Subramanian VA, McCabe JC, Geller CM: Minimally invasive direct coronary artery bypass grafting: Two-year experience. Ann Thorac Surg 64:1648–1655, 1997.
71. Magovern JA, Mack MJ, Landreneau RJ, et al: The minimally invasive approach reduces the morbidity of coronary artery bypass (Abstract). Circulation 94:I–52, 1996.
72. Lazzara RR, McLellan BA, Kidwell FE, et al: Intraoperative angiography during minimally invasive direct coronary artery bypass operations. Ann Thorac Surg 64:1725–1727, 1997.
73. Izzat MB, Yim APC: MIDCABG: Lessons learned from routine "on-table" angiography. Ann Thorac Surg 64:1872–1874, 1997.
74. Gayes JM, Emery RW: The MIDCAB experience: A current look at evolving surgical and anesthetic approaches. J Cardiothorac Vasc Anesth 11:625–628, 1997.

75. Schaff HV, Cable DG, Rihal CS, et al: Minimal thoracotomy for coronary artery bypass: Value of immediate postprocedure graft angiography (Abstract). Circulation 94:I–51, 1996.
76. Emery RW, Emery AM, Flavin TF, et al: Revascularization using angioplasty and minimally invasive techniques documented by thermal imaging. Ann Thorac Surg 62:591–593, 1996.
77. Jacobsohn E, Aronson S, Young C, et al: Perfusion echocardiography during minimally invasive coronary bypass (Abstract). Anesth Analg 84:S90, 1997.
78. Aronson S, Lee BK, Wiencek JG, et al: Assessment of myocardial perfusion during CABG surgery with two-dimensional transesophageal contrast echocardiography. Anesthesiology 75:433–440, 1991.
79. Westaby S: Coronary surgery without cardiopulmonary bypass: Rationale and evolution of technique. *In* Emery RW, Arom KV, Fonger JD, et al (eds): Techniques for Minimally Invasive Direct Coronary Artery Bypass (MIDCAB) Surgery. Philadelphia, Hanley & Belfus, 1997, pp 3–8.
80. Chaney MA: Intrathecal and epidural anesthesia and analgesia for cardiac surgery. Anesth Analg 84:1211–1221, 1997.
81. Shennib H, Mack MJ, Lee AGL: A survey on minimally invasive coronary artery bypass grafting. Ann Thorac Surg 64:110–115, 1997.
82. Clements F, Wright SJ, de Bruijn N: Coronary sinus catheterization made easy for port-access minimally invasive cardiac surgery. J Cardiothorac Vasc Anesth 12:96–101, 1998.
83. Falk V, Walther T, Diegeler A, et al: Echocardiographic monitoring of minimally invasive mitral valve surgery using an endoaortic clamp. J Heart Valve Dis 5:630–637, 1996.
84. Siegel LC, Peters WS, St. Goar, et al: Anesthetic considerations for port-access cardiac surgery (Abstract). Anesth Analg 82:SCA79, 1996.
85. Toomasian JM, Peters WS, Siegel LC: Extracorporeal circulation for port-access cardiac surgery. Perfusion 12:83–91, 1997.
86. Siegel LC, Stevens JH, St. Goar, et al: Intraoperative monitoring of patients undergoing port-access coronary artery bypass grafting (Abstract). Anesthesiology 85:A160, 1996.
87. Winkelmann J, Aronson S, Young CJ, et al: Retrograde-delivered cardioplegia is not distributed equally to the right ventricular free wall and septum. J Cardiothorac Vasc Anesth 9:135–139, 1995.
88. Cosgrove DM III, Sabik JF: Minimally invasive approach for aortic valve operations. Ann Thorac Surg 62:596–597, 1996.
89. Navia JL, Cosgrove DM III: Minimally invasive mitral valve operations. Ann Thorac Surg 62:1542–1544, 1996.
90. Cohn LH, Adams DH, Couper GS, Bichell DP: Minimally invasive aortic valve replacement. Semin Thorac Cardiovasc Surg 9:331–336, 1997.
91. Chitwood WR Jr, Wixon CL, Elbeery JR, et al: Video-assisted minimally invasive mitral valve surgery. J Thorac Cardiovasc Surg 114:773–782, 1997.
92. Hearn CJ, Kraenzler EJ, Wallace LK, et al: Minimally invasive aortic valve surgery: Anesthetic considerations. Anesth Analg 83:1342–1344, 1996.

Chapter 53

Echocardiography in Minimally Invasive Cardiac Surgery

Mohammad Bashar Izzat, Fabio Capasso, Vincenzo Lucchetti, and Gianni D. Angelini

Less invasive approaches to cardiac surgical procedures are being developed in an effort to decrease patient morbidity and enhance postoperative recovery in comparison to conventional methods.[1, 2] It is crucial that an acceptable level of patient safety be maintained when such new methods are applied, and echocardiography plays an important role in this context. Selecting suitable candidates for a procedure, or selecting the best procedure for a particular patient, is based on several factors, including the echocardiographic findings. Echocardiography also plays an integral part in intraoperative and postoperative care strategy. In our program, a detailed transesophageal echocardiographic (TEE) assessment is routinely performed before commencing surgery, and we consider the availability of echocardiography in the operating room and the intensive care unit a prerequisite to performing minimally invasive cardiac surgery.[2, 3]

Echocardiography in Off-Pump Coronary Artery Grafting

Echocardiographic findings are important in confirming the suitability of a particular patient for off-pump surgery and in ruling out the existence of a concurrent cardiac pathology (e.g., mitral valve incompetence or left ventricular aneurysm) that may require a change in the surgical management.[3] Echocardiography's most critical role in off-pump surgery is intraoperative, however. Performing coronary artery anastomoses on the beating heart usually involves the temporary occlusion of the targeted coronary artery in order to achieve a bloodless operative field, with the possibility of causing regional ischemia and hemodynamic compromise. Moreover, heart displacement and use of cardiac stabilizers can produce abrupt variations in left ventricle (LV) chamber geometry and some mechanical wall motion abnormalities.

Intraoperative TEE allows continuous and sensitive monitoring of global and regional LV function, extent of ischemia, and hemodynamic effects of heart manipulations, and it guides the surgeon in decision-making during surgery. It can also be used to examine segments that were hypokinetic preoperatively to evaluate the success of the grafting procedure.

Left Ventricular Segmental Wall Motion Analysis. Segmental wall motion abnormalities precede, and may occur in the absence of, ST-segment changes indicative of ischemia on the electrocardiogram (ECG). TEE, for this purpose, is a more sensitive and specific monitor of myocardial ischemia than ECG. In practice, the two techniques are used not in competition but in concert. The severity of wall motion abnormalities corresponds to the degree of perfusion abnormality. At 50% reduction in coronary flow, hypokinesia develops; dyskinesia takes place with a 90% to 95% reduction in flow.

Segmental wall motion analysis can be performed through the transgastric short-axis view at the level of the papillary muscles and through the long-axis view at the same level by 90 degrees rotation of a multiplane probe. The LV is divided into 16 segments, and each is graded by qualitative visual estimation on a scale of 1 to 4, 1 being normal and 4 being dyskinesia. Wall motion score is calculated preoperatively, during coronary occlusion, and after reperfusion. A worsening of segmental wall motion and wall thickening of at least two classes is diagnostic of ischemia. Analysis of all 16 segments of the LV is essential, because distant areas that are perfused through collateral circulation may be affected by coronary occlusion. Throughout the procedure, the probe is maintained in a stable position so that apparent segmental changes do not erroneously result from scanning a neighboring segment transiently.

The myocardial response to temporary coronary occlusion varies according to the degree of native vessel disease and collateral circulation. Upon snaring a chronically occluded native left anterior descending artery (LAD), wall motion remains unchanged from baseline, without hemodynamic compromise. If a stenotic LAD supplying an occluded right coronary artery is snared, extensive wall motion abnormalities are commonly seen within 15 seconds of coronary occlusion. Using a coronary shunt in such cases returns wall motion to baseline.

Compression coronary stabilizers can produce localized myocardial asynergy (Fig. 53–1), whereas the Octopus device causes a restricted akinetic area in the stabilized region (Fig. 53–2). These changes do not usually cause significant impairment of LV function. Yet their identification is important to differentiate these asynergies from those caused by impairment of perfusion upon coronary occlusion.

Left Ventricular Function Analysis. Early detection of imminent depression of LV function is a useful function of TEE monitoring. Left ventricular ejection fraction can be serially calculated before and during surgery by the area-length single-plane method, obtained from the midesophageal four-chamber view. Cardiac output can also be reliably measured by TEE through Doppler estimation of pulmonary artery blood flow.[4]

Left ventricular systolic dP/dt correlates global LV contractility to pressure increase during isovolumic systole. In the presence of mitral regurgitation, depressed LV func-

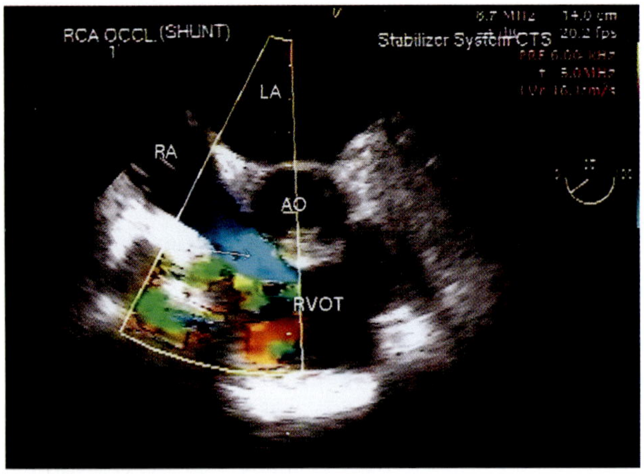

Figure 53–1. Transesophageal echocardiographic basal short-axis view in the middle esophageal position in a patient undergoing off-pump right coronary artery grafting. Cardiac displacement and the compression stabilizer (CTS) have caused moderate narrowing of the right ventricular inlet.

tion is associated with a slower rise in LV pressure and hence the velocity of the mitral regurgitant jet. Doppler envelop of the regurgitant jet, therefore, reflects LV systolic pressure, and integrating the onset will be a measure of left ventricular dP/dt.

Left Ventricular Changes With Cardiac Displacement. During extreme cardiac dislocation, as during grafting of obtuse marginal coronary artery branches, heart chambers can lose their normal shape and uniform concentric contraction pattern. Therefore, even in the absence of perfusion impairment, the LV can present several dyskinetic segments as a consequence of the changes in timing and velocity of myocardial excursion. This loss in kinetic synchrony may herald total failure of LV global contraction.

Mild to moderate, but occasionally severe, mitral regurgitation may also result from distortion of LV geometry (Fig. 53–3), and this can be worsened by posteromedial papillary muscle dysfunction following right coronary artery snaring. This additional hemodynamic load is particularly important, considering the already ischemic and dislocated heart, and can explain a sudden change in certain hemodynamic parameters such as central venous or pulmonary capillary wedge pressure.

TEE, therefore, is useful in detecting a variety of changes and in avoiding sudden hemodynamic collapse. The heart should always be examined after it has been stabilized in the new position, and multiple interrogations through transgastric and midesophageal views are performed because good-quality images are often difficult to obtain owing to surgical swabs or air interposition between the heart and the transducer.

Echocardiography in Minimally Invasive Intracardiac Surgery

Intraoperative TEE, already established in the care of cardiac surgical patients, assumes an even greater role in the setting of minimally invasive intracardiac surgery.[2] TEE subsitutes for the surgeon's ability to directly visualize or feel the ventricles to confirm adequate heart decompression and to avoid ventricular distention. For this purpose, the echocardiographer can monitor the size of the left ventricular cavity through the transgastric short-axis view and can alert the surgeon about the need for additional ventricular venting maneuvers. Similarly, TEE monitoring is used to indicate the adequacy of ventricular filling when weaning the patient from cardiopulmonary bypass.

Of particular importance is the ability of TEE to assist and direct the de-airing of the heart. Evacuation of air from heart chambers is troublesome when a minimally invasive approach is used because the standard de-airing maneuvers cannot be performed. With TEE, air is detected within heart chambers, great vessels, pulmonary veins, or left atrial appendage, and its removal is confirmed before the aortic cross-clamp is released (Fig. 53–4).

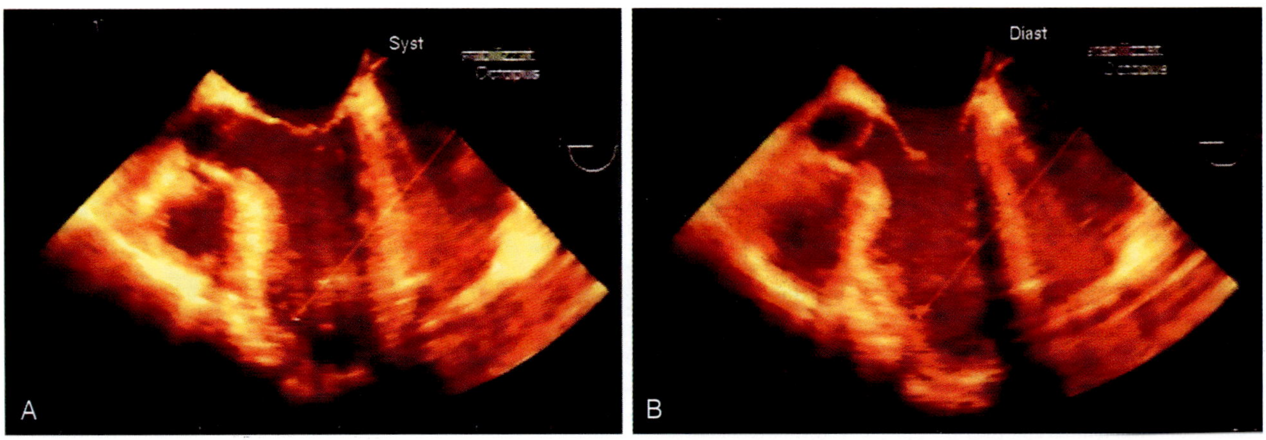

Figure 53–2. Transesophageal echocardiographic short-axis view in a patient undergoing off-pump grafting of left internal mammary artery (LIMA)–to–left anterior descending artery (LAD). Applying the Octopus system to the LAD has immobilized the septum (*arrow*), although it still increased in thickness in systole. (*A*) systole, and (*B*) diastole.

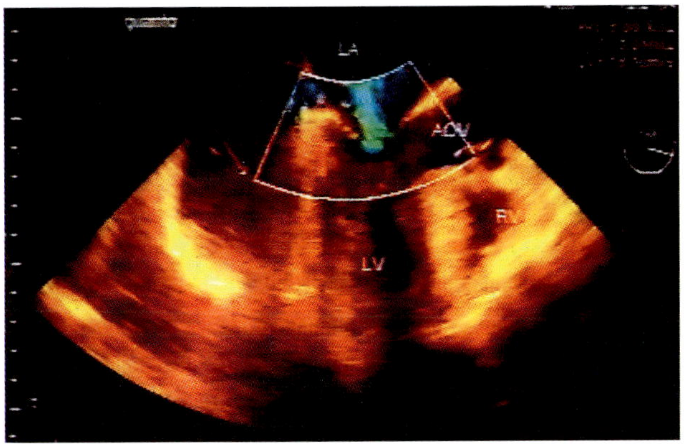

Figure 53–3. Transesophageal echocardiographic longitudinal two-chamber view in a patient undergoing off-pump posterior descending coronary artery grafting. A surgical glove filled with saline is used to dislocate the heart (*arrow*), distorting its geometry and causing moderate mitral incompetence.

Intraoperative TEE has several other applications as well. The insertion of a retrograde cardioplegia catheter in the coronary sinus is particularly difficult when an upper mini-sternotomy incision is performed, owing to the limited access and the inability to feel its position. TEE can guide and verify the correct positioning of the catheter by visualizing the coronary sinus and the catheter on the midesophageal transverse plane. As with conventional cardiac operations, TEE is also routinely used to verify successful mitral and tricuspid valve repair procedures before removing the arterial cannula (Fig. 53–5).

Echocardiography in Port Access Surgery

In the Port-Access approach, it is crucial to perform a detailed preoperative TEE assessment of the entire thoracic aorta because of the need for peripheral cardiopulmonary bypass cannulation, retrograde aortic perfusion, and the additional manipulations associated with the insertion and placement of endovascular aortic balloon clamps. The presence of extensive aortic atherosclerotic plaques can cause serious embolization during operative manipulation, and its presence, extent, and severity should be taken into account (Fig. 53–6).This has also been implicated in the infrequently reported iatrogenic acute aortic dissection.[5] Furthermore, the port access approach is contraindicated in the presence of a dilated ascending aorta, and retrograde cardioplegia should be used when aortic incompetence is present.

Several steps in the setup of the port access cardiopulmonary bypass system can be performed under fluoroscopy control. TEE, however, is a less cumbersome and equally effective method that also reduces the risk of radi-

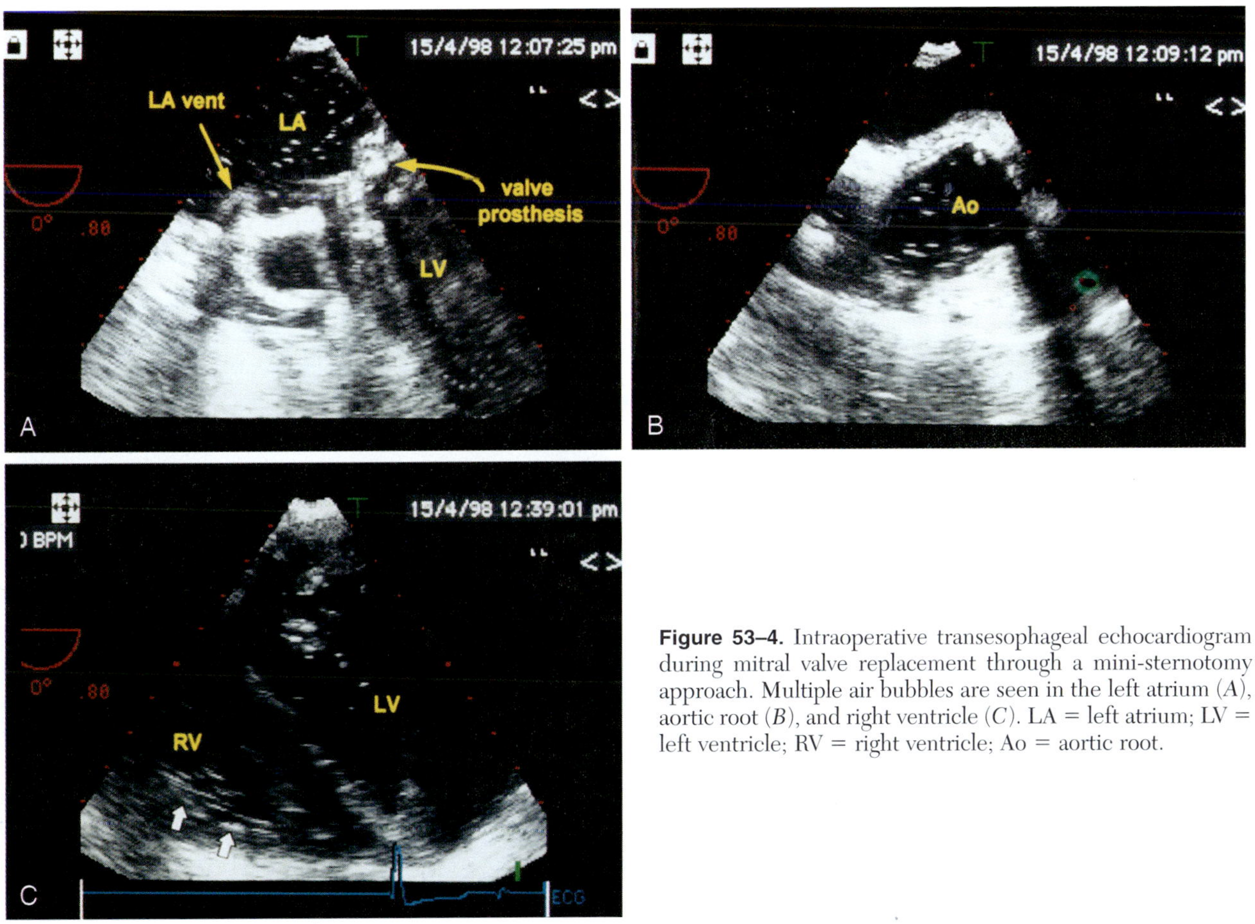

Figure 53–4. Intraoperative transesophageal echocardiogram during mitral valve replacement through a mini-sternotomy approach. Multiple air bubbles are seen in the left atrium (*A*), aortic root (*B*), and right ventricle (*C*). LA = left atrium; LV = left ventricle; RV = right ventricle; Ao = aortic root.

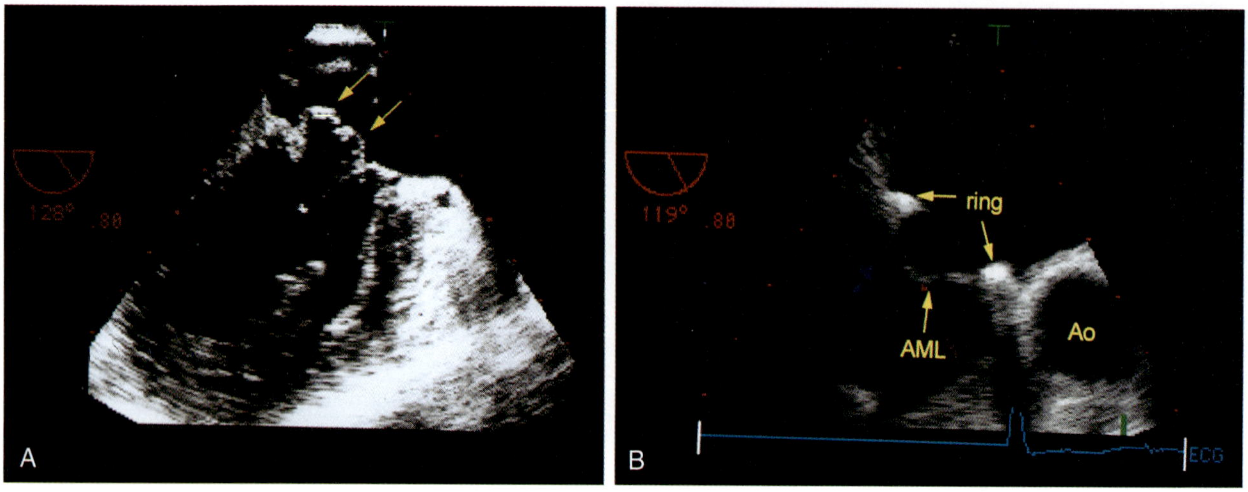

Figure 53–5. Intraoperative transesophageal echocardiogram. There is (*A*) prolapsed middle segment of the posterior leaflet of the mitral valve and (*B*) good result following quadrangular excision and ring annuloplasty.

ation exposure to both patient and staff. At the start of the procedure, the correct positioning of the venous cannula in the right atrium and the retrograde cardioplegia catheter in the coronary sinus can be assisted and verified by TEE. The endopulmonary vent catheter is placed by the anesthetist through the right internal jugular vein using pressure control, and its position is confirmed by TEE. The endovascular aortic balloon clamp is advanced up the descending aorta and into the ascending aorta, and the balloon is usually placed 2 cm above the aortic valve; its position is confirmed by TEE (Fig. 53–7).[6] Throughout the operative procedure, TEE is continuously used to monitor the correct positioning of the balloon, because of its tendency to migrate.

Similar to other minimally invasive intracardiac operations, intraoperative TEE is used to confirm the adequacy of ventricular decompression at the start of surgery, and heart chamber de-airing at its conclusion. Even though the risk is small, the availability of intraoperative TEE means that iatrogenic injuries to the aorta, such as acute aortic dissection, are readily recognizable.

Postoperative Echocardiography

As with conventional cardiac surgery, echocardiography is used routinely in patient care following minimally invasive heart operations. Echocardiography can significantly enhance the cardiac surgeon's diagnostic and therapeutic accuracy. It can monitor myocardial function, detect complications, and guide therapy.

After a minimally invasive procedure, we take special care to obtain an immediate TEE study whenever hemodynamic instability occurs. Unlike with conventional surgery, the pericardial sac usually remains closed, and

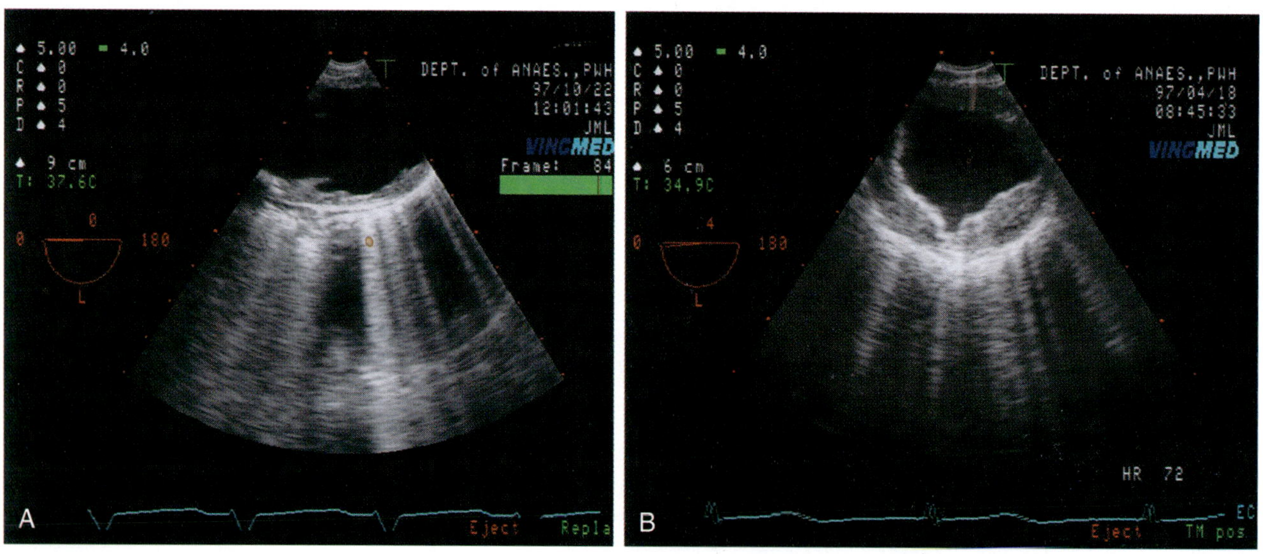

Figure 53–6. Intraoperative transesophageal echocardiogram of the aorta, showing severe atheromatous changes of the aortic arch (*A*) and the descending aorta (*B*).

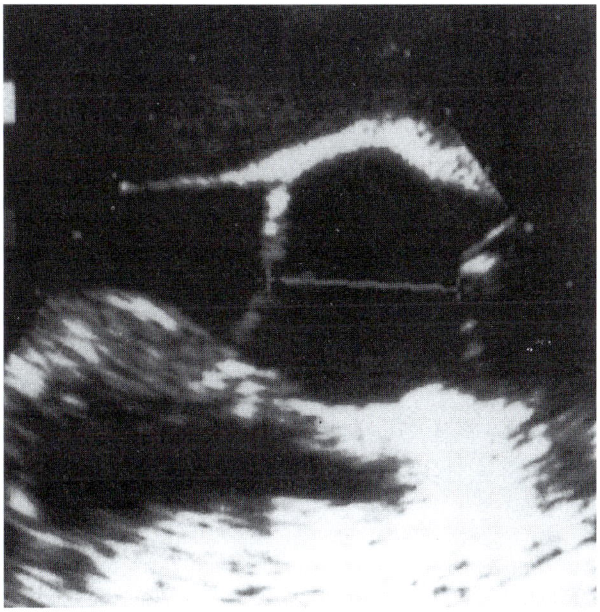

Figure 53–7. Intraoperative transesophageal echocardiogram of the aortic root (long-axis view, 130 degrees) showing the position of the endovascular aortic balloon clamp at a distance of 2.6 cm from the aortic annulus. (From Mohr FW, Falk V, Diegeler A, et al: Minimally invasive port-access mitral valve surgery. J Thorac Cardiovasc Surg 115:567–576, 1998.)

dramatic hemodynamic instability can develop with only a small pericardial collection (Fig. 53–8). This is particularly important because, in the case of hemodynamic collapse, rapid heart decompression or internal cardiac massage is not easily achievable in the absence of a prior sternotomy.[2, 3]

Various Doppler echocardiographic methods have been used for evaluating the success of grafting with minimally invasive techniques, both in the operating room and postoperatively (see Chapter 69). Transcutaneous Doppler echocardiography is the main noninvasive method currently used for the postoperative assessment of left internal mammary artery (LIMA) grafts. Two approaches can be used to visualize the conduit: suprasternal (to visualize the LIMA at its origin from the subclavian artery), and parasternal (through its course along the intercostal spaces).

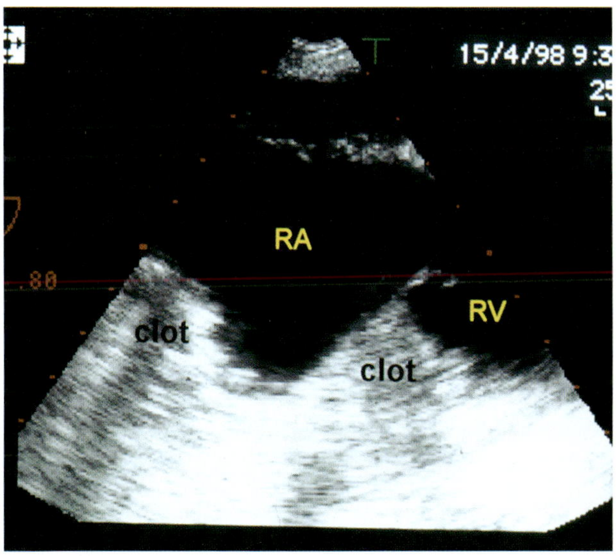

Figure 53–8. Postoperative transesophageal echocardiogram following aortic valve replacement through a mini-sternotomy approach. A relatively small intrapericardial clot anterior to the right atrium (RA) and right ventricle (RV) has caused cardiac tamponade and hemodynamic instability.

Using Doppler analysis, the ungrafted LIMA has a characteristic flow velocity pattern with a prevalent systolic component, a negative end-systolic peak (which is not always present), and a small diastolic component (Fig. 53–9*A*). When anastomosed to LAD, the flow velocity pattern becomes biphasic with an important diastolic component (Fig. 53–9*B*). LIMA flow velocity pattern, however, is directly related to the characteristics of the coronary bed to which the graft is connected. Therefore, the diastolic component is related to the resistance to graft flow: the severity of LAD stenosis and the state of the myocardium, which is LAD dependent. Furthermore, the flow velocity pattern can be affected by modification of systemic arterial pressure, change in heart rate, and use of inotropes or vasodilators.

Documenting the presence of the biphasic flow velocity pattern indicates that the LIMA-to-LAD anastomosis is patent. However, to determine whether the anastomosis is restrictive during higher flow conditions, the flow velocity pattern is examined during the Azoulay maneuver using the ratios between diastolic and systolic velocities, as proposed by Gallina and Calafiore.[7]

The Azoulay maneuver consists of two steps. First, the patient's legs are lifted up by an assistant, and second, the patient is required to actively hold this position for a few seconds. Acute hypervolemia follows as the circulating volume in both legs is suddenly emptied into the upper body circulation. As a consequence, heart rate and cardiac out put transiently increase; this causes an increase of blood flow to both the muscular circulation (systolic phase of the LIMA flow pattern) and the coronary circulation (diastolic phase of the LIMA flow pattern).

From comparing postoperative angiograms and Doppler flow velocity evaluations at rest and during the Azoulay maneuver, the following guidelines were suggested to predict the quality of LIMA-to-LAD grafts: If peak and mean diastolic/systolic velocity ratios at rest were equal to or greater than 1, or were less than 1 at rest but increased to 1 or more during the Azoulay maneuver, this indicates that the anastomosis is not restrictive. However, when ratios are less than 1 both at rest and during the Azoulay maneuver, this indicates graft malfunction or an occluded graft.[7]

The Future

In addition to the established role that echocardiography plays in conventional cardiac surgery, its part in new minimally invasive approaches to cardiac operations is an additional strong argument in favor of training cardiac surgeons in echocardiography.[8, 9] Echocardiography is no longer a "special interest" for some cardiac anesthetists and fewer cardiac surgeons; it is now an integral part of the operative

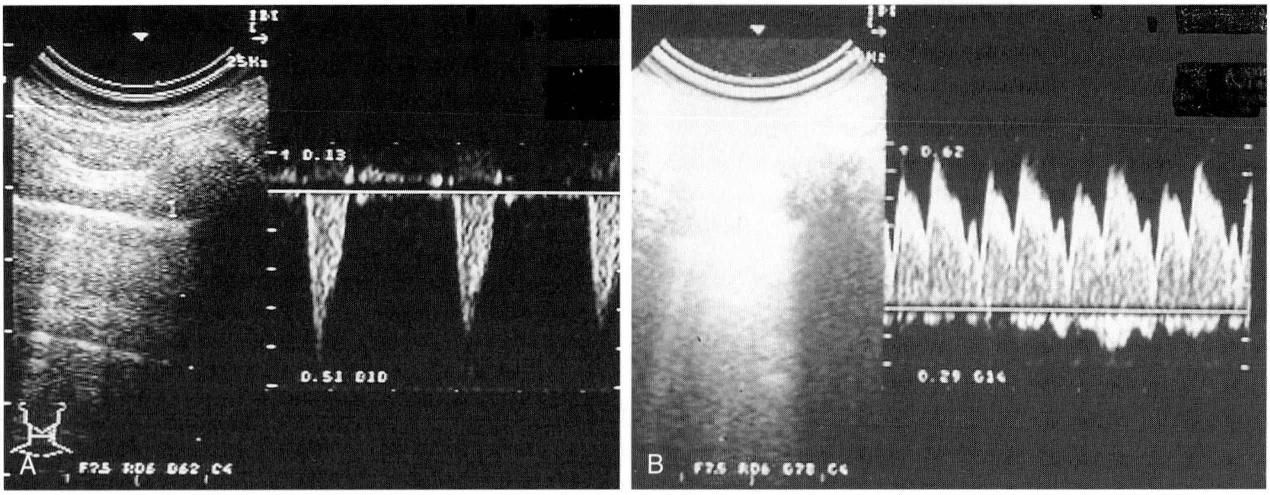

Figure 53–9. Characteristic Doppler flow velocity pattern of the left internal mammary artery before (*A*) and after (*B*) grafting to the left anterior descending artery.

procedure per se. It is clear that upcoming cardiac surgeons, on their way to establishing less invasive techniques for heart operations in their everyday practice, should be routinely trained in the specifics of echocardiography.

References

1. Izzat MB, Yim APC: Minimally invasive cardiac surgery, a fleeting fancy or a lasting prospect [Editorial]? Int J Cardiol 59:223–225, 1997.
2. Izzat MB, Yim APC: Intracardiac surgery. *In* Mack MJ, Cohn WE, Landreneau RJ, Fonger J (eds): Minimally Invasive Cardiac Surgery. St. Louis, MO, QMP Publishers (in press).
3. Izzat MB, Yim APC: Echocardiography in minimally invasive cardiac surgery. *In* Izzat MB, Sanderson JE, Sutton MSJ (eds): Echocardiography in Adult Cardiac Surgery. Oxford, UK, SIS Medical Media (in press).
4. Izzat MB, Regragui IA, Wilde P, et al. Transesophageal echocardiographic measurement of cardiac output in cardiac surgical patients. Ann Thorac Surg 58:1486–1489, 1994.
5. Reichenspurner H, Gulielmos V, Wunderlich J, et al: Port-access coronary artery bypass grafting with the use of cardiopulmonary bypass and cardioplegic arrest. Ann Thorac Surg 65:413–419, 1998.
6. Mohr FW, Falk V, Diegeler A, et al: Minimally invasive port-access mitral valve surgery. J Thorac Cardiovasc Surg 115:567–576, 1998.
7. Gallina S, Calafiore AM: Doppler echocardiography and the MIDCAB procedure. *In* Izzat MB, Sanderson JE, Sutton MSJ (eds): Echocardiography in Adult Cardiac Surgery. Oxford, UK, ISIS Medical Media (in press).
8. Izzat MB, Wilde P, Bryan AJ, Angelini GD: Surgeon-echocardiographers: The way forward. Int J Cardiol 56:209–210, 1996.
9. Izzat MB, Wilde P, Hutter JA, Angelini GD: Should transesophageal echocardiography be part of the cardiac surgeon's repertoire? Eur J Cardiothorac Surg 9:52–53, 1995.

COMMENTARY

Peter Wilde

Many important advances in medicine have taken place in the past by appropriate juxtaposition of skills and techniques that have previously been unrelated or only distantly related. The areas of cardiac surgery and echocardiography may well be a developing example of such a phenomenon.

The authors describe a number of important areas in which echocardiography, both transthoracic and transesophageal, is of benefit in the treatment of patients by minimally invasive cardiac surgery. This builds on existing experience with conventional surgery using cardiopulmonary bypass. The use of TEE is, for example, already well established in the surgical management of mitral valve repair or in the preoperative management of aortic dissection.

Running through this chapter is a persistent theme of closer integration of echocardiographic data and the practical steps taken by surgeons. The authors suggest a way of improving the quality of their work by establishing a new stream of data about patients in the perioperative period, adding to direct vision and touch, hemodynamic and physiologic monitoring, and preoperative data.

This augurs well, but we must take care with two particular areas. First, who will do the echocardiography? Echocardiography is a sophisticated and demanding technique, requiring knowledge of anatomy, pathology, cardiology, surgery, physics, and technology, as well as considerable practical and manual skills. It cannot be learned without considerable time and application. Is it right to expect the surgeon, already fully committed, to supervise the echo technique? Similarly, can the anesthetist spare the necessary time and attention to perform echo studies at the critical moments of the procedure, or do we need an additional person, highly trained and expensive, to add to the surgical team? Answers to these questions are many in current practice.

Second, if we are to recommend the addition of another sophisticated and expensive layer of technology to cardiac surgery, we must make sure that it is justified. We should look forward to objective assessments of the value of these potentially synergistic techniques by clinical trials and other means.

There are various separate professional bodies in different countries that are concerned with the development and advancement of both echocardiography and cardiac surgery. We can only hope that through the good offices of these organizations, acting in concert, we will be able to determine the future of this developing area.

Chapter 54

Alternative Incisions for Cardiac Surgery

Kit V. Arom and Robert W. Emery

Minimally invasive cardiac surgery represents a significant change in the way cardiac surgeons approach heart disease. The basic premise is that by having only a small skin incision, the patient will experience less tissue injury, a less painful and quicker overall recovery, and a shorter hospital stay. If minimally invasive cardiac surgery is to be widely accepted, the operation must be easy enough to perform with good exposure using instruments and equipment that already exist, and it must be as safe and efficacious as a standard procedure via conventional exposure.

Because the skin incision currently made for minimally invasive cardiac surgery is about 8 to 10 cm long and is significantly smaller than the heart itself, it is imperative for surgeons to develop new incisions for various areas of the chest wall through which targets, both intracardiac and extracardiac, can be reached. These incisions must be small enough to provide adequate exposure and ensure surgeon comfort while minimizing the risk of complication from limited exposure.

This chapter addresses the technical details of each approach designed for specific areas of the heart, the feasibility of reaching target areas via limited exposure, and whether the conventional technique of arterial and venous cannulation can be kept in the chest, thereby avoiding groin cannulation.

Mini-Thoracotomy Incisions

Mini-thoracotomy incisions can be carried out in various positions, depending on the location of the target artery or valve. When entering the pleural or mediastinal cavity, excision of the rib or costal cartilage is uncommon. However, in obese patients, patients with narrow intercostal spaces, patients with deep chests, or those with well-developed thoracic muscle mass, removal or dislocation of a specific rib or cartilage may be required.

Left Anterior Mini-Thoracotomy

A skin incision of 8 to 10 cm is made along the inframammary crease and curved upward medially, parallel to the lower end of the sternum (Fig. 54–1). The incision length is immaterial in terms of recovery time, although it is of concern and of interest to most patients. In women, the incision should be just below the inframammary crease and positioned more medially to minimize the possibility of infection. The pectoralis major is mobilized cephalad for access to the fourth intercostal space. The intercostal muscle of the fourth interspace is first divided laterally and then addressed medially; particular care must be taken until the internal mammary artery (IMA) pedicle is identified. The fourth and occasionally fifth sternochondral joints are then disconnected (Fig. 54–2). Cartilage excision is rarely necessary, thus eliminating the paradoxical movement and chest deformity commonly seen in slim patients.[1] To achieve increased access, mobilization of the intercostal muscle more laterally may be required if one is dealing with a laterally placed left anterior descending (LAD) or diagonal artery. This left anterior thoracotomy incision allows good exposure to the LAD, the diagonal artery, and occasionally the intermediate artery if the heart is not overly hypertrophied.

Right Anterior Mini-Thoracotomy

This incision is used for aortic and mitral surgery and for coronary artery bypass surgery when the right IMA is anastomosed to the main trunk of the right coronary artery. Exposure of the main trunk of the right coronary artery, not beyond the acute margin of the heart, can be accomplished on the right side of the chest wall with an incision similar to the one described earlier. But because the right atrioventricular groove is a midline structure located farther away from the anterior chest wall, in certain cases it is necessary to retract the pericardium more laterally upward to present the target artery close to the skin incision. In many circumstances, the mini-sternotomy incision provides better exposure to the right coronary system.

For aortic valve procedures, the right anterior mini-thoracotomy is usually carried out by making a skin incision into the third intercostal space, with dislocation of the second costosternal junction. The aortic root and the aortic valve can be visualized adequately with generous pericardial retraction. Maximal exposure of the valve can be obtained with both arterial and venous cannulae introduced through the groin. Left ventricular venting through the right superior pulmonary vein is difficult with this approach, and trans–right atrial retrograde cardioplegia is impossible.

For mitral valve procedures, the incision is similar to a port access approach.[2] The fourth or fifth intercostal space is usually used to enter the right pleural cavity, depending on the location of right heart shadow as seen posteroanterior on the chest x-rays. The third or fourth sternocostal junction can be dislocated, if necessary, for better exposure. Whenever an aortic cross-clamp with existing instrumentation is impossible, a specially designed aortic cross-clamp (Scanlen International, St. Paul, MN) can be used, or the procedure can be performed with a fibrillating heart. Both right superior pulmonary vein venting and trans–atrial retrograde cardioplegia are feasible with this approach. This incision can also be used for tricuspid valvular disease, atrial septal defects, and high ventricular septal defects.

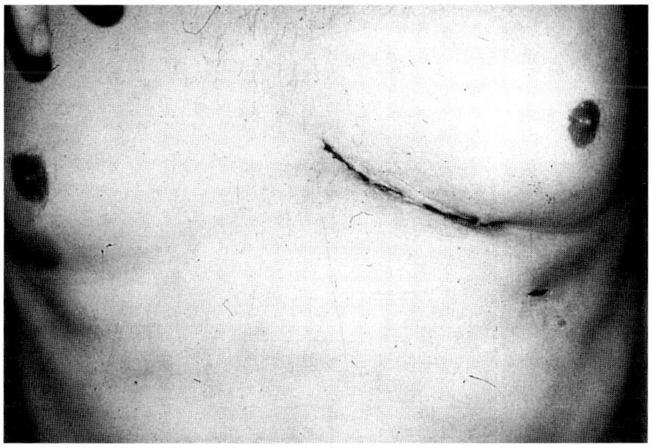

Figure 54–1. The skin incision is made along the inframammary crease. The first costicartilage and rib are exposed, and the pleural cavity is entered through the fourth intercostal space.

Left Lateral Mini-Thoracotomy

An incision approximately 10 cm long is made between the anterior and posterior axillary lines. The level of the intercostal incision for lateral minimally invasive direct grafting varies, depending on the circumstances. Usually, incisions of the intercostal muscle are carried out more medially without cutting into the serratus anterior muscle. The incision is used primarily for the intermediate artery and first obtuse marginal branch of the circumflex artery, accessed through the third or fourth intercostal space by collapsing the left lung. With generous pericardial retraction, the left atrial appendage and its adjacent area can be brought up near the chest wall to facilitate exposure of the target artery.

Left Posterolateral Mini-Thoracotomy

The approach to the main circumflex system and its branches can be accomplished via this incision. This incision is somewhat longer, measuring approximately 12 cm to just below the tip of the scapula. Muscle-sparing technique should be carried out whenever possible, and removal of the specific rib may be necessary for better exposure. Exposure of the main circumflex artery and its obtuse marginal branches usually requires entering through the fifth, sixth, or even seventh intercostal space, depending on the location of the target arteries. The incision is carried more anteriorly if the left IMA is planned for the conduit but more posteriorly toward the paraspinatus muscle if a free graft radial artery or saphenous vein conduit will be used between the target artery and the descending aorta.

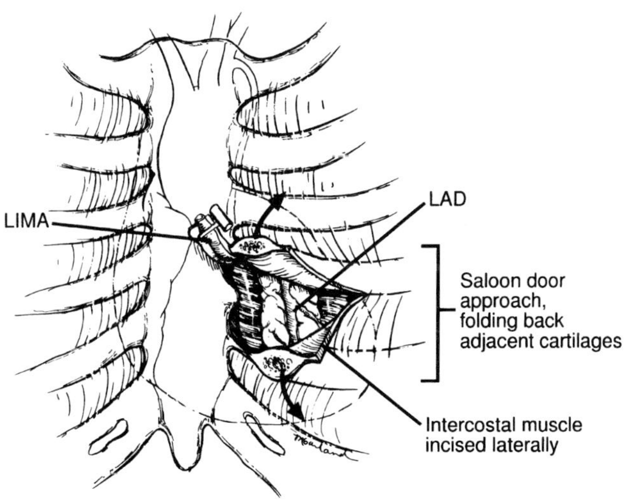

Figure 54–2. The muscle of the fourth intercostal space is incised laterally first; then the surgeon works medially until the left internal mammary artery pedicle is identified. The fourth and occasionally the fifth costosternal joints are dislocated.

Inferior Subxiphoid Incision

An upper midline incision from the body of the xiphoid down to a point halfway to the umbilicus is preferred over a right subcostal incision, if the right gastroepiploic artery is being considered as a conduit. After the anterior mediastinum and the peritoneal cavity are entered, the attachment of the diaphragm at the right anterior chest wall is separated and pulled downward anteriorly with heavy suture material. Care must be taken to avoid injury to the liver while passing a big needle through the diaphragm. The distal right coronary and proximal half of the posterior descending coronary arteries can be adequately exposed and grafted with this approach. Occasionally, the posterolateral branches of the right coronary artery can be reached as well but are often too deep to get adequate exposure.

Mini-Parasternal Incisions

Both left and right parasternal approaches have been used for minimally invasive coronary artery bypass surgery and valve procedures. These approaches provide good exposure but can cause the postoperative complication of chest wall instability.

Mini-Parasternal Approach for Coronary Artery Bypass Surgery

Currently, coronary artery bypass procedures involve predominantly IMA grafting to the anterior wall vessels, such as the LAD and main trunk of the right coronary artery. Both the LAD and the main trunk of the right coronary artery traverse a course adjacent to the respective sternal border, so that the parasternal approach generally overlies the coronary artery. With an approach from either left or right, the suspensory mechanism of the pericardium remains largely intact, maintaining the heart and vessels in a readily accessible anterior position. Taking the left or right IMA down is also easier with this technique than with the thoracotomy approaches. Because IMA rests just underneath the perichondrium, removal or dislocation of the third, fourth, and fifth costal cartilages should expose almost the entire length of the IMA.[3] The conduit can be taken down and anastomosed to the target artery with ease. By applying traction from appropriately positioned sutures through the main body of the pericardium, the target artery can be maneuvered to both a central and an anterior position. When adequately adjusted, the coronary artery can be accessed for grafting without any sense of restriction. Incision of the intercostal muscle laterally and additional anterior and medial leverage from the pericardial traction sutures allow access to the diagonal artery as well.[1] This parasternal approach has one major disadvantage: in slender patients with less muscle and subcutaneous tissue, it may potentiate the development of chronic paradoxical movement along the parasternal area.

Mini-Parasternal Incision for Valvular Surgery

Approach to the mitral, tricuspid, and aortic valves can be accomplished through the right parasternal approach as pioneered by the Cleveland Clinic group.[4, 5] Cardiopulmonary bypass is accomplished via a groin cannulation technique, facilitating excellent visualization of aortic, mitral, and tricuspid valve lesions. The right IMA has to be sacrificed, however, to obtain maximal exposure. This maneuver has drawn criticism from cardiac surgeons.

The right parasternal approach to the mitral valve requires a 10-cm skin incision, resection of the third and fourth costal cartilages, and ligation of the right IMA to provide excellent exposure. Cardiopulmonary bypass is achieved with femoral arterial and venous cannulation and direct cannulation of the superior vena cava.[5] Exposure of the valve is equally good either through the left atriotomy parallel to the atrioventricular groove or with the trans–right atrial approach through the atrial septum. Insertion of retrograde cardioplegia cannula and right superior pulmonary vein venting are also feasible with this approach.

The right parasternal approach to the aortic valve requires the same length skin incision and complete excision of the second and third costal cartilages. Like with the parasternal approach to the mitral valve, the right IMA can be either sacrificed or left intact and retracted laterally for better exposure of the aortic root.[6] With this approach, the left ventricular vent via the superior pulmonary vein is difficult, and trans–right atrial cannulation of the retrograde cardioplegia cannula is impossible.

Mini-Sternotomy

As an alternative approach to complete sternotomy, Arom and colleagues first reported mini-sternotomy for off-pump coronary artery bypass surgery.[7] In June 1996, at the first meeting on minimally invasive direct coronary artery bypass (MIDCAB) in Minneapolis, two different approaches for aortic and mitral valve surgery via partial sternotomy incisions were described.[8, 9] Later, Konertz and colleagues reported 19 cases of valvular surgery using a similar approach.[10]

Mini-sternotomy is defined as a small skin incision (10 to 12 cm long) with a partial sternotomy (Fig. 54–3). It is important to differentiate the complete sternotomy from the partial sternotomy incision. A complete sternotomy incision is about 12 in. (30 cm) long and is spread about 10 in. (25 cm) apart. For mini-sternotomy, the skin incision is about 10 to 12 cm long, and the bone is partially incised. The sternal spreading is no more than 6 to 8 cm.

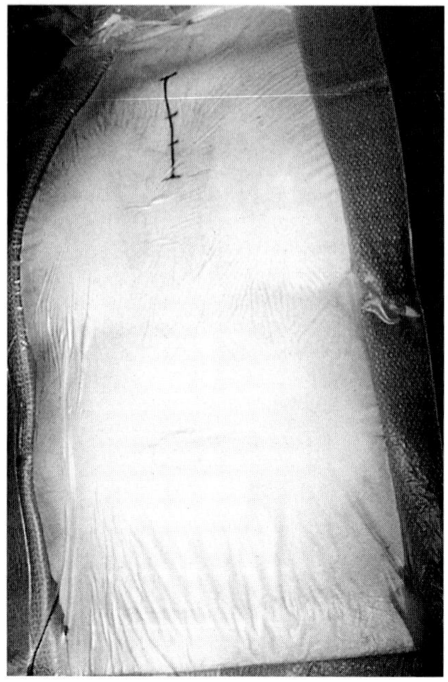

Figure 54–3. The skin incision for the mini-sternotomy approach is usually about 10 cm long and is on top of the area planned for partial sternotomy.

Proponents of the left anterior small thoracotomy incision approach have overstated the complications of the complete median sternotomy and assume that a partial sternotomy incision will lead to the same postoperative course of healing and complications as a complete sternotomy. Mini-sternotomy incisions, however, prove to have fewer postoperative complications resulting from stretching or damaging of the muscles, ribs, cartilages, and shoulder joints, which commonly occurs with complete sternotomy. The mini-sternotomy incision provides good exposure for aortic and mitral valve surgery, but the exposure and presentation for left-sided arterial branches may not be as good as with a thoracotomy incision. The partial sternotomy incision provides improved visualization for takedown of the IMAs, however, and in most circumstances, the entire length of the LAD can be easily visualized. The mini-sternotomy technique can benefit surgeons who have recently learned to perform coronary artery bypass surgery on a beating heart.[7]

Skin Incision

The skin incision is about 10 cm long or half the length of the sternum, whichever is shorter. The site of the skin incision depends on the location of the planned partial sternotomy. In general, after the skin incision is made, a generous undermining of the subcutaneous tissue is carried out in both caudad and cephalad directions (Fig. 54–4). For the upper mini-sternotomy, the skin incision is made approximately four fingerbreadths below the sternal notch down to the area near the fourth intercostal space. The subcutaneous tissue is undermined cephalad to expose the sternal notch and caudad to the right or left sixth intercostal space.

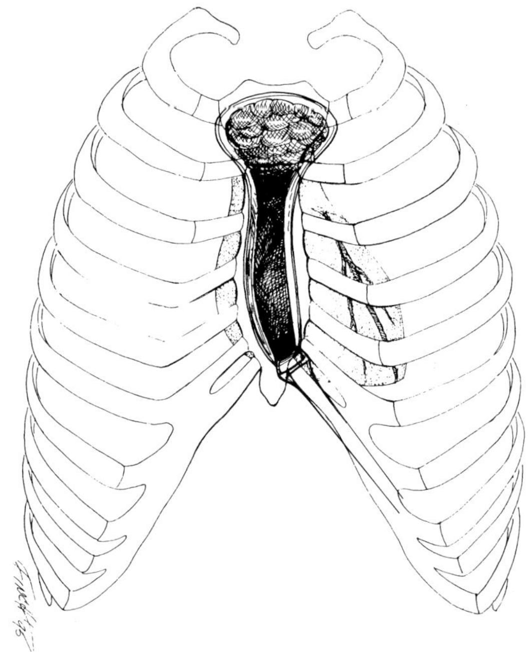

Figure 54–4. After the skin incision is made, a generous undermining of the subcutaneous tissue is carried out in both cephalad and caudad directions.

For the lower mini-sternotomy, the skin incision is made from the area near the fourth inter-costal space down near the last costosternal junction. Again generous undermining of the subcutaneous tissue is carried out.[9]

Sternal Incision

The pathway of the sternal incision varies with the procedure (Fig. 54–5). With this approach it is impossible to take the sternal saw from the sternal notch down, because of limitations from the skin flap and the location of the sternal notch. Therefore, it is necessary to start the saw from the desired intercostal space at the specific costosternal angle medial to the IMA. A Kelly clamp is used to create an entry site between the IMA and the sternal border before insertion of the tip or hook of the saw. The saw is then carried cephalad to the limit of the skin incision. At this point, if one wants to keep the benefit of the small skin incision, a Striker oscillating saw (Hall Surgical, Carpenteria, CA) can be used to go underneath the skin to complete the sternotomy. Adding more length to the skin incision at this end does not increase the advantages of the exposure.[9]

Upper Partial Sternotomy. Gundry and colleagues reported a similar approach to the aortic and mitral valves, but their recommended incision is somewhat shorter and begins just below the sternal notch and extends down to the third intercostal space. The partial sternotomy begins from the sternal notch and "t-off" at the third or fourth intercostal space, depending on the location of the aortic root on intraoperative transesophageal echocardiogram.[8] This incision is higher and closer to the sternal notch, making it somewhat less cosmetically appealing to women. The mitral valve is approached only via the dome of the left atrium, and insertion of retrograde cardioplegia and a right superior pulmonary vein vent is difficult.

Right Upper Partial Sternotomy. A J-shaped incision for aortic valve surgery that starts at the fourth intercostal space is described by Arom and colleagues. A similar incision is used for mitral valve surgery but begins one intercostal space lower. In both cases, the sternotomy incision is terminated at the sternal notch.[9]

Left Partial Sternotomy. This incision is used mainly for MIDCAB surgery; the reversed J incision starts from the left sixth intercostal space and extends all the way up to the sternal notch or goes from the last costoxiphoid angle on the left upward, exiting at the left first intercostal space. The latter incision provides better exposure for the inferior aspect of the heart, but spreading the sternum is more difficult. Similarly, lower partial sternotomy can also be carried out on the right side.

Exposure of Specific Structures

The Delacroix retractor (Delacroix-Chevalier, Paris, France) is useful for these techniques. The length of both IMAs can be taken down in their entirety, and the first branch divided (Fig. 54–6). The same retractor can be left in place for the anastomosis between the left IMA and the LAD. Otherwise, the retractor is replaced with Cooley's retractor (V. Mueller Division, Baxter Healthcare Corp., McGraw Park, IL) for right IMA to distal right coronary

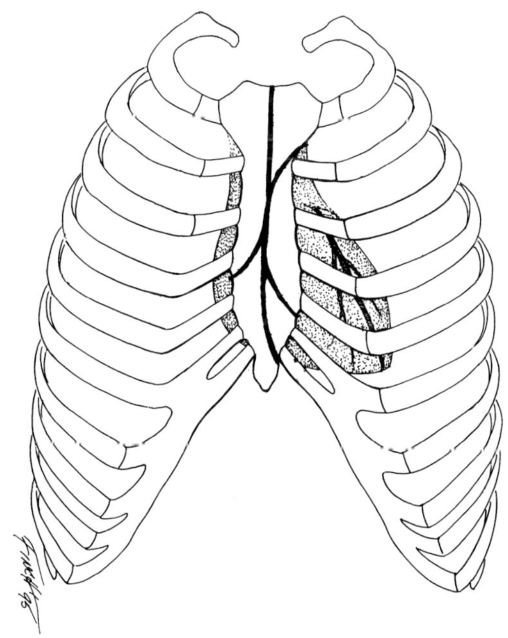

Figure 54–5. For a left partial sternotomy, the reversed J incision is started from the left sixth costosternal angle up to the sternal notch or from the last costosternal angle upward, exiting at the left first intercostal space (C incision). For a right partial sternotomy, a J-shaped incision starts at the fourth or fifth costosternal angle for aortic and mitral valve surgery and terminates at the sternal notch.

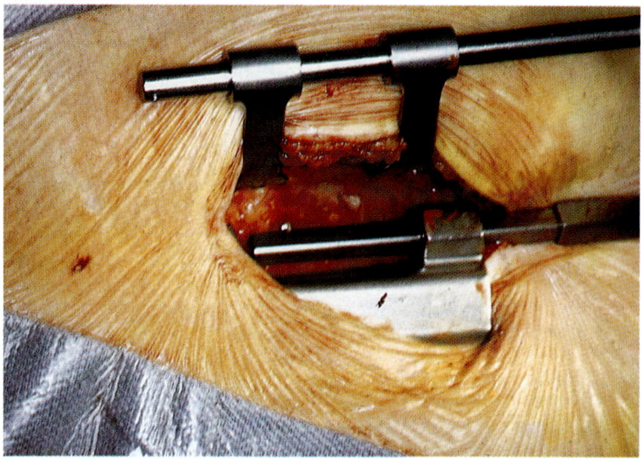

Figure 54–6. Partial sternotomy incision with Delacroix-Chevalier retractor in place. The entire length of both internal mammary arteries can be taken down in their entirety and the first branch divided.

artery anastomosis or for aortic and mitral valve procedures. Whenever exposure of the specific target is difficult owing to limitations resulting from a small skin incision and/or the intact sternum, the Favaloro internal mammary retractor can be placed across the table and the patient to elevate part of the intact sternum and manubrium.[11]

Exposure of the Coronary Artery. Exposure of the right and left coronary system is described elsewhere in this chapter.

Exposure of the Aortic and Mitral Valves. With a retractor in place, the opening is about 6 by 6 cm (Fig. 54–7), which allows enough room for aortic and right atrial cannulation using the same cannulae and the same cannulation technique as for the full sternotomy approach.[12, 13] With a sternotomy starting at the fifth or sixth costosternal angle, the retrograde cardioplegia cannula is placed in the usual fashion. A coronary pressure waveform is necessary to confirm the position, because finger-guiding the tip of the cannula into the coronary sinus is no longer feasible. The left ventricular vent through the right superior pulmonary vein can be inserted without difficulty. The pursestring suture is applied at its usual site on the aortic arch near the takeoff of the innominate artery, and atrial cannulation with a single two-stage venous cannula is accomplished via the right atrial appendage (Fig. 54–8). Although the same aortic cross-clamp has been used, a newly designed clamp (Scanlen International, St. Paul, MN) improves exposure. Exposure of the aortic valve should follow the conventional approach, but for mitral valve procedures, an approach via the dome of the left atrium is preferred.[12]

The mini-sternotomy incisional approach has proved to be useful when learning to perform coronary anastomoses on a beating heart. For limited valvular surgeries, this exposure is adequate in spite of using the same cannulae and cannulation techniques as for complete sternotomy approaches. The mini-sternotomy approach has also been reported to be feasible in more complex aortic root and hemi–aortic arch procedures.[14]

Conclusion

This chapter has described the various small incision techniques used on the chest wall to gain limited but adequate access to different areas of the heart. With specific attention to detail, this technique can be safely used to achieve excellent long-term cosmesis (Fig. 54–9) and outcome results with reduced resource utilization. The previously described approaches for minimally invasive cardiac surgery may someday replace the conventional technique currently used.

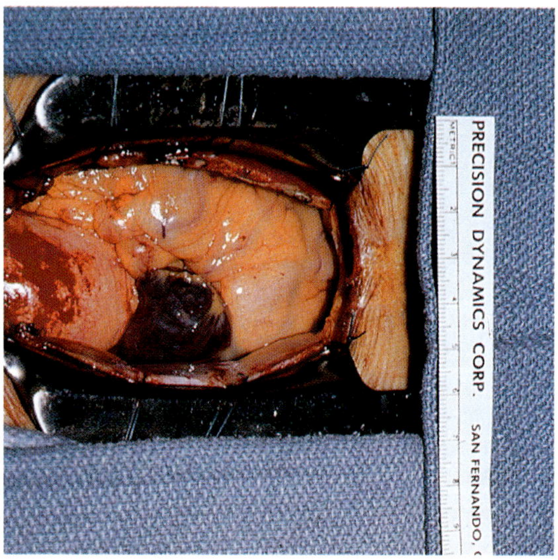

Figure 54–7. Adequate exposure of the aortic root and right atrium via a J-shaped partial sternotomy incision. The opening is approximately 6 by 6 cm.

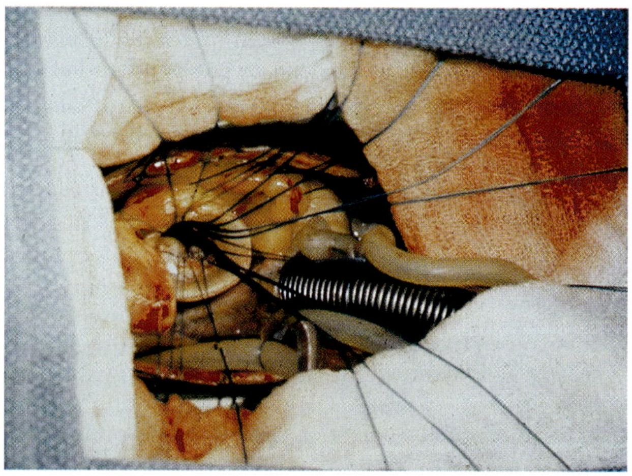

Figure 54–8. Good exposure is obtained during aortic valve surgery in spite of all the cannulation (aortic, right atrial, right superior pulmonary vein vent, and transatrial retrograde cardioplegia) carried out through this opening. Exposure is also excellent for mitral valve surgery.

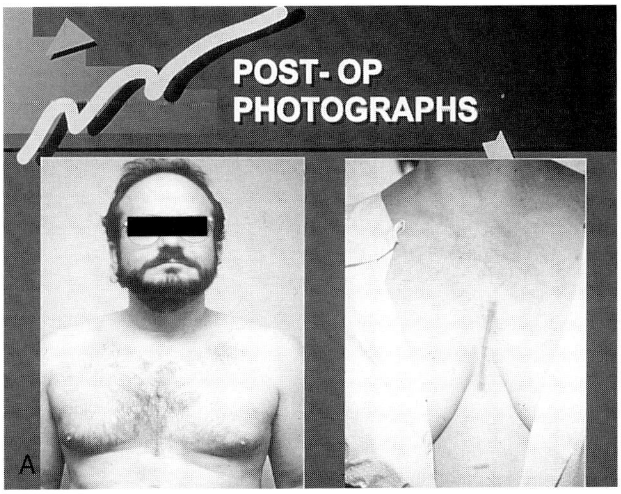

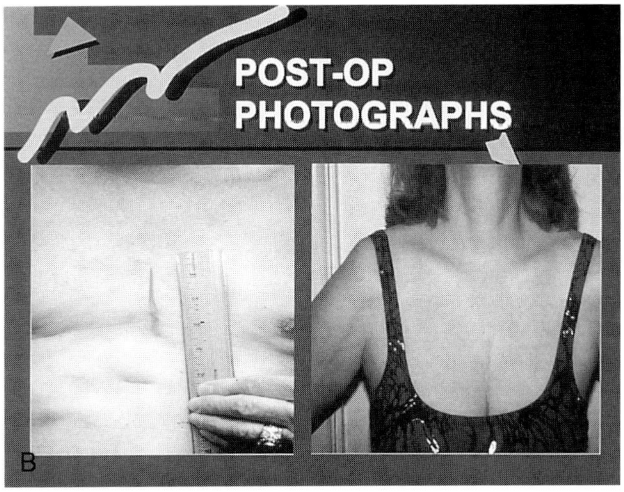

Figure 54–9. *A*, Postoperative skin incisions in four patients. *B*, Note the length of the incision and the distance from the sternal notch.

References

1. Robinson MC: "Saloon-door" parasternal approach in MIDCAB. *In* Emery RW (ed): Techniques for Minimally Invasive Direct Coronary Artery Bypass (MIDCAB) Surgery. Philadelphia, Hanley & Belfus, 1997, pp 49–53.
2. Fann JI, Pompili MF, Burdon TA, et al: Minimally invasive mitral valve surgery. Semin Thorac Cardiovasc Surg 9:320–330, 1997.
3. Stanbridge RDL, Hadjinikolaou LK, Cohen AS, et al: Minimally invasive coronary revascularization through parasternal incisions without cardiopulmonary bypass. Ann Thorac Surg 63: S53–S56, 1997.
4. Cosgrove DM, Sabik JF: Minimally invasive approach for aortic valve operations. Ann Thorac Surg 62:596–597, 1996.
5. Navia JL, Cosgrove DM: Minimally invasive mitral valve operation. Ann Thorac Surg 62:1542–1544, 1996.
6. Cohn LH, Adams DH, Couper GS, Bichell DP: Minimally invasive aortic valve replacement. Semin Thorac Cardiovasc Surg 9:331–336, 1997.
7. Arom KV, Emery RW, Nicoloff DM: Mini-sternotomy for coronary artery bypass grafting. Ann Thorac Surg 61:1271–1272, 1996.
8. Gundry SR, Shattuck CH, Sardari FF, Bailey LL: Cardiac operations in adults and children by ministernotomy: Facile minimally invasive cardiac surgery. Presented at the 33rd annual meeting of the Society of Thoracic Surgeons, San Diego, CA, February 3, 1997.
9. Arom KV, Emery RW, Nicoloff DM: Ministernotomy for cardiac surgery. *In* Emery RW (ed): Techniques for Minimally Invasive Direct Coronary Artery Bypass (MIDCAB) Surgery. Philadelphia, Hanley & Belfus, 1997, pp 43–48.
10. Konertz W, Waldenberger F, Schmutzler, et al: Minimal access valve surgery through superior partial sternotomy: A preliminary study. J Heart Valve Dis 5:638–640, 1996.
11. Doty DB: Full spectrum cardiac surgery through a minimal incision: Mini-sternotomy (lower half) technique. Ann Thorac Surg (in press).
12. Arom KV, Emery RW: Minimally invasive mitral operations, comments to the editor. Ann Thorac Surg 63:1209–1222, 1997.
13. Tam RKW, Almeida AA: Minimally invasive aortic valve replacement via hemi-sternotomy. Ann Thorac Surg (in press).
14. Svensson LG: Minimal-access "J" or "j" sternotomy for valvular, aortic, and coronary operations or reoperations. Ann Thorac Surg 64:1501–1503, 1997.

COMMENTARY

Denton A. Cooley

In the present era of increasingly less invasive cardiac surgery, surgeons must choose an incision that, though limited in size, affords adequate exposure for performing a safe, precise operation. Many types of incisions may be used; however, some are associated with less successful outcomes than others. Drs. Arom and Emery describe the different types of incisions that are being used by surgeons for minimally invasive surgery.

In the early years of cardiac surgery, transverse and intercostal incisions were used routinely, although they were associated with complications. When the sternum is transected, as in a transverse incision, both internal thoracic arteries may be lost. In my experience with intercostal incisions, patients reported severe pain, in some cases because of damage to the intercostal nerve. The median sternotomy replaced both of these earlier techniques, providing exposure to all cardiac chambers and major arteries. Because the intercostal nerves were not damaged, it was also less painful. Unfortunately, some surgeons used wide, rectangular retraction in performing this procedure, which caused brachial plexus injuries and increased pain in some patients. These complications can be avoided by making the retraction pyramidal rather than rectangular, narrowing the cephalad portion of the incision.

With the advent of minimally invasive procedures, the reputation of the standard median sternotomy has suffered.

In my opinion, however, parasternal incisions offer few, if any, advantages over the median sternotomy and may result in inadequate or impaired exposure of the cardiac chambers. In many instances, costal cartilages are divided or excised, which may cause severe postoperative pain or herniation of the lung. Of all the techniques for minimal exposure, I believe that the best is the mini-sternotomy. This approach allows for cannulation of the right atrium and the distal ascending aorta, and it usually provides good exposure of the mitral valve. The incision used in performing the standard median sternotomy, however, is not much more invasive than that used in a mini-sternotomy and guarantees complete exposure.

As we continue to develop challenging new approaches to established cardiac procedures, surgeons should focus on the cardiac needs of the patient and place only a modest emphasis on cosmesis. Just because an operation *can* be performed by a special approach does not necessarily mean that it *should* be performed in that manner. Good surgical judgment must always prevail.

COMMENTARY

Zohair Al-Halees

There is no doubt that minimal access cardiothoracic surgery is here to stay. We surgeons will have to modify our thinking and techniques, and we will have to acquire new skills. However, we should not compromise the quality and safety of our work just to get on the bandwagon.

Currently, we are in the evolutionary phase of developing techniques and refinements in instruments. Some confusion still exists as to what constitutes a minimally invasive cardiac procedure. Is it a small skin incision? Is it avoiding division of the sternum completely? Is it avoiding the use of cardiopulmonary bypass? Why do we do it? Is it because of cosmetic reasons? Is it less painful? Are the recovery and outcome better? These questions and many others will have to be answered as more experience is gained and more time is available for follow-up.

Table 54–1 summarizes the different incisions used in minimal access cardiac surgery. It is obvious that conventional median sternotomy remains the only versatile incision that provides access for more or less all cardiac procedures. Historically, the median sternotomy incision revolutionized cardiac surgery and allowed the vast progress we have witnessed in open-heart surgery since its inception. This should not be forgotten.

With some modification, the median sternotomy incision can be made more cosmetic and less painful, and its use does not necessarily mean that cardiopulmonary bypass is required. The skin incision can be made smaller with undermining of subcutaneous tissues. It can be made submammary with elevation of bilateral breast flaps, providing an excellent cosmetic result. Most of the pain from the median sternotomy incision is related to excessive separation of the divided sternal blades with the retractor. Limiting this separation and being careful not to break any ribs will result in less pain. I believe, however, that thoracotomy incisions are not less painful. I personally operated on a physician through a median sternotomy to redo a left internal thoracic artery to LAD bypass graft that had been done through a mini left anterior thoracotomy. This patient had no doubt that the median sternotomy incision was much less painful than the mini left anterior thoracotomy.

Not only are all other incisions small, but they also provide limited access as well. One should therefore use such an approach only in selected cases with appropriate indications and with the proper setup. For example, one should not abandon the concept of complete revascularization in coronary artery disease surgery and treat only the "culprit" lesion and ignore other diseased vessels. This can be accepted only if the center is ready to perform new "hybrid" procedures, such as minimally invasive coronary revascularization and angioplasty to revascularize the remaining coronary arteries. This concept is new and has not stood the test of time.

Table 54–1. Incisions Used in Minimal Access Cardiac Surgery

Incision	LAD	RCA	CX	MV	AV	TV	ASD	VSD	Complex
Classic median sternotomy	+	+	+	+	+	+	+	+	+
Left anterior mini-thoracotomy	+	−	−	−	−	−	−	−	−
Right anterior mini-thoracotomy	−	±	−	+	+	+	+	+	−
Left lateral mini-thoracotomy	−	−	+	−	−	−	−	−	−
Left posterolateral mini-thoracotomy	−	−	+	−	−	−	−	−	−
Inferior subxiphoid	−	+	−	−	−	±	±	±	−
Mini-parasternal									
Left	+	+	−	−	−	−	−	−	−
Right	−	+	−	+	+	+	+	+	−
Mini-sternotomy									
Upper	Has to be modified, depending on the target vessel or the valve procedure						+	+	−
Lower									
Partial right									
Partial left									

Chapter 55

Instrumentation for Minimally Invasive Cardiac Surgery

Hani Shennib

Minimally invasive cardiac surgery techniques are predicted to represent 25% of all cardiac surgical procedures by the year 2000.[1] Initially, the limiting factors for the expansion of minimally invasive cardiac surgery were the lack of innovations in instrumentation and the discrepancy between the push by cardiac surgeons to develop minimally invasive technology and the lukewarm reception by industry based on its marketing potential. Today, the situation is different. Numerous companies have embraced minimally invasive cardiac surgery and are well positioned to produce exciting new instruments in a rapidly growing market. In addition to the traditional cardiac industry, several new start-up companies with a focus on designing technology for minimally invasive coronary artery bypass and valve surgery and left ventricular support systems will contribute to the advancement of novel concepts in cardiac surgery. The exponential increase in scientific meetings, abstracts, and articles on minimally invasive cardiac surgery attests to the fact that we are at a turning point in the history of cardiac surgery.

This chapter examines the evolution of instrumentation for minimally invasive cardiac surgery and some ideas currently in development. For simplicity, the chapter is divided into sections on instrumentation for specific procedures and tasks, even though many of the tools are interchangeable and can be used for tasks they were not originally designed for. In general, minimally invasive surgical instruments can be divided into those used for coronary artery bypass graft surgery, valve and intracardiac procedures, and general enabling technology. The latter includes technology to improve visualization through smaller incisions, for example, video assistance, robotics and computer-assisted technology, and minimal access cardiopulmonary bypass and left ventricular support.

Instrumentation for Coronary Artery Bypass Graft

Even though initial interest focused on the minimally invasive direct coronary artery bypass (MIDCAB) graft procedure with preferred access through a left anterior thoracotomy, it is clear that this can be performed on only a minority of patients in whom the culprit lesion involves primarily the left anterior descending coronary artery (LAD). The majority of patients have multivessel involvement and require access through some form of limited or full sternotomy, a longer thoracotomy, or a paramedian incision. Because of the potential benefit to patients of having surgery on a beating heart, a variety of instruments to stabilize the coronary artery have been designed and validated[2–4] and are currently marketed. In a recent survey, most cardiac surgeons perceived stabilization of the target segment of coronary artery for the purpose of anastomosis as the most challenging component of the MIDCAB procedure. Currently, the mechanical stabilizer developed by CTSI (Cupertino, CA) is most widely applicable to single-vessel coronary artery bypass graft (CABG) (Fig. 55–1). It gives excellent stabilization of anteriorly located arteries. Its impact on the performance of a good and safe anastomosis has been validated by data from the CTS registry, which consists of over 1500 patients. Angiographic follow-up confirmed anastomotic patency in over 95% of the cases. Its major disadvantage is that it is disposable, resulting in added operative costs. Other equally effective disposable stabilizers are made by US Surgical (Fig. 55–2). Partially reusable disposable stabilizers are currently marketed by Johnson and Johnson, and completely reusable stabilizers are manufactured by Genzyme (Fig. 55–3), Scanlan, and several other companies. An alternative method of stabilization is based on the concept of suction traction of the epicardium. This has been popularized by Medtronic (Octopus) (Fig. 55–4). The Octopus stabilizer provides superb coronary artery stability for multivessel anastomosis, particularly when performing posterior descending and obtuse marginal coronary artery anastomosis. Its disadvantage is that it takes some time and effort to set and is bulky, imposing on the surgical field and making surgeons and assistants uncomfortable with their positions. This is most evident when performing MIDCAB minithoracotomy. For this indication, it is suggested that the stabilizer handles be inserted through separate stab incisions. An alternative stabilizer for multivessel anastomosis is the MVS-CTSI system, which is based on the same concept as the original CTS stabilizer but has an additional joint at the ankle. This permits stabilization of the coronary arteries positioned on a widely obtuse angle. Forthcoming designs of the Medtronic Octopus stabilizer will feature reduced size and greater facility of assembling the stabilizer intraoperatively.

Because coronary artery anastomosis on the beating heart depends not only on a steady targeted coronary artery but also on a bloodless field and good myocardial protection, other tools to keep the coronary arteriotomy bloodless, such as the hemodified blower and coronary artery occluders and shunts (Fig. 55–5), are gaining acceptance. Even though, theoretically, it makes sense to maintain blood flow and minimize the risk of ischemia during occlusion, experience has shown that minimal reversible or no ischemic changes are observed during coronary artery occlusion and anastomosis on the beating heart.

Access through a sternotomy for multivessel anastomosis is generally well tolerated for anterior, lateral, right, and

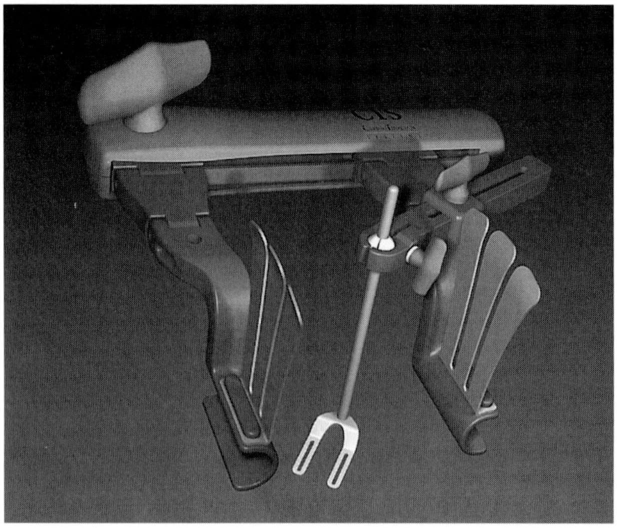

Figure 55–1. Disposable mechanical stabilizer. (Courtesy of CTS Inc., Cupertino, CA.)

distal posterior descending artery anastomoses. When there is a need to access the deep obtuse marginal and posterior ventricular branches, subluxation of the heart during such exposure may result in hemodynamic instability. The Octopus device permits gentle subluxation of the heart, and with the addition of the Trendelenburg position, it is possible to access relatively posterior vessels with acceptable hemodynamic changes. Occasionally, however, instability precludes CABG on the beating heart. The development of less invasive cardiopulmonary bypass or left ventricular assisted devices to permit comfortable cardiac subluxation maneuvers is imminent.

A variety of conduits may be used for the purpose of performing CABG on a beating heart. The most popular and consistently used is the left internal mammary artery (LIMA) pedicle. The LIMA is usually accessed through a left mini-thoracotomy when a MIDCAB procedure to graft the LAD is contemplated. Internal mammary artery (IMA) harvest in this particular situation can be done entirely under direct visualization using chest wall retractors designed by CTS, US Surgical, Johnson and Johnson, Medtronic, and others. There is, however, some difficulty visualizing the uppermost part of the LIMA under direct vision, and many surgeons prefer to use video-assisted techniques to reach this part and ensure complete mobilization. Several surgeons have advocated totally endoscopic mobilization of the IMA; the advantages are avoidance of the vigorous retraction of the ribs required with direct visualization, avoidance of potential rib fractures and cartilage dislocation, and probably less postoperative pain. The limiting factor for totally endoscopic IMA harvest is the time

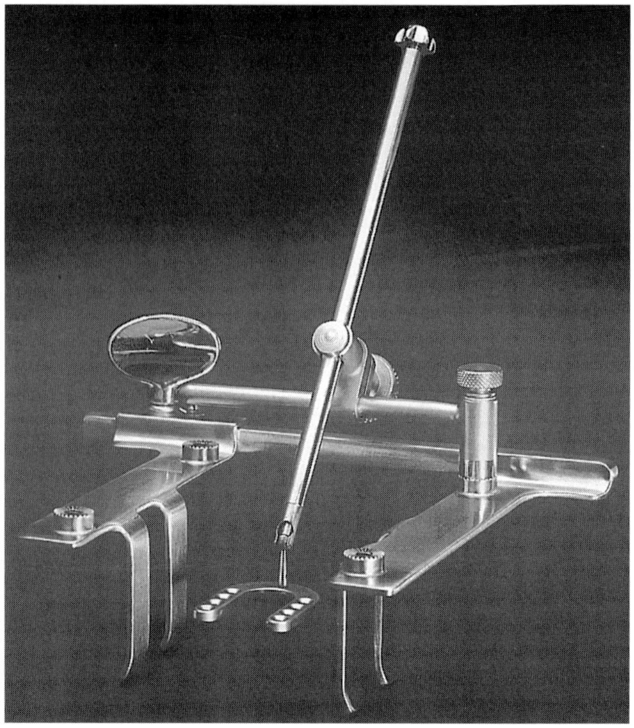

Figure 55–3. Completely reusable mechanical stabilizer. (Courtesy of Genzyme Surgical Products, Tucker, GA.)

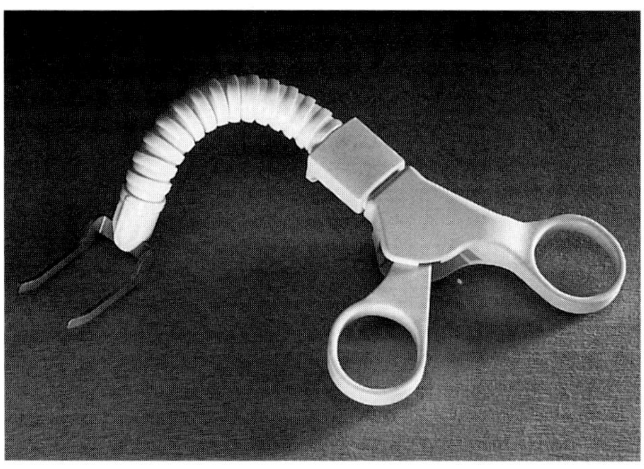

Figure 55–2. Disposable mechanical stabilizer. (United States Surgical, Norwalk, CT. Copyright © 1999 United States Surgical. All rights reserved. Reprinted with the permission of United States Surgical.)

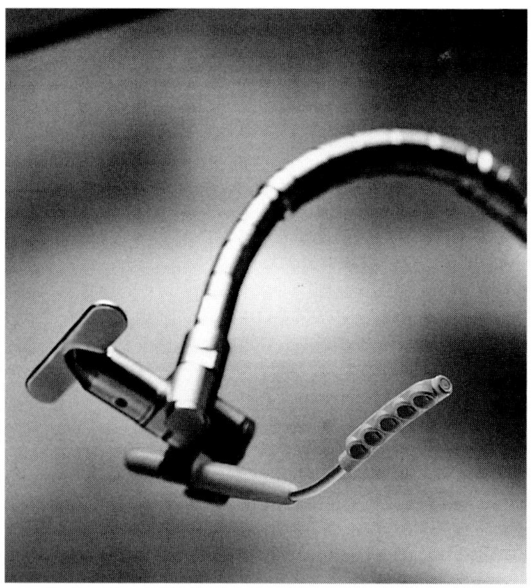

Figure 55–4. Octopus suction traction. (Courtesy of Medtronic, Inc., Minneapolis, MN.)

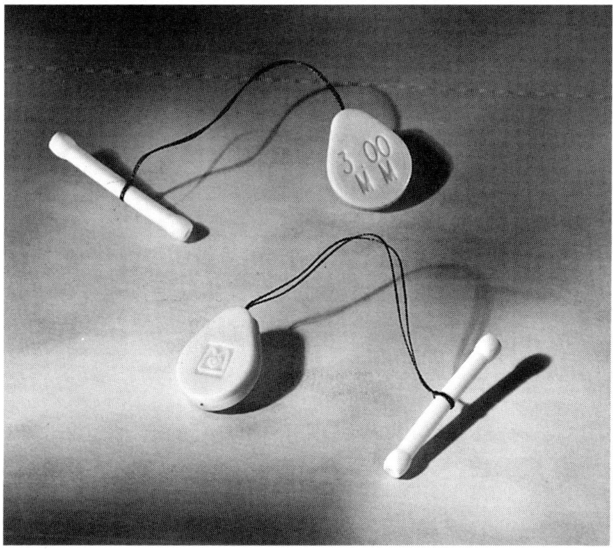

Figure 55–5. Coronary artery occluders and shunts. (Courtesy of Chase Medical Inc., Richardson, TX.)

and setup necessary. In addition, many cardiac surgeons are not trained in the use of endoscopic devices. But with the rapid progression of minimally invasive cardiac procedures, it will become essential for all surgeons to adapt and acquire endoscopic skills in the future. The development of instruments to facilitate performance of the anastomosis, such as the one-shot anastomotic stapler developed by US Surgical (Fig. 55–6), will likely reduce operative time and potentially render CABG access less invasive.

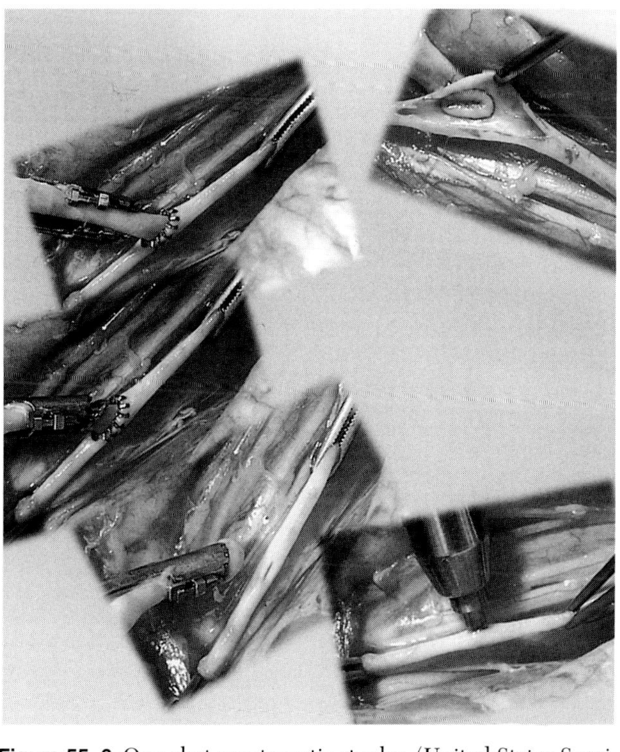

Figure 55–6. One-shot anastomotic stapler. (United States Surgical, Norwalk, CT. Copyright © 1999 United States Surgical. All rights reserved. Reprinted with the permission of United States Surgical.)

Instrumentation for Valve Surgery

The initial focus on technology for minimally invasive surgery has been on access instrumentation. These instruments are geared toward creating a platform that lies over or within the chest incision and permits the installation of retractors on it. This also facilitates the insertion of instrumentation, without impingement of the awkward and rigid chest wall. The limiting factor for the development of such instrumentation is the diversity of chest wall incisions used to access the aortic and mitral valves and for other intracardiac repairs. With the return of some form of ministernotomy as the preferred approach to aortic and mitral valve surgery, it is likely that a focused effort will be made to improve access platforms. Several endoretractors have been designed to provide direct visualization of the mitral valve apparatus. Indirect visualization using advanced visualization technology such as that developed by VISTA (Fig. 55–7) is likely to become popular and to provide great assistance in performing mitral valve surgery as well as other intracardiac procedures. The added advantage of three-dimensional vision may facilitate valve repair and improve its quality.

Perhaps the most desired and potentially exciting development in minimal access valve surgery is in the field of valve fastening into the implantation location. The avoidance of suturing techniques will contribute significantly to the facility of valve surgery and reduce operative time as smaller access incisions evolve. A stitcher that creates a pledgeted mattress suture to fix the new valve annulus (Fig. 55–8) will likely reduce the time required for valve implantation and permit access through smaller incisions.

Cardiopulmonary Bypass and Left Ventricular Support

One of the most important benefits of minimally invasive cardiac surgery has been our critical review of conventional methods for supporting the circulation and arresting the heart. We are now more aware of the serious deleterious effects of cardiopulmonary bypass in its current form. Although we recognized some of the serious neuropsycho-

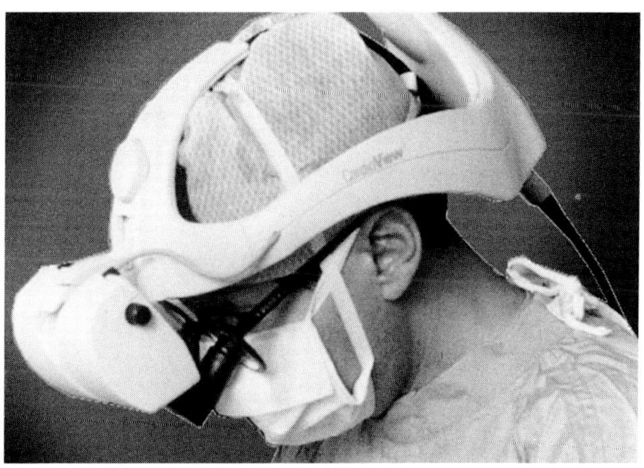

Figure 55–7. Indirect visualization with a head-mounted display. (Courtesy of VISTA Medical Technologies, Inc., Westborough, MA.)

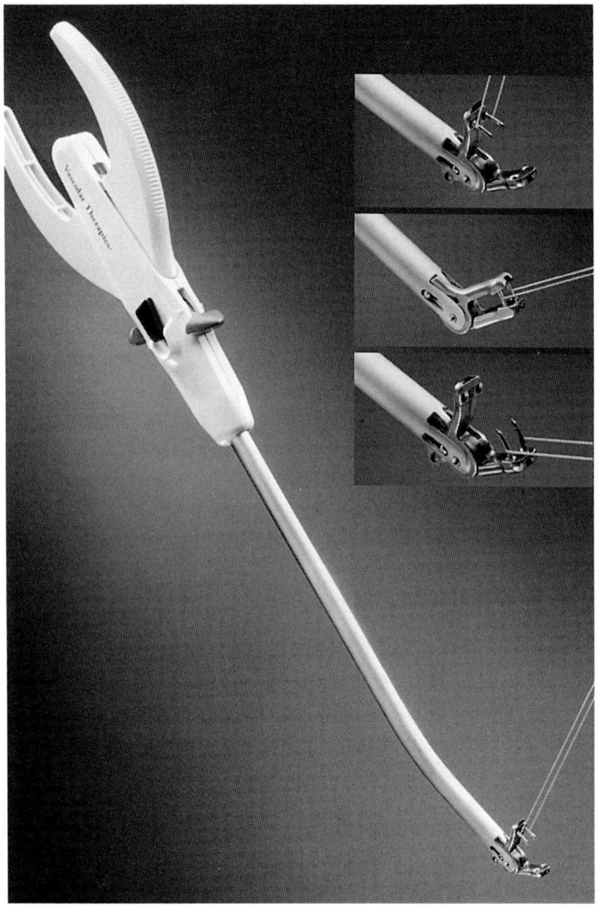

Figure 55–8. Endoscopic stitcher for placement of annular stitches. (United States Surgical, Norwalk, CT. Copyright © 1999 United States Surgical. All rights reserved. Reprinted with the permission of United States Surgical.)

logical defects in the past, nothing was done about them until surgery on the beating heart regained popularity. For such surgery, some form of left ventricular assistance may be necessary when reaching out to posterior and far lateral coronary arteries to perform the anastomosis. Similarly, when abrupt hemodynamic compromise occurs in the course of CABG surgery on the beating heart, a rapid bailout left ventricular support system would be advantageous. The hemopump (Medtronic) was initially experimented with. Cannulation was attempted from the ascending aorta into the left ventricle, which often required insertion of the cannula through a graft anastomosed to the ascending aorta. Similar concepts based on a rotator pump positioned in the left ventricle and ejecting into the root of the aorta are currently in the development phase. Ideally, those would also be suitable for peripheral cannulation. As smaller-caliber pumps are developed, it will be essential to ascertain that this is not at the expense of flow or blood destruction.

More modern versions of traditional cardiopulmonary bypass are also under development. These consist of shorter circuits, with a decreased requirement for anticoagulants. It is likely that a simplified pump will be positioned on the operating table in the proximity of the surgeon, resulting in reduced contact area between the blood and the cardiopulmonary bypass system and direct surgeon control of the apparatus, further reducing cost and labor.

Similarly, cannulation systems that will facilitate insertion of arterial perfusion cannulae into the ascending aorta as opposed to through groin arteries will avoid the early complications associated with retrograde arterial perfusion and the passage of arterial cannulae through the descending thoracic aorta and abdominal aorta. A transthoracic aortic cannula that will permit arterial perfusion administration of cardioplegia and balloon occlusion of the ascending aorta is forthcoming. These advances will render cardiopulmonary bypass apparatus more patient-friendly and likely minimize the trauma associated with it.

References

1. Shennib H, Mack MJ, Lee AGL: A survey on minimally invasive coronary artery bypass grafting. Ann Thorac Surg 64:110–115, 1997.
2. Calafiore AM, Angelini A, Izzat MB: Minimally invasive coronary artery bypass grafting. Ann Thorac Surg 62:1545–1548, 1996.
3. Calafiore A, Teodori G, Giammarco G, et al: Midterm results after minimally invasive coronary surgery (LAST operation). Presented at Annual Meeting of the American Association of Thoracic Surgeons, Washington, DC, 1997.
4. Shennib H, Lee A, Akino J: A safe and effective method of coronary artery stabilization for coronary artery bypass on a beating heart. Ann Thorac Surg 63:988–992, 1997.

COMMENTARY

Piet W. Boonstra

Minimally invasive cardiac surgery will play an important role by the beginning of the new millennium. However, it is difficult to quantify the degree to which conventional procedures will be replaced by new minimally invasive procedures. In this respect, a major role will be played by training centers. After all, cardiac surgery has reached established and reproducible results; its indications are clear and defined. Why change? Moreover, is it fair that today's patients pay the price of failure and complications for the good of tomorrow's patients? We have a great responsibility. On the one side, we must encourage research on these new topics. On the other side, we have to monitor the results critically and train new surgeons. And in the meantime, we must not forget that our commitment is to treat our patients as well as we can.

Regarding minimally invasive cardiac surgery, it is my firm opinion that the key issue is and will remain the avoidance of cardiopulmonary bypass. I foresee a great expansion in off-pump coronary surgery and in the development of instruments for this type of surgery. There will probably be two tendencies: multiple minimally invasive video-assisted approaches with specific indications for different surgical strategies, and a return to the "good-old" midline sternotomy to handle patients with multivessel disease with a single surgical approach. Whatever the preferred surgical access, developments in stabilizing tools and video-assistance devices will play the main role.

As far as minimally invasive surgery is concerned, the industry has made a big commitment that has not yet paid off in improved clinical results. Is it wise to overload patients with longer pump runs and the health care system with increased costs only to reduce the length of the surgical incision? Or to move the incision from the midline to somewhere else that is not the sternum? The state of the art in minimally invasive valve surgery is still fighting with its great enemy, which is also its only ally: cardiopulmonary bypass. It is difficult to imagine valve surgery without cardiopulmonary bypass. In this sense, all possible improvements in cardiopulmonary bypass and ventricular support systems should be rewarded with maximal scientific attention, because this will be one of the major factors in the improvement of cardiac surgery.

In conclusion, at the beginning of the new millennium, our commitment will be both to encourage and control the evolution of beating heart coronary surgery and to invest in research focused on extra- and intracorporeal assistance devices. If we succeed in combining these two apparently opposite tendencies, we will accomplish our mission: better health care available to more patients.

Chapter **56**

Minimally Invasive Direct Coronary Artery Bypass

Antonio Maria Calafiore and Giuseppe Vitolla

Vassili Kolessov,[1] in 1967, described in detail how to graft on a beating heart the left anterior descending artery (LAD) using the left internal mammary artery (LIMA) through a left anterior thoracotomy in the fifth intercostal space (see Chapter 49). The LIMA was harvested under direct vision for a short length (up to the second intercostal space), the LAD was preconditioned, and the connection was accomplished with interrupted sutures (mean anastomotic time, 6 minutes). Postoperative electrocardiogram showed, in one case, ST elevation, which Kolessov interpreted as LIMA spasm and treated with sublingual nitroglycerin. Basically, Kolessov described all the technical and functional aspects of the procedure as it is performed today.

Kolessov's operation was forgotten for a long time. In 1994 Federico Benetti[2] reproposed the same procedure, using the thoracoscope for LIMA harvesting. Other surgeons, such as Acuff, Robinson, Subramanian, and others,[3–5] followed with different surgical approaches and different methods for LIMA harvesting.

In this chapter we describe our surgical technique and our results with this procedure for LAD grafting on 528 patients. The surgical approach is a left anterior small thoracotomy, or LAST.

Surgical Technique

Anesthesia is induced with fentanyl and sodium thiopental and is maintained with fentanyl and droperidol. Muscular relaxation is obtained with pancuronium bromide. A Carlens tube was used in the beginning of our experience to avoid left lung ventilation, but its use has been discontinued. At the beginning of the procedure, a continuous infusion of diltiazem (10 mg/hr) is begun; small boluses (10 mg) are injected, when necessary, to obtain a heart rate of 45 to 50 bpm. In the final part of the operation, a mixture of IV_2O_2 and O_2 is used, to allow rapid awakening of the patient.

The patient is positioned on the operating table supine. The chest is opened via a LAST in the fourth intercostal space (N = 264, 50%), fifth intercostal space (N = 245, 46.4%), or both (N = 19, 3.6%). In the beginning of our experience, we preferred the fifth intercostal space, but now the choice depends on the surgical anatomy of the LAD, detectable at angiography (intramyocardial position, distal size, and so forth). When both intercostal spaces were opened, it was because it was necessary to find a suitable anastomotic site. The pleural cavity is always opened. The ribs are then retracted. No costal cartilage is resected, but sometimes the chondrosternal joint breaks by itself; if so, it is reconstructed during wound closure.

The first step is the opening of the pericardium, to check the feasibility of the procedure. The LIMA is then identified and dissected. Early in our experience,[6] we harvested a short segment of the LIMA. More recently, with increasing experience and new instruments, a much longer segment can be harvested if necessary. The conduit is harvested distally up to the bifurcation and proximally, for the length necessary to reach the LAD (Fig. 56–1). For this purpose, in the last 201 cases, we used a new retractor (Cardio Thoracic System, Cupertino, CA) that pulls up the chest wall and exposes the LIMA clearly; the conduit can be easily dissected, skeletonized, or pedicled up to the first rib if necessary (Fig. 56–2). Heparin (1 mg/kg) is then given, and the distal LIMA is ligated and transected. Five milliliters of a solution with papaverine (1 mg/ml) is injected into the distal tip, which is then clipped to allow a pharmacologic dilatation of the conduit. A second retractor, to be used for the distal anastomosis, is then positioned. The LAD is occluded proximally and distally using a 4–0 Prolene suture with a 25-mm needle, passed deeply to surround the vessel. To avoid any direct compression of the suture on the coronary wall,[6] both needles are passed through a small piece of silicone tubing. Both 4–0 sutures are gently snared to ensure an operative field that is as bloodless as possible. A stabilizer with two feet (Cardio Thoracic System, Cupertino, CA, USA), connected to the retractor, is positioned parallel to the LAD and pushed down gently. The up-and-down movement of the heart is antagonized, and as a consequence, the LAD remains steady and its movements are nearly abolished. The distal LIMA is prepared as usual; the LAD is dissected and incised. The anastomosis is performed using two 8–0 Prolene sutures with a 6-mm needle (Fig. 56–3).[6] Both of them are passed three times at the heel and at the apex; the LIMA is then pulled down to reach the LAD. The two edges of the vessels now face each other, and the anastomosis is completed with two running sutures from both sides. The LIMA and the LAD are then unclamped, and hemostasis is checked. In the past, heparin was reversed with protamine (1:1), but we do not reverse the heparin anymore. A drain is positioned in the chest, along with a small catheter, to infuse an analgesic drug (bupivacaine). The wound is closed as usual.

Six patients (1.1%) had associated surgery: five had carotid endarterectomy, and one had carotid endarterectomy and femorofemoral bypass for lower leg gangrene.

The LAD occlusion time was 25.3 ± 8.0 minutes, and the anastomotic time was 18.3 ± 5.8 minutes; the operation time was 2.1 ± 0.5 hours. The LIMA was directly anastomosed to the LAD in 483 patients (in two, a Y graft with an inferior epigastric artery [IEA] was used to graft a

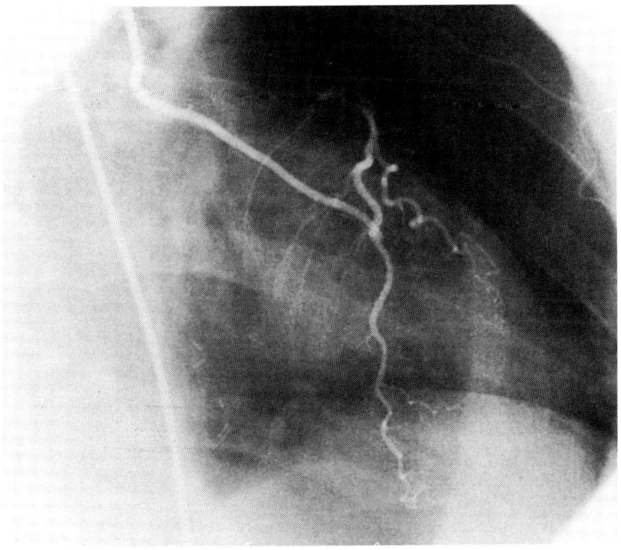

Figure 56–1. Angiography after a left anterior small thoracotomy. A length of the left internal mammary artery is harvested to reach the left anterior descending artery with a gentle curve.

diagonal branch), an IEA was used between the LIMA and the LAD in 41 patients (Fig. 56–4), and a saphenous vein was used in three patients; in one patient, an IEA was used as a bridge from the in situ LIMA to the LAD. The necessity of elongating the LIMA to reach a lateral LAD has decreased over time and with increasing experience. In the last 100 patients, an IEA was used in only three cases ($P < 0.05$ in comparison with the remaining patients).

The great majority of the patients were extubated in the operating room or during the first 2 hours in the intensive care unit (N = 369, 69.9%). Mean bleeding was 148.6 ± 190.7 ml in the first 12 hours; however, 9 patients (1.7%) had a redo for bleeding, and 10 (1.9%) were transfused. Mean creatine-kinase myocardial brain international unit (CKMB) peak was 20.0 15.2 UI, and mean stay in the intensive care unit was 4.1 ± 4.3 hours. Postoperative atrial fibrillation developed in 42 patients (7.9%) and was quickly reversed by amiodarone. Pericarditis, necessitating further hospitalization, was present in 3 patients (0.7%), and 12 patients (2.3%) had some delayed chest wound healing. Two patients showed late lung herniation through the wound, owing to pectoralis muscle dehiscence. Both required further suturing of the chest wall. Mean postoperative hospital stay was 66 ± 29 hours, often owing to delay in the control angiography; nevertheless, 349 patients (66.1%) were discharged within the first 2 postoperative days.

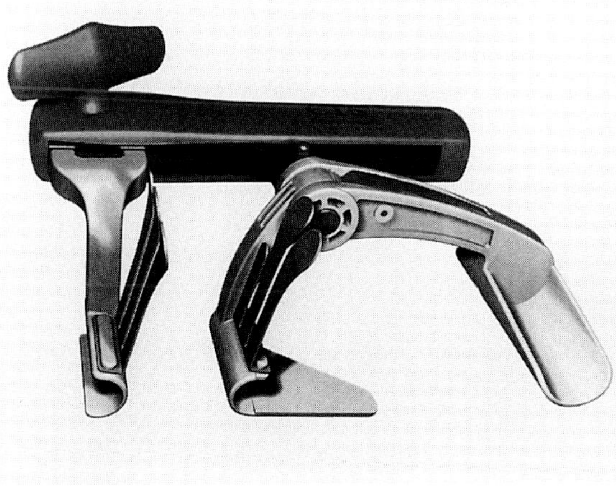

Figure 56–2. The new instruments available (Cardio Thoracic System, Cupertino, CA) allow the harvesting of a much longer segment of the left internal mamary artery.

Technical Concerns

Total or Partial LIMA Harvesting. The relationship between the heart and the thoracic wall is different after a median sternotomy than after a LAST. In the first situation, as both lungs are displaced and the pericardium is opened, the heart moves down, away from the chest wall. For this reason, the LIMA harvesting must be complete, because the LAD is far from the graft and the graft must be as long as possible.[7] To obtain this length, the first part of the LIMA (from the subclavian origin to the first rib) must be detached from the wall, because it is directed upward; otherwise, it is too short in its natural position.

In the second situation, the relationship between the LIMA and the chest wall is not modified. The distance from the LIMA to the LAD, as measured by us in 130 cases, was 3.39 ± 1.59 cm—nearer at the fourth intercostal space (3.01 ± 1.50 cm) and farther away at the fifth intercostal space (3.81 ± 1.64 cm). The mean length of the harvested LIMA necessary to reach the LAD was, in the same series, 8.04 ± 2.29 cm (8.02 ± 2.31 cm at the fourth intercostal space and 8.07 ± 2.17 cm at the fifth intercostal space); 76.9% of the LADs needed a LIMA length of 9 cm or less to be grafted—82.2% at the fourth intercostal space, and 70.6% at the fifth intercostal space. Therefore, from a technical point of view, the total length of the LIMA is not needed to reach the LAD. On the contrary, harvesting of the distal LIMA portion (up to the bifurcation) is more important than harvesting of the first 2 cm, because to reach the LAD, the LIMA has to move as a pendulum.

If the LIMA is only partially harvested, the possibility of flow competition with the LAD territory, owing to persistence of undivided LIMA branches, has to be explored. The LIMA, like all muscular arteries, has a mainly systolic flow, with a small percentage of diastolic flow (diastolic-systolic flow ratio <0.3). When this artery is grafted to the LAD, the flow pattern changes abruptly as the diastolic component, which is LAD related, becomes predominant. As muscular flow is mainly systolic and coronary flow is mainly diastolic, competition of flow cannot exist, because they occur in two different hemodynamic phases.

We demonstrated this aspect in the catheterization laboratory.[8] Thirty patients were selected. The LIMA was totally harvested in 15 of them after a median sternotomy and partially harvested in the remaining 15 after a LAST. The flow reserve was measured by positioning a flow probe in the distal third of the totally harvested LIMA, and after the last branch but before the LAD anastomosis in the partially harvested LIMA. Adenosine (12 to 14 mg) was injected into the LIMA at its origin from the subclavian artery. Acute LAD hyperemia caused an increase in the di-

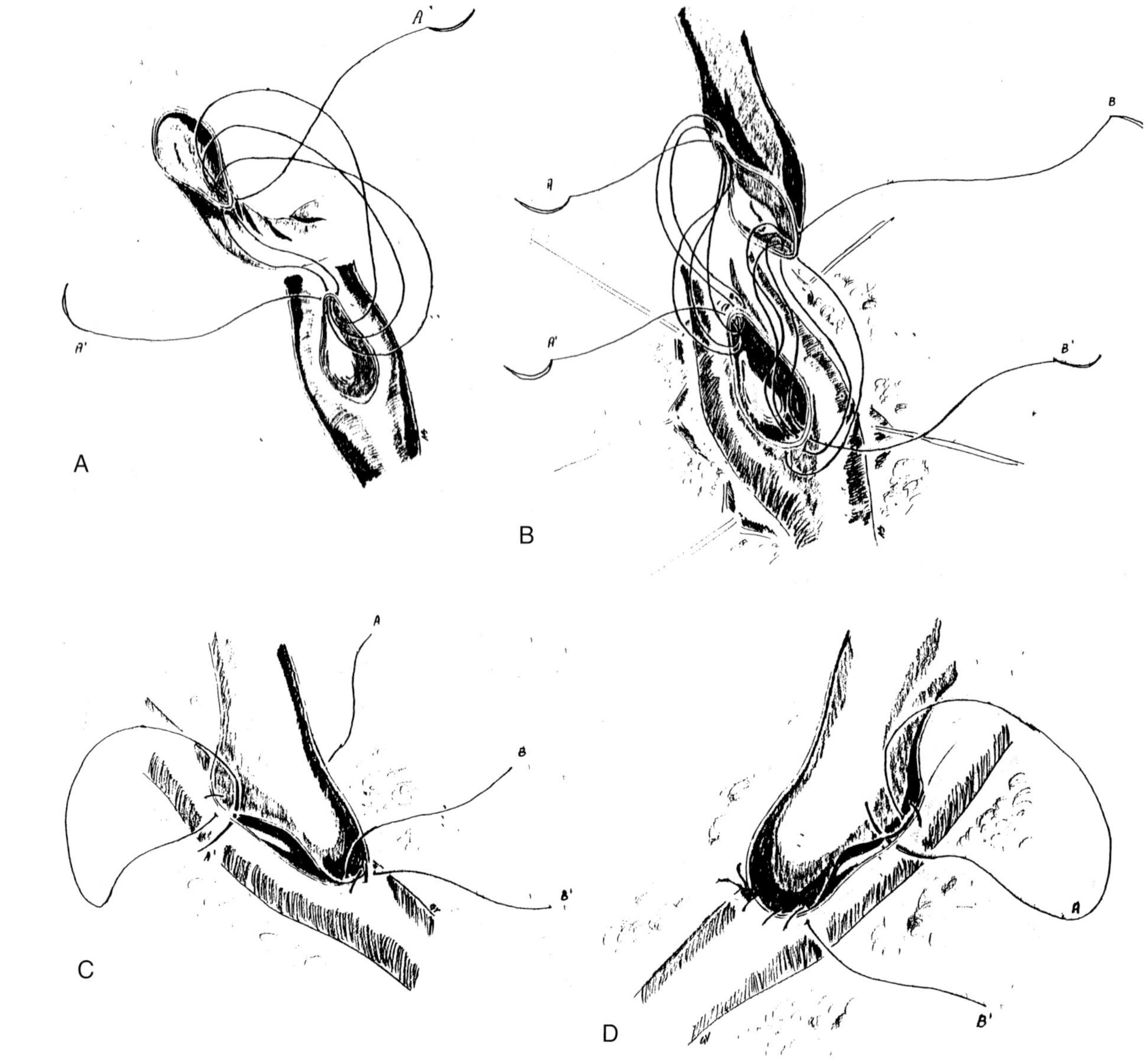

Figure 56–3. The anastomosis is performed using two 8–0 Prolene sutures with a 6-mm needle. Both sutures are passed three times at the heel (*A*) and at the apex (*B*); the left internal mammary artery is then pulled down to reach the left anterior descending artery. The anastomosis is completed with two running sutures from both sides (*C, D*).

astolic flow. The hyperemic basal average peak velocity (flow reserve) was the same in both groups (2.6 ± 0.5 vs. 2.6 ± 0.3, P = ns).

Kern and colleagues[9] reported an interesting case in which a large pectoralis branch of the LIMA was found undivided at angiography performed 7 years after surgery. Flow velocity was measured in the main LIMA, in the LIMA after the branch, and in the pectoralis branch. In the main LIMA, the flow velocity was systolic and diastolic (diastolic-systolic ratio 0.62); both velocities increased two and three times, respectively, after adenosine-induced acute hyperemia. In the LIMA beyond the pectoralis branch bifurcation, the flow pattern shifted to predominantly diastolic (diastolic-systolic ratio 1.25); after adenosine injection, diastolic velocity increased 3.5 times and systolic velocity 2.5 times. In the pectoralis branch, the flow velocity was predominantly systolic (diastolic-systolic ratio 0.4); adenosine increased both systolic and diastolic components, but to a lesser extent than the increases observed in the main LIMA and in the LIMA distal to the pectoralis branch. The hyperemic basal average peak velocity (flow reserve) was 2.5 in the main LIMA, 3.1 in the distal LIMA, and 1.6 in the pectoralis branch. These findings show that a chest wall branch of the LIMA, even if large, makes a minimal contribution to flow diversion during the diastolic phase of the cardiac cycle.

LAD Occlusion. Extensive experience with off-pump coronary surgery via a median sternotomy[10, 11] has shown that the distal portion of the LAD can be occluded for long time without harmful effects. In fact, via a LAST, the anastomotic site is distal to the second diagonal branch. Transesophageal echocardiography studies demonstrate that wall abnormalities occur in only about 50% of cases, are

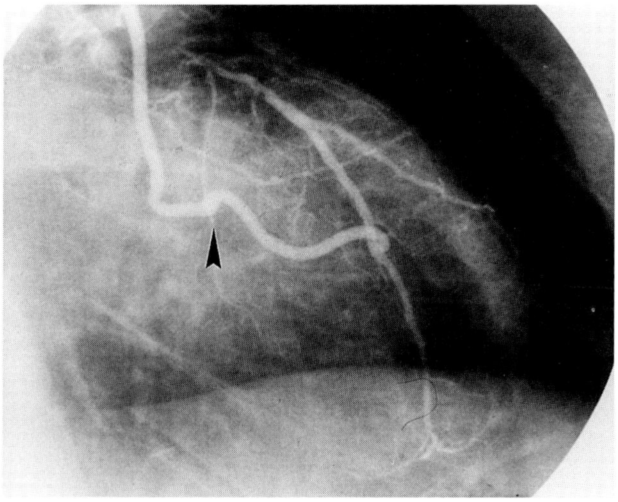

Figure 56–4. The left internal mammary artery (LIMA) was elongated with an inferior epigastric artery (IEA) to reach a laterally located left anterior descending artery. The *arrow* indicates the end-to-end anastomosis between the LIMA and the IEA.

limited to the apical portion of the free wall or of the septum, do not cause hemodynamic impairment or ventricular arrhythmia, and, more importantly, are immediately reversible. We do not use ischemic preconditioning, as our large clinical experience has shown that if nothing happens in the first 7 to 10 minutes of occlusion, nothing will happen. For this reason, we prefer to occlude the LAD and then prepare the LIMA and stabilize the operative field.

LAD Stabilization. If LAD movements are reduced, the anastomosis will be easier and the final results more predictable. LAD stabilization can be achieved using intravenous drugs or mechanical tools. Perioperatively, adenosine or esmolol is frequently used. Adenosine induces asystole for a few seconds, and during this time the surgeon can pass one or two bites; use of ventricular temporary pacing is advisable. Esmolol is a β-blocker with a short half-life and can be used as a continuous infusion or as a bolus. We prefer to use diltiazem, a calcium blocker, because of its many positive effects: it lowers the heart rate, reduces cardiac hypercontractility (negative inotropic effect), and enhances collateral coronary circulation (diltiazem is a powerful coronary vasodilator).

Mechanical LAD stabilization is, however, the most important factor in achieving a perfect anastomosis. Many companies manufacture such instruments, including the stabilizer we have used since April 1996 (Cardio Thoracic System, Cupertino, CA)[12] and the Octopus (Medtronic, Minneapolis, MN).[13] Good results can be obtained with every kind of instrument, even a homemade one (e.g., a fork).

In a small percentage of patients (<5%), the problem is how to manage the very lateral LAD. We initially proposed LIMA elongation with the IEA, to be used in selected cases. Our results were satisfying, with an angiographic patency rate of 95.4%. However, with greater experience and new instruments, we can now reach every LAD without the need to elongate the LIMA.

Quality Control of the Anastomosis

Echo Doppler Flow Assessment. The flow velocity pattern can be easily detected by the echo Doppler as the LIMA remains in its anatomic position for a few centimeters. The increase in the diastolic component at rest means that the anastomosis is patent, but not if the anastomosis is restrictive. A pharmacologic stress test, using adenosine, dobutamine, or dipyridamole, can be helpful to evaluate the quality of the anastomosis, but these tests are not easy to perform, require some organization, and are often difficult to repeat.

The solution was found by applying the Azoulay maneuver.[14] In this maneuver, there are two steps: one passive, one active. In the first step, the passive one, the patient's legs are lifted up by an assistant; in the second step, the active one, the patient has to remain in the same position for a few seconds, performing an isometric exercise. Acute hypervolemia is induced, with an increase in cardiac output and heart rate. If the echo Doppler flow velocity is recorded at rest and during the Azoulay maneuver, an increase in the diastolic flow velocity can be observed (Fig. 56–5). Correlating different Doppler patterns and angiography, we found that:

1. If a patient has a basal peak systolic-diastolic velocity ratio (PSDVR) or mean diastolic-systolic velocity ratio (MDSVR) equal to or greater than 1, the anastomosis is nonrestrictive (FitzGibbon's[15] grade A); this was true in every case that showed this pattern.
2. If both basal ratios are less than 1 but during the Azoulay maneuver the PSDVR or MDSVR increases to 1 or greater, the anastomosis is nonrestrictive (grade A); this was true in every case that showed this pattern.
3. If all the ratios are less than 1 but at least one is greater than 0.60, the anastomosis is restrictive (grade B) but not occluded. In the five patients who showed this pattern, in only one case was the anastomosis nonrestrictive (grade A).
4. If every ratio is 0.60 or less, the anastomosis or the conduit can be occluded. In the single patient who showed this pattern, the conduit was occluded at angiography.

Angiography. In 324 patients (61.4%) a postoperative angiography was performed during the first year after surgery. According to the FitzGibbon classification[15] (Table 56–1), the anastomosis was grade A + B in 307 cases (patency rate 94.7%) and grade A in 293 cases (perfect patency rate 90.4%). Based on cumulative results from angiography and echo Doppler, a patent anastomosis was obtained in 511 patients (96.8%) and a nonrestrictive anastomosis in 497 patients (94.2%). However, if we consider the last 300 patients, angiographic results are improving. In this series, 182 angiographies were performed; 180 anastomoses were grade A + B (98.9%, $P < 0.001$ vs. the global series) and 176 grade A (96.7%, $P < 0.001$). The total patency rate (angiography plus echo Doppler) was 99.3% (298 of 300, $P < 0.001$ vs. the global series), and 294 patients had nonrestrictive anastomoses (98%, $P < 0.05$ vs. the global series).

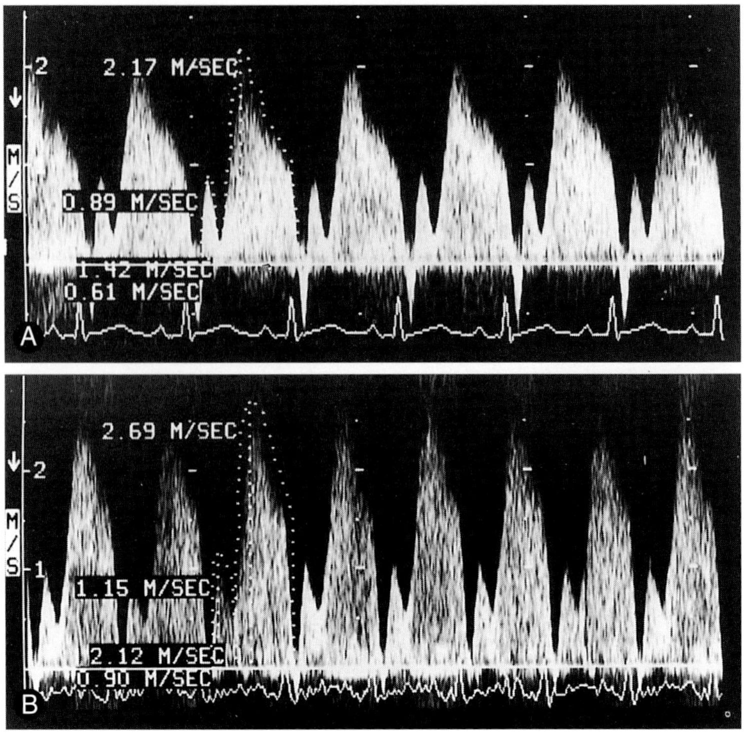

Figure 56–5. Echo Doppler flow velocity assessment at rest (*A*) and during the Azoulay maneuver (*B*). The huge increase in the diastolic flow velocity is characteristic of a nonrestrictive anastomosis.

A favorable unexpected event occurred: six patients who had anastomotic or conduit malfunction at the control angiography showed reversal of the anomalies after an interval of 115 ± 78 days. This was probably owing to small clots, which can disappear after a few weeks, or to adventitial hematomas, which also can reverse. What we learned is that no decisions have to be made in the early days after surgery. If any angiographic anomaly exists, we wait 2 or 3 months and then reapeat the angiography. Based on this experience, we decided not to reverse heparin at the end of the procedure, hoping to limit this phenomenon; however, we have no data to support this hypothesis, even though the solution seems reasonable.

Thirty-nine patients underwent a new angiographic control study more than 1 year after surgery (mean 17.6 ± 5.3 months) to evaluate the stability of the anastomosis over time and to check the development of LAD irregularities or stenosis in the proximal and distal occlusion sites. No patient showed any modification in shape of the anastomosis or of the LAD. Recently, a study by Perrault and colleagues showed that the hemostatic technique of snaring the proximal and distal LAD with double looping of suture over silicone tubing, with sufficient tension to achieve a clear operative field, does not cause endothelial dysfunction.[16]

Table 56–1. FitzGibbon Classification of Anastomosis Quality

Grade	Description
A	Excellent graft with unimpaired runoff
B	Stenosis reducing the caliber of the proximal or distal anastomoses or trunk to <50% of the grafted coronary artery; overall B grade is determined by the lowest of the three specific site grades
O	Occlusion

Clinical Results

At a mean follow-up of 18.3 ± 9.1 months, 517 patients (97.9%) were alive and asymptomatic with or without medical treatment; 487 patients (92.2%) were alive and asymptomatic without repeat surgical or cardiologic intervention on the LAD. Actuarial survival and event-free survival are shown in the Figure 56–6. For the purpose of the curve, events were defined as deaths (any cause), acute myocardial infarction in the LAD territory, or necessity of further revascularization (by surgery or catheterization) because of anastomotic or conduit malfunction.

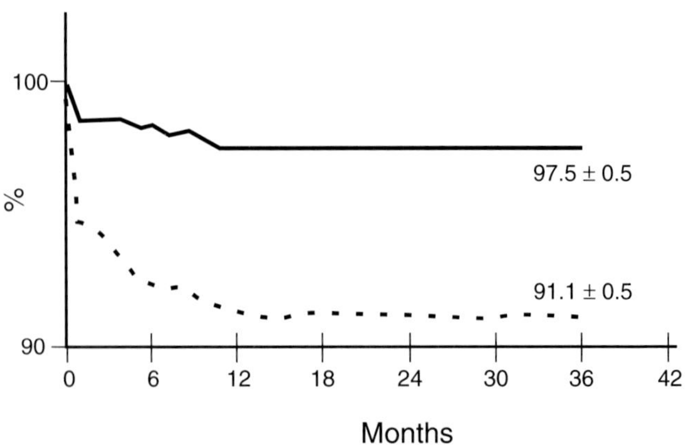

Figure 56–6. Survival (————) and event-free survival (------------) curves after 36 months.

Interestingly, no patient had a perioperative or late myocardial infarction in the target area. This means that LAD occlusion did not cause any harmful effect and that the anastomotic technique was effective, as no LAD damage was caused in any patient.

Conclusions

The LAST operation is a procedure that, in single-LAD disease, can provide acceptable results. Even though 36 months is not enough to define the role of this surgical procedure, our results allow us to assume that, in single-LAD disease, the LAST operation is at least comparable with the two procedures that are already standardized: LAD stenting and conventional surgery. A learning curve has to be considered; however, with the experience achieved by different teams and the development of new instruments, its duration can be shortened and perhaps eliminated. Randomized studies will give us the information we need to provide the best treatment for every patient.

In multiple-vessel disease, the LAST procedure can be helpful in selected patients, provided they need only a graft on the LAD; patients with major preoperative risk factors can benefit to a greater extent. However, as in every cardiac procedure, selection of patients is the most important issue.

References

1. Kolessov VI: Mammary artery—coronary artery anastomosis as method of treatment for angina pectoris. J Thorac Cardiovasc Surg 54:535–544, 1967.
2. Benetti FJ, Ballester C: Use of thoracoscopy and a minimal thoracotomy, in mammary-coronary bypass to left anterior descending artery, without extracorporeal circulation: Experience in 2 cases. J Cardiovasc Surg 36:159–161, 1995.
3. Acuff TE, Landreneau RJ, Griffith BP, Mack MJ: Minimally invasive coronary artery bypass grafting. Ann Thorac Surg 61:135–137, 1996.
4. Robinson MC, Gross DR, Zeman W, Stedje-Larsen E: Minimally invasive coronary artery bypass grafting: A new method using an anterior mediastinotomy. J Card Surg 10:529–536, 1995.
5. Subramanian V, Stelzer P: Clinical experience with minimally invasive coronary artery bypass grafting (CABG). Eur J Cardiothorac Cardiovasc Surg 10:1058–1063, 1996.
6. Calafiore AM, Di Giammarco G, Teodori G, et al: Left anterior descending coronary artery grafting via left anterior small thoracotomy without cardiopulmonary bypass. Ann Thorac Surg 61:1658–1665, 1996.
7. Calafiore AM, Teodori G, Di Giammarco G, et al: Left internal mammary elongation with inferior epigastric artery in minimally invasive coronary surgery. Eur J Cardiothorac Cardiovasc Surg 12:393–398, 1997.
8. Luise R, Teodori G, Di Giammarco G, et al: Persistence of mammary artery branches and blood supply to the left anterior descending artery. Ann Thorac Surg 63:1759–1764, 1997.
9. Kern MJ, Bach RG, Donohue TJ, et al: Role of large pectoralis branch artery in flow through a patent left internal mammary artery conduit. Cathet Cardiovasc Diagn 34:240–244, 1995.
10. Benetti FJ, Naselli G, Wood M, Geffner L: Direct myocardial revascularization without extracorporeal circulation: Experience in 700 patients. Chest 100:312–316, 1991.
11. Buffolo E, Silva de Andrade JC, Rodrigues Branco JN, et al: Coronary artery bypass surgery without cardiopulmonary bypass. Ann Thorac Surg 61:63–66, 1996.
12. Boonstra PW, Grandjean JG, Mariani MA: Local immobilization of the left anterior descending artery for minimally invasive coronary bypass grafting. Ann Thorac Surg 63:S76–S78, 1997.
13. Borst C, Jansen EW, Tulleken CA, et al: Coronary artery bypass without cardiopulmonary bypass and without interruption of native coronary flow using a novel anastomosis site restraining device ("Octopus"). J Am Coll Cardiol 27:1536–1564, 1996.
14. Calafiore AM, Teodori G, Di Giammarco G, et al: Minimally invasive coronary artery bypass grafting on a beating heart. Ann Thorac Surg 63 (suppl 6):S72–S75, 1997.
15. Fitzgibbon GM, Kafka HP, Leach AJ, et al: Coronary bypass graft fate and patient outcome: Angiographic follow-up of 5,065 grafts related to survival and reoperation in 1,388 patients during 25 years. J Am Coll Cardiol 28:616–626, 1996.
16. Perrault LP, Menasch P, Bidouard JP, et al: Snaring of the target vessel in less invasive bypass operations does not cause endothelial dysfunction. Ann Thorac Surg 63:751–755, 1997.

COMMENTARY

William R. Mayfield

The authors are to be congratulated for their substantial contribution to the initiation and progress of minimal access cardiac surgery. Their series of patients is among the largest and best studied in the world. As described, they routinely perform internal mammary artery (IMA) harvest under direct vision via a left anterior mini-thoracotomy. This approach often requires resection or dislocation of costal cartilage for adequate visualization. Only a short length of IMA is mobilized—enough to reach the LAD. Furthermore, the incision must be large enough both to visualize the IMA and to operate on the heart.

My own preference is for a totally thoracoscopic technique for IMA takedown, which has been performed in over 200 patients. This technique has several advantages, the principal one being that the entire length of the IMA from the first to the sixth rib can be mobilized. The artery thus lies nicely against the mediastinum medially to the lung, preventing the tendency to kink at the chest wall or behind the inflated lung. Furthermore, this avoids putting any tension on the anastomosis and the associated risk of graft avulsion. Another advantage is that the procedure can be performed through a smaller thoracotomy. There is no need for upward distraction on the chest wall, nor for disarticulation of the costochondral junction. This method is easy to perform. Residents are able to learn the technique rapidly, and LIMA usage at my institution is over 98%. We have recently started using 5-mm endoscopes, and the development of 3-mm cardiac endoscopic instruments should facilitate the procedure and decrease trauma to the intercostal nerves.

It is remarkable how many heart operations have been

performed endoscopically; IMA harvest, coronary anastomoses, mitral valve repair and replacement, intracardiac repair of congenital heart defects, patent ductus arteriosus closure, and removal of intracardiac foreign bodies. Moreover, robotic technology and three-dimensional visualization are appearing as enhancements to endoscopic techniques. It is appropriate here to recognize that all this work has been built on the efforts of the authors and their contemporaries.

COMMENTARY

Mohammad Bashar Izzat

Minimally invasive direct coronary artery bypass (MIDCAB) is still in evolution, and the technique is continually being subjected to refinement. Preparation of the IMA presents a challenge, owing to both poor exposure and limited access. The authors advocate preparing the IMA through the incision under direct vision with the use of dedicated chest wall retractors, whereas others harvest the IMA thoracoscopically. The latter, however, is time-consuming and technically demanding and requires the use of special endoscopic surgical instruments.

I prefer not to harvest the IMA exclusively thoracoscopically but to use video assistance to improve exposure of the operative field. With this method, conventional surgical instruments are inserted through the incision to dissect the IMA under video guidance. This technique is expeditious, does not require former training in video-assisted surgery, and is cost-effective. Compared with IMA preparation under direct vision, this technique negates the need for excessive spreading of the ribs, which is the main source of postoperative pain.

Whichever technique an individual surgeon prefers, full mobilization of the IMA should be achieved so that the length of the IMA is not limited. Hence, IMA avulsion or kinking at its attachment to the chest wall (when incompletely mobilized) is prevented, and concerns of IMA steal through side branches, albeit largely theoretical, are alleviated.

COMMENTARY

Erik Fosse

The resurgence of off-pump coronary vascularization is due to an increasing awareness of the deleterious effects of cardiopulmonary bypass. Although extracorporeal technology today is safe and allows surgery to be performed on severely ill patients, 6% of elderly patients have persistent cerebral dysfunction following cardiopulmonary bypass.[1] The inflammatory response due to extracorporeal circulation is also well documented and may be the cause of postpump organ failure.[2]

During the past decade, a number of devices such as blowers, stabilizers, improved endoscopic equipment, and dedicated internal mammary artery (IMA) harvesting equipment have emerged, all facilitating off-pump surgery and particularly the left anterior small thoracotomy approach. Open-heart surgery today has a low complication rate when mortality and perioperative infarction are considered.[3] It is therefore important that any new techniques do not lead to an increase in complications, while the patency rates obtained during surgery on cardiopulmonary bypass are retained.

The present study demonstrates that in single-vessel disease, off-pump surgery through a small anterior thoracotomy can indeed be performed without any increase in mortality and perioperative infarction. Randomized studies comparing on- and off-pump surgery must be performed to improve neuropsysiologic outcome.

The left anterior thoracotomy approach is suitable for patients with single-vessel disease in the left anterior descending (LAD) artery. In some cases, IMA-to-LAD anastomosis through a small thoracotomy has been combined with percutaneous transluminal coronary angioplasty (PTCA) preoperatively, perioperatively, or immediately postoperatively in cases in which disease is present in two of three vessels, a so-called hybrid procedure.[4, 5] So far, the number of hybrid procedures worldwide has been limited, probably because the procedure requires structural changes in hospitals and, in the present hospital setting, is not cost-effective. Thus, the left small anterior thoracotomy approach is presently suited only for selected patients. Today, an increasing number of patients with stenoses in the LAD are normally treated with PTCA and stenting. Even in occluded vessels, PTCA and stenting can be performed successfully. The advantage of PTCA compared with off-pump coronary surgery is that it is an even less invasive procedure that enables the patient to leave the hospital the day after the procedure, and no anesthesia is required. The disadvantages are, of course, that long-term patency with PTCA and stent has not been documented, and so far this cannot compete with a functional IMA graft.

Today, most patients referred for single-vessel IMA-to-LAD grafting are patients with an occluded LAD in whom PTCA is not possible or in whom PTCA has been tried unsuccessfully. Long-term quality-of-life studies must be implemented to allow recommendation of one treatment above the other. An increasing number of patients are now undergoing off-pump coronary artery bypass grafting through a median sternotomy using stabilizers. Full revascularization including the posterior vessels can be achieved without the use of cardiopulmonary bypass in most patients.

Another concept that is challenged by the new methods is the term *full revascularization.* As it has been demonstrated that the IMA-to-LAD graft is the most significant factor for freedom from symptoms and extended life expectancy following coronary surgery.[6] What does a graft to a small posterior vessel mean when LAD circulation is restored by a functional IMA graft? The increasing experience with off-pump surgery will probably give more answers to this.

Again, patency rate, mortality, and perioperative infarction must be monitored with these techniques, preferably in randomized studies. In the present study, the authors have an excellent patency rate comparable with published results of on-pump surgery. However, in coronary surgery today, an increasing number of patients with poor vessel quality and long-standing occlusions are accepted for surgery; therefore, to compare outcome of off-pump surgery with that of historic materials is unsatisfactory. Randomized trials must be performed to test its relative efficacy. The present article, however, gives a good indication that this type of surgery can be performed with more or less the same results as conventional coronary surgery on the beating heart.

References

1. Roach GW, Kanchuger M, Mangand CM, et al: Adverse cerebral outcomes after coronary bypass surgery. N Engl J Med 335:1857–1863, 1996.
2. Gillinov AM, Devaleria PA, Winkelstein JA, et al: Complement inhibition with soluble complement receptor type 1 in cardiopulmonary bypass. Ann Thorac Surg 55:619–624, 1993.
3. Øvrum E, Tangen G, Åm Holen E: Facing the era of minimally invasive coronary grafting: Current results of conventional bypass grafting for single-vessel disease. Ann Thorac Surg 64:159–162, 1997.
4. Angelini GD, Wilde P, Salerno TA, et al: Integrated left anterior small thoracotomy and angioplasty for multivessel coronary artery revascularization. Lancet 347:757–758, 1996.
5. Barstad RM, Fosse E, Vatne K, et al: Intraoperative evaluation of bypass anastomosis during MIDCAB. The value of intraoperative coronary angiography. Ann Thorac Surg 64:1835–1839, 1997.
6. Loop FD, Lytle BW, Cosgrove DM, et al: Influence of the internal-mammary-artery graft on 10-year survival and other cardiac events. N Engl J Med 314:1–6, 1986.

Chapter 57

The H-Graft MIDCAB

William E. Cohn

The term *H-graft* refers to a short segment of conduit, either artery or vein, interposed between the target coronary artery and the side of the in situ nonmobilized mammary artery (Fig. 57–1). Postoperative angiograms have a characteristic H appearance (Fig. 57–2). Although this type of graft requires two anastomoses, the ease of those anastomoses, the avoidance of mammary artery harvest, and the excellent visualization without chest wall retraction make the H-graft an attractive alternative approach for performing minimally invasive direct coronary artery bypass (MIDCAB) in selected patients.

Standard MIDCAB was first reported by Benetti and associates[2] in November 1995, and since that time, the number of procedures performed has increased exponentially. Although many variations of MIDCAB have been described, the standard approach involves dissection of the left internal mammary artery (LIMA) through a small left anterior thoracotomy, immobilization of the left anterior descending coronary artery (LAD), and anastomosis of the end of the LIMA to the side of the LAD on the beating heart without cardiopulmonary bypass.[1, 4, 17] The avoidance of cardiopulmonary bypass is attractive from the standpoint of decreasing potential postoperative morbidity. The economic advantages owing to decreased length of stay and resource utilization as well as the market appeal have contributed to the procedure's rapid growth in popularity.[7]

Although the advantages of standard MIDCAB are considerable, there are disadvantages as well. Harvesting the LIMA through a left anterior mini-thoracotomy can be technically demanding. When the proximal LIMA is inadequately mobilized, the graft courses dorsally from the chest wall, medial to the edge of the left lung, and then laterally to the LAD. In this position the graft lie may be affected by respiratory motion, resulting in the development of graft tension or kinking in the early postoperative period, which may compromise intermediate-term patency. Furthermore, the retraction required to visualize the cephalad portion of the LIMA through a limited access incision results in significant musculoskeletal trauma.

In our initial experience of 32 standard MIDCAB procedures, we routinely obtained angiograms within 24 to 48 hours of surgery in all patients with normal renal function. Although the clinical results were good, a number of patients (6 of 32) had sharp bends or kinks that were clearly not present at the time of wound closure. Two of these patients in whom the kinks were believed to be flow limiting underwent limited access reoperation for revision.[18] Others have reported similar experiences after standard MIDCAB.[11, 14]

Our early experience was also marked by impressive postoperative incisional pain in nearly all patients. The irony of severe pain after a "less invasive" operation was somewhat disappointing to both patient and surgeon. Others have confirmed this experience informally, and although this paradoxically increased pain was thought to be due in part to the shorter, lighter anesthetic, the issue of a vigorously retracted anterior thoracotomy could not be disregarded. Based on our consideration of these issues, we devised the H-graft technique for minimally invasive arterial bypass of the LAD.

Technical Details of the H-Graft MIDCAB Procedure

The procedure is performed from the left side of the supine patient. After adequate anesthetic, a single-lumen endotracheal tube is placed. All patients in our series had a transesophageal echocardiographic probe passed, and Swan-Ganz catheters were not routinely used. The patient is prepped and draped as for a conventional coronary artery bypass graft.

A 6- to 7-cm incision is centered over the fourth rib medial to the nipple. The pectoralis muscle is incised, as are the intercostal muscles above and below the fourth costal cartilage. The intercostal muscles are initially left intact medially to avoid injury to the mammary artery and vein. Careful dissection is carried out deep to the posterior perichondrium 1 cm lateral to the costochondral junction, so that the rib can be divided without violating the left pleura. We prefer a fine right-angle clamp and a sliding rib cutter for these maneuvers. Once the rib is divided, the costal cartilage can be gently rotated anteriorly and medially, to allow dissection of the posterior surface. The dissection is continued medially to the chondrosternal joint, which is disarticulated by incising the fibrous capsule with electrocautery, and the cartilage and perichondrium are removed in their entirety. The LIMA lies immediately deep to the cartilage 1 cm lateral to the chondrosternal joint such that a 1.5- to 2-cm segment of vessel is exposed by this maneuver. This limited exposure is adequate for obtaining proximal and distal control of the mammary artery, allowing the proximal H-graft anastomosis to be constructed. No further mammary dissection is required. No branches of the mammary are disrupted.

While the thoracotomy is being performed, an assistant harvests a segment of conduit. The radial artery is currently our graft of choice, but we have had good results with saphenous vein as well.

After LIMA exposure, while harvesting of the conduit is being completed, the pericardium is incised and the cut edges are sutured to the skin to bring the heart forward, rotating the LAD into view. A T-shaped pericardial incision is used, combining a 5- to 6-cm horizontal incision and a 4-cm vertical incision parallel with and just lateral to the in situ LIMA. The LAD is identified and immobilized as had been described for standard MIDCAB.[4] Systemic heparin is given to maintain the activated clotting time greater than

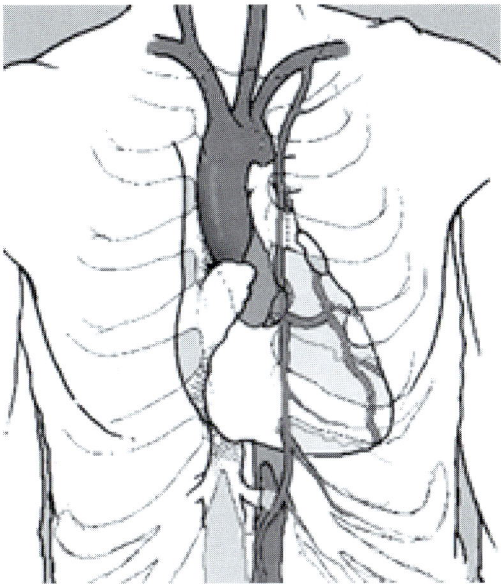

Figure 57–1. Diagram demonstrating a short horizontal H-graft interposed between the in situ left internal mammary artery and the left anterior descending coronary artery.

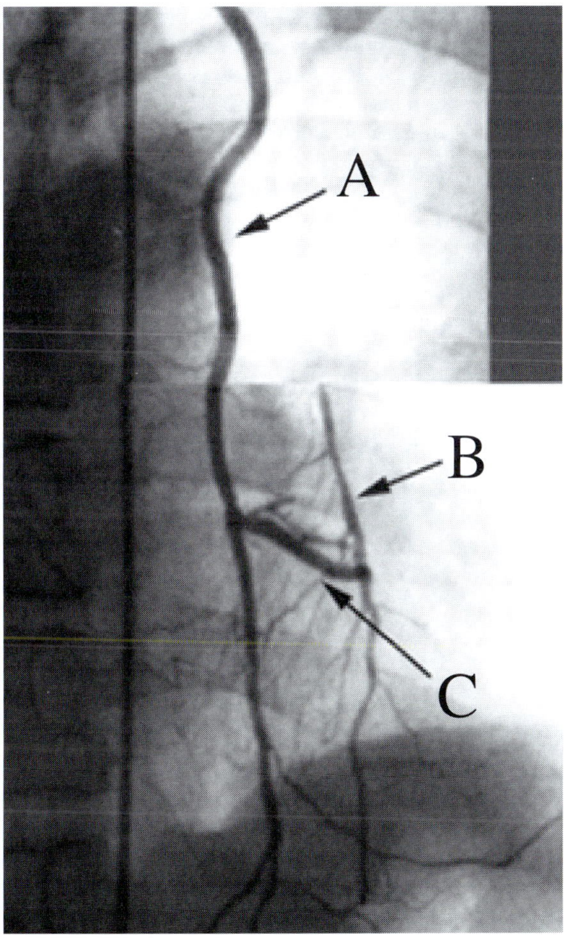

Figure 57–2. Characteristic appearance of a postoperative angiogram in an H-graft patient. A, In situ left internal mammary artery with terminal musculophrenic and superior epigastric branches. B, Left anterior descending coronary artery. C, H-graft.

300 seconds, and the flow through the LAD is temporarily stopped using silicon-elastic vessel loops proximal and occasionally distal to the point of anastomosis. Although a number of coronary artery stabilizers are commercially available, I prefer the Genzyme system, the platform of which was developed at Beth Israel Deaconess Medical Center in Boston (Fig. 57–3). The unique geometry of this stabilizer allows gentle anteroposterior compression of the coronary artery by applying lateral tension on the silicone-elastic tapes (Fig. 57–4). The LAD is opened longitudinally, and the slightly spatulated end of the graft is sutured to the LAD arteriotomy. To facilitate a tension-free, nonkinking graft lie, we prefer to construct the anastomosis in such a fashion that the H-graft is oriented perpendicularly with respect to the LAD, using a running 8–0 polypropylene single-suture technique. Performing the critical distal anastomosis is facilitated by the fact that the short segment of graft is completely untethered and can be moved about to provide optimal exposure of each aspect of the anastomosis.

After completion of the anastomosis, flow is restored through the LAD, and the presence and amount of back-bleeding through the graft are noted. Thus a crude intraoperative assessment of distal anastomotic patency is made possible. Brisk, pulsatile backflow suggests a good anastomosis and, even in the presence of a tight proximal LAD stenosis or occlusion, has been uniformly present in our experience. Additionally, a coronary probe can be passed down the graft across the completed anastomosis, or a syringe and blunt needle can be attached to the free end of the H-graft, permitting injection and resistance assessment. None of these intraoperative quality checks is possible with standard MIDCAB.

The graft is then measured to a point on the short segment of exposed LIMA that will permit a straight, relaxed path for the conduit (Figs. 57–5 and 57–6). The graft may come off precisely at a right angle or have a slightly obtuse angle relative to the in situ LIMA. This direct measure-

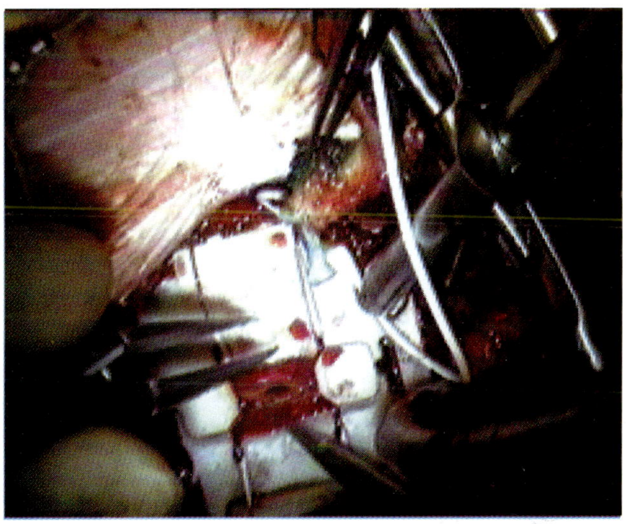

Figure 57–3. The Cohn Cardiac Stabilizer™ shown applied to the left anterior descending coronary artery through a small anterior thoracotomy. (Courtesy of Genzyme Surgical Products, Cambridge, MA.)

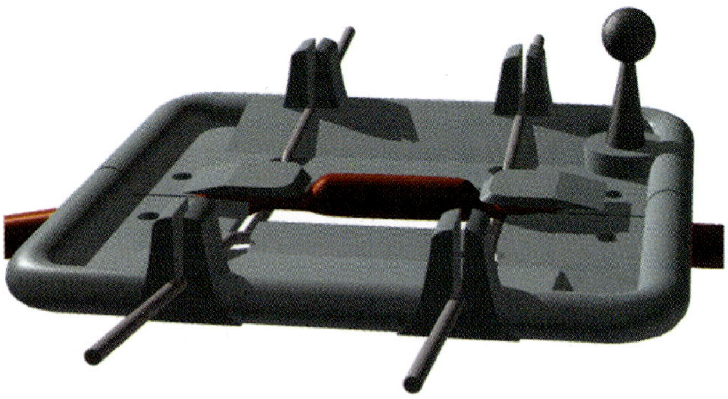

Figure 57–4. Computer-generated image demonstrating how the lateral tension applied to the silicone elastic tape results in gentle anteroposterior compression of the coronary artery.

ment is performed after releasing the pericardial stays and during full-volume lung ventilation. This precludes the addition of any but the most minimal redundancy in length. In addition, the horizontal orientation of the graft reduces the risk of postoperative kinking, as it lies parallel with respect to the motion of the medial edge of the left lung.

Local control of the LIMA is obtained with microvascular spring clamps proximal and distal to the point of H-graft attachment. In our experience, dividing the lateral mammary vein is beneficial, as it allows the anastomosis to be constructed on the lateral aspect of the in situ LIMA. Early in our experience with the LIMA arteriotomy, we created focal dissections in two patients. We have since recognized the importance of obtaining proximal and distal control of the LIMA with microvascular spring clamps before incising the vessel wall. This provides a distended segment of artery that can be readily opened without injury to the back wall. Once nicked, the segment rapidly decompresses, decreasing the risk of intramural hematoma or dissection.

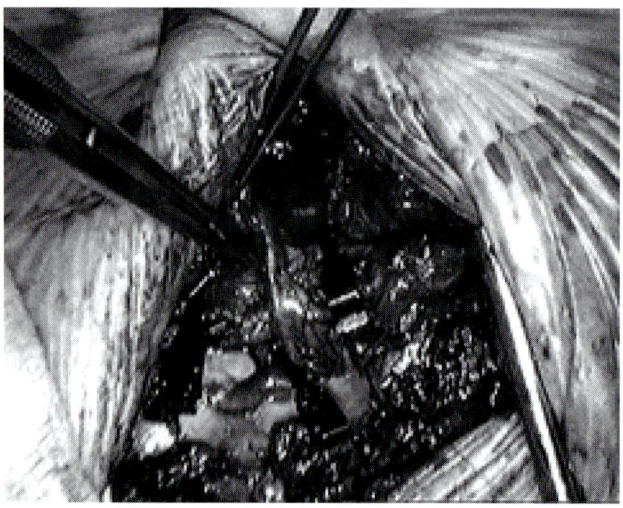

Figure 57–5. Operative photograph showing measurement of the H-segment before division of the graft and construction of the proximal anastomosis. Delicate microvascular spring clamps are used for vascular control. A, Segment of radial artery sutured to the left anterior descending artery. B, In situ left internal mammary artery. C, Sternal facet of resected fourth costal cartilage.

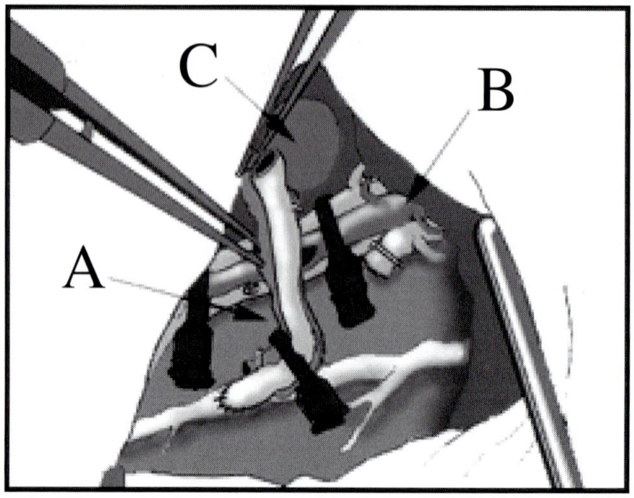

Figure 57–6. Diagram corresponding to the photograph in Figure 57–3.

After completion of the proximal anastomosis, again using running 8–0 monofilament, the clamps are removed and a flow probe is used to assess flow through the H segment. The audible Doppler signal should demonstrate a dramatic augmentation and prolongation of the diastolic phase, as with any coronary graft. Quantitative or transit time Doppler flows are generally 40 cc/min or greater. The wounds are then closed, the heparin is reversed, intercostal blocks are administered with 0.25% bupivacaine, and the patient is extubated in the operating room. A small left pleural tube is placed if the left pleura is entered. A flat, perforated, closed suction drain is placed intrapericardially if the pleura is intact.

Patient Selection

The determination of H-graft MIDCAB suitability in individual patients ultimately will depend on intermediate- and long-term patency results in larger series. For the moment, however, the H-graft MIDCAB, in contrast to the standard MIDCAB, requires less dissection, provides excellent visualization, permits better intraoperative assessment of distal anastomotic patency, facilitates construction of a tension-free nonkinking graft, and is associated with less postoperative pain owing to a reduction in chest wall retraction. Thus, if long-term patency approaches that of a conventional LIMA-to-LAD bypass, the procedure may prove to be an attractive alternative to standard MIDCAB in all patients.

The H-graft MIDCAB may be well suited for several types of patients even if long-term patency falls short of standard LIMA-to-LAD bypass. Because of the shorter operative time and decreased dissection and musculoskeletal trauma, it is an attractive approach in the elderly and other high-risk patients. The procedure is also useful in patients in whom mammary artery harvest would be technically demanding, as in obese patients or those with left pleural adhesions due to previous operations or other pleural processes. Avoiding mammary harvest is advantageous in patients who have received chest wall radiation and in patients with impaired coagulation.

The H-graft MIDCAB approach may also be beneficial in young patients with multivessel disease in whom only the LAD stenosis is severe enough to warrant a bypass or in those in whom a hybrid strategy is selected, combining a graft to the LAD with a catheter-based intervention to a second lesion in another vessel. Many of these patients will require multivessel surgical revascularization at some point in their lives, and this subsequent operation will be greatly facilitated in patients initially managed with H-graft MIDCAB. After H-graft MIDCAB, the in situ LIMA is relatively untouched, and with ligation and division of the H segment (which may be possible, depending on the patient's coronary anatomy at the time of reoperation and bypass support), the heart can be freed and the mammary dissected for routine use. Alternatively, the in situ LIMA can be readily mobilized proximal to the origin of the H-graft, and the distal LIMA divided. The right-angle geometry, once freed from the sternum, allows adequate laxity to expose the lateral and posterior lateral surfaces of the heart while preserving the graft to the LAD.

Choice of Conduit

Initially, we enthusiastically used the right inferior epigastric artery (RIEA), first reporting its exclusive use in eight patients.[6] Our enthusiasm was based in part on the fact that the H-graft, owing to its short length, could be constructed out of the proximal half of the RIEA. Compared with the distal half, this portion has relatively few side branches, is of generous diameter, and is histologically somewhat similar to the LIMA. Proximal inferior epigastric artery (IEA) luminal diameter ranges from 1.9 to 3.3 mm, as determined by evaluation of digitized images obtained from postoperative angiograms.[6] In addition, there are several published series documenting good intermediate-term patency for the IEA when used as an aortocoronary graft,[3, 12, 20] as well as when used as part of a LIMA composite.[5] Our intermediate results with the IEA have been variable, as described later.

Our current conduit of choice is the radial artery, but we have used saphenous vein in elderly patients and in patients in whom the radial artery is of poor quality. Because of the relative proximity between the in situ LIMA and the LAD, only a short segment of conduit, generally 3 to 6 cm, is required to perform the operation. Thus it is possible to limit the radial harvest incision to the proximal third of the forearm, preserving distal ulnar-to-radial collaterals and staying far from the superficial cutaneous nerves at the wrist. If saphenous vein is used, a segment of adequate length in which there are no branches or valves can be identified in the calf. As in the forearm, only a short incision on the lower leg is necessary to satisfy the limited conduit requirements.

Our Experience

Patient Selection. From December 1996 through July 1998, 34 patients at the Beth Israel Deaconess Medical Center underwent bypass grafting of the LAD with a variety of conduits. In 13 patients, the RIEA was used. Subsequently, 15 patients underwent grafting of the LAD with a short segment of radial artery and 6 with reversed saphenous vein. Twenty patients had critical stenoses involving only the LAD. Fourteen patients had at least one other vessel with critical stenosis. Eleven of these 14 patients were thought to be high-risk candidates for conventional coronary artery bypass graft with cardiopulmonary bypass. The remaining three were believed to be good candidates for a hybrid approach, combining H-graft MIDCAB with a catheter-based intervention on an additional coronary lesion.

Among these 34 patients, there were 15 females. The mean age was 67 years (range, 44 to 93 years). There were eight octogenarians. Twenty-six patients had unstable angina preoperatively, and eight had positive exercise tolerance tests despite maximal medical therapy. Seventeen patients had previously undergone catheter-based interventions.

Early Postoperative Results. Thirty-one of these 34 patients underwent postoperative angiography within 24 hours of surgery. In two patients, acute occlusion was diagnosed. Two additional patients had nonocclusive narrowing at the proximal anastomosis requiring limited access revision. In all four of these patients from the first half of our series, there was focal LIMA dissection at the lateral arteriotomy. In two of these patients, the dissection was identified intraoperatively but was inadequately repaired with fine tacking sutures. The remaining 27 patients had widely patent grafts with rapid filling of the LAD in each case. All patients with patent grafts who had operation for unstable symptoms had resolution of those symptoms. Nine patients underwent postoperative thallium stress testing, with normalization of the LAD territory in each case. There were no perioperative infarctions and no evidence of postoperative cardiac ischemia. Seven patients experienced transient atrial fibrillation that responded to procainamide.

Four of our first 13 patients in whom the IEA was used returned 2 to 4 months postoperatively with recurrence of angina. Subsequent angiography demonstrated narrowing of the IEA in three patients and complete occlusion in the fourth (Fig. 57–7). In each, initial postoperative angiography had demonstrated a widely patent graft. Although three additional patients in whom the IEA was used were recatheterized 10 to 14 months postoperatively with widely patent grafts, we no longer advocate the use of this conduit for the H-graft MIDCAB (Fig. 57–8). We have subsequently used radial artery (n = 15) and saphenous vein (n = 6) for the H-graft segment. These patients have been followed for 2 to 14 months with no recurrence of angina.

Mammary Steal: Misnomer or Myth?

Perhaps the most intriguing possible disadvantage is the potential for diversion of significant LIMA flow to noncoronary vascular beds subtended by the many nonligated branches of the in situ LIMA. There are a small number of anecdotal reports in the cardiac surgical literature describing patients who have undergone LIMA-to-LAD bypass and in whom persistent LAD territory ischemia was thought to be present as a result of undivided first and second intercostal branches.[8, 10, 13, 15, 16] This condition has been inaccurately referred to as mammary steal.

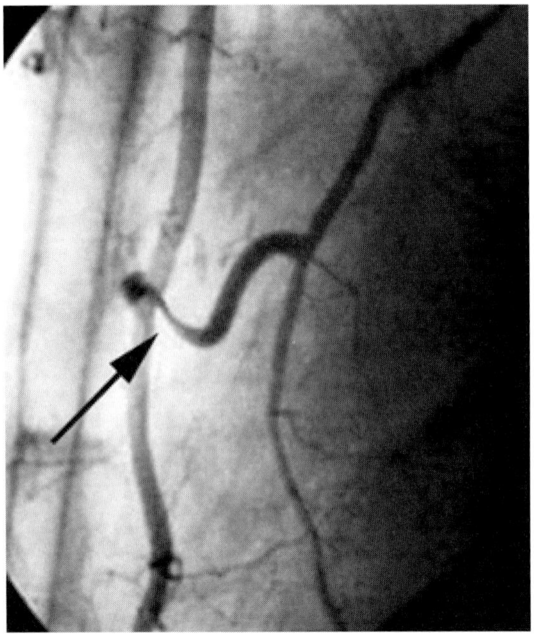

Figure 57–7. Inferior epigastric H-graft angiogram obtained 3 months postoperatively in a patient with return of angina. There is tight focal stenosis of the proximal portion of the inferior epigastric segment (*arrow*).

Arterial steal is a well-known phenomenon that has been described for several arteries and organ systems. Steal may develop in the presence of hemodynamically significant stenosis involving a common arterial trunk shared by two distinct organs or anatomic locations. If the two organs have vascular resistances or collateral blood supplies that differ significantly, blood may flow in a retrograde direction from one organ, through the common trunk, to the other. This "stolen" blood may result in signs or symptoms of arterial insufficiency. One such syndrome is subclavian steal, in which retrograde blood flow from the brain to the arm through the vertebral artery develops as a result of subclavian stenosis manifesting as vertebral basilar insufficiency.

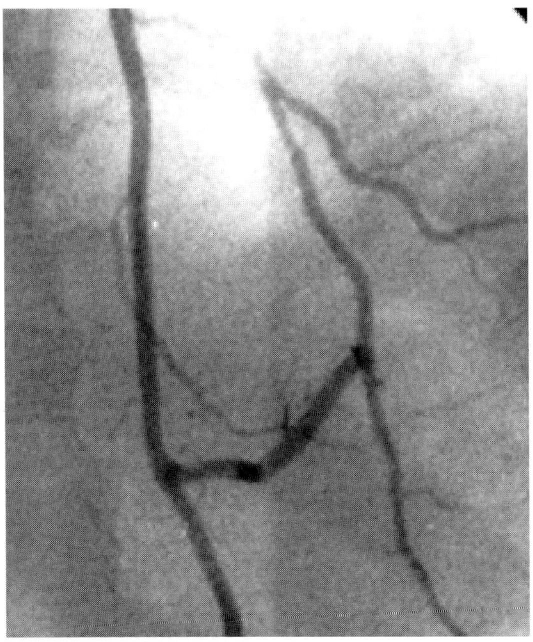

Figure 57–8. Inferior epigastric H-graft angiogram obtained 14 months postoperatively in a clinically well patient.

The term *mammary steal* is a misnomer, as it implies retrograde LIMA flow from the heart to the chest wall by way of the retained intercostals. In order for this to occur, the vascular resistance of the intercostal bed would have to be substantially less than that of the coronary circulation. Such a condition is highly unlikely to occur. If graft flow to the heart is compromised in the presence of retained intercostals, it would be as a result of fractionation of a limited antegrade flow reserve. We describe this theoretical condition as "critical branch diversion." Several arguments can be made, however, that this condition does not exist.

Acutely, we recognize that the predominance of arterial flow to skeletal muscle occurs during systole, whereas coronary flow is primarily during diastole. This is observable with intraoperative Doppler examination, and diastolic reversal of flow in the in situ LIMA distal to the H-graft has been observed on postoperative angiograms in some patients. Preliminary H-graft flow dynamics in a canine model from our institution suggest that, absent significant proximal LIMA stenosis, flows down the branches of the in situ LIMA and through the H-graft segment are determined only by the resistance of their vascular beds, and that antegrade flow reserve is not the limiting factor. In addition, distal LIMA flow reserve as determined by Doppler flow wire measurement during adenosine-induced coronary hyperemia has been shown to be independent of the degree of mammary mobilization and intercostal branch division.[9]

Another argument is based on the well-recognized process of mammary maturation. It has been observed angiographically that LIMA grafts enlarge within the first several weeks postoperatively. We assume that this is in response to the decrease in vascular resistance that results from replacing the intercostal and terminal mammary beds with that of the coronary artery and the increased LIMA flow that results. This results in a gradual dilatation or maturation of the LIMA graft, much in the way the radial artery dilates in response to increased flow after creation of an arteriovenous fistula at the wrist for hemodialysis access. In construction of the H-graft, the coronary vascular bed does not replace that of the in situ LIMA; rather, it is added to it in parallel. As the net resistance of two vascular beds in parallel is lower than that of either bed, the flow down the in situ H-graft LIMA is maximized, which may accentuate the maturation process. The fact that the LIMA is completely in situ may facilitate maturation as well.

Perhaps the most compelling argument against the existence of critical branch diversion, however, is evident in patients who have undergone successful H-graft MIDCAB. Despite the retention of all intercostal branches, as well as the terminal musculophrenic and superior epigastric branches, none of these patients has demonstrated any clinical signs of graft insufficiency. All patients with isolated LAD stenosis have experienced relief of angina after H-grafting. Furthermore, several patients have undergone postoperative thallium stress tests that revealed normalization of LAD territory ischemia in each case.

Advantages and Disadvantages

There are several potential disadvantages to the H-graft procedure. The operation necessitates a second small incision for harvest of radial artery or saphenous vein, and it requires a second anastomosis for attachment of the proximal end of the H-segment to the LIMA. Although the second (proximal) anastomosis is composed of relatively large-caliber, motionless, nondiseased arteries, it demands technical precision. Furthermore, some find the right-angle orientation of the two anastomoses to be aesthetically displeasing. It should be noted, however, that the coronaries arise from the ascending aorta at essentially right angles, as do the septals from the LAD and the renals from the aorta. Finally, the intermediate- and long-term radial artery and saphenous vein patency in this particular situation has not been demonstrated, and longer follow-up with larger series will be required and will ultimately determine the utility of the procedure.

To reiterate, when compared with the standard end-to-side LIMA-to-LAD MIDCAB, the immediate and delayed advantages of H-graft MIDCAB are:

- Reduction in postoperative pain, in the absence of chest wall retraction or rib spreading
- Expedience of the MIDCAB procedure by eliminating the LIMA harvest
- Elimination of potential complications associated with limited access LIMA harvest, including injury to the artery, inadequate mobilization, and bleeding from the LIMA bed
- Avoidance of left pleural entry, permitting two-lung full-volume ventilation throughout the procedure, which may be of benefit in patients with marginal pulmonary reserve
- Creation of a tension-free nonkinking graft lie
- Facilitation of the critical distal anastomosis
- Facilitation of any future operation

Conclusion

H-graft MIDCAB is a technically simple operation that offers considerable advantages for both patient and surgeon. Additional data are needed to determine the intermediate- and long-term patency of the various conduits, but our early results suggest that it is a useful procedure to have in one's minimally invasive bypass armamentarium.

References

1. Acuff TE, Landreneau RJ, Griffith BP, Mack MJ: Minimally invasive coronary artery bypass grafting. Ann Thorac Surg 61:135–137, 1996.
2. Benetti FJ, Ballester C, Sani G, et al: Video assisted coronary bypass surgery. J Card Surg 10:620–625, 1995.
3. Buche M, Schoevaerdts JC, Louagie Y, et al: Use of the inferior epigastric artery for coronary bypass. J Thorac Cardiovasc Surg 103:665–670, 1992.
4. Calafiore AM, Giammarco GD, Teodori G, et al: Left anterior descending coronary artery grafting via left anterior small thoracotomy without cardiopulmonary bypass. Ann Thorac Surg 61:1658–1665, 1996.
5. Calafiore AM, Di Giammarco G, Teodori G, et al: Radial artery and inferior epigastric artery in composite grafts: Improved midterm angiographic results. Ann Thorac Surg 60:517–523, 1995.
6. Cohn WE, Suen HC, Weintraub RM, Johnson RG: The "H" graft: An alternative approach for performing minimally invasive direct coronary artery bypass. J Thorac Cardiovasc Surg 115:148–151, 1998.
7. Doty JR, Fonger JD, Nicholson CF, et al: Cost analysis of current therapies for limited coronary artery revascularization. Circulation 96(suppl 9):16–20, 1997.
8. Hartz RS, Heuser RR: Embolization of IMA side branch for post-CABG ischemia. Ann Thorac Surg 63:1765–1766, 1997.
9. Luise R, Teodori G, Di Giammarco G, et al: Persistence of mammary artery branches and blood supply to the left anterior descending artery. Ann Thorac Surg 63:1759–1764, 1997.
10. Pelias A, Del Rossi A: A case of post operative internal mammary steal. J Thorac Cardiovasc Surg 90:174–176, 1985.
11. Possati G, Gaudino M, Alessandrini F, et al: Systematic clinical and angiographic follow-up of patients undergoing minimally invasive coronary artery bypass. J Thorac Cardiovasc Surg 115:785–790, 1998.
12. Puig LB, Ciongolli W, Cividanes GV, et al: Inferior epigastric artery as a free graft for myocardial revascularization. J Thorac Cardiovasc Surg 99:251–255, 1990.
13. Sbarouni E, Corr L, Fenech A: Microcoil embolization of large intercostal branches of internal mammary artery grafts. Cathet Cardiovasc Diagn 31:334–336, 1994.
14. Schaff HV, Cable DG, Rihal CS, et al: Minimal thoracotomy for coronary artery bypass: Value of immediate postprocedure graft angiography. Circulation 94:1–51, 1996.
15. Schmid C, Heublein B, Reicheli S, Dorst HG: Steal phenomenon caused by a parallel branch of the internal mammary artery. Ann Thorac Surg 50:463–464, 1990.
16. Spanos PK, Bisbos AD, Arditis II: Treatment of internal thoracic artery steal syndrome with supraclavicular approach. J Thorac Cardiovasc Surg 115:464–465, 1998.
17. Subramanian VA, McCabe JC, Geller CM: Minimally invasive direct coronary artery bypass grafting: Two-year clinical experience. Ann Thorac Surg 64:1648–1655, 1997.
18. Suen HC, Johnson RG, Weintraub RM, et al: Minimally invasive direct coronary artery bypass: Our experience with 32 patients. Int J Cardiol 62:S95–S100, 1997.
19. van Son JA, Smedts F, Vincent JG, et al: Comparative anatomic studies of various arterial conduits for myocardial revascularization. J Thorac Cardiovasc Surg 99:703–707, 1990.
20. Vincent JG, van Son JAM, Skotnicki SH: Inferior epigastric artery as a conduit in myocardial revascularization: The alternative free arterial graft. Ann Thorac Surg 49:323–325, 1990.

Chapter 58

Combined Minimally Invasive Coronary Artery Bypass and Angioplasty: An Integrated Approach

Clinton T. Lloyd, Antonio M. Calafiore, Peter Wilde, Alan J. Bryan, Leonardo Paloscia, Chris Monk, and Gianni D. Angelini

Minimally invasive direct coronary artery bypass (MIDCAB) grafting is rapidly evolving as an accepted modality for the treatment of occlusive coronary artery disease. Following the initial suggestion of Benetti in 1994 that the procedure could be performed through a small left thoracotomy,[5] Calafiore and associates presented their series of 155 patients who had grafts of the left internal mammary artery (LIMA) to the left anterior descending (LAD) coronary artery using the left anterior small thoracotomy (LAST) incision.[9] Since then, a number of approaches have been proposed and described. These include a right mini-thoracotomy for access to the right coronary artery,[24] subxiphisternal incision for harvest and anastomosis of the gastroepiploic artery,[16] and thoracoscopic, video-assisted bypass grafting via port access.[25] The problem with any of these approaches is that they provide access to only a single diseased vessel, thus limiting patient suitability or compromising adequacy of revascularization.

Parallel to the growth in minimally invasive coronary bypass grafting has been the expansion of interventional cardiovascular procedures.[7] The increase in the use of percutaneous transluminal coronary angioplasty (PTCA) has been accompanied by the introduction of methods to decrease the atheroma within the lumen, such as directional atherectomy and laser angioplasty. More notably, the use of stenting has seen a dramatic rise in recent years. Technical refinements with better deployment of the stent, improved adjunctive pharmacologic treatment, and a better understanding of the mechanisms involving restenosis have helped minimize occlusion rates. However, despite these advances, and given that angioplasty allows multiple-vessel revascularization in selected cases, its limitation remains its restriction to appropriate and accessible lesions.

Our institutions have developed an integrated, or hybrid, procedure that combines the benefits of minimally invasive coronary grafting with the versatility of angioplasty. This presents a novel treatment for multivessel coronary artery disease and allows treatment of high-risk patients. This approach remains controversial and has not been assessed in a large randomized trial. Here, we discuss some of the issues encountered in our experience.

Angioplasty Versus Bypass Grafting

Since its advent in the late 1970s, PTCA has been used as an alternative to coronary bypass grafting. The concept of a nonsurgical method of revascularization with early recovery and reduced costs is appealing, but it is not suitable for all patients owing to inaccessible or anatomically difficult coronary lesions. Coronary artery bypass grafting (CABG) also relies on the existence of reasonably sized vessels to be grafted. In practice, the risks and benefits of each procedure govern the choice of method for a particular patient. A number of randomized studies comparing PTCA with CABG have shown a similar incidence of death and myocardial infarction at 1, 3, and 5 years.[20, 27] PTCA was as effective as CABG in the treatment of angina, although further revascularization was required more often with PTCA. CABG does, however, compare more favorably with respect to 5-year survival in the diabetic subgroup of patients.

Restenosis remains the Achilles' heel of PTCA. Intimal thickening has been responsible for approximately 30% of the loss of luminal diameter 6 months after coronary interventions, whereas shrinkage of the dilated segment accounted for the rest.[19] In an effort to prevent this shrinkage, stents are deployed to maintain the enlarged diameter mechanically, thereby reducing the restenosis rate in the early period by 25 to 30%.[14, 22] The problems remain in the late period, with intimal encroachment through the stent accounting for all the late reduction in luminal diameter.[13] Intimal hyperplasia also affects coronary bypass grafts, particularly vein grafts, in which the cumulative attrition rate is 15 to 20% at the end of the first year. The occlusion rate is 2 to 3% per year between 1 and 5 years and increases 5% per year, with 50% occluded at the end of 10 years.[11] By comparison, the LIMA graft, which is almost always used in MIDCAB procedures, has a long-term patency of 92 to 97% in the first year and 88 to 93% at 10 years.[4, 26]

Subacute and acute stent thromboses following PTCA pose further problems necessitating some means of anticoagulation. This is the result of the thrombogenic effect of the foreign stent material or perhaps the inadequate deployment of the stent itself.[12] Pharmacologic prevention has typically been through systemic administration, and a number of compounds are under clinical evaluation. Aspirin, which is almost uniformly used, blocks the formation of thromboxane A_2, which mediates platelet aggregation and degranulation. Alone, however, it does not prevent early thrombosis. Ticlopidine blocks the binding of fibrinogen to the platelet glycoprotein IIb/IIIa receptor, and abciximab, a newer drug, is a monoclonal Fab fragment directed against the same receptor. Early results indicate that stent thrombosis rates are reduced with the use of ticlopidine[21]; more importantly, with abciximab there is a significant reduction in nonfatal myocardial infarction and the need for repeat intervention at 30 days.[28] The protective effects of these agents on stent thrombosis are offset by the risks of systemic anticoagulation, in particular, hemorrhage. This risk of hemorrhage becomes of greater clinical significance when anticoagulation is used at the time of surgery, as discussed later.

Experience

We initially published our experience with 6 patients and their early follow-up in 1996, and all of them had successful outcomes.[2] Although the series was small, we believed that this approach was suitable for selected patients and continued to use this technique at our institutions. Friedrich and associates subsequently reported 2 of their patients who had similar good results.[15] Both patients had minimally invasive grafting of the LIMA to the LAD and PTCA to the right coronary artery, and angiography was used to assess the graft before PTCA. Izzat and associates presented 11 patients who had complete revascularization in multivessel coronary artery disease with the staged approach.[17] The early results were again encouraging, with all patients free of angina at a mean follow-up of 11.4 months. Late angiographic assessment of the graft and angioplasty site was not performed in any of these studies. We reviewed 18 patients in the late follow-up period. Half the patients had elective angiography, which showed patency of both the graft and the angioplasty vessel, and these patients were free of angina. These numbers are still small, but the results warrant larger studies.

Preoperative Considerations

The hybrid procedure which was developed as a means of extending the benefits achieved through minimally invasive surgery clearly lends itself to certain patient groups. Patient selection plays a critical role in the success of the procedure.

Patient Selection

A number of factors should be considered.

Age. We initially reported operating on a group of patients between 49 and 87 years of age. Although there are no contraindications for any particular age, certain groups may be more appropriate. Younger patients may be suitable because the avoidance of median sternotomy enables safer reoperation should there be progression of coronary disease requiring a second surgical intervention. Elderly patients who would otherwise have been refused surgery on the basis of the increased morbidity associated with the extracorporeal circulation are also candidiates for the hybrid procedure.

Coexistent Morbidity. Patients who have coexistent morbidity are considered at increased risk of systemic effects of cardiopulmonary bypass (CPB) and would thus benefit from the minimal invasiveness of the procedure. Such conditions include poor left ventricular function, impaired respiratory function, compromised renal function, significant concomitant carotid artery stenosis, or a recent stroke. Coexistent malignant disease is also considered a relative contraindication for CPB.

Previous Cardiac Surgery. Conventional reoperative CABG using CPB carries a relatively high mortality and morbidity. This is of particular concern when a patent vein graft exists in the midline behind the sternum. A minimal access approach avoids the risks of reopening on the midline, and angioplasty allows intervention on the native coronary vessels as well as on diseased grafts.

Coronary Anatomy and Disease

Nature of the Vessel. The LAD artery should have a diameter greater than 1.5 mm to ensure adequate runoff. Angiographic assessment should exclude the possibility of an intramyocardial or heavily calcified artery, which would preclude grafting.

Nature of the Lesion. Diffusely diseased vessels with angiographically complex lesions are contraindications to angioplasty. These include distant and complex type C lesions, chronic totally occluded arteries, and small tortuous vessels. Lesions should obviously be amenable to balloon angioplasty, and very tight stenoses may be difficult to access. When the LAD artery is involved with an isolated type C stenosis, minimally invasive bypass grafting has been shown to be superior to PTCA with regard to the need for further revascularization.[22]

Operative Considerations

Surgical Technique

The method we use for the MIDCAB procedure has been described in detail previously (see Chapter 56).[10] A LAST incision is made through the fourth or fifth intercostal space. We do not advocate the routine excision of costal cartilage, because adequate exposure can be gained with retraction of the ribs alone. Once hemostasis is secured, the pericardium is incised vertically, at which point the LAD artery is visualized directly below. At this stage, accessibility of the LAD artery anastomosis site needs to be evaluated (see section on Coronary Anatomy and Disease). Dissection and mobilization of the LIMA from the chest wall are carried out with the aid of a retractor (CTS MIDCAB System, Cupertino, CA). This allows good visualization to the level of the second intercostal space superiorly, or, with the aid of a thoracoscope introduced through the left fourth intercostal space, at the anterior axilliary line. This allows proximal dissection as high as the first intercostal space and distal dissection to the inferior border of the fifth rib. After heparinization, the LIMA is divided, and topical diluted papaverine is applied to prevent vasoconstriction while the anastomosis site is prepared. To provide a bloodless field during construction of the anastomosis, the proximal and distal portions of the LAD artery are snared with 4–0 Prolene (Ethicon, Somerville, NJ) with a rubber tubing snugger to prevent damage to the coronary artery.[24] Esmolol, a short-acting intravenous β-blocker, is used to slow the heart (50 to 75 bpm). The anastomosis is constructed with continuous 7–0 to 8–0 Prolene, and upon completion, the diastolic flow in the LIMA graft is demonstrated by standard Doppler echocardiography to confirm patency and adequacy of the anastomosis.[3, 10] The wound is then closed with a pleural drain and an intercostal catheter for postoperative analgesia.

Angioplasty Technique

The timing of angioplasty is discussed later. Standard access for PTCA is achieved via cannulation of the femoral artery with the insertion of a hemostatic sheath and the use of a 6 or 8 French guiding catheter. An initial diagnostic angiography is performed with the objectives of assessing the quality of the LIMA-to-LAD graft and confirming the anatomy of the lesions for angioplasty. The angioplasty is performed using a 6 or 8 French guiding catheter. The lesions are initially cannulated with a 0.014-in. steerable guide wire, followed by balloon dilatation with or without additional stenting. The decision for stent deployment depends on the operator's assessment of the lesion following initial balloon dilatation and whether the procedure is done as a simultaneous or delayed procedure (see later). Heparinization is used throughout the procedure, with the activated clotting time maintained over 300 seconds. Once the PTCA is completed, the patient is started on antiplatelet therapy. We use aspirin when angioplasty alone is performed and aspirin in conjunction with ticlopidine when stents have been deployed.

Simultaneous Versus Delayed Surgery

The decision to perform both procedures either during the same anesthesia or with a delay period depends on a number of factors. Having initially performed the PTCA simultaneously, we have more recently opted for a delayed approach, with the surgery preceding the angioplasty. We recognize, however, that there may be reasons for patients who have had only partially successful angioplasty to undergo minimally invasive surgery later.

Simultaneous. The advantages of the simultaneous approach are only a single operation for the patient and complete revascularization at the one visit. The graft and anastomosis can be assessed at the time of operation, and patient discomfort during angioplasty is minimized. One disadvantage with this approach is the necessity of operating in the unfamiliar and often crowded environment of the catheterization suite (Fig. 58–1). A second disadvantage is the potential risk, following the use of stents, of anticoagulant-induced hemorrhage from both the anastomotic site and the surgical incision. In our institutions, aspirin and ticlopidine are used for the prevention of acute and subacute thrombosis associated with the stent. These drugs have been shown to be as efficacious alone as when combined with heparin and oral anticoagulants in reducing stent thrombosis, but the risk of hemorrhage is still a problem. A potential solution to the problem may be the introduction of heparin-bonded stents that provide local thromboresistance without the need for systemic anticoagulation. In the pilot phase of the Benestent II study, in which heparin-bonded stents were used, no (sub)acute thrombosis was observed in 203 patients.[23]

Delayed. The advantage of a delayed procedure is the ability of carrying out both interventions under ideal circumstances (i.e., in the normal operating environment). The potential for ischemic complications during angioplasty should be reduced with a well-functioning LIMA graft. The most important reason for delaying the procedure is the ability of deploying stents and providing simultaneous anticoagulation without concern for bleeding. The disadvantage, however, is the recovery of the patient from the MIDCAB procedure with potentially incomplete revascularization before proceeding to angioplasty a few days later. It also automatically prolongs the hospital stay and recovery time. The optimal time before angioplasty is patient dependent, but we prefer to allow a minimum of 24 to 48 hours after surgery.

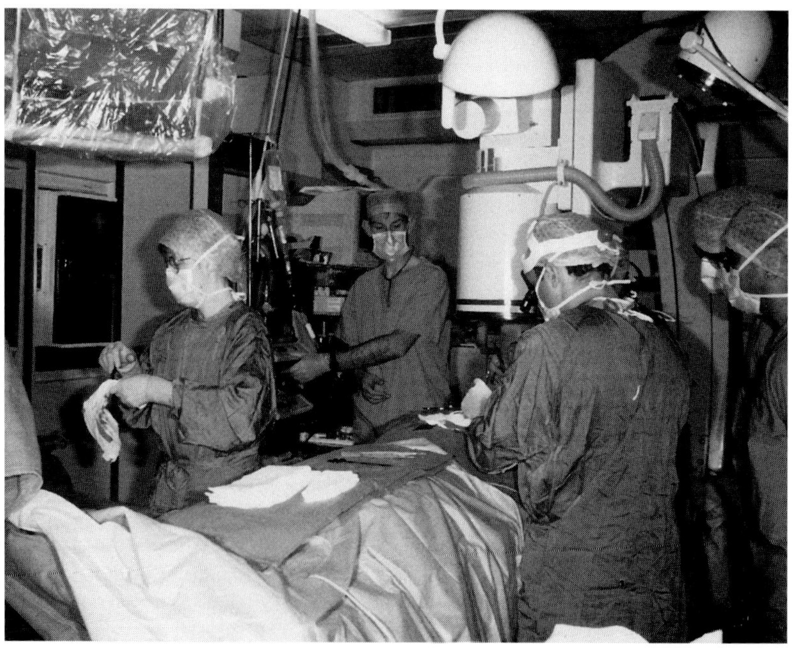

Figure 58–1. Simultaneous combined left anterior small thoracotomy and percutaneous transluminal coronary angioplasty performed in the cardiac catheterization laboratory.

Postoperative Care

Following surgery, all patients are admitted to the cardiac intensive care unit for monitoring. We keep patients intubated and ventilated until hemodynamic and gaseous exchange stability is achieved, but extubation is generally earlier than for on-bypass midline sternotomy procedures. Routine investigations, such as blood samples for coagulation, chest radiographs, and electrocardiograms are performed. The LIMA graft is usually assessed again in the early postoperative period by Doppler echocardiography, in which flow is compared with that in the ungrafted right internal mammary artery. The pleural drains and intercostal catheter are removed the following day. The time of discharge is again dependent on whether a simultaneous or a delayed procedure is performed.

Results

As with the evolution of any new surgical technique, our practice changed as experience with the procedure was gained. Most notable was the change from using the simultaneous to the delayed approach for the reasons mentioned previously. In total, we have operated on 18 patients, with complete revascularization in all individuals. Of the 18, 9 were operated on in Bristol, United Kingdom, and 9 in Chieti, Italy. The mean age for the group was 63.2 years and ranged from 35 to 87 years. Four patients had impaired left ventricular function with an ejection fraction of less than 50%, and most (78%) had two-vessel disease at initial angiography (Fig. 58–2A). Four of the 18 patients had been selected for the procedure because they were considered at increased risk from the effects of CPB, namely, they had significant carotid artery disease, cancer, chronic obstructive airways disease, or severely impaired left ventricular function.

All patients had grafting of the LIMA to LAD coronary artery (see Fig. 58–2B) through a LAST incision. In total, 21 additional coronary arteries were angioplastied, with stenting in 10 of these (see Fig. 58–2C to E). The sites of angioplasty included the right coronary artery, the diagonal artery, and the circumflex artery and its marginal branches. This was performed as a simultaneous procedure in 4 patients and as a delayed procedure in 14.

Mortality for the procedure was 0%. One patient required reoperation following ischemic changes during the recovery period. This patient had undergone simultaneous grafting of the LIMA to LAD coronary artery and angioplasty with stent deployment to the first obtuse marginal branch of the circumflex artery. Repeat angiography con-

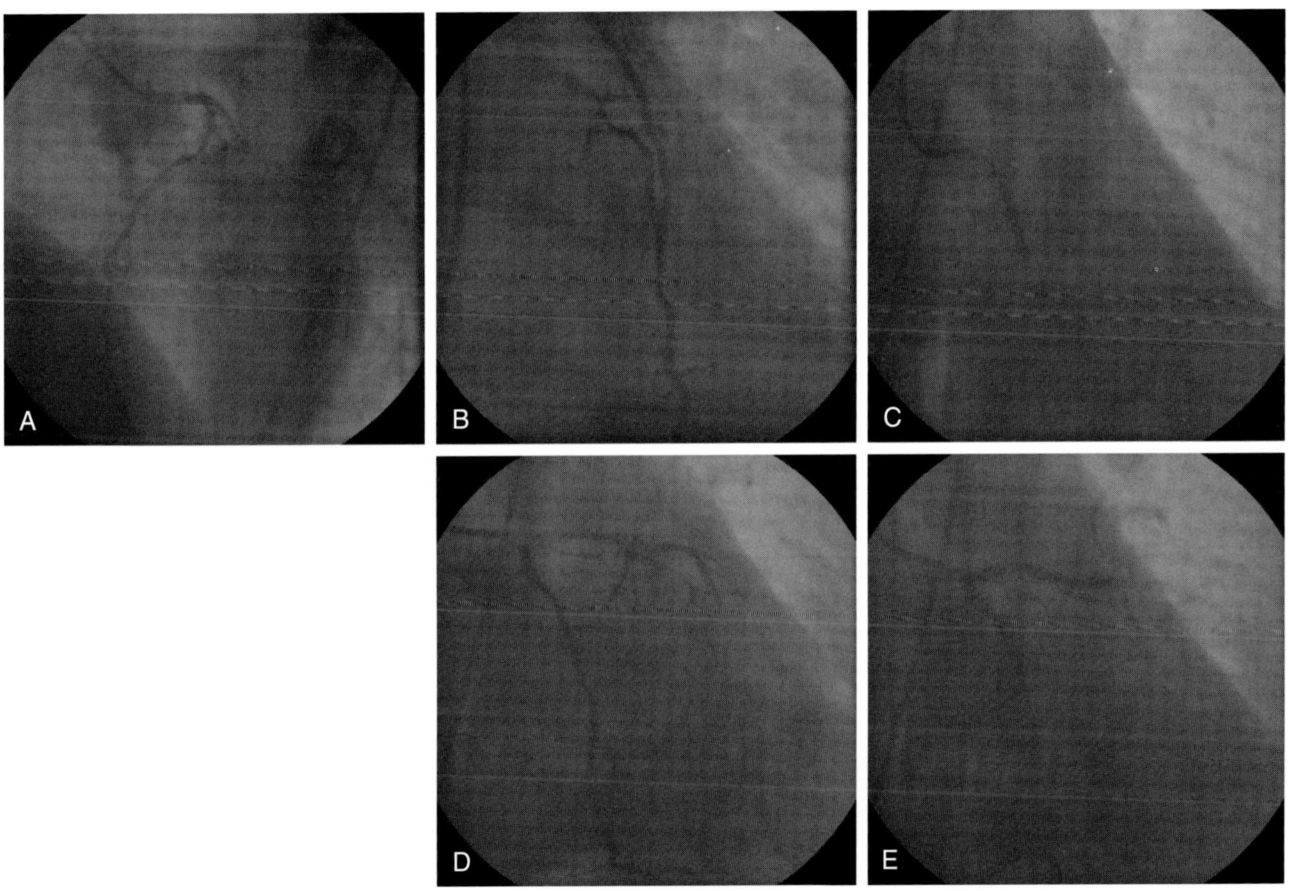

Figure 58–2. *A*, Preoperative coronary angiogram showing disease in the proximal left anterior descending coronary artery and proximal circumflex coronary artery. *B*, Postoperative coronary angiogram before percutaneous transluminal coronary angioplasty showing patent left internal mammary artery to left anterior descending coronary artery. *C*, Coronary angiogram showing stenosed circumflex artery lesion before dilatation, with the balloon visible through the stenotic segment, *D*, during and *E* after dilatation and stent deployment.

firmed that the cause of the ischemia was related to thrombosis of the stent in the obtuse marginal artery. This was thought to be related to inadequate anticoagulation with the reduced heparin dose. In view of the potential risk of bleeding with further anticoagulation, we elected to reoperate on this patient with conventional CPB and venous grafting to the obtuse marginal branch. The patient made a good recovery.

The remaining patients did well with no other associated morbidity and no wound infections. The mean intensive care stay was 14.7 hours, with a range of 2.5 to 26 hours, and the mean hospital stay was 5 days (range 3 to 7 days).

Long-term follow-up included functional assessment and angiography. Seventeen patients are symptom free and on no antianginal medication. The remaining patient has improved from New York Heart Association grade IV to grade I. Nine patients underwent elective angiography at a mean of 6 months. All showed patency of the LIMA-to-LAD graft, and all the angioplasty sites remain free from stenosis.

Future Prospects

The combined procedure is still in its infancy. Although it clearly provides a means whereby at-risk patients can achieve multivessel revascularization through minimally invasive interventions, its role in patients who are not necessarily at increased risk is less well defined. In addition, the technique is now in competition with off-pump coronary revascularization through a median sternotomy, which is becoming widely used in several centers around the world.[6, 8] This too allows multiple-vessel grafting, but also in selected patients. A limiting factor with this technique is accessibility. Distal circumflex lesions are difficult to graft without compromising left ventricular function, especially in patients with marked left ventricular impairment. The combined use of the off-bypass procedure for accessible lesions with subsequent angioplasty for inaccessible lesions may provide another treatment option.

References

1. Alessandrini F, Gaudino M, Glieca M, et al: Lesions of the target vessel during minimally invasive myocardial revascularisation. Ann Thorac Surg 64:1349–1353, 1997.
2. Angelini G, Wilde P, Salerno T, et al: Integrated left small thoracotomy and angioplasty for multivessel coronary artery revascularization. Lancet 347:757–758, 1996.
3. Barnea O, Santamore W: Intraoperative monitoring of IMA flow: What does it mean? Ann Thorac Surg 63(suppl):S12–S17, 1997.
4. Barner H, Standeven J, Reese J: Twelve year experience with internal mammary artery for coronary artery bypass. J Thorac Cardiovasc Surg 90:668, 1985.
5. Benetti F: Symposium on myocardial protection: Looking towards the 21st century. Chicago, IL, October 1994.
6. Benetti F, Naselli G, Wood M, Geffner L: Direct myocardial revascularization without extracorporeal circulation: Experience in 700 patients. Chest 100:312–316, 1991.
7. Bittl J: Advances in coronary angioplasty. N Engl J Med 335:1290–1302. 1996.
8. Buffallo E, de Andrade J, Branco J, et al: Coronary artery bypass grafting without cardiopulmonary bypass. Ann Thorac Surg 61:63, 1996.
9. Calafiore A, Angelini G, Bergsland J, Salerno T: Minimally invasive coronary artery bypass grafting. Ann Thorac Surg 62:1545–1548, 1996.
10. Calafiore A, Di Giammarco G, Teodori G, et al: Left anterior descending coronary artery grafting via left anterior small thoracotomy without cardiopulmonary bypass. Ann Thorac Surg 61:1658–1665, 1996.
11. Campeau L, Enjalbert M, Lesperance J, et al: Atherosclerosis and late closure of aortocoronary saphenous vein grafts: Sequential angiographic studies at 2 weeks, 1 year, 5 to 7 years and 10 to 12 years after surgery. Circulation 68(suppl II):II-1s–II-7s, 1983.
12. Colombo A, Hall P, Nakamura S, et al: Intracoronary stenting with anticoagulation accomplished with intravascular ultrasound guidance. Circulation 94:1519–1527, 1995.
13. Dussaillant G, Mintz G, Pichard A, et al: Small stent size and intimal hyperplasia contribute to restenosis: A volumometric intravascular ultrasound analysis. J Am Coll Cardiol 26:720–724, 1995.
14. Fischman D, Leon M, Baim D, et al: A randomized comparison of coronary stent placement and balloon angioplasty in the treatment of coronary artery disease. N Engl J Med 331:496–501, 1994.
15. Friedrich G, Bonatti J, Dapunt O, et al: Preliminary experience with minimally invasive coronary-artery bypass surgery combined with coronary angioplasty. N Engl J Med 336:1454–1455, 1997.
16. Grandjean J, Mariani M, Ebels T: Coronary reoperation via small laparotomy using right gastroepiploic artery without CPB. Ann Thorac Surg 61:1853–1855, 1996.
17. Izzat M, Yim A, Mehta D, et al: Staged minimally invasive direct coronary artery bypass and percutaneous angioplasty for multivessel coronary artery disease. Int J Cardiol 62(suppl I):S105–S109, 1997.
18. Mariani M, Boonstra P, Grandjean J, et al: Minimally invasive coronary artery bypass grafting versus coronary angioplasty for isolated type C stenosis of the left anterior descending artery. J Thorac Cardiovasc Surg 114:434–439, 1997.
19. Mintz G, Pompa J, Pichard A, et al: Intravascular ultrasound predictors of restenosis after angioplasty after percutaneous transcatheter revascularization. J Am Coll Cardiol 27:1678–1687, 1996.
20. Pocock S, Henderson R, Rickards A, et al: Meta-analysis of randomised trials comparing coronary angioplasty with bypass surgery. Lancet 346:1184–1189, 1995.
21. Schomig A, Neumann F, Kastrati A, et al: A randomized comparison of antiplatelet and anticoagulant therapy after placement of coronary artery stents. N Engl J Med 334:1084–1089, 1996.
22. Serruys P, de Jaegere P, Kiemeneij F, et al: A comparison of balloon expandable stent implantation with balloon angioplasty in patients with coronary artery disease. N Engl J Med 331:489–495, 1994.
23. Serruys P, Emanuelsson H, van der Giesen W, et al: Heparin-coated Palmaz-Schatz stents in human coronary arteries: Early outcome of the Benestent-II pilot study. Circulation 93:412–422, 1996.
24. Stanbridge R, Hadjinikolaou L, Cohen A, et al: Minimally invasive coronary revascularization through parasternal incisions without cardiopulmonary bypass. Ann Thorac Surg 63(suppl): S53–S56, 1997.
25. Stevens J, Burdon T, Peters W, et al: Port access coronary artery bypass grafting: A proposed surgical method. J Thorac Cardiovasc Surg 111:567–573, 1996.
26. Tector A, Kress D, Downey F, et al: Complete revascularization with internal thoracic artery grafts. Semin Thorac Cardiovasc Surg 8:29, 1996.
27. Bypass Angioplasty Revascularization Investigation (BARI) In-

vestigators: Comparison of coronary bypass surgery with angioplasty in patients with multivessel disease. N Engl J Med 335:217–225, 1996.

28. EPIC Investigators: Use of monoclonal antibody directed against the platelet glycoprotein IIb/IIIa receptor in high risk coronary angioplasty. N Engl J Med 330:956–961, 1994.

COMMENTARY

John E. Sanderson

The prospect of performing coronary artery bypass grafting (CABG) without the traditional median sternotomy scar or cardiopulmonary bypass (CPB) is extremely attractive not only to cardiologists but also to patients. The sternotomy scar is unsightly, frequently disfiguring, and often especially disliked by women. Although healing is usually good, occasionally deep-seated infection can be particularly disfiguring. CPB also has its complications, although the shorter bypass times with current practice have made it less of a problem. But the adverse cerebral complications that may affect 6% of elderly patients are worrisome.[1] Therefore, the prospect of being able to graft the left internal mammary artery (LIMA) to the left anterior descending (LAD) artery through a small incision is particularly appealing. However, it is not entirely clear how this operation fits into the management of patients who have coronary disease, even if combined with percutaneous transluminal coronary angioplasty (PTCA).

What Patients Are Suitable for Combined MIDCAB and PTCA?

Unlike minimally invasive direct coronary artery bypass (MIDCAB) alone, the combined procedure is clearly designed for patients with multivessel disease. However, immediate problems are apparent. For management purposes, patients with two- or three-vessel disease fall largely into two broad categories: Those who have such severe diffuse disease that angioplasty is technically impossible and who require full (three- to four-vessel) revascularization with CABG, and those patients who have isolated stenosis in two or three vessels that can be tackled by PTCA. In fact, the LAD is the easiest artery to tackle by PTCA and is usually the one cardiologists can handle most effectively. Therefore, the number of patients who have disease in the LAD that is technically inappropriate for PTCA but who have lesions suitable for PTCA in the other two arteries is going to be relatively small. The other group of patients who might be candidates are those who have contraindications to major surgery or CPB, such as renal disease or advanced age. There may be a few patients in this group who would be considered under normal circumstances for full revascularization by CABG but in whom a single LIMA graft may produce good symptomatic relief, and an optional PTCA can be done to the other two arteries, if necessary, to improve the result. Again, this is going to be a relatively small number of patients. This debate has been further complicated by the development of coronary bypass grafting without CPB.[2] It appears that many surgeons are now able to obtain satisfactory results without using CPB.[2, 3] Therefore, this procedure may also be suitable for those patients who have contraindications to bypass. Another development, the use of a smaller median sternotomy incision that still allows full revascularization,[4] may also be preferred over a combined MIDCAB and PTCA.

Is the Quality of the Anastomosis With Minimally Invasive Surgery as Good as With Conventional Surgery?

This is a concern for cardiologists. There is clearly a long learning curve while surgeons develop the skills necessary for operating on a beating heart. Doubts have been raised that an anastomosis done via a minimally invasive procedure is not as good as that done via conventional surgery. A minimal requirement would be for the surgeon to check the anastomosis by LIMA angiogram immediately after the surgery and before the patient leaves the operating theater. In my institution, LIMA grafts are checked on the table. A solution to the problem of the learning curve may be the development of robotic techniques and real-time manipulation of thoracoscopic images producing a "virtual cardiac arrest image."[2]

Two Procedures or One? A major drawback to the combined technique is that patients find it difficult to understand why, having undergone an operation (be it minimally invasive or not), they have to have another procedure to cure their problem. In discussing this with patients, it has become apparent that the choice between having a median sternotomy but full revascularization in one sitting or having an operation with a small incision but undergoing PTCA later is a finely balanced one. The advantages of the minimally invasive procedure are greatly reduced in this context.

PTCA Before or After Surgery? There are many arguments from the cardiologist's point of view that suggest that MIDCAB should follow PTCA. In patients who have multivessel disease, it makes more sense if the cardiologist is allowed to tackle the arteries with PTCA first. If the result to the LAD is suboptimal, the patient can be referred for minimally invasive LIMA grafting. Increasingly, multivessel disease can be tackled quite effectively by angioplasty. But it would be useful to have a surgical technique for those cases in which the LAD result is suboptimal, especially if it is a minimally invasive procedure, which would be more acceptable to a patient who has already undergone a "failed" angioplasty than a full traditional CABG procedure.

In summary, minimally invasive techniques are exciting and are clearly more acceptable to patients than the threatening and frighteningly large median sternotomy scar. However, until complete three-vessel revascularization can be carried out by a minimally invasive procedure, it is likely to be marginalized, and off-pump CABG through a small sternotomy incision is likely to be preferred by the patient and the referring cardiologist. Also, I do not see the combined procedure of MIDCAB and PTCA being applicable to many patients. Its value would be to patients who had failed PTCA to the LAD artery. Furthermore, the "goalposts" are constantly moving. PTCA, especially with stenting, is markedly successful.[5] Multivessel disease and even left main stem stenosis can be effectively tackled. The restenosis rate is now much lower, and new techniques are in the pipeline that will reduce it even further.[5] Thus, the role of surgery is increasingly for those who have severe, diffuse, three-vessel disease, especially those who have poor left ventricular function, in whom PTCA is technically impossible. For these particular patients, it is unlikely that a single LIMA graft will be satisfactory. The combined MIDCAB and PTCA approach might be acceptable for patients who have other severe medical conditions or for frail elderly patients who have persistent and intractable angina.

References

1. Roach GW, Kanchuger M, Mangano CM, et al: Adverse cerebral outcomes after coronary bypass surgery. N Engl J Med 335:1857–1863, 1996.
2. Borst C, Jansen EWL, Grundeman PF: Less invasive coronary artery bypass grafting: Without cardiopulmonary bypass and via reduced surgical access. Heart 77:302–303, 1997.
3. Buffolo E, De Andrade JCS, Branco JNR, et al: Coronary artery bypass grafting without cardiopulmonary bypass. Ann Thorac Surg 61:63–66, 1996.
4. Hartz RS: Minimally invasive heart surgery. Circulation 94:2669–2670, 1996.
5. King SB: The development of interventional cardiology. J Am Coll Cardiol 31:64B–88B, 1998.

Chapter 59

Off-Pump Coronary Artery Surgery

Enio Buffolo

The location of the coronary arteries in the subepicardium allows myocardial revascularization without cardiopulmonary bypass (CPB). The first attempt to revascularize the left anterior descending coronary artery (LAD) with the left internal mammary artery (LIMA) was performed by Kolessov[28] in the former Soviet Union. The operation was performed on a beating heart via a left thoracotomy using mechanical suture (see Chapter 49). With the advent of CPB technology, myocardial revascularization on a beating heart was abandoned in favor of coronary anastomoses performed under the ideal conditions of a quiet field provided by CPB and cardioplegia.

The first consecutive series of direct surgical revascularization of coronary arteries performed in a beating heart were published by Trapp and Bisarya[43] in 1975 and reported by Ankeney[4] in the same year. However, this initial experience was soon abandoned, owing to technical difficulties and also because it was felt that distal perfusion of the coronary circulation was needed during occlusion of the coronary artery.

The first large experience in coronary surgery without CPB was reported by our group[14] in 1982 and almost simultaneously by Benetti[9] in Argentina. Lower morbidity and mortality and reduced costs of the procedure were subsequently reported by different centers, and the procedure was particularly useful in high-risk patients.[5, 10, 12, 15–18, 23, 29, 33, 34] Despite initial uncertainty regarding the quality of the anastomoses and the benefits of the procedure,[32, 44] this alternative technique of direct myocardial revascularization has received increasing acceptance by other groups with results comparable to those initially reported by us.[14] The advent of mini-thoracotomy to perform LIMA anastomoses to the LAD on a beating heart, as originally proposed by Benetti[11] and popularized by Calafiore and colleagues,[20] represents one of the most important developments in coronary artery surgery in recent years.[1, 19, 21, 22, 31, 35, 37, 40–42] This operation is limited to patients with single LAD lesions, and there were concerns about the initial learning curve associated with the procedure.

It was also observed that the quality of the anastomosis was not the same as that with a regular sternotomy approach,[19] leading to the development of stabilizers,[13, 26, 39] flow occluders, and other devices, including video-assisted dissection of the LIMA.[11, 31, 35] With the advent of minimally invasive direct coronary artery surgery, some groups explored the possibility of performing LIMA-to-LAD anastomosis and treating the other coronary arteries by percutaneous angioplasty or stent.[3] This is an attractive approach because it combines the "gold standard" treatment of an important coronary artery (LAD) with percutaneous intervention to provide effective myocardial revascularization via a less invasive approach and at a lower cost (see Chapter 58). Irrespective of immediate and long-term results, revascularization of the myocardium has entered a new era. Comparative studies of surgical revascularization and angioplasty will have to be re-evaluated owing to recent technological progress.

Adverse Effects of Cardiopulmonary Bypass

Despite recent technological developments, CPB is still considered a controlled shock. The circulation of blood outside its natural endothelium is responsible for the inflammatory reaction, which leads to liberation of complement and cytokines-tumor necrosis factor alpha (TNF-α)[8] or lead to vasoplegic syndrome with occasional serious sequelae.[25] The inflammatory response leads to capillary permeability, sequestration of neutrophils, and microembolism.[7, 36] Transesophageal echocardiographic and transcutaneous Doppler studies show that cerebral embolization occurs in 10% of patients at the time of cannulation, aortic clamping, and declamping.[6] We have also shown a decreased incidence of postoperative complications in elderly patients in whom CPB was not used, especially complications related to the central nervous system.[18] A recent survey of 162 surgeons showed that when given a choice between avoiding sternotomy or avoiding CPB, 81% favored avoiding CPB.[40] This is a strong indication that the concept of minimally invasive coronary surgery is related to avoidance of CPB and not to the length of the skin incision.

Myocardial revascularization without CPB further reduces the need for blood transfusions and their inherent risks. Paradoxical septal motion is less frequently observed after non-CPB sugery, in contrast to surgery in which CPB is used.[2]

Indications

At our center, coronary revascularization without CPB is restricted to approximately 22% of patients who undergo coronary artery revascularization. Figure 59–1 shows the incidence of non-CPB sugery during 16 years' experience. Note that despite extensive use of angioplasty of one or more coronary vessels, a large number of patients experience failure of the procedure, restenosis, and malplacements of stents and enter the surgical series. Basically, what determines the feasibility of coronary surgery without CPB is analysis of the preoperative angiogram. Candidates are patients with lesions affecting the LAD, diagonal artery, or right coronary artery (RCA).

With few exceptions, we accept incomplete revascularizations, leaving a stenotic circumflex branch untreated.

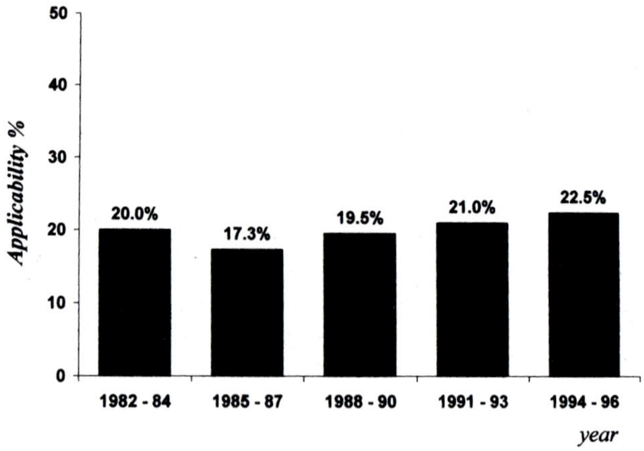

Figure 59–1. Applicability of off-pump myocardial revascularization at 3-year intervals during our 16-year experience.

Other surgeons, however, are able to bypass the circumflex coronary artery using special exposure techniques.[30]

Figure 59–2 shows the number of grafts performed without CPB. In the majority of cases (53.4%), two grafts were performed. The number of grafts ranged from 1 to 5 (mean, 1.7) grafts per patient. Any type of conduit can be used.

We routinely perform LIMA–LAD and vein grafts to other coronary arteries. Table 59–1 shows the conditions that are particularly useful for grafting without CPB. In general, the sicker the patient, the more beneficial it is if CPB is not used, such as in the elderly and those with serious comorbidities. Poor left ventricular function is also a good indication for the procedure. Our recent data using multivariate analysis show that ejection fraction below 0.40 is not a risk factor when myocardial revascularization is performed without CPB. During reoperation, the procedure is useful to bypass the LAD and RCA, because there is little movement owing to previous adhesions (see Chapter 68). Calcification of the ascending aorta is an absolute indication for this procedure, using the LIMA as a composite arterial graft. Because bleeding is usually not a problem and is minimal, Jehovah's Witnesses, who do not permit blood transfusion, can benefit from this procedure.

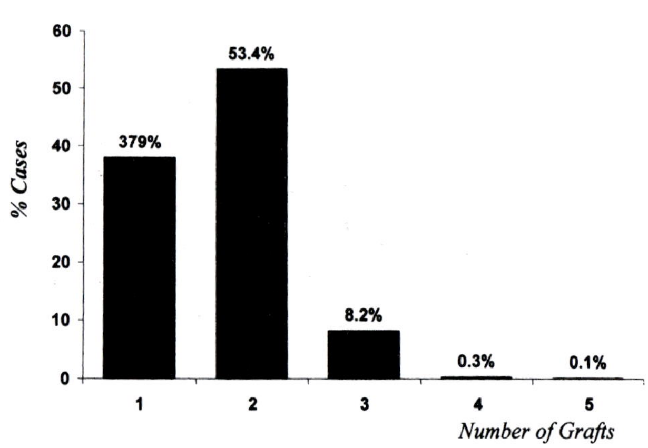

Figure 59–2. Number of grafts per patient, ranging from one to five. Observe that more than 50% of the patients received two grafts, with a mean of 1.7 grafts per patient. Any type of conduit can be used.

Table 59–1. Clinical Situations in Which Grafting Without Cardiopulmonary Bypass Is Useful

Elderly patients
Renal insufficiency
Emphysema
Cerebrovascular accident
Poor ventricular function
Reoperations
Calcified ascending aorta
Jehovah's Witnesses

Operative Technique

Different approaches can be used, such as sternotomy (complete or partial) or mini-thoracotomy. We prefer a limited skin incision for complete median sternotomy as used in recent years by our group (Fig. 59–3).

For the LAD and diagonal artery, we use the technique described by Calafiore and colleagues.[20] Our experience with this approach started in 1995, and only 60 patients have been operated on owing to selection criteria.

In this chapter we describe the procedure via median sternotomy. Before surgery, the angiogram is reviewed and the number of grafts is planned. Although a perfusionist is always present in the operating room, the CPB circuit is not set up. After a 12-cm incision, a median sternotomy is performed. The LIMA is then dissected, avoiding opening the left pleura. Simultaneously, another conduit (saphenous vein, epigastric or radial artery) is harvested. Heparin (2 mg/kg) is administered before occlusion of the coronary artery. The artery to be bypassed is then controlled with a piece of silicone tube applied in a segment where there is no plaque (Fig. 59–4). When the coronary artery is already totally occluded, no drugs are used. Otherwise, 5 mg of verapamil is given intravenously to decrease the arterial pressure, heart rate, and oxygen consumption. We do not precondition the heart, as we believe that this is unnecessary for up to 17 minutes of coronary blood flow interruption. For an RCA without critical

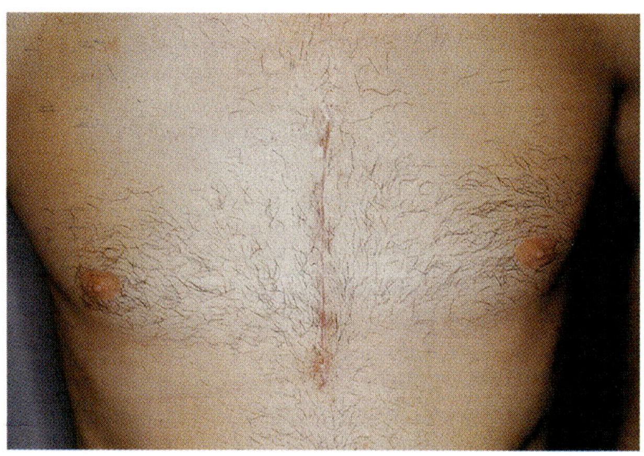

Figure 59–3. This photo shows a 12-cm incision that permits complete opening of the sternum and complete revascularization, treating not only the left anterior descending artery but also the diagonal and right coronary arteries.

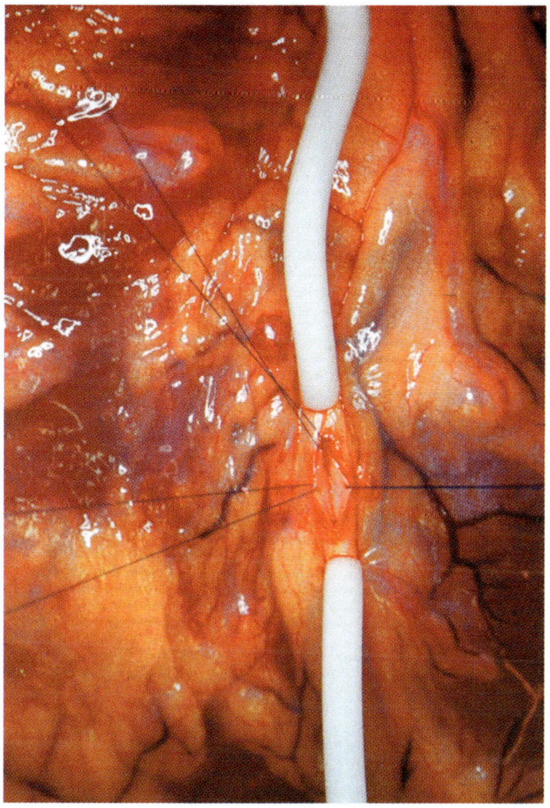

Figure 59–4. A surgeon's view of the left anterior descending coronary artery, the length of the coronary incision, and the delicate silicone devices used to interrupt coronary blood flow.

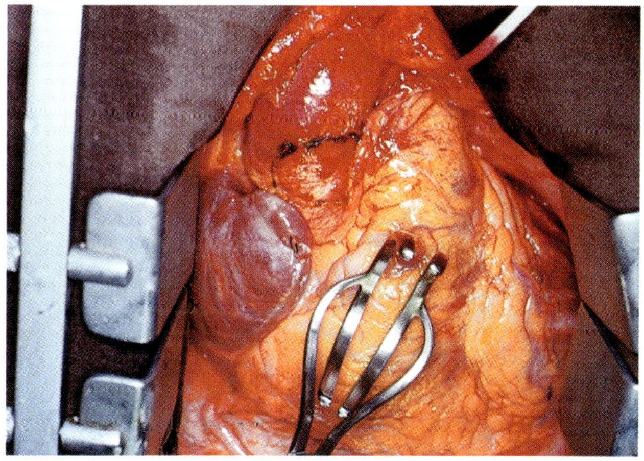

Figure 59–5. A special clamp is used for tangential clamping of the ascending aorta during proximal anastomoses.

stenosis, we use a distal shunt from the ascending aorta if bradycardia or hypotension occurs. For the LAD anastomosis, we elevate the heart with a sponge placed dorsolaterally in the pericardium and use suture retraction of the pericardium anterior to the phrenic nerve. The septal region is then exposed. Fenestrated sponge facilitates the procedure, with exposure of the artery via a small orifice. This prevents the surgeon from having to deal with a moving target. For the RCA, we use the Trendelenburg position and traction sutures at the marginal border of the right ventricle. All anastomoses are performed with 7–0 running prolene suture. Should arrhythmias or hypotension occur, the distal coronary artery is perfused with a shunt as previously described. The proximal anastomoses are performed in the ascending aorta via a partial clamp (Fig. 59–5) and 6–0 running prolene suture. At completion of the anastomoses, protamine is administrated (1 : 1) and the mediastinum is closed, leaving behind a chest drain.

The patient is transferred to the intensive care unit for one day and is usually discharged home on the fifth postoperative day.

Results

Mortality and morbidity are reduced when CPB is not used, especially in high-risk patients.[5, 16–18, 24, 33] In our hospital, of 1886 patients operated on without CPB from September 1981 to October 1997, there were 47 hospital deaths (mortality rate of 2.4%). This is an acceptable risk, considering the characteristics of our patients, the teaching environment, and the fact that for some patients the procedure was considered only when CPB was contraindicated.

During the same period, 9382 consecutive patients were operated on using extracorporeal circulation. The mortality was 5.2% ($P \leq .05$) with the same surgeons. An unpublished study from our center shows that CPB is an isolated risk factor in myocardial revascularization. Postoperative morbidity is less compared with conventional coronary artery surgery. Table 59–2 shows some postoperative complications in a prospective series of 709 patients operated on during 1995. Note the lower complication rate in patients revascularized without CPB. We believe that reproducible results can be achieved, with excellent patency rates with this procedure. This is applicable to surgeons who have experience with conventional coronary surgery.

We compared prospectively 60 patients undergoing LIMA–LAD anastomosis with CPB (30 patients) and without CPB (30 patients) and found an identical patency rate of 93.4% in both groups studied just before hospital discharge[38] (Figs. 59–6 and 59–7).

Table 59–2. Incidence of Major Postoperative Complications With and Without Cardiopulmonary Bypass (CPB)

Complication	With CPB (509 cases)		Without CPB (200 cases)	
Perioperative myocardial infarction	18	(3.5%)	2	(1.0%)
Arrhythmias	25	(5.6%)	5	(2.5%)
Cerebrovascular accident	3	(0.6%)	0	(0.0%)
Acute renal failure	8	(1.5%)	0	(0.0%)
Gastrointestinal bleeding	7	(1.4%)	2	(1.0%)
Excessive bleeding	16	(3.0%)	3	(1.5%)
Prolonged intubation	40	(7.8%)	9	(4.5%)
Vasoplegic syndrome	10	(2.1%)	2	(1.0%)
	127	(24.9%)	23	(11.5%)

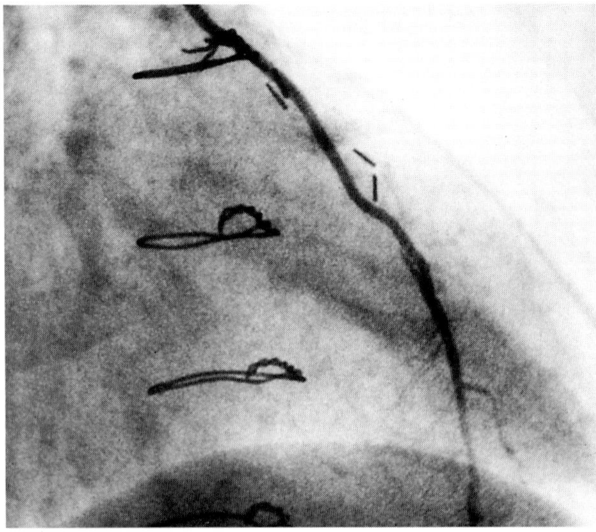

Figure 59–6. One-year postoperative study showing left internal mammary artery–left anterior descending artery (LIMA–LAD) anastomosis.

Costs

Costs are reduced when CPB is not used, considering the equipment that is not utilized. Time in the intensive care unit is decreased, and costs of total hospitalization are reduced. Fewer postoperative complications also reduce costs, allowing treatment of more patients with the same resources and decreasing the waiting list for coronary artery surgery.

In summary, there is growing interest in coronary revascularization without CPB, and it may become the procedure of choice in patients with coronary artery disease. Technological advancements will facilitate the procedure. The teaching of new residents and young surgeons will eliminate the learning curve, allowing for predictable results. In the future, it is possible that CPB will be used only in selected patients undergoing revascularization.

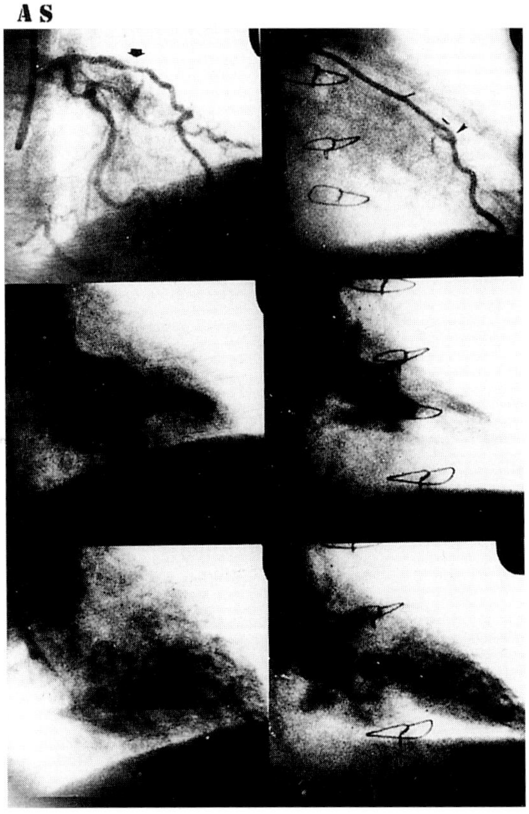

Figure 59–7. Left internal mammary artery–left anterior descending artery (LIMA–LAD) anastomosis and normal postoperative left ventricular function.

References

1. Acuff TE, Landreneau RJ, Griffith BP, et al: Minimally invasive coronary artery bypass grafting. Ann Thorac Surg 61:135–137, 1996.
2. Akins CW, Boucher CA, Pohost GM: Preservation of interventricular septal function in patients having coronary artery bypass grafts without cardiopulmonary bypass. Am Heart J 107:304–309, 1984.
3. Angelini GD, Wilde P, Salerno TA: Integrated left small thoracotomy and angioplasty for multivessel coronary artery revascularization. Lancet 347:757–758, 1996.
4. Ankeney JL: To use or not to use pump oxygenator in coronary bypass operations. Ann Thorac Surg 19:108–109, 1975.
5. Arsiwala S, Bedi HS, Sharma VK, et al: Coronary artery bypass grafting without cardiopulmonary bypass. Indian Heart J 42: 453–454, 1990.
6. Barbut D, Yao FS, Hager BA, et al: Comparison of transcranial Doppler ultrasonography and transesophageal echocardiography to monitor emboli during coronary artery bypass surgery. Stroke 27:87–90, 1996.
7. Blauth CL, Arnold JV, Schulemberg WE, et al: Cerebral microembolism during cardiopulmonary bypass. J Thorac Cardiovasc Surg 95:668–676, 1988.
8. Brasil LA, Gomes WJ, Buffolo E, et al: Ativação da citocina (TNF-α) e resposta clínica induzida pela circulação extracorpórea. Rev Bras Cir Cardiovasc 11:188–200, 1996.
9. Benetti FJ: Direct coronary surgery with saphenous vein bypass without either cardiopulmonary bypass or cardiac arrest. J Cardiovasc Surg 26:217–222, 1985.
10. Benetti FJ, Naselli G, Wood M, et al: Direct myocardial revascularization without extracorporeal circulation. Chest 100:312–316, 1991.
11. Benetti FJ: Video assisted coronary bypass surgery. J Card Surg 10:620–625, 1995.
12. Bergsland J, Hasnan S, Lewin NA: Coronary artery bypass grafting without cardiopulmonary bypass: An attractive alternative in high risk patients. Eur J Cardiothorac Surg 11:876–880, 1997.
13. Borst C, Jansen WEL, Tulleken CAF, et al: Coronary artery bypass grafting without cardiopulmonary bypass and without interruption of native coronary flow using a novel anastomoses site restraining device "octopus." J Am Cell Cardiol 27:1356–1364, 1996.
14. Buffolo E, Andrade JCS, Succi JE, et al: Revascularização direta do miocrdio sem circulação extracorpórea. Descrição da técnica e resultados iniciais. Arq Bras Cardiol 38:365–373, 1982.
15. Buffolo E, Andrade JCS, Succi JE, et al: Direct myocardial revascularization without extracorporeal circulation: Technique and initial results. Tex Heart Inst J 12:33–41, 1985.
16. Buffolo E, Andrade JCS, Branco JNR: Myocardial revascularization without extracorporeal circulation. Eur J Cardiothorac Surg 18:504–508, 1990.
17. Buffolo E, Andrade JCS, Branco JNR: Coronary artery bypass

grafting without cardiopulmonary bypass. Ann Thorac Surg 61: 63–66, 1996.
18. Buffolo E, Summo H, Aguiar LF: Myocardial revascularization in patients 70 years of age and older without the use of extracorporeal circulation. Am J Geriatr Cardiol 6:6–8, 1997.
19. Buffolo E, Teles C, Aguiar LF, et al: Left anterior small thoracotomy and left anterior descending anastomoses: Immediate postoperative angiographic analysis (Abstract). J Am Cell Cardiol 29:716, 1997.
20. Calafiore AM, Gianmarco GD, Teodori G: Left anterior descending coronary artery grafting via left anterior small thoracotomy without cardiopulmonary bypass. Ann Thorac Surg 61:1658–1665, 1996.
21. Calafiore AM, Teodori G, Gianmarco G, et al: Left internal mammary elongation with inferior epigastric artery in minimally invasive coronary surgery. Eur J Cardiothorac Surg 12:393–396, 1997.
22. Emery RW, Arom KV, Nicoloff DM: Ministernotomy for coronary artery bypass grafting. Ann Thorac Surg 61:1271–1272, 1996.
23. Fanning WJ, Kakos GS, Williams TE Jr: Reoperative coronary artery bypass grafting without cardiopulmonary bypass. Ann Thorac Surg 55:486–489, 1993.
24. Folliguet TA, Laborde F, Temkine J: Coronary artery revascularization without extracorporeal circulation: Indications and results. Eur J Cardiothorac Surg 11:870–875, 1997.
25. Gomes WJ, Carvalho ACC, Buffolo E, et al: Vasoplegic syndrome: A new dilemma. J Thorac Cardiovasc Surg 107:942–943, 1994.
26. Izzat MB, Yim APC: Cardiac stabilizer for minimally invasive direct coronary artery bypass. Ann Thorac Surg 64:570–571, 1997.
27. Kirklin JK, Westaby S, Blackstone EH, et al: Complement and the damaging effects of cardiopulmonary bypass. J Thorac Cardiovasc Surg 86:845–857, 1983.
28. Kolessov VL: Mammary artery coronary anastomosis as method of treatment for angina pectoris. J Thorac Cardiovasc Surg 54:535–544, 1967.
29. Laborde F, Abdelmequid I, Piwnica A: Aorto-coronary bypass without extracorporeal circulation. Eur J Cardiothorac Surg 3:152–154, 1989.
30. Lobo GJ, Oliveira FM, Ciarline C, et al. Cirurgia de revascularização do miocárdio através de minitoracotomia esquerda. Rev Bras Cir Cardiovasc 11:143–147, 1996.
31. Mack M, Acuff T, Yong P, et al: Minimally invasive thoracoscopically assisted coronary artery bypass surgery. Eur J Cardiothorac Surg 12:20–24, 1997.
32. Messmer BJ: Coronary surgery without extracorporeal circulation: Benefit or additional risk for the patient? Eur J Cardiothorac Surg 4:5, 1990.
33. Moshkovitz Y, Mohr R: Coronary artery bypass without cardiopulmonary bypass: The pros and cons. Isr J Med Sci 29: 716–720, 1993.
34. Moshkovitz Y, Lusky A, Mohr R: Coronary artery bypass without cardiopulmonary bypass: Analysis of short term and mid term outcome in 222 patients. J Thorac Cardiovasc Surg 110:979–987, 1995.
35. Nataf P, Lima L, Benarim S, et al: Video assisted coronary artery bypass surgery: Clinical results. Eur J Cardiothorac Surg 11: 865–869, 1997.
36. Parker FB, Masvasti MA, Bove EL: Acute neuropsychological consequences of coronary artery bypass surgery: The role of atherosclerose emboli. Thorac Cardiovasc Surg 33:207–209, 1985.
37. Robinson MC, Gross DR, Zeman W, et al: Minimally invasive coronary artery bypass grafting: A new method using anterior mediastinotomy. J Card Surg 10:529–536, 1995.
38. Rota CA: Perviabilidade da anastomose da mamária com a descendente anterior em pacientes operados com e sem circulação extracorpórea. São Paulo, Brazil, Tese Mestrado Escola Paulista de Medicina, 1993.
39. Shennib H, Lee AGL, Akin J: Safe and effective method of stabilization for coronary artery bypass grafting on the beating heart. Ann Thorac Surg 63:988–992, 1997.
40. Shennib H, Mack M, Lee AGL: A survey on minimally invasive coronary artery bypass grafting. Ann Thorac Surg 64:110–115, 1997.
41. Stanbridge RL, Symmons GV, Banwell PE: Minimal access surgery for coronary artery revascularization. Lancet 346:837, 1995.
42. Subramanian VA, Sani G, Benetti FJ, et al: Minimally invasive coronary artery bypass surgery: A multicenter report of preliminary clinical experience. Circulation 92:645, 1995.
43. Trapp WG, Bisarya R: Placement of coronary artery bypass graft without pump oxygenator. Ann Thorac Surg 19:1–9, 1975.
44. Ullyot DJ. Look Ma, no hands. Ann Thorac Surg 61:10–11, 1996.
45. Westaby S: Coronary surgery without cardiopulmonary bypass. Br Heart J 73:203–205, 1995.

COMMENTARY

Sami Kabbani

Dr. Buffolo makes a good argument for coronary artery bypass grafting (CABG) without cardiopulmonary bypass (CPB), at least in certain subsets of patients. He is to be credited, along with Dr. Benetti from Argentina, for popularizing a procedure that is clearly here to stay. Some of the points he brings up, however, are open to question.

Not all surgeons would agree that CPB, in its present form, is as injurious to the patient as suggested in this chapter. Disposable materials, minimally reactive surfaces, membrane oxygenators, improvements in myocardial protection and blood conservation, and the new application of centrifugal pumps have all combined to make CPB extremely well tolerated by most patients, including those with adverse clinical situations. Nor are these salutary developments expected to stop at the present stage. Surface modification of components with heparin (or other compounds) and efficient pulsatile pumps are only two other refinements anticipated to improve on the already auspicious state of CPB. As for neuropsychological sequelae (perhaps the most dreaded complications of CPB), a recent study failed to show any difference in their incidence between "on-" and "off-bypass" patients undergoing CABG.[1]

That CABG without CPB reduces operative cost cannot be denied, but that it offers lower mortality and morbidity than the conventional procedure is unlikely. Reported short- and medium-term postoperative graft patency rates have often been poorer in "off-" than in "on-bypass" cases.[2, 3] It only stands to reason that coronary anastomosis can be better achieved in a quiet, dry field than on a moving, bloody target. Stabilization devices and intraluminal shunts have helped reduce this difficulty but have not eliminated it, and it is more acute the earlier the surgeon is on that infamous learning curve.

In a symposium on minimally invasive coronary bypass in New York in January 1997 featuring nine live operative demonstrations by leaders in the field, two of the immediate follow-up angiograms demonstrated anastomotic occlusions. Poorer patency rates may also be the consequence of certain methods of temporary occlusion of the target vessel.[4] Naturally, clinical outcome, morbidity, and mortality have to conform to statistics of graft patency. Indeed, the present results of single CABG using standard CPB are impeccable and are hard to improve upon.[5, 6] Any benefits afforded by excluding CPB have to be carefully balanced against the decrease in quality of the all-important coronary anastomosis.

Finally, I disagree with the principle of accepting incomplete revascularization just to avoid CPB. Untreated significant occlusions are known to be the main reason for early postoperative morbidity and reoperation.

So where does this leave off-bypass coronary surgery? Obviously, the economic factor, which I am told was the major reason behind resorting to this method in Brazil and Argentina in the first place, is an important issue in developing countries. It is becoming an important issue in this era of cost containment in developed nations as well. Acceptable results of CABG can be obtained for much less cost. However, one caveat here is that less-than-ideal bypasses can eventually cause more complications and require more interventions,[7] so that the cost-effectiveness edge may be abolished in the long run. This advantage will also be offset by surgeons who see hybrid procedures (off-bypass CABG plus percutaneous transluminal coronary angioplasty) as the way of the future. Cost reduction, in any case, should never be attained at the expense of a carefully executed, complete, and durable operation.

Beyond expense curtailment, CABG without CPB could benefit certain subsets of patients—not so much those who can be harmed by (or refuse) blood transfusion, because standard CABG can be achieved without homologous blood transfusion[8]; not so much those with calcified aortas, because aortic atheromas can be detected by intraoperative transesophageal echocardiography and, if possible, avoided[9]; but to the rest of the categories of patients with comorbidities mentioned in Dr. Buffolo's chapter, especially the elderly and those with poor ventricles or failing kidneys. But even in those special situations, a clear decision about the preference for CABG without CPB cannot be reached without a prospective randomized study, properly executed and supported by postoperative angiography.

It will be interesting, over the next few years, to watch the developments of two tendencies in cardiac surgery, each vying to outdo the other: minimizing the objections to CPB on the one hand (e.g., by inhibiting endothelial and blood activation during CABG,[10] or by reperfused blood leukocyte and platelet depletion)[11] and maximizing the quality of off-pump coronary anastomosis on the other (e.g., by conducting it under controlled intermittent asystole[12] and subjecting it to quality control with intraoperative angiography). Whatever the outcome, it behooves us to recall the point made by Dr. Cooley at the 1997 AATS meeting: "Our goal should be to fit the operation to the patient, not the patient to the operation."

References

1. Browne S, Westaby S, Taggart DP: Neuropsychological and respiratory injury following CABG surgery with and without cardiopulmonary bypass. 11th annual meeting of the EACTS, Copenhagen, Denmark, Sept 28–Oct 1, 1997.
2. Calafiore AM: Mid-term results after minimally invasive coronary surgery (LAST operation). 77th annual AATS meeting, Washington, DC, May 4, 1997.
3. Mack M, Magovern JA, Scruggs G, et al: Results of immediate angiography for graft patency in minimally invasive coronary artery bypass surgery. 34th STS meeting, New Orleans, LA, Jan 26–28, 1998.
4. Pagni S, Qaqish NK, Senior DG, et al: Anastomotic complications in minimally invasive coronary bypass grafting. Ann Thorac Surg 63(suppl 6): S64, 1997.
5. Boylan MJ, Lytte BW, Loop FD, et al: Surgical treatment of isolated left anterior descending coronary stenosis. J Thorac Cardiovasc Surg 107:657, 1994.
6. Ovrum E, Tangen G, Am Holen E: Facing the era of minimally invasive coronary grafting: Current results of conventional bypass grafting for single-vessel disease. Ann Thorac Surg 64: 159, 1997.
7. Gundry SR, Ramano M, Shatuk OH, et al: Seven-year follow-up of coronary artery bypasses performed with and without cardiopulmonary bypass. 77th annual AATS meeting, Washington, DC, May 4, 1997.
8. Helm RE, Rosengart TK, Gomez M, et al: Comprehensive multimodality blood conservation: 100 consecutive CABG operations without transfusion. Ann Thorac Surg 65:125, 1998.
9. Trehan N, Mishra M, Dhole S, et al: Significantly reduced incidence of stroke during coronary artery bypass grafting using transesophageal echocardiography. Eur J Cardiothorac Surg 11:234, 1997.
10. Baufreton C, Jansen PGM, LeBesnerais P, et al: Heparin coating with aprotinin reduces blood activation during coronary artery operations. Ann Thorac Surg 63:50, 1997.
11. Boyle EM, Pohlman TH, Johnson MC, et al: Endothelial cell injury in cardiovascular surgery: The systemic inflammatory response. Ann Thorac Surg 63:277, 1997.
12. Robinson MC, Thielmeier KA, Hill BB: Transient ventricular asystole using adenosine during minimally invasive and open sternotomy coronary artery bypass grafting. Ann Thorac Surg 63(suppl 6):S30, 1997.

Chapter 60

Myocardial Function and Metabolism During Beating Heart Coronary Revascularization

Malcolm J. Underwood, Vincenzo Luchetti, Fabio Capasso,
Mohammed Saadeh Suleiman, and Gianni D. Angelini

Myocardial revascularization without cardiopulmonary bypass on the beating heart is becoming increasingly popular.[3] To perform the anastomosis in a bloodless field, temporary occlusion of the coronary artery is required. This has raised concerns regarding the potential risk of ischemic damage to the warm, metabolically active myocardium normally supplied with blood by the target coronary vessel. It also has been suggested that preconditioning the heart with a short period of ischemia and reperfusion may be beneficial,[14] and surgeons performing off-pump revascularization are in a prime position to instigate this technique.

In our institutions, there has been increasing interest in performing myocardial revascularization on the beating heart. The aforementioned concerns convinced us to investigate the effect of temporary coronary occlusion on myocardial metabolism and function and also ascertain whether there was any benefit to preconditioning the at-risk myocardium before performing the coronary anastomosis. Furthermore, the use of an intracoronary shunt to maintain blood flow during construction of the anastomosis was investigated.

Assessment of Myocardial Damage

A range of different methods of assessing myocardial injury are available, and each has advantages and disadvantages.[2] Biochemical markers of myocardial damage can be used as surrogate markers of clinical outcome, and their use minimizes the number of patients required to perform a valid statistical analysis of differences. Serum markers offer a simple, easily accessible clinical and research tool and allow accurate diagnosis of perioperative myocardial infarction and identification of more subtle forms of myocardial injury. In our studies, we used the assessment of troponin I release, as described later. However, the measurement of systemic levels of markers is limited by the fact that they can only represent the cumulative effects of perioperative events on myocardial injury and do not allow the timing of the injury to specific operative interventions. More acute changes in myocardial function can be derived by evaluating the degree of myocardial ischemia that occurs at specific time points intraoperatively. This can be achieved by sampling serum directly from myocardial effluent blood via a coronary sinus catheter. In our investigations, this technique was also used with respect to troponin I generation.

Sampling of myocardial tissue directly can be used to investigate changes in cellular metabolic function and structural changes associated with ischemia and reperfusion. In our work, left ventricular biopsies were taken to assess changes in intracellular substrates (adenosine triphosphate [ATP], adenosine diphosphate [ADP], lactate, and amino acids), alteration of which has been implicated in myocardial ischemia.[12]

During conduction of these studies, particularly the investigation of the use of intracoronary shunts, we also used continuous perioperative transesophageal echocardiography (TEE) to provide indications of overall left ventricular function.

Troponin I

The troponins (T, C, and I) are a group of intimately related regulatory proteins located in striated muscle.[6] In acute myocardial injury, there is a biphasic release of troponins T and I into the serum. Troponin in the cell, presumed to originate from the cytoplasm, is released 3 to 5 hours after loss of membrane function. A late phase of continued release of troponin for 5 days or more follows and is thought to be associated with destruction of the contractile apparatus and cell death.[7]

Troponin I is solely confined to the myocardium and has been shown to be a highly specific marker for the detection of myocardial injury.[8] In our studies, troponin I was measured in systemic venous samples for a period of 48 hours postoperatively and also immediately perioperatively in blood samples obtained directly from a cannula positioned in the coronary sinus.

Intracellular Myocardial Metabolites

After long periods, impaired coronary flow leads to myocardial damage and necrosis. However, after short periods of ischemia, damage can occur after reperfusion of the ischemic area. Ischemia alone, or ischemia and reperfusion, is associated with profound metabolic derangement and disruption of the cellular ionic homeostasis, the end result of which is an alteration in contractile activity.[13]

During ischemia, the heart is deprived of oxygen and of important substrates, such as lactate and glucose. This results in reduced energy production (anaerobic metabolism). In addition, ischemia depletes the citric acid cycle of several of its intermediates and influences secondary metabolism. As a result of this, the concentration of several metabolites is altered (e.g., ATP, ADP, lactate, glutamate), and these changes are used as markers of ischemia and reperfusion injury.[11] ATP is the main provider of energy for myocardial cellular function. Preservation of the concentration of ATP in left ventricular biopsy specimens has been used to indicate the effectiveness of myocardial protection.[10] Under physiologic conditions, lactate is one of the major fuels for energy production. However, during ischemia, and as a result of anaerobic metabolism, myocardial lactate extraction is replaced by production, whose levels can also be used as a surrogate marker for myocardial ischemia.[13]

Amino acids, such as aspartate and glutamate, are important for secondary metabolism. During anaerobic metabolism, the myocardium utilizes these amino acids, and this is associated with alanine production. Therefore, the extent of changes in such amino acid concentrations in the myocardium provides evidence as to the extent of the ischemic stress placed on the myocardium. In our studies, analysis was made of concentrations of 10 adenine nucleotides and related compounds, lactate, glycogen, 15 amino acids, ATP, and ADP in ventricular biopsy samples taken intraoperatively at appropriate time intervals.

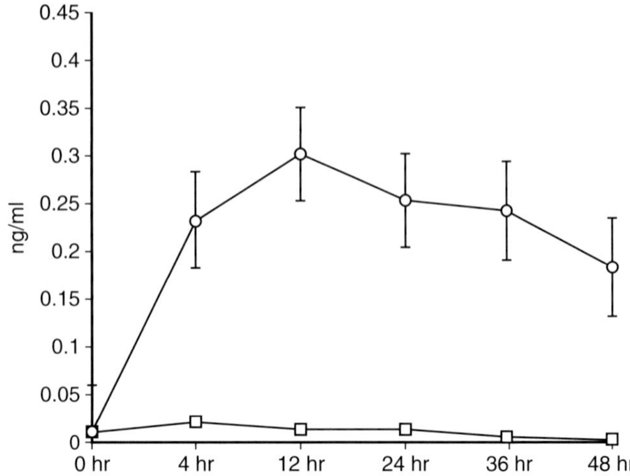

Figure 60–1. Release of troponin I over time. □ = Minithoracotomy group, ○ = Bypass group.

Transesophageal Echocardiography

Transesophageal echocardiography (TEE) is a sensitive indicator of segmental wall motion abnormalities that may occur during myocardial ischemia, and it is more sensitive than ECG.[9] One of the simpler semiquantitative schemes for analyzing wall motion is the generation of a wall motion index score.[4] This technique involves dividing the left ventricle into a predefined number of segments, each of which is then graded on a score for wall motion ranging from 1 (normal) to 4 (dyskinesis). The total wall motion score or index can then be calculated with higher numbers representative of increasing degrees of ventricular dysfunction. Furthermore, the ejection fraction can also be calculated using standard methods,[5] with the probe in the midesophageal position orientated at zero degrees so as to obtain a view to include the ventricular apex.

Myocardial Injury During Vessel Occlusion

Postoperative Release of Serum Troponin I

Serum levels of troponin I were analyzed in a series of patients undergoing revascularization of the left anterior descending coronary artery via a mini-thoracotomy. These levels were compared with those of a control group of patients undergoing conventional revascularization with normothermic cardiopulmonary bypass and intermittent antegrade warm blood cardioplegia.[1] All patients had well-preserved left ventricular function and were comparable with respect to other preoperative characteristics. No patient had clinical or electrocardiographic evidence of perioperative myocardial infarction.

Preoperative troponin I concentrations were undetectable in both groups. In the control (on-bypass) group, a significant rise in troponin I levels was observed 4 hours postoperatively, peaking at 12 hours. This remained elevated 48 hours following the operation (Fig. 60–1).[1] In contrast, in the off-pump group, troponin I levels were significantly lower, peaking at 4 hours and declining rapidly thereafter (see Fig. 60–1).[1]

This study suggests that ischemic or reperfusion injury to the myocardium as indicated by serum troponin I levels may not be important after temporary occlusion of the left anterior descending coronary artery during off-pump revascularization. Furthermore, troponin I release in this minimally invasive group was significantly less than that produced by the global insult resulting from conventional revascularization.

Coronary Sinus Troponin I Levels

Although troponin I is a sensitive marker of ischemia in the serum, the release is slow, requiring several hours for peak levels to be seen. It is not known whether troponin I can be released in situ and whether short periods of ischemia followed by reperfusion (preconditioning) affect local release. With this in mind, we studied a further series of patients undergoing revascularization via a median sternotomy, without the use of cardiopulmonary bypass, and measured troponin I levels in samples obtained directly from the coronary sinus. Ischemia was induced by occlusion of the left anterior descending coronary artery, and hearts were subjected to two cycles of 3 minutes of ischemia followed by 3 minutes of reperfusion. Blood samples were collected before ischemia (control), 3 minutes after ischemia, 10 seconds after reperfusion, 3 minutes after reperfusion for each cycle of preconditioning, at the end of the anastomosis, and 10 seconds, 3 and 10 minutes after reperfusion.

Preischemic levels of troponin I in the coronary sinus were 0.077 ± 0.026 ng/ml (range 0.0 to 0.15). A transient release was seen in five of the six patients studied (range 1.5 to 5.0 ng/ml). The timing of this release was different for all patients. In four patients, the release was seen during the first cycle of ischemia and reperfusion (at the end of ischemia in two, after 10 seconds of reperfusion in the third, and after 3 minutes of reperfusion in the fourth). The release in the fifth patient was seen in the second cycle (end of ischemia). Only one patient showed more than transient release. However, following ischemia (anastomosis) and reperfusion, there was no significant release of troponin I. This was similar to the control group (without preconditioning) (Figs. 60–2 and 60–3).

This work demonstrates that short periods of ischemia

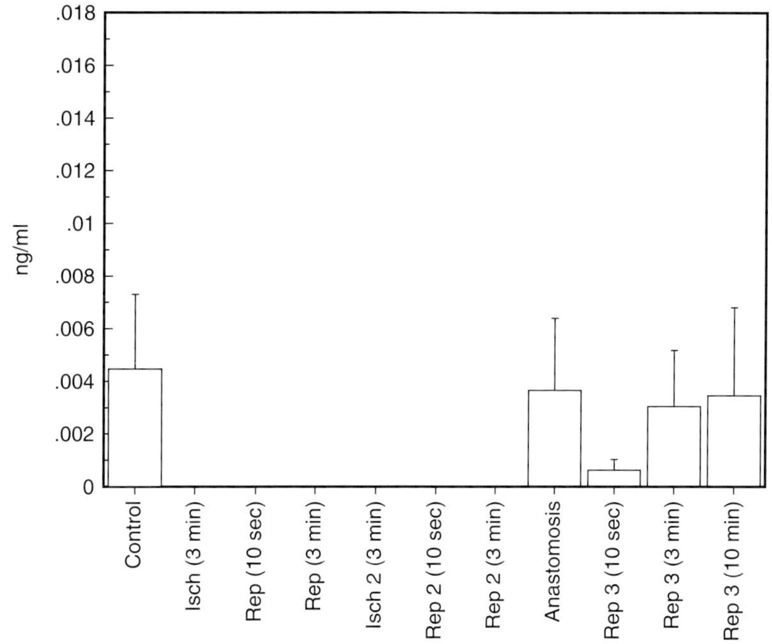

Figure 60–2. Release of troponin I during revascularization without bypass: not preconditioned.

and reperfusion in patients undergoing revascularization on the beating heart can induce a transient in situ release of troponin I. However, return to baseline levels was seen in all patients following completion of the anastomosis, and the relevance of in situ troponin I release to concomitant myocardial tissue damage is not yet known. The release of troponin I in situ during the preconditioning phase may be related to an overall prolongation of the ischemic time and suboptimal reperfusion in between via the stenosed native coronary artery.

In view of these findings, we performed a further study to assess the effects of periods of myocardial ischemia and reperfusion using direct biochemical markers of myocardial damage.

Intracellular Metabolites

Patients undergoing coronary artery bypass surgery without the use of cardiopulmonary bypass were randomized into two groups. After median sternotomy and mobilization of the internal mammary artery, the left anterior descending coronary artery was identified and snared proximally and distally. In group 1, the anastomosis between the mammary and coronary arteries was performed immediately, whereas in group 2, this was preceded by 3 minutes of preconditioning followed by 3 minutes of reperfusion. Myocardial tissue samples were taken from the anterior wall of the left ventricle using a Trucut needle. Samples were taken immediately after the pericardium was opened and after 3 minutes of reperfusion upon completion of the

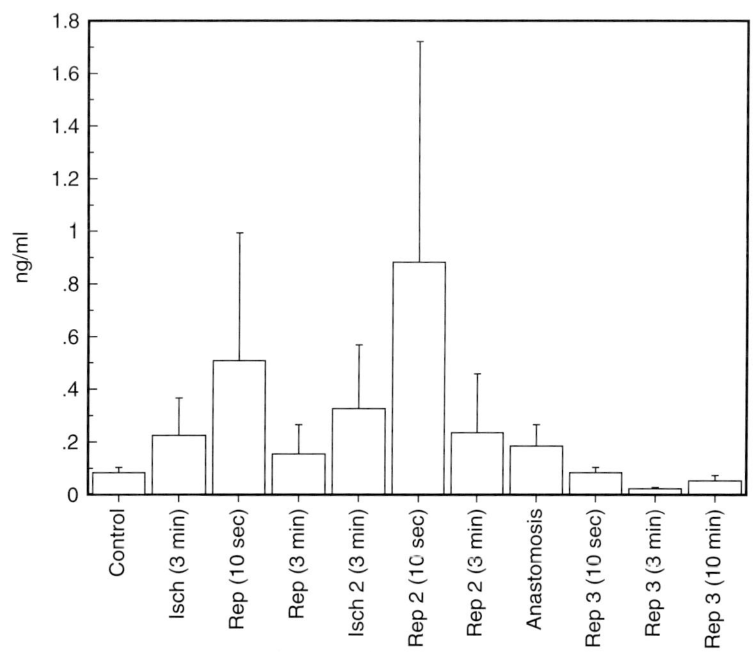

Figure 60–3. Release of troponin I during revascularization without bypass: preconditioned.

anastomosis. These samples were immediately frozen and analyzed for intracellular substrates (ATP, ADP, lactate, and amino acids). There was no difference in the ischemic times taken for the anastomosis in each group (group 1, 12 ± 1.2 minutes; group 2, 11 ± 1.3 minutes).

No difference was observed in levels of any of the measured markers over time, and preconditioning did not confer any benefit (Table 60–1). Indeed, all values remained within "normal" limits as defined by the levels in the control biopsies.

These data indicate that myocardial damage, assessed by intramyocardial biochemical markers, does not occur during temporary occlusion of the left anterior descending coronary artery for periods up to 14 minutes. This suggests that there must be adapting mechanisms by which the myocardium can continue to function. One explanation is the presence of a collateral circulation capable of providing some degree of perfusion during the period of coronary occlusion. We also did not find any evidence of a beneficial effect of preconditioning in these patients.

The chronic nature of the coronary disease in these patients may have contributed to a progressive preconditioning, capable of protecting against tissue damage and inducing favorable metabolic changes, such as preservation of ATP and intracellular amino acids, and a reduction in lactate production. This may well explain the absence of biochemical injury detected in the control group and also the lack of any additional beneficial effect of a further period of preconditioning intraoperatively.

Transesophageal Assessment of Left Ventricular Function During Vessel Occlusion

Use of Intracoronary Shunts

Although the results of the studies assessing the effect of temporary coronary occlusion as a marker of myocardial metabolism were encouraging, we also thought it was important to measure an indicator of ventricular function during the conduct of beating heart surgery. Also, it is possible during beating heart surgery to introduce an intracoronary shunt via the arteriotomy incision, which maintains blood flow in the native coronary artery during construction of the anastomosis.

In this study, TEE was used to monitor global and regional wall motion, and the left ventricular wall motion score index (WMSI) and ejection fraction (EF%) were calculated by multiplane TEE during construction of the left internal mammary to the left anterior descending coronary artery anastomosis, as previously described. WMSI was assessed preoperatively, at 1, 3, and 6 minutes during the construction of the anastomosis, and after 5 minutes of reperfusion. EF% was calculated preoperatively, 5 minutes into the construction of the anastomosis, and 5 minutes after reperfusion. Twenty patients underwent the operation without the use of an intracoronary shunt, and 17 patients had the anastomosis performed after a shunt had been inserted into the coronary artery.

There was no difference in the preoperative and perioperative characteristics in the two groups. During construction of the anastomosis, after a shunt had been placed, there was no change seen in WMSI and ER%; however, a significant decline was seen in the group of patients in whom the anastomosis was constructed without a shunt being used (Figs. 60–4 and 60–5). On reperfusion, all the analyzed parameters returned to baseline. These data suggest that although the biochemical markers of myocardial injury we measured showed no changes during coronary artery occlusion, significant effects could be demonstrated in terms of wall motion and overall ventricular function. These are only temporary, and all functional indices return to normal after the anastomosis has been completed. This information and the biochemical data we have accumulated indicate that any adverse effects on the myocardium are rapidly normalized and are not followed by any permanent sequelae representing myocardial ischemia or infarction. These data also show that assessment of ventricular function using TEE is a more sensitive indicator of temporary myocardial dysfunction than hemodynamic parameters and continuous ECG monitoring.

Despite the normalization of myocardial function after completion of the anastomosis, as demonstrated by these data, some concerns still exist. These are particularly relevant to the occlusion of a mildly stenosed coronary vessel, which, despite the presence of coronary disease, may well perfuse a significant area of myocardium, and occlusion of which may lead to serious hemodynamic consequences. Placement of an intracoronary shunt in these circumstances, however, should allow myocardial perfusion to be maintained during performance of the anastomosis without adverse consequences.

Table 60–1. Values for Biochemical Markers*

	Nonpreconditioned		**Preconditioned**	
	Control	Reperfusion	Control	Reperfusion
ATP	2.68 ± 0.3	2.40 ± 0.25	2.78 ± 0.13	2.60 ± 0.25
ADP	1.07 ± 0.17	1.26 ± 0.26	1.25 ± 0.2	1.3 ± 0.13
ATP/ADP	2.9 ± 0.60	2.42 ± 0.42	2.95 ± 0.78	2.02 ± 0.16
Lactate	22.53 ± 8.4	22.3 ± 5.8	25.9 ± 5.2	27.9 ± 5.3
Amino Acids†	31.3 ± 1.8	31.5 ± 1.7	34.2 ± 1.8	30.47 ± 1.67

* Data expressed as mean ± SEM. Biochemical markers (μmol/g wet weight).

† The total intracellular free amino acid pool includes 15 essential and nonessential amino acids, as well as the nonprotein amino acid taurine. ADP = adenosine diphosphate; ATP = adenosine triphosphate.

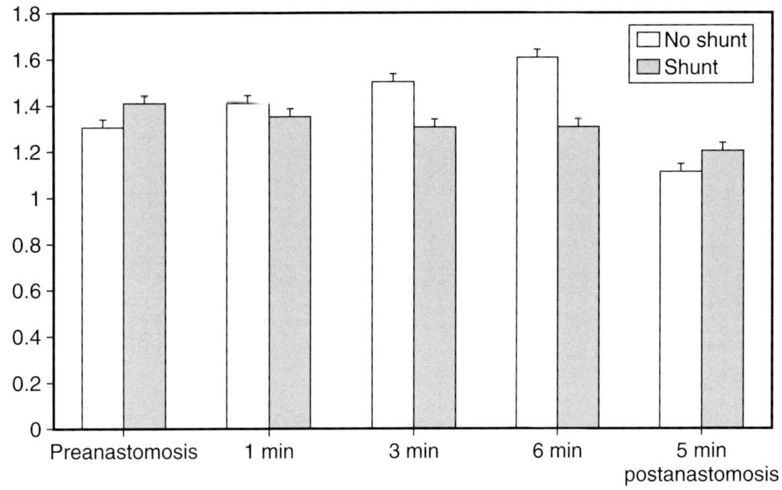

Figure 60–4. Wall motion index assessed by transesophageal echocardiography: effect of intracoronary shunt.

Conclusions

Despite the fact that coronary bypass grafting using cardiopulmonary bypass is a safe procedure (overall mortality 0.8% in our departments), significant morbidity remains, and along with cost containment, this has provided the impetus to develop techniques that enable the procedure to be performed off pump. A major consideration, however, has been the potential for myocardial damage to occur during the temporary coronary artery occlusion that is necessary when the coronary anastomosis is performed.

The work carried out in our institutions has shown that myocardial damage, assessed by postoperative systemic troponin I release, is less after short periods of coronary occlusion during coronary revascularization performed via a mini-thoracotomy than in patients undergoing conventional surgery with cardioplegic arrest with warm blood cardioplegia. We also have evidence that myocardial injury, quantified by the measurement of myocardial metabolites, is insignificant during short periods of coronary occlusion, and no additional benefit is obtained with a period of ischemic preconditioning.

However, our study demonstrated that coronary artery occlusion produces a temporary impairment of left ventricular function (possibly associated with coronary sinus troponin I release), although all parameters return to baseline after completion of the anastomosis.

These functional abnormalities may be avoided by the placement of an intracoronary shunt, which maintains coronary blood flow during construction of the anastomosis. We would recommend use of a shunt as an option when operating on patients who have unstable angina or poor left ventricular function, or in cases in which a long time to perform the anastomsis is anticipated. We also believe that the information regarding myocardial function provided by intraoperative TEE is extremely useful, and we recommend its use in all cases, so that changes in ventricular contractility can be continuously monitored and any deterioration recognized early (see Chapter 53).

There is no doubt that the performance of off-pump surgery is beneficial in selected cases, and from the studies we have performed, there is no evidence of permanent myocardial damage related to temporary coronary occlusion. In more controversial cases, utilization of a coronary shunt maintains myocardial perfusion, and techniques such as this will continue to develop and add to the armamentarium of the surgeon dedicated to performing coronary surgery without the use of cardiopulmonary bypass.

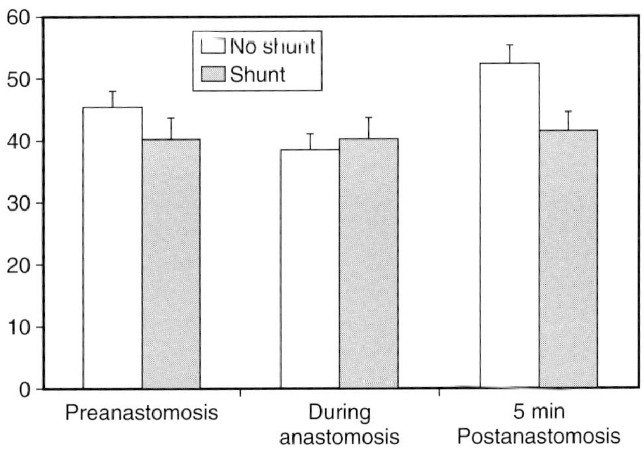

Figure 60–5. Ejection fraction assessed by transesophageal echocardiography: effect of intracoronary shunt.

References

1. Birdi I, Caputo MD, Hutter JA, et al: Troponin I release during minimally invasive coronary artery surgery. J Thorac Cardiovasc Surg 114:509–510, 1997.
2. Birdi I, Bryan AJ, Angelini GD: Detection and prevention of myocardial damage during open heart surgery. Heart 76:189–190, 1996.
3. Buffalo E, Andrande JCDS, Branco JNR, et al: Coronary artery bypass grafting without cardiopulmonary bypass. Ann Thorac Surg 61:63–66, 1996.
4. Clements FM, de Bruijn NP: Perioperative evaluation of regional wall motion by transoesophageal two-dimensional echocardiography. Anaesth Analg 66:249–261, 1987.
5. Fisher HA, Stahl JA, Budd JH, et al: Transoesophageal echocardiography: Procedures and clinical applications. J Am Coll Cardiol 18:1333–1348, 1991.
6. Katus H, Scheffold MD, Remppis A, et al. Proteins of the troponin complex. Lab Med 23:311–317, 1992.
7. Katus H, Schoeppenthau M, Tanzeem A, et al: Non-invasive as-

sessment of perioperative myocardial cell damage by circulating troponin T. Brit Heart J 65:259–264, 1991.
8. Saggin L, Gorza L, Ausoni S, et al: Troponin I switching in the developing heart. J Biol Chem 264:16299–16302, 1989.
9. Smith JS, Cahalan MK, Benefiel DJ, et al: Intraoperative detection of myocardial ischaemia in high risk patients: Electrocardiography versus two-dimensional echocardiography. Circulation 72:1015–1021, 1985.
10. Stahl R, Soller BR, Hsi C, et al: Decreasing myocardial pH reflects ischaemia during continuous warm retrograde cardioplegic arrest. Ann Thorac Surg 58:1645–1650, 1994.
11. Suleiman MS, Fernando HC, Dihmis W, et al: A loss of taurine and other amino acids from the ventricles of patients undergoing bypass surgery. Brit Heart J 69:241–245, 1993.
12. Suleiman MS, Dihmis WC, Caputo M, et al: Changes in the myocardial concentration of glutamate and aspartate during coronary artery surgery. Am J Physiol 272:1065–1069, 1997.
13. Yau TM, Ikonomidis, JS, Weisel RD, et al: Ventricular function after normothermic versus hypothermic cardioplegia. J Thorac Cardiovasc Surg 105:833–844, 1993.
14. Yellon DM, Alkhulaifi AM, Pugsley WB: Preconditioning of the human myocardium. Lancet 342:276–277, 1993.

COMMENTARY

Andrew S. Wechsler

This chapter by Dr. Underwood and his colleagues is highly provocative. It uses investigational methods, difficult to apply in the clinical setting, to answer important questions for which the authors are to be highly commended. The advent of minimally invasive, direct coronary artery bypass grafting and its many variations has raised interesting questions. Are the effects of global ischemia in hearts supported by cardiopulmonary bypass greater or less than the effects of local ischemia in hearts actively working and not supported by cardiopulmonary bypass? Does minimally invasive coronary artery bypass (MIDCAB) have a beneficial effect simply by avoiding cardiopulmonary bypass? If there are advantages of MIDCAB, are these the consequences of avoiding cardiopulmonary bypass, aortic cross-clamping, or a combination of both?

In an attempt to address some of these issues, these interesting studies have more or less demonstrated the following:

1. In contrast to conventional coronary artery bypass graft (CABG), MIDCAB was not associated with troponin I release when sampled from venous blood.
2. Small amounts of troponin I were found in coronary sinus samples, at unpredictable times, in patients undergoing a preconditioning protocol during MIDCAB.
3. Adenosine triphosphate (ATP) concentration did not change significantly in myocardial samples taken from either preconditioned or non–preconditioned hearts during MIDCAB.
4. Regional wall motion scores worsened during MIDCAB, but, performed without the benefit of a shunt, did not occur during the use of the shunt, and similar observations were made with regard to changes in ejection fraction.

All these observations are of interest and importance, but they do not eliminate the need for further investigation. There are some interesting, internal inconsistencies in the data, which are provocative. For example, if interruption of blood flow was sufficient to alter regional wall motion scores and ejection fraction, why was that not translated into a reduction in ATP? Under closer scrutiny, this may not be as great an inconsistency as it appears. The ATP samples were somewhat on the low side, and I would have been happier to have seen them expressed as ATP content per milligram of protein nitrogen or dry weight. This would help eliminate concerns raised by the amount of blood in the tissue or edema at the time of sampling. If we assume that there were no major changes at the ATP level, how might one explain the diminished shortening? Presumably, this is the consequence of regional ATP decrements, possibly at the site of potassium channels. Regional decreases in ATP content in the potassium channels result in opening of potassium channels and collapse of the action potential. This is a protective early event of ischemia in that the collapsed action potential diminishes calcium entry into the cell, because the plateau phase of the action potential essentially disappears. The consequence of this is a contraction with decreased force. This physiologic reality would be entirely consistent with the observations made by the authors.

The preconditioning studies are more complex. Because the authors demonstrated that there was minimal troponin I release following occlusion and reperfusion in the course of performing a MIDCAB, there was a relatively insignificant event for which preconditioning might be beneficial. Preconditioning has been demonstrated to diminish myonecrosis; observations regarding myocardial stunning are much less certain. Even as regards myocardial stunning, data provided by the authors on regional wall motion and ejection fraction suggest that no stunning was present. Thus, in the absence of a distinctly measurable endpoint, it is not possible to determine whether preconditioning was induced or not. Part of the frustration in making that assessment is the high level of surgical expertise applied in the study, in which anastomotic time, even in beating hearts, was kept in the vicinity of 12 minutes. In early studies using canine models, Jennings and Reimer[1] demonstrated that it required at least 16 minutes of coronary occlusion in awake dogs before the earliest signs of irreversible subendocardial injury were discernible. Thus, the ischemic times may simply have been too short to demonstrate any potential benefit of a preischemic preconditioning protocol.

In reviewing an earlier study performed by the authors of this chapter, I was struck by their release of troponin I into the venous blood and their persistence, in association with routine cardiopulmonary bypass, in employing cross-clamping and cardioplegia under normothermic conditions. One can either address the importance of their observation in demonstrating myocardial injury that may be immutable, or, alternatively, one can focus on the fact that regional occlusion of an isolated off-pump MIDCAB produced no suggestion of myocardial injury. The duration of the coronary occlusion was consistently below the duration thought to produce injury, and these studies further supported the accuracy of those experimental observations. This chapter provides much food for thought. It tackles directly the question of whether the heart can withstand temporary coronary occlusion without injury. As yet, there is no evidence suggesting the safety of this technique when used by surgeons who require significantly longer periods of interrupted coronary blood flow, although data provided by the authors suggest that the use of an intraluminal shunt may allow prolongation of the ischemic interval beyond the 12 minutes used in this study. It would have been interesting to have examined troponin release and extent of wall motion score abnormality in a regressed fashion against the time of clamping. Perhaps re-evaluation of the data can provide that information to the readers.

Reference

1. Jennings, RB, Reimer KA: Lethal myocardial ischemic injury. Am J Pathol 102:241–255, 1981.

Chapter 61

Role of Cytokines in Coronary Artery Bypass Grafting With or Without Cardiopulmonary Bypass

Song Wan, Mohammad Bashar Izzat, and Anthony P. C. Yim

The role of cardiopulmonary bypass (CPB) in the development of postoperative morbidity has been extensively investigated over the past two decades. It is well known that CPB is associated with a systemic inflammatory response that can contribute to postoperative complications.[61] Many factors during CPB, either material-dependent (i.e., the exposure of blood to nonphysiological surfaces and conditions) or material-independent (i.e., surgical trauma, ischemia-reperfusion to the organs, and changes in body temperature), are incriminated in inducing this response. It has been documented that these factors can trigger complement activation and the release of endotoxin and cytokines, which can induce cellular activation along with the expression of adhesion molecules, oxygen-free radicals, arachidonic acid metabolites, platelet-activating factor, nitric oxide, and endothelins (Fig. 61–1). This complex chain of events may result in bleeding disorders, as well as altered respiratory, renal, neurologic, and hepatic function, which may ultimately lead to multiple organ failure.[61] Therefore, avoiding the use of CPB ("off-pump") during coronary artery bypass grafting (CABG) is believed to be associated with less risk of postoperative morbidity.

Minimally invasive direct CABG has been shown to be beneficial in primary CABG,[6, 7, 21, 48] reoperative CABG,[4, 13] and high-risk patients with multivessel coronary artery disease.[26] Off-pump CABG through a median sternotomy is also associated with less postoperative arrhythmia and fewer pulmonary and neurologic complications compared with conventional surgery.[5] Underwood and colleagues noted that the degree of myocardial injury is reduced after off-pump operation, as reflected by a lower level of cardiac troponin I in the peripheral blood (minimally invasive direct CABG group) and in the coronary sinus blood (off-pump surgery through median sternotomy) (see Chapter 60).

To improve our understanding of the benefits of off-pump surgery, we have studied cytokine reactions associated with the procedure. This chapter reviews the current knowledge on cytokine responses to CPB and summarizes our initial data.

Cytokine Responses to Cardiopulmonary Bypass

Recent clinical investigations have indicated that both pro- and anti-inflammatory cytokines play a key role in the inflammatory cascade associated with CPB.[62] Proinflammatory cytokines, such as tumor necrosis factor α (TNF-α) and interleukin (IL)-6 and IL-8, may contribute to myocardial dysfunction and hemodynamic instability after CPB.[9, 22, 36, 62] In particular, they can significantly alter myocardial contractility[3, 14, 22] or profoundly influence the peripheral circulation, reducing vascular tone and thus resulting in postoperative low systemic vascular resistance.[36, 41] Notably, these cytokines do not need to circulate because the myocardium is capable of synthesizing biologically active TNF-α, IL-6, and IL-8.[32, 59] Local release of TNF-α in the myocardium may be involved in myocardial stunning after CPB.[14] Some of these effects may be mediated by an increased production of nitric oxide within cardiac myocytes.[3, 14] Cytokines also exert a direct damaging effect on other organs and contribute to the development of postoperative multiple organ failure.[8, 18, 43] Finally, the release of cytokines under CPB conditions may be involved in postoperative immunologic alterations.[62]

Ischemia-reperfusion is an important trigger for cytokine release.[58] TNF concentration can be detected only after aortic unclamping in patients undergoing conventional CABG.[27] In fact, TNFα,[22] IL-6,[22, 58] and IL-8[42, 58] levels correlated significantly with the duration of cardiac ischemia. Furthermore, we have found that the heart, but not the lungs, is a main source of these three cytokines during CPB.[59]

Conversely, the release of an anti-inflammatory cytokine, IL-10, mainly from the liver during CPB,[63] is potentially protective.[12, 62] IL-10 can either directly inhibit the release of proinflammatory cytokines[38] or indirectly exert anti-inflammatory effects by triggering the release of an IL-1 receptor antagonist and TNF-soluble receptors.[35]

Cytokine Responses to Off-Pump Coronary Artery Bypass Graft (CABG)

Unlike conventional CABG, there is no increase in leukocyte count, plasma levels of elastase (the marker of leukocyte activation), β-thromboglobulin (the marker of platelet degranulation), and C3a, when minimally invasive direct CABG is performed.[21] This may contribute to the reduced blood loss, shorter postoperative ventilatory support, and hospital stay after minimally invasive direct CABG operations.[21] Reduced production of TNF-α, along with its receptors and IL-6, has also been observed in patients undergoing minimally invasive direct CABG,[48] which was associated with reduced endothelial cell activation and less myocardial injury when compared with patients undergoing CABG with CPB.[69] Conversely, however, the acute phase response was shown to be similar in patients undergoing multivessel CABG with CPB.[17]

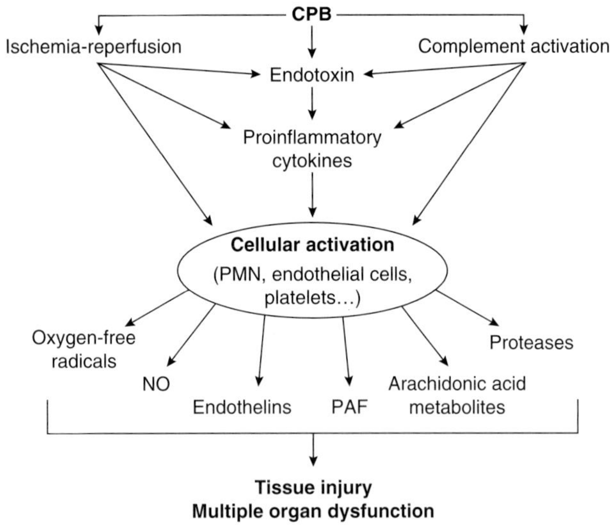

Figure 61–1. Schematic representation of the inflammatory response to cardiopulmonary bypass (CPB). NO = nitric oxide; PAF = platelet-activating factor; PMN = polymorphonuclear. (From Wan S, LeClerc JL, Vincent JL: Inflammatory response to cardiopulmonary bypass: Mechanisms involved and possible therapeutic strategies. Chest 112:676–692, 1997.)

In light of these findings, we[65] conducted a prospective study to compare the production of cytokines in patients undergoing CABG through median sternotomy with or without CPB. In this study, therefore, only one parameter was investigated—the use of CPB.

Forty-four consecutive patients who had multivessel coronary artery disease underwent complete revascularization. Patients were selected for off-pump CABG whenever technically feasible. There were no differences between the two groups of patients with respect to age, gender ratio, symptoms, or functional class. No patients received corticosteroids before, during, or after surgery.

Cardiopulmonary Bypass

The extracorporeal circuit consisted of a roller pump (Sarns 9000, 3M Health Care, Ann Arbor, MI) and a membrane oxygenator (Turbo, 3M Health Care, Ann Arbor, MI). Standard systemic heparinization (3 mg/kg) was performed and an activated clotting time of greater than 480 seconds was maintained during CPB. The pump flow was set at 2.4 L/min/m^2. Patients were not cooled during CPB and they received intermittent antegrade normothermic (35 to 37°C) blood cardioplegia, which was a mixture of 400 to 600 ml of oxygenated blood with graduated doses of potassium-magnesium solution (added to blood by a syringe pump). On discontinuation of CPB, heparin was neutralized with protamine sulfate.

Off-Pump Technique

Traction sutures were applied to pericardial edges, displacing the heart anteriorly. For exposure of the left anterior descending artery or its diagonal branches, additional pericardial traction sutures were inserted anterior to the left phrenic nerve to rotate the heart, and a moist sponge was placed behind its laterodorsal aspect, bringing the coronary artery into the operative field. For exposure of obtuse marginal or right coronary branches, two wet cotton tapes were passed through the transverse sinus with their right ends secured to the surgical drape. The two loose lengths of tape were then used to lift and rotate the heart toward the surgeon, as well as to stabilize the coronary artery. Patients were given heparin (1 mg/kg), and two 4-0 Prolene sutures (Ethicon, Scotland) were used to occlude the coronary artery temporarily on either side of the anastomosis site. Heparin was neutralized with protamine sulfate after all anastomoses were completed.

Cytokine Measurements

Blood samples were collected from each patient before surgery, at the end of the procedure, and 2, 4, 8, 24, and 48 hours thereafter. Samples were immediately cooled to 4°C and centrifuged (3000 g for 10 minutes at 4°C). Plasma was stored at −70°C until assay. TNF-α, IL-6, IL-8, and IL-10 levels were determined by means of commercially available enzyme-linked immunosorbent assays (R & D Systems, Minneapolis, MN). Plasma levels of the MB isoenzyme of creatine kinase (CK-MB) and cardiac troponin-I, a highly specific marker of myocardial injury, were also measured after surgery.

There was no death or major complication in either group. The duration of CPB and aortic cross-clamping in the CPB group was 91 ± 7 and 49 ± 4 min (mean ± SEM), respectively. The number of grafts was 2 ± 0.2 in the off-pump group and 3 ± 0.2 in the CPB group.

TNA-α levels were equally low in both groups. The mean values of TNF-α never exceeded 10 pg/ml in either group throughout the study period. IL-6 levels increased in both groups after surgery. However, no significant differences were noted between the two groups regarding serial IL-6 measurements (Fig. 61–2), which were in agree-

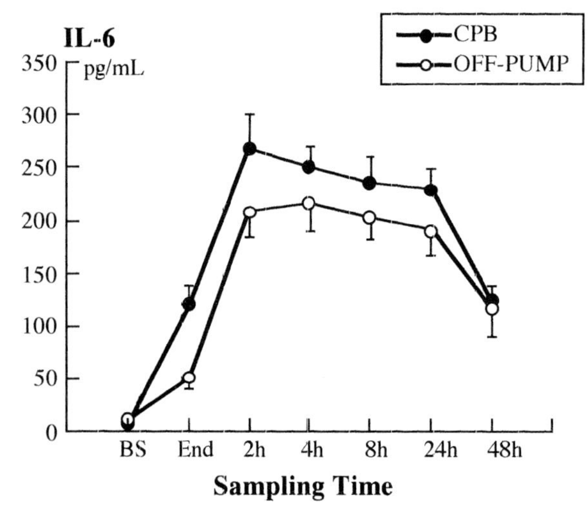

Figure 61–2. Plasma levels of interleukin (IL)-6 in patients undergoing coronary artery bypass grafting (CABG) with or without cardiopulmonary bypass (CPB). Data are mean ± SEM. (From Wan S, Izzat MB, Lee TW, et al. Avoiding cardiopulmonary bypass in multivessel-CABG reduces cytokine response and myocardial injury. Ann Thorac Surg [in press]).

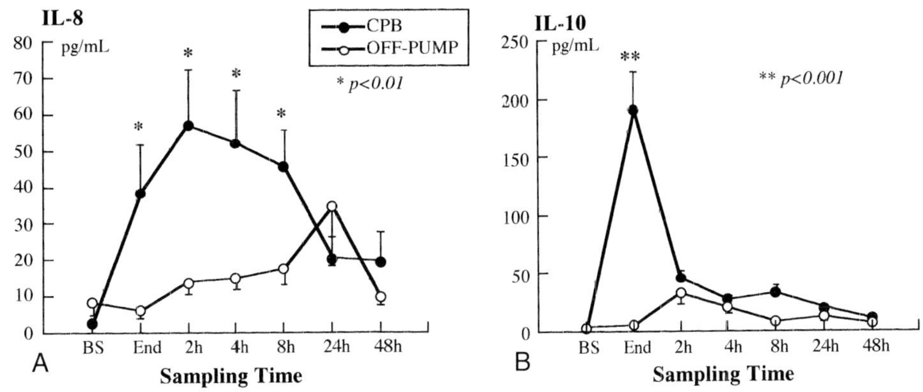

Figure 61–3. Plasma levels of IL-8 and IL-10 in patients undergoing CABG with or without CPB. Data are mean ± SEM. The Mann-Whitney *U* test was used for comparison between two groups. (From Wan S, Izzat MB, Lee TW, et al. Avoiding cardiopulmonary bypass in multivessel-CABG reduces cytokine response and myocardial injury. Ann Thorac Surg [in press]).

ment with a recent observation.[17] After surgery, IL-8 levels were significantly elevated in the CPB group but not in the off-pump group (Fig. 61–3A). Moreover, IL-10 production shortly after operation was also markedly increased in the CPB group but remained low in the off-pump group (Fig. 61–3B). Although postoperative CK-MB values tended to be lower in the off-pump group, the intergroup differences were not statistically significant. Nevertheless, cardiac troponin-I levels increased in the CPB group only and not in the off-pump group (Fig. 61–4). Moreover, cardiac troponin-I values 24 hours after surgery correlated strongly with IL-8 levels 4 hours after surgery (Fig. 61–5).

Off-Pump Coronary Artery Bypass Grafting: The Role of Reduced Interleukin-8 Production

Our data indicate that when compared with conventional CABG, off-pump surgery is associated with reduced cytokine responses as suggested by the lower release of IL-8 and IL-10. The degree of postoperative myocardial injury is also lower after an off-pump procedure.

Although it has no significant hemodynamic effects, IL-8 is an important chemokine known to attract, activate and control trafficking[46] of neutrophils[2, 15] and T lymphocytes. IL-8 can also stimulate histamine release.[46] In animal models, the release of IL-8 is induced only after reperfusion of the ischemic myocardium.[25, 34] Furthermore, administration of anti-IL8 antibodies prevents lung ieschemia-reperfusion injury[50] or acid-induced injury.[16] Clinical studies have also indicated that the myocardium is an important source of IL-8 during reperfusion after long ischemic periods[42, 58] or acute myocardial infarction.[40, 59] Because neutrophil activation and adherence to the vascular endothelium is a critical step in ischemia-reperfusion injury, the lower myocardial injury seen after off-pump surgery in our study, as well as in other studies (see Chapter 60), may be explained by the lower IL-8 production associated with the procedure.

In the meantime, it is noteworthy that cytokines are likely to act both individually and within a network of interrelated and interacting signals.[62] It has been shown that the production of IL-10 can be enhanced by proinflamma-

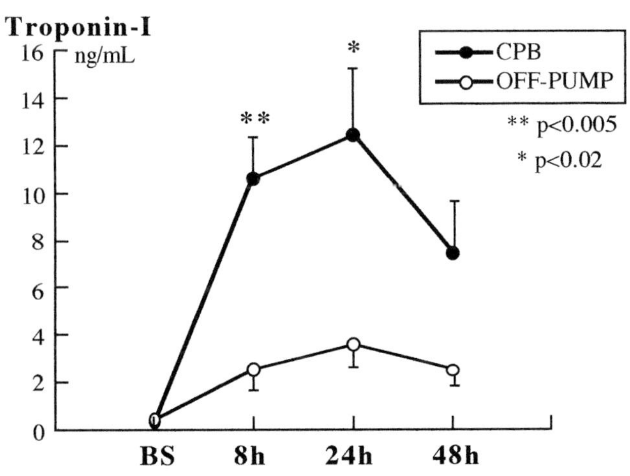

Figure 61–4. Plasma levels of cardiac troponin-I in patients undergoing CABG with or without CPB. Data are mean ± SEM. The Mann-Whitney *U* test was used for comparison between two groups. (From Wan S, Izzat MB, Lee TW, et al. Avoiding cardiopulmonary bypass in multivessel-CABG reduces cytokine response and myocardial injury. Ann Thorac Surg [in press]).

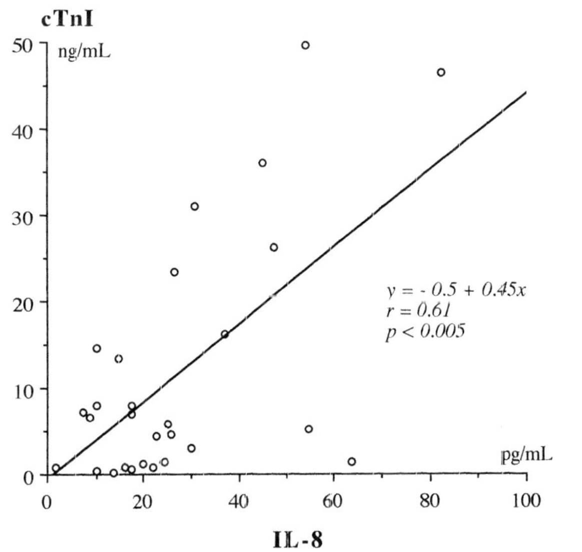

Figure 61–5. Relationship between cardiac troponin-I values 24 hours after surgery and IL-8 levels 4 hours after surgery in patients undergoing CABG with and without CPB. (From Wan S, Izzat MB, Lee TW, et al. Avoiding cardiopulmonary bypass in multivessel-CABG reduces cytokine response and myocardial injury. Ann Thorac Surg [in press]).

tory cytokines such as TNF-α,[55, 67] a cycle that provides a negative feedback to TNF-α production. In the current study, the lower release of IL-10 during off-pump surgery may be related to the reduced production of IL-8. Therefore, the balance between the pro- and anti-inflammatory responses may be even more crucial in reducing the damaging effects of CPB.

A Better Pump: Therapeutic Strategies During Cardiopulmonary Bypass (CPB)

Apart from avoiding the use of CPB, a number of therapeutic strategies aiming at modulating the inflammatory reactions associated with CPB may also be considered to reduce the incidence and the severity of postoperative complications. For instance, intraoperative leukocyte depletion has been shown to reduce pulmonary dysfunction after CPB.[20, 39] Since the inflammatory response is multifactorial, combined therapies may be more efficient than a single intervention to improve outcome.

A variety of interventions targeted at interfering with the cytokine response associated with CPB have been proposed and are described in the following sections.

Steroid Pretreatment

Corticosteroids can inhibit the release of proinflammatory cytokines, including TNF-α,[27, 53, 54] IL-1β,[11] IL-6,[33, 54] and IL-8.[11, 33, 53, 54] In addition, they also greatly enhance the production of anti-inflammatory cytokine IL-10.[50, 60, 63] These effects may reduce the inflammatory response after CPB and may improve the postoperative recovery.[10, 23, 27, 54] The timing of steroid administration, before rather than after CPB, is important to achieve these benefits.[60]

The Use of Aprotinin

Low-dose aprotinin may blunt CPB-induced systemic TNF-α release,[24] but the effects of aprotinin on the inflammatory response to CPB might be dose-dependent.[2, 49] In fact, high-dose aprotinin not only may preserve platelet function[51, 56, 57] but also may inhibit complement activation, neutrophil elastase release, and kallikrein production.[57] Aprotinin prime in combination with heparin-coated CPB circuits has been found to reduce postoperative morbidity and the length of stay in the intensive care unit.[29] In patients undergoing reoperative heart transplantation, aprotinin was shown to reduce not only postoperative bleeding but also the inflammatory response, which was associated with improved net fluid balance, pulmonary function, and right-sided heart function.[45]

Heparin Coating of Cardiopulmonary Bypass Circuits

A crucial factor triggering the inflammatory response to CPB is the exposure of blood to nonphysiologic surfaces. Heparin coating of CPB circuits has been demonstrated to improve its biocompatibility by reducing complement and granulocyte activation, inhibiting platelet adhesion, and preserving platelet function.[61] The use of heparin-coated CPB circuits can also inhibit the release of proinflammatory cytokines[19, 44, 52, 68] as well as anti-inflammatory cytokine IL-10[64] and soluble TNF receptors.[68] Thus, by limiting material-dependent blood activation and the subsequent reactions on the different target organs, heparin coating of CPB circuits may inhibit both pro- and anti-inflammatory responses associated with CPB. This may contribute to the reduction in myocardial injury as reflected by a lower release of cardiac troponin-I 12 and 24 hours after heart and heart-lung transplantation.[64] An improved postoperative recovery has been observed in patients undergoing primary CABG with heparin-coated circuits.[1, 28]

Intraoperative Ultrafiltration

Proinflammatory cytokines, such as TNF-α and IL-6, can be removed by intraoperative ultrafiltration in children undergoing CPB.[30, 31, 37, 66] These effects appeared to result in less postoperative inflammatory reaction.[31] Nevertheless, IL-10 was also removed, and this phenomenon may be deleterious.[31] Future study is needed to determine the best choice of filter material, pore size, hemofiltration rate, and the timing of the procedure.[47]

Summary

Off-pump CABG has been shown to be a valuable alternative to conventional surgery. Although evidence in favor of this approach is continually growing, stepwise investigation is essential to explore the underlying mechanisms. Off-pump CABG is associated with reduced release of cytokines, in particular IL-8, which may, in turn, reduce the degree of postoperative myocardial injury as well as the inflammatory response.

Conversely, CPB itself can also be improved. A solid understanding of the pathophysiology involved in the inflammatory response to CPB may lead to the development of better therapeutic strategies. Both pharmacologic interventions and modification of techniques or mechanical devices may have beneficial clinical implications.

References

1. Aldea GS, Doursounian M, O'Gara P, et al: Heparin-bonded circuits with a reduced anticoagulation protocol in primary CABG: A prospective, randomized study. Ann Thorac Surg 62:410–418, 1996.
2. Ashraf S, Tian Y, Cowan D, et al: "Low-dose" aprotinin modifies hemostasis but not proinflammatory cytokine release. Ann Thorac Surg 63:68–73, 1997.
3. Barry WH: Mechanisms of immune-mediated myocyte injury. Circulation 89:2421–2432, 1994.
4. Boonstra PW, Grandjean JG, Mariani MA: Reoperative coronary bypass grafting without cardiopulmonary bypass through a small thoracotomy. Ann Thorac Surg 63:405–407, 1997.
5. Buffolo E, Gerola LR: Coronary artery bypass grafting without cardiopulmonary bypass through median sternotomy and minimally invasive procedure. Int J Cardiol 62(suppl I):S89–93, 1997.
6. Calafiore AM, Angelini GD, Bergsland J, Salerno TA: Minimally invasive coronary artery bypass grafting. Ann Thorac Surg 62: 1545–1548, 1996.

7. Calafiore AM, Di Giammarco G, Teodori G, et al: Midterm results after minimally invasive coronary surgery (LAST operation). J Thorac Cardiovasc Surg 115:763–771, 1998.
8. Casey LC: Role of cytokines in the pathogenesis of cardiopulmonary-induced multisystem organ failure. Ann Thorac Surg 56:S92–96, 1993.
9. Deng MC, Dasch B, Erren M, et al: Impact of left ventricular dysfunction on cytokines, hemodynamics, and outcome in bypass grafting. Ann Thorac Surg 62:184–190, 1996.
10. Engelman RM, Rousou JA, Flack JE III, et al: Fast-track recovery of the coronary bypass patient. Ann Thorac Surg 58:1742–1746, 1994.
11. Engelman RM, Rousou JA, Flack JE III, et al: Influence of steroids on complement and cytokine generation after cardiopulmonary bypass. Ann Thorac Surg 60:801–804, 1995.
12. Eppinger MJ, Ward PA, Bolling SF, Deeb GM: Regulatory effects of interleukin-10 on lung ischemia-reperfusion injury. J Thorac Cardiovasc Surg 112:1301–1306, 1996.
13. Fanning WJ, Kakos GS, Williams TE Jr: Reoperative coronary bypass grafting without cardiopulmonary bypass. Ann Thorac Surg 55:486–489, 1993.
14. Finkel MS, Oddis CV, Jacob TD, et al: Negative inotropic effects of cytokines on the heart mediated by nitric oxide. Science 257:387–389, 1992.
15. Finn A, Naik S, Klein N, et al: Interleukin-8 release and neutrophil degranulation after pediatric cardiopulmonary bypass. J Thorac Cardiovasc Surg 105:234–241, 1993.
16. Folkesson HG, Matthay MA, Hebert CA, Broaddus VC: Acid aspiration-induced lung injury in rabbits is mediated by interleukin-8-dependent mechanisms. J Clin Invest 96:107–161, 1995.
17. Fransen E, Maessen J, Dentener M, et al: Systemic inflammation present in patients undergoing CABG without extracorporeal circulation. Chest 113:1290–1295, 1998.
18. Goldstein DJ, Moazami N, Seldomridgė JA, et al: Circulatory resuscitation with left ventricular assist device support reduces interleukins 6 and 8 levels. Ann Thorac Surg 63:971–974, 1997.
19. Gu YJ, van Oeveren W, Akkerman C, et al: Heparin-coated circuits reduce the inflammatory response to cardiopulmonary bypass. Ann Thorac Surg 55:917–922, 1993.
20. Gu YJ, deVries AJ, Boonstra PW, van Oeveren W: Loukocyte depletion results in improved lung function and reduced inflammatory response after cardiac surgery. J Thorac Cardiovasc Surg 112:494–450, 1996.
21. Gu YJ, Mariani MA, van Oeveren W, et al: Reduction of the inflammatory response in patients undergoing minimally invasive coronary artery bypass grafting. Ann Thorac Surg 65:420–424, 1998.
22. Hennein HA, Ebba H, Rodriguez JL, et al: Relationship of the proinflammatory cytokines to myocardial ischemia and dysfunction after uncomplicated coronary revascularization. J Thorac Cardiovasc Surg 108:626–635, 1994.
23. Hill GE, Snider S, Galbraith TA, et al: Glucocorticoid reduction of bronchial epithelial inflammation during cardiopulmonary bypass. Am J Respir Crit Care Med 152:1791–1795, 1995.
24. Hill GE, Alonso A, Spurzem JR, et al: Aprotinin and methylprednisolone equally blunt cardiopulmonary bypass-induced inflammation in humans. J Thorac Cardiovasc Surg 110:1658–1662, 1995.
25. Ivey CL, Williams FM, Collins PD, et al: Neutrophil chemoattractants generated in two phases during reperfusion of ischemic myocardium in the rabbit: Evidence for a role for C5a and interleukin-8. J Clin Invest 95:2720–2728, 1995.
26. Izzat MB, Yim APC: Minimally invasive LAD revascularisation in high-risk patients with three-vessel coronary artery disease. Int J Cardiol 62(suppl I):S101–104, 1997.
27. Jansen NJG, van Oeveren W, v.d. Broek L, et al: Inhibition by dexamethasone of the reperfusion phenomena in cardiopulmonary bypass. J Thorac Cardiovasc Surg 102:515–525, 1991
28. Jansen PGM, te Velthuis H, Huybregts RAJM, et al: Reduced complement activation and improved postoperative performance after cardiopulmonary bypass with heparin-coated circuits. J Thorac Cardiovasc Surg 110:829–834, 1995.
29. Jansen PGM, Baufreton C, Le Besnerais P, et al: Heparin-coated circuits and aprotinin prime for coronary artery bypass grafting. Ann Thorac Surg 61:1363–1366, 1996.
30. Journois D, Pouard P, Greeley WJ, et al: Hemofiltration during cardiopulmonary bypass in pediatric cardiac surgery: Effects on hemostasis, cytokines, and complement components. Anesthesiology 81:1181–1189, 1994.
31. Journois D, Israel-Biet D, Pouard P, et L: High-volume, zero-balanced hemofiltration to reduce delayed inflammatory response to cardiopulmonary bypass in children. Anesthesiology 85:965–976, 1996.
32. Kapadia S, Lee J, Torre-Amione G, et al: Tumor necrosis factor-α gene and protein expression in adult feline myocardium after endotoxin administration. J Clin Invest 96:1042–1052, 1995.
33. Kawamura T, Inada K, Okada H, et al: Methylprednisolone inhibits increase of interleukin 8 and 6 during open heart surgery. Can J Anaesth 42:399–403, 1995.
34. Kukielka GL, Smith CW, LaRosa GJ, et al: Interleukin-8 gene induction in the myocardium after ischemia and reperfusion in vivo. J Clin Invest 95:89–103, 1995.
35. McBride WT, Armstrong MA, Crockard AD, et al: Cytokine balance and immunosuppressive changes at cardiac surgery: Contrasting response between patients and isolated CPB circuits. Br J Anaesth 75:724–733, 1995.
36. Menasché P, Haydar S, Peynet J, et al: A potential mechanism of vasodilation after warm heart surgery: The temperature-dependent release of cytokines. J Thorac Cardiovasc Surg 107:293–299, 1994.
37. Millar AB, Armstrong L, van der Linden J, et al: Cytokine production and hemofiltration in children undergoing cardiopulmonary bypass. Ann Thorac Surg 56:1499–1502, 1993.
38. Moore KW, O'Garra A, de Waal Malefyt R, et al: Interleukin-10. Ann Rev Immunol 11:165–190, 1993.
39. Morioka K, Muraoka R, Chiba Y, et al: Leukocyte and platelet depletion with a blood cell separator: Effects on lung injury after cardiac surgery with cardiopulmonary bypass. J Thorac Cardiovasc Surg 111:45–54, 1996.
40. Neumann F-J, Ott I, Gawaz M, et al: Cardiac release of cytokines and inflammatory responses in acute myocardial infarction. Circulation 92:748–755, 1995.
41. Ohkawa F, Ikeda U, Kanbe T, et al: Effects of inflammatory cytokines on vascular tone. Cardiovasc Res 30:711–715, 1995.
42. Oz MC, Liao H, Naka Y, et al: Ischemia-induced interleukin-8 release after human heart transplantation: A potential role for endothelial cells. Circulation 92(suppl II) 428–432, 1995.
43. Partrick DA, Moore FA, Moore EE, et al: The inflammatory profile of interleukin-6, interleukin-8, and soluble intercellular adhesion molecule-1 in postinjury multiple organ failure. Am J Surg 172:425–431, 1996.
44. Plötz FM, van Oeveren W, Hultquist KA, et al: A heparin-coated circuit reduces complement activation and the release of leukocyte inflammatory mediators during extracorporeal circulation in a rabbit. Artif Organs 16:366–370, 1992.
45. Prendergast TW, Furukawa S, Beyer AJ III, et al: Defining the role of aprotinin in heart transplantation. Ann Thorac Surg 62: 670–674, 1996.
46. Rollins BJ: Chemokines. Blood 90:909–928, 1997.
47. Saatvedt K, Lindberg H, Geiran OR, et al: Ultrafiltration after cardiopulmonary bypass in children: Effects on hemodynamics, cytokines and complement. Cardiovasc Res 31:596–602, 1996.

48. Schulze CJ, Wildhirt SM, Böhm DH, et al: Evaluation of the inflammatory response after minimally invasive coronary artery bypass grafting (MIDCAB) versus conventional CABG (Abstract). Presented at the 1st annual meeting of the International Society for Minimally Invasive Cardiac Surgery, June 25–27, 1998.
49. Segahye MC, Duchateau J, Grabitz RG, et al: Influence of low-dose aprotinin on the inflammatory reaction due to cardiopulmonary bypass in children. Ann Thorac Surg 61:1205–1211, 1996.
50. Sekido N, Mukaida N, Harada A et al: Prevention of lung reperfusion injury in rabbits by a monoclonal antibody against interleukin-8. Nature 365:654–657, 1993.
51. Shinfeld A, Zippel D, Lavee J, et al: Aprotinin improves hemostasis after cardiopulmonary bypass better than single-donor platelet concentrate. Ann Thorac Surg 59:872–876, 1995.
52. Steinberg BM, Grossi EA, Schwarz DS, et al: Heparin bonding of bypass circuits reduces cytokine release during cardiopulmonary bypass. Ann Thorac Surg 60:525–529, 1995.
53. Tabardel Y, Duchateau J, Schmartz D, et al: Corticosteroids increase blood interleukin 10 levels during cardiopulmonary bypass in men. Surgery 119:76–80, 1996.
54. Teoh KHT, Bradley CA, Gauldie J, Burrows H: Steroid inhibition of cytokine-mediated vasodilation after warm heart surgery. Circulation 92(suppl II) 347–353, 1995.
55. van der Poll T, Jansen J, Levi M, et al: Regulation of interleukin 10 release by tumor necrosis factor in humans and chimpanzees. J Exp Med 180:1985–1988, 1994.
56. van Oeveren W, Harder MP, Roozendaal KJ, et al: Aprotinin protects platelets against the initial effect of cardiopulmonary bypass. J Thorac Cardiovasc Surg 99:788–797, 1990.
57. Wachtfogel YT, Kucich U, Hack CE, et al: Aprotinin inhibits the contact, neutrophil, and platelet activation systems during simulated extracorporeal perfusion. J Thorac Cardiovasc Surg 106:1–10, 1993.
58. Wan S, Marchant A, DeSmet JM, et al: Human cytokine responses to cardiac transplantation and coronary artery bypass grafting. J Thorac Cardiovasc Surg 111:469–477, 1996.
59. Wan S, DeSmet JM, Barvais L, et al: Myocardium is a major source of proinflammatory cytokines in patients undergoing cardiopulmonary bypass. J Thorac Cardiovasc Surg 112:806–811, 1996.
60. Wan S, DeSmet JM, Antoine M, et al: Steroid administration in heart and heart-lung transplantation: Is the timing adequate? Ann Thorac Surg 61:674–678, 1996.
61. Wan S, LeClerc JL, Vincent JL: Inflammatory response to cardiopulmonary bypass: Mechanisms involved and possible therapeutic strategies. Chest 112:676–692, 1997.
62. Wan S, LeClerc JL, Vincent JL: Cytokine responses to cardiopulmonary bypass: Lessons learned from cardiac transplantation. Ann Thorac Surg 63:269–276, 1997.
63. Wan S, LeClerc JL, Schmartz D, et al. Hepatic release of interleukin-10 during cardiopulmonary bypass in steroid-pretreated patients. Am Heart J 1997;133:335–9
64. Wan S, LeClerc JL, Antoine M, et al: Heparin-coated circuits reduce myocardial injury in heart or heart-lung transplantation: Ann Thorac Surg (in press).
65. Wan S, Izzat MB, Lee TW, et al. Avoiding cardiopulmonary bypass in multivessel-CABG reduces cytokine response and myocardial injury. Ann Thorac Surg (in press).
66. Wang MJ, Chiu IS, Hsu CM, et al: Efficacy of ultrafiltration in removing inflammatory mediators during pediatric cardiac operations. Ann Thorac Surg 61:651–656, 1996.
67. Wanidworanun C, Strober W: Predominant role of tumor necrosis factor-α in human monocyte IL-10 synthesis. J Immunol 151:6853–6861, 1993.
68. Weerwind PW, Maessen JG, van Tits LJH, et al: Influence of Duraflo II heparin-treated extracorporeal circuits on the systemic inflammatory response in patients having coronary bypass. J Thorac Cardiovasc Surg 110:1633–1641, 1995.
69. Wildhirt SM, Schulze C, Boehm DH, et al: Myocardial cell damage and lipid peroxidation after minimally invasive (MIDCAB) versus conventional CABG (Abstract). Presented at the 1st annual meeting of the International Society for Minimally Invasive Cardiac Surgery, June 25–27, 1998, Minneapolis, MN.

COMMENTARY

Andrew S. Wechsler

In this article, the authors have attempted to find biochemical markers that might help understand why patients undergoing off-pump coronary bypass may have more rapid recovery and less morbidity than patients undergoing cardiopulmonary bypass. A cohort of 44 patients is somewhat vaguely described. Some were assigned to off-pump coronary bypass grafting and the others received conventional bypass grafting. Cytokines were used as a marker of the inflammatory response. Interestingly, TNF-α and IL-6 levels were the same in both groups, and relatively minor changes in IL-8 and IL-10 were noted. Because both groups of patients underwent sternotomy, the authors attribute the different cytokine concentration from the peripheral bloodstream taken up to 24 hours postoperatively to be the consequence of the use of CPB.

This is an intuitively logical argument, but there may be other factors involved that are of equal importance. For example, the authors acknowledge that the heart has been identified as an organ generating interleukins under conditions of ischemia and reperfusion. When one examines the difference in operative technique, those patients undergoing conventional CPB had an average of one additional graft and about 42 minutes of global ischemic time. Perhaps the initiator of the cytokine response is ischemia and reperfusion of the myocardium more than the use of CPB. This does not in any way negate the observation that there was a difference in the inflammatory cytokine response between the two groups, but it does raise the question as to whether one can blame the CPB circuit for the difference.

I am surprised that the difference in inflammatory response between the two groups was so small. Perhaps the bypass times were not long enough to generate a strong inflammatory response. Perhaps the ischemic time was too short. Perhaps the hearts were too well protected. It would have been of great interest to know if there were vast differences in the local concentration of cytokines between the two groups (e.g., in the coronary venous effluent). Were the patients in one way or another different? There was probably a reason that only two bypasses were performed in the off-pump group versus three bypasses in the on-pump group. Do other factors such as age and gender enter into the differences? We must be careful not to attribute too readily explanations that are intuitively correct but for which there may be alternative hypotheses. Cytokine expression is complex and, as the authors aptly point out, there are strong interactions between cytokines. Could the dose of heparin have been a factor? Perhaps most important of all is to challenge the most fundamental hypothesis of the authors, which is that use of off-pump bypass is associated with a more rapid and less morbid postoperative course. No data were given that supports this contention in this particular writing. In my personal experience and that of our group operating on a large number of patients using both on and off CPB techniques, those patients that undergo off-pump bypass who are in generally good health do not fare significantly differently from those patients in whom CPB is used. Good operative candidates in good health who undergo two vessel coronary bypass grafting are generally able to leave the hospital about 3 days after their operation. This is not much different from patients who undergo median sternotomy for purposes other than cardiac surgery, for example, thymectomy.

I enjoyed this provocative article because it stimulated me to think about all the reasons that might account for different hospital courses in patients operated on using one or the other of the techniques employed in this study. As we dissect further and further, I believe we will learn that the explanations are multifactorial, but it may require large groups of patients to do so. For now, readers may enjoy this chapter and determine for themselves whether the cup is half full or half empty.

COMMENTARY

Willem van Oeveren and Y. John Gu

Cytokine responses to CPB have recently received considerable attention. In this chapter, Wan and colleagues compared the release of some cytokines in patients undergoing either conventional or "off-pump" CABG. Reduced IL-8 production was observed in the off-pump group, and this may be related to less myocardial injury in these patients. In the same group of patients, however, IL-6 production increased shortly after surgery and reached levels almost as high as those in the CPB group, indicating that factors other than CPB can trigger the release of IL-6. Median sternotomy may well be involved in inducing IL-6 production, given that it was used in both groups. This is in line with our recent finding of significantly lower IL-6 levels in patients undergoing off-pump CABG through minithoracotomy compared with median sternotomy (4.8 ± 1.8 pg/ml versus 16.1 ± 6.1 pg/ml by the end of operation). It seems that a smaller surgical wound may be associated with less pronounced IL-6 production.

The authors propose that ischemia-reperfusion can be an important trigger for cytokine release, and this hypothesis is supported by TNF release after aortic unclamping and by the correlation between cytokine levels and the duration of ischemia. However, the CPB circuit may also be an important cofactor in cytokine production. We noted that clamping the aorta before blood had passed the CPB circuit reduces the inflammatory reaction. It is also possible that the initial "priming" of inflammatory cells and complement activation in the CPB circuit aggravates the subsequent responses to surgical trauma, cooling-warming, ischemia-reperfusion, and so on.

In their current study, the authors considered that the use of CPB was the only independent variable. Nevertheless, the cardioplegic arrest of the heart in the CPB group should be considered another important variable. It might be interesting to measure cytokine production after CABG using other techniques of myocardial protection. In addition, IL-8 production may be a useful marker in determining the quality of myocardial preservation methods, particularly when blood cardioplegia is used.

Overall, it seems that the off-pump technique results in reduced inflammatory reaction, not only directly by reducing blood-material interaction but also indirectly by eliminating major material-independent triggers. This may also explain the relative benefits of off-pump surgery compared with "surface-treated" CPB circuits.

Chapter 62

Pharmacologic and Mechanical Stabilization During Minimally Invasive Coronary Artery Surgery

M. Clive Robinson and Salik Jahania

Since the early reports of minimally or less invasive coronary artery bypass grafting (CABG) in 1995,[1–3] several fundamental defining features have emerged. These characteristics have centered around smaller incisions that reduce the degree of surgical trauma, coronary artery grafting on the beating heart without cardiopulmonary bypass, and elimination of aortic manipulation from instrumentation or cannulation. Initially, the main endeavors were limited vessel off-pump grafting via small thoracotomy incisions and anastomosing of the internal mammary artery to the left anterior descending or right coronary arteries. More recently, renewed attention to multivessel off-pump grafting via partial or full sternotomy have been included.

Vital to these procedures are effective methods for optimizing myocardial physiology during cardiac displacement for access and for myocardial immobilization during grafting. Pharmacologic control involves interventions for reducing myocardial oxygen needs during ischemia, enhancing ischemic tolerance, and providing therapy to moderate myocardial contractility so that conditions for mechanical stabilization during grafting on the beating heart are improved.

Also under evaluation are new concepts related to inhibition of the injurious effects of metabolites known to be associated with myocardial injury during ischemia and infarction. For actual cardiac immobilization, mechanical techniques are currently the most important, and they employ either suction devices or localized pressure to the myocardium.

Although available techniques and therapy continue to improve significantly, minimally invasive coronary surgery is currently in a state of developmental infancy. Existing methods and techniques are largely adaptations of conventional surgical principles to use in confined anatomic spaces. For truly minimal invasiveness, methods must change drastically, and to qualify as viable alternatives, the procedures must, in many situations and categories of coronary artery disease, provide the benefits of surgical arterial revascularization with a degree of invasiveness that bears comparison with catheter-based methods. Progression to this state will include a transition to imaged surgery and radical new methods of instrumentation—most likely controlled robotically, along with development of new safety nets. Pharmacologic and mechanical methods of myocardial control, both for optimized physiology and immobilization, will be critical to this process.

Pharmacologic Control

Optimizing Myocardial Physiology

Well beyond the needs of conventional CABG, beating heart off-pump grafting involves dynamically controlled pharmacologic therapy. Many aspects of this therapy are independently important, but they also frequently serve as adjuvant therapy to mechanical methods of stabilization. Effective anastomotic site presentation and control involve the ability to select appropriately and use effectively a number of these methods. The anesthesiologist's initiative and management are integral to this process, and minimally invasive coronary surgery has become a specialty area for the cardiac anesthesiologist.

Methods of Preventing Ischemia

During flow interruption in the isolated artery during grafting, inevitable degrees of ischemia occur. These ischemic intervals may be as short as 6 to 12 minutes, but they can range from 20 to 25 minutes. It appears that at least in patients who have chronic coronary artery disease, the myocardium has a substantial, although largely undetermined, tolerance for episodes of ischemia. Variable degrees of transient coronary flow reduction are frequent events during the everyday activities of patients who have ischemic heart disease. In many respects, the ischemic intervals during off-pump coronary artery isolation are comparable with the usually self-limiting, noninjurious ischemia that occurs frequently in coronary patients.

There is now quite a large body of observational experience regarding these intervals, in both minimally invasive direct coronary artery bypass grafting (MIDCAB) and catheter-based procedures. These have been assessed in the setting of comprehensive cardiac monitoring using continuous electrocardiography, transesophageal echocardiography, pulmonary artery pressures, and continuous systemic venous oxygen saturation measurements. Much has been learned from these data and, in a general way, such ischemic intervals appear well tolerated and of little consequence. With diligent and appropriate management of the off-pump grafting situation, these changes can be either totally pre-empted or minimized further, allowing grafting to be completed safely and without undue time constraint. As a result, acute decompensation has become an infrequent event and has not occurred in our last 60 MIDCAB cases.

Of relevance in surgical revascularization is that part of the tolerance of ischemia may also relate to the more distally placed site of vessel isolation during grafting compared with the level of flow interruption in native coronary disease or that induced by catheter methods. A smaller area of myocardium may be affected, and the response, therefore, may be correspondingly less profound. For prevention or reduction of myocardial ischemia during off-pump grafting, several routine pharmacologic protocols are now established as described below.

Reducing Myocardial Oxygen Requirements

Preoperative and intraoperative β-blockade therapy is used to reduce (dP/dt) and heart rate. Patients should continue oral β blockers, including their dose on the morning of operation. Also useful are calcium channel blockers, including diltiazem, infused at a rate of 5 mg per hour. Intraoperative infusions of short-acting β blockers, such as esmolol in doses of 50 to 100 μg/kg per minute, are titrated to optimal effect. Attenuation of myocardial ischemia associated with coronary occlusion during percutaneous balloon catheter ablation has been shown with ultra–short-acting β blockers.[4] The most effective agent with the least cardiodepressant side effect is diltiazem infused at a rate of 5 mg per hour. Afterload reduction is as well an important aspect of diminishing myocardial work and, therefore, oxygen use. Systolic blood pressure should be maintained in a well-defined range that is neither unduly high nor low. Intravenous nitrates are a vital part of this control therapy. Deepening the level of anesthesia and allowing the systemic temperature to decrease by 1 to 2 degrees may be useful in contributing to this aspect of myocardial management. All these methods are dynamically adjusted so as to provide optimal myocardial physiology in this situation.

Enhancing Ischemic Tolerance

Preconditioning the human myocardium for tolerance of ischemia and prevention of stunning remains somewhat elusive and empiric, although the concept has been definitively demonstrated in a variety of animal models.[5–7] In the human situation, a number of clinical observations support preconditioning. The data usually cited relate to the improvement of myocardial contractility and increased ease of defibrillation noted in patients who have successive reperfusion intervals during coronary grafting with intermittent ischemic arrest. Observation of decreasing S-T segment changes seen with progressive balloon inflation during percutaneous transluminal coronary angioplasty (PTCA) has also been described.[8]

There are many series in the literature noting reduced infarct size in patients who have previous unstable angina versus those who have an infarction occurring as the initial event. Both pharmacologic and ischemic methods of preconditioning have been described, and the response is probably maximally beneficial when the two methods are used in combination. The difficulty in demonstrating preconditioning in patients centers, no doubt, around difficulties in quantitating the impact of collateral circulation, size variations in the myocardium perfused by a given vessel (area at risk), and severity and duration of the obstructing lesion. Nonetheless, several articles relating to preconditioning of the human myocardium in a clinical setting have been published.[9–11]

Ischemic preconditioning routines in patients generally follow those proposed in animal studies as described by Downey.[12] Sequential routines aiming at 5 minutes of tolerated ischemia with 5 minutes of reperfusion are carried out. Pharmacologic preconditioning agents have included adenosine, norepinephrine, β blockers, and a variety of other substances. In our own practice of off-pump grafting, we infuse adenosine intravenously at 0.3 mg/kg over 20 minutes before vessel isolation. An additional part of this preconditioning routine includes use of β blockers with infusion of esmolol. The regionally and transiently ischemic myocardium in MIDCAB offers a particularly useful model for future analysis of many aspects of preconditioning.

New Concepts in Averting Injury From Acute Ischemia or Infarction

The effects of sodium-hydrogen exchange blockers on the ischemic myocardium have been evaluated. With anaerobic myocardial cell metabolism during ischemia, the cellular hydrogen ion concentration increases. As a result, the sodium-hydrogen system and, secondarily, the sodium-calcium exchange system are activated.[13] Intracellular calcium levels become elevated, and it is this change that promotes cell death. At least theoretically, any agent that inhibits the sodium-hydrogen exchange system can prevent sodium and calcium overload within the cell, and eventually, prevent or limit cell death.[14] Clinical trials of this principle are currently in progress involving patients receiving PTCA or CABG for unstable angina or infarction. The outcome of this new strategy as a further method of promoting ischemic tolerance will be watched closely.

Various methods of preventing ischemia and maintaining myocardial stability during off-pump grafting involve active and quite complex protocols. Diligent attention to hemodynamic monitoring and early response to correct changes are vital in offsetting both the signs and progression of ischemia. This dynamic process is summarized in Table 62–1. With these measures, the visible evidence of ischemia is reduced to the order of 10 to 20%, most of

Table 62–1. Optimizing Myocardial Physiology

Reduction of Myocardial Oxygen Needs
Reduction of dP/dt
Reduction of heart rate
Afterload reduction
Deepening anesthesia
Systemic temperature fall by 1 degree
Diligent monitoring and hemodynamic control
Enhancing Ischemic Tolerance
Pharmacologic preconditioning
Ischemic preconditioning
Combination
New Concepts of Sodium-Hydrogen Ion Exchange Inhibition

which is transient and modest. The broadening experience of MIDCAB has confirmed that with the above measures the occurrence of ischemia is uncommon and unlikely to be of any consequence, and, as a result, the anastomosis can be completed without undue time constraint.

Pharmacologic Immobilization of the Heart

Satisfactory immobilization of the anastomotic site is critical for CABG. The three principal methods relevant in this area are the production of a quiescent beating heart with relaxed contractility, the induction of bradycardia, and the induction of transient ventricular asystole with pacing back up.

Production of a Globally Quiescent Heart

Pharmacologic therapy for reduction of dP/dT is of vital importance in providing a quiet surgical field as well as for reducing myocardial oxygen consumption. With moderated contractility, heart displacement and immobilization are all facilitated and, in particular, the effectiveness of mechanical stabilizers is dramatically enhanced. To achieve this, coordination between the surgeon and the anesthesiologist is necessary based on data from direct observation of the heart, echocardiography, and hemodynamic monitoring. Concentrated effort and time are required to produce such a quiescent state, and, when achieved, the heart is seen to have an easy, loping action. Pharmacologic agents include clonidine 5 mg on the morning of the operation. Intraoperative titrated infusions of β blockers and calcium channel blockers and nitrates are given. Deepening anesthesia also contributes to this goal.

Induction of Bradycardia

Although initially widely used to facilitate actual anastomotic suturing, induction of bradycardia for this purpose is now regarded as a relatively unimportant part of the off-pump method. Agents used most widely were β blockers, particularly the ultra–short-acting agents, such as esmolol. However, considerable variation exists in their rate-lowering effect, and undue hemodynamic depression may occur. The expected bradycardia of 35 to 40 beats per minute in our experience was achieved and adequately tolerated in only approximately 40% of cases. In many cases, rate may change little, yet hemodynamic compromise may develop. Further, even with induction and tolerance of a heart rate in the vicinity of 35 to 40 beats per minute, in the absence of other stabilization measures, the technical demands of suturing still remain excessive.

Transient Ventricular Asystole With Pacing Backup

Individual suture placement times during cardioplegic coronary grafting are 4 to 5 seconds. The coronary arteriotomy requires 8 to 12 seconds. This time requirement for suturing extrapolates to a heart rate in the vicinity of 15 beats per minute. Because of the inability of predictably achieving such a low rate, and because of the uncertainty of the patient's tolerating it hemodynamically, our group[15] developed the alternative of pharmacologically induced transient complete heart block and ventricular asystole with adenosine and dual or ventricular chamber pacing as backup. Both components of this technique—complete heart block and ventricular asystole—are equally important for safe suturing, because during the asystolic interval the heart must be reliably immobilized and free of escape beats.

Complete Heart Block and Ventricular Asystole Induced by Adenosine

The experience accumulated with this agent is now comprehensive, and our actual technique, dose, administration, and route have been published previously.[16] Adenosine is a biologically occurring nucleoside present in all body cells, which has a half-life of less than 10 seconds. After intravenous injection, there is rapid elimination of adenosine from the blood by erythrocytes and vascular endothelial cells, with conversion by adenylate deaminase to the metabolites adenosine monophosphate and inosine. When given as a rapid central intravenous bolus in doses in the range of 0.2 to 0.4 mg/kg, reliable induction of block and asystole for 5 to 12 seconds occurs. In our early MIDCAB experience, we repeated adenosine boluses up to 8 to 10 times per anastomosis, and this was our main method of cardiac stabilization. To control the asystolic interval to the minimum necessary, pacing backup was used, and the systemic hypotensive effect of adenosine was corrected by using a bolus dose of 100 to 200 μg of neosynephrine. The reflex tachycardia associated with the hypotensive interval is largely minimized by the baseline β blockade.

In our experience, use of β blockers and also deepening anesthesia have appeared effective in suppressing ventricular escape during the pause. With the advent of mechanical stabilizers, however, particularly when used in combination with pharmacologic moderation of myocardial contractility, the routine need for adenosine has been largely eliminated. Nonetheless, we continue to use this technique for difficult toe and heel sutures, grafting small arteries, and hemostatic suture placement for anastomotic bleeding.

Extended Ventricular Asystole With Pacing Control—Experimental Study

Other alternatives have been described, including induction of extended ventricular asystole with pacing control of heart action and transient cessation of pacing for a static surgical field. In a sheep model experiment, Khanna and Cullen[17] induced sustained intervals of complete heart block and ventricular asystole using direct lidocaine infiltration into the area of the bundle of His. Cardiac function was maintained with ventricular or dual pacing and transient cessation of pacing enabled a controlled pause and immobile field for suturing. In their small animal experience using an injection of 2 ml of 2% lidocaine, ventricular escape activity was minimal and pacing response reliable. Concerns with this technique include potential injury to intracardiac structures during injection and to late conduction system dysfunction.

At the First Annual Meeting of the International Society for Minimally Invasive Cardiac Surgery, held in Minneapolis in June 1998, Dr. F. Duyalongsod of Duke University described the use of an unrevealed combination of agents infused directly via an indwelling catheter in the right coronary artery that has resulted in consistent and sustained asystole during which heart function was maintained by pacing. Pacing termination again allowed a pause for suturing. Reversal of the effects of this agent was also feasible. Should this drug combination prove safe and reliable, the technique may be accepted for widespread use not only in off-pump CABG but as an alternative to cardioplegic arrest. The technique will obviate the need for aortic clamping. A further extension of this basic principle could perhaps include use of electrophysiology catheters and radio frequency ablation or temporary freezing of the bundle region for production of the previously described effect. This, however, is likely to be less reliable, and, again, potentially damaging to the conduction system.

Although these techniques are novel, they carry the risk of several potentially adverse effects. The first relates obviously to the hypotensive interval associated not only with the asystolic pause but also with the systemic hypotension produced by adenosine or other substances. Any hypotensive episode is followed by the physiologic responses of vasoconstriction and tachycardia, although the latter is usually controlled with β blockers. Added to this, the technique often includes infusion of a vasoconstrictor for expediting blood pressure recovery. With repetitive use in individual patients and also broader clinical use, this may correlate with an increased incidence of multiorgan ischemia, including aggravation of the myocardial ischemia already associated with the isolated graft artery and possibly the gastrointestinal tract, kidney, and brain. This has not been seen in our experience with adenosine, however.

The second potential problem is the incidence of breakthrough extrasystoles and the risk of repolarization arrhythmias. Acetylcholine was used initially for controlled induction of asystole, which enables early coronary angiography. Repolarization arrhythmias and extrasystoles were a major problem with that method. Again, in our experience with adenosine in patients who have received adequate amounts of β blocker and anesthesia, extrasystoles were uncommon and no significant repolarization arrhythmias occurred. Delivery of these agents into the right coronary artery would no doubt enable improved dose response curves and substantially reduce systemic effects. Another concern relates to the persistently beating atria in the presence of ventricular standstill. This leads to progressive ventricular dilatation with raised wall tension and possible impairment of coronary flow. A final issue is the actual facility of grafting onto a heart that is alternating through a process of beating and pausing. These interesting methods may, however, with further refinement, establish themselves widely in these operations and also have applications in other areas of cardiovascular medicine in cardiac imaging.

Methods of pharmacologic control are comprehensive and include therapy for myocardial ischemic protection as well as for surgical field immobilization. They represent one component of several interventions required to achieve a satisfactory environment for completion of safe and accurate grafting off pump.

Mechanical Control

The rapid advance in the development of mechanical stabilization devices has established them as the most important current method of achieving satisfactory anastomotic field immobilization. Two basic principles are common: The regional immobilization by suction devices, of which the Octopus is currently the most widely used, and which is fully described (see Chapter 63); and local pressure devices, which most commonly use a foot-shaped or rectangular frame. Many varieties and modifications are available, and others no doubt will emerge with future design. The foot device applies local pressure on the epicardium on either side of the grafted vessel. This effectively dissipates the propagated systolic wave and immobilizes the graft site within a bridge of myocardium. Immobilization is enhanced further by using a closed rectangular frame that also compresses the coronary artery and facilitates control of bleeding from the arteriotomy. As described earlier, mechanical immobilization methods are greatly facilitated by pharmacologic control of myocardial contractility. For maximal stability, the foot device should be applied at right angles to the epicardial surface. Care should be taken to avoid protrusion of the ends of the foot into the beating myocardium. The immobilized segment is often visible on transesophageal echocardiography as an akinetic area. With effective pharmacologic control and careful positioning of the mechanical device, adequate coronary artery immobilization is achieved.

As in many aspects of minimally invasive coronary surgery, mechanical immobilization of the heart is in an early stage of development, and, no doubt, other effective and more sophisticated systems will emerge.

References

1. Benneti RJ, Ballester C, Sani G, et al: Video assisted coronary artery bypass surgery. J Card Surg 10:620–625, 1995.
2. Robinson MC, Gross DR, Seman W, et al: Minimally invasive coronary artery bypass grafting: A new method using an anterior mediastinotomy. J Card Surg 10:529–536, 1995.
3. Subramanian VA, Sani G, Benneti FJ, et al: Minimally invasive direct coronary bypass surgery: A multi-center report of preliminary clinical experience. Circulation 92:1–645, 1995.
4. Labovitz AJ, Barth C, Costello R, et al: Attenuation of myocardial ischemia during coronary occlusion by ultrashort acting beta adrenergic blockade. Am Heart J 5:1247–1351, 1991.
5. Miyamae M, Fujiwara H, Kida M, et al: Preconditioning improves energy metabolism during reperfusion but does not attenuate myocardial stunning in porcine hearts. Circulation 88:223–234, 1993.
6. Cohen M, Liu G, Downey J: Preconditioning causes improved wall motion as well as smaller infarcts afer transient coronary occlusion in rabbits. Circulation 84:341–349, 1991.
7. Lasley RD, Zhou Z, Hegge JO, et al: Adenosine attenuates in vivo myocardial stunning with minimal effects on cardiac energetics. Basic Res Cardiol 93:303–312, 1998.

8. Leesar M, Stoddard M, Ahmed M, et al: Preconditioning of human myocardium with adenosine during coronary angioplasty. Circulation 95:2500–2507, 1997.
9. Lee T, LaFaro R, Reed G: Pretreatment of human myocardium with adenosine during open heart surgery. J Card Surg 10: 665–676, 1995.
10. Alkhulaifi AM, Yellon DM, Pugsley WB. Preconditioning the human heart during aorto-coronary bypass surgery. Eur J Cardiothorac Surg 8:270–276, 1994.
11. Lasley RD, Mentzer RM: Preconditioning and its potential role in myocardial protection during cardiac surgery. J Card Surg 10:349–353, 1995.
12. Cohen M, Liu G, Downey J. See Reference 6.
13. Scholz, W, Albus U: Potential of selective sodium-hydrogen exchange inhibitors in cardiovascular therapy. Cardiovasc Res 29:184–188, 1995.
14. Conti R: New concept for treatment of acute myocardial ischemia. Clin Cardiol 21:A32, 1998.
15. Robinson MC, Thielmeier K, Hill B: Transient ventricular asystole using adenosine during minimally invasive and open sternotomy coronary artery bypass grafting. Ann Thorac Surg 63: S30–S34, 1997.
16. Robinson MC, Thielmeier K, Hill B: See Reference 16.
17. Khanna R, Cullen HC: Coronary artery surgery with induced temporary asystole and intermittent ventricular pacing: An experimental study. Card Surg 4:231–236, 1996.

COMMENTARY

Robert W. Emery

Drs. Robinson and Jahania present an excellent in-depth view of current methods of myocardial stabilization during the conduct of off-pump bypass surgery. The first and most important of several issues stressed by the authors is that minimally invasive off-pump coronary artery surgery is a team effort. Excellent communication between the surgical team and the anesthesia team is imperative. A cooperative effort minimizes any untoward myocardial side effects or untoward patient effects that might occur during regional ischemia and fosters a milieu for construction of a patulous anastomosis. Performance of various maneuvers by both anesthesiologist and surgeon, as well as delivery of any pharmacologic therapy, must be coordinated with the knowledge of other individuals to maximize the safety and efficiency of the operation. Moreover, regional myocardial ischemia is well tolerated with proper preparation; an exception to this rule is a large right coronary system. In the majority of cases, this allows anastomotic construction in an orderly yet timely fashion. Finally, mechanical stabilization, although still an adjunct, has become the most important means of offering a quiet field in which to perform coronary anastomosis. Multiple methods of regional and global stabilization may be necessary for working in concert to achieve the quiescent field desired. This is particularly the case when the surgery is directed away from the anterior descending artery, requiring application of myocardial traction as well as stabilization.

The concept of myocardial stabilization is in its infancy, and we can expect new and interesting developments over the next several years, especially as we enter the field of robotically enabled cardiovascular surgery.

Chapter 63

Off-Pump Coronary Artery Bypass Grafting Using the "Octopus" Device*

Erik W. L. Jansen, Jaap R. Lahpor, Arno P. Nierich, Pieter R. Stella, Egidius van Aarnhem, and Johan J. Bredée

In 1964, Kolesov[1] successfully performed left internal thoracic artery (ITA) grafting to the left anterior descending artery (LAD) on the beating heart through a left thoracotomy access (see Chapter 49). In the following years, only South American surgeons Benetti and Buffolo and associates[2, 3] persisted in off-pump coronary artery bypass grafting, CABG, guided by surgical-technical and economic motives (see Chapter 59). Difficulties in stabilizing the anastomosis site by using stay sutures and vessel loops alone prevented widespread application. Recently, the aspiration toward minimally invasive thoracic surgery has induced the development of specific local cardiac wall stabilizers. These stabilizers play a fundamental role in safe off-pump CABG.

This chapter describes the clinical and angiographic outcomes of off-pump CABG with the Octopus tissue stabilizer. An outline of the properties and capacities of suction fixation are presented.

Methods

The Octopus tissue stabilizer is described extensively elsewhere.[4, 5] The device (Fig. 63–1) consists of two paddles with four or five suction domes, each of which has an internal diameter of 6 mm. Each paddle is fixed by an articulating arm attached to the rail of the operating table or to opposite rails (Fig. 63–2). The shorter the arm (paddle and articulating arm), the better the stiffness. Preparation is carried out in the "thaw" mode of the arm. Once both paddles are selected and adjusted to the cardiac surface by prebending the malleable segment with two thumbs, suction is activated in each paddle separately. The arm is then "frozen" by tightening the bolt moderately. Immobilization in the x and y direction to 1 × 1 mm is effective when suction has reached −400 mm Hg. Additional immobilization in the z direction is achieved by slightly stretching the epicardium. The epicardium is stretched by subtly spreading the paddles, which, in turn, results in a residual target motion of about 1 × 1 × 1 mm.[4] Finally, when immobilization is accomplished, the target site is presented by moving both paddles simultaneously in the frozen mode. In animal experiments, the current practice of using the table rails and the two-arm system has proved effective and versatile with respect to different surgical approaches.

Clinical experience with the Octopus stabilizer dates from September 1995. By January 1998, 1639 patients underwent complete revascularization for isolated coronary artery disease. The off-pump technique was used with the Octopus method in 150 patients (9%). More recently, this number has increased to 14%. The preoperative characteristics of these patients are summarized in Table 63–1. The inclusion and exclusion criteria have been reported elsewhere.[6] Briefly, patients were included who had invalidating angina according to the New York Heart Association (NYHA) class III and class IV based on subtotal and total isolated proximal coronary artery disease (>70% angiographic diameter stenosis) refractory to medical treatment and catheter-based procedures. Patients who had unstable angina (Braunwald classes IIc and IIIc), those who had diffuse disease requiring long anastomoses, those who required more than four anastomoses or endarterectomies, or those who had a suspected intramyocardial LAD were excluded. Poor left ventricular function was not an exclusion criterion, except when exposure of the target vessel would mean considerable displacement of the heart, for example, posterior wall exposure through sternotomy access. Posterior wall revascularization was performed only in patients who had one dominant circumflex branch. In 8 high-risk patients, conventional on-pump CABG procedures were considered contraindicated because of complicated previous cardiac surgery, poor left ventricular function (2 patients), or associated disease (3 patients). Two patients who had a left ventricular ejection fraction less than 20% were operated on using intra-aortic balloon pumping (IABP). In the protocol, the following intraoperative data were sampled online, event-related, and stored in a computer: mean arterial blood pressure, heart rate, transit time of cardiac output, cardiac index, mixed venous oxygen saturation, and ST segment changes in lead V_5. All patients were prepared as for conventional CABG to enable conversion of strategy if necessary. Normothermia was maintained with a warm-water blanket. General anesthesia consisted of intravenous propofol and high-dose sufentanil-citrate. More recently, in the absence of coagulation disorders, a combination of general and regional thoracic anesthesia was used and consisted of intravenous propofol with low-dose sufentanil-citrate and bupivacaine 0.5% respectively. This facilitates perioperative management—blockade of the hormonal stress response, regional chemical sympathetic blockade, thoracic vasodilation of the coronary arteries (and collaterals), better control of circulation, improved analgesia, and improved postoperative respiratory function.[7]

* The study was supported by grants from the Netherlands Heart Foundation (No. 1993/43.028) and the University Hospital, Utrecht (No. 1995/B903).

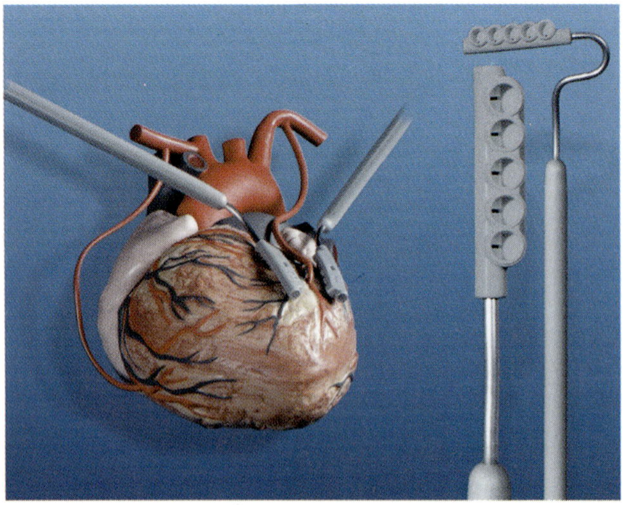

Figure 63–1. The Octopus tissue stabilizer on a heart model with two internal thoracic artery grafts. The straight and preformed paddles are shown. The straight version is used for a lengthwise approach, and the preformed paddles are used for a more perpendicular approach to the vessel. Note the asymmetrical configuration and malleable segment for adjustment to the surface of the heart.

Surgical Access and Grafting

The surgical technique is described in detail elsewhere.[5, 6] The surgical access routes are shown in Figure 63–2. Briefly, limited access (i.e., the small left anterior thoracotomy and subxiphoid laparotomy) was used for one-vessel disease. Full access (i.e., sternotomy and posterior thoracotomy) were used for two- and three-vessel disease. The anterior and inferior cardiac walls were easy to expose. Posterior wall exposure (tilting of the heart), however, required fluid supplementation and redistribution of blood volume (Trendelenburg maneuver).[8] Sometimes inotropic drug support was also necessary to maintain an adequate cardiac index and arterial blood pressure. For technical reasons (a wide-angled fork), the sternotomy approach was also used for three sequential diagnonal/LAD artery grafts. The left posterolateral thoracotomy was used for one- and two-vessel grafting. This approach is particularly useful in patients undergoing reoperation, in whom sternotomy is contraindicated. Because the heart stays in its pericardial cradle, hemodynamics are not compromised.

After immobilization, the patient was given heparin (1.5 mg/kg) intravenously. The coronary artery was then occluded for 5 minutes to evaluate signs of ischemic dysfunction. Five minutes of reperfusion was then carried out for preconditioning before occlusion of the artery to construct the anastomosis. The coronary artery was dissected free over 15 mm to allow a 4-mm arteriotomy between two atraumatic microvascular clamps (Acland clamps, S & T Marketing, Neuhausen, Switzerland). This type of grafting is depicted in Figure 63–3.

Revascularization Assessment Criteria

Electrocardiograms were recorded at least twice during admission, and serial myocardial fractions of creatine kinase (CK-MB) were determined six times up to 48 hours after surgery. Perioperative myocardial infarction was diagnosed in the presence of one or both of the following criteria: CK-MB levels greater than 50 IU, development of new Q waves, or both. Repeat angiography was scheduled for all patients 6 months after the procedure. The mean follow-up was 13 months, with a range of 2 to 30 months. Follow-up information was collected through direct patient contact and from the referring cardiologist. Clinical outcome was assessed according to the Canadian Cardiovascular Society (CCS) and NYHA and by exercise testing at 3 months.

Statistical Analysis

All data are presented as mean ± SD or as a median and range. An unpaired Student t-test was used to compare intraoperative mean values, using limited and full access techniques.

Results

The Octopus tissue stabilizer immobilized and presented the target site effectively through all access routes. The operative data are summarized in Table 63–2. Inadvertent detachment of the suction paddles never occurred during anastomosis suturing. Prompt treatment of false air suction by longitudinal or axial adjustment of the paddle to the epicardium prevented detachment.

Suturing of a bleeding suction hematoma[9] was necessary in 1 of 2740 lesions (0.03% of 274 anastomoses with 2 × 5 × 274 lesions). The hematomas tended to resolve within 10 minutes, and, moreover, most were restricted to the fatty tissue accompanying the vessels. Temporary segmental occlusion of the coronary artery occasionally caused 1- to 2-mm ST segment changes that lasted a few minutes. The effect on hemodynamics of local cardiac wall immobilization by suction was low.[7] Intraoperative continuous inotropic drug support (dopamine, >2 μg/kg) was necessary in 46 patients (31%). In 44% of sternotomy cases, dopamine was required for exposure of the posterior wall. Conversion to cardiopulmonary bypass (CPB) was necessary in 3 patients (2%) (in 1 patient because of hemodynamics compromised by ischemia). The procedure was converted to CPB without aortic cross-clamping. In 2 patients, conversion to CPB was necessary for an underrated coronary pathologic condition. Conversion to CPB was avoided in another patient in whom occlusion of the right coronary artery was not tolerated, using a temporary aortocoronary shunt. In 3 patients, a sternotomy was performed along with an anterior thoracotomy because of underrated LAD artery disease combined with insufficient conduit length. In these patients, grafting was performed during CPB. With respect to harvesting the arterial conduits, damage to the left ITA occurred three times (all female patients) early in the series. The damage could be repaired in 2 patients.

Postoperative Course

There was no operative mortality. In the majority of patients, recovery was fast and uneventful. Extubation was performed in 96% of patients in the first hours after surgery, and the stay in the intensive care unit was 24 hours.

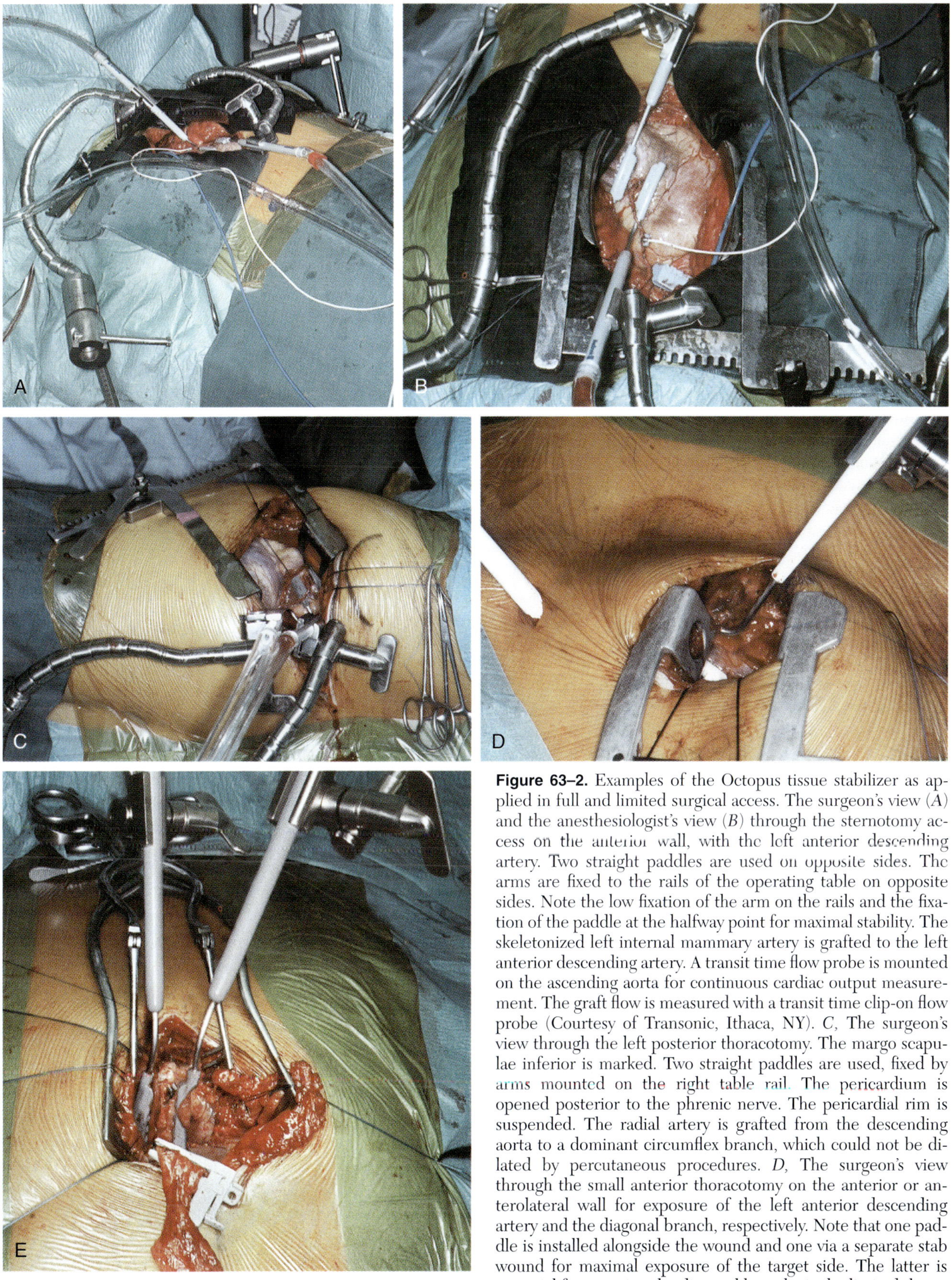

Figure 63–2. Examples of the Octopus tissue stabilizer as applied in full and limited surgical access. The surgeon's view (*A*) and the anesthesiologist's view (*B*) through the sternotomy access on the anterior wall, with the left anterior descending artery. Two straight paddles are used on opposite sides. The arms are fixed to the rails of the operating table on opposite sides. Note the low fixation of the arm on the rails and the fixation of the paddle at the halfway point for maximal stability. The skeletonized left internal mammary artery is grafted to the left anterior descending artery. A transit time flow probe is mounted on the ascending aorta for continuous cardiac output measurement. The graft flow is measured with a transit time clip-on flow probe (Courtesy of Transonic, Ithaca, NY). *C,* The surgeon's view through the left posterior thoracotomy. The margo scapulae inferior is marked. Two straight paddles are used, fixed by arms mounted on the right table rail. The pericardium is opened posterior to the phrenic nerve. The pericardial rim is suspended. The radial artery is grafted from the descending aorta to a dominant circumflex branch, which could not be dilated by percutaneous procedures. *D,* The surgeon's view through the small anterior thoracotomy on the anterior or anterolateral wall for exposure of the left anterior descending artery and the diagonal branch, respectively. Note that one paddle is installed alongside the wound and one via a separate stab wound for maximal exposure of the target side. The latter is essential for exposing the diagonal branch via the limited thoracotomy by rotation of the heart. The arms are fixed to opposite sides of the table. *E,* The view caudally through a small subxiphoid laparotomy on the inferior wall of the heart for exposure of the distal right and the proximal right posterior descending artery. The arms are fixed to opposite sides of the table. The gastroepiploic artery has been prepared and the distal right coronary artery is occluded temporarily with a microvascular Acland clamp.

Table 63–1. Patient Characteristics

		n	%
Sex			
Male		111	74
Female		39	26
Age (yr)		60 ± 10 (range 35–81 years)	
NYHA class			
I		0	0
II		3	2
III		134	89
IV		13	9
One-vessel disease		88	59
Two-vessel disease		52	35
Three-vessel disease		10	6
LVEF >40%		127	85
20–40%		21	14
<20%		2	1
Not suitable for PTCA		113	75
Previous PTCA		37	25
failed	21		
restenosis	16		
Hypercholesterolemia		70	47
Previous myocardial infarction		54	36
Smoking history		43	29
Diabetes mellitus		18	12
Prior stroke		14	9
Previous cardiac surgery		12	8
Peripheral vascular disease		9	6

LVEF = left ventricular ejection fraction; PTCA = percutaneous transluminal coronary angioplasty.

Complications

The median peak CK-MB was 13 U/L (range 2 to 257 U/L). Myocardial infarction occurred in 7 patients (5%): 2 of these patients required IABP for low cardiac output. Myocardial infarction related to the grafted vessel occurred in 1 patient in whom conversion to sternotomy was necessary. One patient required percutaneous transluminal coronary angioplasty of an ungrafted artery (identification error) and 5 days' continuation of preoperatively initiated intra-aortic balloon pumping because of intraoperative myocardial infarction. In another patient, distal tapering of the right ITA required revision to a free graft, again performed off-pump using the Octopus method. This tapering was detected on routine angiography performed during admission of the first 10 patients.

One patient suffered prolonged respiratory insufficiency caused by kyphoscoliosis with extremely restricted lung function. Reversible ischemic neurologic deficits occurred in 2 patients who had pre-existing cerebrovascular insufficiency, in whom a free ITA anastomosis had been constructed on the ascending aorta. The procedure had been converted to CPB in 1 of these 2 patients. None of the patients experienced mental disorders. In 5 of the first 10 patients in the anterior thoracotomy group, an early pericarditis was observed electrocardiographically. This was probably related to a dry gauze pad that was used to improve exposure. The median postoperative length of the hospital stay was 5 days in the limited-access group and 7 days in the full-access group. Within 1 month after surgery, 97% of patients had resumed their premorbid activities. The postoperative data are summarized in Table 63–3.

Follow-Up

There was a 100% complete follow-up. Two patients died. One patient, a 74-year-old man, died because of a fatal intracerebral bleeding episode after a repeat 6-month angiography (with all grafts patent). The second patient, who had poor left ventricular function without residual ischemia, died because of presumably fatal arrhythmia despite an internal defibrillator inserted because of proven sustained ventricular tachycardia. At the 13-month follow-up (range 3 to 30 months), 99% of the surviving patients were in CCS class I. There was one successful late balloon angioplasty of an anastomosis site.

Exercise testing was performed 6 months after operation in 92% of patients, including 3 patients who refused recatheterization. Signs of ischemia were present in 2 patients. Six-month follow-up angiography was performed in

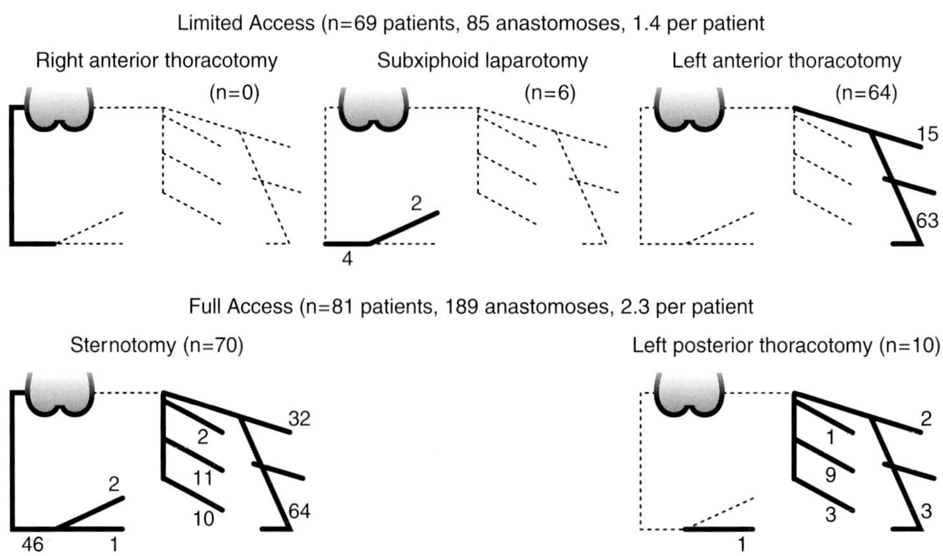

Figure 63–3. Types of access and bypassed vessels.

Table 63–2. Operative Data

	Limited Access (n = 69 Patients)	Full Access (n = 81 Patients)	*P* Value
Arterial grafts	53 (98%)	82 (94%)	
Total distal anastomoses	85	189	
with arterial grafts	63 (98%)	101 (94%)	
Sequential anastomoses per graft	16 (23%)	40 (26%)	
Anastomoses per patient (average)	1.4	2.3	
Left ITA harvesting time (minutes)	44 ± 13	24 ± 8	*P* <.0001
Right ITA harvesting time (minutes)	—	23 ± 7	
Anastomosis time (minutes)	18 ± 8	15 ± 5	NS
Immobilization-presentation time per anastomosis (minutes)*	42 ± 14	30 ± 9	*P* <.0001
Surgery time (minutes)	183 ± 45	231 ± 40	*P* <.0001
Conversion to CPB	1†	1† + 1‡	
Conversion to full access	3†	—	

* Including coronary artery preparation time, 5 minutes preconditioning ischemia, and 5 minutes reperfusion.
† For technical reasons.
‡ Because of ischemia.
ITA = internal thoracic artery; CPB = cardiopulmonary bypass; NS = not statistically significant.

Table 63–3. Postoperative Data (0 to 30 Months Follow-Up)

	Limited Access n (%)	Full Access n (%)
Mortality		
operative	0 (0)	0 (0)
late	1 (1)	1 (1)
Operative myocardial infarction	3 (4)	4 (5)
Low output requiring IABP	0 (0)	2 (2)
Reinterventions (during admission)		
bleeding	0 (0)	1 (1)
revision of anastomosis*	0 (0)	1 (1)
PTCA of ungrafted vessel†	0 (0)	1 (1)
Reversible ischemic neurologic deficit	1 (1)	1 (1)
Paroxysmal atrial fibrillation	9 (13)	14 (17)
Acute noninfectious pericarditis‡	8 (12)	1 (1)
Pleural effusion	5 (7)	4 (5)
Gastrointestinal bleeding	0 (0)	2 (1)
Wound infection	1 (1)	0 (0)
Use of blood products (patients)	8 (12)	19 (23)
Postoperative hospital stay (median, range)	5 (2–31)	7 (3–44)
Readmissions	12§	1†
Coronary reinterventions after initial discharge	1‖	0

* Revision of the right internal thoracic artery to the right coronary artery because of too much tapering of the distal graft.
† Patient who had poor left ventricular function.
‡ Five patients were among the first 10 patients; see §.
§ Four patients for pain associated with pericarditis.
‖ Balloon angioplasty of anastomosis site.
IABP = intra-aortic balloon pumping; PTCA = percutaneous transluminal coronary angioplasty.

87 of the first 100 (87%) patients, representing 149 of 172 anastomoses. Of these, nine anastomoses could not be visualized because selective injection of the grafts (four gastroepiploic arteries [GEPAs], two free ITAs, and two right ITAs) failed. The overall patency rate was 95%. Six anastomoses were occluded, related to sequential grafting in the early experience. All single left ITA grafts to the LAD artery were patent.

Discussion

The key to successful off-pump CABG is mechanical stabilization, whether by pressure or by suction fixation. Each method has its specific applications. Retractor-mounted pressure fixation has been used increasingly, with excellent results in a large series using single left ITA grafting to the LAD artery via anterior thoracotomy.[10] The two-arm stabilizer that is mounted on the rails of the operating table, as described in this chapter, proved to be an effective immobilization and presentation method for all major coronary arteries; a versatile method, with any incision, and effective even in a closed-chest approach[4]; and without adverse effects. In this experience, suction fixation was used through an anterior thoracotomy (including 23% sequential diagonal grafts/LAD grafts), subxiphoid approach, or thoracotomy and sternotomy for two- and three-vessel grafting. Stabilization by suction was well tolerated hemodynamically because it compromises a small quantity of myocardium containing the target vessel. Therefore, it may also be considered in patients who have poor left ventricular function.

Exposure of the posterior wall was tolerated provided that dislocation was performed slowly and by avoiding kinking of the inflow tract of the heart. Fluid redistribution (Trendelenburg maneuver)[8] or administration, along with inotropic drug support (dopamine in 44% of patients), helped maintain arterial pressure. This might also be explained by the small quantity of myocardium that is fixed while the remaining myocardium is unrestrained. Still, selection of candidates for posterior wall revascularization through sternotomy is strict. Apart from the posterior wall revascularization, the left ventricular dysfunction seems to be a relative exclusion criterion.

The accuracy of the immobilization was reflected in a 95% patency rate. Optimal exposure of the anastomosis site by two microvascular clamps may be fundamental. The clinical outcome of off-pump CABG is promising. The median hospitalization was relatively short (5 to 7 days, a reduction of ±2 days in our institution), and premorbid activities were resumed within one month. At 3- to 30-month follow-up, 99% of 148 patients were in the CCS class I. These results encouraged us to expand the off-pump CABG procedure to 13% in early 1998.

Advantages of Off-Pump Bypass Surgery

The major advantage to off-pump bypass surgery is avoiding CPB and global cardiac arrest. Thus, neuropsychological deficits caused by malperfusion, microemboli from CPB, and atheromatous emboli from manipulation of the aorta may be avoided.[11] In our experience, no stroke with permanent deficit and no delirium occurred. Using the Society of Thoracic Surgery Registry format, off-pump CABG had significantly fewer overall neurologic complications ($P < .001$) and less delirium ($P < .01$) compared with a comparable group in our institution matched for age, elective surgery, and surgeon. The rapid psychosomatic recovery of the patients was striking, and cognitive functions appeared to be well preserved in these patients but were not formally tested. Undoubtedly, there is morbidity, reflecting the learning curve—for example, acute sterile pericarditis leading to early readmissions. The results justify that off-pump CABG be considered in patients who have associated disease, especially cerebrovascular insufficiency, and also in elderly patients in whom in-hospital mortality may be as high as 11.5%.[12]

Limitations

Patients who have diffuse coronary artery disease requiring long anastomoses and multiple (more than four) grafts and those with an intramyocardial LAD artery are unsuitable candidates. The globally arrested heart allows more time-efficient bypass grafting when compared with installing a stabilizer for each vessel separately.

The standard of comparison will be on-pump CABG using the left ITA to the LAD artery as single-vessel CABG[13] and multivessel CABG, the latter with a long-term 96% patency rate of the left ITA.[14] Using arterial grafts, in this series 96% favorable long-term patency may be expected. Although there is a learning curve for this type of CABG on the beating heart, the initial results are encouraging and seem to be cost-effective. Randomized studies have been initiated in our institution to compare off-pump CABG using the Octopus with conventional CABG with CPB and to percutaneous transluminal coronary angioplasty with stenting.

Conclusion

By effective local cardiac wall immobilization, the Octopus tissue stabilizer facilitated limited and full-access CABG without CPB for selected patients who had single- and multiple-vessel disease.

ACKNOWLEDGMENTS

The authors gratefully acknowledge the assistance of Dr. H Wesenhagen, HJ Mansvelt Beck, JP van der Brugge, T Maikoe, and J de Witte.

References

1. Kolesov VI: Mammary artery–coronary artery anastomosis as method of treatment for angina pectoris. J Thorac Cardiovasc Surg 54:535–544, 1967.
2. Benetti FJ, Naselli G, Wood M, Geffner L: Direct myocardial revascularization without extracorporeal circulation. Experience in 700 patients. Chest 100:312–316, 1991.
3. Buffolo E, Andrade JCS, Branco JNR, et al: Coronary artery bypass grafting without cardiopulmonary bypass. Ann Thorac Surg 61:63–66, 1996.
4. Borst C, Jansen EWL, Tulleken CF, et al: Coronary artery bypass grafting without cardiopulmonary bypass and without interruption of native coronary flow using a novel anastomosis site restraining device ("Octopus"). J Am Coll Cardiol 27:1356–1364, 1996.
5. Jansen EWL, Lahpor JL, Borst C, et al: Off-pump coronary bypass grafting: How to use the "Octopus" tissue stabilizer. Ann Thorac Surg 66:576–579, 1998.
6. Jansen EWL, Borst C, Lahpor JL, et al: Coronary artery bypass grafting without cardiopulmonary bypass using the "Octopus" method: Results in the first 100 patients. J Thorac Cardiovasc Surg 116:60–67, 1998.
7. Desborough JP: Thoracic epidural analgesia in cardiac surgery. Anesthesia 51:805–807, 1996.
8. Gründeman PF, Borst C, van Herwaarden JA, et al: Hemodynamic changes during displacement of the beating heart by the Utrecht "Octopus" method. Ann Thorac Surg 63:S88–92, 1997.
9. Jansen EWL, Gründeman PF, Borst C: Mechanical techniques for local cardiac wall stabilization. *In* Mack M, Landreneau R, Cohen R (eds): Minimally Invasive Cardiac Surgery. St. Louis, Quality Medical Publishing, (in press).
10. Calafiore AM, Di Giammarco G, Teodori G, et al: Left anterior descending coronary artery grafting via left anterior small thoracotomy without cardiopulmonary bypass. Ann Thorac Surg 61:1658–1665, 1996.
11. Moody DM, Brown WR, Challa VR, et al: Brain emboli associated with cardiopulmonary bypass: A histologic and magnetic resonance imaging study. Ann Thorac Surg 59:1304–1306, 1995.
12. Peterson ED, Cowper PA, Jollis JG et al: Outcomes of coronary artery bypass graft surgery in 24,461 patients aged 80 years or older. Circulation 92(suppl II):85–91, 1995.
13. Ovrum E, Tangen G, Holen EA: Facing the era of minimally invasive coronary grafting: Current results of conventional bypass grafting for single-vessel disease. Ann Thorac Surg 64:159–162, 1997.
14. Loop FD, Lytle BW, Cosgrove DM, et al: Influence of left internal mammary artery graft on 10 year survival and other cardiac events. N Engl J Med 314:1–6, 1986.

COMMENTARY

Enio Buffolo

The idea of immobilizing the surface of the heart with special devices focused extraordinary interest on myocardial revascularization in a beating heart.

Despite the fact that surgeons have responded to this challenge for many years and have accumulated experience without the aid of a stabilizer, we consider this device to be helpful in the modern era of less invasive myocardial revascularization.

The concept of a stabilizer was originally developed for use in the left anterior small thoracotomy approach, but with increasing experience it has been possible to expand its use to the sternotomy approach.

Our group and many others have increased the applicability of the "non-pump" technique of myocardial revascularization because of the possibility of exposing and stabilizing marginal branches.

At the beginning of our experience, the applicability of this approach was 20%, but by 1997 it had reached 36.1%.

The creation of the Utrecht Octopus device was of great importance in the development of this type of myocardial revascularization, because with immobilization of the coronary arteries, suturing of the same quality as that which is used in conventional anastomosis in an arrested heart can be performed more easily, and many steps of the learning curve can be eliminated.

Basically, we agree with Dr. Jansen's recommendations, and we avoid extracorporeal circulation in critically ill patients who have significant comorbidities.

Because we are working in the Southern Hemisphere (Brazil), the majority of published papers have projected the point of view our initial experiences with this surgery were prompted by cost-saving considerations. This concept is wrong. We use off-pump myocardial revascularization because we think it is a superior treatment of coronary insufficiency. Lower cost is a consequence and not the original purpose.

Dr. Jansen mentioned the preconditioning principle before starting the anastomosis. I am not sure that this is important, especially for the left anterior descending, diagonal, and marginal branches. I do not judge it necessary unless at least 15 minutes of coronary blood flow interruption is to occur.

There may be problems in dominant right coronary arteries without tight stenosis. Coronary occlusion for longer periods may cause hypotension and heart block. In these cases, we have ready access to a device to perfuse the distal right coronary artery if necessary.

Finally, I fully agree with Dr. Jansen's experience that the postoperative recovery of patients operated on without CPB is far better than that of a control group in the same institution. There is earlier recovery, fewer neurologic, pulmonary, and other complications, and earlier hospital discharge.

Chapter 64

Limited Incision Coronary Surgery With Cardiopulmonary Bypass Support

Pyng Jing Lin, Jaw-Ji Chu, and Chau-Hsiung Chang

Coronary artery bypass grafting is classically carried out with median sternotomy. However, the poor cosmetic effect and possible complications of median sternotomy are occasionally troublesome.

Surgical invasiveness determines the severity of postoperative physiologic derangement and its effect on recovery.[54] The benefits of a minimally invasive approach with less surgical trauma have been adopted by an increasing number of surgical specialties.[33] Technologic advances allow miniaturized incisions to be made during surgery. Minimally invasive laparoscopic and thoracoscopic surgical techniques can be applied to replace well-established, safe, and minimally complicated standard procedures such as cholecystectomy for gallstones or bullectomy for pneumothorax, without compromising treatment and safety.[33] In recent years, the concept of minimally invasive surgery has been introduced in the milieu of cardiac surgery.[1, 5, 10, 11, 13, 14, 16, 17, 23, 27–29, 53] These surgeries have been performed through minithoracotomy with or without cardiopulmonary bypass support. The aim of these surgeries is to lessen incisional pain, minimize incisional length, enhance functional recovery, and shorten hospital stay.[37]

Limited Incision Coronary Surgery for One-Vessel Disease

Limited incision coronary surgery for one-vessel coronary artery disease had been performed in the beating heart without extracorporeal circulation by snaring the coronary artery and reducing blood pressure and heart rate pharmacologically through limited left anterior thoracotomy.[1, 5–7, 11, 12, 20, 24, 35, 36, 44, 51, 54] The left internal thoracic artery is harvested either under direct vision or with the assistance of a thoracoscope.[5] The anastomosis between the left internal thoracic artery and the left coronary artery is performed under direct vision with or without the assistance of a stabilizer.[8, 9, 19, 43] This has resulted in a great deal of enthusiasm and is gaining acceptance among cardiac surgeons and cardiologists. However, limited access and the beating heart restrict the indications for this operation to severe disease of the left anterior descending coronary artery. The vast majority of patients who undergo coronary artery bypass grafting, usually those who have triple-vessel disease, cannot benefit from this kind of minimally invasive procedure.

Limited Incision Coronary Surgery With Femorofemoral Cardiopulmonary Bypass and Fibrillatory Arrest

In cardiac surgery, cardiopulmonary bypass can be performed through cannulation of the femoral artery and vein[21, 25, 26] with excellent results. Limited incision cardiac surgery for correction of coronary artery disease or intracardiac lesions can be performed with the use of femorofemoral cardiopulmonary bypass.[13–15, 17, 27–31, 38, 39, 46, 53] Cardiopulmonary bypass can be established through cannulation of the femoral artery and femoral vein and can provide satisfactory perfusion of all vital organs, including the brain. Using modern vascular techniques and good suture material, the complications of femoral cannulation can be reduced to a minimum. However, in patients who have peripheral vascular occlusive disease, these techniques should not be used.

Infusion of a cardioplegic solution is the standard procedure for myocardial protection. Continuous coronary perfusion with fibrillatory arrest is currently used as a method of myocardial protection.[2–4] The aorta is not cross-clamped and the heart is protected by continuous coronary perfusion with fibrillatory arrest, without the infusion of a cardioplegic solution. Topical cooling of the heart can be applied to facilitate fibrillation of the heart, enhance myocardial protection, and avoid deep hypothermia. Fibrillatory arrest can provide a quiet and steady operative field. For short cardiac procedures, the myocardial function is well preserved. In the early experience with limited incision coronary surgery, this method also provided good myocardial protection.[13–15, 27–30, 53]

Our experience of limited incision coronary surgery for revascularization in patients with one- or two-vessel coronary artery disease using continuous coronary perfusion with fibrillatory arrest demonstrated that the stenotic coronary arteries can be revascularized with left internal thoracic arterial grafts or right gastroepiploic arterial grafts in a steady and motionless operative field.[29] In our series, continuous coronary perfusion with fibrillatory arrest also provided prompt cardiac arrest and decompression of the heart. Indeed, fibrillatory arrest is a simple and effective method of myocardial protection that can be applied in uncomplicated coronary artery surgery. All practicing cardiac surgeons can, without any special training, perform limited incision coronary surgery under continuous coronary perfusion with fibrillatory arrest.

Limited Incision Coronary Surgery With Port Access Endovascular Cardiopulmonary Bypass System

Limited incision coronary surgery with endovascular cardiopulmonary bypass has been used in animal experiments, cadaver studies, and patients.[3, 18, 40–42, 46, 47, 49, 50] This system includes the following:

1. Femorofemoral cardiopulmonary bypass
2. Transfemoral endoclamp device for endovascular

aortic occlusion, delivery of cardioplegic solution, and left ventricular decompression
3. Transjugular endovascular pulmonary artery venting catheter
4. Transjugular endovascular coronary sinus perfusion catheter for retrograde delivery of cardioplegic solution

Port access technology allows endovascular aortic occlusion, cardioplegia delivery, and left ventricular decompression. The endoaortic clamp is a triple-lumen catheter with an inflatable balloon at its distal end. Antegrade cardioplegia is accomplished through a central lumen, which also acts as an aortic root vent. A second lumen is used as an aortic root pressure monitor, and a third lumen is used for balloon inflation to provide aortic occlusion. Experimental and clinical studies have demonstrated the feasibility of port access coronary artery bypass grafting and port access mitral valve procedures. Endovascular cardiopulmonary bypass using the endoaortic clamp is effective in achieving cardiac arrest and myocardial protection so that anastomosis of the internal mammary artery to the coronary artery can proceed in a still and bloodless field. Intracardiac procedures, such as mitral valve replacement or repair, have been successfully performed clinically. The port access system effectively achieves cardiopulmonary bypass and cardioplegic arrest, thereby enabling the surgeon to perform cardiac procedures in a minimally invasive fashion.[18] However, this system, which needs multiple vascular access sites, fluoroscopic equipment in the operating room, and multiple monitoring systems,[45] is presumably expensive.

Limited Incision Coronary Surgery With Cardiopulmonary Bypass and Cardioplegic Arrest

Limited incision coronary surgery can be performed in one- or two-vessel disease through limited left anterior thoracotomy[1, 3, 5–7, 11, 12, 18, 20, 24, 35, 36, 40–42, 44, 46, 49, 51, 54] or parasternal incision,[48] with or without extracorporeal circulation. The limited incision coronary surgical technique has only recently been used in left main or triple-vessel disease.[31] It was performed through a left parasternal minithoracotomy, and the stenotic coronary arteries were bypassed with saphenous vein grafts and an internal thoracic arterial graft under femorofemoral cardiopulmonary bypass. However, the saphenous vein grafts were harvested by conventional methods using long incisions on the legs. Lately, the use of video-assisted endoscopy in the harvesting of saphenous vein grafts [22, 34, 52] has significantly shortened the length of the leg incisions. Our experience in limited incision coronary surgery through a left parasternal minithoracotomy in combination with minimally invasive harvesting of saphenous vein grafts demonstrates that limited incision coronary surgery can be performed safely and effectively in patients who have left main or triple-vessel disease.[32, 55, 56]

Surgical Technique

After induction of general anesthesia, transesophageal echocardiographic monitoring is set up and the regional wall motion abnormality is determined. The patient is placed in a supine position, exposing the groin and lower limbs. Left parasternal minithoracotomy (length 8 to 12 cm, Figs. 64–1*A* and 64–2*A*) is performed and the costal cartilages of the third and fourth ribs are resected.[31, 32, 55, 56] Care must be taken not to damage the underlying left internal thoracic artery. The left internal thoracic artery is identified beside the sternal border and is mobilized from the first to the fifth intercostal space under direct vision (see Fig. 64–1*A*). After mobilization of the internal thoracic arterial graft, the pericardium is opened and the position of the left anterior descending artery identified. The accessibility of an internal thoracic arterial graft to the left anterior descending artery is evaluated.

In the meantime, a greater saphenous vein graft is harvested from the lower limb using a minimally invasive technique.[56] Two small incisions (3 to 4 cm in length) are made on the medial side of the thigh (see Fig. 64–1*B*). The saphenous vein is identified and harvested under di-

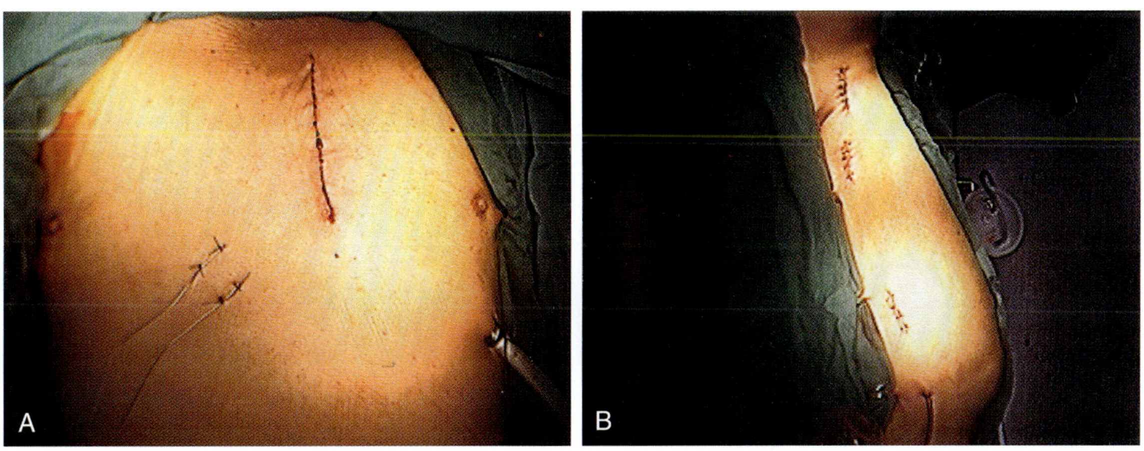

Figure 64–1. Limited incision coronary surgery of a patient with left main coronary artery stenosis. *A*, Left parasternal minithoracotomy (length 9 cm). *B*, Two small incisions (each 4 cm in length) on the left thigh for harvesting the saphenous vein graft using the minimally invasive technique. Another 4-cm groin incision was made to isolate the left common femoral artery and vein.

rect vision. Using conventional surgical instruments and the Vario Retractor System (Aesculap AG, Tuttlingen, Germany), which provides integrated cold light for illumination and retraction, it is possible to dissect the saphenous vein from the surrounding tissue without damage to the vein graft. A 35-cm greater saphenous vein is harvested through these two small incisions.

A 4-cm groin incision (see Fig. 64–1*B*) is made to isolate the left common femoral artery and vein (see Fig. 64–2*B*). Systemic heparinization (250 U/kg) is carried out at this time.

The ascending aorta is isolated from the main and right pulmonary arteries, is encircled with umbilical tape and pulled into the operative field (see Fig. 64–2*C*). Proximal anastomosis of the saphenous vein graft to the ascending aorta can be performed at this time.[31, 32, 55, 56] A partial clamp (Kay Clamp, Pilling, Fort Washington, PA) is then applied on the proximal part of the ascending aorta. A hole is made in the ascending aorta. Proximal anastomosis of the saphenous vein graft to the ascending aorta is performed under direct vision. However, the proximal anastomosis of the saphenous vein graft to the ascending aorta can also be performed after all distal anastomoses have been completed.

Cardiopulmonary bypass is established through cannulation of the left femoral artery and the left femoral vein in most of our patients. Cannulation of the right atrium can also be performed to increase venous drainage. To avoid a groin incision in some patients, cannulation of the ascending aorta, main pulmonary artery, and right atrium is performed for cardiopulmonary bypass.[56] A double-lumen aortic root cannula (DPL, Inc., Grand Rapids, MI) is then inserted at the aortic root for delivery of cardioplegic solution and venting of the left ventricle (see Fig. 64–2*C*). A membranous oxygenator (Maxima Plus oxygenation system, Medtronic, Inc., Cardiopulmonary Division, Anaheim, CA) is used. Systemic hypothermia (rectal temperature 27.4 ± 1.0°C) begins immediately after the start of cardiopulmonary bypass. Topical cooling of the heart is not used. The aorta is cross-clamped at the distal part of the ascending aorta (see Fig. 64–2*C*). The myocardium is protected by a cold blood cardioplegic solution, which is infused into the aortic root at this point and after each distal anastomosis is completed. The heart soon undergoes arrest and is cooled and decompressed by venting through the aortic root cannula (see Fig. 64–2*D*).

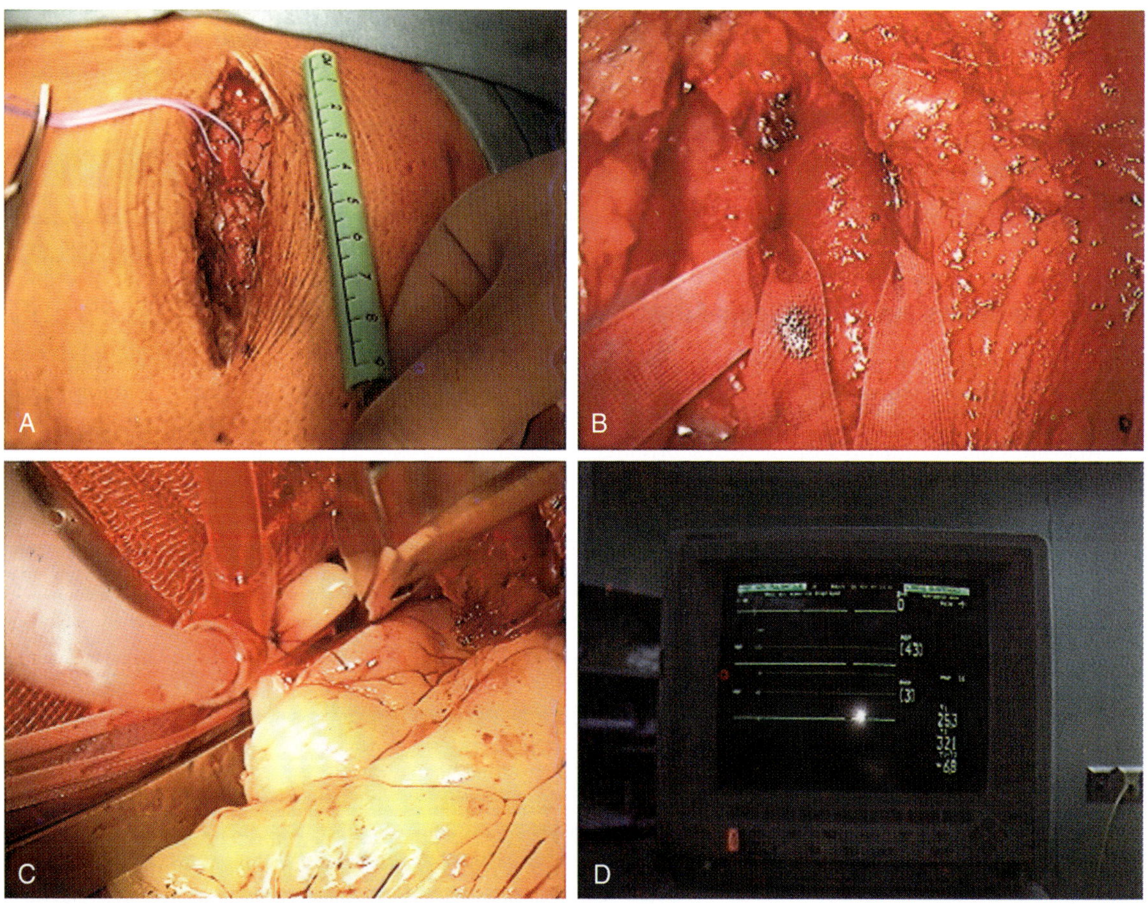

Figure 64–2. Limited incision coronary surgery with cardiopulmonary bypass and cardioplegic arrest. *A,* Left parasternal minithoracotomy with excision of the costal cartilages of the third and fourth ribs. The internal thoracic arterial graft was isolated and looped. *B,* The left femoral artery and femoral vein were isolated and looped. *C,* The ascending aorta was encircled and pulled into the operative field. A double-lumen aortic root cannula was inserted at the aortic root for delivery of cardioplegic solution and venting of the left ventricle. The aorta was cross-clamped at the distal part of the ascending aorta. *D,* The heart was arrested soon after delivery of blood cardioplegic solution into the aortic root.

The saphenous vein graft is grafted sequentially to the posterior descending branch, obtuse marginal branch (Fig. 64–3), and diagonal branch (see Fig. 64–4*A* and *B*) with a running suture under direct vision. The internal thoracic arterial graft is then anastomosed to the left anterior descending artery while rewarming is started (see Fig. 64–4*C* and *D*). The anastomotic areas are steady and clear because of cardioplegic arrest and aortic cross-clamping, making the anastomosis easy and smooth.

After all anastomoses are completed, proximal anastomosis of the saphenous vein graft to the ascending aorta can be performed, if it has not been performed before cardiopulmonary bypass. Warm blood cardioplegic solution is then infused into the aortic root before removal of the aortic cross-clamp. Sinus rhythm should recover spontaneously and cardioversion is not necessary in most patients. Cardiopulmonary bypass is terminated after rewarming of the patients. The pericardium is not closed. A small dose of sodium nitroprusside is infused. Intra-aortic balloon pumping or cardiotonic drugs are necessary in some patients who have poor ventricular function before operation. Temporary pacemaker wires and pleural drain-age are set up routinely (see Fig. 64–1*A*). Hemostasis and closure of the incisions are easily achieved.

Patient Information

From November 1996 to November 1997, 75 patients (63 men and 12 women) aged 35.7 to 81.6 years old (63.1 ± 9.5 years old, mean ± SD) were operated on in our institution for left main or triple-vessel coronary artery disease using limited incision coronary surgery. The predicted mortality based on the Society of Thoracic Surgeons National Cardiac Surgery database was 0.5 to 22.9% (4.0 ± 4.4%). In 15 patients, predicted mortality was greater than 5%.

Three to five distal anastomoses (3.6 ± 0.5) were performed in each patient. The aortic cross-clamping time was 62 to 137 minutes (83 ± 12). The duration of extracorporeal circulation ranged from 88 to 168 minutes (118 ± 22). Transesophageal echocardiography performed after termination of extracorporeal circulation showed improvement of the regional wall motion abnormality from the original impairment in all patients. All patients regained consciousness without any neurologic deficit shortly after arriving at the intensive care unit. In most patients, the endotracheal tube was removed on the operative night or in the early morning of the first postoperative day. The cardiotonic drugs and intra-aortic balloon pumping were discontinued within 24 hours after operation. Two patients died of myocardial failure. There were no chest wound infections. One minor groin infection was

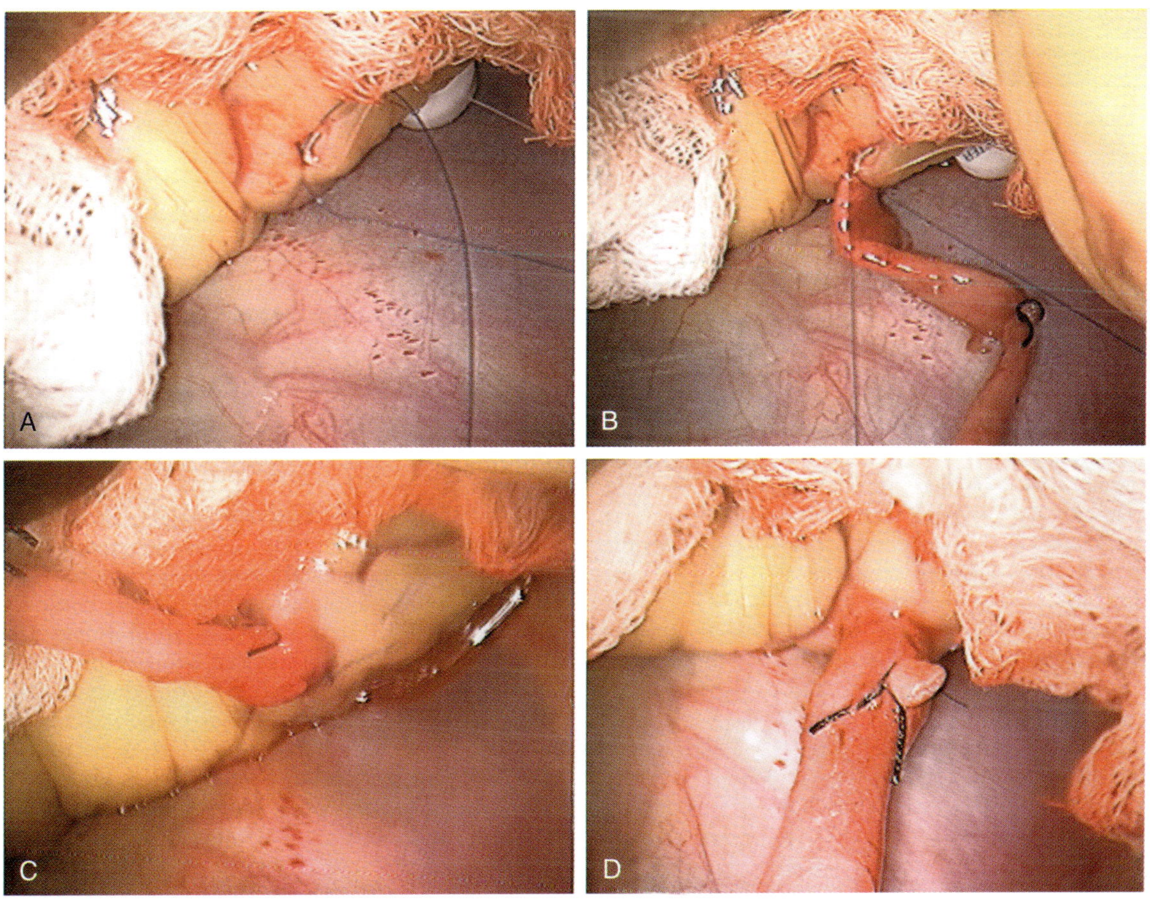

Figure 64–3. Distal anastomosis of the saphenous vein graft. *A*, An arteriotomy was made on the obtuse marginal branch. *B*, The saphenous vein grafts were anastomosed to the obtuse marginal branches under direct vision. *C*, Completion of the anastomosis. *D*, Hemostasis was accomplished easily under direct vision.

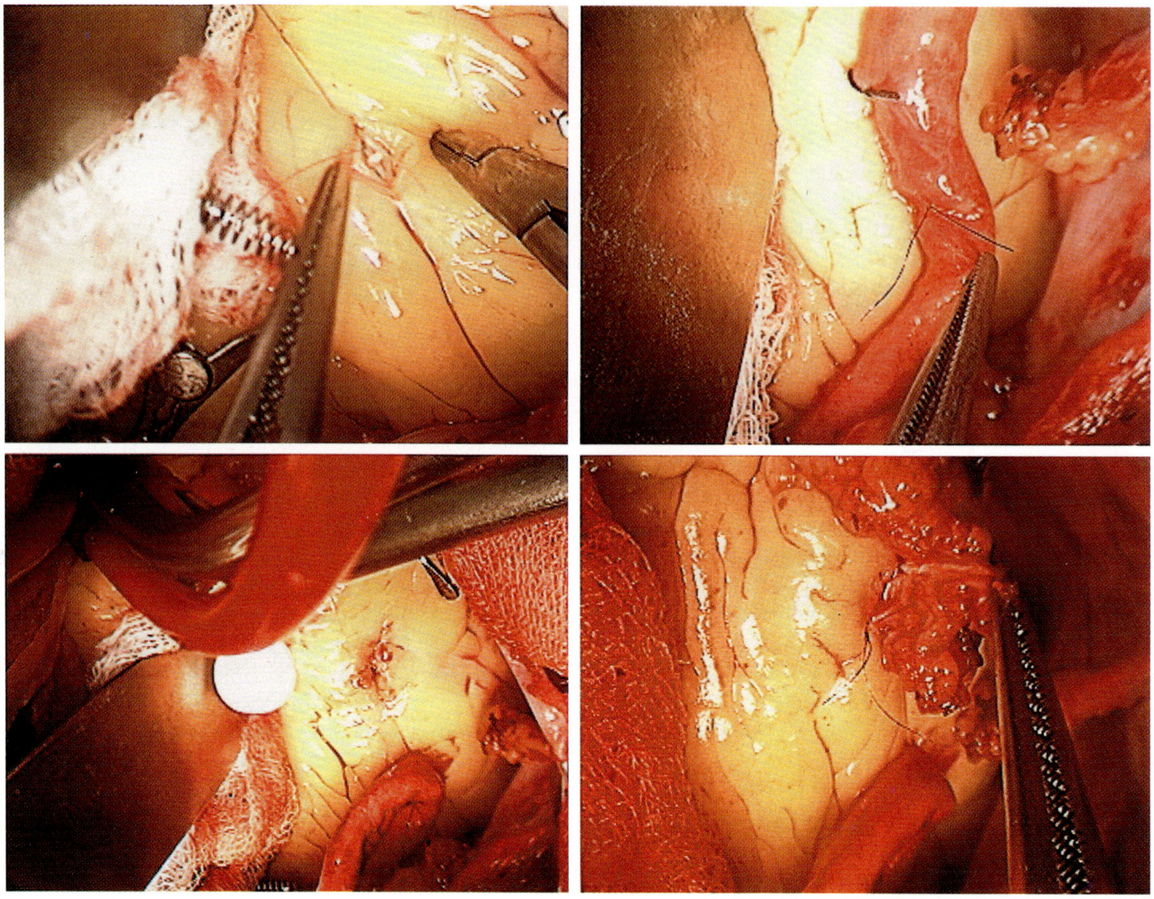

Figure 64–4. Distal anastomosis of the saphenous vein graft and left internal thoracic artery. *A*, An arteriotomy was made on the diagonal branch. *B*, Completion of the anastomosis between the saphenous vein grafts and the diagonal branch. *C*, An arteriotomy was made on the left anterior descending artery. *D*, Completion of the anastomosis between the left internal thoracic artery and the left anterior descending artery.

treated conservatively. The postoperative hospital stay was 3 to 33 days (6.8 ± 3.6). Follow-up (1.0 to 5.6 months, mean 2.9) was completed in all patients, without angina, lower limb vascular complications, or late deaths. Fifteen patients signed permission for coronary angiography, which showed patent grafts. Transthoracic echocardiographic examinations showed adequate left ventricular performance with an ejection fraction of 34 to 75% (66 ± 9%). All the survivors were found to be New York Heart Association functional class I or II. All patients were satisfied with the cosmetic result and healing of the minithoracotomy incision.

When compared with patients who underwent coronary artery bypass grafting via median sternotomy in the same period, the aortic cross-clamp time and cardiopulmonary bypass time were significantly longer in the patients in whom a limited incision approach was used. There was no difference between these two groups of patients in terms of distal anastomoses (average 3.6 in both groups), use of cardiotonic drugs, intra-aortic balloon pumping, transfusion of blood products, duration of chest tube insertion, wound infection rate, and hospital mortality. However, the length of incision, duration of endotracheal intubation, timing of first oral intake, amount of drainage on the day of operation, incidence of parenteral injection of narcotics, pain score, intensive care unit stay, length of hospitalization, and return to normal activity were significantly less in patients who underwent limited incision coronary surgery.

Comment

In our limited incision coronary surgery, techniques vary in four major ways from those of classic coronary artery bypass grafting approached via median sternotomy and from those of minimally invasive direct vision coronary artery bypass surgery. First, a median sternotomy is avoided. With the operative method that we have presented, there is good access to the left anterior descending artery, diagonal branches, obtuse marginal branches, and posterior descending branch while the heart is relaxed, decompressed, arrested, and protected. In this way, limited incision coronary surgery can be expanded to applications in surgical revascularization in left main or triple-vessel coronary disease.

Second, a groin incision for cannulation of the femoral artery and vein can be avoided in selected patients. In limited incision coronary surgery, simple femoro-femoral cardiopulmonary bypass can establish satisfactory perfusion of all vital organs. However, the possibility of vascular complications in the lower limbs, although slight, is always present. Aortoatrial cardiopulmonary bypass is familiar to most cardiac surgeons. In our series, an aortopulmonary arterial–right atrial cardiopulmonary bypass was performed in 12 patients, indicating that this technique can be performed in limited incision coronary surgery to avoid a groin incision and its possible complications.

Third, cardioplegic arrest is established with blood cardioplegia. Cardioplegic arrest is the standard method of myocardial protection. A double-lumen aortic root cannula is easily inserted at the aortic root for delivery of the cardioplegic solution and for venting the left ventricle. With the heart relaxed, decompressed, arrested, and protected, access to, and anastomosis of, all portions of the coronary arteries is easy, and the aortic cross-clamp time can be reasonably extended. In our series using blood cardioplegia for myocardial protection, there was no low cardiac output in most patients postoperatively, and only two patients died of myocardial failure.

Fourth, there is minimally invasive harvesting of the saphenous vein graft. Traditionally, saphenous vein grafts have been harvested through long incisions on the lower limbs. The poor cosmetic results and possible wound complications make harvesting of saphenous vein grafts an unpleasant procedure. Recently, video-assisted endoscopic harvesting of saphenous vein grafts has become a reality.[22, 34, 52] However, it is technically demanding and requires expensive disposable equipment. In our series, minimally invasive harvesting of the saphenous vein graft was performed under direct vision with the reusable Vario Retraction System, which provides illumination and retraction. Most cardiac surgeons are familiar with this technique. The saphenous vein graft can be harvested with good quality and adequate length.

Conclusion

Limited incision coronary surgery is technically feasible and can be performed easily and safely. Multiple grafting with internal thoracic arterial graft and saphenous vein grafts was accomplished using the following:

1. Left parasternal minithoracotomy
2. Minimally invasive harvesting of the saphenous vein graft
3. Aortopulmonary arterial–right atrial or femorofemoral cardiopulmonary bypass
4. Cardioplegic arrest with blood cardioplegia.

Our experience demonstrates that limited incision coronary surgery can offer decreased postoperative pain, a shortened hospital stay, excellent cosmetic healing, and fast functional recovery.

References

1. Acuff TE, Landreneau RJ, Griffith BP, Mack MJ: Minimally invasive coronary artery bypass grafting. Ann Thorac Surg 61:135–137,1996.
2. Akins CW: Noncardioplegic myocardial preservation for coronary revascularization. J Thorac Cardiovasc Surg 88:174–181, 1984.
3. Akins CW, Carroll DL: Even-free survival following nonemergency myocardial revascularization during hypothermic fibrillatory arrest. Ann Thorac Surg 43:628–633, 1987.
4. Akins CW: Early and late results following emergency isolated myocardial revascularization during hypothermic fibrillatory arrest. Ann Thorac Surg 58:1205–1206, 1994.
5. Benetti FJ, Ballester C: Use of thoracoscopy and a minimal thoracotomy, in mammary-coronary bypass to left anterior descending artery, without extracorporeal circulation. Experience in 2 cases. J Cardiovasc Surg 36:159–161, 1995.
6. Benetti F, Mariani MA, Sani G, et al: Video-assisted minimally invasive coronary operations without cardiopulmonary bypass: A multicenter study. J Thorac Cardiovasc Surg 112:1478–1484, 1996.
7. Boonstra PW, Grandjean JG, Mariani MA: Reoperative coronary bypass grafting without cardiopulmonary bypass through a small thoracotomy. Ann Thorac Surg 63:405–407, 1997.
8. Boonstra PW, Grandjean JG, Mariani MA: Improved method for direct coronary grafting without CPB via anterolateral small thoracotomy. Ann Thorac Surg 63:567–569, 1997.
9. Boonstra PW, Grandjean JG, Mariani MA: Local immobilization of the left anterior descending artery for minimally invasive coronary bypass grafting. Ann Thorac Surg 63(suppl):S76–78, 1997.
10. Burke RP, Chang AC: Video-assisted thoracoscopic division of a vascular ring in an infant: A new operative technique. J Cardiac Surg 8:537–540, 1993.
11. Calafiore AM, Angelini GD, Bergsland J, Salerno TA: Minimally invasive coronary artery bypass grafting. Ann Thorac Surg 62:1545–1548, 1996.
12. Calafiore AM, Teodori G, Di Giammarco G, et al: Minimally invasive coronary artery bypass grafting on a beating heart. Ann Thorac Surg 63(suppl):S72–75, 1997.
13. Carpentier A, Loulmet D, Carpentier A, et al: First open heart operation (mitral valvuloplasty) under videosurgery through a minithoracotomy. C R Acad Sci Paris 319:219–223, 1996.
14. Chang CH, Lin PJ, Chu JJ, et al: Surgical closure of atrial septal defect: Minimally invasive cardiac surgery or median sternotomy? Surg Endosc 12:820–824, 1998.
16. Chu JJ, Chang CH, Lin PJ, et al: Video-assisted thoracoscopic surgery for interruption of patent ductus arteriosus in adult. Ann Thorac Surg 63:175–179, 1997.
17. Cosgrove DM III, Sabik JF: Minimally invasive approach for aortic valve operations. Ann Thorac Surg 62:596–597, 1996.
18. Fann JI, Pompili MF, Stevens JH, et al: Port-access cardiac operations with cardioplegic arrest. Ann Thorac Surg 63(suppl): S35–S39, 1997.
19. Izzat MB, Yim AP: Cardiac stabilizer for minimally invasive direct coronary artery bypass. Ann Thorac Surg 64:570–571, 1997.
20. King RC, Reece TB, Hurst JL, et al: Minimally invasive coronary artery bypass grafting decreases hospital stay and cost. Ann Surg 225:805–811, 1997.
21. Kirklin JW, Barratt-Boyes BG: Cardiopulmonary bypass established by peripheral cannulation. *In* Kirklin JW, Barratt-Boyes BG (eds): Cardiac Surgery, 2nd ed. New York: Churchill Livingstone, 1993, pp 110–111.
22. Kyo S, Kaneko K, Nishikiori Y, et al: Endoscopic harvesting of saphenous vein for coronary artery bypass grafting: Development of new technique. Circulation 94(suppl):I-476.
23. Laborde F, Noirhomme P, Karam J, et al: A new video-assisted thoracoscopic surgical technique for interruption of patent ductus arteriosus in infants and children. J Thorac Cardiovasc Surg 105:278–280, 1993.
24. Landreneau RJ, Mack MJ, Magovern JA, et al: "Keyhole" coronary artery bypass surgery. Ann Surg 224:453–462, 1996.

25. Lin PJ, Chang CH, Tan PPC, et al: Protection of the brain by retrograde cerebral perfusion during circulatory arrest. J Thorac Cardiovasc Surg 108:969–974, 1994.
26. Lin PJ, Chang CH, Tan PPC, et al: Prolonged circulatory arrest in moderate hypothermia with retrograde cerebral perfusion: Is brain ischemic? Circulation 94(suppl II):169–172, 1996.
27. Lin PJ, Chang CH, Chu JJ, et al: Video-assisted mitral valve surgeries. Ann Thorac Surg 61:1781–1787, 1996.
28. Lin PJ, Chang CH, Chu JJ, et al: Video-assisted cardiac surgery: Preliminary experience in one center. Circulation 94(suppl):I-174, 1996.
29. Lin PJ, Chang CH, Chu JJ, et al: Video-assisted coronary artery bypass grafting during hypothermic fibrillatory arrest. Ann Thorac Surg 63:1113–1117, 1997.
30. Lin PJ, Chang CH, Chu JJ, et al: Minimally invasive cardiac surgical technique in the closure of ventricular septal defect: An alternative approach. Ann Thorac Surg 65:165–170, 1998.
31. Lin PJ, Chang CH, Chu JJ, et al: Minimal access surgical techniques in coronary artery bypass grafting for triple vessel disease. Ann Thorac Surg 65:407–412, 1998.
32. Lin PJ, Chang CH, Chu JJ, et al: Minimally invasive coronary surgery in women. Chinese Med J 111:302–305, 1998.
33. Liu HP, Chang CH, Lin PJ, et al: Video-assisted thoracic surgery—The Chang Gung experience. J Thorac Cardiovasc Surg 108:834–840, 1994.
34. Lumsden AB, Eaves FF 3rd, Ofenloch JC, Jordan WD: Subcutaneous, video-assisted saphenous vein harvest: Report of the first 30 cases. Cardiovasc Surg 4:771–776, 1996.
35. Mack MJ, Acuff TE, Casimir Ahn H, et al: Video-assisted coronary bypass grafting on the beating heart.63(suppl):S100–S103, 1997.
36. Mack MJ, Brown DL, Sankaran A: Minimally invasive coronary bypass for protected left main coronary stenosis angioplasty. Ann Thorac Surg 64:545–546, 1997.
37. Magovern JA, Mack MJ, Landreneau RJ, et al: The minimally invasive approach reduces the morbidity of coronary artery bypass. Circulation 94(suppl):I-52, 1996.
38. Navia JL, Cosgrove DM III: Minimally invasive mitral valve operations. Ann Thorac Surg 62:1542–1547, 1996.
39. Reitz BA, Stevens JH, Burdon TA, et al: Port-access coronary artery bypass grafting: Lessons learned in a phase I clinical trial. Circulation 94(suppl):I-52, 1996.
40. Schwartz DS, Ribakove GH, Grossi EA, et al: Port-access coronary artery bypass grafting with cardioplegic arrest: A canine study. Circulation 94(suppl):I-52, 1996.
41. Schwartz DS, Ribakove GH, Grossi EA, et al: Minimally invasive cardiopulmonary bypass with cardioplegic arrest: A closed chest technique with equivalent myocardial protection. J Thorac Cardiovasc Surg 111:556–566, 1996.
42. Schwartz DS, Ribakove GH, Grossi EA, et al: Single and multivessel port-access coronary artery bypass grafting with cardioplegic arrest: Technique and reproducibility. J Thorac Cardiovasc Surg 114:46–52, 1997.
43. Shennib H, Lee AG, Akin J: Safe and effective method of stabilization for coronary artery bypass grafting on the beating heart. Ann Thorac Surg 63:988–992, 1997.
44. Shennib H, Mack MJ, Lee AG: A survey on minimally invasive coronary artery bypass grafting. Ann Thorac Surg 64:110–115, 1997.
45. Siegel LC, St. Goar FG, Stevens JH, et al: Monitoring considerations for port-access cardiac surgery. Circulation 96:562–568, 1997.
46. St Goar FG, Siegel LC, Stevens JH, et al: Catheter based cardioplegic arrest facilitates port-access cardiac surgery. Circulation 94(suppl):I-52, 1996.
47. St Goar FG, Stevens JH, Burdon TA, et al: Closed-Chest CABG clinical characteristics: potential for procedural synergy in managing CAD. J Am Coll Cardiol 27(suppl A):392A, 1996.
48. Stanbridge RD, Symons GV, Banwell PE: Minimal-access surgery for coronary artery revascularization (Letter). Lancet 346: 837, 1995.
49. Stevens JH, Burdon TA, Peters WS, et al: Port-access coronary artery bypass grafting: A proposed surgical method. J Thorac Cardiovasc Surg 111:567–573, 1996.
50. Stevens JH, Burdon TA, Siegel LC, et al: Port-access coronary artery bypass with cardioplegic arrest: Acute and chronic canine studies. Ann Thorac Surg 62:435–441, 1996.
51. Subramanian VA: Less invasive arterial CABG on a beating heart. Ann Thorac Surg 63(suppl):S119–121, 1997.
52. Tevaearai HT, Mueller XM, von Segesser LK: Minimally invasive harvest of the saphenous vein for coronary artery bypass grafting. Ann Thorac Surg 63(suppl):S119–S121, 1997.
53. Tsai FC, Lin PJ, Chang CH, et al: Video-assisted cardiac surgery: Preliminary experience in reoperative mitral valve surgery. Chest 110:1603–1607, 1996.
54. Westaby S, Benetti FJ: Less invasive coronary surgery: Consensus from the Oxford meeting. Ann Thorac Surg 62:924–931, 1996.
55. Wu YC, Chang CH, Lin PJ, et al: Minimally invasive approach for coronary artery bypass surgery. Int J Cardiol 62 (suppl): S111–S117, 1997.
56. Yeh CS, Chang CH, Lin PJ, et al: Totally minimally invasive cardiac surgery for coronary artery disease. Eur J Cardiothorac Surg 14 (suppl):S43–S47, 1998.

COMMENTARY

Alan J. Bryan

Lin and associates from Taiwan report their experience using a limited access approach, cardiopulmonary bypass and fibrillatory arrest in a cohort of 75 patients. Multiple grafts were performed in a range of patients, with two deaths. In some patients, femoral cannulation was avoided. The prolongation of ischemic time and cardiopulmonary bypass time in the minimally invasive group are acknowledged. There are the usual claims for reduced intensive care stay, hospital stay, and return to normal activity. While this may be true, in the absence of any attempt at randomization or the presentation of numerical data, these claims must be considered unsubstantiated.

These authors are to be congratulated for their ingenuity, and their methods represent a further alternative in the range of less invasive approaches. What is in doubt is whether the increased complexity in association with the small incision really does lead to patient benefit.

Chapter 65

Ministernotomy for Coronary Artery Bypass Surgery

Kit V. Arom and Robert W. Emery

Today, coronary artery bypass surgery with a beating heart can be performed through small incisions on various areas of the chest wall through which the target artery can be reached. The small incisions provide adequate exposure to the target area of the heart, but sometimes the limited exposure can lead to difficulty in recognizing the surface anatomy.

As an alternative to the left anterior small thoracotomy (LAST) incision, a small skin incision and partial sternotomy to access the heart for minimally invasive direct coronary artery bypass (MIDCAB) surgery was introduced by Arom and associates in 1996.[1] The skin incision for this approach is approximately 8 to 12 cm long, and the sternum is partially divided and spread approximately 6 to 8 cm apart. Compared with a LAST incision, this approach may not prove superior for access to the left anterior descending (LAD) artery and diagonal artery, but it does offer better visualization of the surface anatomy of the heart, and in many instances the entire LAD artery can be reached. The appropriate target on the distal LAD artery can be chosen for anastomosis, an advantage that sometimes cannot be accomplished via the LAST incision. Conversion to cardiopulmonary bypass is feasible with this approach, in which the right atrial appendage and adjacent aorta can be cannulated quickly without groin cannulation. This approach also appears to be better than right anterior thoracotomy for right MIDCAB surgery, and the ministernotomy incision can benefit surgeons who are learning to perform surgery on a beating heart.

The definition of minimally invasive cardiac surgery is still unclear. At the 1996 meeting on minimally invasive direct coronary artery bypass surgery in Montreal, Canada, the participating cardiac surgeons were asked to define minimally invasive cardiac surgery. Eighty-one percent felt that the absence of the use of cardiopulmonary bypass was the defining factor, whereas 19% considered the use of median sternotomy a more important component.[2] Despite the use of the sternotomy incision for the past several decades, some cardiac surgeons still believe that it requires a longer healing process and produces more postoperative complications than does a thoracotomy.

It is important to differentiate "complete sternotomy" from "partial sternotomy," because these two approaches use different incisions, have different healing processes, and probably have different postoperative complications. The fact is that the complete sternotomy incision is approximately 1 ft (30 cm) long and is spread about 10 in. (25 cm) apart. For ministernotomy, the skin incision is approximately 10 to 12 cm long, the sternum is partially incised, and the spreading of the sternum is not more than 6 to 8 cm.[3] The ministernotomy incision has proved to result in fewer postoperative complications from stretching or damaging of the ribs, cartilages, and shoulder joints, which commonly occur with complete sternotomy. The time needed for partial sternotomy to heal has not been determined, but partial sternotomy for MIDCAB procedures appears to be no different from that for thymectomy, in which patients are discharged and resume activity in about half the time that it takes patients who undergo conventional heart surgery. We believe that patients who undergo coronary artery bypass surgery using a partial sternotomy approach can resume activity sooner.

Skin Incision

The skin incision is approximately 10 cm long or half the length of the sternum, whichever is shorter (Fig. 65–1). The site of the skin incision is dependent on the location of the planned partial sternotomy and is usually made on top of the sternal incision. To reach the left coronary artery, either a left upper or left lower partial sternotomy is appropriate. For left upper partial sternotomy, the skin incision is made about four fingerbreadths caudal to the sternal notch down to an area near the fourth intercostal space. The subcutaneous tissue is generously undermined cephalad to expose the sternal notch and caudad to the left sixth intercostal space. (See Chapter 54.)

For left and right lower sternotomy, the skin incision is made from the area near the third intercostal space down near the last costosternal junction with generous undermining of the subcutaneous tissues at both ends.

Sternal Incision

With the ministernotomy approach, it is impossible to start the sternal saw at the sternal notch downward because of the limitation presented by the skin flap and the location of the sternal notch away from the skin edge. Therefore, it is necessary to start the saw at the desired left intercostal space at the specific costosternal angle, medial to the left internal mammary artery. A Kelly clamp is used to create an entry site between the internal mammary artery (IMA) and the sternal border before insertion of the tip of the Hall saw (Hall Surgical, Carpentaria, CA). The saw is then carried cephalad to the limit of the skin incision. If one desires to maintain the benefit of a small skin incision, a Striker oscillating saw (Hall Surgical, Carpentaria, CA) can be used subcutaneously at this point to complete the sternotomy. Adding more length to the skin incision at this end does not increase the advantages of exposure.

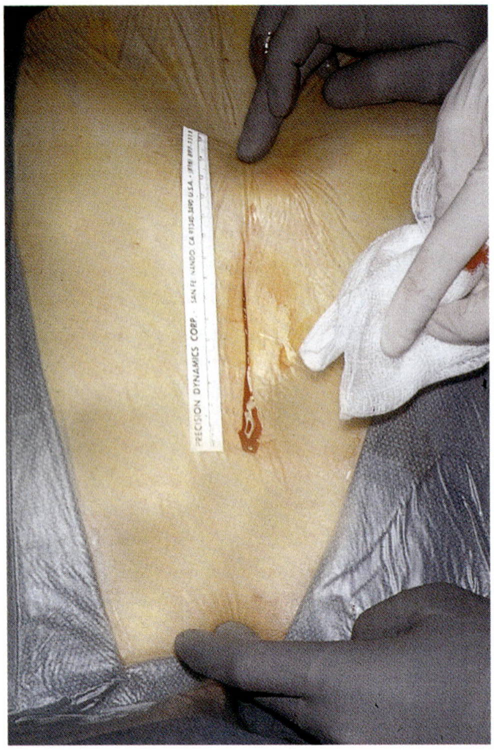

Figure 65–1. Ministernotomy skin incision. The incision is usually approximately 10 cm long and is made on top of the sternal incision.

Left Partial Sternotomy. The *reversed J sternotomy* incision starts from the sixth costosternal angle and extends to the sternal notch or begins at the last costoxiphoid angle on the left and extends upward, exiting at the first left intercostal space (a C incision) (Fig. 65–2). These two incisions give good exposure to the LAD artery and possibly the diagonal artery. The latter incision provides better exposure to the inferolateral aspect of the heart; however, spreading of the sternum is more difficult with this incision.

Right Lower Partial Sternotomy. The incision or the J sternotomy incision can be performed on the right side in the same manner as the left partial sternotomy described earlier.

Internal Mammary Artery Harvesting

Most harvesting of the IMA is carried out by direct visualization through a limited ministernotomy incision, in a manner similar to the conventional approach through a complete sternotomy. However, when the partial sternotomy incision exits at the first left intercostal space, the approach to the first branch and origin of the IMA may be difficult; therefore, a video-assisted technique may be necessary. In general, a partial sternotomy incision provides the best approach to the IMA compared with the LAST and parasternal incisions. The first branch of the IMA can be divided, and the IMA can be taken down entirely, including the most distal part of the artery (Fig. 65–3). The dissection of the IMA via this approach is not differentiated from the conven-tional technique used in complete sternotomy (see Fig. 65–3).

Heart and Coronary Artery Presentation

The presentation of the target artery close to the sternal opening is crucial for this approach. Placement and maneuvering of the pericardial traction sutures, particularly on the left side, enable optimal positioning of the vessels for grafting. When the main trunk of the right coronary artery near the midline is the target artery, the approach is easy. To approach the LAD and diagonal arteries, the left side of the pericardium is generously pulled up, and the left ventricle is briefly elevated and rotated counterclockwise by placing a homemade "tampon" (Fig. 65–4) or the commercially available, inflatable retrocardiac dual-chamber device of Cardiac Instruments (Cardiac Instruments, Plymouth, MN) (Fig. 65–5). Octopus suction stabilization devices (Medtronic, Inc., Eden Prairie, MN) can also be used for a lateral target presentation (Fig. 65–6). The search for the LAD artery is sometimes difficult, and this artery can be confused with a large right ventricular branch coming across the right ventricular outflow tract. The juncture of the left side of the pulmonic root and the left ventricular outflow tract should always be identified as landmarks for the normal course of the LAD artery.

Surgical Technique and Intraoperative Safety Net

The patient is placed in the supine position with conventional double-lung anesthesia. Blood pressure is controlled with anesthetic agents and nitroglycerin (0.5 μg/kg/min); occasionally, a small dose of sodium nitroprusside has been

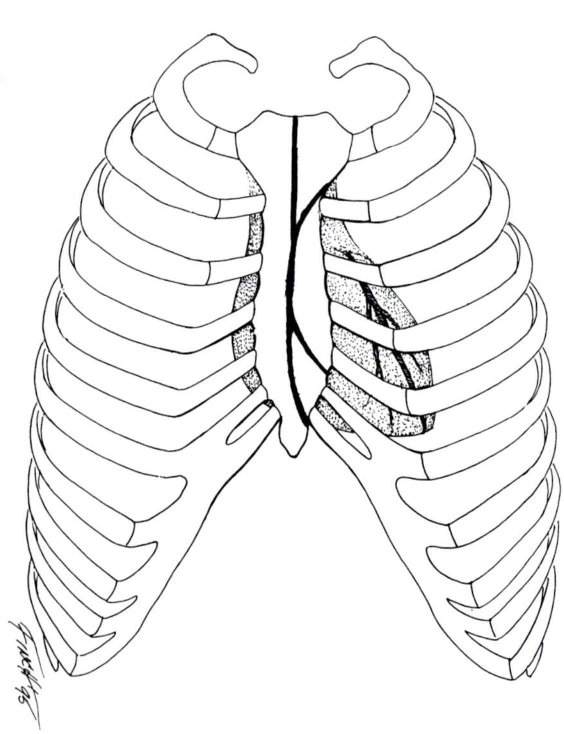

Figure 65–2. The two most common partial sternotomy incisions to expose the left coronary artery system. A reverse J incision starts from the left fifth or sixth costosternal angle and extends upward to the sternal notch. A C incision starts from the last costoxiphoid angle and extends upward, exiting at the first left intercostal space.

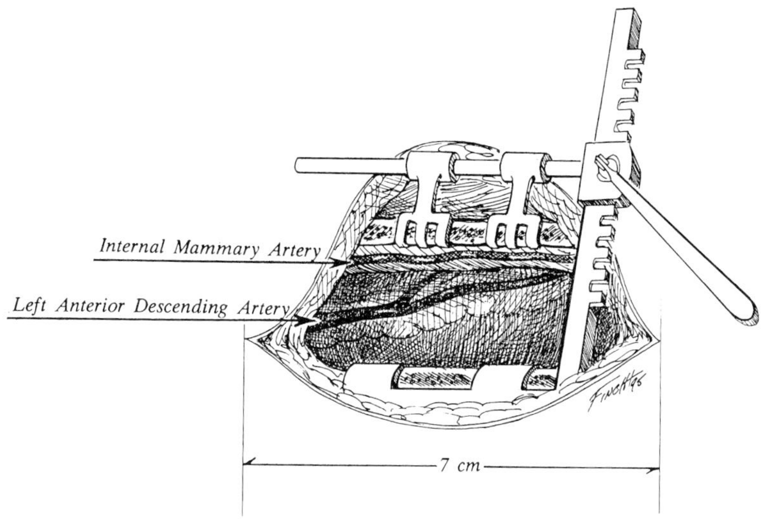

Figure 65–3. Exposure through a reversed J partial sternotomy approach with the Delacroix-Chevalier retractor in place. The left internal mammary artery is well visualized and is taken down in the usual fashion.

added to maintain arterial blood pressure at about 80 mm Hg. Infusion of esmolol hydrochloride may become necessary to minimize myocardial oxygen consumption, thereby reducing the heart rate to less than 60 beats per minute. Occasionally, a 6-mg bolus of adenosine is given every 5 minutes to create brief sinus arrest and provide myocardial protection. Ischemic preconditioning[4] of the left coronary artery system was used in early cases but has recently been abandoned. However, ischemic preconditioning may be necessary for the right coronary artery, in which hemodynamic instability often occurs during right coronary artery occlusion.

The intraoperative "safety net" begins during review of the angiogram and before making the skin incision. The distal LAD artery must be at least 1.5 mm and must not be calcified. The septal perforator and intramyocardial LAD artery need to be identified on review of the angiogram. The large septal perforator needs to be avoided during encircling of the LAD artery for anastomosis. An intramyocardial course of the LAD artery seen on angiography is an absolute contraindication for the procedure. External defibrillator patches should always be applied to the appropriate sites on the chest wall. Priming of the cardiopulmonary bypass circuit, putting two pursestring sutures at the right atrial appendage and adjacent aorta, and inserting the guide wires through the groin for emergent percutaneous cardiopulmonary bypass[5] have now been abandoned. In our experience, continued cardiac output is the most helpful measurement for predicting life-threatening hemodynamic instability. When the cardiac output begins to drop while the heart is being rotated and positioned during the coronary artery occlusion, or if it continues to decrease after manipulation is completed, ventricular fibrillation will certainly occur. The other monitoring parameters are of less importance; this includes a prolonged ST elevation,

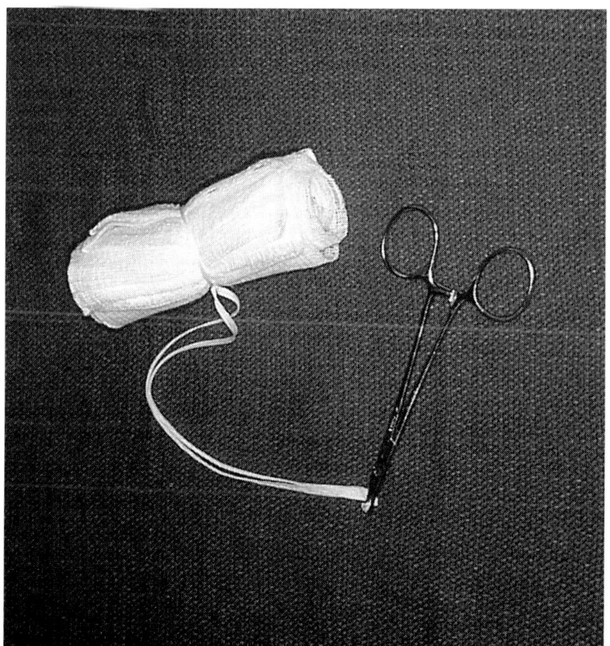

Figure 65–4. Photograph of a homemade "tampon." One 4 × 4 sponge is tied in the middle with umbilical tape. The tail end of the tape is used for pulling the device out.

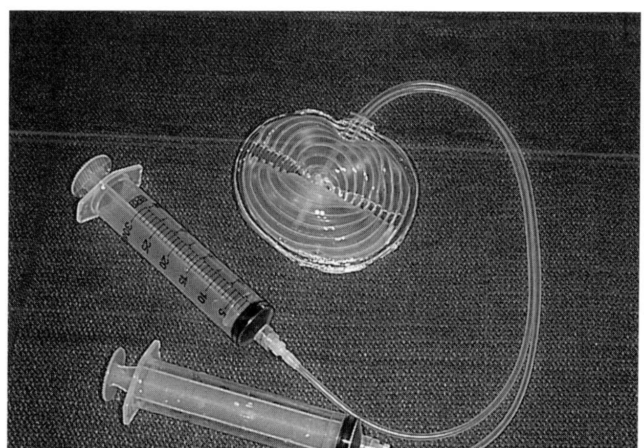

Figure 65–5. Inflatable retrocardiac presentation device. The dual-chamber positioner can be inflated separately or together for better presentation of the target artery.

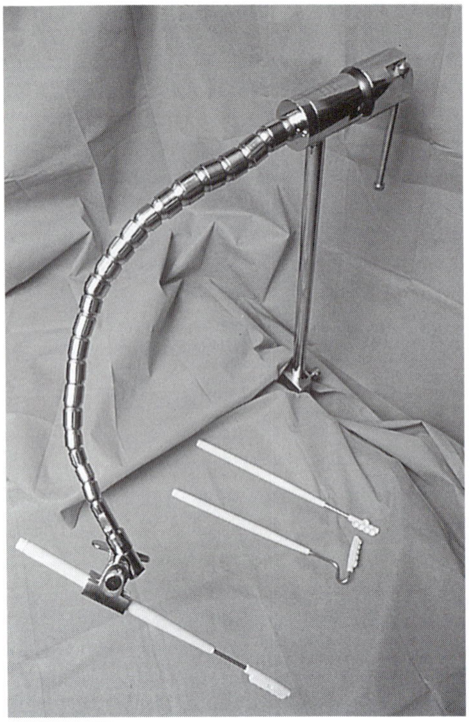

Figure 65–6. The Utrecht Octopus device. This device consists of a system of suction cups on two fixed handles that are positioned on either side of the target artery. This system offers not only immobilization but also variable degrees of target presentation as well. The drawback of this device is the size of the system, which does not work well with small access sites.

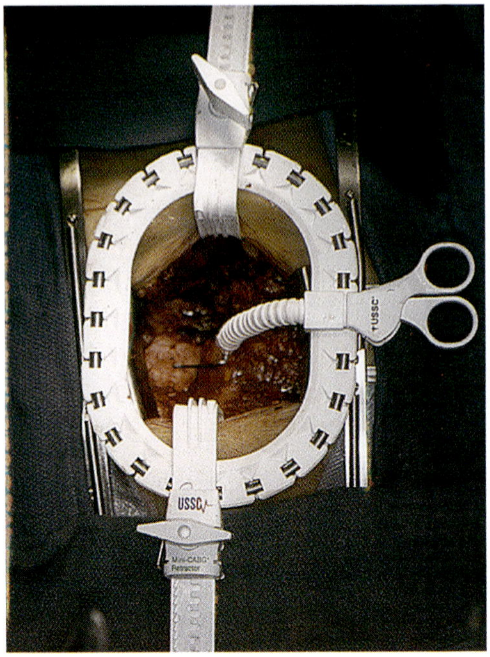

Figure 65–7. Partial sternotomy incision with sternal spreader. A 15-cm disposable universal-based retractor is placed on top of the sternal spreader and is secured in place with two retractors placed in the opposite direction. The compression stabilizer footplate is placed at the desired location.

which seems to be less sensitive and is not a good predictor of life-threatening ventricular arrhythmias.

Vessel Stabilization and Anastomosis

Like the thoracotomy approach, the ministernotomy requires good local wall immobilization of the target artery. Many different technologies have been developed, to allow local wall immobilization, including various *disposable* platform compression devices from USSC (United Surgical Supply Corp., Norwalk, CT) and CTS (Cardiothoracic Surgery System, Cupertino, CA) as well as *reusable* devices developed by Genzyme (Genzyme Surgical Products, Tucker, GA) and Scanlen (Scanlen International, St. Paul, MN) and suction stabilization apparatus from Cardiac Instruments (Cardiac Instruments, Inc., Plymouth, MN) and Medtronics (Medtronics, Inc., Eden Prairie, MN). All these devices can be used via a ministernotomy approach; however, the disposable USSC compression stabilizing device seems to fit well with the sternal spreader. This stabilizer arm is short and stable enough to immobilize different target areas of the anterior surface of the heart. To use this device, the Delacroix-Chevalier retractor has to be replaced with a Cooley sternal spreader or modified Ankeney retractor with one pair of the foot blades removed. The O-ring platform (15-cm disposable universal-base retractor) is placed on top of the sternal retractor and secured with two disposable retractors (3 or 5 cm) placed in opposite directions. The compression stabilizer footplate can be directed to various areas on the anterior wall of the heart (Fig. 65–7). This compression stabilization device does not work as well as the suction stabilization device for lateral targets, for which the suction device provides better presentation of the heart.

Vessel stabilization can be accomplished with suture material, either Silastic or 4–0 Prolene, doubled loop proximal and distal to the site of arteriotomy.[6] It is important not to pull this suture up too tightly, and at no time should stitches be used for cardiac presentation. The suture is pulled just enough to gently immobilize and occlude the flow during

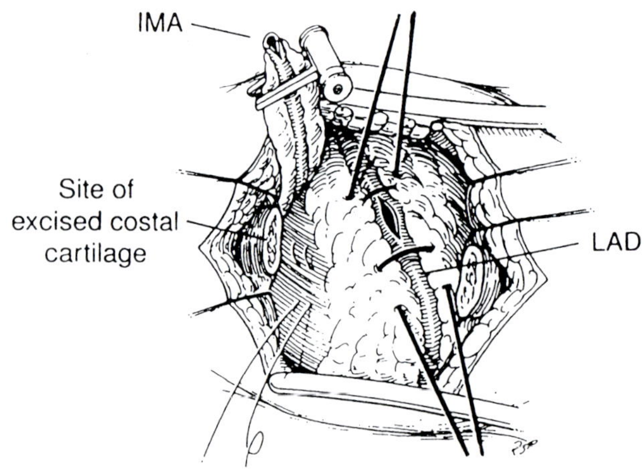

Figure 65–8. Vessel stabilization can be accomplished with suture material. It is important not to pull this suture too tightly, and at no time should stitches be used for cardiac presentation.

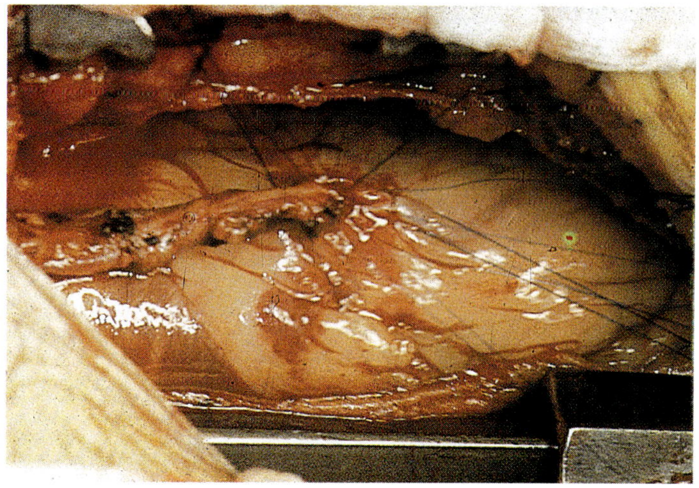

Figure 65–9. Anastomosis and course of the conduit. The pericardium is incised proximally toward its attachment to the great vessels (not shown) for better alignment of the conduit.

the anastomosis. This technique is used at many institutions because costs are reduced considerably when compared with the disposable stabilizing devices (Fig. 65–8).

After a small dose of heparin (1 mg/kg or 1000 U/kg) is given, the flow can be occluded and the subsequent anastomosis can be performed with either running or interrupted stitches. We prefer the interrupted technique, which we believe causes less microdamage at the suture lines during the anastomosis with a beating heart. Eight interrupted sutures of 7–0 Prolene are used; the details of suturing technique have been previously described.[7]

The patency of the anastomosis and the alignment of the conduit can be checked with limited angiography on the operating table, before the chest is closed, via a radial artery approach. Correction can then be made before leaving the operating room. The pericardium is incised proximally toward its attachment to the great vessel, for better alignment of the conduit, (Fig. 65–9) and is partially approximated distally, keeping the conduit away from overexpansion of the lung. The 24 French catheter or 19 Fr Blake silicone drain (Blake, Johnson & Johnson, Arlington, TX) is used instead of a large-bore draining tube.

Occasionally, the continuous epidural anesthesia catheter is inserted after surgery is completed and coagulation has returned to baseline. The patient is extubated in the operating room, with more than half of patients bypassing the intensive care unit, and is discharged on postoperative day 3 or 4. Patients are allowed to return to work in less than 4 weeks. At 3 months' follow-up, the small skin incision is well healed and is located away from sternal notch, providing excellent cosmesis (Fig. 65–10).

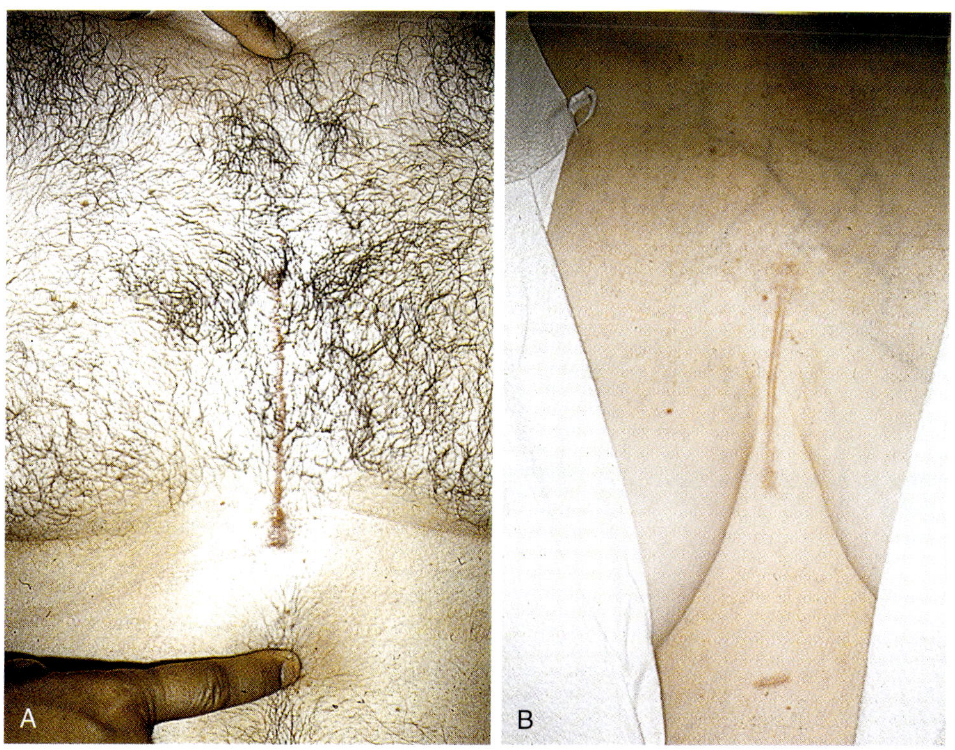

Figure 65–10. *A,B,* Two postoperative photographs of the skin incision. The incision is short and is located low enough to provide excellent long-term cosmesis.

Table 65–1. Preoperative Patient Demographics

Variable	Group A (%) (Low Risk N = 42)	Group B (%) (High Risk N = 10)
Age (mean age in yr)	58 ± 8.7	69 ± 8.4*
Male	26 (62)	4 (40)
NYHA classifications		
Unknown	2 (5)	0 (0)
I	2 (5)	0 (0)
II	4 (9)	0 (0)
III	19 (45)	2 (20)
IV	15 (36)	8 (80)
COPD	3 (7)	4 (40)
Prior CVA	0 (0)	3 (30)
Diabetes	8 (19)	6 (60)
Hypercholesterolemia	27 (64)	5 (50)
Morbid obesity	5 (12)	1 (10)
PVD	2 (5)	5 (50)
Renal failure	1 (2)	2 (20)
Prior MI	20 (48)	7 (70)
<6 hr	1 (2)	0 (0)
1–7 d	5 (12)	1 (10)
8–21 d	1 (2)	1 (10)
>21 d	13 (31)	5 (50)
Ejection fraction	62 ± 9	50 ± 20

* *P* value <.05.
NYHA = New York Heart Association; COPD = chronic obstructive pulmonary disease; CVA = cerebrovascular accident; PVD = peripheral vascular disease; MI = myocardial infarction.

Our Limited Clinical Experience

From June 1995 to February 1998, we performed 52 consecutive ministernotomy procedures for coronary artery bypass surgery at our institutions. We divided the patients into two groups for study purposes. Group A consisted of healthy low-risk patients with single LAD artery or right coronary artery lesions, or a combination, who met the criteria for this technique. Group B consisted of high-risk patients who were not good candidates for conventional cardiopulmonary bypass procedures. There were 42 patients in group A and 10 patients in group B. Patient data were collected, analyzed, and reported according to The Society of Thoracic Surgery National Cardiac Surgery Database guidelines. Using their preoperative risk module, a preoperative risk of 0.8% was identified for group A; the risk for group B was 11%. Group B patients were older, with more patients in New York Heart Association functional class III and IV when compared with Group A. Group B patients also had more incidents of previous cerebrovascular accidents, more renal failure, more obstructive pulmonary disease, and severe peripheral vascular disease. The preoperative patient demographics and preoperative variables are listed in Tables 65–1 and 65–2.

The total operating and ischemic times were the same in both groups. Blood loss in both groups was less than 500 ml, and no blood or blood products were given to any of the patients. Some of these intraoperative variables and

Table 65–2. Preoperative Variables

Variable	Group A (%) (Low Risk N = 42)	Group B (%) (High Risk N = 10)
STS predicted risk*	0.8 ± 0.6	10.9 ± 9.1†
Diseased number of vessels		
LM only	0 (0)	1 (10)
Single	27 (64)	0 (0)
Double	14 (34)	3 (30)
Triple	1 (2)	6 (60)
Incidence		
First Operation	41 (98)	6 (60)
Reoperation	1 (2)	4 (40)
Status		
Elective	35 (84)	8 (80)
Urgent	4 (9)	2 (20)
Emergent	3 (7)	0 (0)

* STS predicted risk = The Society of Thoracic Surgeons predicted risk of operative mortality.
† *P* value <.05.
LM = left main.

Table 65–3. Intraoperative Variables

Variable	Group A (%) (Low Risk N = 42)	Group B (%) (High Risk N = 10)
Operative blood loss (ml)	454 ± 284	462 ± 274
Ischemic time (min)	16 ± 7	17 ± 10
Skin-to-skin time (min)	143 ± 35	182 ± 53
Single vessel bypassed (%)	32 (76)	7 (70)
Double vessel bypassed (%)	10 (24)	3 (30)

Table 65–4. Postoperative Variables

Variable	Group A (%) (Low Risk N = 42)	Group B (%) (High Risk N = 10)
Intubation (hr)	7.2 ± 8	13.4 ± 15
ICU stay (hr)	31 ± 72	50 ± 62
8-hr chest tube loss (ml)	267 ± 207	162 ± 123
Reoperation for bleeding	0 (0)	0 (0)
Perioperative MI	1 (2)	1 (10)
Stroke	1 (2)	0 (0)
Renal failure requiring dialysis	0 (0)	0 (0)
New atrial fibrillation	9 (21)	1 (10)
Thoracentesis	2 (5)	0 (0)
Postoperative length of stay	5.1 ± 2.1	5.2 ± 2.1
Readmission within 30 d	2 (5)	1 (10)
Operative mortality	1 (2)	2 (20)

MI = myocardial infarction.

differences in surgical approach are listed in Table 65–3. Postoperatively, all patients in group B were admitted to the intensive care unit, whereas only about half of the patients in group A were admitted. The rest of the patients went to the recovery room and then to the step-down unit. The postoperative length of stay averaged 5 days for both groups. The readmission rate was about 5% for group A and 10% for group B. The main reasons for readmission were left pleural effusion, atrial fibrillation, and planned admission for other surgical procedures. The 30-day operative mortality rate was 2% in group A and 20% in group B. The cause of death was not related to the technical aspect of the procedure. The details of postoperative demographics are listed in Table 65–4. All the survivors were closely tracked at 3-month intervals, and 80% of the patients were free of angina at the time of our latest follow-up.

Conclusion

In conclusion, this chapter describes another approach for MIDCAB via a limited partial sternotomy gathered from our own experiences and concentrated primarily on the technical aspects, for which the details of each step are outlined. It is hoped that this information will be helpful to fellow cardiac surgeons who are embarking on the field of minimally invasive cardiac surgery.

References

1. Arom KV, Emery RW, Nicoloff DM: Mini-sternotomy for coronary artery bypass grafting. Ann Thorac Surg 61:1271–1272, 1996.
2. Shenib H, Mack MJ, Lee AGL: A survey on minimally invasive coronary artery bypass grafting. Ann Thorac Surg 64:110–115, 1997.
3. Arom KV, Emery RW, Nicoloff DM: Ministernotomy for cardiac surgery. *In* Emery RW (ed): Techniques for Minimally Invasive Direct Coronary Artery Bypass (MIDCAB) Surgery. Philadelphia, Hanley & Belfus, 1997, pp 43–48.
4. Mentzer RM, Lasley RD: Ischemic preconditioning. *In* Emery RW (ed): Techniques for Minimally Invasive Direct Coronary Artery Bypass Surgery. Philadelphia, Hanley & Belfus, 1997, pp 113–118.
5. Arom KV, Emery RW, Nicoloff DM: Conversion to complete sternotomy. *In* Emery RW (ed): Techniques for Minimally Invasive Direct Coronary Artery Bypass (MIDCAB) Surgery. Philadelphia, Hanley & Belfus, 1997, pp 73–76.
6. Robinson MC: "Saloon-door" parasternal approach in MIDCAB. *In* Emery RW (ed): Techniques for Minimally Invasive Direct Coronary Artery Bypass (MIDCAB) Surgery. Philadelphia, Hanley & Belfus, 1997, pp 49–53.
7. Emery RW, Arom KV, Lillehei TJ, et al: Suture techniques for MIDCAB surgery. *In* Emery RW (ed): Techniques for Minimally Invasive Direct Coronary Artery Bypass (MIDCAB) Surgery. Philadelphia, Hanley & Belfus, 1997, pp 87–91

COMMENTARY

Antonio M. Calafiore

Partial sternotomy for LAD artery grafting without cardiopulmonary bypass is an alternative to full sternotomy. Nevertheless, clinical experience is limited, and data on surgical effectiveness are lacking. The ability to expose the entire LAD artery does not seem to me a crucial issue, because the LAD artery can be snared safely only below the second diagonal branch. An interesting aspect of partial sternotomy, however, would be the possibility of grafting the posterior descending coronary artery with the right gastroepiploic artery.

For single LAD artery grafting, using the left anterior small thoracotomy (LAST) approach has a specific rationale, for the LAD artery is not in the midline but on the left side of the heart. In the LAST approach, the incision is located directly over the LAD artery; hence, even a lateral LAD artery (which occurs in as many as 15% of patients) can be easily reached. Conversion to cardiopulmonary bypass cannot be achieved as quickly as through a partial sternotomy; however, such conversion is uncommon.

It is not clear to me what the rationale behind using partial sternotomy in single LAD artery grafting is. I also fail to understand why this approach is better than a full median sternotomy in combined LAD and right coronary artery disease when off-pump grafting is planned. I have never encountered problems with healing of a median sternotomy when cardiopulmonary bypass is not used. Even though the cosmetic result of partial sternotomy is better, this has never been the primary goal of cardiac surgery over and above the success of the grafting procedure.

I believe that the indications for partial sternotomy and the angiographic results of coronary grafting through this approach should be investigated and reported.

Chapter 66

Port Access Coronary Artery Bypass Grafting

John S. Ikonomidis, James I. Fann, Thomas A. Burdon, and Mario F. Pompili

As video-assisted technology continues to improve, a minimally invasive approach has become the preferred means of managing many general and thoracic surgical disorders.[8, 10] This progress in less invasive surgery has been extended to the field of cardiac surgery with the introduction of alternative techniques.[1–4, 6, 7, 9, 11–18, 20–22] In addition to the need for defining the optimal means of exposure, considerations that are unique to a minimally invasive approach to cardiac surgery include the possible need for cardiopulmonary bypass, myocardial protection, and ventricular decompression.

This chapter reviews the development of port access coronary bypass grafting, a technique that employs an endovascular system that achieves cardiopulmonary bypass and cardioplegic arrest, thus permitting the surgeon to perform various cardiac procedures in a still and bloodless field through smaller alternative incisions.[6, 7, 12–15, 17, 18, 21, 22] The following discussion reviews the history, technical considerations, and results of coronary artery bypass grafting using port access technology.

Historical Background

In 1993, Peters devised a method of minimally invasive cardiac surgery using a unique aortic balloon catheter that provides aortic occlusion, delivery of cardioplegia, and aortic root venting.[11] This novel design has been modified and is the basis for an effective, percutaneously accessible endovascular system for cardiopulmonary bypass with cardioplegic arrest. Using this system, the surgeon can perform various open heart operations, including coronary revascularization and intracardiac procedures (e.g., valve surgery), using a smaller chest incision and avoiding a median sternotomy.

Some investigators, notably those at Stanford University and New York University, sought to validate this technique in experimental models. Schwartz and associates evaluated the effectiveness of the port access system in providing myocardial protection during cardioplegic arrest.[17] Based on indexes of left ventricular contractility, including maximal elastance, end-diastolic stroke work, preload recruitable stroke work, and stroke work end-diastolic length relationship, no difference was found between dogs who underwent port access cardiopulmonary bypass and those who underwent conventional cardiopulmonary bypass ($n = 6$ in each group).[17] Because of its capability to deliver cardioplegic solution, leading to prompt diastolic arrest and myocardial cooling, the port access system achieved equivalent myocardial protection.

Peters and colleagues retrospectively analyzed the results of closed chest cardiopulmonary bypass and cardioplegia in 54 dogs.[13] Endoaortic clamping was used in all animals, and the heart was arrested with cardioplegia delivered via the aortic root. Seventeen animals had cardiac arrest maintained via cardioplegic administration retrograde through the coronary sinus. The mean cardiopulmonary bypass time was 111 ± 27 (mean ± SEM) minutes and the cardiac arrest time was 66 ± 21 minutes. The results showed safe and reproducible institution of closed chest cardiopulmonary bypass with adequate myocardial protection as evidenced by no change in preoperative (2.9 ± 0.70 L/min) and postoperative (2.9 ± 0.65) cardiac outputs.

In a series of experiments, Stevens and associates demonstrated the feasibility of port access coronary revascularization.[21, 22] After harvesting the internal mammary artery graft thoracoscopically, peripheral cardiopulmonary bypass and cardioplegic arrest were achieved using the port access endovascular system, thereby allowing an internal mammary artery–to–coronary artery anastomosis to be performed in a still and bloodless field with the aid of an operating microscope. After the coronary anastomosis, the animals were successfully weaned from cardiopulmonary bypass. The mean aortic clamp time was 61 minutes, and the mean cardiopulmonary bypass time was 104 minutes. The early patency rate of the internal mammary artery graft was 93%. Bilateral internal mammary harvesting has also been shown to be feasible in the canine model, thus creating the potential for the port access technique to be used in multivessel coronary artery disease.[12, 18]

Human cadaver studies showed that when compared with the dog, the endoaortic clamp was easier to position in the ascending aorta because of its increased length. However, the decreased anteroposterior diameter of the human chest made approaching the internal mammary artery extremely difficult using a completely closed-chest technique using multiple thoracic ports and a stereomicroscope for the coronary anastomosis.[21] Therefore, the currently used approach employs a mini–anterior mediastinotomy to achieve better visualization and access to the coronary arteries.[14, 21] A Food and Drug Administration–regulated phase I clinical trial was performed at Stanford University between April 1995 and February 1996,[14] with subsequent controlled clinical trials introduced at New York University[15] and elsewhere. This technique has spread to more than 100 centers in the United States. Use of the minithoracotomy modification appears to allow the port access approach to be extended to multivessel coronary bypass grafting in humans.[6, 12, 15] Further, this approach may also allow proximal graft anastomoses to the ascending aorta.

Patient Selection

At present, most patients with single- or double-vessel coronary artery disease can be considered candidates for port access coronary bypass procedures. Triple and quadruple bypass operations have been performed less frequently in carefully selected situations. Potential contraindications to this technique include renal insufficiency (which would make femoral vessel cannula insertion difficult or impossible), and a diffusely diseased ascending aorta (which would make inflation of the endoaortic balloon potentially hazardous). Aortic insufficiency is not a contraindication to port access surgery because the heart may be arrested with retrograde cardioplegia, and the antegrade cardioplegia infusion port of the endoaortic clamp can be used as an aortic root vent during the procedure (Fig. 66–1).

Technical Considerations

Anesthesia and Monitoring

The anesthesiologist plays a critical role in port access operations. After general induction of anesthesia, a double-lumen endotracheal tube or a left bronchial blocker is placed to allow collapse of the left lung during harvesting of the internal mammary artery. Special catheters are then placed percutaneously via the right internal jugular vein.

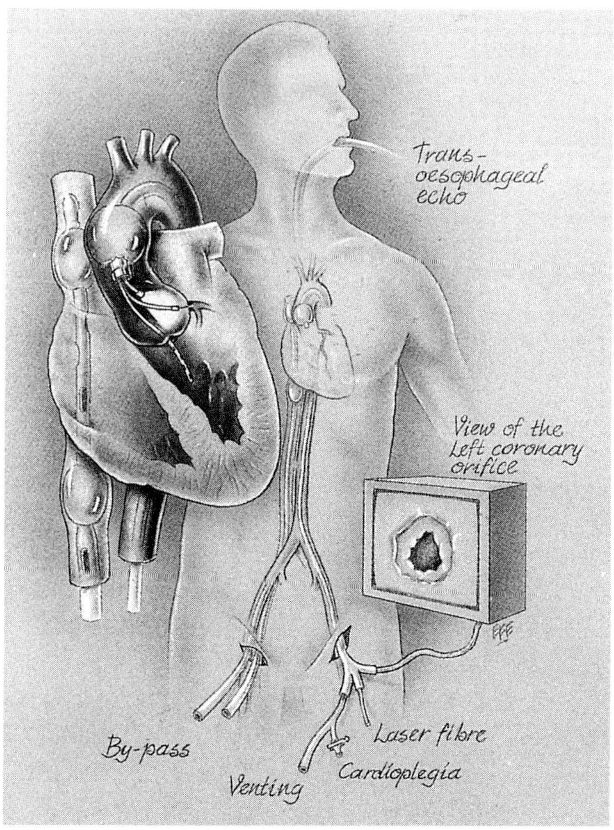

Figure 66–1. Peters' concept of peripheral cardiopulmonary bypass, cardioscopy, and laser angiosurgery. After ascending aortic balloon catheter placement, cardioplegia, and venting, cardioscopy may be achieved through a separate lumen of the endovascular catheter. The proposed system allows controlled laser ablation of coronary stenoses under direct vision. (From Peters WS: Minimally invasive cardiac surgery by cardioscopy. Austraas J Cardiac Thorac Surg 2:152–154, 1993.)

The first is the endovascular coronary sinus catheter, which is advanced into the coronary sinus under fluoroscopic or transesophageal echocardiographic guidance. This catheter, which is used for delivery of retrograde cardioplegia, is not always required because adequate cardiac arrest can be obtained by delivering cardioplegia antegrade via a port on the endovascular clamp that empties between the endoaortic balloon and the aortic valve. A second catheter that is used in selected patients is the endovascular pulmonary vent. This catheter is used to decompress the heart and keep the surgical field dry. Therefore, the anesthesiologist must have expertise in operative echocardiography. Transesophageal echocardiography (TEE) is also used to assess the ascending aorta for atheromas that may preclude passage of the endoaortic clamp (Fig. 66–2). In addition, TEE is used to monitor catheter position during the procedure.[5, 19]

The anesthesiologist can indirectly and continuously monitor the position of the endovascular clamp through placement of bilateral radial artery catheters.[15] The pressures in the radial artery lines should remain equal throughout the clamping time. If the right radial artery pressure is seen to decrease relative to that of the left radial artery, it may indicate distal migration of the balloon endoclamp with occlusion of the innominate artery, mandating repositioning of the balloon. Other monitoring strategies include surveillance of endoaortic balloon pressure and pulsed-wave Doppler examination of the right carotid, right temporal, or right middle cerebral artery.[19]

Incisions and Vascular Conduits

A left or, less commonly, right anterior thoracotomy (5 to 8 cm in length) is made in the inframammary skin fold, followed by resection of the fourth costal cartilage. The internal mammary artery can be mobilized comfortably from under the first to the fifth costal cartilage with the aid of a specially designed chest retractor and specifically angled instruments designed for this dissection.

Saphenous vein or radial artery free grafts can be harvested concurrently for use in multivessel graft procedures.

Establishing Cardiopulmonary Bypass and Cardioplegic Arrest

The left common femoral artery and vein are prepared for cannulation at the level of the inguinal ligament. After systemic heparinization, venous drainage is accomplished using a thin-walled 24 to 28 French × 65 cm catheter inserted at the saphenofemoral junction to the right atrium via the femoral vein.[23, 24] An endoarterial reinfusion catheter is inserted into the common femoral artery. This catheter contains a Y-connector that allows arterial reinfusion from one side and insertion of the endoaortic clamp coaxially through the other side via a hemostatic valve (Fig. 66–3). The endoaortic clamp is a peripherally inserted triple-lumen catheter with an inflatable balloon at its distal end.[6, 7, 12–15, 17, 18, 21–24] The balloon is positioned via guide wire in the ascending aorta using fluoroscopy and transesophageal echocardiography; it serves as an intraluminal aortic "clamp" (Fig. 66–4). The lumen used for balloon in-

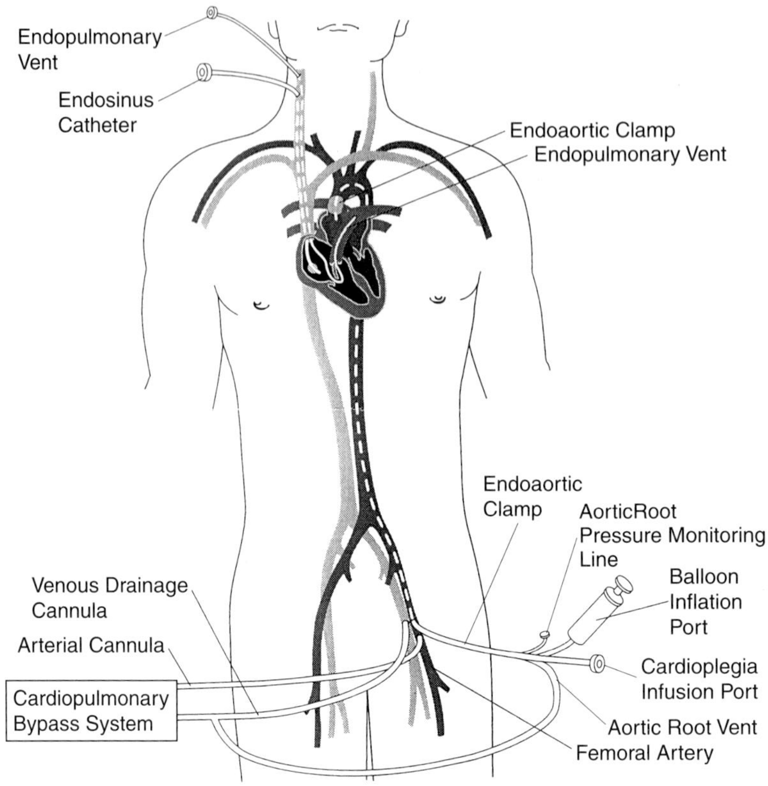

Figure 66–2. Port access cardiopulmonary bypass system. The endopulmonary vent and endosinus catheter are placed percutaneously. Peripheral cardiopulmonary bypass is achieved via femoral cannulation. The endoaortic clamp is passed through the side port of the arterial cannula and directed into the ascending aorta. After inflation of the balloon, antegrade cardioplegia is delivered via the central lumen, thereby achieving cardioplegic arrest. Retrograde cardioplegia may be delivered via the endosinus catheter.

flation is connected to a manometer to monitor balloon pressure. Cardioplegic solution is delivered through a central lumen; this lumen also acts as an aortic root vent after delivery of cardioplegia. A third, smaller lumen serves as an aortic root pressure monitor (Fig. 66–5). Percutaneously placed through the jugular vein and passed into the

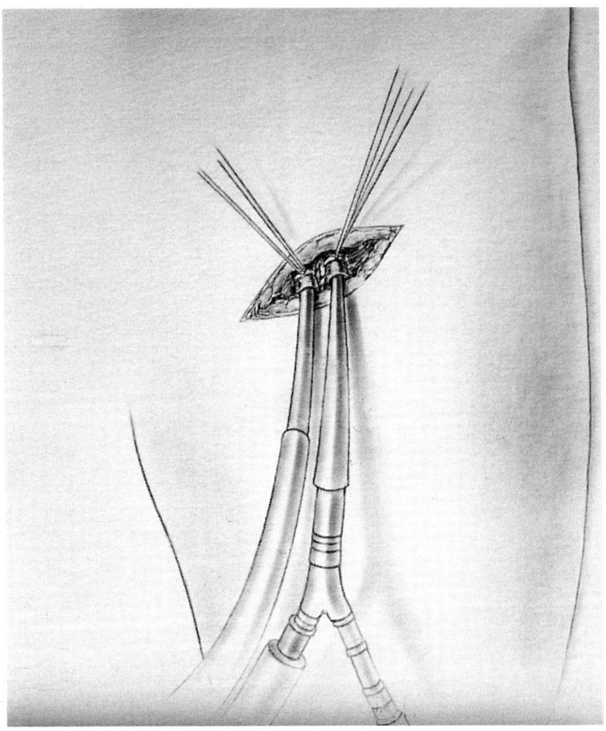

Figure 66–3. Current technique of cardiopulmonary bypass requires surgical exposure of the femoral artery and vein. The side port on the arterial cannula permits subsequent passage of the endoaortic clamp. (From Fann JI et al: Port-access multivessel coronary artery bypass grafting. Op Tech Card Thorac Surg 3:16–31, 1998.)

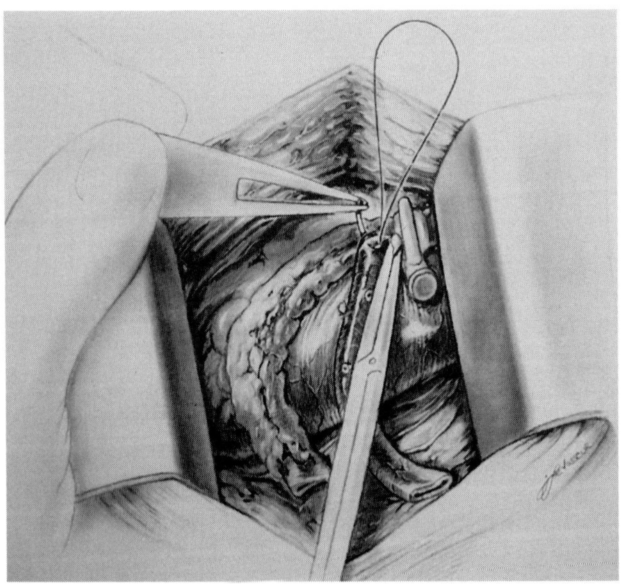

Figure 66–4. For port access multivessel coronary artery bypass grafting, a radial artery can be harvested from the nondominant arm and anastomosed in an end-to-side fashion to the internal mammary artery. (From Fann JI et al: Port-access multivessel coronary artery bypass grafting. Op Tech Card Thorac Surg 3:16–31, 1998.)

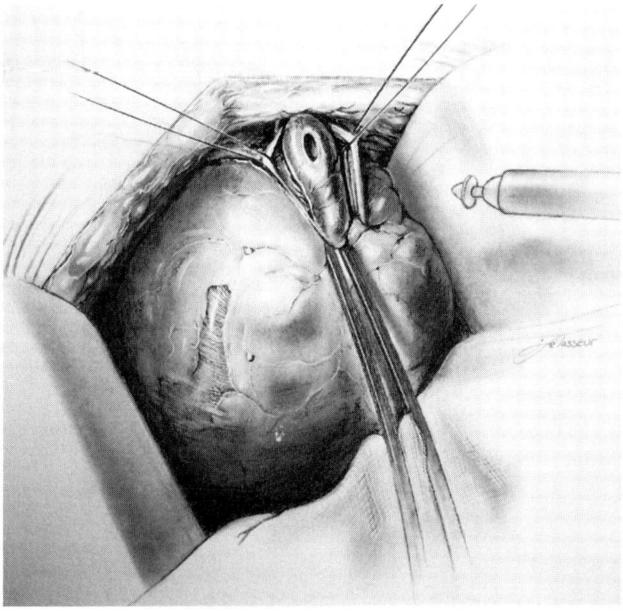

Figure 66–5. For port access multivessel coronary artery bypass grafting, a side-biting clamp can be placed on the exposed ascending aorta while it is on cardiopulmonary bypass and an end-to-side anastomosis can be performed with a reversed saphenous vein graft. Cardioplegic arrest is achieved by inflating the endoaortic balloon and starting cardiplegia delivery. (From Fann JI et al: Port-access multivessel coronary artery bypass grafting. Op Tech Card Thorac Surg 3:16–31, 1998.)

pulmonary artery, the pulmonary artery venting catheter assists in ventricular decompression.

Cardiopulmonary bypass is instituted using a standard circuit. Venous drainage can be kinetically assisted with, for example, a Biomedicus pump, maintaining the siphon pressure between 40 and 90 mm Hg.[23, 24]

The endoaortic clamp is properly positioned with the aid of TEE, and contrast ascending aortography is performed under fluoroscopy.[5, 19] The aortic occlusion balloon is then inflated using a mixture of saline and contrast dye (20 to 30%). A small amount of the dye is infused into the aortic root to visualize occlusion and proper position.

Cardioplegia can be instituted in an antegrade or retrograde direction. Retrograde cardioplegia can be infused via the percutaneously placed coronary sinus catheter at a flow rate of 200 to 250 ml/min, keeping the coronary sinus pressure in the 30- to 50-mm Hg range.[23, 24] Antegrade cardioplegia is administered at flow rates of 250 to 300 ml/min, keeping the aortic pressure at 60 to 90 mm Hg.[23, 24] Prompt clearance of the contrast material previously injected into the aortic root after balloon inflation provides evidence that cardioplegia is being adequately delivered. Myocardial temperature can be measured directly with a myocardial probe inserted via the thoracotomy.

Construction of Bypass Grafts

Distal coronary anastomoses are constructed in standard fashion with continuous 6–0 or 7–0 monofilament polypropylene suture. Usually, the inferior wall undergoes bypass before the lateral wall, and the lateral wall undergoes bypass before the anterior wall (Fig. 66–6). Recent experience with port access coronary revascularization has been extended experimentally and clinically into multivessel coronary artery bypass grafting.[7, 13, 15] For instance, in two-vessel port access coronary artery bypass grafting, a radial artery graft can be harvested and anastomosed in an end-to-side fashion to the internal mammary artery creating a T-graft.[6, 15] After establishing cardiopulmonary bypass and cardioplegic arrest in the manner described, the heart is retracted and the radial artery is anastomosed to the obtuse marginal artery, after which the internal mammary artery is anastomosed to the left anterior descending artery. The endoaortic clamp is deflated, and the patient is weaned from cardiopulmonary bypass.

Results

Clinically, Reitz and colleagues reported the outcome of the initial 10 patients who underwent port access coronary revascularization as part of a Food and Drug Administration–regulated phase I trial.[14] All procedures, which involved grafting the left internal mammary artery to the left anterior descending artery, were performed at Stanford University between April 1995 and February 1996. The average age of the patients was 55.6 years, with eight of male gender. In three patients, internal mammary harvesting was performed entirely with the aid of an endoscope. Because of technical difficulties associated with the use of multiple thoracic ports and prolonged operating room

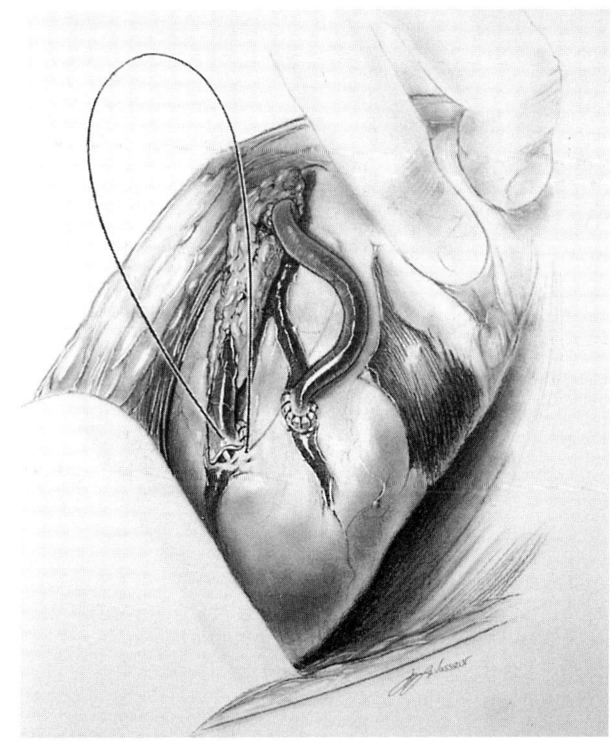

Figure 66–6. For port access multivessel coronary artery bypass grafting, anastomosis of the distal radial artery graft, the vein graft, or both, is performed before anastomosis of the left anterior descending artery, as is the case in the conventional setting. (From Fann JI et al: Port access multivessel coronary artery bypass grafting. Op Tech Card Thorac Surg 3:16–31, 1998.)

times, the mini–anterior thoracotomy approach was used in the remaining seven patients. Peripheral cardiopulmonary bypass was employed, and the endoaortic clamp provided ascending aortic occlusion, cardioplegic arrest, and sufficient myocardial protection. There were no operative deaths or early mortality; however, conversion to an open procedure was required in three patients because of early thrombosis of the graft, kinking of the internal mammary pedicle at the pericardial edge, and trauma to the distal internal mammary artery during dissection. In the seven patients in whom conversion to an open procedure was not required, the mean hospital stay ranged from 2 to 6 days. At follow-up, all patients were alive, and 9 of 10 patients have functioning grafts.

Ribakove and colleagues reported the first 6 months' experience with port access coronary bypass at New York University.[15] Twenty-five men and six women with a mean age of 60 years were evaluated. Seventeen patients underwent single bypass surgery, nine patients underwent double bypass surgery, and five patients underwent triple bypass surgery. All patients received an internal mammary artery graft (harvested via anterior mediastinotomy) to the left anterior descending coronary artery, with a radial artery free graft ($n = 9$) or saphenous vein graft ($n = 5$) when additional bypasses were necessary. The left internal mammary artery was used as the proximal anastomotic site for these extra grafts. No conversion to an open procedure was necessary, and there were no deaths, strokes, or myocardial infarctions. In-hospital complications included one early operation for pulmonary embolus and graft revision. One patient required an angioplasty for occlusion of a Y-graft to the right coronary artery. Two patients received reoperation for bleeding or tamponade. Postoperative coronary angiograms were performed in 29 of 31 patients and showed an overall graft patency rate of 98%. The median hospital stay was 5 days, and the average length of time before resumption of full activity was 3 weeks.

To date, there are no published data comparing port access coronary bypass grafting in a prospective randomized manner to the conventional open technique.

Summary

Minimally invasive cardiac surgery has generated a tremendous amount of enthusiasm in the cardiology and cardiac surgery communities. Coronary revascularization on a beating heart, which has been used effectively in the past in selected patients, has been reintroduced as an alternative to the conventional approach. In order to further minimize the invasiveness of coronary revascularization, a small anterior thoracotomy or mediastinotomy has been used to access the region of pathology. This beating heart approach primarily has been applicable to patients with single-vessel coronary artery disease. In spite of its real and potential advantages, coronary artery bypass grafting without cardiopulmonary bypass is technically more demanding, may not be possible in some patients, and may have less reproducible results. An endovascular or port access technique for cardiopulmonary bypass and cardioplegic arrest has been developed for use in cardiac surgery. This peripherally based system achieves aortic occlusion, delivery of cardioplegia, and left ventricular decompression. It enables the surgeon to perform coronary revascularization and various cardiac procedures effectively in a less invasive fashion than is possible with conventional median sternotomy. Although the initial experience with this technique is encouraging, prospective randomized studies are required to compare this technique with the conventional open coronary revascularization technique. The goals of this procedure are to provide a safe, effective operation; less tissue trauma and pain for the patient; and a shorter hospital stay and shorter time to resumption of regular activity. It is hoped that continued technical advances in the field of minimally invasive cardiac surgery will facilitate the conduct of more diverse cardiac procedures, increase patient safety, and contribute to long-term results that are comparable to and, in some aspects, superior to conventional open techniques.

References

1. Acuff TE, Landreneau RJ, Griffith BP, et al: Minimally invasive coronary artery bypass grafting. Ann Thorac Surg 61:135–137, 1996.
2. Benetti FJ, Ballester C, Sani G, et al: Video assisted coronary bypass surgery. J Card Surg 10:620–625, 1995.
3. Boonstra PW, Grandjean JG, Mariani MA: Improved method for direct coronary grafting without CPB via anterolateral small thoracotomy. Ann Thorac Surg 63:567–569, 1997.
4. Calafiore AM, DiGiammarco G, Teodori G, et al: Left anterior descending coronary artery grafting via left anterior small thoracotomy without cardiopulmonary bypass. Ann Thorac Surg 61:1658–1665, 1996.
5. Falk V, Walther T, Diegeler A, et al: Echocardiographic monitoring of minimally invasive mitral valve surgery using an endoaortic clamp. J Heart Valve Dis 5:630–637, 1996.
6. Fann JI, Peters WS, Burdon TA, et al: Port-access two-vessel coronary revascularization in the dog (Abstract). J Am Coll Cardiol 29 (suppl A): 466A, 1997.
7. Fann JI, Pompili MF, Stevens JH, et al: Port-access cardiac operations with cardioplegic arrest. Ann Thorac Surg 63:S35–S39, 1997.
8. Landreneau RJ, Mack MJ, Hazelrigg SR, et al: Video-assisted thoracic surgery: Basic technical concepts and intercostal approach strategies. Ann Thorac Surg 54:800–807, 1992.
9. Nataf P, Lima L, Regan M, et al: Minimally invasive coronary surgery with thoracoscopic internal mammary artery dissection: Surgical technique. J Card Surg 11:288–292, 1996.
10. Mack MJ, Aronoff RJ, Acuff TE, et al: Present role of thoracoscopy in the diagnosis and management of diseases of the chest. Ann Thorac Surg 54:403–409, 1992.
11. Peters WS: Minimally invasive cardiac surgery by cardioscopy. Australas J Thorac Cardiovasc Surg 2:152–154, 1993.
12. Peters WS, Burdon TA, Siegel LC, et al: Port-access bilateral internal mammary artery grafting for left main coronary disease: Canine feasibility study. J Card Surg 12:1–7, 1997.
13. Peters WS, Siegel LC, Stevens JH, et al: Closed chest cardiopulmonary bypass and cardioplegia: Basis for less invasive cardiac surgery. Ann Thorac Surg 63:1748–1751, 1997.
14. Reitz BA, Stevens JH, Burdon TA, et al: Port-access coronary artery bypass grafting: Lessons learned in a phase I clinical trial (Abstract). Circulation 94 (suppl I): I-52, 1996.
15. Ribakove GH, Galloway AC, Grossi EA, et al: Port-access coronary artery bypass grafting. Semin Thorac Cardiovasc Surg 9:312–319, 1997.
16. Robinson MC, Gross DR, Zeman W, et al: Minimally invasive

coronary artery bypass grafting: A new method using an anterior mediastinotomy. J Card Surg 10:529–536, 1995.
17. Schwartz DS, Ribakove GH, Grossi EA, et al: Minimally invasive cardiopulmonary bypass with cardioplegic arrest: A closed chest technique with equivalent myocardial protection. J Thorac Cardiovasc Surg 111:556–566, 1996.
18. Schwartz DS, Ribakove GH, Grossi EA, et al: Single and multivessel port-access coronary artery bypass grafting with cardioplegic arrest: Technique and reproducibility. J Thorac Cardiovasc Surg 114:46–52, 1997.
19. Siegel LC, St. Goar FG, Stevens JH, et al: Monitoring considerations for port-access cardiac surgery. Circulation 96:562–568, 1997.
20. Shennib H, Lee AGL, Akin J: Safe and effective method of stabilization for coronary artery bypass grafting on the beating heart. Ann Thorac Surg 63:988–992, 1997.
21. Stevens JH, Burdon TA, Peters WS, et al: Port-access coronary artery bypass grafting: A proposed surgical method. J Thorac Cardiovasc Surg 111:567–573, 1996.
22. Stevens JH, Burdon TA, Siegel LC, et al: Port-access coronary artery bypass with cardioplegic arrest: Acute and chronic canine studies. Ann Thorac Surg 62:435–441, 1996.
23. Toomasian JM, Peters WS, Siegel LC, et al: Extracorporeal circulation for port-access cardiac surgery. Perfusion 12:83–91, 1997.
24. Toomasian JM, Williams DL, Colvin SB, et al: Perfusion during coronary and mitral valve surgery utilizing minimally invasive port-access technology. J Extra-Corporeal Technol 29:66–72, 1997.

COMMENTARY

Denton A. Cooley

Dr. Ikonomidis and colleagues present an interesting description of a minimally invasive technique for myocardial revascularization using port access coronary bypass grafting. Although the authors describe many theoretical and some practical advantages for the patient, several disadvantages of this technique deserve consideration.

Technically, the port access method presents many challenges. First, the procedure requires cannulation of the femoral artery and vein through an incision in the groin. Most patients who have coronary artery occlusive disease, however, have generalized atherosclerosis, so the femoral artery and other potential cannulation sites may themselves be occluded. In addition, passing a large-bore cannula through the femoral and iliac veins may cause thrombosis. Even positioning the aortic occluder in the ascending aorta (which may also be diseased) requires careful attention, mostly on the part of the anesthesiologist, because the occluder could become dislodged during the procedure. Finally, placing the catheters in the desired position for port access grafting requires more contrast medium than does catheter placement for a conventional coronary bypass; the excess medium could compromise a patient's renal function.

In terms of cost, the port access method requires equipment that may not be available in some operating rooms, such as video equipment, transesophageal ultrasonography and, possibly, fluoroscopy. The method also necessitates extended time in the operating room, which is the most expensive service in most hospitals. After adding the cost of disposable surgical items, the port access method actually becomes less cost-effective than conventional coronary bypass.

Beyond these logistical considerations lie more abstract ones. It behooves us to recall why conventional cardiopulmonary bypass was used in the first coronary artery bypass graft procedures. Surgeons felt more comfortable operating on quiet, bloodless coronary vessels, and cardiologists required even minor branches of the coronary circulation system to be bypassed to achieve complete revascularization. Now, however, cardiologists may suggest only a single internal mammary artery graft to the left anterior descending coronary artery, which is performed through a minimally invasive incision. If such a graft is tenable, they may attempt to repair right and circumflex stenoses using angioplasty, thus eliminating the need for more invasive surgery.

Ultimately, surgeons should be technically capable of performing vascular anastomoses on the beating heart. In many centers, including our own, minimally invasive bypass procedures are successfully performed with the heart beating. Because such procedures are entirely feasible, and in light of the preceding concerns, I believe that, with a few exceptions, port access coronary bypass grafting should be reserved for intracardiac surgery.

COMMENTARY

Alan J. Bryan

The development of port access coronary artery bypass grafting has been of enormous interest to cardiac surgeons around the world. Its development from drawing board to animal laboratory to operating theater has been a model of scientific evaluation. The only difference has been the huge commercial investment riding on its success.

The port access system is wonderfully innovative but suffers somewhat from its complexity, and exactly how minimally invasive it is is open to debate. It does, after all, incorporate femoral cannulation, cardiopulmonary bypass, and cardioplegic arrest, albeit in association with a smaller chest incision. It is now possible to carry out coronary artery bypass grafting to multiple sites using these techniques in selected patients.[1] All the standard advantages associated with a standard cardiac surgical approach are present, that is, a still, bloodless, decompressed operating field. In addition, the accepted adjuncts to modern cardiac surgery, including retrograde cardioplegia, the extended use of arterial grafts, and so on, appear to be possible.[2] The clinical results from the major centers appear excellent, with acceptable morbidity and mortality. A note of caution is important, however, because it is apparent that intensive case selection precedes the use of these techniques, and a true picture has yet to emerge.

If the techniques are proven, we must ask why their use remains limited. Is this for fiscal reasons? Is it because the techniques are so complicated that cardiac surgeons are reluctant to abandon techniques with a proven track record? Or is it because there are remaining concerns about the current techniques that leave a degree of skepticism among many cardiac surgeons that the proponents of this technique have so far failed to answer? There are concerns that the use of femoral cannulation is a backward rather than a forward step, and there remains the specter of retrograde dissection, a potentially catastrophic complication not addressed in this chapter. Indeed, some of the early proponents of this technique have reverted to central cannulation techniques. The complexity of the technique, the routine use of TEE, and the financial aspects of these approaches have already been alluded to. There is a nagging concern that target vessels and selected conduits may be tailored to a minimal access approach rather than to what is predicted to be in the best long-term interests of the patient. Finally, there is the continuing lack of prospective controlled data to demonstrate reduced hospital stay and enhanced recovery.

This is undoubtedly a technology in evolution, and let us hope that these techniques can be developed and safely applied to a large proportion of cardiac surgical patients. In the meantime, despite the obvious commercial disadvantages, it is my view that further evaluation of these techniques by reference centers is justified before their widespread use is encouraged.

References

1. Gulielmos V, Kraut M, Wagner FM, et al: Minimally invasive surgical technique for the treatment of multi-vessel coronary artery disease. Ann Thorac Surg 65:1331–1334, 1998.
2. Ribakove GH, Miller JS, Anderson RV, et al: Minimally invasive port-access coronary artery bypass grafting with early angiographic follow up: Initial clinical experience. J Thorac Cardiovasc Surg 115:1101–1110, 1998.

COMMENTARY

Mohammad Fouda

The term *minimally invasive cardiac surgery* has been, and still is, used indiscriminately by a number of investigators worldwide. It is important to define *minimally invasive cardiac surgery* in a precise scientific and linguistic manner, because we are setting the cornerstones for this evolving branch of cardiac surgery. Multiple-vessel off-pump grafting through limited or full sternotomy or through thoracotomy should not be classified under the same heading as port access surgery, which I tend to consider *minimal access invasive surgery.* I believe that the morbidity of port access surgery, including that of cardiopulmonary bypass, in addition to the potential peripheral vascular complications due to peripheral cannulation and the use of aortic occlusion balloons, indicates that the only clear advantage of these procedures is the small size of the incision.

To move from this narrow field of minimal access surgery to the broader field of minimally invasive coronary grafting, I believe that the use of cardiopulmonary bypass should be avoided, and devices for mechanical stabilization of the beating heart must be improved. This may or may not be combined with the use of smaller incisions. Only then will we be heading in the right direction toward achieving the right definition of minimally invasive cardiac surgery.

Chapter 67

Axial Blood Flow Pumps: An Alternative to Cardiopulmonary Bypass for Coronary Surgery

Urban Lönn and Henrik Casimir-Ahn

Coronary artery bypass grafting (CABG) supported by cardiopulmonary bypass (CPB) evolved into a practical technique during the late 1960s and has become the state of the art, with low morbidity and mortality.[1–3] There are, however, several concerns related to CPB in high-risk patients. Negative factors attributed to CPB include blood trauma leading to coagulopathy, need for full heparinization, complement activation and leukocyte-mediated inflammatory reaction leading to pulmonary and renal dysfunction, hemodilution with volume overload, and gastrointestinal damage with gut mucosal ischemia.[4–11] Blood transfusions, when necessary, add the risk of transmission of hepatitis or human immunodeficiency virus (HIV).[12] The concomitant use of aortic cross-clamping with cardiac arrest causes ischemic damage with temporary or permanent ventricular impairment.[13] CPB is not mandatory, however, because revascularization surgery is performed on the surface of the closed heart.

Beating heart surgery has generated a lot of interest since the introduction of minimally invasive direct coronary artery bypass (MIDCAB) surgery. This procedure is not new, however. In 1967, the Russian surgeon Kolesov described a left anterior thoracotomy by which he performed an anastomosis between the left mammary artery and the left descending coronary artery without extracorporeal circulation.[14] Buffolo, Benetti, and Pfister and associates reported beating heart bypass surgery through a midline sternotomy in over 1500 patients[15–17] as an alternative to the "gold standard," i.e., use of CPB, aortic cross-clamping, and cardioplegic arrest. This procedure is technically more demanding, and concerns have been raised about long-term results. MIDCAB surgery has become a more common procedure, even though no results regarding long-term efficiency have been reported.

Ventricular assist devices (VADs) (Fig. 67-1) have been successfully used to support patients during CABG. These techniques avoid the risks of CPB and an artificial oxygenator, because the patient's own lungs are functioning. Decompression of the heart is effective and allows the surgeon to reach vessels that are inaccessible by the MIDCAB approach.

Clinical use of the Hemopump (Medtronic/DLP Inc., Grand Rapids, MI), a temporary cardiac assist device, was first reported by Frazier and associates.[18] It was the result of a research program started in the early 1970s by Dr. Richard Wampler, who, during irrigation work in Egypt, came up with the idea of using the principle of the Archimedes screw to move liquid (Fig. 67–2). This led to the construction of the Hemopump.[19, 20] The operating principle is a one-site cannulation and introduction of a minimally invasive pump into the aorta. Through a cannula mounted on the pump and positioned in the left ventricle, the system can suck blood out of the heart and expel it into the systemic circulation. The system has been used primarily as a left ventricular assist device (LVAD) in patients with postcardiotomy heart failure, where it has proved to be an excellent device.[21–26] Other indications for this pump include circulatory support in high-risk percutaneous transluminal coronary angioplasty (PTCA), using the percutanous version of the Hemopump[27, 28]; while awaiting heart transplant[29, 30]; and during CABG, replacing the heart-lung machine.[31]

We found the idea of replacing CPB with the Hemopump through a midline sternotomy an attractive way to perform less invasive CABG. This might enable surgery on an unloaded heart and make multiple grafts feasible.

Operating Principles of the Hemopump

The Hemopump consists of a catheter-mounted, minimally invasive axial blood flow pump; a small extracorporeal electromagnetic motor; a purge set assembly; and a console that provides power to the pump and purge set assembly (Fig. 67–3). The system is based on the principle of the Archimedes screw, whereby a rotating screw within a tube can transport liquid. The moving part of the pump (rotor) is positioned at the top of an approximately 1-meter-long metallic wire (drive cable). The drive cable is covered by a polyurethane sheet. At the proximal end, a magnet is connected to the drive cable. One end of a plastic tube (pump cannula) that is open at both ends is placed over the rotor. The magnet is placed within the motor, which is connected to the console. The electromagnetic motor makes the drive cable and rotor spin. The purge set assembly is connected to the sheet covering the drive cable, providing blood-seal integrity and hydrodynamic lubrication. The maximum rotating speed of these pumps varies from 25,000 to 48,000 revolutions/min, depending on the size of the pump used. The system allows blood to be sucked out of the left ventricle and expelled into the aorta. This is achieved by placing the pump cannula's distal tip (inflow) transvalvularly into the left ventricle. The proximal end (outflow) of the cannula with the rotor is located in the aorta (Fig. 67–4).

The first version of the Hemopump was designed to be placed through a cutdown in the groin into the femoral artery, and then guided into the right position with fluoroscopy. This pump, labeled HP-21, had a cannula length of 26.2 cm and a diameter of 7.9 mm. The maximal flow capacity was around 3 L/min, against a pressure head of 70 mm Hg. The speed of the pump could be altered from 17,000 to 25,000 revolutions/min. Initial clinical experi-

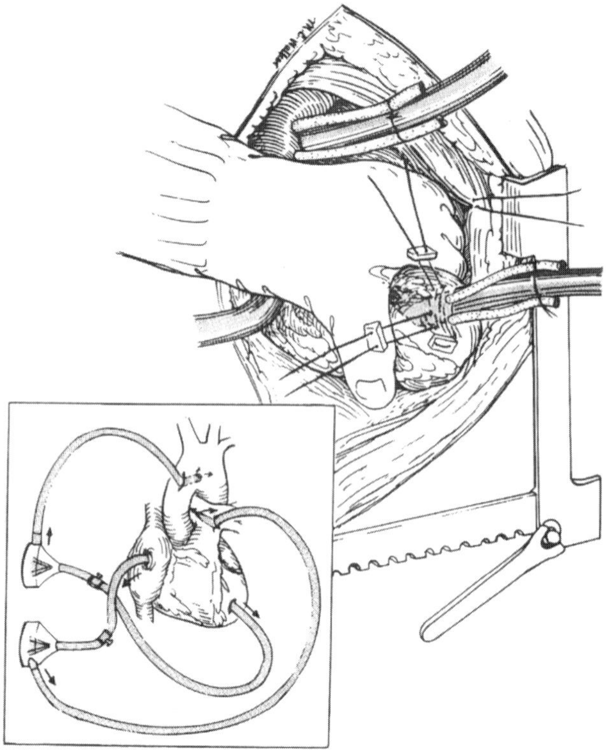

Figure 67–1. Schematic illustration of setup for ventricular-device-supported coronary artery bypass graft. Bio-Medicus systems aspirate blood from the left ventricle and the right atrium. The blood is pumped back into the aorta and the pulmonary artery. (From Sweeney MS, Frazier OH: Device-supported myocardial revascularization: Safe help for sick hearts. Ann Thorac Surg 54:1065–1070, 1992. (Courtesy of Medtronic/DLP, Inc., Grand Rapids, MI.)

ence with this pump showed a 23% failure to insert the device owing to arteriosclerosis of the pelvic arteries. Another pump (HP-31) was introduced in the beginning of the 1990s. The changes included redesign of the rotor and a shorter cannula (9.5 cm). This increased pump outflow by 1.5 L/min. Access is through a graft sutured to the ascending aorta, thus the chest needs to be open. A third version of the Hemopump (HP-14) was recently introduced. It is a percutanous system, designed to be placed through an introducer and a guide wire from the femoral artery. The diameter of this pump is only 4.6 mm, making it possible to use with this approach. Outflow is limited to approximately 2 L/min at a maximum speed of 48,000 revolutions/min (Fig. 67–5).

The first study presenting the Hemopump as an alternative to CPB during CABG was published in 1992 by Sweeney and Frazier.[31] They used the device as an LVAD in combination with a Bio-Medicus pump on the right side to perform beating heart coronary surgery in critically ill patients (Fig. 67–6). In a few patients, the Hemopump acted as the only means of circulatory support. In addition to the circulatory support, they used the short-acting β-blocker esmolol to reduce the contractility of the heart, enhancing the precision of the anastomosis. They concluded that this technique is safe and offers real advantages in the management of critically ill patients.

We have been using the Hemopump as an LVAD in patients who have postcardiotomy shock for the past 6 years and have been impressed with the system's capability to fully unload a failing left ventricle while sustaining adequate blood flow to the body and preserving multiorgan function.[26, 32] In this group of patients we were able to wean and discharge 58%. In a subgroup of patients (54%) in which early intervention was applied, 85% were discharged from the hospital. Based on the knowledge we had gained using the Hemopump as an LVAD in the "failure to wean" situation, together with the method described by Sweeney and Frazier, we decided to try to refine the use of the Hemopump as a circulatory support system in place of CPB during CABG. Our hypothesis was that we should be able to use the Hemopump as the only means of circulatory support during these procedures. We proceeded in three steps:

1. An animal trial
2. A small pilot study in humans
3. A prospective randomized trial toward the goal—HP-supported CABG vs. the gold standard (CPB with cold cardioplegic arrest)

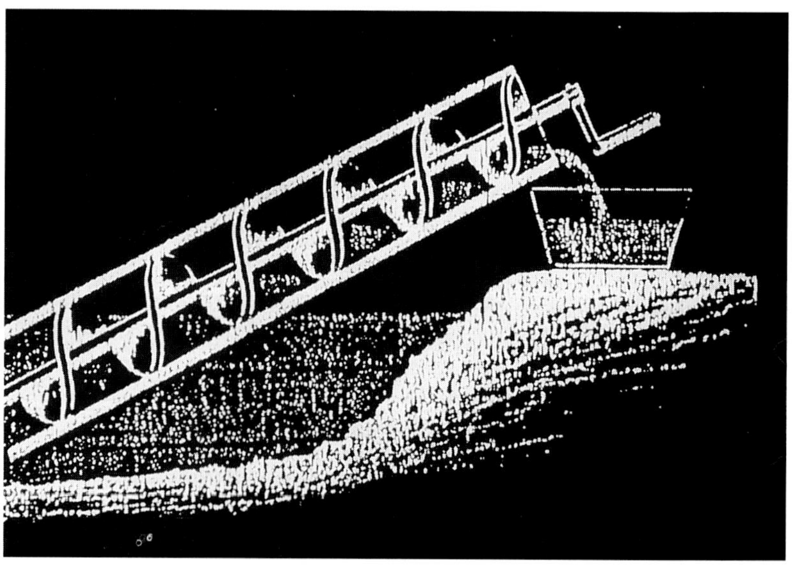

Figure 67–2. Schematic illustration of the Archimedes screw.

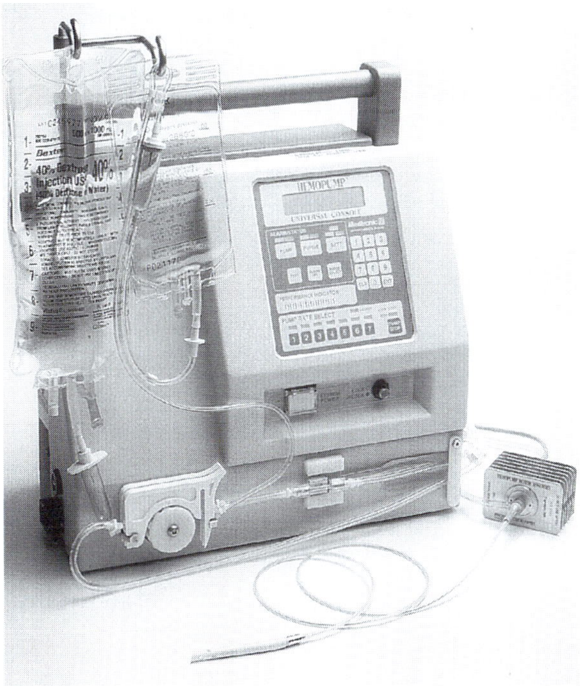

Figure 67–3. The Hemopump temporary cardiac assist system. Components included are the drive console, purge assembly, electromagnetic motor, and pump assembly (in this picture, an HP-31). (Courtesy of Medtronic/DLP, Inc., Grand Rapids, MI.)

Method

An animal model was set up to evaluate whether our hypothesis was valid. We used 12 pigs with a mean weight of 56 kg. They were all prepared in a standard fashion for bypass surgery, including complete hemodynamic monitoring. After a midline sternotomy, the left or right internal mammary artery (IMA) was dissected and prepared for grafting. The Hemopump was inserted into the abdominal

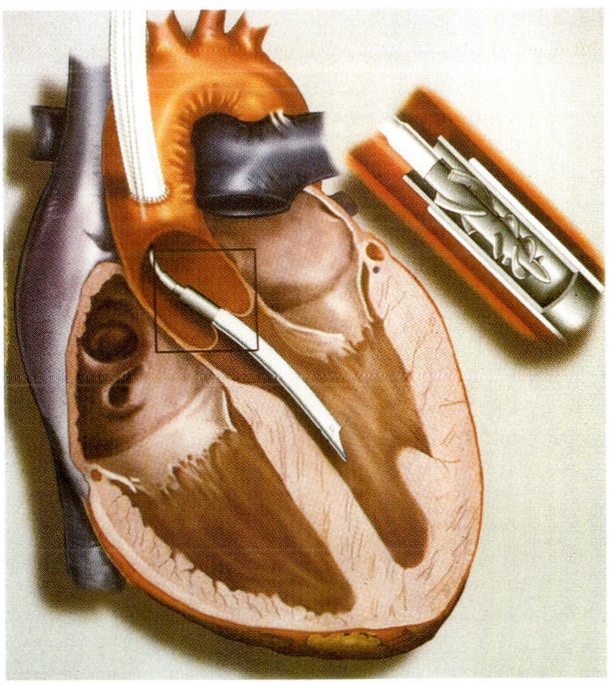

Figure 67–4. Hemopump HP-31 (sternotomy cannula) in position within the heart through a graft anastomosed to the ascending aorta. A cross-section of the pump housing is also shown. (Courtesy of Medtronic/DLP, Inc., Grand Rapids, MI.)

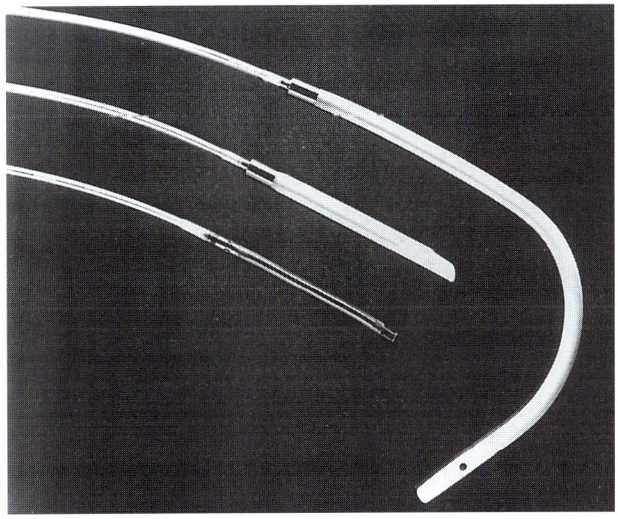

Figure 67–5. The three different Hemopumps. *Top,* HP-21; *middle,* HP-31 (sternotomy cannula); and *bottom,* HP-14. (Courtesy of Medtronic/DLP, Inc., Grand Rapids, MI.)

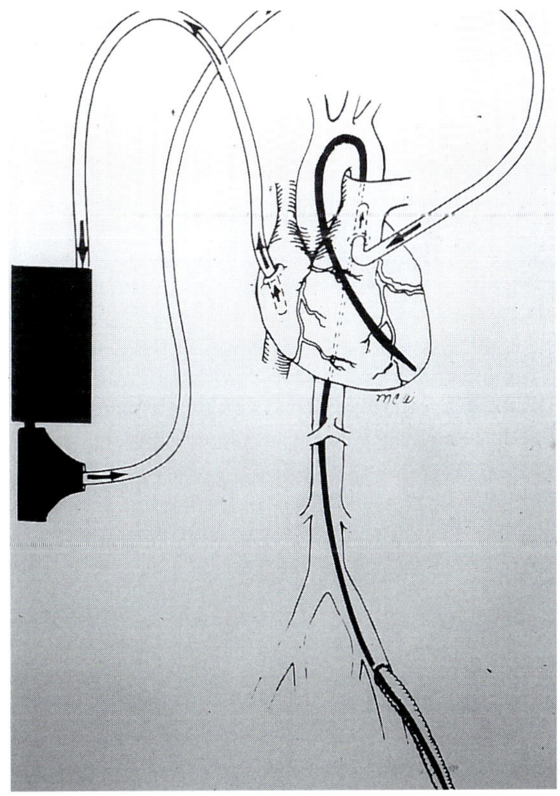

Figure 67–6. Setup for ventricular assist device–supported coronary artery bypass graft as described by Sweeney and Frazier.[31] An HP-21 in the left ventricle is inserted via the femoral artery, and a Bio-Medicus system is aspirating blood from the right atrium of the heart and pumping it back into the pulmonary artery.

aorta using a retroperitoneal approach and brought over a guide wire into the left ventricle. Radiographs were used to confirm correct positioning. During Hemopump support, a bolus dose 0.5 to 5 mg/kg of esmolol was given before incremental titration from 100 to 600 μg/kg per minute over 15 to 20 minutes. The infusion was held constant when the heart became flaccid enough to allow surgery. The IMA was sutured to the distal part of the left anterior descending artery (LAD) after occlusion with "lasso" sutures placed proximal and distal to the anastomotic site. The esmolol infusion was stopped when the anastomosis was completed using 7–0 polypropylene suture. The Hemopump was withdrawn to the aorta after a weaning period of 20 to 30 minutes. Hemodynamic measurements were done periodically (Fig. 67–7). At the end of the experiment, patency of the anastomosis was verified with a 1.5-mm metallic probe.

A subsequent pilot study in humans was carried out. Five patients, four men and one woman with a mean age of 64.8 years (range 54 to 78 years) who were scheduled for CABG procedures, were selected for this study. Four patients had single-vessel disease involving the LAD. Three of them had LAD occlusions, and 1 had a significantly long stenosis that was not suitable for PTCA. The fifth patient had two-vessel disease. A midline sternotomy was performed, and the pericardium was opened to visualize the area of intervention. At this point the decision was made as to the patient's suitability for this surgical strategy.

The IMA was dissected in a standard fashion while the Hemopump was prepared and primed. A catheter was placed into the pulmonary artery for measurement of pulmonary pressure and mixed venous saturation. The patients were given 7500 U of heparin. A 12-mm Hemashield graft (Boston Scientific, Oakland, NJ), 15 cm long, was cut at a 45-degree angle at one end. This end was sutured about 5 cm cephalad to the sinus of Valsalva, with the edge of the graft pointing toward the aortic valves. All patients had a No. 31, 24-French Hemopump cannula placed through the graft into the left ventricle (Figs. 67–8 to 67–10).

Adequate positioning of the pump was ascertained by on-off tests and feeling the position of the pump housing by a smooth compression of the aorta just distal to the aortic valves. The pump speed was gradually increased to the highest velocity over 1 minute. A bolus dose of 1 mg/kg esmolol was given to the patient, followed by a continuous infusion starting with 300 μg/kg per min. The esmolol infusion was titrated up to a dose at which the surgeon judged that the heart was flaccid enough to perform bypass surgery without difficulty (Fig. 67–11). Before every increase in infusion speed, an additional bolus dose of 0.5 mg/kg of esmolol was given. The average esmolol dose at surgery was 560 μg/kg per min (range, 400 to 700). Proximal and distal to the anastomotic site of the coronary artery, vessel loops were placed to prevent bleeding. Four patients received the IMA-to-LAD graft as the only intervention. The fifth patient had an IMA-to-LAD graft, one vein graft to the first diagonal branch of the LAD, and one vein graft to the right coronary artery. The esmolol infusion was stopped just before completion of bypass surgery, and at least 15 minutes of reperfusion were maintained with the Hemopump on full speed before weaning the patient off the circulatory support.

Before surgery **After surgery** **+30min** **+60min** **+90min**

Hemopump on
I------------------I
Esmolol
I--------------I
1 **2** **3** **4** **5**

Figure 67–7. Schematic illustration of the experimental protocol. Hemodynamic measurements were carried out before and after bypass surgery. The Hemopump was used to decompress the heart and as circulatory support. Esmolol administration was started before surgery and stopped after grafting.

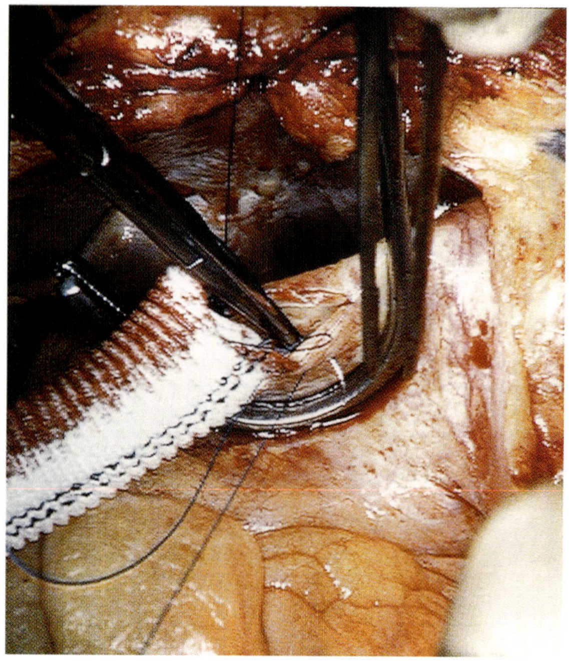

Figure 67–8. A 12-mm Hemashield graft is sutured to the ascending aorta approximately 5 cm distal to the sinus of Valsalva.

A randomized study was then performed to validate this procedure. Thirty-two patients who had stable angina scheduled for CABG were selected. Because previous experience had shown us that there might be problems reaching the middle branches of the circumflex artery when using the Hemopump technique, patients needing bypass to this area were excluded. The patients were prospectively randomized into two groups. Patients in the control group underwent CPB and aortic cross-clamping with cold ischemic arrest. Those in the study group were operated on with the heart empty and beating by means of Hemopump support. Both groups received routine pre- and postoperative care. A Swan-Ganz catheter was placed before anesthesia, allowing hemodynamic monitoring as well as real-time measurements of mixed venous oxygen saturation. A midline sternotomy was performed, and the pericardium was opened to visualize the areas of intervention.

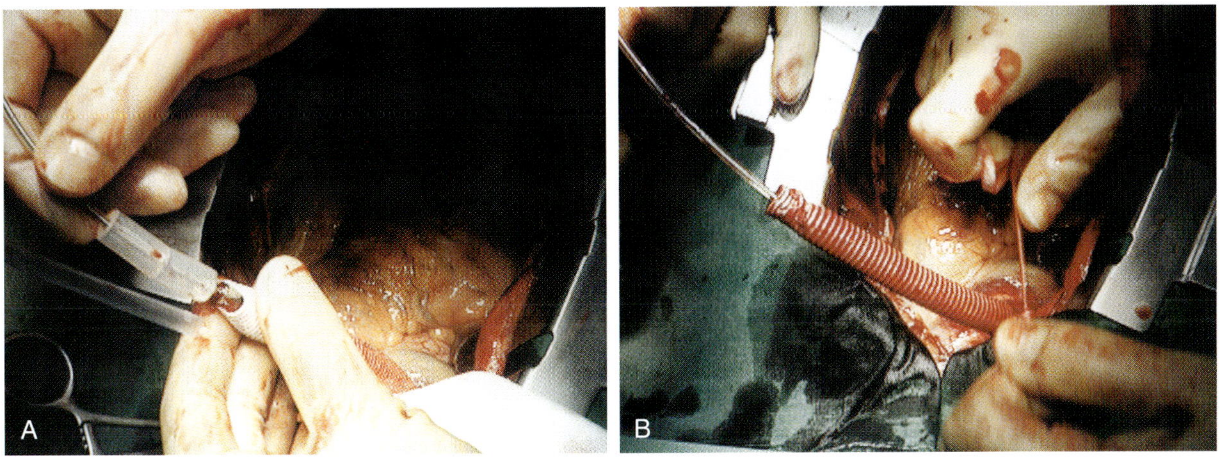

Figure 67–9. *A*, Two silicon graft plugs are positioned around the drive cable into the graft, securing the system in place during the procedure. *B*, The graft plugs are fixed firmly with cotton bands.

CPB Group

Patients randomized to CPB had standard cannulation of the right atrium and the ascending aorta. Cold crystalloid cardioplegia (Plegisol, Abbott), aortic cross-clamping, and mild hypothermia (32 to 34°C) were used. The CPB circuit involved a non-heparin-coated membrane oxygenator and a hard-shell venous reservoir (Sorin Biomedica Cardio, Saluggea, Italy). Heparin was given to achieve an activated clotting time (ACT) not less than 400 sec. The operation was then performed in a standard fashion. Hemodynamic recordings were made before anesthesia, after induction of anesthesia, after termination of CPB, on arrival at the intensive care unit (ICU), 6 hours postoperatively, and at discharge from the intensive care unit (ICU).

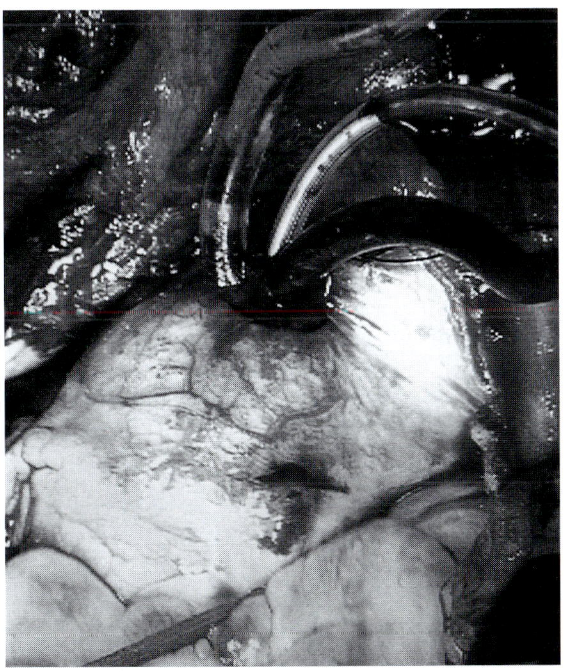

Figure 67–10. Alternatively, the Hemopump can be positioned and secured by a double pursestring suture.

Hemopump Group

Heparin was given at a dose of 5000 to 10,000 U to achieve an ACT of about 200 sec. The hemodynamic response was measured before anesthesia, after induction of anesthesia, at a steady-state level with maximal esmolol effect during surgery, after removal of the Hemopump, on arrival at the ICU, 6 hours postoperatively, and at discharge from the ICU. The esmolol infusion was stopped just before completion of bypass surgery, and reperfusion was maintained for at least 15 minutes with the Hemopump at full speed before weaning the patient off circulatory support. After weaning, the Hemopump was withdrawn into the graft, a sidebiter was placed just proximal to the insertion site, the graft was removed, and the arteriotomy was sutured with two layers of running 4–0 Prolene.

Two different techniques were used for the vein grafts. Either the distal anastomosis was completed first and then connected to the aorta in a standard fashion, or the proximal anastomosis was sutured first, at the same time as the graft for the Hemopump was placed. With this approach, flow to the native coronary artery could be established as soon as each distal anastomosis was done.

In both groups blood chemistry data were obtained the day before surgery and the morning after surgery in the ICU, except for plasma-free hemoglobin and troponin T, which were only measured postoperatively. To determine heart muscle damage, the enzyme aspartate aminotrans-

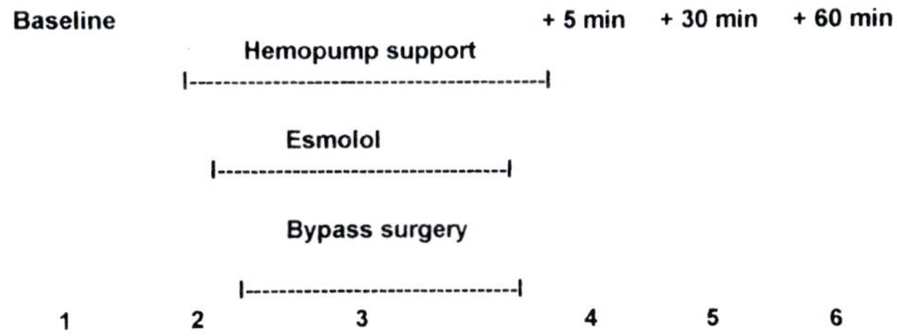

Figure 67–11. Schematic illustration of the procedure. With the Hemopump on full speed, esmolol administration was started. Bypass surgery was performed when the heart was sufficiently decompressed and flaccid. Hemodynamic measurements were carried out intermittently (1–6).

ferase (AST) was measured together with troponin T. Renal function was assessed by means of serum creatinine, and platelet consumption was assumed to be the difference between pre- and postoperative counts.

Results

In the animal trial, 7 of 12 pigs went through the whole procedure and were weaned off the Hemopump without complications. Five of the first seven animals died owing to right ventricular failure in association with esmolol administration. A bolus dose of 1 to 5 mg/kg proved to be too high for these animals. All animals survived when we reduced the initial dose to 0.5 mg/kg and started the infusion with 100 μg/kg per minute. None of these animals had right ventricular failure. There were significant differences in esmolol dose-response curves among the surviving animals (Fig. 67–12).

Temporary ST elevations were observed during occlusion of the LAD, but there were no adverse hemodynamic reactions. There was complete resolution of the esmolol effect within 20 to 30 minutes, and no antagonist was needed. No significant hemodynamic differences were observed during the procedure (Figs. 67–13 and 67–14). We did not measure cardiac index during Hemopump support because of the unreliability of values obtained by the thermodilution technique during Hemopump assist. Mixed venous saturation was good throughout the experiment in these animals. All anastomoses proved to be patent after the experiment.

In the pilot study in humans, all patients came through the procedure uneventfully. They stayed in the ICU for an average of 1.2 days. Total hospital stay averaged 9 days. Average time on Hemopump support was 56 minutes. All patients were separated from the Hemopump within 5 minutes after the final anastomosis. The ACT averaged 219 seconds after the initial bolus dose of heparin and leveled out to 192 seconds at steady state. Protamine was given to all patients when the Hemopump was withdrawn. The patients were back to normal ACT levels (mean, 129 sec) 60 minutes after Hemopump removal.

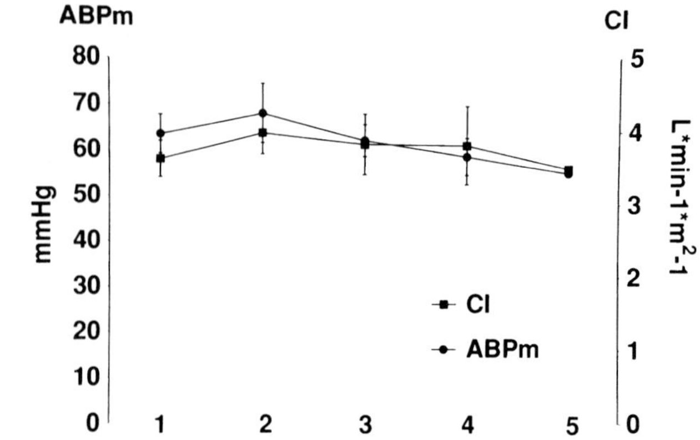

Figure 67–13. Combined data from the surviving animals depicting cardiac index (CI) and mean arterial blood pressure (ABPm). No significant differences were observed during the experiment.

The hemodynamic response measured by mean arterial blood pressure (MAP), mean pulmonary artery pressure (MPAP), and central venous pressure (CVP) is shown in Figure 67–15. There was a significant fall in MAP from baseline to steady-state measurements (P = .0002). All patients were back to baseline values 30 minutes after pump removal. MPAP did not change significantly during the procedure. CVP showed a significant rise between the baseline and steady-state recordings (P = .04). Baseline measurements were attained 30 minutes after pump removal. Heart rate and mixed venous saturation did not change significantly during the operation (Fig. 67–16).

Median blood loss during the first 12 postoperative hours, including intraoperative bleeding, was 545 ml (range, 250 to 1090 ml). None of the patients needed blood transfusion. Urinary output was not a problem in these patients, and we did not observe any renal impairment. In an attempt to quantify heart damage during the procedure, AST and alanine aminotransferase (ALT) were registered the morning after surgery. The values averaged 1.1 μkat (range, 0.64 to 1.40) and 0.43 μkat (range, 0.24 to 0.75), respectively (reference value, <0.8 μkat). Perioperative echocardiograms did not show any signs of acute infarction.

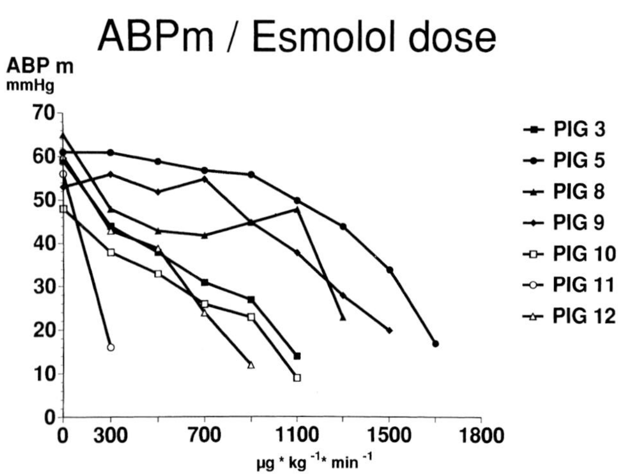

Figure 67–12. Dose-response curves for the surviving seven animals, showing mean blood pressure (ABPm) response to changes in esmolol dose. Large variations were observed among animals.

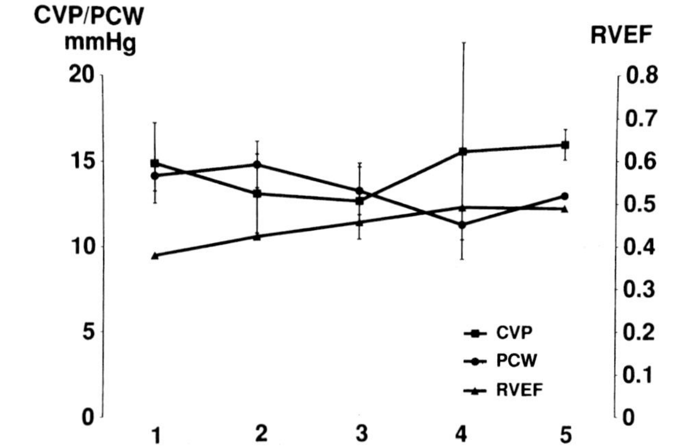

Figure 67–14. Combined data from all seven surviving pigs on central venous pressure (CVP), pulmonary capillary wedge pressure (PCW), and right ventricular ejection fraction (RVEF). No significant differences were observed during the procedure.

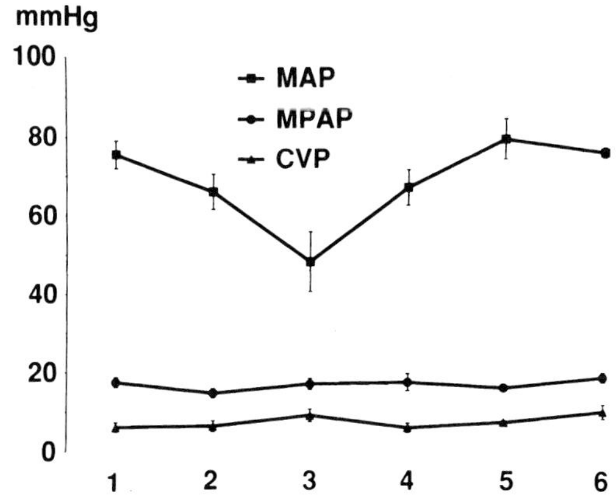

Figure 67–15. Recording of mean arterial blood pressure (MAP), mean pulmonary artery pressure (MPAP), and central venous pressure (CVP) during the procedure. MAP fell significantly when Hemopump and esmolol were combined. A concomitant increase of CVP was observed. The baseline values were attained 30 minutes after the Hemopump and esmolol were stopped.

In the prospective randomized trial, statistically more grafts were placed in the CPB group than in the Hemopump group (2.5, range 1 to 4; vs. 1.8, range 1 to 3; $P = .03$). The average aortic cross-clamp time in the CPB group was 34.1 minutes (range, 15 to 75 minutes). Time on cardiac support and total operating time did not differ between the groups. Intraoperative bleeding was statistically different, however. In the Hemopump group, mean blood loss was 312 ml (range, 150 to 500 ml) compared with 582 ml (range, 350 to 1150 ml) in the CPB group ($P = .0003$).

Total fluid balance, including all fluids given or lost (crystalloids, colloids, urine output, evaporation), did not differ between the groups.

There was no statistical difference in the mean time to extubation between the groups: mean for the Hemopump group, 6.5 hours compared with 29.8 hours for the CPB group. The median time was 6 hours vs. 10 hours. Mean time spent in the ICU was 1.1 days for the Hemopump group and 1.9 days for the CPB group, which did not differ statistically. Four patients needed inotropic support in

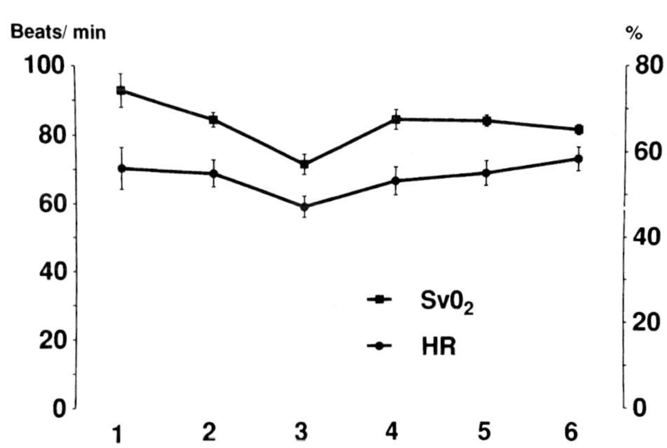

Figure 67–16. Recording of heart rate (HR) and mixed venous saturation (Svo_2) during the procedure. A trend similar to the variables in Figure 67– was observed. The changes were not statistically significant. Svo_2 did not fall below 50%.

the CPB group, compared with one in the Hemopump group. Total length of stay in the hospital averaged 8 days in both groups.

There were no statistical differences in the levels of ASAT, serum creatinine, or platelets pre- and postoperatively between the groups. The level of troponin T as a sensitive marker of heart muscle ischemia during surgery differed between the groups; the mean value in the Hemopump group was 0.23 μg/L, compared with 1.17 μg/L in the CPB group ($P = .004$). From a hemodynamic point of view, there were no differences during or after the procedure.

Discussion

Since the introduction of the MIDCAB procedure, operating on the beating heart has become an alternative in selected patients for many thoracic surgeons. It is, however, more demanding than the gold standard, especially if it is done through a very small incision. We believe that the method described here constitutes an intermediate step in the process of converting classic coronary artery surgery to a closed chest procedure. The question of whether sternotomy or CPB should be the first procedure to go has not yet been answered. For us, it was a natural step to move into the field of less invasive coronary bypass surgery by first excluding CPB while retaining the convenience of full sternotomy. In this way, the limitations of MIDCAB surgery, with access to only one or two vessels per incision, can be avoided, and control of the operative field is optimal.

Esmolol, a β1-selective β-blocker that is metabolized in the red blood cells with a half-life of 9 minutes, is excreted in an inactive form via the urine.[33–35] The efficacy and safety of esmolol in the treatment of supraventricular tachyarrhythmias are well documented.[33, 34] A bolus dose of about 1 mg/kg has often been used in these studies. The drug has also been safely used in patients who have myocardial ischemic conditions.[35, 36] When used in patients with severe left ventricular dysfunction, esmolol was associated with significant reduction of both left and right ventricular ejection fractions.[37] These changes were accompanied by increases in end-diastolic volumes, as well as a reduction in cardiac output. The hemodynamic abnormalities showed considerable interindividual variability and returned to near baseline levels 10 to 30 minutes after the infusion was stopped.[12] Esmolol is also known to increase right atrial pressure.[38] These findings are in accordance with our experience in the laboratory. The left ventricle is effectively supported and decompressed by the Hemopump. The pressures on the right side are often increased in association with Hemopump support. This phenomenon may increase when esmolol is added. Therefore, it is important to carefully monitor the right-side pressures and pulmonary vascular resistance. In the seven animals that went through the protocol, we could control these variables.

In the human application, it proved to be very important to reconfirm the position of the Hemopump after manipulation of the heart, as it had a tendency to be sucked into the left ventricle. Palpation of the device in the aortic root was easily done, and there was no need for fluoroscopic control. One potential benefit of Hemopump-supported CABG is a reduced need for blood transfusions. The blood loss in our pilot patients averaged 562 ml, and no transfusions were given. However, massive bleeding from the aorta can be coped with more effectively when CPB is used. Some kind of blood preserving system for intra- and postoperative autotransfusion is essential to exploit fully the potential of Hemopump-supported CABG. Even if there is a need for transfusions in 25 to 75% of patients when CPB is used, a simple but strict protocol can reduce this need to less than 5%.[39]

Avoidance of full heparinization is a potential advantage with Hemopump-supported CABG. We used 7500 to 10,000 U of heparin, and there was no oozing of blood at the end of the operation. Similar results can probably be achieved using heparin-coated CPB.

The aorta is not cross-clamped, and the heart is perfused with its own blood at normothermia, avoiding global myocardial ischemia. This is another approach to the warm heart surgery advocated by several proponents of blood cardioplegia in the clinical setting.[40] Warm blood cardioplegia appears to be beneficial in operations on hearts that are metabolically depleted or acutely ischemic.[41] CABG supported by a Hemopump may be an alternative way of handling patients who have ongoing ischemia or poor ventricular function. Besides offering good "myocardial protection," an effective VAD is already in place if needed. In patients who have compromised hearts, improved outcomes may be possible because intervention is early and the heart is maintained in an unloaded state postoperatively, with coronary perfusion improved by operation. There are also data indicating reduction of acute infarcts when mechanical ventricular decompression is created.[42–44]

Temporary occlusion of the coronary vessels has not caused problems in previous series of CABG without CPB.[15–17] Occlusion of the coronary arteries is usually well tolerated during PTCA without any cardiac decompression. The absence of ST changes during Hemopump-supported CABG may be explained by the combined use of ventricular unloading and high doses of β-blocker, creating a global left ventricle preconditioning.

In the randomized trial, in both groups, we followed our standard clinical protocol regarding anesthesia and postoperative follow-up. We did not expect any differences in time on the ventilator and hospital stay for these patients. If we modified our anesthesia protocol and used short-acting substances, the patients could probably be extubated while in the operating room or soon after. A critical factor is the preservation of normothermia. A significant number of these patients could probably be sent home on the third or fourth postoperative day if we used a "fast-track" protocol, but this was not evaluated. We hope to address this in future trials. The reason for the significant difference in the number of grafts placed in these groups is unclear, but all patients received bypass to the intended vessels based on preoperative angiograms.

The most suitable candidates for this procedure are patients with impaired left ventricular function or acute ongoing ischemia, because myocardial ischemia is reduced using this technique and if the heart should fail, an LVAD is already in place. Hemopump-supported CABG was shown to be a safe and feasible method compared with the gold standard. Potential benefits include less intraoperative bleeding and less ischemia of the heart muscle. The procedure takes no longer to perform, and time of intraoperative cardiac support does not differ. No device-related complications have been seen. Esmolol is an important adjuvant that facilitates precise surgery.

A crucial issue in beating heart CABG surgery is graft patency. We performed follow-up angiography of the left IMA in 11 patients operated on with this method (Fig. 67–17). All patients had IMA-to-LAD grafts. Median follow-up time was 314 days (range, 111 to 401 days). All patients had contrast medium passing through the IMA to the LAD. In 8 of 11 patients, there was rapid and adequate filling of the LAD. In 1 patient, a suspected stenosis of the anastomosis was detected; the stenosis was classified as not significant. In 3 of 11 patients there was a narrow and thin IMA with little contrast passing to the LAD, and the anastomosis could not be evaluated. Two of these patients had large anterior wall infarctions with akinesia of that area preoperatively. Both patients also had LAD occlusion and poor retrograde filling of the LAD preoperatively. The filling of LAD was better after surgery in one of these patients, however. The third patient had peripheral coronary artery disease. All patients were angina free after surgery.

A more comprehensive follow-up investigation would include a complete coronary and graft angiography. But because angiography is connected with some morbidity and mortality[46, 47] and we wanted to expose the patients to minimal risk, we preferred a less invasive investigation. We selected the IMA grafts because anastomoses using arterial grafts are generally more delicate to perform.

Closed chest bypass surgery by means of endoscopic technique will be a reality in the near future. We have developed and published a method of performing totally endoscopic bypass surgery in calves.[48] The method proposed for this approach is built on four distinct tools that are mandatory for closed chest surgery: visualization (we use the VISTA 3D system, enabling endoscopic suturing); local wall immobilization with the Octopus system; percutanous Hemopump support via groin access to facilitate the surgery and as a safety net during the procedure; and

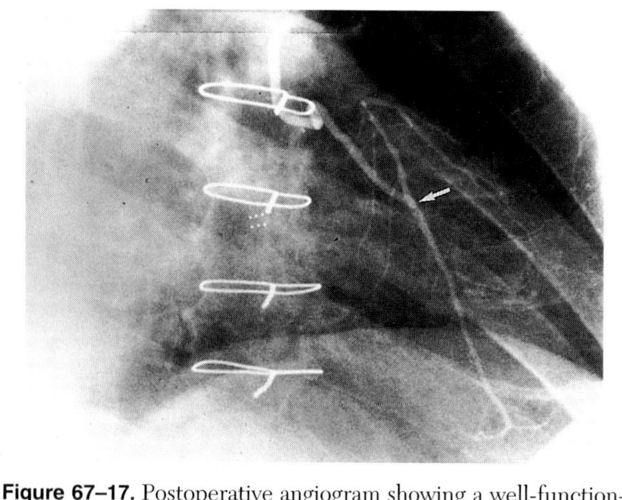

Figure 67–17. Postoperative angiogram showing a well-functioning left internal mammary artery sutured to the left descending coronary artery.

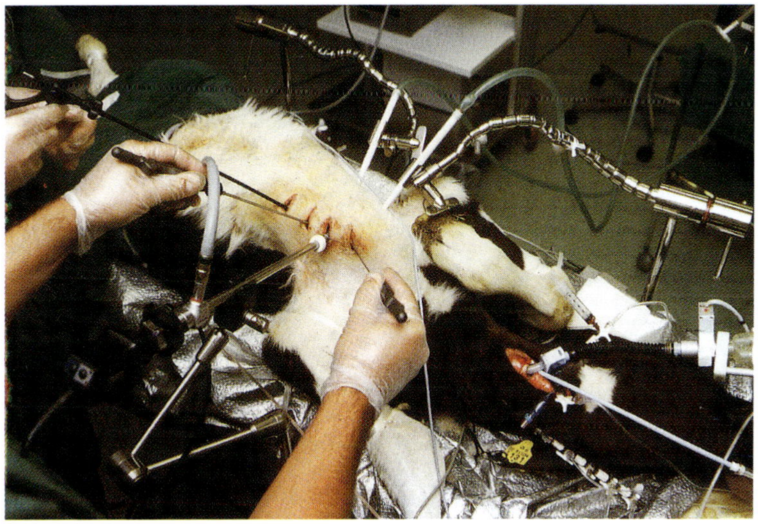

Figure 67–18. Experimental setup for total endoscopic bypass surgery, including the percutanous Hemopump inserted through the right carotid artery, the Octopus immobilization device, a three-dimensional visualization technique, and special surgical instruments.

special endoscopic surgical instruments, including the harmonic scalpel (Fig. 67–18).

Summary

CABG on the beating heart with Hemopump support is an alternative to conventional bypass surgery for multivessel grafting. The combination of the Hemopump and some kind of local wall immobilization device, such as the Octopus system,[49] the introduction of intravascular shunts,[50] and a specially designed device that blows a mixture of saline and carbon dioxide promise the ability to totally revascularize the beating heart. This can be seen as a natural step toward future techniques involving closed chest surgery. This method, including totally endoscopic CABG on the beating heart, has recently been reproduced in humans by our group. Our current clinical protocol does not include any ventricular assistive device or robotic system. This project is an ongoing collaboration among the heart centers in Linkoping, Sweden, and Helsingfors, Finland.

References

1. Favaloro RG: Saphenous vein graft in the surgical treatment of coronary artery disease: Operative technique.J Thorac Cardiovasc Surg 58:178–185, 1969.
2. Brandrup-Wognsen G: Coronary artery bypass grafting: Mortality and morbidity during two years of follow up. Thesis, Dept of Cardiothoracic Surgery, Sahlgrenska University Hospital, Göthenburg, Sweden, 1995.
3. Ovrum E, Tangen G, Am Holen E: Facing the era of minimally invasive coronary grafting: Current results of conventional bypass grafting for single-vessel disease. Ann Thorac Surg 64: 159–162, 1997.
4. Kirklin JK: Prospects for understanding and eliminating the deleterious effects of cardiopulmonary bypass (Editorial). Ann Thorac Surg 51:529–531, 1991.
5. Hammerschmidt DE, Stroncek DF, Bowers TK, et al: Complement activation and neutropenia occurring during cardiopulmonary bypass. J Thorac Cardiovasc Surg 81:370–377, 1981.
6. Kirklin JK, Westaby S, Blackstone EH, et al: Complement and damaging effects of cardiopulmonary bypass. J Thorac Cardiovasc Surg 86:845–857, 1983.
7. Westaby S: Organ dysfunction after cardiopulmonary bypass: A systemic inflammatory reaction initiated by the extracorporeal circuit. Intensive Care Med 13:89–95, 1987.
8. Leitman MI, Paull DE, Barie PS, et al: Intraabdominal complications after cardiopulmonary bypass operations. Surg Gynecol Obstet 165:251–254, 1987.
9. Castillo CF, Harringer W, Warshaw AL, et al: Risk factors for pancreatic cellular injury after cardiopulmonary bypass. N Engl J Med 325:382–387, 1991.
10. Komai H, Yamamoto F, Tanaka K, et al: Increased lung injury in pulmonary hypertensive patients during open heart operations. Ann Thorac Surg 55:1147–1152, 1993.
11. Lindsay CHJ, Rees GM, Kovacs IB: Inhibition of platelet function by heparin. J Thorac Cardiovasc Surg 105:816–822, 1993.
12. Love TR, Hendren WG, O'Keefe DD, et al: Transfusion of predonated autologous blood in electric cardiac surgery. Ann Thorac Surg 43:508–512, 1987.
13. Kirklin JW, Barrat-Boyes BG: Cardiac Surgery. New York, Wiley and Sons, 1986.
14. Kolesov VI: Mammary artery–coronary artery anastomosis as method of treatment for angina pectoris. J Thorac Cardiovasc Surg 54:535–544, 1967.
15. Buffolo EA, Andrade JCS, Branco JNR, et al: Myocardial revascularization without extracorporeal circulation: Seven year experience in 593 cases. Eur J Cardiothorac Surg 4:504–508, 1990.
16. Benetti FJ, Naselli G, Wood M, et al: Direct myocardial revascularization without extracorporeal circulation: experience in 700 patients. Chest 100:312–316, 1991.
17. Pfister AJ, Zaki MS, Garcia JM, et al: Coronary bypass without cardiopulmonary bypass. Ann Thorac Surg 54:1085–1092, 1992.
18. Frazier OH, Wampler RK, Duncan JM, et al: First human use of the Hemopump, a catheter-mounted ventricular assist device. Ann Thorac Surg 49:299–304, 1990.
19. Wampler RK, Moise JC, Frazier OH, et al: In vivo evaluation of a peripheral vascular access axial flow blood pump. ASAIO Trans 34:450–454, 1988.
20. Butler KC, Moise JC, Wampler RK: The Hemopump—a new cardiac prosthesis device. IEEE Trans Biomed Eng 37: 193–196, 1990.
21. Lönn U, Wulff J, Keck K-Y, et al: Flow characteristics of the Hemopump: An experimental in vitro study. Ann Thorac Surg 63:162–166, 1997.
22. Frazier OH, Nakatani T, Duncan JM, et al: Clinical experience with the Hemopump. ASAIO Trans 35:604–606, 1989.

23. Wiebalck AC, Wouters PF, Waldenberger FR, et al: Left ventricular assist with an axial flow pump (Hemopump): Clinical application. Ann Thorac Surg 55:1141–1146, 1993.
24. Meyns BP, Sergeant PT, Daenen WJ, et al: Left ventricular assistance with the transthoracic 24Fr Hemopump for recovery of the failing heart. Ann Thorac Surg 60:392–397, 1995.
25. Dreyfus GD: Hemopump 31, the sternotomy Hemopump: Clinical experience. Ann Thorac Surg 61:323–328, 1996.
26. Lönn U, Peterzén B, Granfeldt H, et al: Hemopump treatment in patients with postcardiotomy heart failure. Ann Thorac Surg 60: 1067–1071, 1995.
27. Scholz KH, Figulla HR, Schweda F, et al: Mechanical left ventricular unloading during high risk coronary angioplasty: First use of a new percutaneous transvalvular left ventricular assist device. Cathet Cardiovasc Diagn 31:61–69, 1994.
28. Dubois-Rande JL, Deleuze P, Dupoy P, et al: Assessment of a percutaneous Hemopump in high risk coronary angioplasty patients. ASAIO J 40:M486–M488, 1994.
29. Baldwin RT, Radovancevic B, Duncan JM, et al: Quality of life in long time survivors of the Hemopump left ventricular assist device. ASAIO Trans 37:M422–M423, 1991.
30. Meyns B, Vanermen H, Vanhaecke J, et al: Hemopump fails as a bridge to transplantation in postinfarction ventricular septal defect. J Heart Lung Transplant 13:1133–1137, 1994.
31. Sweeney MS, Frazier OH: Device-supported myocardial revascularization: Safe help for sick hearts. Ann Thorac Surg 54: 1065–1070, 1992.
32. Peterzén B, Lönn U, Babic A, et al: Postoperative management of patients with Hemopump support after coronary artery bypass grafting. Ann Thorac Surg 62:495–500, 1996.
33. The Esmolol vs. Placebo Multicenter Study Group: Comparison of the efficacy and safety of esmolol, a short-acting beta blocker, with placebo in the treatment of supraventricular tachyarrhythmias. Am Heart J 111:42–48, 1986.
34. The Esmolol vs. Placebo Multicenter Study Group: Intravenous esmolol for the treatment of supraventricular tachyarrhythmia: Results of a multicenter, baseline-controlled safety and efficacy study in 160 patients. Am Heart J 112:498–505, 1986.
35. Blanski L, Lutz J, Laddu A: Esmolol, the first ultra-short-acting intravenous beta-blocker for use in critically ill patients. Heart Lung 17:80–89, 1988.
36. Kirshenbaum JM, Kloner RF, McGowan N, Antman EM: Use of an ultrashort-acting beta-receptor blocker (esmolol) in patients with acute myocardial ischemia and relative contraindications to beta-blockade therapy. J Am Coll Cardiol 12: 773–780, 1988.
37. Iskandrian AS, Bemis CE, Hakki AH, et al: Effects of esmolol on patients with left ventricular dysfunction. J Am Coll Cardiol 8:225–231, 1986.
38. Bateman GRJ, Czer TM, Conklin LS, Matloff JM: Comparison of esmolol and nitroprusside for acute post-cardiac surgical hypertension. Am J Cardiol 59:887–891, 1987.
39. Øverum E, Holen EÅ, Abdelnoor M, Øystese R: Conventional blood conservation techniques in 500 consecutive coronary artery bypass operations. Ann Thorac Surg 52:500–505, 1991.
40. Lichtenstein SV, Ashe KA, el-Dalati H, et al: Warm heart surgery. J Thorac Cardiovasc Surg 101:269–274, 1991.
41. Guyton RA: Warm blood cardioplegia: Benefits and risks (Editorial). Ann Thorac Surg 55:1071–1072, 1993.
42. Shiiya N, Zelinsky R, Deleuze PH, et al: Effects of Hemopump support on left ventricular unloading and coronary blood flow. ASAIO Trans 37:M361–M362, 1991.
43. Hering JP, Schroder T, Uhlig P, et al: Myocardial support and protection during regional myocardial ischemia using the Hemopump assist device. Thorac Cardiovasc Surg 39:257–262, 1991.
44. Smalling RW, Cassidy DB, Barrett R, et al: Improved regional myocardial blood flow, left ventricular unloading, and infarct salvage using an axial-flow, transvalvular left ventricular assist device: A comparison with intra-aortic balloon counterpulsation and reperfusion alone in a canine infarction. Circulation 85: 1152–1159, 1992.
45. Lönn U, Peterzén B, Granfeldt H, Casimir-Ahn H: Coronary artery operation supported by the Hemopump: An experimental study on pig. Ann Thorac Surg 58:516–518, 1994.
46. de Bono D, on behalf of the Joint Audit Committee of the British Cardiac Society and Royal College of Physicians of London: Complications of diagnostic cardiac catheterisation: Results from 34,041 patients in the United Kingdom: Confidential enquiry into cardiac catheter complications. Br Heart J 70:297–300, 1993.
47. Noto TJ Jr, Johnson LW, Krone R, et al: Cardiac catheterization 1990: A report of the Registry of the Society for Cardiac Angiography and Interventions (SCA&I). Cathet Cardiovasc Diagn 24:75–83, 1991.
48. Mack MJ, Acuff TE, Casimir-Ahn H, et al: Video-assisted coronary bypass grafting on the beating heart. Ann Thorac Surg 63(suppl 6):S100–S103, 1997.
49. Grundeman PF, Borst C, van Herwaarden JA, et al: Hemodynamic changes during displacement of the beating heart by the Utrecht Octopus method. Ann Thorac Surg (suppl 6):S88–S92, 1997.
50. Rivetti LA, Gandra SM: Initial experience using an intraluminal shunt during revascularization of the beating heart. Ann Thorac Surg 63:1742–1747, 1997.

COMMENTARY

Antonio M. Calafiore

The Hemopump was originally designed as an LVAD. However, early models could provide only a low cardiac output (2 L/min), and this limited its clinical application to high-risk PTCA. Such cases are now uncommon, and the Hemopump is rarely needed for this purpose. The new model described in this chapter is capable of supporting the entire cardiac output; hence it can be used for postcardiotomy circulatory support. To unload the left ventricle during elective or urgent CABG using the Hemopump is an interesting idea that deserves investigation. However, many questions remain to be answered.

Any comparison of the stated indications for the Hemopump and those for off-pump surgery should point out that the need for any ventricular support device for LAD or right coronary artery grafting is questionable. Indeed, off-pump CABG has been used for such cases for a long time, with good results. Off-pump CABG is also useful in patients with atherosclerosis of the ascending aorta, which is increasingly common. The need for aortic insertion of the Hemopump limits its use in this subgroup of patients.

One problem that has not been addressed is that of grafting the obtuse marginal branches of the circumflex artery. The difficulty in reaching these vessels with the Hemopump makes it less attractive, because it allows only limited revascularization of the heart.

The great advantage of off-pump CABG is preventing further damage to end organs that are already affected by various pathologies. Even when we use CPB in our practice, we use warm systemic perfusion and intermittent antegrade warm blood cardioplegia, a technique associated with excellent early postoperative and midterm outcomes. Do we know that using the Hemopump has less damaging effects than warm heart surgery? The Hemopump can be part of the surgical armamentarium in coronary surgery, but its role has not yet been defined.

COMMENTARY

Mehmet Oz

CPB causes a well-described systemic inflammatory response. To avoid these potential detrimental effects, off-pump CABG has been attempted on the beating heart. With the use of an LVAD during CABG, the heart can be made flaccid with β-blockade, with continued support of the systemic circulation. The hemodynamic and hematologic consequences of left heart bypass are reported in this comprehensive chapter that reviews both animal and clinical data. The potential benefits of LVAD support as opposed to unsupported beating heart surgery include easy accessibility to all distal vessels, less cardiac motion during the anastomoses, guaranteed hemodynamic stability, and avoidance of the inflammation associated with CPB. Limitations to this technology include the reality that some lateral wall vessels may be difficult to reach, especially if right ventricular function is already compromised, and some patients have relative contraindications to full sternotomy or aortic cannulation.

We have pursued an investigation similar to that of our Swedish colleagues using a miniature axial flow pump in a sheep CABG model. The pump weighs 45 g and is connected to standard venous and arterial cannulas. Left-sided inflow and brachiocephalic outflow are employed. A pump speed of 14,000 revolutions/min resulted in a flow of 5.63 ± 0.18 L/min and provided 75% of the left ventricular output during a 2-hour pump run. This resulted in complete capture of the aortic pressure tracing (mean, 56.3 mm Hg) with a 15.5 mm Hg augmentation in the esmolol-depressed ventricle. Reductions in left ventricular end-diastolic pressure and left ventricular end-systolic pressure resulted in a 66% reduction in left ventricular external work under baseline conditions and an 83% reduction in the β-blocked ventricle. Myocardial oxygen demand was reduced 16% after axial flow unloading in the esmolol-depressed condition. Right ventricular pressures, pulmonary artery flow, left ventricular filling, and oxygenation were adequate in the esmolol-depressed animal and remained unchanged throughout the experiment. No changes in hematocrit, total bilirubin, lactate dehydrogenase, or plasma free hemoglobin were detected after 2 hours of assistance. We concluded that axial flow left heart bypass results in acceptable hemodynamics with no hemolysis and may provide an alternative to CPB during CABG.

Unanswered questions include the optimal cannulation technique, including full consideration of left ventricular apical cannulation. In addition, novel agents, such as nitric oxide, may prove useful in providing selective pulmonary vasodilatation in the event of right ventricular inadequacy, especially in the setting of pulmonary hypertension. This area is fertile for future investigation.

Chapter 68

Reoperative Minimally Invasive Direct Coronary Artery Bypass (MIDCAB) Coronary Grafting

James D. Fonger

Coronary bypass grafting since the 1970s has primarily involved the use of saphenous vein grafts as the new bypass conduit for surgical revascularization. In more recent years, the long-term limitation of saphenous vein grafts exposed to arterialized pressures has become increasingly apparent.[1–3] This has resulted in the burgeoning population of patients who are now presenting for reoperative coronary grafting. It has also given rise to increasing enthusiasm for the use of arterial conduits in coronary bypass grafting, particularly for patients who have a significant life expectancy.[4–8]

These reoperative coronary patients may have had only vein grafts placed previously or may have been grafted with a combination of arterial and venous conduits. In addition, there are other patients who have previously undergone congenital or valvular cardiac procedures who develop coronary disease later in life. Conventional reoperative coronary surgery requires re-entry into the scarred mediastinum in patients who may have had both progression of their native coronary disease and, often, the development of progression of other comorbidities as well.

Conventional reoperative coronary bypass grafting at experienced centers is now performed with excellent results considering the additional risks that are often involved.[9–14] However, the technical challenges and physiologic insult are not trivial and still may pose significant challenges. Regardless of the amount of grafting that needs to be accomplished, resternotomy, cardiac dissection, cannulation, and the establishment of cardiopulmonary bypass support with cardioplegic arrest are still employed. Although multiple vessel regrafting is frequently employed once these steps have been accomplished, many patients have only one or two coronary sites that actually cause recurrent anginal symptoms or that threaten survival.

Minimally invasive direct coronary artery bypass (MIDCAB) grafting is a simplified operative approach to coronary revascularization. This procedure developed out of the coronary grafting experience without cardiopulmonary bypass support through a sternal incision. This was done for many years, primarily in developing countries, as a strategy to conserve the resources required to provide cardiopulmonary bypass. Avoiding cardiopulmonary bypass in a segment of the coronary bypass surgery population ensured that resources would be available to provide cardiopulmonary bypass support in at least all valvular and congenital cardiac cases.[15–17] In 1994, this off-pump coronary bypass experience was further enhanced with the notion that a small directed incision might be all that was required to achieve limited coronary revascularization of one or two vessels of a beating heart. A pedicled arterial conduit was also required to obviate the need for additional exposure necessary for a proximal anastomosis.[18, 19] The development and adoption of MIDCAB grafting has evolved into what is now a safe, effective, and reliable strategy for limited surgical coronary revascularization performed in experienced centers.[20]

The MIDCAB approach is currently employed mostly for primary grafting of one or two coronary arteries. Patients who have this type of problem are often unable to have a catheter-based intervention, or they may have undergone prior interventions that have failed. Other patients may be young and interested specifically in the longevity of a surgically placed arterial graft. Conventional bypass grafting for one- or two-vessel disease in such patients is a reasonable alternative, albeit with a slightly longer postoperative recovery and an additional neurocognitive risk. However, patients facing reoperative coronary grafting may face a greater risk with a conventional surgical option. Reduction of this procedural risk with MIDCAB grafting is most dramatic in the reoperative population, allowing coronary grafting to be offered even to some patients who would not have been candidates for any additional conventional surgical treatment of their recurrent angina. Regardless of the risk, the limited dissection required to accomplish reoperative MIDCAB grafting makes this truly a focal therapy for a focal problem.

Advantages of Reoperative MIDCAB Grafting

MIDCAB grafting offers a number of advantages to patients facing reoperative coronary revascularization. Most notable is the ability to undergo coronary bypass surgery through a small directed incision instead of a conventional sternotomy, without exposure to the cardiopulmonary bypass circuit. Less recognized are the additional advantages of not manipulating the ascending aorta and using an arterial conduit instead of a saphenous vein for the bypass grafting. Together, these four features comprise the key advantages of the reoperative MIDCAB approach.

In the patient who has undergone prior cardiac surgery, a smaller directed incision clearly disposes of the need for a resternotomy. The advantage of this in patients who have undergone prior valvular or congenital cardiac surgery is that the risk of aortic or right ventricular damage upon reentry is avoided. However, the largest group of reoperative candidates by far are those facing repeat coronary grafting, and in this group the advantages can be even more significant.

Reoperative coronary grafting in the late 1990s is most often performed in the setting of previous coronary grafting that includes a left internal mammary artery (LIMA) to the anterior surface of the heart, along with vein grafts to the other coronary distributions. This has usually resulted in failure of one or more vein grafts by the time of reoperation, with a patent LIMA graft below the healed sternal incision. The open left pericardial edge and mediastinal fat often cause the proximal portion of the LIMA to be pushed medially and to heal in that position immediately below the sternum after the initial operative procedure (Fig. 68–1). At reoperation, this patent LIMA is often the only remaining reliable blood supply to the myocardium, and it sustains the patient, making its protection and preservation of paramount importance.[21]

Conventional reoperations using resternotomy place the patent LIMA graft and the other underlying structures at risk upon re-entry. In addition, the ascending aorta is usually recannulated, re–cross-clamped, and then partially reclamped in the process of replacing old vein grafts with proximal anastomoses for new venous conduits. The neurocognitive consequences of these maneuvers are just beginning to be appreciated.[22–25] However, the greatest risk of all may be the manipulation of atheromatous debris within old vein grafts. This can cause sudden hemodynamic collapse during the initial cardiac dissection, which is refractory to inotropes and requires the immediate institution of cardiopulmonary bypass support.

Cardiopulmonary bypass is not required for reoperative MIDCAB grafting unless an unexpected conversion has taken place. Conversion may occasionally be required for deteriorating hemodynamics, bleeding, or inability to achieve adequate exposure for safe and effective grafting. Postoperative bleeding with MIDCAB grafting is reduced, because the cardiac dissection is much less extensive and there is no hemodilution associated with priming the bypass circuit. The absence of a systemic inflammatory response to the prosthetic bypass circuit improves immediate postoperative pulmonary function, and the dose of heparin required during grafting is generally about one third of that required for conventional reoperations. The shift from phasic to mean blood flow and pressures is avoided with the MIDCAB approach, reducing the risk of perioperative stroke.[26–28] This also means that patients who might normally require a concomitant carotid endarterectomy because of this risk can often undergo reoperative MIDCAB grafting without this additional procedure.

Employing a MIDCAB approach for repeat coronary grafting clearly reduces a number of these risks in patients who require limited revascularization of one or two coronary arteries. Small directed incisions can now be employed for grafting any of the coronary locations around the heart with a new arterial conduit. Only a small area of the heart is re-exposed, and patent diseased vein grafts are left undisturbed. The ascending aorta is also not manipulated, and the anterior surface of the heart is only exposed if the prior anterior graft has failed and the left anterior descending (LAD) or diagonal artery is the intended site of reoperative MIDCAB grafting.

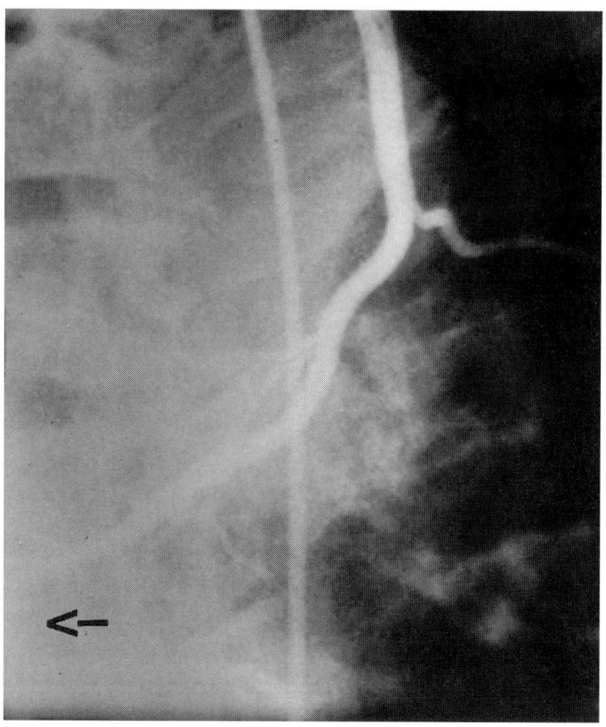

Figure 68–1. Left internal mammary artery directly below the healed sternal table (*arrow*). The artery was scarred into position by pressure that pushed medially from the pericardium and left lung postoperatively.

Disadvantages of Reoperative MIDCAB Grafting

Patients who present for reoperative coronary grafting have had a number of additional years in which to undergo progression of their native coronary disease. This often means they have sustained subsequent myocardial infarctions with further diminished left ventricular function and, therefore, increased perioperative risk. This progression of disease may also mean that the target vessel is of poor quality for grafting or not identifiable at all. Undiseased branches can also be mistaken for their diseased counterparts when there is significant epicardial scarring or suboptimal exposure. Transmyocardial laser revascularization is a good default therapy to have available in the operating room if it appears that effective grafting may not be possible because of these issues.[29–32]

Being able to operate on elderly, very sick patients is clearly a double-edged sword. As our initial clinical experience demonstrated, these patients were at greater risk from their comorbidities than from the coronary grafting itself. Exacerbated pre-existing pulmonary and renal failure were the two most common causes of noncardiac morbidity and mortality in patients who commonly had good cardiac recovery after their grafting. In cases of elderly patients, family members often made appropriate decisions not to persist with prolonged ventilation or chronic dialysis when unexpected problems arose in these organ systems. Overall perioperative mortality can actually be higher with MIDCAB than with conventional reoperative grafting, because this expanding patient population is inherently at higher risk.[33, 34]

Reoperative Anterior MIDCAB Grafting

The general setup for reoperative MIDCAB grafting is similar to that for primary MIDCAB procedures. Double-lumen endotracheal intubation is used whenever the procedure may involve entering a pleural cavity. External adhesive defibrillation pads are routinely placed on the patient and connected to the defibrillator. The circulating nurse remains near the defibrillator during portions of the procedure in which cautery is used near the heart. Preparing and draping allow for either the planned MIDCAB incision or a sternotomy, should that be required. Both groins are prepared but not dissected. A pulmonary artery catheter capable of measuring both continuous cardiac outputs and mixed venous oxygen saturations is used in high-risk patients to help with intraoperative and postoperative clinical management.

The anterior surface of the heart is the target approached least often for reoperative MIDCAB revascularization. This region may not have been grafted originally; a previously placed graft may have failed; or the previous grafting may have mistakenly been performed on a diagonal branch of the LAD coronary artery leaving the LAD artery itself untreated (Fig. 68–2). Options for all reoperative grafting situations include placing a new graft distal to the earlier anastomosis, placing the new graft into the hood of the old graft directly over the anastomosis, or grafting a previously ungrafted branch in that region (Fig. 68–3). In selected cases in which the old conduit is only diseased or damaged distally, another option is to remove the old conduit from the coronary artery, resect the damaged portion, and recycle the graft by reanastomosing it to the original arteriotomy (Fig. 68–4). None of these strategies requires extensive redissection of the heart.

When the previous grafting has used saphenous vein, revascularization is usually accomplished with a pedicled LIMA, which is harvested via a direct (nonthoracoscopic) approach. However, when the LIMA has already been used and is occluded, an alternate free or pedicled arterial conduit is required. The most effective solution in this setting is to harvest the right gastroepiploic artery (GEA) as a pedicled conduit via a short, vertical, epigastric, abdominal incision. A three-inch transverse counterincision is made in the left fourth intercostal space to expose the intended LAD target. The GEA is then routed anterior to the stomach and liver, tunneling it beneath the left costal margin into the site exposed by the intercostal counterincision. An anastomosis can then be fashioned by placing the hood of the GEA onto the LAD end to the side in a retrograde configuration (Fig. 68–5). This approach requires two small incisions but only one anastomosis, with the patient

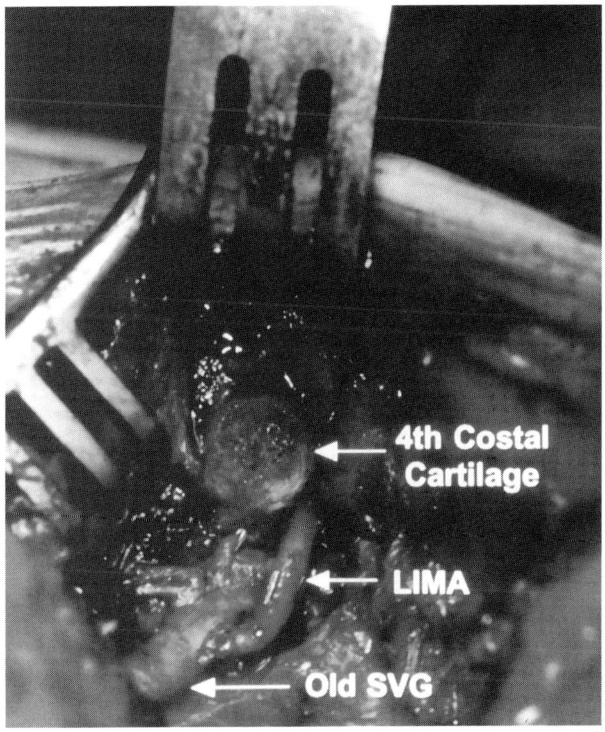

Figure 68–3. Left internal mammary artery anastomosed into the mid-portion of the old vein graft distal to the ostial stenosis through the left fourth intercostal space.

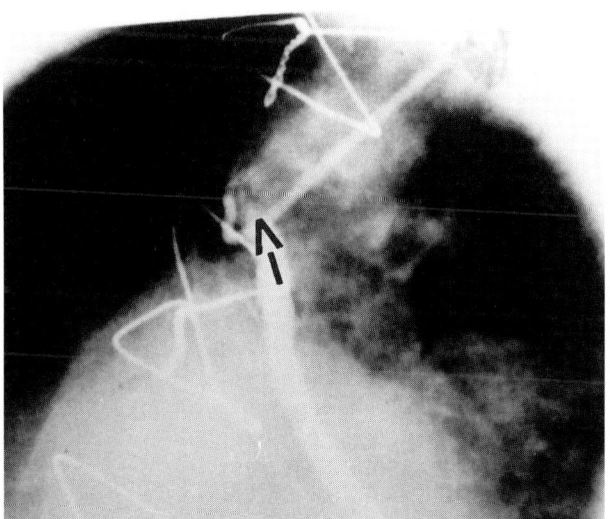

Figure 68–2. Ostial stenosis (*arrow*) of proximal anastomosis of old saphenous vein graft supplying multiple distal sites on the left ventricle.

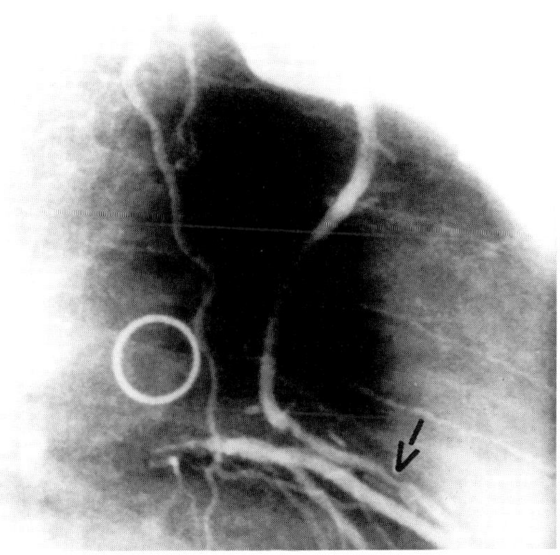

Figure 68–4. Previously grafted left internal mammary artery with a damaged distal end (*arrow*) that was resected with the left internal mammary artery reanastomosed through a fourth intercostal space incision.

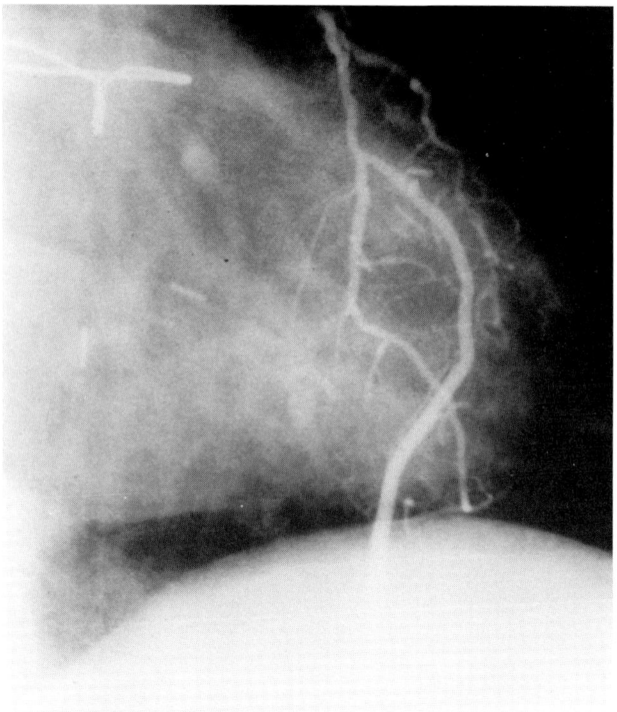

Figure 68–5. One-month postoperative angiogram of the right gastroepiploic artery anastomosed retrograde to the left anterior descending coronary artery.

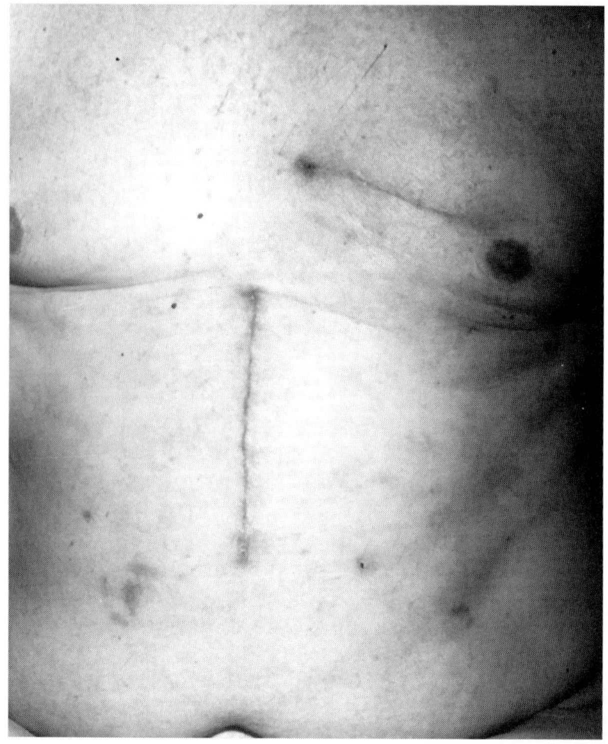

Figure 68–6. Epigastric and left fourth intercostal space incisions required to accomplish the approach shown in Figure 68–5.

remaining in the supine position throughout the procedure (Fig. 68–6).

A less commonly used solution to this problem is harvesting the radial artery from the nondominant forearm and grafting it to the LAD through a small anterior intercostal incision. The free end of the conduit is then tunneled into a pocket laterally and the patient repositioned right side down for a left posterior thoracotomy. A short, posterior left thoracotomy in the sixth intercostal space allows the graft to be found at the apex of the incision and directed posteriorly with an end-to-side proximal anastomosis fashioned on the descending thoracic aorta. In the reoperative setting, the ascending aorta is generally not easily accessible through the intercostal incision because of adhesions. The location required for identification of the LAD is too far from the ascending aorta for exposure without left and downward retraction of the heart and the mediastinum. This is not feasible when all these tissues have been scarred into place from previous cardiac surgery.

Reoperative Inferior (Subxiphoid) MIDCAB Grafting

The right GEA has been used with excellent results for primary and reoperative conventional grafting of the distal right coronary circulation since the 1980s with excellent results.[35–37] Reoperative patients may present with isolated new or recurrent right coronary disease that is refractory to medications and not amenable to a catheter-based intervention. This is sometimes accompanied by additional issues involved with re-entering a sternal incision that was complicated at the time of initial healing. A limited approach to the inferior surface of the heart may be very desirable in these settings. If the proximal right coronary artery is the only site of disease, then a reoperative MIDCAB graft, placing the right internal mammary artery (RIMA) to the mid-right coronary through a limited right anterior thoracotomy is usually the approach of choice. However, if there is any evidence of mid- or further distal right disease, then the subxiphoid approach using the GEA is the most effective reoperative strategy (Fig. 68–7). This approach can be used to graft the distal right, posterior descending, or posterolateral branches of the right coronary artery. Unlike other arterial conduits, such as the LIMA and the radial artery, the GEA is not easily used as a sequential conduit to more than one target because of its size, tapered configuration, and numerous side branches.

It is generally a good idea, especially in the reoperative setting, to expose the coronary artery and confirm that there is an adequate coronary target before harvesting the GEA conduit. The proposed target may be too small, too diseased, or hidden directly beneath the posterior descending coronary vein when grafting distally in the right circulation. However, this distal location also improves toleration of temporary coronary occlusion without shunting during the sewing of the anastomosis. The best target can be selected if there is more than one graftable branch, because grafting to a second site is not easily done using the GEA.

Exposure of the inferior surface of the heart is accomplished through a short, vertical, epigastric incision from the xiphisternum halfway down to the umbilicus. The peritoneum is entered over the liver and opened upward to enter the pericardium. Reoperative dissection anterior to the heart and below the sternum is not done. This spares anteriorly placed old vein grafts from re-entry and allows the sternum to pull the heart out of the chest. With a conven-

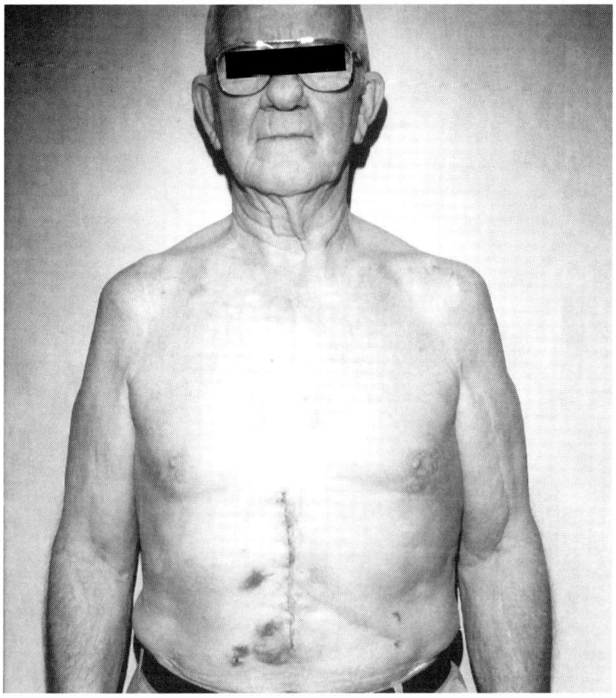

Figure 68–7. Fifth coronary bypass operation in this patient is done through an epigastric incision using the right gastroepiploic artery rather than using a fifth trans-sternal approach.

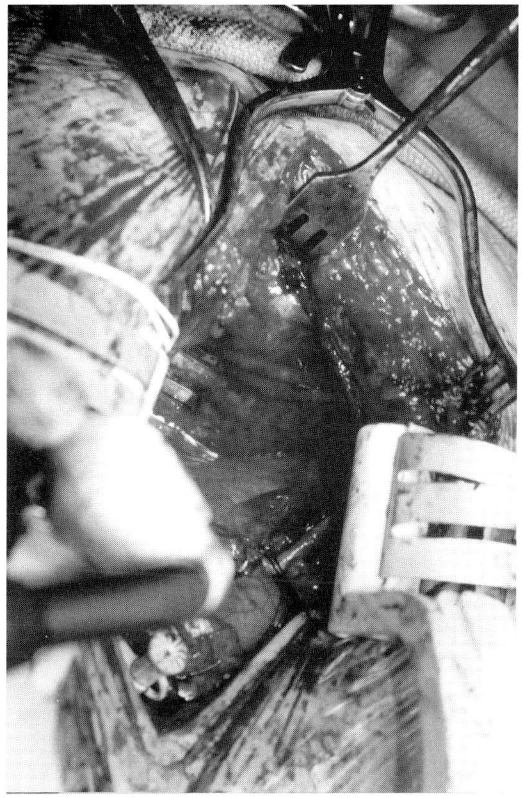

Figure 68–8. Exposure of the inferior surface of the heart through the subxiphoid approach.

tional internal mammary artery (IMA) retractor based at the left shoulder, the lower sternal table is retracted vertically and craniad after removal of the xiphisternum, and the heart is elevated into the wound. The diaphragm is dissected off the inferior surface of the heart, allowing the inferior pericardial space to open up like a book. The target site and old vein grafts can then be identified, and a decision can be made about the feasibility of grafting. Exposure can be enhanced by the release of the diaphragm from the undersurface of the costal margins bilaterally and with caudal pericardial retraction across the abdomen, securing the diaphragm to the abdominal wall with pericardial sutures. If further exposure is required, an additional releasing incision can be made vertically in the diaphragm downward toward the inferior vena cava through the tendinous diaphragm, leaving the muscular layer intact. The diaphragm is never completely divided because it must retract the abdominal viscera. With the proposed coronary target evaluated, attention is redirected to harvesting the GEA (Fig. 68–8).

The limited abdominal dissection generally only visualizes the liver, the stomach, and the transverse colon. Only the stomach is exteriorized, and this is facilitated by previous placement of a nasogastric tube with suction. If the patient is known to have a generalized vasculopathy with carotid, renal, aortic, or peripheral vascular disease, then consideration needs to be given to conducting a preoperative angiographic evaluation of the ostial patency of the celiac axis. The GEA conduit should be palpated gently before harvest to confirm a satisfactory pulse and to rule out the rare instance of GEA atherosclerosis, which would probably be a contraindication to its use. Harvesting the GEA as a pedicle is begun by entering the lesser sac below the GEA and separating the omentum from the GEA along its length. The gastric branches, from the greater curvature of the stomach to the GEA, are divided and ligated or stapled, freeing the pedicle proximally almost to the pancreas. This assures that the maximal caliber of conduit is used for the graft, because it tapers much more than the IMA along its course. Harvesting the GEA in this fashion results in a reliable pedicle, which will be long enough to reach any target on the bottom of the heart or the distal LAD. Final preparation includes intraluminal injection of the GEA through a 24-gauge angiocatheter with a mixture of papaverine and verapamil (60 mg papaverine and 10 mg verapamil in syringe with 50 ml of normal saline solution). This dilates the conduit and guards against subsequent spasm during manipulation.

The GEA conduit is routed over the left lobe of the liver, the stomach, and the diaphragm, with an end-to-side antegrade anastomosis fashioned within the pericardium to the proposed target site. The length of the conduit is trimmed to eliminate any redundant GEA, which might kink or require the anastomosis to be unnecessarily distal in a small-caliber region of the tapered GEA conduit. Automated mechanical stabilization from below is very stable; pushing against the backstop of the septum with minimal ventricular deformity. Respirations can be held during stitch placement and the pedicle tacked to the epicardium when finished to ensure the proper anastomotic configuration. Intraoperative transit time ultrasound is used routinely before closure for measuring volumetric flow through the new graft and for confirming that it functions well with appropriate diastolic augmentation of the spectral velocity trace (Fig. 68–9). The average flow measured

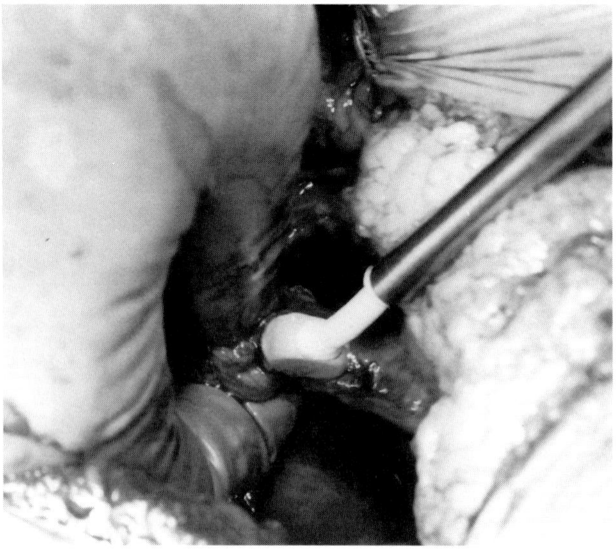

Figure 68–9. Transit time ultrasound probe placement on the right gastroepiploic artery (*arrow*) over the left lobe of the liver before closure of the wound.

immediately after grafting the GEA to the distal right coronary circulation is 15 ml per minute (Fig. 68–10). The greater curvature of the stomach and abdomen are checked once again for bleeding, and a small suction drain is directed across the abdomen into the pericardium and pleural space, if it has been entered. Soft tissue is closed routinely without pacing wires, and prophylaxis with oral calcium channel blockade is continued for 1 month postoperatively. The epigastric incision is well tolerated by patients, who routinely experience early mobility and discontinuation of nasogastric suction the following morning.

Our initial experience with 74 patients, involving 41 reoperative cases (55%), has been reported previously and includes our entire learning curve for this approach.[38] This series was done without the benefit of automated mechanical stabilization, coronary blowers, current coronary occlusion techniques, or the technical lessons we are now able to outline above. This series resulted in an initial clinical patency of 87.3%, which rose to 95.2% after selected patients required a subsequent catheter-based intervention through the GEA graft. Relief of symptoms was ultimately achieved in 88.3%, with or without medications. More recently, there has been clinical patency without intervention in the last 15 GEA grafts, suggesting continued improvements in this evolving approach (Fig. 68–11). In the primary setting, this incision also allows simultaneous grafting of the LIMA to the LAD artery. In the reoperative setting, when the LIMA to the LAD artery remains patent, this approach is sometimes combined with a free radial artery graft placed through a separate posterolateral thoracotomy to an obtuse marginal coronary artery (see the following paragraph on the lateral approach). The simplicity of the subxiphoid approach combined with the high frequency of mid-right coronary disease, which obviates use of the RIMA as a pedicled graft, should result in greater rates of adoption for the subxiphoid approach as more clinical data become available.

Reoperative Lateral MIDCAB Approach

The other clinical scenario that is often encountered in the reoperative coronary bypass patient is that of a patent LIMA to the LAD with either new or recurrent disease in an obtuse marginal branch of the circumflex coronary distribution. When this location is unsuitable for catheter-based intervention and the patient is refractory to medical management, surgical regrafting becomes necessary. The right coronary artery may be uninvolved, previously grafted, or subtending a region that is infarcted or ungraftable. A conventional reoperative approach requires the safe exposure of the LIMA graft as the reoperative dissection is carried from the front around to the left side of the heart. Grafting is then done with a free segment of saphenous vein or radial artery, which needs to be anastomosed to the ascending aorta proximal to the takeoff of the carotid circulation. These accepted risks of reoperative grafting can be obviated with a lateral approach to the circumflex coronary through a small directed posterior left thoracotomy incision.[39–44]

The lateral MIDCAB approach is almost always performed on patients who are undergoing reoperative grafting. As with all MIDCAB approaches, adhesive external defibrillation pads are routinely placed outside the intended operative field. After administration of general anesthesia with double-lumen intubation, the radial artery conduit is harvested from the nondominant forearm with the patient in the supine position. The radial artery is harvested as a free graft, with a pedicle of neighboring veins and fascia dissected by the Harmonic scalpel, which avoids

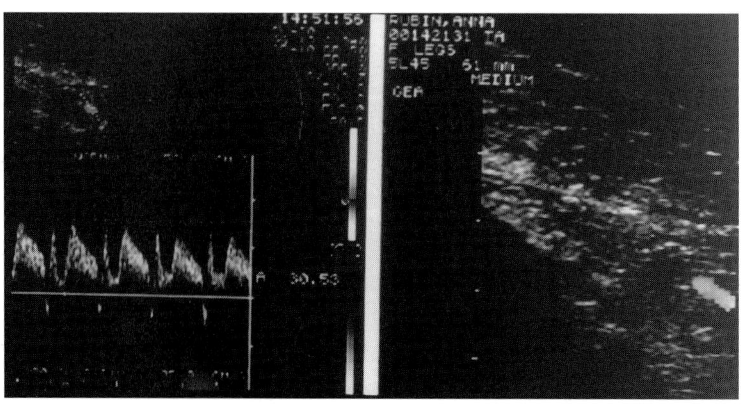

Figure 68–10. Typical waveform obtained with marked diastolic augmentation of flow.

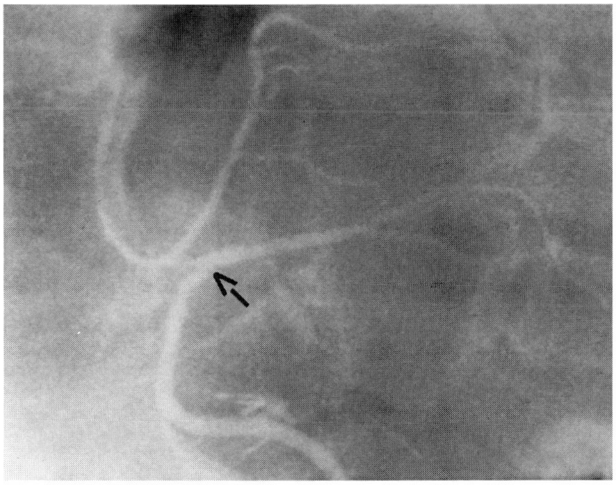

Figure 68–11. Three-month postoperative angiography of the right gastroepiploic artery graft (*arrow*) demonstrating caliber similar to that of the distal right posterior descending coronary artery.

undue thermal damage or spasm. The patient is then repositioned right side down for a left posterolateral thoracotomy (Fig. 68–12). Because of this positioning, the lateral MIDCAB approach is generally not combined with other MIDCAB incisions or operations. If the right radial artery or saphenous vein is used for the conduit, the harvesting of the conduit can be performed with the patient in the thoracotomy position while the chest is being opened concurrently.

The thoracotomy is usually done through a six-inch incision in the sixth intercostal space placed in a very posterior location on the lateral chest wall. If a high ramus branch is the grafting target, the fifth space can be considered. When a low posterolateral branch is to be grafted, the seventh space is sometimes used after retracting the diaphragm out of the way with stay sutures. The entire operation is conducted in the posterior portion of the left chest posterior to the left phrenic nerve and caudal to the hilum of the lung. Therefore, a more extensive thoracotomy is generally not helpful in accomplishing the grafting. When the pleural cavity has been entered, the inferior pulmonary ligament is divided and the collapsed left lung is packed up into the apex of the chest. The hilar fascia is also divided up to the level of the inferior pulmonary vein to create a path for the graft over to the descending thoracic aorta.

The pericardium is divided longitudinally, parallel to and below the left phrenic nerve. The coronary target is mechanically stabilized, exposed, and locally occluded after partial systemic heparinization. The conduit is anastomosed to the coronary artery in a standard end-to-side antegrade fashion and sized to facilitate its reaching the descending thoracic aorta. Grafts must be sized long enough to allow movement of the mediastinum away from the aorta during respiration. Moreover, shortening must be anticipated during the healing process. The course of the graft is planned so as not to be too close to the inferior pulmonary vein. This prevents kinking during left-lung reexpansion. The proximal anastomosis is performed in a standard fashion on the descending thoracic aorta, with a side-biting clamp leaving a radiopaque marker as an aid to future angiographic visualization of the graft (Fig. 68–13). Graft flow is routinely measured by transit time ultrasound to confirm adequate graft performance before chest closure. This is particularly important with the lateral MIDCAB approach, because the graft cannot be subse-

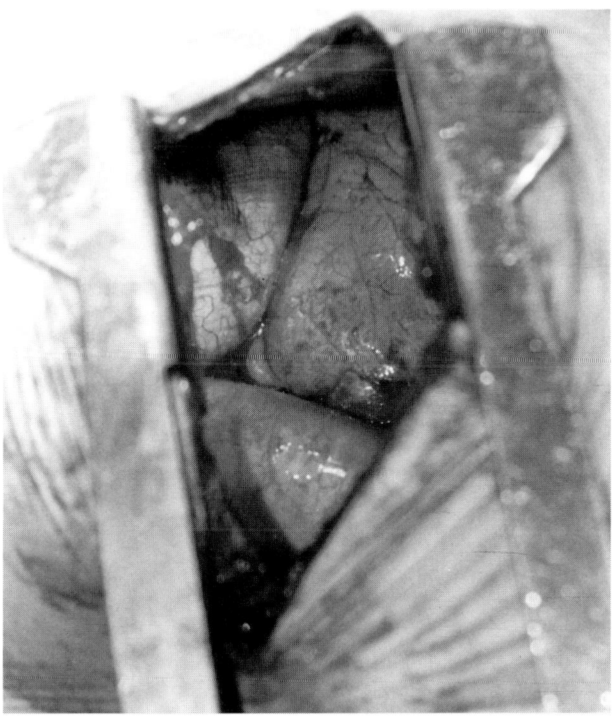

Figure 68–12. Operative field through a limited posterolateral thoracotomy in the sixth interspace.

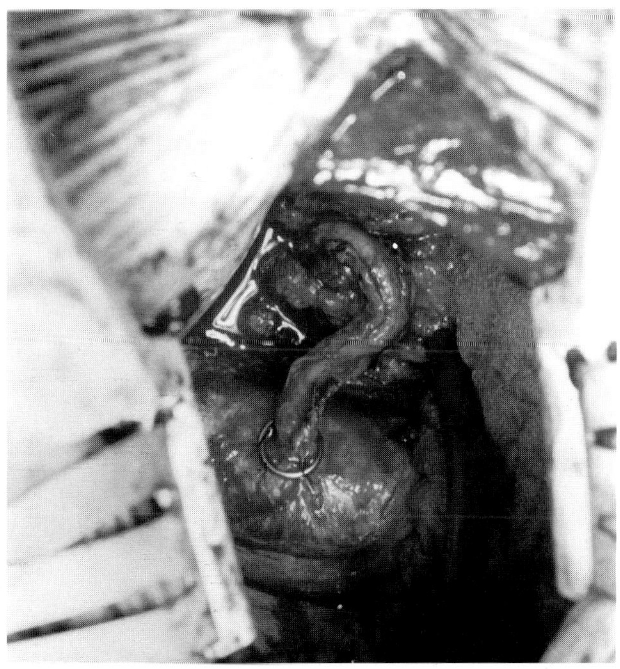

Figure 68–13. Final position of a radial artery graft from the descending thoracic aorta to the main circumflex coronary artery in the atrioventricular groove marked with a radiopaque ring.

quently inspected by transcutaneous Doppler ultrasound as is done with the anterior and subxyphoid MIDCAB grafts (Fig. 68–14). Given a native coronary target of adequate caliber, the average expected flow for a radial artery conduit in this configuration is roughly 35 ml per minute. The lung is reexpanded, a chest tube and intercostal nerve block are placed, and the chest is closed in a standard fashion (Fig. 68–15).

Our initial experience using full thoracotomy, saphenous vein conduits, and retrograde coronary anastomosis has undergone continuous evolution to the technique outlined above (Fig. 68–16). However, some cautions or limitations to the current technique still exist. If the lateral wall coronary target is intramyocardial, there are often no landmarks to aid in identifying the correct location for myocardial dissection and grafting. The coronary target courses somewhere across the lateral wall but is not located over an identifiable anatomic site, such as the septum or atrioventricular groove, as in other approaches. If the intended obtuse marginal branch is not marked by a previously placed diseased vein graft, it may not be found, or it can easily be mistaken for another obtuse marginal branch, possibly resulting in the grafting of the wrong marginal branch. As with all MIDCAB approaches for limited symptomatic revascularization, if the coronary target cannot be found or is ungraftable, it is important to have transmyocardial laser revascularization (TMR) readily available in the operating room for treating the region.

The primary limitation of graft performance with the lateral exposure, as with all MIDCAB approaches, is the quality of the native coronary artery target. This is particu-

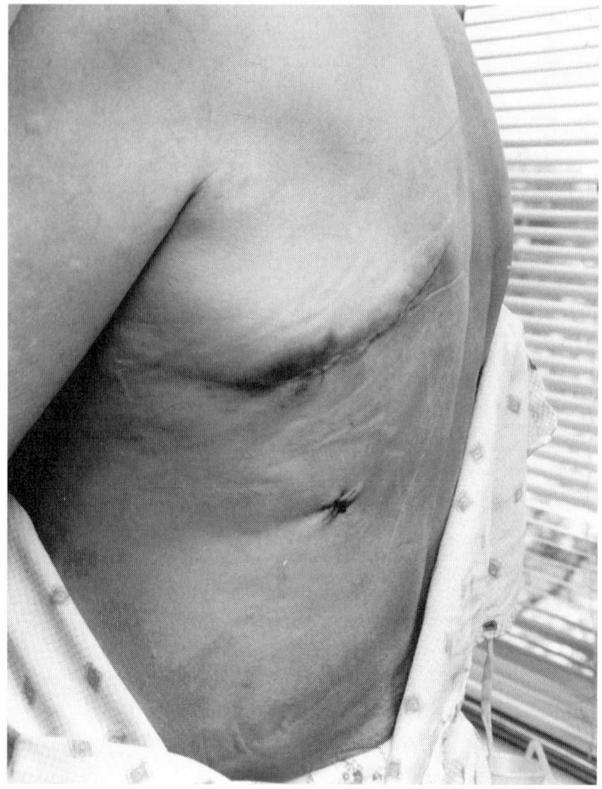

Figure 68–15. Posterior position of the final lateral minimally invasive direct coronary artery bypass skin incision.

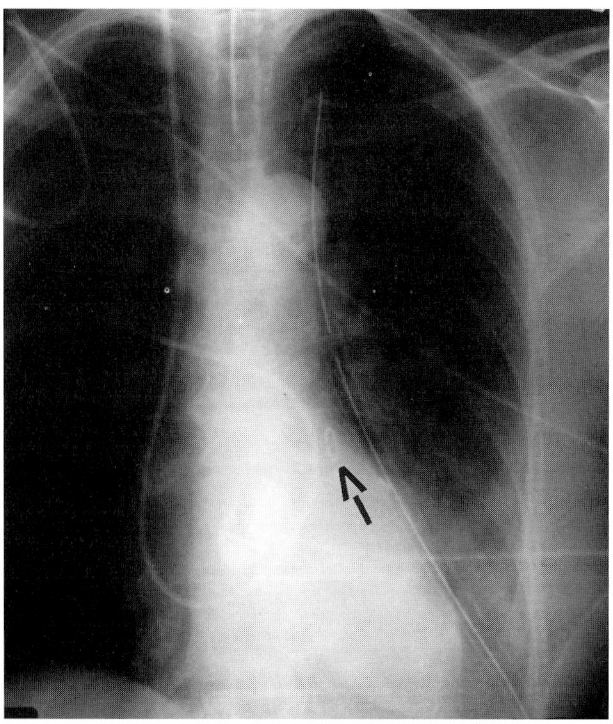

Figure 68–14. Position of the radiopaque marker (*arrow*) on a routine postoperative chest radiograph midway down the left side of the mediastinum.

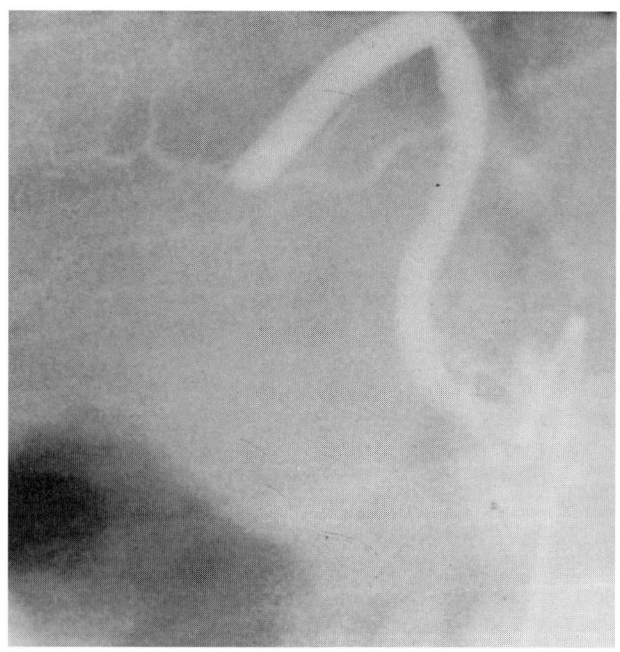

Figure 68–16. A saphenous vein graft used in an early lateral minimally invasive direct coronary artery bypass (MIDCAB) procedure demonstrating a marked size discrepancy compared with the native obtuse marginal coronary artery.

larly important in lateral MIDCAB grafting, in which multiple branches off the circumflex artery are smaller than other coronary targets. The graft failures we have experienced since our exclusive adoption of the radial artery conduit have been in situations in which graft outflow is restricted by the small caliber of the coronary target. Over the past 3 years, 20 radial artery conduits have been placed through a lateral MIDCAB approach, and 80% of those were reoperative coronary cases. Three grafts placed to small marginal branches have failed, which means there were patency and relief of symptoms without further reinterventions in 85% of cases (Fig. 68–17). Case selection and availability of TMR will continue to improve these results with the lateral approach. Radial artery conduits have been recatheterized as long as 2 years after lateral MIDCAB grafting during recatheterization for new right coronary disease, demonstrating excellent midterm performance (Fig. 68–18).

It is also important to note that the limited posterior MIDCAB incision through the sixth interspace is the most painful of all the small directed incisions, and it should be accompanied by liberal intercostal rib blocks and other analgesia for the first few days after surgery. Nevertheless, the discomfort is justified by the mitigation of reoperative risk in patients who have patent anterior and right-sided grafts.

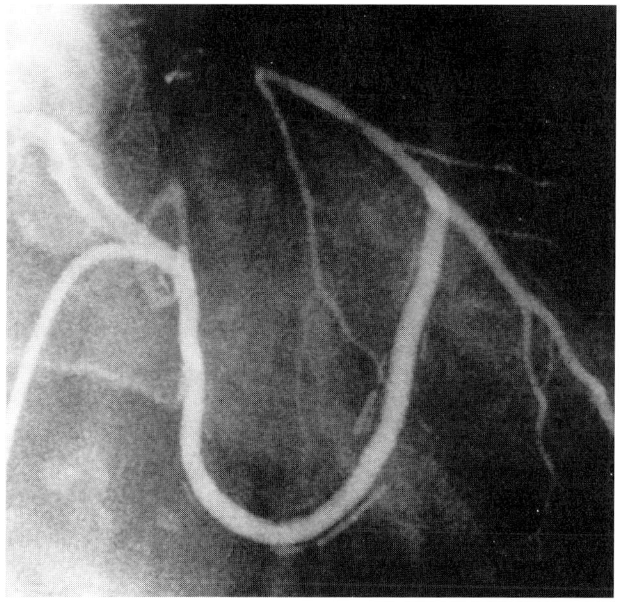

Figure 68–18. Radial artery graft 2 years after placement through a lateral minimally invasive direct coronary artery bypass (MIDCAB) approach during catheterization for new right coronary disease.

Reoperative MIDCAB Without Conversion

Patients about to undergo MIDCAB grafting are routinely informed about the remote possibility that their case will be converted to a sternal incision, cardiopulmonary bypass support, or both, during the course of their operation. This generally is done because of some technical, anatomic, or physiologic reason that was not appreciated or anticipated preoperatively. Despite the disappointment of the patient, the patient's family, and the surgeon, if the safety or efficacy of the grafting might be compromised, everyone concerned understands the importance of having this option available. Fortunately, with recent advances in experience and technique, the conversion rate in high-volume MIDCAB centers is now often less than 1%.

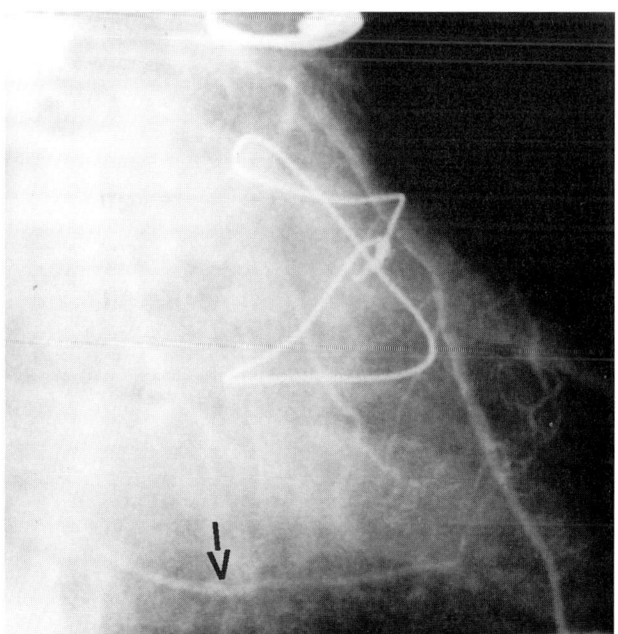

Figure 68–17. Example of a native obtuse marginal coronary artery (*arrow*) that failed to provide adequate outflow to support a patent radial artery graft 2 months after surgery.

There is a small but important subset of reoperative coronary patients who are considered to be too high risk to be offered conventional reoperative coronary grafting under any circumstances. Reasons for this have included extremely advanced age, significant comorbidities, or previous sternal wound complications that preclude sternal re-entry or cardiopulmonary bypass support. Nevertheless, the overall medical condition of these patients is such that they can tolerate a general anesthetic and a limited surgical incision. This may mean that these candidates are at a tolerable—albeit high—risk for reoperative MIDCAB grafting. However, conversion in this setting would not be a reasonable option, because it would not be a strategy that would serve to further reduce operative risk. In these patients, conversion would actually increase the risk of the procedure.

Given these circumstances, reoperative MIDCAB grafting can be offered specifically as MIDCAB without conversion. Detailed preoperative discussions are held with the patient, the patient's family, and referring doctors about the fact that the option of conversion will not be offered under any circumstances, and this is a condition of proceeding with the operation. Everyone understands that if the grafting cannot be adequately accomplished, the wound will be closed and the procedure will be terminated. If the patient becomes unstable during the surgery, standard supportive medical measures, which may include an intra-aortic balloon pump, will be employed without resorting to sternotomy or cardiopulmonary bypass. This helps to clarify both expectations and operative management for everyone involved in these high-risk cases.

MIDCAB without conversion allows a small additional subset of reoperative patients to be considered for some sort of surgical coronary grafting. Although the coronary regrafting is generally successful, our experience has been that overall mortality is considerably higher in this group than in the standard MIDCAB population. Mortality is usually related to one of the associated medical conditions or the patients' inability to tolerate postoperative problems, such as bleeding, in their frail condition. Nevertheless, most of these patients have a relatively uneventful perioperative course and an expeditious recovery. The result is a meaningful relief of symptoms and a gratifying surgical result for a group of patients who previously did not have any surgical option for regrafting their coronary arteries.

Summary

The burgeoning population of reoperative coronary patients continues to represent unique and challenging problems for interventionists as well as for cardiac surgeons. Reoperative MIDCAB grafting is currently a fast-growing segment of the minimally invasive cardiac surgical experience and represents a new and powerful tool for helping surgeons better manage reoperative coronary surgical patients. The limited dissection and manipulation required for safe and effective accomplishment of reoperative MIDCAB grafting truly makes this a focal therapy for a focal problem.

References

1. Lytle BW, Loop FD, Thurer RL, et al: Isolated left anterior descending coronary atherosclerosis: Long-term comparison of internal mammary artery and venous autografts. Circulation 61: 869–874, 1980.
2. Jones JW, Ochsner JL, Mills NL, et al: A Clinical comparison between patients with saphenous vein and internal mammary artery as a coronary graft. Thorac Cardiovasc Surg 80:334–341, 1980.
3. Myojin K, Weiss G, Mee R, et al: Functional comparison of coronary bypass grafts of the saphenous vein and internal mammary artery. Thorac Cardiovasc Surg 79:713–717, 1980.
4. Dietl CA, Madigan NP, Menapace FJ, et al: Results of coronary artery bypass grafting using multiple arterial conduits. Cardiovasc Surg 34:513–516, 1993.
5. Lytle BW, McElroy D, McCarthy P, et al: Influence of arterial coronary bypass grafts on the mortality in coronary reoperations. J Thorac Cardiovasc Surg 107:675–683, 1994.
6. Siclari F, Heublein B, Schaps D: Total arterial revascularization of the heart using both mammary arteries and the right gastroepiploic artery. J Card Surg 5:309–314, 1990.
7. Calafiore AM, Di Giammarco G, Luciani N, et al: Composite arterial conduits for a wider arterial myocardial revascularization. Ann Thorac Surg 58:185–190, 1994.
8. Calafiore AM, Di Giammarco G, Teodori G, et al: Radial artery and inferior epigastric artery in composite grafts: Improved midterm angiographic results. Ann Thorac Surg 60:517–524, 1995.
9. Christenson JT, Schmuziger M, Simonet F: Reoperative coronary artery bypass procedures: Risk factors for early mortality and late survival. Eur Cardiothorac Surg 11:129–133, 1997.
10. Weintraub WS, Jones EL, Craver JM, et al: In-hospital and long-term outcome after reoperative coronary artery bypass graft surgery. Circulation 92(suppl 9):II50–II57, 1995.
11. He GW, Acuff TE, Ryan WH, et al: Determinants of operative mortality in reoperative coronary artery bypass grafting. Thorac Cardiovasc Surg 110:971–978, 1995.
12. Kaul TK, Fields BL, Wyatt DA, et al: Reoperative coronary artery bypass surgery: Early and late results and management in 1300 patients. Cardiovasc Surg (Torino) 36:303–312, 1995.
13. Kron IL, Cope JT, Baker LD Jr, et al: The risks of reoperative coronary artery bypass in chronic ischemic cardiomyopathy: Results of the CABG Patch Trial. Circulation 96(suppl 9):II-1–II-25, 1997.
14. Weintraub WS, Jones EL, Morris DC, et al: Outcome of reoperative coronary bypass surgery versus coronary angioplasty after previous bypass surgery. Circulation 95:868–877, 1997.
15. Benetti FJ: Direct coronary surgery with saphenous vein bypass without either cardiopulmonary bypass or cardiac arrest. J Cardiovasc Surg 26:217–222, 1985.
16. Buffolo E, de Andrade JCS, Branco JNR, et al. Coronary artery bypass grafting without cardiopulmonary bypass. Ann Thorac Surg 61:63–66, 1996.
17. Pfister AJ, Zaki M, Garcia JM, et al: Coronary artery bypass without cardiopulmonary bypass. Ann Thorac Surg 54:1085–1092, 1992.
18. Robinson M, Gross D, Zeman W, et al: Minimally invasive coronary artery bypass grafting: A new method using an anterior mediastinotomy. J Card Surg 10:529–536, 1995.
19. Subramanian VA, Sani G, Benetti FJ, Calafiore AM. Minimally invasive coronary bypass surgery: A multi-center report of preliminary clinical experience. Circulation 92(suppl I):1654, 1655, 1995.
20. Calafiore AM, Di Giammarco G, Teodori G, et al: Left anterior descending coronary artery grafting via left anterior small thoracotomy without cardiopulmonary bypass. Ann Thorac Surg 61:1658–1665, 1996.
21. Nkere UU, Whawell SA, Sarraf CE, et al: Pericardial trauma and adhesions in relation to reoperative cardiac surgery. Thorac Cardiovasc Surg 43:338–346, 1995.
22. Sotaniemi KA: Long-term neurologic outcome after cardiac operation. Ann Thorac Surg 59:1336–1369, 1995.
23. McKhann GM, Goldsborough MA, Borowicz LM Jr, et al: Predictors of stroke risk in coronary artery bypass patients. Ann Thorac Surg 63:516–521, 1997.
24. Mills SA: Cerebral complications of cardiopulmonary bypass. *In* Wechsler AS (ed): Systemic Effects of Cardiopulmonary Bypass. New York, Cahners, 1993.
25. Roach GW, Kanchuger M, Mangano CM, et al. Adverse cerebral outcomes after coronary bypass surgery. N Engl J. Med 335:1857–1863, 1996.
26. Edmunds LH Jr: Why cardiopulmonary bypass makes patients sick: Strategies to control the blood-synthetic surface interface. *In* Karp: Advances in Cardiac Surgery vol. 6, Baltimore, Mosby–Year Book, 1995.
27. Edmunds LH Jr: Systemic inflammatory responses secondary to cardiopulmonary bypass. In Wechsler AS (ed): Systemic Effects of Cardiopulmonary Bypass. New York, Cahners, 1993.
28. Khuri SF: Hemostatic complications of cardiopulmonary bypass. *In* Wechsler AS (ed): Systemic Effects of Cardiopulmonary Bypass. New York, Cahners, 1993.
29. Frazier OH, Kadipasaoglu KA, Radovancevic B, et al: Transmyocardial laser revascularization in allograft coronary artery disease. Ann Thorac Surg Apr;65:1138–1141, 1998.
30. Frazier OH, Kadipasaoglu KA, Cooley DA: Transmyocardial laser revascularization. Does it have a role in the treatment of ischemic heart disease? Tex Heart Inst J 25:24–29, 1998.

31. Trehan N, Mishra M, Bapna R, et al: Transmyocardial laser revascularization combined with coronary artery bypass grafting without cardiopulmonary bypass. Eur J Cardiothorac Surg Aug;12:276–284, 1997.
32. Saatvedt K, Dragsund M, Nordstrand K: Transmyocardial laser revascularization and coronary artery bypass grafting without cardiopulmonary bypass. Ann Thorac Surg 62:323–324, 1996.
33. Doty JR, Salazar JD, Fonger JD, et al: Reoperative MIDCAB grafting: Three-year clinical experience. Eur J Cardiothorac Surg (in press).
34. Allen KB, Matheny RG, Robison RJ, et al: Minimally invasive versus conventional reoperative coronary artery bypass. Ann Thorac Surg 64:616–622, 1997.
35. Suma H, Wanibuchi Y, Terada Y, et al: The right gastroepiploic artery graft: Clinical and angiographic midterm results in 200 patients. J Thorac Cardiovasc Surg 105:615–623, 1993.
36. Suma H: Optimal use of the gastroepiploic artery. Semin Thorac Cardiovasc Surg 8:24–28, 1996.
37. Antona C, Zanobini M, Pompilio G, et al: Role of right gastroepiploic artery in myocardial revascularization with arterial grafts. Cardiovasc Surg 4:217–221, 1996.
38. Fonger JD, Doty JR, Salazar JD, et al: Initial experience with MIDCAB grafting using the gastroepiploic artery. Ann Thorac Surg (in press).
39. Uppal R, Wolfe WG, Lowe JE, et al: Right thoracotomy for reoperative right coronary artery bypass procedures. Ann Thorac Surg 57:123–125, 1994.
40. Grosner G, Lajos TZ, Schimert G, et al: Left thoracotomy reoperation for coronary artery disease. J Card Surg 5:304–308, 1990.
41. Ungerleider RM, Mills NL, Wechsler AS: Left thoracotomy for reoperative coronary artery bypass procedures. Ann Thorac Surg 40:11–15, 1985.
42. Burlingame MW, Bonchek LI, Vazales BE: Left thoracotomy for reoperative coronary bypass. J Thorac Cardiovasc Surg 95: 508–510, 1988.
43. Faro RS, Javid H, Najafi H, et al: Left thoracotomy for reoperation for coronary revascularization. Thorac Cardiovasc Surg 83: 453–455, 1982.
44. Knight JL, Cohn LH: Left thoracotomy and femoro-femoral bypass for reoperative revascularization of the posterior coronary circulation. J Card Surg 2:343–349, 1987.

COMMENTARY

William R. Mayfield

According to the 1997 Society of Thoracic Surgeons Database,[1] reoperative coronary artery bypass grafting represents 8% of coronary artery bypass surgeries performed in the United States, or 25,000 cases per year. Although no single factor is responsible for the increased risk associated with reoperative surgery, it is generally conceded that manipulation of diseased grafts or injury to the heart at repeat sternotomy may contribute to morbidity and mortality. Massive hemorrhage resulting from injury to the aorta, coronary bypass grafts, right atrium or ventricle, innominate vein or lung is certainly associated with a high risk of mortality.[2] Several other factors may also adversely influence the risk of reoperation. These include more than one reoperation, ascending aortic aneurysm, conditions enlarging the right atrium or ventricle, right ventricular outflow patch or conduit, and previous mediastinitis with sternal osteomyelitis.[3]

A variety of techniques and procedures have been designed to reduce the risk of reoperative coronary surgery, such as use of a thoracotomy incision or application of femoral-femoral cardiopulmonary bypass before performance of sternotomy. It is within this context that Dr. Fonger's reoperative minimally invasive direct coronary artery bypass (MIDCAB) surgery is an effective tool. MIDCAB avoids the need for resternotomy, reduces the need for dissection, limits graft manipulation, and avoids aortic cross clamping. It may even allow otherwise high-risk patients who have poor ventricular function to undergo repeat revascularization safely. Dr. Fonger has described the operative technique in detail, and has distinguished himself by the liberal use of the gastroepiploic artery. Off-pump, single-vessel reoperative MIDCAB is certainly an appropriate and desirable procedure in selected patients.

Other new alternative approaches for reoperative coronary surgery are constantly being developed. Our own method is to use video-assisted visualization and lysis of retrosternal adhesions for a safe resternotomy. With this technique, the heart is retracted away from the sternum with an integrated retractor-endoscope, and is freed from the sternum by use of cautery under video guidance. When this is completed, routine sternotomy is performed, and injury to intrathoracic structures is avoided.[4]

As Dr. Fonger states, given the large number of patients who have vein grafts and who are now returning for redo surgery, the new safer techniques for reoperative coronary surgery should be in every surgeon's armamentarium.

References

1. Society of Thoracic Surgeons National Cardiovascular Surgery Database, 1997.
2. Machiraju MJ: Technical complications during redo cardiac surgery. *In* Redo Cardiac Surgery in Adults. Southampton, NY, CME Network, 1997.
3. Loop F: Catastrophic hemorrhage during sternal reentry. Ann Thorac Surg 37:271–272, 1984.
4. Mayfield WR: Endoscopic repeat sternotomy. Heart Surg Forum 1:26–29, 1998.

Chapter 69

Graft Assessment in Off-Pump Coronary Artery Bypass Surgery

Mohammad Bashar Izzat, Randall K. Wolf, Wassim Atassi, and Anthony P. C. Yim

Quality assessment is fundamental to the development of a new surgical procedure and is a prerequisite for its acceptance by the community. The role of the new minimal access and off-pump coronary artery bypass techniques in clinical practice will ultimately depend on verifying their success, measured in terms of graft patency compared with the conventional technique.[11, 12]

It is generally believed that the patency rate for left internal mammary artery (LIMA) grafts to the left anterior descending (LAD) coronary artery using the conventional technique is around 90% at 10 years. It is also believed that patency rates for arterial conduits, in particular the LIMA, change very little after the initial postoperative period. This implies that the majority of graft failures occur early, most likely owing to technical errors. Hence, if technical problems with a new method are identified early and corrected, it follows that graft patency can be improved.[24] This is particularly important during the early phase of the learning curve with any new technique. Evaluating the success of grafting is therefore best performed soon after completion of the grafting procedure. Ideally, this should be accomplished in the operating room, so that any graft abnormality can be recognized and corrected by the surgeon.

Although the ideal noninvasive graft assessment modality is yet to be discovered, minimal access and off-pump coronary artery surgery have already focused our attention on the importance of documenting graft patency.[12, 24]

Anatomic Assessment

Intraoperative Angiography

Despite encouraging technological advances in noninvasive scanning and in physiologic measurements of blood flow in the coronary vessels, catheter-based coronary angiography remains the "gold standard" for graft assessment.[12, 21] For immediate postprocedure angiography, the patient has to be transferred from the operating room to the catheter laboratory and, when necessary, back to the operating room for re-exploration. This is impractical, and time is wasted as both the catheter laboratory and the operating room staff must stand by.[14] Performing operative procedures in the catheter laboratory also presents problems.[2] Angiographic assessment is therefore best performed immediately in the operating room. This enables the surgeon to detect, explain, and correct angiographic abnormalities before the patient leaves the operating room, eliminating the need for early reoperation.[13–15]

With current operating room designs, intraoperative coronary angiography can be performed with a fixed fluoroscopy unit installed in the operating room or with a portable unit. High-quality portable units with good image definition are now available and are relatively inexpensive compared with fixed units.[15] Ultimately, however, the trend toward performing more hybrid procedures means that operations will be performed in dedicated combined cardiac catheterization and surgery suites with ideal angiographic facilities.[3]

Intraoperative angiography of the LIMA can be performed through selective catheterization of the mammary artery via femoral, brachial, or radial artery cannulations (Fig. 69–1).[7, 13, 15] Although these techniques are straightforward and easy to learn, they are more commonly performed by cardiologists than by cardiac surgeons. Recently, we proposed alternative techniques that allow the direct injection of contrast medium into the LIMA. In one method, the most distal coronary anastomosis is performed in a side-to-side fashion, leaving the end of the LIMA graft available for cannulation and retrograde injection of contrast medium (Fig. 69–2).[25, 26] This retrograde technique avoids cannulation of the more proximal LIMA. Another technique is suitable for multiple arterial grafting procedures through median sternotomy.[16] In this method, the proximal end of the free radial artery graft is anastomosed to the side of the proximal LIMA in an inverted-Y fashion before the anastomosis to the LAD is performed. Contrast medium is then injected directly into the free distal end of the radial artery. Straight anterior and lateral views clearly define the patency of both radial and LIMA grafts, the anastomoses, and the distal and proximal runoff into the LAD (Fig. 69–3). The radial artery is then used to revascularize the lateral and/or inferior wall of the left ventricle.

These techniques are simple and expeditious and do not require any ancillary personnel other than the radiographer to capture the images. An additional advantage is that only a small volume of contrast medium (usually 3 to 5 ml) is required, whereas a much larger volume is ordinarily used while locating the mammary artery takeoff from the subclavian artery.[16] This is clinically relevant in the patients who have failure, who are now routinely considered for surgery without cardiopulmonary bypass by many surgeons.

Immediate angiograms are occasionally difficult to interpret. Certain abnormalities on the immediate postoperative angiogram may be due to transitory localized edema or small thrombus formation that may resolve spontaneously, resulting in normal postoperative angiograms several months later.[4] Despite the present paucity of knowledge

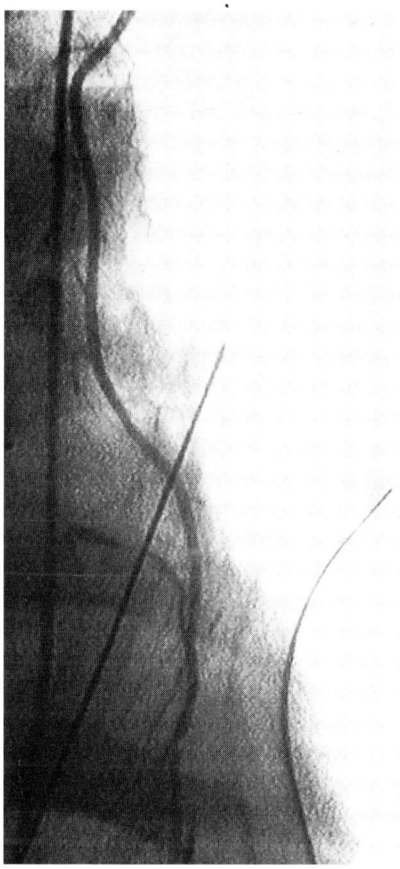

Figure 69–1. "On-table" angiography of a left internal mammary artery–to–left anterior descending artery graft (a minimally invasive direct coronary artery bypass [MIDCAB]) performed using a standard portable unit.

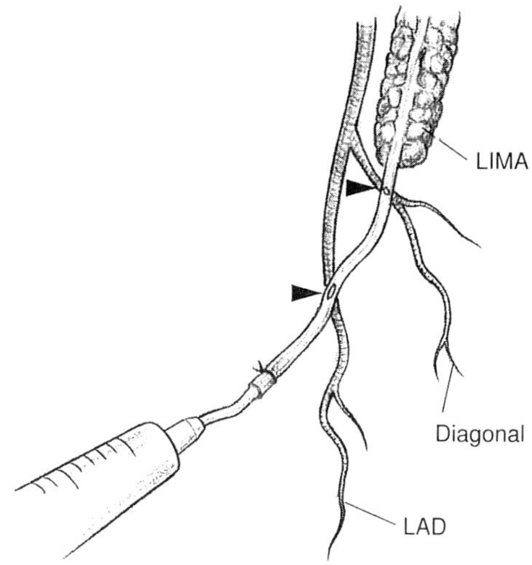

Figure 69–2. Technique of direct intraoperative angiography for the left internal mammary artery (LIMA), which was sequentially anastomosed to the left anterior descending artery (LAD) and a diagonal branch. (From Wolf RK, Ohtsuka T, Takamoto S (eds): Illustrated Minimally Invasive Coronary Artery Bypass Grafting. Tokyo, Chugai Igaku-sha, 1998.)

on the "normal" early angiographic appearance, angiography remains the best method of determining the success of coronary grafting procedures (Fig. 69–4).

Thermal Imaging

Thermal imaging is a unique technology, based on detection of infrared radiation. Small differences in surface temperature between the coronary arteries and the myocardium can be detected and analyzed to create a real-time visual image of the coronary anatomy on video display, hence producing thermal coronary angiography (TCA).

Use of thermal imaging was first reported in cardiac surgery in 1971,[22] but the image resolution with early equipment did not allow for clear visualization of anatomic structures. With newer thermal imaging technology, differences in surface temperature as small as 0.2 to 0.4°C can be detected, making the thermal resolution much better, and digital subtraction of frames has also helped to enhance image contrast. Indeed, TCA has been demonstrated to document the success or failure of myocardial revascularization reliably with the conventional technique.[20]

Use of TCA to document graft and anastomosis patency in off-pump coronary surgery is made difficult by the fact that, unlike the practice in conventional surgery, myocar-

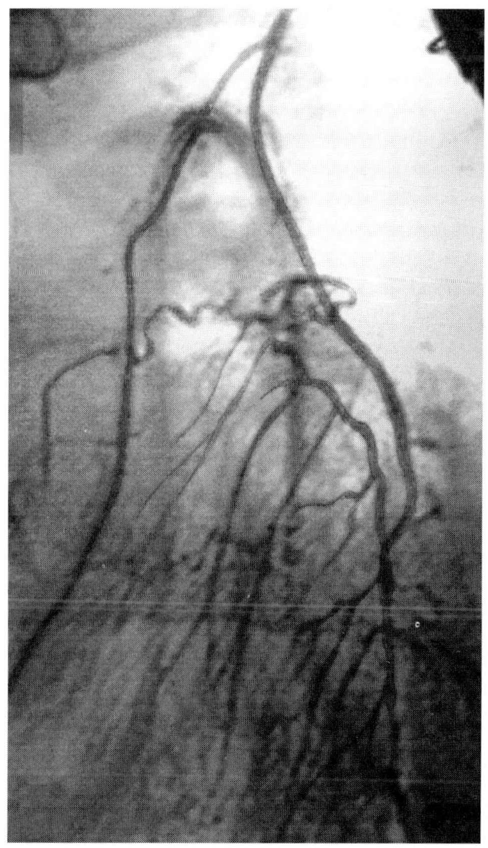

Figure 69–3. Intraoperative direct angiography of the composite radial artery–left internal mammary artery (LIMA) graft, with good result. (From Izzat MB, El-Zufari MH, Yim APC: Intraoperative direct LIMA angiography for beating heart operations. Ann Thorac Surg 66:1431, 1432, 1998.)

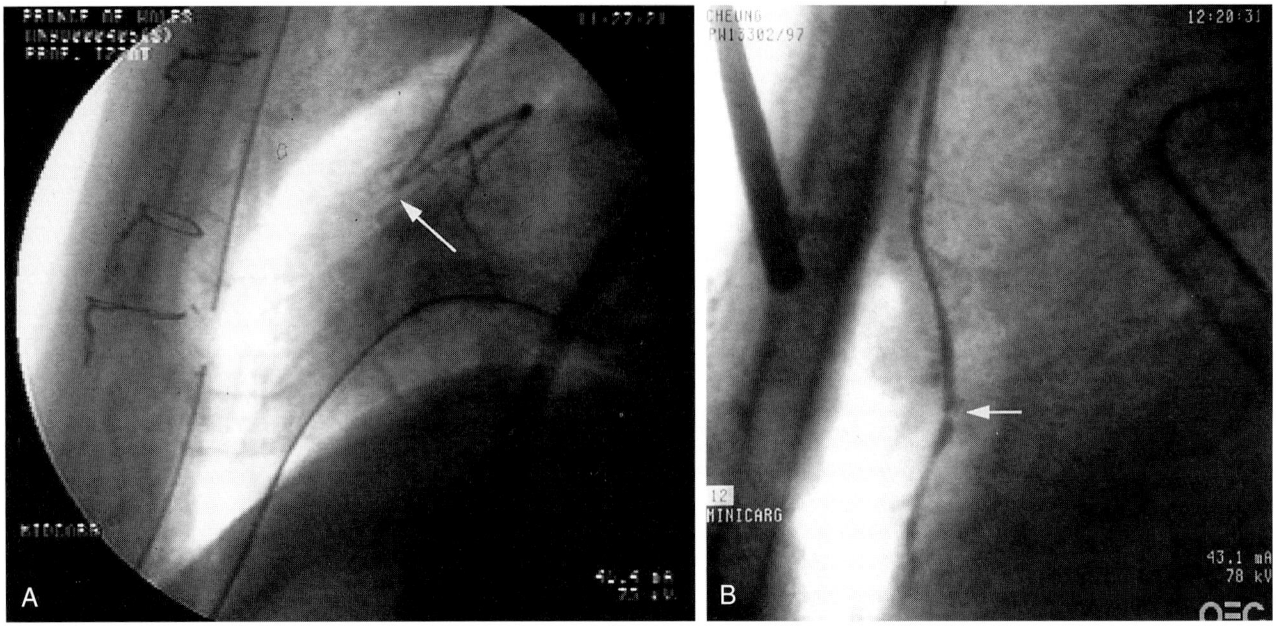

Figure 69–4. *A,* Intraoperative angiography of a left internal mammary artery–to–left anterior descending artery (LIMA-to-LAD) graft revealing absent distal flow into the LAD (*arrow*). *B,* Angiography of a LIMA-to-LAD graft (minimally invasive technique) (MIDCAB) that was lengthened using a segment of the saphenous vein. Stenosis of the LIMA–to–saphenous vein anastomosis is seen (*arrow*) (OEC 9600 imaging system).

dial cooling is not used. Nevertheless, satisfactory outline of LIMA-to-LAD graft anatomy can occasionally be obtained by employing topical cooling of the myocardial surface with cold saline (Fig. 69–5).[8] Often, however, image definition is inadequate owing to small temperature gradients or the presence of a thick layer of epicardial fat. Vein or radial artery grafts can be imaged without cooling the myocardium by injecting cold saline (25°C) directly down the graft, which is clinically safe.

TCA imaging has been shown to detect LIMA strictures, torsion, and traumatic wall disruption or dissection during conventional "open" harvesting.[20] It is possible that this technology may be applicable to the minimally invasive LIMA harvesting methods as well.

Although TCA is relatively expensive, it has significant advantages: It is easy to perform, totally noninvasive, and does not involve exposure to radiation or use of contrast agents. Current research indicates that flow quantification through thermal imaging may also become possible in the near future.

Angioscopy

Currently available angioscopes can be as small as 0.7 mm in diameter and have several components that function together to permit intraluminal vessel imaging. The system is usually disposable and includes an outer sleeve and an inner catheter that function as a monorail system to deliver the imaging system and light source to the location in the blood vessel. The imaging system is made up of a fiberoptic imaging bundle that contains several thousand individual fibers and a light source that provides high-intensity light that does not create thermal injury.

To perform LIMA graft angioscopy, the full percutaneous system is introduced through femoral or brachial punctures, and selective cannulation of LIMA takeoff from

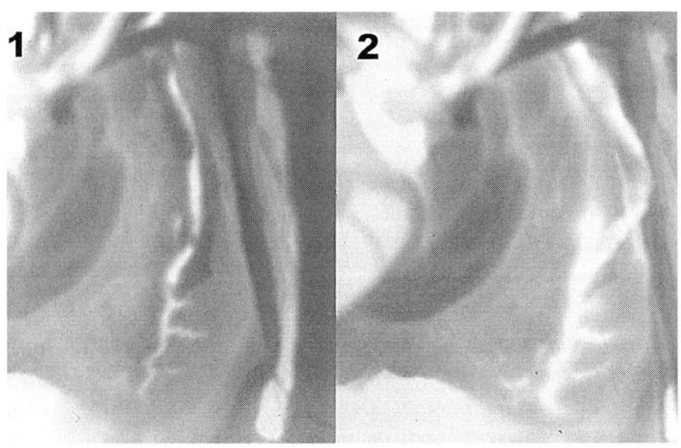

Figure 69–5. Thermal angiography of a left internal mammary artery–to–left anterior descending artery (LIMA-to-LAD) graft (off-pump through median sternotomy) after cooling of the myocardial surface with cold saline. A satisfactory outline of both the LIMA and the LAD system is obtained (*1*), followed 5 seconds later by rewarming of the mammary pedicle and myocardial surface (*2*).

the left subclavian artery is performed. A blood-free field is necessary for intraluminal imaging and is obtained using a combination of an occlusive cuff on the tip of the catheter to interrupt antegrade blood flow and the injection of warmed saline via a power injector. Once correct positioning of the catheter is confirmed by fluoroscopy, angioscopic examination is conducted during brief periods of interruption of blood flow to minimize myocardial ischemia.

Another method of performing LIMA graft angioscopy is similar to that detailed for intraoperative direct angiography and is suitable for multiple arterial grafting procedures through a median sternotomy. In this method, the proximal end of the free radial artery graft is anastomosed to the side of the proximal LIMA in an inverted-Y fashion before the anastomosis to the LAD is performed. The angioscope is then introduced directly into the free distal end of the radial artery, and both the radial and LIMA grafts, the anastomoses, and the LAD can be studied. The radial artery is then used to revascularize the lateral, inferior, or both parts of the wall of the left ventricle. Angioscopy of a free arterial or vein graft can be performed by introducing the angioscope directly into the proximal free end of the vessel and advanced to the completed anastomosis.[17]

Excellent images of the completed anastomoses can be obtained, and atherosclerotic plaques, adherent thrombi, and localized intimal flaps are all readily visualized.[17, 23] The effect of these morphologic abnormalities on the short- and long-term success of grafting has not been established, however. To date, angioscopic assessment of coronary artery bypass grafts performed on the beating heart have not been performed.

Physiologic Assessment

Physiologic assessment can be performed using a range of technologies. Various Doppler ultrasound methods have been used in coronary artery bypass graft assessment, both in the operating room and postoperatively. Although this can provide useful physiologic data that can predict graft patency, it has not yet been able to provide precise anatomic data. However, further modifications of these techniques are anticipated in the near future.

Transcutaneous Doppler Echocardiography

Transcutaneous Doppler echocardiography is the main noninvasive method currently used for the postoperative quality assessment of LIMA grafts performed with the minimally invasive direct coronary artery bypass (MIDCAB) technique. Two approaches can be used to visualize the conduit: suprasternal (to visualize the LIMA at its origin from the subclavian artery) and parasternal (through its course along the intercostal spaces) (Fig. 69–6).

Using Doppler analysis, the ungrafted LIMA has a characteristic flow velocity pattern with a prevalent systolic component, a negative end-systolic peak (which is not always present), and a small diastolic component (Fig. 69–7*A*). When anastomosed to the LAD, the flow velocity pattern becomes biphasic with an important diastolic component (Fig. 69–7*B*).[9] The LIMA flow velocity pattern, however, is directly related to the characteristics of the coronary bed to which the graft is connected. Therefore, the diastolic component is related to the resistance to graft flow: the severity of LAD stenosis and the state of the myocardium, which is LAD dependent. Furthermore, the flow velocity pattern can be affected by modification of systemic arterial pressure, change in heart rate, and use of inotropes or vasodilators.

Documenting the presence of the biphasic flow velocity pattern indicates that the LIMA-to-LAD anastomosis is patent. However, to determine whether the anastomosis is restrictive during higher flow conditions, the flow velocity

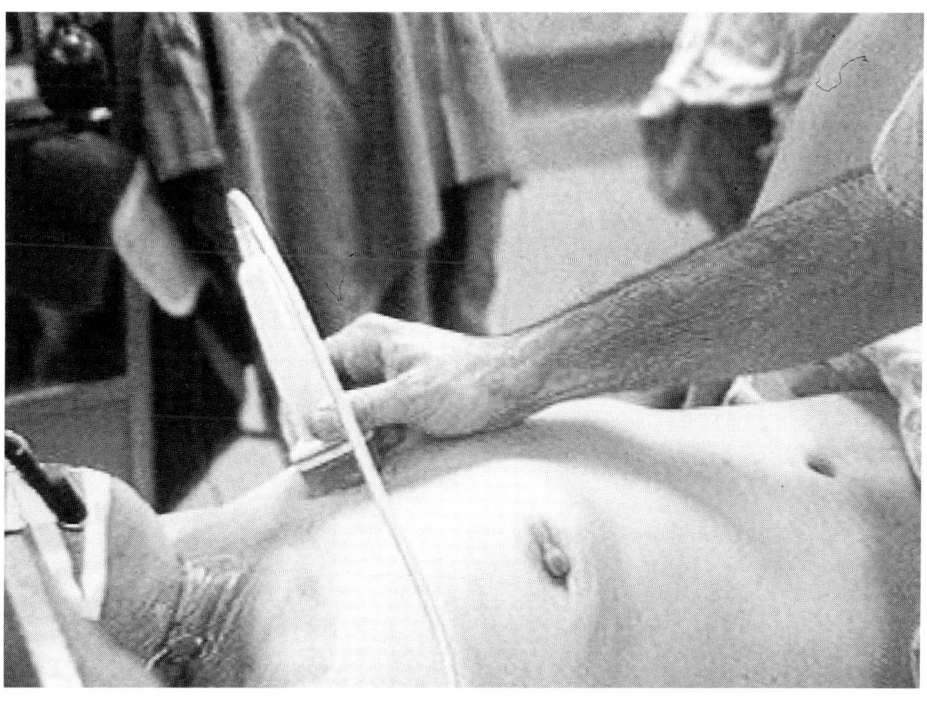

Figure 69–6. The parasternal approach for transcutaneous Doppler assessment of left internal mammary artery–to–left anterior descending artery (LIMA-to-LAD) grafts. The LIMA conduit is visualized through its course along the intercostal spaces.

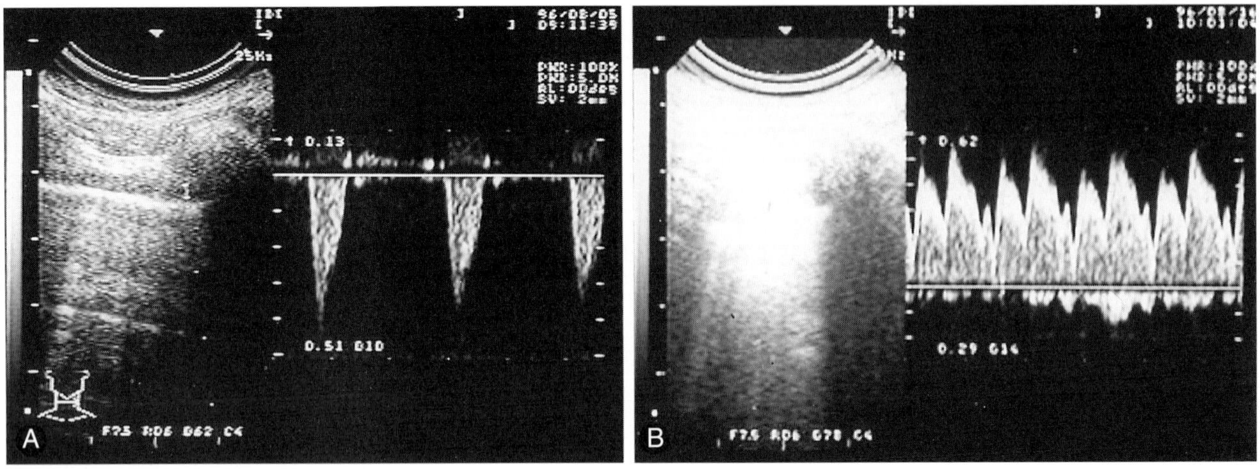

Figure 69–7. Characteristic Doppler flow velocity pattern of the left internal mammary artery before (*A*) and after (*B*) grafting to the left anterior descending artery (LAD).

pattern is examined during the Azoulay maneuver, using the ratios between diastolic and systolic velocities as proposed by Calafiore.[4, 9]

The Azoulay maneuver consists of two steps. First, the patient's legs are lifted up by an assistant, and second, the patient is required to hold this position actively for a few seconds. Acute hypervolemia follows as the circulating volume in both legs is suddenly emptied into the upper body circulation. As a consequence, heart rate and cardiac output increase transiently; this causes an increase of blood flow to both the muscular circulation (systolic phase of the LIMA flow pattern) and the coronary circulation (diastolic phase of the LIMA flow pattern).

From comparing postoperative angiograms and Doppler flow velocity evaluations at rest and during the Azoulay maneuver, the following guidelines were suggested to predict the quality of LIMA-to-LAD grafts[4, 9]: If peak and mean diastolic-systolic velocity ratios at rest are equal to or greater than 1, or are less than 1 at rest but increase to 1 or more during the Azoulay maneuver, this indicates that the anastomosis is not restrictive. However, when ratios are less than 1, both at rest and during the Azoulay maneuver, this indicates graft malfunction or an occluded graft.

Ultrasonic Transit Time Flow Volume Sensor

This noninvasive hand-held device is positioned directly on the conduit under study intraoperatively. The probe head houses two ultrasonic transducers that simultaneously direct ultrasonic waves upstream and downstream through each measurement cycle and subtract the transit times of both waves, resulting in an estimate of flow volume. This measurement is independent of flow velocity, probe alignment, and flow turbulence.[6] Using this ultrasonic transit time sensor, an average intraoperative flow volume of 30 ml/min was recorded in the mammary circulation after the MIDCAB procedure, and graft revision was advised if graft flow was less than 5 ml/min.[24]

A principal shortcoming of this "functional" graft assessment is the fact that graft flow depends on both mean arterial blood pressure and resistance in the distal coronary bed. A change in blood pressure can therefore bring about significant variations in flow measurements. Moreover, measured graft flow may still be adequate in the presence of good retrograde flow in the grafted coronary artery but absent distal runoff beyond the anastomosis. Analysis of the diastolic volume curve may add sensitivity to this test.

Other Ultrasound-Based Technologies

High-Frequency Epicardial Echocardiography. This technique was introduced for the intraoperative imaging of coronary arteries, aiming to develop a method for the direct evaluation of the coronary artery lumen and wall in cross-section that could assess the extent of atherosclerosis.[19] Doppler color flow mapping was also shown to identify coronary stenoses in experimental models.[1] This technology has been tested in the evaluation of coronary artery bypass grafts, but mainly in the arrested heart.[10] Anecdotally, in the MIDCAB procedure, an epicardial echocardiogram is difficult to perform because of heart motion while examining small-sized (1 to 2 mm) vessels. Examination during stabilization may improve the test, but it may also interfere with flow in the native coronary bed. Nevertheless, if epicardial echocardiography can achieve the predictive ability of Duplex scans in peripheral vascular disease, it may become a valuable tool in the intraoperative assessment of off-pump coronary artery surgery.

Intravascular Ultrasound (IVU). IVU can give precise information on the characteristics of the vessel wall, although the perpendicular direction of imaging can preclude visualization of some stenoses. IVU has been able to demonstrate technical problems in saphenous vein grafts intraoperatively. However, the relatively large catheter diameter and the need for selective catheterization of the LIMA origin currently preclude its use in evaluating mammary conduits. Future advances in IVU technology may bring this method into the operating room.

Doppler Flow Wire. This technique was developed to assess the severity of coronary artery stenoses through measurements of blood flow velocities. Using a Doppler angioplasty guide wire, velocity data are acquired with a forward-directed ultrasound beam and processed in real time. Basal and hyperemic velocities can be recorded, and a coronary flow reserve ratio can also be calculated. In a pilot study, we evaluated the Doppler flow wire passed directly through the distal anastomosis during MIDCAB procedures. The flow wire accurately demonstrated augmented velocities in LIMA grafts to the LAD. It has the distinct advantage of measuring velocities downstream or distal to the anastomosis. The flow wire can be removed from the anastomosis easily, even after the anastomosis has been completed. Further evolution of this technique is promising and may include direct epicardial flow wire measurements.

The Future

Research continues in an attempt to find a graft assessment method that is noninvasive, suitable for intraoperative use, and capable of yielding precise anatomic and physiologic information. It is likely that the solution will involve a combination of anatomic and physiologic evaluation using two or more different technologies, such as combining Doppler flow wire with thermal imaging. For now, it is vital that the success of grafting through any new operative modality be verified using the gold standard technique, that is intraoperative angiography.[11, 12] Such data are essential to evaluate the technique and to help individual surgeons in their own learning process. The advent of new coronary artery surgery techniques has already highlighted the importance of documenting graft patency. The development of new graft assessment modalities is likely to lead to an overall improvement in graft patency.

References

1. Aragam JR, Main J, Guerrero JL, et al: Doppler color flow mapping of epicardial coronary arteries: Initial observations. J Am Coll Cardiol 21:478–487, 1993.
2. Angelini GD, Wilde P, Salerno TA, et al: Integrated left small thoracotomy and angioplasty for multivessel coronary artery revascularisation. Lancet 347:757–758, 1996.
3. Barstad RM, Fosse E, Vatne K, et al: Intraoperative angiography in minimally invasive direct coronary artery bypass grafting. Ann Thorac Surg 64:1835–1839, 1997.
4. Calafiore AM, Gallina S, Iaco A: Minimally invasive mammary artery Doppler flow velocity evaluation in minimally invasive coronary operations. Ann Thorac Surg 66:1236–1241, 1998.
5. Calafiore AM, Di Giammarco G, Teodori G, et al: Left anterior descending coronary artery grafting via left anterior small thoracotomy without cardiopulmonary bypass. Ann Thorac Surg 61:1658–1665, 1996.
6. Caver CC, Dame NA: Ultrasonic assessment of internal thoracic artery graft flow in the revascularized heart. Ann Thorac Surg 58:135–138, 1994.
7. Elbeery JR, Chitwood WR: Intraoperative catheterization of the left internal mammary artery via the left radial artery. Ann Thorac Surg 64:1840–1842, 1997.
8. Emery RW, Emery AM, Flavin TF, et al: Revascularization using angioplasty and minimally invasive techniques documented by thermal imaging. Ann Thorac Surg 62:591–593, 1996.
9. Gallina S, Calafiore AM: Doppler echocardiography and the MIDCAB procedure. *In* Izzat MB, Sanderson JE, Sutton MSJ (eds): Echocardiography in Adult Cardiac Surgery. Oxford, Isis Medical Media, 1999.
10. Hiratzka LF, McPherson DD, Brandt B, et al: The role of intraoperative high-frequency epicardial echocardiography during coronary artery revascularization. Circulation 76(suppl V):33–38, 1987.
11. Izzat MB: Invited commentary on Calafiore AM, et al: Minimally invasive mammary artery Doppler flow velocity evaluation in minimally invasive coronary operations. Ann Thorac Surg 66:1241, 1998.
12. Izzat MB, Yim APC: Didn't they do well? [Editorial]. Ann Thorac Surg 64:1–2, 1997.
13. Izzat MB, Yim APC: MIDCABG: Lessons learned from routine "on-table" angiography. Ann Thorac Surg 64:1872–1874, 1997.
14. Izzat MB, Yim APC: Trouble shooting in minimally invasive direct coronary artery bypass. Lancet 350:665–666, 1997.
15. Izzat MB, Yim APC, El-Zufari MH: Routine intra-operative angiography improves the results of off-pump coronary artery grafting. Chest 115:987–990, 1999.
16. Izzat MB, El-Zufari MH, Yim APC: Intra-operative direct LIMA angiography for beating-heart surgery. Ann Thorac Surg 66:1431, 1432, 1998.
17. Keogh BE, Bidstrup BP, Taylor KM, Sapsford RN: Angioscopic evaluation of intravascular morphology after coronary endarterectomy. Ann Thorac Surg 52:766–772, 1991.
18. Lazzara RR, McLellan BA, Kidwel FE, et al: Intraoperative angiography during minimally invasive direct coronary artery bypass operations. Ann Thorac Surg 64:1725–1727, 1997.
19. McPherson DD, Armstrong M, Rose E, et al: High frequency epicardial echocardiography for coronary artery evaluation: In vitro and in vivo validation of arterial lumen and wall thickness measurements. J Am Coll Cardiol 8:600–606, 1986.
20. Mohr FW, Falk V: Thermal coronary angiography: A method for assessing graft patency and coronary anatomy in coronary bypass surgery. Ann Thorac Surg 63:1506–1507, 1997.
21. Rainer WG, Sadler TR, Hilgenberg AD, Kelly TF. Technique and value of operative arteriography in coronary artery bypass operations. J Thorac Cardiovasc Surg 83:358–362, 1982.
22. Senyk J, Malm A, Bornmyr S: Intraoperative cardiothermography: A new method for detecting ischemic areas in the heart muscle and for investigation of the results of revascularization procedures in coronary surgery. Eur Surg Res 3:1–12, 1971.
23. Siegel SB, White GH, Colman PD, Nelson RJ: Intraoperative angioscopy for coronary bypass surgery. J Card Surg 10:210–220, 1995.
24. Wolf RK: MIDCAB: The intra-operative assessment of coronary bypass grafts. *In* Cohen RG, Mack MJ, Fonger JD, et al (eds): Minimally Invasive Cardiac Surgery. St. Louis, Quality Medical Publishers (in press).
25. Wolf RK: A new simple intra-operative angiographic technique for MIDCAB. Utrecht MIDCABG Workshop III, Utrecht, The Netherlands, 1997.
26. Wolf RK, Ohtsuka T, Takamoto S (eds): Illustrated Minimally Invasive Coronary Artery Bypass Grafting. Tokyo, Chugai Igakusha, 1998.

COMMENTARY

W. Gerald Rainer

This chapter covers in a concise but thorough way the various methods that have been used in the past and are currently being used or investigated for assessing the status of the bypass conduit in myocardial revascularization surgery. It is well established that the quality of bypass grafting depends on a number of factors, including but not limited to the surgical technique, the quality of the bypass conduits, the quality of the recipient coronary vessel, and the status of the runoff in the coronary vascular bed distal to the anastomosis.

Professor Izzat and his colleagues have covered the various modalities used in graft assessment. One might automatically believe that in the area of coronary artery bypass surgery, and especially with minimally invasive techniques, the simpler methods might be more appropriate. These methods might include flowmeter determinations and thermal angiography, because they represent the least invasive approaches to assessing blood flow. Certainly, intraoperative arteriography would be more fraught with technical problems, and angioscopy even more so. In the postoperative phase, transcutaneous Doppler echocardiography and echocardiographic techniques might be more worthwhile.

I am always concerned about intravascular damage with any procedure that involves the direct introduction of catheters, wires, or other instruments into the vessel itself. Great harm can be done to the intima of the bypass and recipient vessels by either direct instrumentation or the chemical effect of contrast media introduced for the purpose of arteriography or flow determination.

I certainly agree with the authors that a safe method for assessing flow in the bypass graft conduit and into the distal myocardium *at the time of surgery* is of great importance in the assessment of the revascularization technique. This takes into account all the variables mentioned earlier and allows corrective measure to be taken if necessary. This may be more important in the minimally invasive approach to revascularization than in conventional coronary bypass graft surgery.

Chapter 70

Quality of Life Assessment for Minimally Invasive Coronary Surgery

Buu-Khanh Lam and Inderjit S. Gill

Avoidance of cardiopulmonary bypass (CPB), shortening of hospital stay, faster return to work, and reduction of costs are all goals that have contributed to the upsurge of minimally invasive coronary surgery (MICS). Innovative and novel approaches have shifted the scientific spotlight onto this new field of cardiac surgery. Early results are favorable, but the focus should not be limited to technical results.[7, 33, 34] Indeed, the aim should be to evaluate all aspects of this new field, including the patients' quality of life (QOL) after undergoing MICS. We intuitively assume that MICS patients have a better early postoperative QOL compared with their counterparts who have undergone conventional coronary artery bypass grafting (CABG). Is this really the case? Is morbidity lessened? Is mortality the same? Is there a faster return to functional level? Do MICS patients recover faster and better in the first postoperative year? Do they truly benefit from avoidance of CPB and sternotomy? All these questions are valid and require objective answers.

Defining and measuring QOL has always been a great challenge. QOL is a multidimensional concept that has been advocated to define more precisely the experience of recovering from major health-care events. Objective indicators of QOL, such as decrease in morbidity, improved survival, lack of angina, exercise tolerance, and return to work are important, but increasing emphasis has been placed on examining the role of subjective perceptions of both physical and psychological well-being. Indeed, the most frequently quoted attributes defining subjective QOL were levels of of life satisfaction, happiness, and physical well-being.[17] Simply put, patients have regained their QOL once they consider that their lives have been restored to normal. Good health and QOL are now defined as much by objective physiologic parameters as they are by subjective perceptions. The physiologic elements are:

- Maximal oxygen uptake (V_{O_2}max), defined as the point at which oxygen uptake reaches a plateau despite further increases in work rate, has been proposed as an objective measure of cardiorespiratory function.[3, 20] It is also one of the most powerful predictors of prognosis in patients who have congestive heart failure and in those who have coronary artery disease.[23, 28] Weber and associates used gas exchange analysis to objectively stratify patients according to the American Heart Association functional classifications. Their stratification ranged from functional class A (no to mild impairment) to functional class D (severe impairment) based on their V_{O_2}max (Table 70–1).[40]
- V_{O_2}peak rather than V_{O_2}max is reported in the literature if a leveling-off criterion cannot be achieved.[9]
- Oxygen uptake efficiency slope (OUES), derived from the relationship between oxygen uptake and minute ventilation during incremental exercise,[3] is the index usually used if patients are unable to achieve a maximal effort.
- Resting and peak metabolic rates are defined by metabolic equivalents (METS).
- Anaerobic threshold, although not a direct measure of cardiovascular function, indicates the level of exercise below which long-lasting physical activity can be performed and above which exhaustion may occur.
- Oxygen pulse is determined by the product of stroke volume and arterial-venous oxygen difference.
- Minute ventilation is observed.
- Forced expiratory volume in 1 second (FEV_1) and functional vital capacity (FVC) are evaluated along with other secondary cardiopulmonary parameters.

At the University of Ottawa Heart Institute, we principally use V_{O_2}peak and percent predicted of V_{O_2}peak as the significant physiologic measures of a patient's cardiorespiratory capabilities. The rationale for using gas exchange analysis obtained by cardiopulmonary exercise testing is twofold: First, it offers an accurate and objective QOL assessment via the measurement of a patient's cardiovascular functional capacity. Second, we believe that gas exchange analysis is of greater clinical significance than values derived from protocols based on the cardiovascular functional capacity of healthy individuals. In the event that gas exchange analysis is not used, caution must be employed when interpreting test results and making inferences concerning the patient's functional capacity and magnitude of impairment.

Patients' self-reported data have been used extensively in recent years as subjective outcome measures in randomized trials of medical and surgical treatments and in large sample studies of the health status of normal and clinically defined populations.[16, 18, 19] Reliable and valid scales have been developed that are sensitive to changes in clinically significant dimensions of patient experience.[22, 27, 38, 42] In addition to excellent psychometric performance, other beneficial characteristics of many of the new instruments include brevity, ease of administration, and ease of interpretation. The use of standardized measures also allows meaningful comparisons across a spectrum of health conditions and study populations. A variety of generic and disease-specific self-report instruments are now being used by health policy analysts, clinical researchers, and care providers to assess patient health status, to track and model changes in disease conditions, and to evaluate and improve treatment procedures.[24, 32] Table 70–2 presents a partial list of subjective QOL assessment tools. Table 70–3

Table 70–1. Assessment of Functional Impairment

Severity of Impairment	Functional Class	Vo_2max (ml/kg per min)	METS
None to mild	A	>20	>5.7
Mild to moderate	B	16–20	4.6–5.7
Moderate to severe	C	10–16	2.9–4.5
Severe	D	<10	<2.9

METS = metabolic equivalents

From Weber KT, Janicki JS, McElroy PA: Determination of aerobic capacity and the severity of chronic cardiac and circulatory failure. Circulation 76(suppl): VI–40, 1987.

illustrates the SF-36 questionnaire used at our institution.[39]

Institutional Experience

We have been performing MICS at the University of Ottawa Heart Institute since January 1996, and our experience encompasses 94 minimally invasive direct coronary artery bypass (MIDCAB) cases and 30 off-pump coronary artery bypass (OPCAB) cases. MIDCAB patients were operated through a left anterior mini-thoracotomy; patients who had left anterior descending and diagonal disease benefited most from this approach. Our MIDCAB technique has been previously described.[12] All our OPCAB patients underwent sternotomy, because the majority of them required two or more grafts, with one of them being either the right coronary artery or a marginal branch. Better exposure and less hemodynamic compromise were achieved with this approach. Our OPCAB technique consisted mainly of off-pump surgery through a sternotomy with the help of either the Cardio Thoracic Systems (CTS) or Octopus stabilizers. To date, there has been no mortality in either group.

Since the introduction of MICS, some concerns have been raised regarding the technical accuracy of distal anastomosis performed on the beating heart.[31, 41] To resolve these concerns, we performed early (4 to 6 hours) postoperative angiographic follow-up on our first 25 MIDCAB patients. This yielded an overall early patency rate of 97.5%; 81% (21 of 26) of the anastomoses were FitzGibbon grade A, signifying absence of stenosis and unimpaired runoff[11]; 19% (5 of 26) were FitzGibbon grade B (Table 70–4). These results were compared with previous

Table 70–2. Quality of Life Instruments

Instrument	Parameters Assessed	Used in Reference
Nottingham Health Profile	Part 1: physical mobility, pain, sleep, energy, social isolation, and emotional reactions Part 2: job, housework, relationships at home, sex life, interests, hobbies, and vacations	6, 36
Spielberger Trait Anxiety Inventory	Level of anxiety	25
SCL-90	Depression, anxiety, somatization scales	25
Satisfaction Life Scale	5-item life satisfaction questionnaire with scoring system	17
Sickness Impact Profile	Sleep, rest, home management, ambulation, social interaction, intellectual function, recreation, and pastimes	17
QOL After Acute MI Questionnaire	26 items regrouped into two dimensions: limitations and emotions	26
Profile of Mood States	65-item 5-point adjective rating scale consisting of six mood factors: hostility, confusion, depression, vigor, tension, and fatigue	13

Table 70–3. SF-36 Quality of Life Questionnaire

Concepts	No. of Items	Summary of Contents
Physical functioning	10	Extent to which health limits physical activities such as self-care, walking, climbing stairs, bending, lifting, and moderate and vigorous exercises
Role functioning—physical	4	Extent to which physical health interferes with work or other daily activities, including accomplishing less than wanted, limitations in the kind of activities, or difficulty in performing activities
Body pain	2	Intensity of pain and effect of pain on normal work, both inside and outside the home
General health	5	Personal evaluation of health, including current health, health outlook, and resistance to illness
Vitality	4	Feeling energetic and full of pep versus feeling tired and worn out
Social functioning	2	Extent to which physical health or emotional problems interfere with normal social activities
Role functioning—emotional	3	Extent to which emotional problems interfere with work or other daily activities, including decreased time spent on activities, accomplishing less, and not working as carefully as usual
Mental health	5	General mental health, including depression, anxiety, behavioral-emotional control, general positive affect

Table 70–4. Patency Rates: MICS Versus CABG (LITA–LAD Grafts)

FitzGibbon Grade	Characteristics	MICS	CABG*
A	Excellent graft with unimpaired run-off	81%	85%
B	Stenosis reducing caliber of distal anastomosis or trunk to <50% of the grafted coronary artery; overall grade B was determined by the lowest of the three specific site grades	19%	10%
O	Occlusion	0%	5%

CABG = coronary artery bypass graft; LAD = left anterior descending artery; LITA = left internal thoracic artery; MICS = minimally invasive coronary surgery.

*From Gill IS, FitzGibbon GM, Higginson LAJ, et al: Minimally invasive coronary artery bypass: A series with early qualitative angiographic follow-up. Ann Thorac Surg 64:710, 1997.

institutional data, and we demonstrated similar patency rates in the left internal thoracic artery (LITA) to left anterior descending artery (LAD) anastomoses of conventional CABG patients (see Table 70–4). A 100% follow-up of our first 51 MIDCAB patients at a mean of 17 months (range, 7 to 28 months) showed no mortality, with a late cumulative patency rate of 93.5% in 60% (30 of 51) of these patients. The anastomoses in these first 51 patients were constructed without the help of stabilizers, but mechanical stabilizers have since been used.

Satisfied with these results, we sought to assess QOL (i.e., cardiopulmonary exercise test and SF-36) in our MICS patients beginning in July 1997. This was carried out at approximately 8 to 12 weeks postoperatively. All MIDCAB and OPCAB patients were eligible. All patients (35 MIDCAB and 12 OPCAB) were approached, but only 20 MIDCAB and 9 OPCAB patients agreed to enter our study. Ten MIDCAB and 3 OPCAB patients were awaiting QOL assessment, and 5 refused to enter, citing lack of time commitment. All entered patients were matched to counterparts who had undergone conventional CABG with CPB. Our results highlight differences in QOL issues that exist between MIDCAB and CABG patients and OPCAB and CABG patients.

MIDCAB Versus CABG

There were no considerable differences between the two populations of patients with regard to their age, New York Heart Association functional status, Canadian Cardiovascular Society anginal class, left ventricular function, and Provincial Acuity Score (PAS). The PAS is a risk index of six variables used to stratify patients preoperatively and to predict their risks of in-hospital mortality, prolonged intensive care unit length of stay, and prolonged hospital length of stay. The index can also be used to compare patient outcomes and resources used among different hospitals and surgeons in the province of Ontario, Canada.[37] Demographic data of these two groups were not significantly different, except for the higher number of patients who had previous myocardial infarction in the CABG group. This did not affect their left ventricular class and overall outcome. There was no mortality in either group. In the MIDCAB group, 1 patient (5%) had a superficial wound infection that resolved with antibiotic treatment. In the CABG group, 5 patients (25%) had postoperative complications: 2 patients developed atrial fibrillation, 1 patient was re-explored for bleeding, 1 patient had low cardiac output syndrome, and 1 patient suffered a perioperative myocardial infarction. Our preliminary data on postoperative atrial fibrillation indicate a significantly lower incidence in the MIDCAB group compared with incidence in the CABG group: 12% versus 32% ($P = .02$).[8]

Length of intubation, intensive care unit stay, and hospital stay were significantly different in the two groups (Table 70–5). Less than 5 hours after surgery, 14 MIDCAB patients (56%) were extubated, 7 (28%) of whom were extubated in the operating room. MIDCAB patients had a shorter intensive care unit stay and were discharged home much earlier than CABG patients.

MIDCAB and CABG patients were brought back for follow-up at a mean of 9.7 ± 9.9 weeks and 14.6 ± 11.6 weeks, respectively (P = NS). Cardiopulmonary exercise tests were performed and the SF-36 administered. Significant differences were found between the groups with regard to the peak oxygen uptake (Vo_2peak) and percent predicted of Vo_2peak; MIDCAB patients reached higher levels of maximal oxygen consumption and best approached their percent predicted values. These differ-

Table 70–5. MIDCAB Versus CABG: Postoperative and Quality of Life Assessment Data

	MIDCAB ±	CABG ±	*P*
Postoperative			
Intubation (hr)	3.5 ± 4.1	12.0 ± 4.1	.001
Intensive care stay (hr)	23.4 ± 6.8	3.5 ± 14.0	.01
Hospital stay (d)	3.7 ± 1.3	7.6 ± 3.7	.001
Physiologic			
Follow-up (wk)	9.7 ± 9.9	14.6 ± 11.6	NS
Vo_2peak (ml/kg/min)	23.6 ± 6.5	19.2 ± 2.9	.01
% expected	82.4 ± 15.6	67.2 ± 9.0	.001
METS	6.7 ± 1.9	5.5 ± 0.9	.01
SF-36 Results			
Physical function	80.7 ± 12.0	62.8 ± 17.6	.001
Role: physical	41.3 ± 40.0	28.8 ± 43.1	NS
Body pain	64.9 ± 20.0	50.5 ± 22.6	.04
General health	69.6 ± 17.0	71.8 ± 13.3	NS
Vitality	59.0 ± 20.2	47.5 ± 21.8	.09
Social function	72.6 ± 29.6	64.0 ± 27.1	NS
Role: emotional	81.3 ± 31.8	65.0 ± 42.6	NS
Mental health	70.4 ± 18.0	77.2 ± 16.0	NS

CABG = coronary artery bypass graft; METS = metabolic equivalents; MIDCAB = minimally invasive direct coronary artery bypass; NS = not significant.

ences correlated with the number of METS achieved by each group (see Table 70–5).

After compilation and scoring, significant differences were also found on the SF-36 self-report tool. The questionnaire consists of 36 items evaluating eight dimensions of physical and mental health. Three physical health scales measure aspects of functional ability, limitations in performance of physical role requirements, and bodily pain. Two mental health scales assess aspects of anxiety and depression and a person's well-being, as well as limitations in the fulfillment of emotional role requirements. Three scales assess aspects of physical and emotional health. These scales evaluate the person's social functioning, feelings of energy or fatigue, and self-perceived general health status. The SF-36 dimensions are all scored along a 0- to 100-point continuum. Lower values signify poorer functioning, and higher values indicate better functioning. Overall, MIDCAB patients scored better than CABG patients in the following (see Table 70–5):

- Physical functioning: fewer physical limitations in performing activities such as self-care, walking, climbing stairs, bending, lifting and moderate to vigorous exercise.
- Body pain index: lower level of pain that did not interfere with daily activities.
- Vitality: although not statistically significant, a trend seemed to indicate that MIDCAB patients had more "pep" and energy.

Table 70–6. OPCAB Versus CABG: Postoperative and Quality of Life Assessment Data

	OPCAB ±	CABG ±	*P*
Postoperative			
Intubation (hr)	5.2 ± 4.3	12.7 ± 4.0	.001
Intensive care stay (hr)	33.8 ± 18.6	35.1 ± 16.8	NS
Hospital stay (d)	5.3 ± 2.3	5.9 ± 1.8	NS
Physiologic			
Follow-up (wk)	12.7 ± 11.9	15.0 ± 9.9	NS
Vo_2peak (ml/kg/min)	22.6 ± 4.9	19.9 ± 2.3	.05
% expected	83.8 ± 15.4	68.4 ± 11.0	.02
METS	6.5 ± 1.4	5.4 ± 0.7	.08
SF-36 Results			
Physical function	88.9 ± 7.0	65.0 ± 23.0	.009
Role: physical	75.0 ± 33.1	33.3 ± 45.1	.04
Body pain	82.7 ± 13.2	58.0 ± 26.0	.02
General health	75.2 ± 14.1	73.9 ± 16.8	NS
Vitality	69.0 ± 17.3	49.4 ± 28.6	.01
Social function	87.7 ± 15.2	73.8 ± 27.4	NS
Role: emotional	88.7 ± 17.0	59.2 ± 43.4	.08
Mental health	77.3 ±18.1	79.6 ± 13.5	NS

CABG = coronary artery bypass graft; METS = metabolic equivalents; NS = not significant; OPCAB = off-pump coronary artery bypass.

OPCAB Versus CABG

Modern cardiac surgery has predominantly been performed through a median sternotomy, which is associated with significant morbidity (wound infection, pain, dehiscence, mediastinitis).[4, 30] MICS circumvents this problem by various approaches: the anterior and posterior mini-thoracotomy, the parasternal approach, the ministernotomy, and the subxiphoid approach.[2, 29, 35] With this QOL study, we sought to determine the net effect of CPB avoidance on the recovery and QOL of cardiac patients. Our secondary goal was to assess the role of the median sternotomy on recovery and QOL.

Of our OPCAB patients, 9 were recruited into our QOL study and were matched to 9 CABG patients. The patients' demographics did not significantly differ. There was no mortality in either group. Atrial fibrillation developed in 9 OPCAB patients. In the CABG group, 4 patients (44.4%) had postoperative complications: 1 patient developed atrial fibrillation, 1 patient had low cardiac output syndrome, 1 patient had a reopening for bleeding, and 1 patient had a myocardial infarction. OPCAB patients were extubated earlier than their counterparts, but intensive care and hospital stays were not significantly different between the two groups (Table 70–6). OPCAB and CABG patients underwent cardiopulmonary exercise testing at 12.7 ± 11.9 weeks and 15.0 ± 9.9 weeks, respectively (P = NS). Significantly noticeable differences were seen with regard to the Vo_2peak and percent predicted Vo_2peak (see Table 70–6). OPCAB patients obtained higher Vo_2peak and percent predicted Vo_2peak values compared with their counterparts, signifying better cardiovascular function and reserve with physical activity.

SF-36 compilation indicated that OPCAB patients scored better than their counterparts in the following scales (see Table 70–6):

- Physical functioning: Despite the sternotomy, OPCAB patients had fewer physical limitations in performing activities such as self-care, walking, climbing stairs, bending, lifting, and moderate to vigorous exercise.
- Role functioning—physical: OPCAB patients' self-perceptions of their health did not interfere with their work or other daily activities.
- Body pain: OPCAB patients seemed to have less pain than their counterparts in the postoperative period, despite the sternotomy. We have postulated that the systemic inflammatory reaction syndrome and microemboli associated with CPB may have lowered nociception thresholds.
- Vitality: Overall, OPCAB patients felt more energetic and full of "pep" than CABG patients.

Conclusion

MICS is a novel technique in the field of cardiac surgery; it is still at an early stage of development and remains to a certain degree experimental. MICS could represent a stepping-stone toward noninvasive or totally endoscopic coronary surgery. Currently, the emphasis is on results; early results by various groups have demonstrated patency rates comparable with those of conventional CABG.[7, 33, 34] Our own experience follows along these lines, with an early patency rate of 97.5% in our MIDCAB population. Late patency rates are encouraging (more than 90% at 2 years), and we anticipate improvement with the development of new stabilizers. Operative mortality was zero in both our MIDCAB and OPCAB groups. The atrial fibrillation rate was significantly lower in the MIDCAB group compared with that of the CABG group. CABG patients tended to have a higher postoperative complication rate. We have established at our institution that MICS can be performed effectively and safely in selected patients. Their immediate (≤6 months) recovery was found to be better than that of conventional CABG patients.

Noninvasive cardiorespiratory physiologic assessment can be carried out in most postoperative patients to ascertain their level of functioning. Gas exchange during exercise, if measured accurately and interpreted correctly, can provide important information concerning the patient's magnitude of cardiovascular and pulmonary impairments beyond what is obtained from a routine exercise test. There are inherent physiologic inaccuracies in estimating Vo_2max from exercise time or work rate. These inaccuracies may cause errors in judgment regarding the patient's clinical management and recommendations for exercise and for recreational and even occupational activities. Indeed, Vo_2 may be overestimated in patients who have impaired cardiac function if the prediction equations used were derived from healthy individuals. It is common practice to use only one standardized predicted Vo_2 for each work stage, such as during the commonly used Bruce protocol; many practitioners are unaware that Bruce (as well as developers of other protocols) provided multiple population-specific prediction equations for the protocol.[5] If the wrong population-specific prediction equation is used, the Vo_2 may be overpredicted at each work stage and at maximal exercise, thus resulting in an erroneous estimation of Vo_2max.

MIDCAB patients' physiologic performance was significantly superior, implying greater cardiovascular reserve and more prompt return to baseline functional status. As for OPCAB patients, despite an adequate convalescence, they demonstrated greater cardiovascular capacity compared with conventional CABG patients. They also had a faster return to functional level with greater life satisfaction. Our OPCAB patients illustrated an important point in MICS: despite the sternotomy, they benefited from the avoidance of CPB. This only emphasizes to a greater degree the adverse effects of CPB and its role as a major contributor to postoperative morbidity and mortality in coronary surgery.

MICS QOL subjective measures indicated a faster and more efficient route to normal life and greater health satisfaction. The validity and reliability characteristics of the SF-36 have well been established, and the instrument is currently being used in more than 150 research studies, as well as in many clinical practice settings.[21, 38] There is currently a large array of instruments used in the literature to measure subjective QOL parameters. This diversity has caused a lack of consensus on subjective QOL assessment standards. Some centers have developed their own QOL assessment instruments, and others have tailored existing ones.[10, 14] This lack of uniformity has often cast doubts on the scientific validity of subjective QOL assessment studies. Nonetheless, we believe that when performed accurately, subjective QOL assessment represents an adjunct to the evaluation of current and new standards of medical practice.

Although this study was a retrospective controlled analysis with a small sample size, it demonstrated for the first time the physiologic and psychological differences that exist between MICS and conventional CABG patients in the early recovery period. We anticipate that these differences will not be significant after the first postoperative year, because most CABG patients are enrolled in cardiac rehabilitation programs and have regained their full functional status by this time.[6, 15] It is our opinion that a prospective study evaluating preoperative and postoperative physiologic and subjective QOL endpoints at regular intervals in the first year would be the best way of ascertaining QOL in MICS patients, or in any other type of minimally invasive surgery.

As mentioned before, with the resurgence of MICS, it has become increasingly important to set new standards or to equal those already existent while keeping in mind the patient's QOL as a central focus. We feel confident that minimally invasive surgery will adhere closely to this principle.

References

1. Allen J: Physical and psychological outcomes after coronary artery bypass graft surgery: Review of the literature. Heart Lung 1:49, 1990.
2. Arom KV, Emery RW: Ministernotomy for cardiac surgery. *In* Emery RW, Arom KV, Fonger D, et al (eds): Techniques for Minimally Invasive Direct Coronary Artery Bypass Surgery, 1st ed. Philadelphia, Hanley & Belfus, 1997, p 43.
3. Baba R, Nagashima M, Goto M, et al: Oxygen uptake efficiency slope: A new index of cardiorespiratory functional reserve derived from the relation between oxygen uptake and minute ventilation during incremental exercise. J Am Coll Cardiol 28:1567, 1996.
4. Bor DH, Rose RM, Modlin JF: Mediastinitis after cardiovascular surgery. Rev Infect Dis 5:885, 1983.
5. Bruce RA, Kusumi R, Hosmer D: Maximal oxygen uptake and normographic assessment of functional aerobic impairment in cardiovascular disease. Am Heart J 85: 546, 1973.
6. Caine N, Harrison S, Sharples L, et al: Prospective study of quality of life before and after coronary grafting. BJM 302:511, 1991.
7. Calafiore AM, Gianmarco GD, Teodori G: Left anterior descending coronary artery grafting via left anterior small thoracotomy without cardiopulmonary bypass. Ann Thorac Surg 61:1658, 1996.
8. Chauhan VS, Gill IS, Wooden KA, et al: Lower incidence of atrial fibrillation after minimally invasive direct coronary artery bypass surgery (MIDCAB) than bypass surgery (CABG). Circulation 96(suppl):1, 1997.
9. Eldridge JE, Ramsey-Green CL, Hossack KF: Effects of the limiting symptom on the achievement of maximal oxygen consumption in patients with coronary artery disease. Am J Cardiol 57:513, 1986.
10. Engblom E, Hamalainen H, Lind J, et al: Quality of life during rehabilitation after coronary artery bypass surgery. Qual Life Res 1:167, 1992.
11. FitzGibbon GM, Burton JR, Leach AJ: Coronary bypass graft fate: Angiographic grading of 1400 consecutive grafts early after operation and of 1132 after one year. Circulation 57:1070, 1978.
12. Gill IS, FitzGibbon GM, Higginson LAJ, et al: Minimally invasive

coronary artery bypass: A series with early qualitative angiographic follow-up. Ann Thorac Surg 64:710, 1997.
13. Gortner S, Jenkins L: Self-efficacy and activity level following cardiac surgery. J Adv Nurs 15:1132, 1990.
14. Hedback B, Perk J, Engvall J, et al: Cardiac rehabilitation after coronary artery bypass grafting: Effects on exercise performance and risk factors. Arch Phys Med Rehabil 71:1069, 1990.
15. Huysmans H, Van Ark E: Predictors of perioperative mortality, morbidity and late quality of life in coronary bypass surgery. Eur Heart J 10(suppl):10, 1989.
16. Kazis L, Clark J, Miller D, et al: Preliminary results from the Veterans Health Study. Presented at the Department of Veterans Affairs Health Services Research and Development annual meeting, Washington, DC, April 21, 1993.
17. King K, Porter L, Norsen L, et al: Patients' perceptions of quality of life after coronary artery surgery: Was it worth it? Res Nurs Health 15:327, 1992.
18. Lohr KN: Applications of health status assessment measures in clinical practice: Overview of the third conference on advances in the health status assessment. Med Care 30(suppl):MS1, 1992.
19. McCarthy M, Shroyer L, Sethi G, et al: Self-report measures for assessing treatment outcomes in cardiac surgery patients. Med Care 33(suppl):OS76, 1995.
20. McConnell T: Value of gas exchange analysis in heart disease. J Cardpulm Rehabil 15:257, 1995.
21. McHorney CA, Ware JE, Rogers WH, et al: The validity and relative precision of MOS short- and long-form health status scales and Dartmouth COOP charts: Results from the medical outcomes study. Med Care 30(suppl):MS253, 1992.
22. McHorney CA, Ware JE, Raczek AE: The MOS 36-item short-form health surveys (SF36). II. Psychometric and clinical tests of validity in measuring physical and mental health constructs. Med Care 31:247, 1993.
23. Morris CK, Ueshima K, Kawaguchi T, et al: The prognostic value of exercise capacity: A review of the literature. Am Heart J 57:513, 1991.
24. Nelson EC, Landgraf JM, Hays RD, et al: The functional status of patient: How can it be measured in physicians' offices? Med Care 28:1111, 1990.
25. Oldenburg B, Martin A, Greenwood J, et al: A controlled trial of a behavioral and educational intervention following coronary artery bypass surgery. J Cardpulm Rehabil 15:39, 1995.
26. Oldridge N, Guyatt G, Jones N, et al: Effects on quality of life with comprehensive rehabilitation after acute myocardial infarction. Am J Cardiol 67:1084, 1991.
27. Patrick DL, Deyo RA: Genetic and disease-specific measures in assessing health status and quality of life. Med Care 27(suppl):S217, 1989.
28. Pawelczyk JA, Hanel B, Pawelczyk RA, et al: Leg vasoconstriction during dynamic exercise with reduced cardiac output. J Appl Physiol 73:1838, 1992.
29. Robinson MC: Parasternal approach in MIDCAB. *In* Emery RW, Arom KV, Fonger D, et al (eds): Techniques for Minimally Invasive Direct Coronary Artery Bypass Surgery, 1st ed. Philadelphia, Hanley & Belfus, 1997, p 49.
30. Saar MG, Gott VL, Townsend TR: Mediastinal infection after cardiac surgery. Ann Thorac Surg 97:88, 1985.
31. Schaff HV, Cable DG, Rimal CS: Minimal thoracotomy for coronary artery bypass: Value of the immediate post-operative angiography. Circulation 94:1, 1996.
32. Steinwachs DM: Application of health status assessment measures in policy research. Med Care 27(suppl):S12, 1989.
33. Subramanian VA, McCabe JC, Geller CC: Minimally invasive direct coronary artery bypass grafting without cardiopulmonary bypass: Two year clinical experience. Society of Thoracic Surgeons 33rd annual meeting, 1997.
34. Subramanian VA, Sani G, Benetti FJ, et al: Minimally invasive coronary bypass surgery: A multi-center report of preliminary experience. Circulation 92:(Suppl I) I-645, 1995.
35. Subramanian VA: MIDCAB grafting via left anterior thoracotomy. *In* Emery RW, Arom KV, Fonger D, et al (eds): Techniques for Minimally Invasive Direct Coronary Artery Bypass Surgery, 1st ed. Philadelphia, Hanley & Belfus, 1997, p 29.
36. Writing Group for the BARI Trial: Five-year clinical and functional outcome comparing bypass surgery and angioplasty in patients with multivessel disease. JAMA 277:715, 1997.
37. Tu J, Jaglal S, Naylor D, et al: Multicenter validation of a risk index for mortality, intensive care unit stay, and overall hospital length of stay after cardiac surgery. Circulation 91:677, 1995.
38. Ware JE: Measures for a new era of health assessment. *In* Stewart AL, Ware JE (eds): Measuring Functioning and Wellbeing: The Medical Outcomes Study Approach. Durham, NC, Duke University Press, 1995.
39. Ware JE: SF-36 Health Survey: Manual and Interpretation Guide. Boston, Health Institute, New England Medical Center, 1993.
40. Weber KT, Janicki JS, McElroy PA: Determination of aerobic capacity and the severity of chronic and circulatory failure. Circulation 76(suppl): VI-40, 1987.
41. Westaby S, Benetti FJ: Less invasive coronary surgery: Consensus from the Oxford meeting. Ann Thorac Surg 62:924, 1996.
42. Wiklund I, Gorkin L, Pawitan Y, et al: Methods of assessing quality of life in the Cardiac Arrhythmia Suppression Trial (CAST). Qual Life Res 1:187, 1992.

Section VIII

Heart Valve Surgery

Chapter 71

Minimally Invasive Heart Valve Surgery: Operative Technique and Results

A. Marc Gillinov, Filip P. Casselman, and Delos M. Cosgrove

Full median sternotomy has been the standard surgical approach to the heart for more than 30 years. Median sternotomy provides excellent and rapid exposure of the heart and great vessels, allows central cannulation for cardiopulmonary bypass (CPB), and facilitates nearly all routine cardiac surgical procedures. Until recently, there has been little impetus for cardiac surgeons to consider alternative operative approaches. With the advent of laparoscopic cholecystectomy and minimally invasive techniques in other surgical fields, cardiac surgeons have started to develop new and potentially less invasive surgical approaches to the heart.

Driving forces behind the current interest in minimal access cardiac surgery include surgeons' intellectual curiosity and desire to provide superior care, publicity in the lay press, patients' requests for smaller incisions and faster recovery, and third-party payers' desire to cut costs. Although there are several different motivations for the development of minimal access cardiac surgery, the result should be new approaches that benefit both patients and surgeons. Potential advantages of new surgical approaches include improved cosmesis; decreased pain, bleeding, and infection; shorter intensive care unit and hospital stays; and reduced cost. However, reduction in size of the operative field increases the technical demands of cardiac surgical procedures.[1] Adequate exposure is essential to successful operative technique, and less invasive approaches to the heart cannot be allowed to compromise the quality of operation (Table 71–1).

Several reports have described less invasive incisions for cardiac valve surgery.[1–14] Most of these approaches use either a partial sternotomy or a thoracotomy. Aortic valve and aortic root procedures have been performed through right parasternal incision,[1, 11, 12] right anterior thoracotomy,[13] transverse sternotomy, and partial sternotomy.[14] Techniques for cannulation vary, but all reports document good results using standard surgical instruments. Minimally invasive mitral valve operations have been performed using right parasternal incision[1, 2] and limited thoracotomy.[3–5] In addition, several groups have reported successful mitral valve surgery using port access techniques and video assistance.[5–9] The latter approaches often require expensive new technology and a considerable learning curve on the part of the surgical team.

Clinical application of minimally invasive techniques for heart valve surgery at the Cleveland Clinic Foundation began January 1, 1996. From January 1, 1996, to July 31, 1997, 444 patients had a variety of valvar procedures performed via minimal access approaches (Table 71–2). Over this 18-month period, there was a gradual evolution of operative technique (Table 71–3). The initial approach to both aortic and mitral valves used a 10-cm right parasternal incision (Fig. 71–1*A*). This technique included resection of the third and fourth costal cartilages. Although safe and effective operations were performed using the parasternal incision, significant disadvantages included occasional difficulty with aortic valve exposure, occasional chest wall instability, sacrifice of the right internal thoracic artery (RITA), frequent need for femoral cannulation, and difficult conversion to median sternotomy. Next, the aortic valve was approached through a transverse sternotomy at the second intercostal space (Fig. 71–1*B*). Although this incision afforded excellent exposure of the aorta, sacrifice of both internal thoracic arteries was an important disadvantage and raised questions concerning wound healing. The current incision of choice for both aortic and mitral surgery is a partial sternotomy (Fig. 71–1*C*). This incision provides excellent exposure for all aortic and mitral valve procedures and allows central cannulation in nearly all instances. When necessary, conversion to full median sternotomy is easily accomplished.

Operative Technique

Mitral Valve Procedures

This approach is used for both mitral valve repair and mitral valve replacement. The patient is positioned on the operating table with both arms tucked. Standard monitoring lines, including a Swan-Ganz catheter if indicated, are placed. Anesthesia is induced with standard techniques, and the patient is intubated with a single-lumen endotracheal tube. A transesophageal echo probe is placed, and defibrillator patches are placed on the chest wall. An 8-cm skin incision is made beginning halfway between the ster-

Table 71–1. Criteria for Acceptable Approaches to Minimal Access Cardiac Valve Surgery

Procedure Requirements

Adequate surgical exposure
Central cannulation for cardiopulmonary bypass
No compromise in surgical procedure
No increase in perioperative morbidity

Patient Advantages

Improved cosmesis
Reduced trauma and pain
Reduced hospital stay
Reduced cost

Table 71–2. Valve Operations Performed via Minimal Access (N = 444)

Aortic (isolated)	156
Mitral (isolated)	231
Tricuspid (isolated)	3
Double valve	21
Valve and CABG	15
Valve and aneurysm	15
Valve and other	3

CABG = coronary artery bypass grafting.

nal notch and the angle of Louis (Fig. 71–2). After raising a soft tissue flap superiorly, the sternum is opened from the sternal notch to the fourth intercostal space. The sternal incision is "T-ed" into the right third or fourth intercostal space (see Fig. 71–1*C*). Care is taken not to damage the right internal mammary artery.

A small Finochietto retractor is placed in the wound and opened. The anterior pericardium is opened slightly to the patient's right and tacked to the drapes with stay sutures. This elevates the heart anteriorly, affording a good view of the aorta, superior vena cava, and right atrial appendage (Fig. 71–3). To help reduce the potential for air emboli, a cannula is sewn to the wound edge and the field is flooded with CO_2 at 6 L/min. This displaces oxygen and nitrogen; bubbles of CO_2 that enter the circulation are rapidly absorbed.[15, 16] After heparinization, the aorta is cannulated with a 20-French Sarns soft-flow cannula. A 20-French right-angle cannula is placed in the superior vena cava, and a second 20-French right-angle cannula is placed through the posterior portion of the right atrial appendage into the inferior vena cava (Fig. 71–4). CPB is initiated with active negative pressure on the hard-shell venous reservoir (−50 mm Hg), and the heart is decompressed. Vacuum-assisted venous drainage reduces priming volume by eliminating the need to prime the venous line. In addition, this technique allows the use of smaller venous cannulas, avoids air locks, and provides a dry operative field. The aorta is cross-clamped, and antegrade cardioplegia is administered. Snares previously placed around the inferior and superior vena cavae are tightened.

The mitral valve is approached trans-septally (Figs. 71–5 and 71–6). The right atrial incision is started at the right atrial appendage and extended cephalad toward the dome of the left atrium and caudad toward the inferior vena cava. Stay sutures are placed on the right atrial wall to aid exposure. A cannula is placed in the coronary sinus for delivery of intermittent retrograde cardioplegia. The interatrial septum is opened through the fossa ovalis, and the incision is extended superiorly onto the dome of the left atrium. Pledgeted stay sutures are placed through the superior portion of the septum and retracted toward the patient's left. Two hand-held retractors are placed at the superior and inferior portions of the interatrial septum. Additionally, a Harrington retractor is placed along the posterior aspect of the septal incision with traction directed toward the surgeon; this maneuver rotates the mitral valve into view. A flail portion of the posterior leaflet of

Table 71–3. Evolution of Minimal Access Valve Surgery at the Cleveland Clinic Foundation

	Incision		
	Right Parasternal	Transverse Sternotomy	Partial Sternotomy
Valves approached	Aortic Mitral	Aortic	Aortic Mitral
Advantages	Good mitral valve exposure	Good aortic valve exposure	Good mitral and aortic valve exposure Familiar operative approach Easy conversion to sternotomy Central cannulation IMAs preserved
Disadvantages	Occasional difficult aortic valve exposure Occasional chest wall instability RITA sacrificed Femoral cannulation often necessary Difficult conversion to sternotomy	No mitral valve exposure Occasional chest wall instability Both ITAs sacrificed Femoral cannulation often necessary Difficult conversion to sternotomy	

ITA = internal thoracic artery; RITA = right internal thoracic artery; IMA = internal mammary artery.

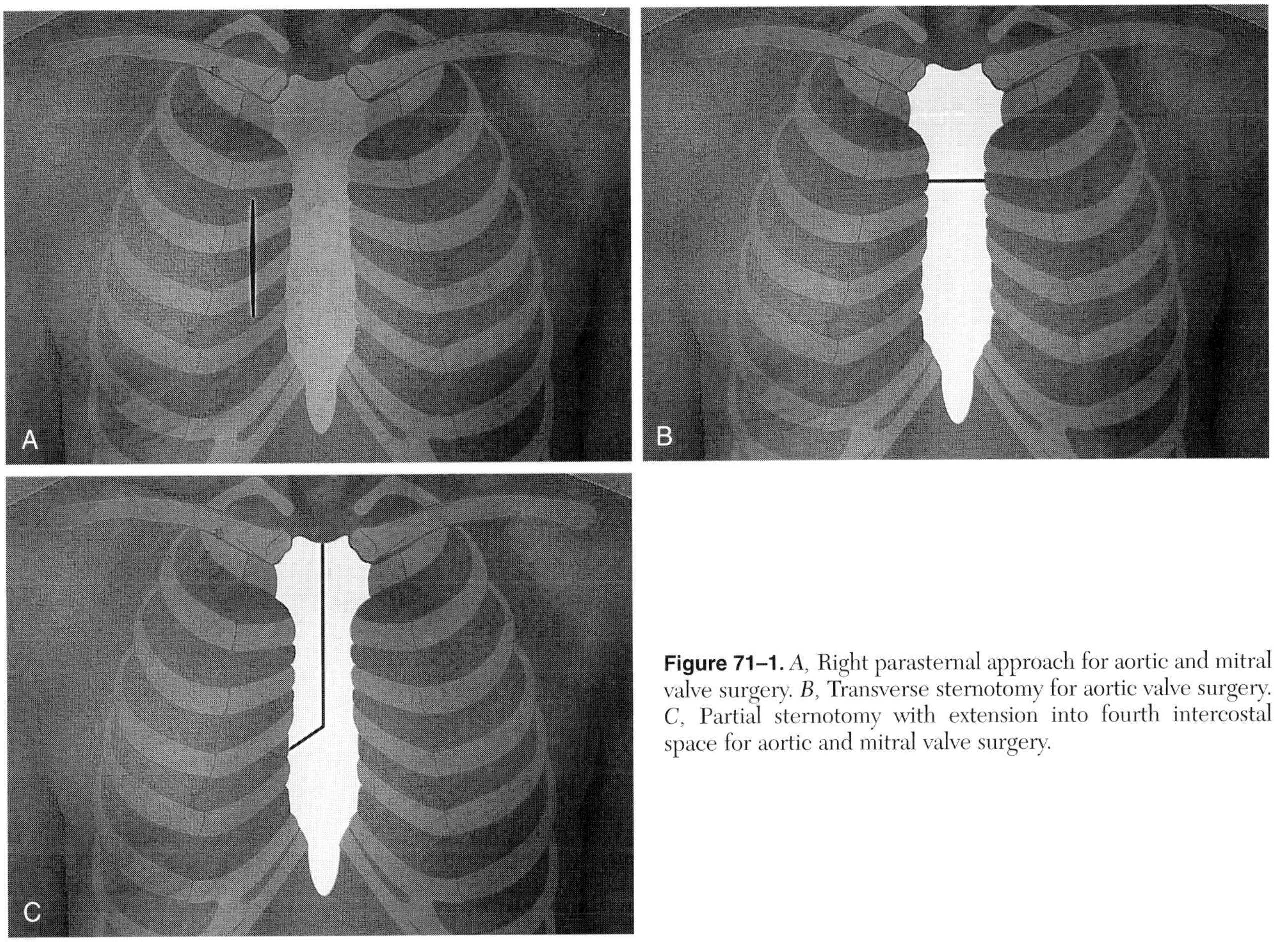

Figure 71–1. *A*, Right parasternal approach for aortic and mitral valve surgery. *B*, Transverse sternotomy for aortic valve surgery. *C*, Partial sternotomy with extension into fourth intercostal space for aortic and mitral valve surgery.

the mitral valve is identified and excised (Fig. 71–7). A standard quadrangular resection and annuloplasty are performed (Fig. 71–8). The incision in the left atrium is closed using continuous 4–0 polypropylene. Before closure of the incision in the interatrial septum, air is evacuated from the left atrium. The incision in the right atrium is closed with running 4–0 polypropylene. De-airing of the left ventricle is facilitated by inflating the lungs and using gentle suction on the cardioplegia cannula in the ascending aorta before and after removal of the aortic cross-clamp. De-airing is guided by transesophageal echocardiography. After normal cardiac function has returned, the cannulas are removed. Four pacemaker wires are applied. Two 28-French chest tubes are placed, one right-angle tube in the right pleural

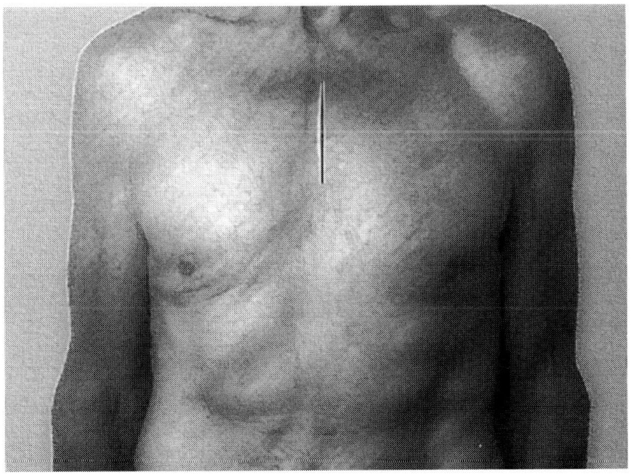

Figure 71–2. Skin incision for partial sternotomy measures 8 cm and extends from midway between the sternal notch and angle of Louis to the third or fourth intercostal space.

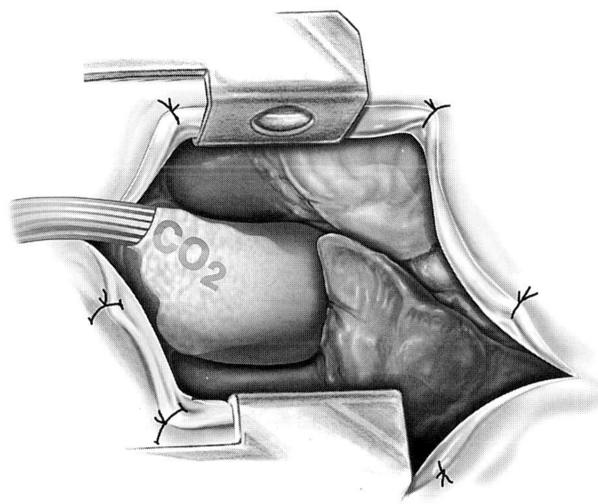

Figure 71–3. Exposure of the ascending aorta and right atrial appendage via partial sternotomy. CO_2 flows onto the operative field at 6 L/min.

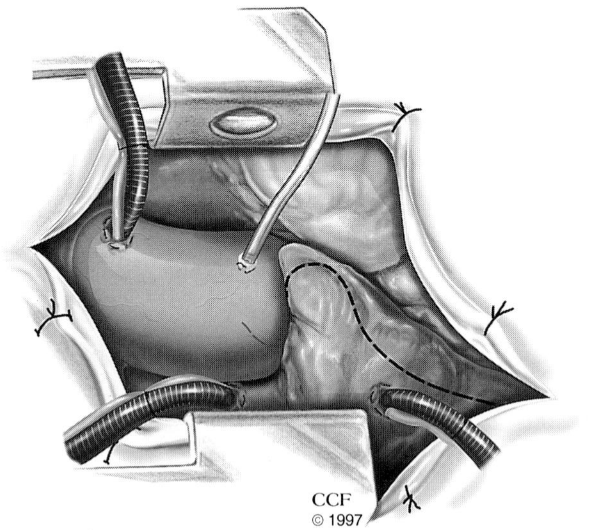

Figure 71–4. Cannulation for mitral valve surgery via partial sternotomy. The planned incision in the right atrium is indicated.

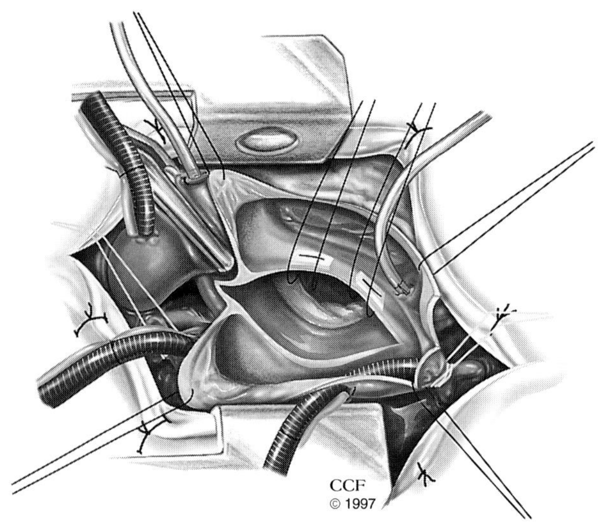

Figure 71–6. Trans-septal approach to the mitral valve. The septum is incised, and the incision is carried over the dome of the left atrium.

space and one straight tube in the mediastinum. The wound is closed in layers. The skin incision is 8 cm long, extending from just above the sternal angle to the fourth intercostal space (Fig. 71–9).

Aortic Valve and Aortic Root Procedures

The skin incision, partial sternotomy, and exposure of the heart and great vessels are identical to those used for surgery of the mitral valve (see Figs. 71–2 and 71–3). The aorta is cannulated at the pericardial reflection, and a single 28-French venous cannula is placed in the right atrial appendage. The retrograde cardioplegia cannula is placed through a stab incision in the right atrium and directed into the coronary sinus. CPB is initiated using vacuum-assisted venous drainage, and the field is flooded with CO_2 as described previously. The aorta is cross-clamped, and an oblique incision is made that is extended into the noncoronary sinus (Fig. 71–10). The incision in the aorta can be varied, depending on the anticipated surgical procedure.

Sutures are placed at the top of each commissure and suspended from the drapes under tension. This serves to elevate the valve, retract the aorta, and preserve normal physiologic orientation of the aortic root. Antegrade cardioplegia can be injected directly into the coronary ostia if it was not given before opening the aortic root (Fig. 71–11). In addition, retrograde cardioplegia is administered intermittently. If the valve cannot be repaired, the leaflets are excised and the annular calcium is debrided. Sutures are placed through the annulus and subsequently

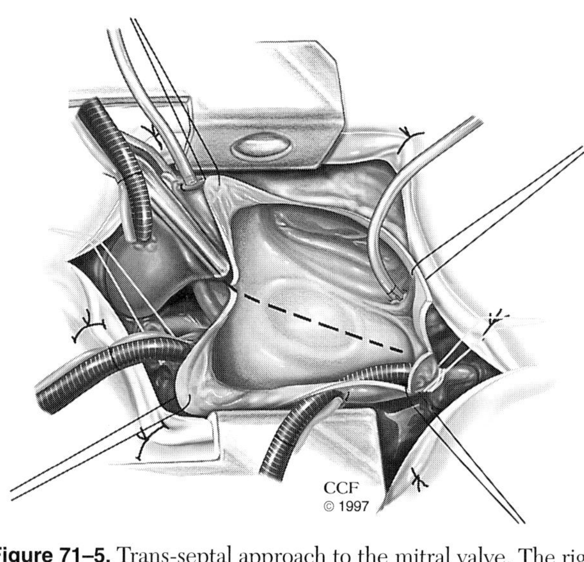

Figure 71–5. Trans-septal approach to the mitral valve. The right atrium is opened and retracted, and the septal incision is indicated.

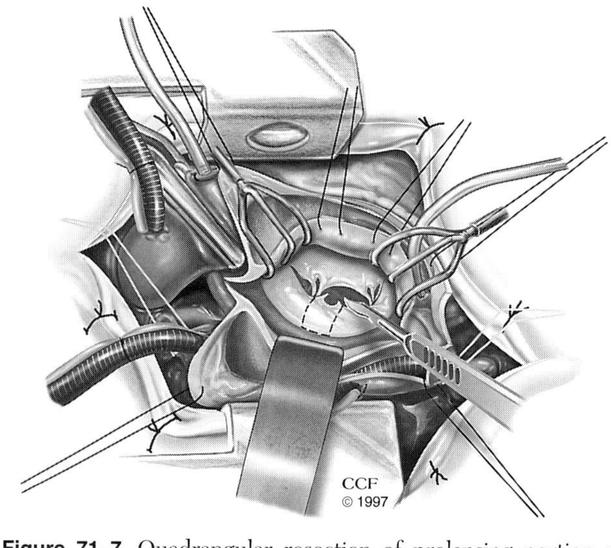

Figure 71–7. Quadrangular resection of prolapsing portion of posterior mitral leaflet via partial sternotomy and trans-septal approach to the mitral valve. Note placement of retractors in the left atrium to expose the mitral valve.

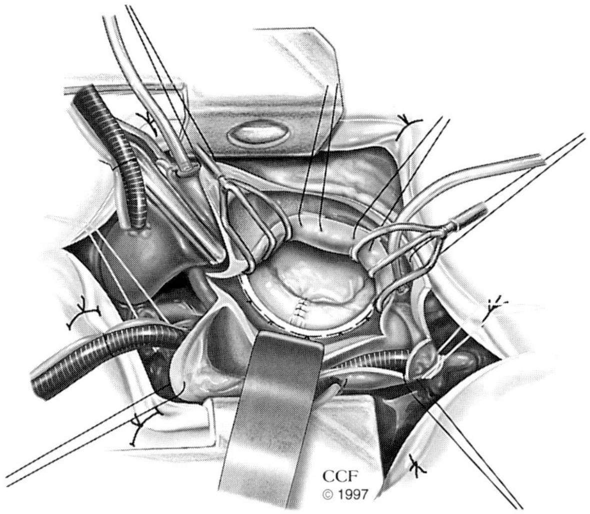

Figure 71–8. Completed mitral valve repair via partial sternotomy with trans-septal approach to the mitral valve. After leaflet repair, measured plication of the posterior annulus is achieved by application of a flexible band.

through the aortic prosthesis and tied (Fig. 71–12). Tension is maintained on the sutures in the valve prosthesis until closure of the aorta has been started. This aids in exposure of the portion of the incision in the noncoronary sinus. The aorta is closed with a single layer of continuous 4–0 polypropylene. Before completion of the aortotomy closure, the lungs are inflated to aid in de-airing. Completeness of de-airing is monitored with echocardiography. At the end of the procedure, the patient is decannulated, and pacing wires are placed as indicated previously (Fig. 71–13).

Results

From January 1996 to July 1997, 444 patients had valve surgery via a minimally invasive approach (see Table 71–2). Of these, 175 patients had aortic valve procedures.

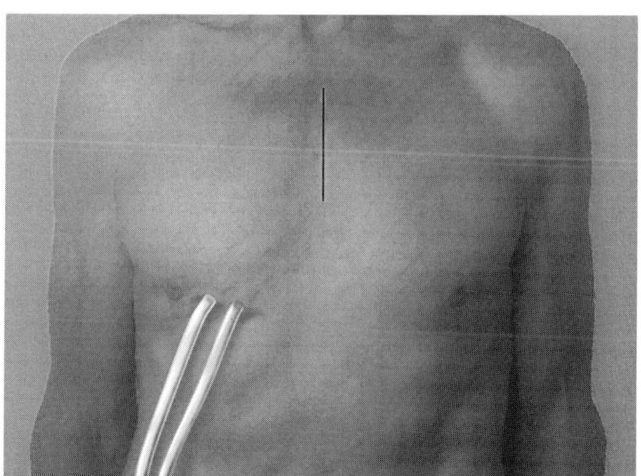

Figure 71–9. After partial sternotomy, the final skin incision is 8 cm long. Two chest tubes are placed, one in the right pleural space and one in the mediastinum.

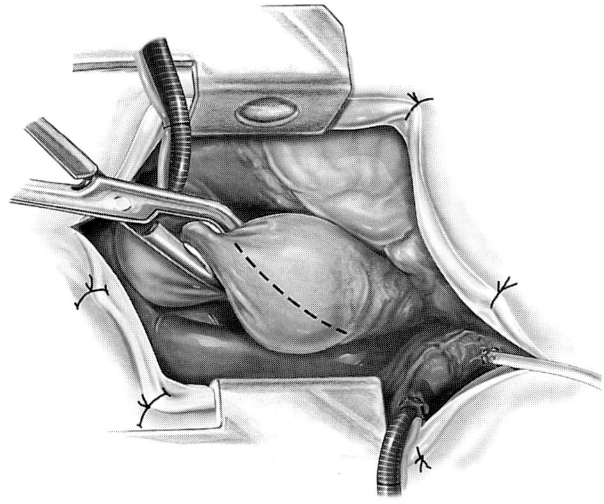

Figure 71–10. Cannulation and exposure of the ascending aorta for aortic valve surgery via partial sternotomy. The planned aortotomy is indicated.

Mean age of the patients having aortic valve surgery was 54.0 ± 1.3 years (range, 18 to 86 years). Seventy percent were in New York Heart Association functional class I or II, and 89% had normal or mildly depressed left ventricular function. Table 71–4 lists the aortic valve procedures performed. All homografts were implanted as aortic roots. Fifty percent of patients were extubated within 6 hours of surgery, and median hospital stay was 5 days. Operative mortality was 1%.

Four patients (2%) undergoing aortic valve procedures required conversion to median sternotomy. Since adoption of the partial sternotomy technique, no patients have required conversion to full sternotomy, and more than 90% of patients have been cannulated centrally in the chest.

Minimally invasive approaches to mitral valve surgery were used in 254 patients. Mean age of these patients was

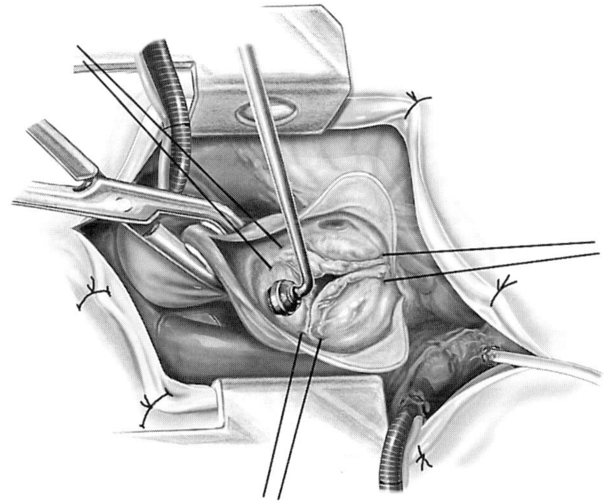

Figure 71–11. The aortic root has been opened and stay sutures placed at the top of each commissure of the aortic valve. Antegrade cardioplegia is administered into the coronary ostia. In the absence of aortic insufficiency, cardioplegia can be administered into the aortic root before aortotomy.

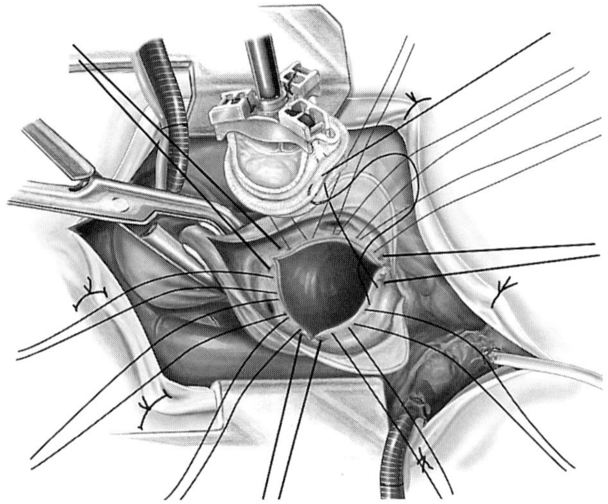

Figure 71–12. Aortic valve replacement via partial sternotomy.

Table 71–4. Aortic Valve Procedures Performed via Minimal Access (N = 175)

Aortic valve replacement*	
Carpentier-Edwards pericardial	58
Homograft	58
St. Jude	13
Aortic valve repair	46

*Four patients had concomitant coronary artery bypass grafting, and 14 patients had repair of an ascending aortic aneurysm.

56.1 ± 0.9 years (range, 21 to 84 years). Seventy-five percent were in New York Heart Association functional class I or II, and 96% had normal or mildly depressed left ventricular function. Eighty-six percent of patients had mitral valve repair, and 14% had mitral valve replacement. In those patients having mitral valve repair, mean degree of mitral regurgitation decreased from 3.7 ± 0.04 preoperatively to 0.43 ± 0.05 postoperatively. Fifty-five percent of patients were extubated within 6 hours of surgery, and median hospital stay was 6 days. There were no operative deaths.

Nine patients (3.5%) undergoing mitral valve surgery had conversion to median sternotomy. Since adoption of the partial sternotomy approach, four patients have required conversion to complete sternotomy because of inadequate exposure; two of these patients had chest wall deformities, including pectus excavatum in one. With the partial sternotomy approach, more than 90% of patients have been cannulated centrally for CPB.

This approach to the mitral valve entails a trans-septal incision carried over the dome of the left atrium. This inevitably results in sacrifice of the artery to the sinoatrial node. Recent experience demonstrates that there are few long-term sequelae associated with this particular incision.[1, 17, 18] Mitral valve exposure is excellent with this approach.

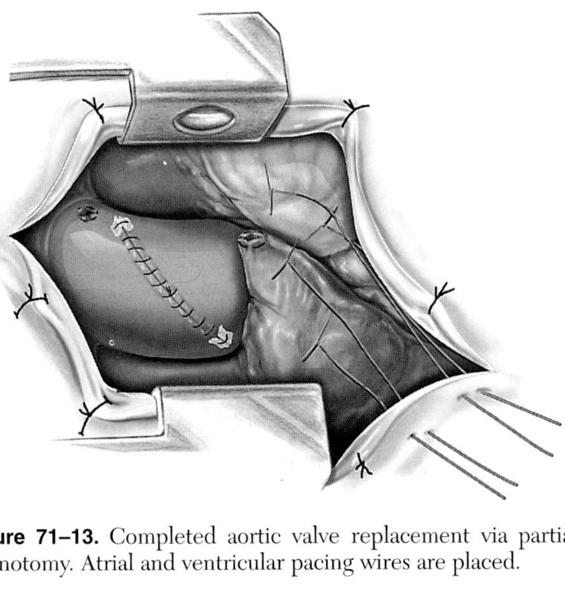

Figure 71–13. Completed aortic valve replacement via partial sternotomy. Atrial and ventricular pacing wires are placed.

Discussion

The current approach to minimally invasive valve surgery at the Cleveland Clinic Foundation is the result of a learning process that began in the autopsy laboratory in 1995 and subsequently evolved in the operating room over a 2-year period. It is likely that improved instrumentation and further innovation will result in continued evolution of minimally invasive approaches to heart valve surgery.

The technique of partial sternotomy for valve surgery has several advantages for both patient and surgeon. This incision affords the surgeon a familiar operative field from which all mitral and aortic valve procedures can be performed. Furthermore, the surgeon is able to use standard surgical instruments and techniques. The ascending aorta and right atrial appendage, which are both upper midline structures, are easily approached through this incision. Therefore, femoral cannulation is avoided in most cases. The internal mammary arteries are preserved. Benefits to the patient include a smaller incision, reduced pain and bleeding, low incidence of wound complications (<1%), and short intensive care unit and hospital stays. When necessary, conversion to full sternotomy is accomplished with ease. Finally, preliminary analysis reveals that minimally invasive valve surgery results in reduced hospital cost.[1]

Current contraindications to partial sternotomy include significant chest wall deformity, history of pericarditis, reoperation, and need to perform associated procedures that require greater exposure of the left side of the heart. It is likely that indications for this approach will broaden with increased experience. Surgeons at Loma Linda have performed redo aortic and mitral valve surgery and a variety of complex congenital cardiac procedures through a partial sternotomy.[14] The latter group has also reduced the size of chest drainage catheters and extubated a large percentage of patients in the operating room, with most patients being discharged home within 4 days. They anticipate hospital stays of 1 to 3 days with this approach, and such a goal is certainly attainable for selected patients.

Whereas several groups have modified traditional approaches to the heart, others have championed port access techniques.[4–6] The feasibility of port access mitral valve surgery has been demonstrated in an animal model and is now being applied in the operating room.[4–6] Current disadvantages of this approach include femoral cannulation with the attendant risk of vascular injury and retrograde dissection, a learning curve for the surgical team, difficulty with knot tying, and increased operating room costs for disposable equipment. However, with further refinement in instrumentation and technique, this may become an attractive option for mitral valve procedures.

Innovative surgeons around the world are developing new, less traumatic approaches to the heart. As surgeons and patients study these new techniques, they should remember that each new surgical procedure must satisfy specific criteria that ensure the integrity of the operation and the safety of the patient. Partial sternotomy meets these requirements, and results demonstrate that it can be used safely and successfully in the treatment of mitral and aortic valvular pathology.

References

1. Cosgrove DM, Sabik JF, Navia J: Minimally invasive valve surgery. Ann Thorac Surg (in press).
2. Navia JL, Cosgrove DM: Minimally invasive mitral valve operations. Ann Thorac Surg 62:1542–1544, 1996.
3. Benetti FJ, Rizzardi JL, Pire L, et al: Mitral valve replacement under video assistance through a minithoracotomy. Ann Thorac Surg 63:1150–1152, 1997.
4. Chitwood WR, Elbeery JR, Moran JF, and the Minimally Invasive Surgery Workgroup: Minimally invasive mitral valve repair using transthoracic aortic occlusion. Ann Thorac Surg 63:1477–1479, 1997.
5. Chitwood WR, Elbeery JR, Chapman WHH, et al: Video-assisted minimally invasive mitral valve surgery: The micro-mitral operation. J Thorac Cardiovasc Surg 113:413–414, 1997.
6. Schwartz DS, Ribakove GH, Grossi EA, et al: Minimally invasive mitral valve replacement: Port-access technique, feasibility, and myocardial functional preservation. J Thorac Cardiovasc Surg 113:1022–1031, 1997.
7. Pompili MF, Stevens JH, Burdon TA, et al: Port-access mitral valve replacement in dogs. J Thorac Cardiovasc Surg 112: 1268–1274, 1996.
8. Lin PJ, Chang CH, Chu JJ, et al: Video-assisted mitral valve operations. Ann Thorac Surg 61:1781–1787, 1996.
9. Carpentier A, Loulment D, Carpentier A, et al: First open heart operation (mitral valvuloplasty) under videosurgery through a minithoracotomy. C R Acad Sci 319:219–223, 1996.
10. Arom KV, Emery RW: Minimally invasive mitral operations. Ann Thorac Surg 63:1219–1220, 1997.
11. Cosgrove DM, Sabik JF: Minimally invasive approach for aortic valve operations. Ann Thorac Surg 62:596–597, 1996.
12. Minale C, Reifschneider HJ, Schmitz E, Uckmann FP: Single access for minimally invasive aortic valve replacement. Ann Thorac Surg 64:120–123, 1997.
13. Benetti FJ, Mariani MA, Rizzardi JL, Benetti I: Minimally invasive aortic valve replacement. J Thorac Cardiovasc Surg 113: 806–807, 1997.
14. Gundry SR, Shattuck OH, Razzouk AJ, et al: Cardiac operations in adults and children via ministernotomy: Facile minimally invasive cardiac surgery. Ann Thorac Surg (in press).
15. Burbank A, Ferguson TB, Burford TH: Carbon dioxide flooding of the chest in open-heart surgery. J Thorac Cardiovasc Surg 50:691–698, 1965.
16. Eguchi S, Sakurai Y, Yamaguchi A: The use of carbon dioxide gas to prevent air embolism during open heart surgery. Acta Med Biol 11:1–13, 1963.
17. El Saegh MM, Aly MA, El Sayegh T, et al: Transseptal approach for mitral valve surgery. Tex Heart Inst J 20:23–27, 1993.
18. Guiraudon GM, Ofiesh JG, Kaushik R: Extended vertical transatrial septal approach to the mitral valve. Ann Thorac Surg 52: 1058–1062, 1991.

COMMENTARY

Alan J. Bryan

It is a pleasure and something of a humbling experience to offer a commentary on the development and clinical experience of the Cleveland Clinic group with respect to minimal access approaches to valve surgery. They are to be congratulated in a number of areas. First, the clinical results presented are uniformly excellent, with a large number of procedures performed with low mortality, early extubation, and short hospital stays. Second, the type of surgical procedure undertaken has not been compromised, with a commendably high proportion of patients undergoing complex aortic valve repair or homograft aortic root replacement and a very high rate of conservative mitral valve procedures. Third, no compromise has been accepted with respect to perfusion, myocardial protection, or risk of air embolism, with avoidance of peripheral cannulation, use of antegrade and retrograde cardioplegia, meticulous de-airing with transesophageal echocardiography monitoring, and CO_2 flooding of the operative field.

This series is also important in a general sense as a model to any clinical surgical investigator. A new approach has been devised and was first evaluated in the autopsy laboratory. This was transferred to the operating room with meticulous attention to detail. Throughout this experience there has been a recognition that these approaches were evolving, and as the clinical series increased, techniques were modified. This is particularly true with respect to the skin incision, which was changed to a partial sternotomy in the most recent group of cases. The merits and demerits of the various approaches are discussed in the text.

What criticisms are there, or what questions remain, with respect to these techniques? Cynics might say that because the preferred approach has now evolved back to a partial sternotomy, the only remaining step is to convert it to a complete median sternotomy to have really good, versatile access for heart surgery. The potential benefits in terms of reduced intensive care unit and hospital stays have proved elusive so far. This is particularly likely to be true in relatively low-risk patients undergoing elective, isolated primary valve surgery in the current era, when hospital stays will be short anyway, even with conventional approaches. The use of CO_2 flooding for de-airing might cause concern about the potential increased risks of systemic air embolism, and data with respect to neurologic and perhaps neuropsychological outcome would be valuable.

Important questions still surround the relative merits of the techniques used by these authors and other groups as compared with use of the Heartport system for valve surgery. At present, these techniques have little role in surgery of the aortic valve or aortic root, because some form of direct access is required. Modifications of conventional techniques can be used, and peripheral cannulation plus endoaortic clamping is unappealing and pointless. For the mitral valve, the situation is somewhat different. Direct access to the ascending aorta is not required, and with video assistance and the Heartport system, mitral valve procedures can be undertaken through a small right thoracotomy.[1] Considering the risks of peripheral cannulation, including retrograde dissection, the increased complexity and expense of the disposable equipment, and the learning curve for surgeons, it remains to be seen whether its widespread use is justified. At present, the beauty of the minimal access techniques described in this chapter is that they can be applied in other units throughout the world with equally good results and without major investments in equipment or expertise.

Reference

1. Carpentier A, Loulmet D, Carpentier A, et al: First open heart operation (mitral valvuloplasty) under video surgery through a mini thoracotomy. C R Acad Sci Paris 319:219–223, 1996.

Chapter 72

Video-Assisted Minimally Invasive Mitral Valve Surgery: Toward an Endoscopic Mitral Operation

W. Randolph Chitwood, Jr.

Minimally invasive cardiac surgery has become more than "just another fad" and is becoming the standard for many single-valve operations. As with any new procedure, criticism and debate exists, as the developmental speed has precluded critical evaluation of most clinical results.[1–3] Despite these concerns, less invasive cardiac valve operations offer promise because they appear to offer the advantage of rapid recovery with reduced costs, while remaining safe. No long-term results are available at present; however, early patient series already suggest excellent operative outcomes with low mortality. Perhaps this success is due to the initiation of a conservative, stepwise approach employing the combination of altered incisions, modified cardiopulmonary perfusion, and direct vision. Cosgrove and associates, among others, pioneered early direct vision approaches.[4–6] Video assistance has provided some surgeons with a new venue for expansion of these minimally invasive valve techniques. Chitwood and associates have been using both two- and three-dimensional videoscopy to replace and repair mitral valves.[7–9] Enhanced video technology, combined with improved surgeon video dexterity, may allow the development of completely endoscopic valve operations.[10] Clearly, our colleagues in general, orthopedic, and gynecologic surgery have mastered extirpative videoscopic operations. Our challenge is to develop fully not only replacement but also reconstructive valve operations performed through true "micro" incisions.

Defining Minimally Invasive Cardiac Surgery

Today, *minimally invasive cardiac surgery* suggests multiple connotations, even among those involved in the development of the field. Some surgeons consider heart surgery without cardiopulmonary bypass to be the only way of defining the term, and others believe that either replacing or downsizing the full sternotomy incision is sufficient. Yet others consider the combination necessary to merit this rubric. In an attempt to provide more precise nomenclature, surgeons worldwide have begun to categorize minimally invasive cardiac operations by (1) incision size and location, (2) the use of cardiopulmonary bypass with cardiac arrest or beating heart surgery, or (3) the type of visualization used as either direct or video-assisted. To fulfill these goals, a new technologic armamentarium has evolved in a short time; for example, cardiopulmonary perfusion for minimal access cardiac surgery has been facilitated by new, smaller high-flow cannulas. Although most minimally invasive valve operations have been performed using direct vision through small incisions, evolving video technology may offer great promise as we progress toward totally endoscopic valve operations.

Minimally Invasive Mitral Valve Surgery—The Early Evolution

The history of minimally invasive valve surgery dates back to 1996, when the Stanford University group performed the first four minimally invasive mitral valve replacements using an intraluminal aortic Endoclamp (Heartport Inc, Redwood City, CA).[11, 12] Falk and Mohr from the University of Leipzig then reported 24 successful mitral valve operations using similar techniques.[8] In 1996, Arom and associates, working independently, also began to perform minimally invasive mitral valve surgery using modified sternal approaches with direct vision.[5, 13–17] These groups rapidly discovered that these operations could be performed with safety, efficiency, and improved patient satisfaction. At a satellite meeting of the 1997 Society for Thoracic Surgeons meeting, Colvin and Galloway at New York University described 27 mitral repairs and replacements performed using direct vision and the port access system with a single mortality.[18] With these early experiences using either the modified minimal access with direct aortic clamping or the port access approach, the field of minimally invasive mitral valve surgery expanded widely in a short time.

Direct Vision Minimally Invasive Mitral Surgery

To date, most aortic and mitral operations have been performed through modified thoracic incisions using direct vision, with or without loupe magnification. Using ministernal and parasternal incisions, Cosgrove and associates have been major proponents of direct-vision minimally invasive mitral surgery.[5, 15, 16, 18] The mini-sternotomy with direct aortic clamping seems reproducible by multiple surgeons. By December 1998, Cosgrove had performed 250 minimally invasive mitral operations using either a mini-sternotomy or a parasternal incision with no mortality.[19] He now prefers a mini-sternotomy with extended right-left atrial incision for wide exposure. In this series, 74% of valves were repaired, and arrest times approximated those of conventional sternotomy operations. The length of hospital stay was short, with 60% of patients being discharged by postoperative day 5. Both complex replacements and repairs were performed, and the reoperative rate for failed repairs was low. Complications, including perioperative bleeding and strokes, were few.

At the 1998 meeting of the American Association of Thoracic Surgery, Cohn reported 100 patients who underwent mitral repairs and replacements using direct vision and a 5 to 8-cm right parasternal incision.[20] A trans-septal cardiac incision was used to approach the mitral valve in these patients. There were no operative deaths and no reoperations for mitral repair failure. Complication rates were low, with strokes occurring in less than 1% of patients. In this series, perfusion and cross-clamp times were slightly longer than with traditional sternotomy technique. However, patient recovery was excellent and the mean length of hospital stay was 5 days, with 40% of patients discharged after only 4 days.

As of October 1997, the group at New York University had performed 113 mitral valve operations using the port access technique with direct vision.[21, 22] Of these operations, 50% were isolated repairs and 32% were replacements. The remainder included complex operations requiring a mitral operation plus another major procedure. Average cardiopulmonary bypass and arrest times were 145 minutes and 93 minutes, respectively. Reoperations for bleeding were necessary in 4.4% of patients, and strokes occurred in 1%. The series mortality rate was 3.5% but rose to 14% with the addition of 21 complex procedures. However, the mortality rate for an isolated mitral valve operation was 1.1% for 92 patients. Technique-related complications were low, with a single aortic dissection. By May of 1998, this group had performed more than 200 mitral operations, with similar mortality and morbidity.

These and other early series suggest that by using direct vision and minimally invasive techniques, complex replacements and repairs can be performed with safety, accuracy, improved patient recovery time, and operative times comparable with traditional operations. Some surgeons believe that retention of direct vision is the major component that has preserved operative quality.

Video-Assisted Minimally Invasive Mitral Valve Surgery

The challenges of videoscopic assistance in mitral surgery may be offset by advantages of an even less traumatic incision. However, video dexterity must be acquired to perfect operations that approximate those performed under direct vision. In early 1996, Kaneko and associates first reported videoscopic assistance during mitral valve surgery performed through an open sternotomy.[23] In February of 1996, Carpentier and colleagues performed the first video-assisted mitral valve repair using a minithoracotomy with cold ventricular fibrillation.[24] Three months later, our group performed the first completely video-assisted mitral valve replacement using a minithoracotomy, a percutaneous transthoracic aortic clamp, and retrograde cardioplegia.[25, 26] Video-assisted atrial septal defect closures and mitral reoperations also have been reported.[27, 28]

At the 1997 meeting of the American Association for Thoracic Surgery, Mohr presented his first 51 minimally invasive mitral operations using the port access method.[9] Early cases were performed using direct vision; however, later surgeries were performed with videoscopic assistance using a three-dimensional videoscopic system. His detailed description of morbidity and mortality (9.8%) stimulated major concerns regarding the potential of retrograde aortic dissections and intra-aortic balloon displacement, which could result in poor myocardial protection and neurologic dysfunction. At the inaugural meeting of the International Society for Minimally Invasive Cardiac Surgery in June 1998, Mohr reported the updated series of 120 video-assisted mitral valve operations. Each operation was performed using videoscopy and a 4-cm incision. Of these, 76 (65%) were repairs. Cardiopulmonary bypass times averaged 112 minutes, with mean cross-clamp times of 50 minutes. With increased team experience, aortic occlusion, cardiopulmonary perfusion, and operative times decreased by approximately 25%. Moreover, in the last half of the series, the operative mortality fell from 9.8 to 4.0%, and there were no retrograde aortic dissections or neurologic complications, suggesting an early learning curve with the port access method. In the latter half of the series, a voice-activated robotic camera control was used to enable instrument tracking and minimize camera cleaning.[29] The Leipzig group found videoscopic assistance helpful for extirpative (replacement) operations; however, complex mitral reconstructions have been significantly more difficult than when performed under direct vision.

At the May 1997 meeting of the American Association for Thoracic Surgery (AATS), our group from East Carolina University presented 31 patients undergoing mitral surgery using two-dimensional telescopic videoscopic assistance.[7] The 30-day operative mortality was similar to 100 previous conventional mitral operations performed through a sternotomy (2.8%), and complications were few. Although perfusion and cross-clamp times were significantly longer than in conventional operations, the patients did well, as described later. In these operations, videoscopic vision clearly was advantageous for both replacements and repairs. In this early series, we were able to perform complex posterior leaflet repairs as well as replacements; however, anterior leaflet repairs were significantly more difficult and limited. Loulmet and associates employed an intra-cardiac "minicamera" when replacing mitral valves through either a mini-thoracotomy or lower ministernotomy.[30] They considered the camera helpful, especially for providing lighting and viewing subvalvular structures; however, two-dimensional visualization was limiting. Currently, three-dimensional digital imaging (Vista), using a headset display, is being evaluated for mitral operations. Early successful cases by Chitwood, Mohr, and Reichenspurner suggest that valve complex reconstructions can be performed solely using three-dimensional imaging. Reichenspurner and colleagues reported 35 mitral valve patients operated on successfully with use of the Vista three-dimensional vision and the port access system with no mortality and the majority of patients undergoing repairs.[31] Thus far, our group has completed eight mitral operations with good results, never having seen the valve directly—that is, the operation was video directed, or truly endoscopic.

The East Carolina University Micro-Mitral Operation

To achieve the potential benefits of video-assisted minimally invasive mitral valve surgery, modifications of conventional operative technology have been applied in the development of a video-assisted mitral valve operation.[7, 25, 26] The operative approach embraces the combined benefits of the following:

1. Mini-thoracotomy
2. Direct transthoracic aortic clamp occlusion
3. Telescopic videoscopic assistance
4. Vortex pump-assisted venous return
5. Peripheral arterial perfusion
6. Instrument development and modification

Perianesthetic Preparation

Although cardiopulmonary bypass can be instituted early with simultaneous lung deflation, we prefer independent left lung ventilation for obtaining early intrathoracic exposure. This is most helpful when using central (atrial) venous cannulation and is required for patients needing transthoracic aortic cannulation. Single-lung ventilation can be effected using either a double-lumen endotracheal tube or a right-sided bronchial blocker. A Swan-Ganz pulmonary catheter is inserted into the right internal jugular vein. The patient is positioned with the right side of the chest elevated 40 degrees and the shoulders tilted back. The right arm can be suspended across the chest on a padded holder or positioned by the side. In the latter instance, the arm must reside behind the posterior axillary line. Smaller, more lateral incisions are facilitated using the latter position. A 6-cm incision line is drawn just anterior to the anterior axillary line in most men and in women with small breasts. For muscular patients and women with larger breasts, the incision is made a bit more lateral. Figure 72–1 shows the correct patient position and location of the incision, as well as the site for the transthoracic cross-clamp and thoracoscopic camera port placement. The right femoral pulse is palpated and a 2-cm transverse incision line is drawn below the inguinal ligament before skin preparation and draping. In early cases, we used a vertical incision; however, the transverse groin crease incision seems to promote better wound healing.

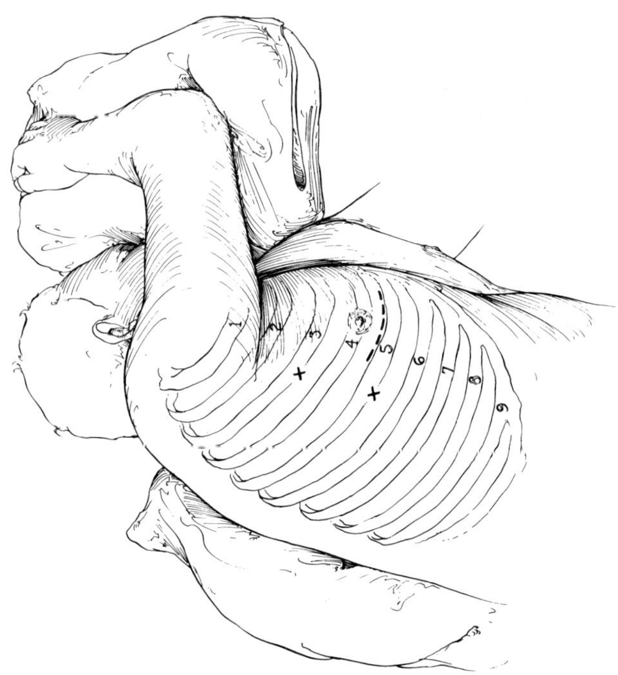

Figure 72–1. Video-assisted micro-mitral operation: Position. The patient is positioned with the right side of the chest elevated to 40 degrees. Generally, the right arm is elevated as shown with the submammary 6-cm incision placed near the midanterior axillary line. The transthoracic cross-clamp is placed in the third intercostal space and the thoracoscopic camera port is placed in the fourth or fifth interspace.

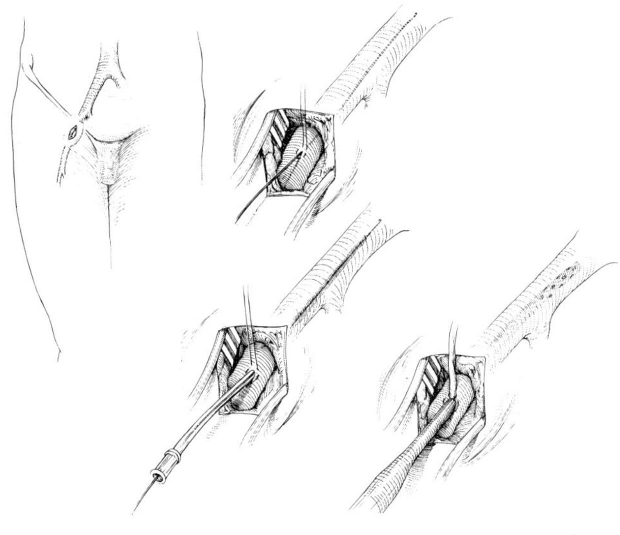

Figure 72–2. Video-assisted micro-mitral operation: Arterial cannulation. A 5–0 monofilament pursestring suture is placed in the exposed femoral artery. Using the Seldinger technique, either a 17 or 19 Fr Bio-Medicus cannula is inserted over a guide wire after serial coaxial dilations. It is important to ensure easy passage of the guide wire into the aorta.

External (Zoll or R2) defibrillator pads are positioned posterior to the right scapula and at the left anterior axillary near the fifth interspace, subtending the greatest cardiac mass. Correct fibrillator patch placement is essential, as direct access to the heart through the mini-thoracotomy is difficult, even when pediatric defibrillator paddles are used. At this time, a transesophageal echocardiographic probe is inserted and the preoperative study performed. Echocardiographic studies are essential to ensure no significant aortic valve insufficiency and complete cardiac air removal as well as to monitor postoperative ventricular function.

Operative Technique

Arterial Cannulation

After the groin incision is made over the right common femoral artery, dissection is carried to the arterial surface. The artery should not be dissected laterally or circumferentially. A longitudinal, oval 5–0 polypropylene pursestring suture is placed in the common femoral portion for perfusion cannulation. After heparinization, the Seldinger guide wire technique is used to pass a 17 to 19 French wire-wound Bio-Medicus arterial cannula through this suture over progressive dilators into the proximal iliac artery (Fig. 72–2). Because no femoral arterial clamps are used, distal perfusion is generally maintained throughout cardiopulmonary perfusion, especially in larger patients. Correct aortic guide wire placement may be confirmed by transesophageal echocardiography. For small or atherosclerotic femoral arteries, central cannulation of the lateral ascending aortic arch can be carried out with the Seldinger method. In this instance, an aortic pursestring suture with pledgets is placed along the right lateral aortic wall, just proximal to the innominate artery and the same cannula that is introduced either through the incision or a thoracoport. Combined thoracoscopic and direct visualization of the aorta is important to guide this less-controlled maneuver. We generally use a 19 French Bio-Medicus cannula for transthoracic aortic cannulation.

Thoracic Incision and Intrathoracic Exposure

A 6-cm submammary skin incision is made with extrapectoral dissection carried to the level of the fourth intercostal space. The intercostal space is entered just above the fourth rib. For obese or muscular patients, the pectoralis muscle fibers should be divided to expose the fourth rib at the costochondral junction and a bony lateral rib segment may be removed. In some instances, we have divided the rib alone. Postincisional pain appears greater when cartilages are spread or removed. Mohr and Falk use a 4-cm incision with excellent results.[29] In the past, we used a Tuffier retractor to deflect soft tissues with almost no rib retraction. However, with large patients, the cephalic retractor blade tends to become dislodged. New "thoracic lift" retractors provide better proximal visualization of the aorta, superior pulmonary vein, and right atrium. Moreover, in large individuals, the upward lift minimizes the tendency for the ribs to spread. Figure 72–3 shows a specially constructed transthoracic cross-clamp used in this approach. Figure 72–4 shows subsequent placement of the transthoracic aortic cross-clamp in the third intercostal space and the 5-mm port and telescopic camera in the fifth interspace.

After the parietal pleura is entered, the right lung should be deflated. As seen in Figure 72–5, the pericardium is opened under direct vision 2 cm anterior to the phrenic nerve. The incision should be carried cephalad, over the superior vena cava to near the aortic reflection. Meticulous care is taken to avoid phrenic nerve injury. Multiple 2–0 retraction sutures are placed to pull the anterior pericardial edge tightly toward the incision. A transthoracic "crochet hook" (Scanlan International, Inc,

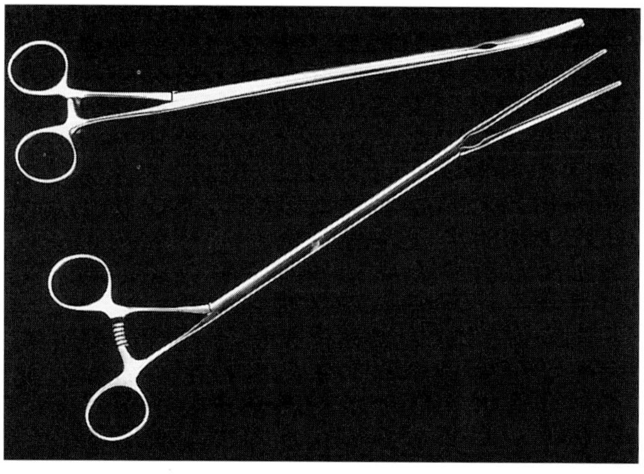

Figure 72–3. Video-assisted micro-mitral operation: Transthoracic cross-clamp (Chitwood). The cross-clamp is designed along a sliding rod mechanism so that it can be placed percutaneously and open completely within the thoracic cavity. The clamp is shown in two tip lengths (Scanlan International, Minneapolis, MN).

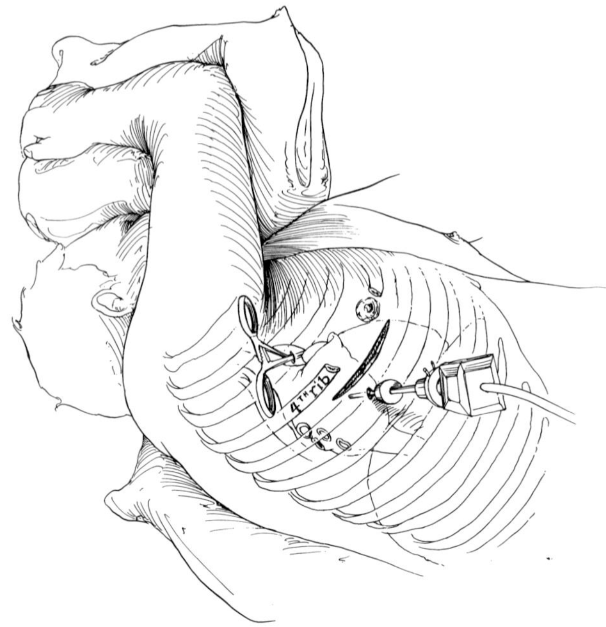

Figure 72–4. Video-assisted micro-mitral operation: Cross-clamp and thoracoscope position. The minithoracotomy has been made in the fourth interspace. A section of rib has been removed. This is not necessary for normal-sized patients. The transthoracic aortic cross clamp is shown in the third intercostal space and the 5-mm port and telescopic camera are through the fifth interspace.

Minneapolis, MN) is used to pull posterior (dorsal) pericardial edge retention sutures through the chest wall. Usually, three sutures are adequate for optimal exposure. Care should be taken to avoid phrenic nerve tension and subsequent injury. Lateral pericardial edge retraction minimizes telescope obstruction and decreases lens contamination. Optimal direct-vision topographic exposure should allow videoscopic access to the base of the aorta,

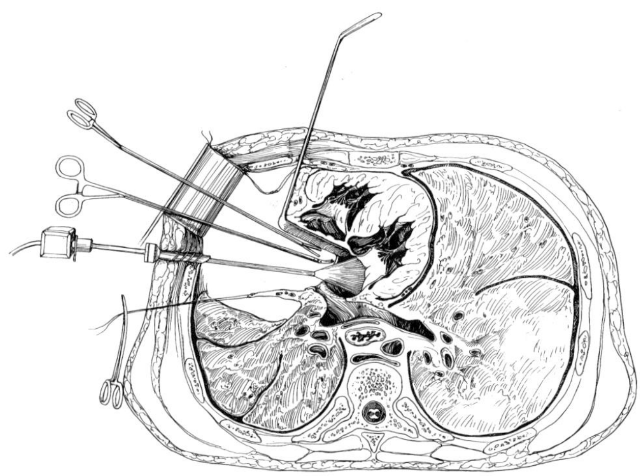

Figure 72–5. Video-assisted micro-mitral operation: Thoracic cross-section. The right lung is shown deflated. After entering the parietal pleura, the pericardium is opened under direct vision 2-cm anterior to the phrenic nerve. Multiple 2–0 retraction sutures are placed to pull the anterior pericardial edge toward the incision tightly. Transthoracic retraction sutures pull the posterior pericardial edge away from the operating site.

atriocaval junction, and the right superior pulmonary vein (Fig. 72–6).

Cardiopulmonary Perfusion Using Assisted Venous Drainage

Assisted venous drainage, using a vortex centrifugal pump (Bio-Medicus), has been helpful in each of our cases. In the early series, we cannulated the right atrium directly through the incision. In this instance, a 2–0 pursestring suture was placed using several felt pledgets to prevent pericannular venous air suction. Usually, the atrial appendage is too cephalad for direct cannulation through the incision. A thin-walled 23 French Bio-Medicus flexible cannula is positioned in the mid–right atrium through the incision. In more recent cases, either a 19 or 21 French venous cannula has been inserted percutaneously into the right femoral vein and passed over a guide wire to the right atrial level. Table 72–1 shows the various cannulation techniques used in our patients. Loulmet and associates designed a two-stage femoral venous cannula that is inserted percutaneously by the Seldinger technique and can be used with or without assisted suction (Fig. 72–7).[30] This cannula is useful for tricuspid valve surgery and atrial septal closures, as the cavae can be isolated. Flege and Wolf reported a jugular venous return method that we have found helpful for aortic surgery; however, it should be applicable to mitral operations as well.[32]

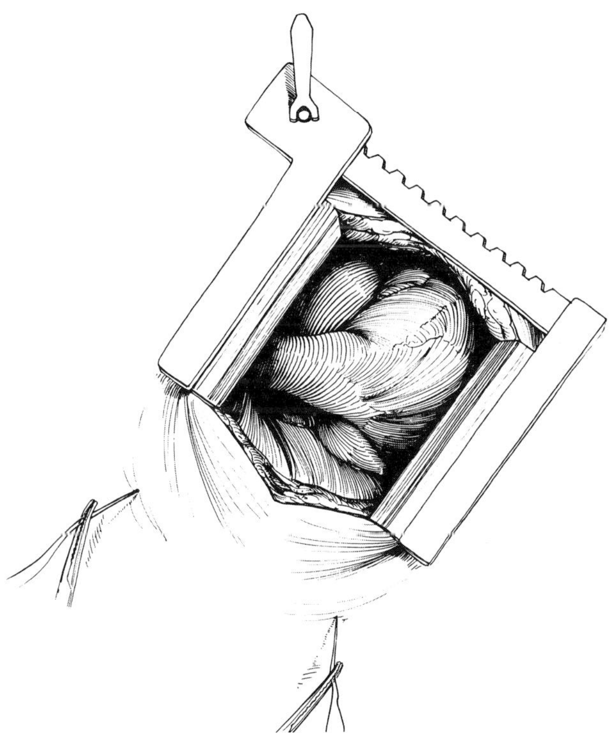

Figure 72–6. Video-assisted micro-mitral operation: topographic view through the minithoracotomy. This view shows the optimal direct-vision topographic exposure, which should allow videoscopic access to the base of the aorta, atriocaval junction, and right superior pulmonary vein. Effective tissue retraction is important, and rib spreading should be minimized. Transthoracic pericardial retraction sutures are seen retained by mosquito clamps.

Table 72–1. Video-Assisted Minimally Invasive Mitral Surgery Cannulation Methods

Peripheral cannulation	
Femoral artery—direct right atrium	n = 31
Femoral artery—femoral vein to right atrium	n = 20
Transthoracic central cannulation	
Direct aorta—direct right atrium	n = 3
Direct aorta—femoral vein to right atrium	n = 1

Visualization and Camera Port Placement

In some patients, direct magnified vision (3.5 × loupes—Design for Vision, Inc.) can be used for part of the intracardiac operation, especially along the posterior leaflet and annulus. To avoid contamination of longer instrument handles, loupes were modified for the longer focal distance to the mitral annulus. In larger patents and when using a smaller thoracic incision (4 cm), most of the operation requires videoscopic visualization. The 5-mm port can be inserted through either the fourth or fifth intercostal space, posterior to the thoracic incision. Before insertion, the surgeon should be sure that the port tip resides anterior to the pericardial edge and parallel to the superior pulmonary vein. The superior pulmonary vein marks the gateway of visualization through the future atriotomy. After application of defogging solution, a 5-mm 0-degree telescopic camera is passed through the port (Fig. 72–8). To date, an assistant has maintained telescopic cleanliness and position in most cases; however, initial experience with robotic camera control has shown great promise for improved instrument tracking.

Transthoracic Aortic Clamp Occlusion and Cardioplegia

Videoscopic assistance is helpful for placement of the aortic cardioplegia-vent needle and essential for aortic clamp positioning. In most instances, cardiopulmonary perfusion

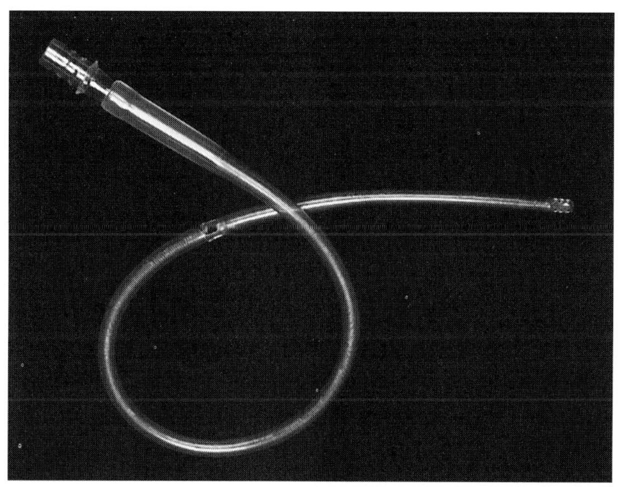

Figure 72–7. Percutaneous femoral vein cannula: two-stage venous return cannula. This cannula, designed by Carpentier, is inserted over a guide wire using serial dilators. It can be used to isolate the superior and inferior venae cavae from the right atrium during mitral, tricuspid, and interatrial surgery (Medtronic-DLP, Inc., Minneapolis, MN).

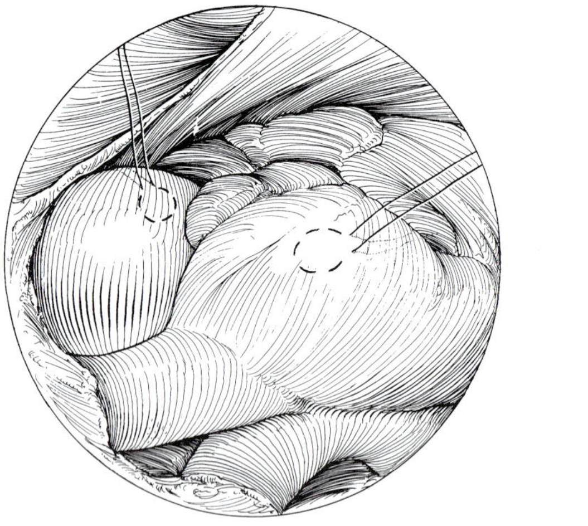

Figure 72–8. Video-assisted micro-mitral operation: videoscopic topography. Thoracoscopic view after insertion of the camera through the port. Pursestring sutures have been placed in the ascending aorta for the cardioplegia needle and, in this instance, the right atrium for central venous cannulation. Peripheral venous cannulation is currently used in most cases. The superior pulmonary vein marks the gateway for left atrial insertion of the thoracoscope after cardiac arrest.

is established before insertion of the aortic cardioplegia pursestring suture and needle. Videoscopically, the pursestring suture is placed along the anterior ascending aorta, just distal to the right coronary origin, and a suction–vent-cardioplegia needle is inserted through either the wound or separate port. A 4-mm incision is made in the third intercostal space, just cephalad to the video port, Figure 72–9 illustrates placement of the transthoracic clamp through the transverse sinus. Under video-assisted guidance, the clamp is positioned with one prong passed behind the ascending aorta through the transverse sinus. Care should be taken to avoid right pulmonary artery, aorta, or left atrial appendage injury during this maneuver. After aortic clamping, the 5-mm telescopic camera should be used to view the complete transverse sinus to ensure correct positioning and complete aortic occlusion. Because the heart and aorta are displaced less than in conventional operations, introduction of air into the aortic root is minimized. If a normal coronary system exists with a large right coronary artery, antegrade cardioplegia can provide excellent myocardial protection. Throughout the period of cardiac arrest, we maintain the systemic perfusion temperature at 26°C. The ambient cardiac temperature in this environment makes colder systemic temperatures preferable because cardiac quiescence is difficult to maintain, even with nearly continuous cardioplegia infusions. At higher temperatures, when retrograde cardioplegia is used, coronary sinus catheter position should be confirmed by transesophageal echocardiography. In this instance, the cannula can be inserted through the incision and directly into the right atrial wall.

Mitral Valve Exposure for Repair and Replacement

The interatrial groove is developed for only 1 to 2 cm. Unlike the sternotomy approach, additional dissection may make atriotomy closure more difficult. A small (3 to 4-cm) left atriotomy is made just medial to the right superior pulmonary vein, and a small ribbon retractor is introduced to provide valve exposure. The retractor is shaped so that "towing in" elevates the interatrial septum and allows the anterior mitral leaflet to hang free as a curtain. Transthoracic retractors, made by Heartport and DSP-Genzyme, are helpful as well. When using these latter retractors, fixation to a self-retaining arm can provide stable position and support. Falk and associates reported the use of similar devices and the AESOP (automated endoscope system for optimal positioning) 3000 robot (Computer Motion, Inc.) for performing solo videoscopic mitral valve surgery.[33] Often smaller atria are easier to manipulate than larger redundant chambers.

Currently, for minimally invasive *mitral valve repairs,* we use both the Carpentier-Edwards Physio annuloplasty ring and the Baxter Cosgrove annuloplasty band. The Cosgrove band extends posteriorly between fibrous trigones, so fewer sutures are required. When the annulus is reduced with ischemic regurgitation, the Cosgrove band is sufficient. However, we prefer the Physio ring for complex

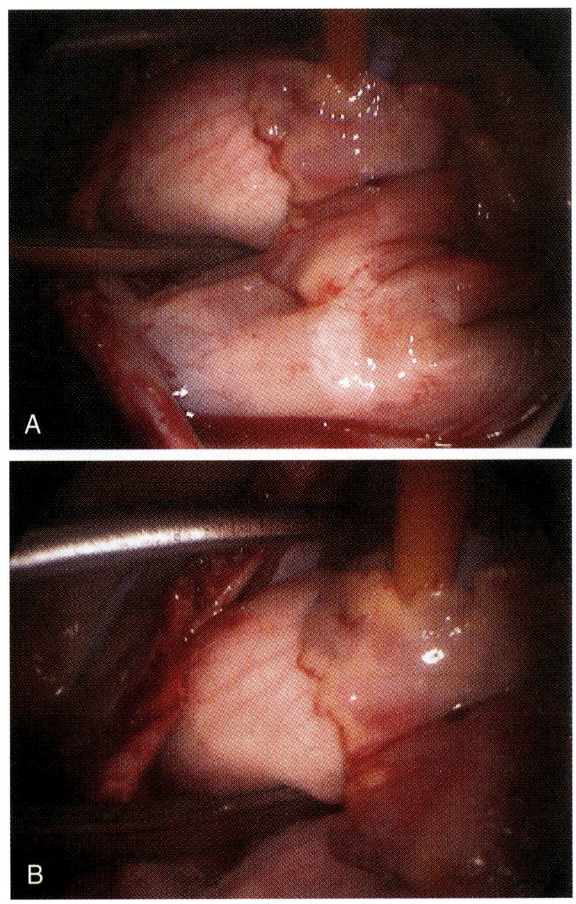

Figure 72–9. Video-assisted micro-mitral operation: intrathoracic cross-clamp placement: videoscopic view. The cross-clamp has been passed through the chest wall. In both *A* and *B,* one prong of the cross-clamp has been passed, under videoscopic control, through the transverse sinus posterior (dorsal) to the aorta. The cardioplegia needle is seen placed in the ascending aorta. *A,* The collapsed right atrium and superior vena are shown in relation to the cross-clamp site. *B,* A closer view shows the anterior prong of the clamp extending across the aorta to touch the pulmonary artery. Optimal clamp position must be ensured before closure.

reconstructions. In large left atria, the lateral walls tend to "fall in," and early placement of commissure sutures helps establish correct anatomic form and orientation. We place annular sutures in a counter-clockwise direction, beginning at either the right fibrous trigone or the commissure. Exposure for subsequent sutures often becomes predicated on retraction of the previous one. The sutures should be arranged serially and suspended tightly from external suture guides. Sutures exiting the posterior incision tend to obstruct telescopic camera vision and are placed last. It is most important to avoid suture fouling and incorrect sequencing, because reorientation through the small incision becomes difficult. Leaflet resections, chordal transpositions, papillary reconstructions, and neochordal substitutions should be carried out after annular sutures are established. The camera is particularly helpful for subvalvular reconstructions or polytetrafluoroethylene chord implantations. In many instances, we place all annular sutures before sizing or beginning a leaflet reconstruction. Occasionally, a posterior annular suture must be replaced during a subsequent annular reconstruction or leaflet resection, or both. Figure 72–10 shows a video-assisted minimally invasive mitral reconstruction from our series.

For minimally invasive *mitral replacements,* we have placed subannular 2–0 sutures with pledgets serially while the anterior leaflet is progressively "snipped" in a counter-clockwise direction. Advancement along the anterior annulus is much like rock climbing. A new suture is placed before releasing the previous hold. The posterior leaflet and subvalvular apparatus are always maintained. In some cases, we make a transition from anterior subvalvular sutures to posterior supraannular everting mattress sutures. To date, we have experienced no perivalvular leakage using this alternate technique. However, care must be taken to avoid mechanical valve leaflet impingement. This method appears to facilitate videoscopic anterior suture placement while providing minimal risk of mechanical leaflet impingement by posterior leaflet tissue. In other cases, the midportion of the anterior leaflet was excised and the anterior chords preserved. Currently, we use rotatable Masters Series St. Jude mechanical prostheses (St. Jude Medical, Inc.), as rotatable valves preserve maximal flexibility. For tissue valve replacement, both leaflets may be left intact with either sub- or supraannular sutures with pledgets selected. Figure 72–11 shows a video-assisted mitral valve replacement in progress.

For both repairs and replacements, anterior sutures usually require videoscopic assistance; however, with 6-cm thoracic incisions, posterior sutures often can be placed by direct vision. Left fibrous trigone and commissure instru-

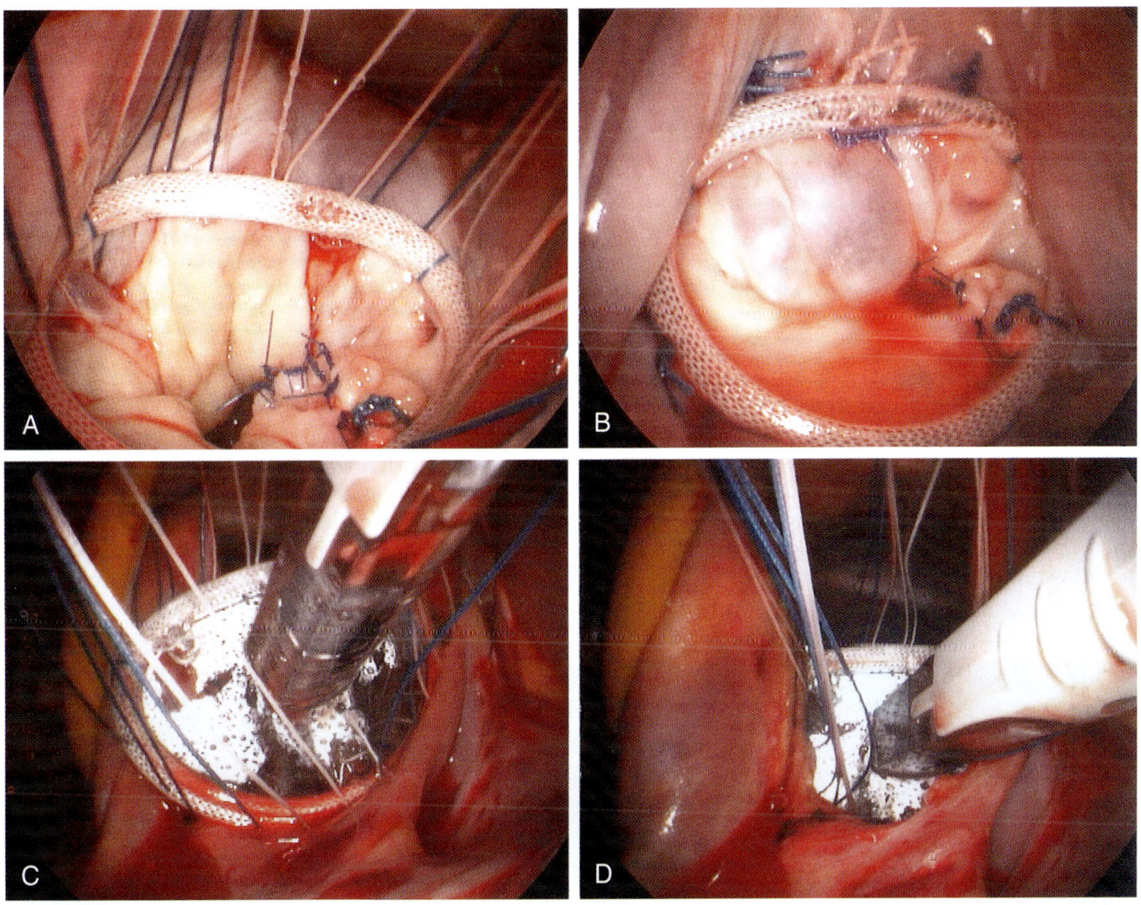

Figure 72–10. Video-assisted micro-mitral repair: quadrangular resection with ring annuloplasty. A completed quadrangular resection of the posterior P_2 segment with ring annuloplasty is shown. The patient had type II mitral insufficiency from ruptured chordae tendineae. *A,* The quadrangular resection is shown to be complete with multiple leaflet sutures. A Carpentier Physio annuloplasty had been lowered into place. *B,* All annuloplasty sutures have been tied and the mitral repair is complete. The saline test shows the valve to be completely competent. *C, D,* A 28-mm Physio annuloplasty ring is lowered through a 3.5-cm atriotomy.

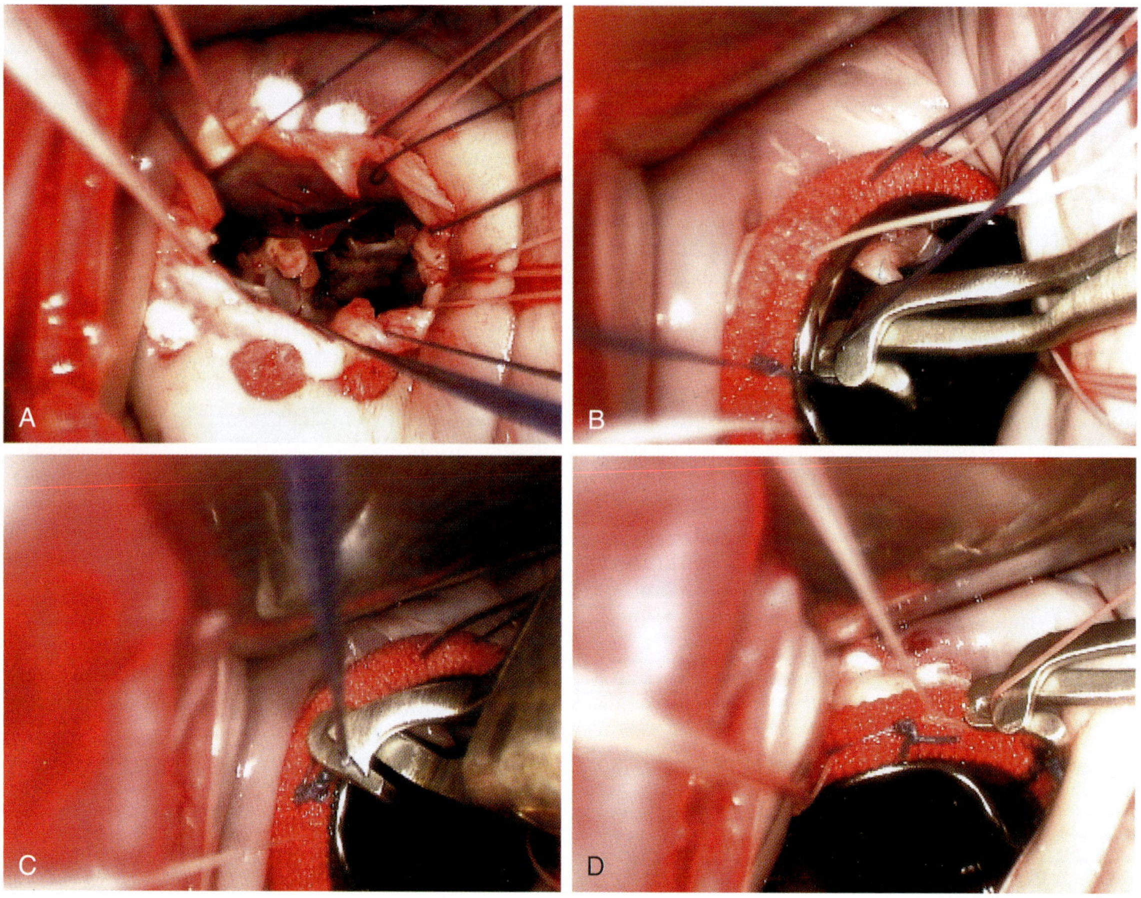

Figure 72–11. Video-assisted micro-mitral replacement: insertion of a bileaflet mechanical prosthesis. *A,* The anterior leaflet has been excised, and supra-annular pledgeted valve sutures have been placed. The posterior leaflet was preserved. *B,* Suture knots are being tied extracorporeally and positioned with a specialized instrument along the St. Jude prosthetic valve sewing annulus. Note the angled instrument offset to allow videoscopic visualization and ensure secure knot placement (Scanlan International, Inc., Minneapolis, MN). *C,* Sutures are cut to predetermined lengths using another specialized instrument.

ment maneuvers are difficult and are best performed using the left hand with a 30-degree telescope. When passing sutures through the mitral annulus, retention of needle position is essential. A short jaw needle holder provides the best needle stability (Fig. 72–12). Varied needle positions and angles are needed for optimal flexibility during suturing. After completion of annular sutures, the extrathoracic prosthesis is lowered into position through the small atriotomy. Care must be taken to prevent the introduction of intracardiac tissue particles as the prosthesis passes tightly through the 3 to 4-cm atriotomy.

The left fibrous trigone suture should be tied first, followed by the right trigone and then the posterior middle suture. We use a specialized instrument to seat the valve and secure suture knots. This device is off-set, like a golf club, to provide valve seating and knot tying with good camera views (see Fig. 72–11). The first two knots must slip to effect tight prosthesis-tissue apposition while avoid-

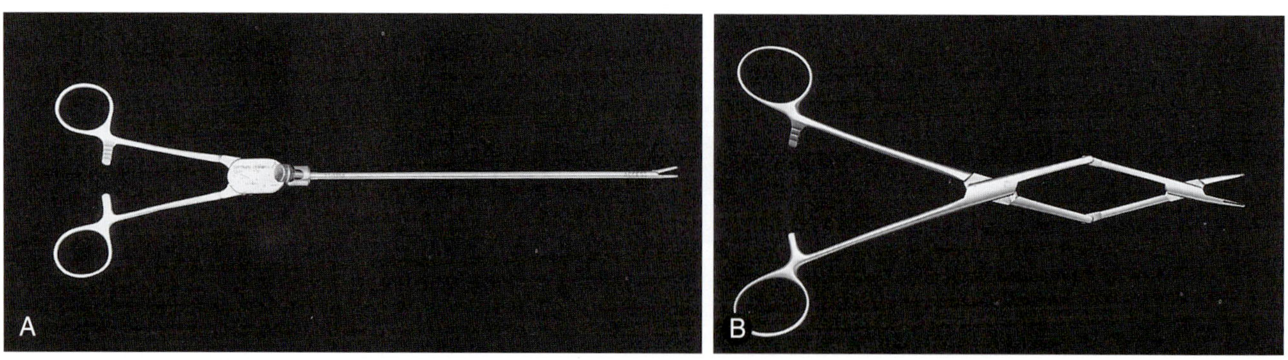

Figure 72–12. Video-assisted micro-mitral valve operation: needle holders. *A,* Landrenau type of needle holder used for videoscopic annular and subvalvular suture placement. *B,* Carpentier needle holder for videoscopic suture placement with calcified or fibrotic annuli and direct-vision atrial closures.

ing suture breakage. Subsequently, all remaining knots are tied and sutures cut by a custom instrument. Such instruments were developed to facilitate this operation and include the transthoracic aortic cross-clamp (see Fig. 72–3), special forceps (Fig. 72–13A–C), the transthoracic "crochet hook" retraction suture puller, and the valve positioner–knot tier (positioner) (Fig. 72–13D) just noted (Scanlan International, Inc., Minneapolis, MN).

Cardiac Air Removal and Cardiopulmonary Bypass Weaning

The left atriotomy should be closed under direct vision with a continuous monofilament suture. Carbon dioxide is much more soluble in blood than in air. Thus, we insufflate this gas into the chest cavity just before the time of atrial closure and then purge the left atrium while ventilating the lungs.[34] This maneuver draws the carbon dioxide into the pulmonary veins, displacing residual air. We have not used a transvalvular vent since employing this method. Before the transthoracic aortic clamp is released, venous return is decreased while both lungs are ventilated and the remaining intracardiac air is evacuated via the atriotomy suture line and the aortic vent. While maintaining aortic venting, the patient is rotated side to side with the head placed in the Trendelenburg position with the right coronary origin compressed. Multiple partial aortic occlusions are performed during cardiac ejection to complete the cardiac air removal, which is confirmed by echocardiography. Following clamp removal, the posterior aorta is inspected for injury using the telescopic camera. The patient is weaned from cardiopulmonary bypass using standard methods. A 30 French Silastic chest tube is placed through the camera port site and the incision is closed. In most patients, temporary pacing wires are not used.

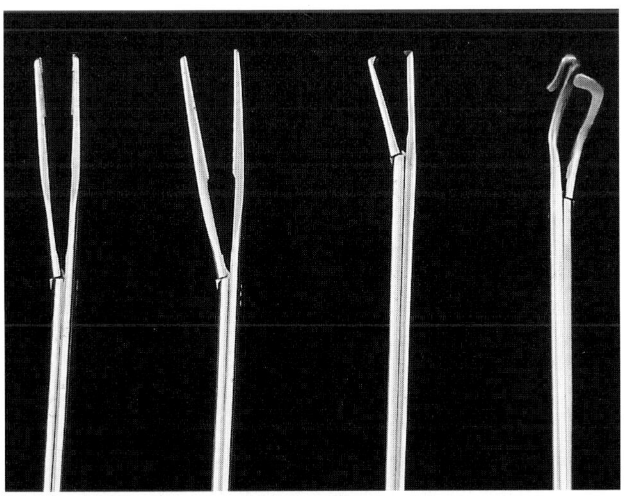

Figure 72–13. Video-assisted micro-mitral valve operation: specialized instruments. Specialized minimally invasive cardiac surgical instruments were designed to facilitate this operation: From left, fine-toothed DeBakey-type forceps tips have been modified to have a diamond platform for intracardiac needle orientation or retrieval; DeBakey forceps have been modified for minimally invasive cardiac surgery; Adson-type coarse forceps were designed to grasp fibrotic rheumatic valve leaflets; the Chitwood knot positioner-tier facilitates videoscopic knot security (Scanlan International, Minneapolis, MN).

Operative Results: The Micro-Mitral Operation

As of May 1998, our group at East Carolina University had performed 55 video-assisted minimally invasive or micro-mitral operations (MMO) with a single death from an arrhythmia 27 days after discharge. Current patient selection criteria are shown in Table 72–2. Demographic data for the series are listed in Table 72–3, and operations performed are listed in Table 72–4. Perioperative clinical data for the series and comparisons with 100 conventional sternotomy patients are listed in Table 72–5. All patients were operated on by one surgeon between May 1996 and May 1998. The previous 100 standard mitral operations were performed by the same surgeon between January 1992 and 1997. Patients requiring concomitant coronary artery bypass grafting were excluded from both series. Statistical comparisons were carried out using a chi-square analysis and a two-tailed t test. Data are shown as ± standard error of the mean (SEM), with a level of significance reported at a *P* valve of equal to or less than .05.

Demographic data (see Table 72–2) suggested similar patient cohorts for age, gender, and functional class. Twenty-one patients who underwent minimally invasive procedures (38%) had mitral valve replacement and 34 patients (62%) had repairs. Five patients who underwent replacement surgery had degenerative disease, and 14 had rheumatic valves. The pathologic conditions in patients who underwent MMO repair were similar to sternotomy repairs and included degenerative changes (n = 27), rheumatic disease (n = 5), and healed endocarditis (n = 2). No patients who underwent MMO had conversion to either a larger incision or a sternotomy. One repair eventuated in a secondary replacement because of increasing insufficiency 1 year after the initial operation.

There were no hospital deaths in MMO patients. However, one New York Heart Association class I patient died suddenly 27 days after discharge of a presumed ventricular arrhythmia (30-day mortality = 1.8%). Autopsy re-

Table 72–2. Video-Assisted Minimally Invasive Mitral Surgery: The Micro-Mitral Operation

Current Patient Selection
Unsuitable Candidates
Prior right-sided chest surgery
Highly calcified mitral annulus
Multiple valve operations
Severe pulmonary hypertension, especially with a small right coronary
Significant untreated coronary disease
Severe peripheral atherosclerosis
Selective Candidates
Repair candidates with significant bileaflet or anterior leaflet prolapse
Suitable Candidates
Patients with primary mitral valve disease
Reoperative mitral valve patients
Obese or large patients
Elderly patients

Table 72–3. Video-Assisted Minimally Invasive Vs. Conventional Sternotomy: Demographic Data

	Video-Assisted Minimally Invasive (n = 55)	Conventional Sternotomy (n = 100)
Age (yr)	59 ± 1.8	59.3 ± 1.4
Range	18–82	29–78
Gender		
Men	27 (49%)	47 (47%)
Women	28 (51%)	53 (53%)
Preoperative functional class (NYHA)		
Class I	3 (5%)	8 (8%)
Class II	25 (46%)	42 (42%)
Class III	24 (44%)	40 (40%)
Class IV	3 (5%)	10 (10%)
Ejection fraction (%)		
>40%	50 (91%)	63 (63%)*
<40%	5 (9%)	37 (37%)*

**P* = .001.
NYHA, New York Heart Association.

Table 72–5. Mitral Valve Surgery—Video-Assisted Vs. Conventional Sternotomy: Perioperative Data

	Video-Assisted Minimally Invasive	Conventional Sternotomy
Cross-clamp time (min)	128 ± 4.5	92 ± 3.6*
Pump time (min)	173 ± 5.7	116 ± 4.4*
PRBC infused (units)	2.2 ± 0.2	3.6 ± 0.4†
Hospital stay (d)	4.8 ± 0.6	8.6 ± 0.5*
ICU stay: if ventilated <48 hr (hr)	25.4 ± 3.8	48.7 ± 8.2†
ICU stay: total group (hr)	29.3 ± 5.3	48.7 ± 8.2
Ventilator period (hr)	12.9 ± 2.1	22.7 ± 5.2
Chest tube drainage (total—ml)	544 ± 68	716 ± 86

**P* = .001
†*P* = .05
PRBC = packed red blood cells; ICU, intensive care unit.

vealed normal prosthesis function. Comparatively, the 30-day mortality for conventional patients was 2.2% (pNS). One late death occurred at 3 months in the MMO group and was related to prosthetic valve endocarditis.

As seen in Table 72–4, cardiopulmonary perfusion and aortic cross-clamp times averaged 173 ± 5.6 and 128 ± 4.5 minutes, respectively. No aortic clamp injuries occurred, and there were no difficulties in weaning patients from bypass. Low-dose dopamine was often started empirically before weaning from bypass; however, none was required for support for more than 6 hours. In several early procedures, the immediate postarrest electrocardiogram showed inferior lead changes, despite meticulous cardiac removal of air. This was before the use of the carbon dioxide air purge. All changes were transient and did not eventuate in complications. Transesophageal echocardiography showed postoperative ventricular function that was similar in each case to preoperative studies.

Both ventilatory and intensive care unit (ICU) times tended to be shorter than with conventional operations (see Table 72–4). MMO patients were extubated 13 hours after surgery and were transferred from the ICU 1.2 days after the operation. For these patients, overall stay in the ICU was significantly shorter than for the sternotomy group (*P* = .05). Overall, MMO patients had a 4.4-day hospital stay, with 81% being discharged between the third and fifth postoperative days (*P* = .001). In the last half of the series, the length of hospitalization fell to 3.5 days. In both series, a similar incidence of new atrial fibrillation occurred postoperatively. Major complications for the MMO group included deep venous thrombosis and phrenic nerve palsy. The latter patient was ventilated for 17 days, representing the only individual requiring respiratory support for more than 48 hours. One 82-year-old patient had transient cerebellar dysfunction with complete recovery. In the MMO group, there were no other neurologic deficits and no re-explorations for bleeding. This compares with 4% re-explorations for bleeding, and a 3% transient stroke rate in our patients undergoing conventional procedures (*P* = .05). Transfusion volumes of packed red cells and frozen plasma were less than in the sternotomy group (*P* = .05). However, 35% of MMO patients received a blood product transfusion.

Table 72–4. Video-Assisted Minimally Invasive Vs. Conventional Sternotomy: Operative Techniques

Operative technique	Video-Assisted Minimally Invasive	Conventional Sternotomy (n = 100)
Valve replacement	21 (38%)	43 (43%)
Valve repair	34 (62%)	57 (57%)
Annuloplasty alone	16 (47%)	27 (47%)
Annuloplasty—quad resection	15 (44%)	17 (30%)
Annuloplasty—chordal replacement	3 (9%)	5 (9%)
Annuloplasty—chordal transfer	0 (0%)	8 (14%)

With the exception of the 2 patients with either deep venous thrombosis and phrenic nerve palsy, all reported little to no perioperative pain and noted rapid return to normal activities. Of all MMO patients, 93% were in functional class I or II after surgery. The first 31 patients were analyzed for economic parameters. In this early series, after cost adjustments for the valve or annuloplasty prosthesis, both charges and costs were found to be 27% and 34% less, respectively, than for conventional sternotomy patients (*P* = .02).[7] Charge and cost reductions resulted primarily from the reduced length of stay.

Conclusions: The Micro-Mitral Operation

The application of the minithoracotomy to minimally invasive valve surgery seems ideal, as the small anterolateral incision provides a direct view of the left atriotomy, while minimizing discomfort. Moreover, with our approach, adequate mitral valve exposure can be obtained without an extended atrial incision, which is usually necessary with the limited sternotomy or parasternal approaches. We believe that minimally invasive atrial incisions (3 to 4-cm) may be an improvement over the larger cardiac access that is necessary with both the parasternal and ministernotomy approaches.

Our transthoracic aortic clamp method appears safe and requires few additional resources or custom disposable supplies. Transthoracic clamp occlusion was not difficult, and antegrade cardioplegia provided excellent cardiac protection. Videoscopic assistance was helpful to avoid injury to the right pulmonary artery and left atrial appendage, as well as to ensure complete occlusion. We did not experience clamp slippage or aortic injury. The Endoclamp, developed by Heartport, provides intraluminal aortic occlusion and antegrade cardioplegia capabilities as well. However, balloon catheter insertion may have a higher potential for aortic dissection and balloon dislodgements.[9] Moreover, in smaller patients and in those who have significant aortoiliac occlusive disease, passage of an intra-aortic catheter may be impossible.

In our 55 patients, videoscopic assistance was always helpful and sometimes essential. In many circumstances, direct exposure of trigonal-commisural regions, the anterior annulus, and intracardiac papillary-chordal structures would have been difficult without videoscopic assistance. Aortic clamping, tissue excision, suture placement, prosthetic valve-ring positioning, and knot tying clearly were facilitated by thoracoscopic vision (see Figs. 72–10 to 72–12). Complex repairs were possible, although anterior leaflet prolapse poses a challenge. Valves that have significant bileaflet prolapse can possibly be treated using video-assisted methods and the leaflet suture apposition technique described by Maisano and associates.[35] Secondary vision was most beneficial in large or obese patients, in those who had a deep thorax, and in individuals who had large left atria. In the video-directed repairs, excellent results were obtained without ever seeing the valve directly. Moreover, videoscopic assistance was of particular help in suturing papillary muscles and in subvalvular reconstructive work.

Despite the potential benefits of video-assisted minimally invasive mitral valve surgery, several concerns arise. First, the lack of three-dimensional perception still limits the full potential of this technique. However, two-dimensional visualization and tactile feedback, transmitted through instruments, appear to have become additive compensatory mechanisms. With practice during sternotomy-based mitral operations, videoscopic dexterity can be learned fairly rapidly with safety. At present, the use of smaller incisions and videoscopic assistance requires longer perfusion and cardiac arrest times. Although both East Carolina University surgeons and the Leipzig group have experienced decreased operative and perfusion times, newer operations eventually must approximate traditional operative standards. The real issue concerns the potential for dispersion of videoscopic methods among contemporary cardiac surgeons.

The decision to repair a mitral valve should not be driven by the operative approach, but by the pathologic condition of the valve. The best mitral operation should have priority over the approach. Quality should never be compromised to minimize hospital cost, improve cosmesis, or lessen temporary discomfort. In this series, the selection criteria were the same for patients having a sternotomy. Most other patient series have reported a predominance of repairs done through less invasive incisions.[4, 14, 16, 22] Our group was pleased with the ability to repair mitral valves using videoscopic assistance. However, indications of patient satisfaction, an early return to work, and discomfort remain difficult to assess retrospectively. Thus, a prospective study using appropriate psychometric measurements is needed to clarify these issues.

These and other results are encouraging and show that both mitral valve replacements and relatively complex repairs can be performed effectively by direct vision and video-assisted methods with good operative results. Moreover, these procedures appear to benefit patients through reduced stays in the ICU, fewer transfusion requirements, less operative discomfort, earlier hospital discharge, and lower cost. Obviously, longer term follow-up is necessary to determine ultimate clinical outcomes.

Robotic Video-Assisted and Directed Mitral Valve Surgery

The combination of new visualization methods with haptic (tactile) feedback could move surgeons toward mitral valve repairs using true microscopic access methods through tiny ports and incisions. Voice-activated robotic camera direction has already been shown to be helpful during minimally invasive mitral valve surgery. Many of us have worked with evolving robotic methods, and it is clear that this enabling technology can provide voice-activated camera manipulation, scaling of instrument motion, camera tracking, flexible intracardiac articulation, and three-dimensional vision. Recently, Mohr and associates and Falk and associates described solo videoscopic mitral operations with the thoracoscopic camera driven by robot.[29, 33] Subsequently, our group used the same robotic device for the first time in the United States to perform a mitral valve repair videoscopically (Fig. 72–14). This device allows accurate camera positioning by the surgeon's voice, with less need for camera cleaning.

Experimentally, we have performed coronary anastomoses and mitral valve repairs that were completely video-directed using an innovative articulated robotic device (Intuitive Surgical Systems, Mountain View, CA.) Using the same device, on May 19, 1998, Carpentier and Loulmet successfully performed the world's first truly robot-assisted mitral valve operation in a patient. In this and two other procedures, they used intracardiac articulated "wrist" instruments, manipulated electronically from a console at a distance from the patient, for repairing valves and placing annuloplasty rings. Later, beginning on May 24, 1998, and using the same system, the Leipzig group performed five additional mitral repairs in patients. They completed repairs with a band annuloplasty and tied all sutures inside the heart robotically. Mohr then did the first successful clinical coronary anastomosis on May 27, 1998, and Loulmet and Carpentier performed the first totally endoscopic coronary artery bypass operation, including internal mammary harvest, 1 month later. The experiences

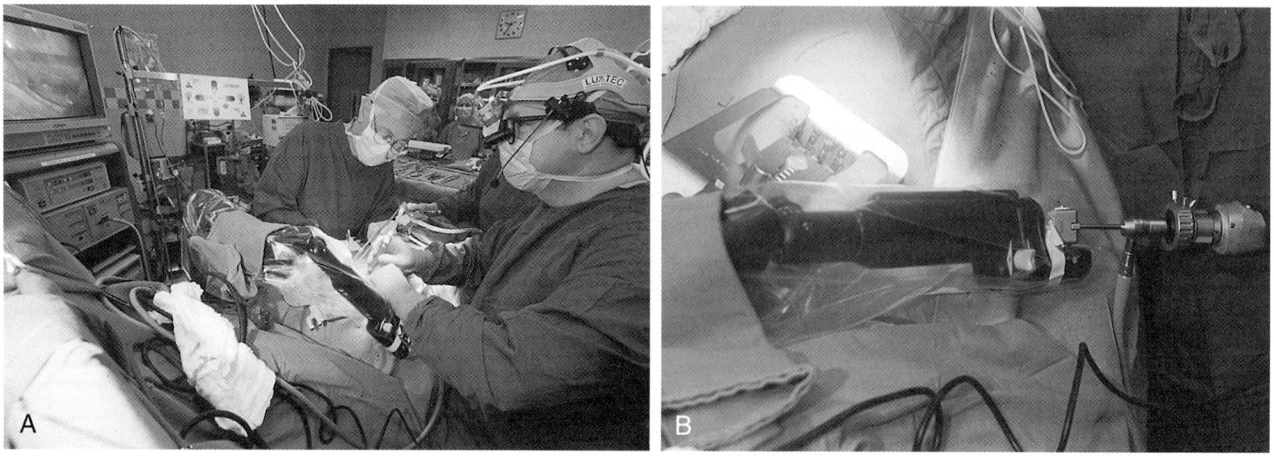

Figure 72–14. Video-assisted micro-mitral valve operation: voice-activated robotic videoscopic assistance. This was the first minimally invasive video-assisted mitral valve operation that was performed in the United States using voice-activated robotic control. Note the surgeon's microphone, which was connected through a voice card microprocessor to computer-activate the AESOP 3000 robot shown in the foreground (Computer Motion, Inc., Goleta, CA).

of Carpentier and Mohr were positive; however, several technologic iterations must evolve before surgeon selection of these complex robotic devices becomes widespread. Moreover, patient acceptance will have to mature in parallel.

Endoscopic Mitral Valve Surgery—Does It Have a Future?

A renaissance in cardiac surgery began with the prospect of minimally invasive operations. In less than 3 years, the specialty has come far. The current enthusiasm of surgeons worldwide, combined with the lightning-like speed of technologic development and communications, appears to be propelling us toward perhaps microinvasive cardiac operations. The advent of true three-dimensional vision with tactile feedback will be a bridge to truly tele-microaccess cardiac operations. To perform mitral reconstructions optimally, extracorporeal surgeons will need improved instruments directed by computer motion and rapid acquisition of videoscopic dexterity. Intrathoracic, fully articulated instruments are on the near horizon and may be the key to video-directed microscopic access for both valve and coronary operations. However, many techniques are evolving so rapidly that multipatient series have not been collected, and data often remain antidotal. We must continue to ask ourselves—Is the new method really benefiting our patients through reduced trauma, similar or fewer complications, more rapid recovery, and similar or better long-term results, compared with traditional operations? To protect these parameters for minimally invasive cardiac surgery, a healthy mix of scientific skepticism and wisdom must be exercised through discussion forums, society meetings, and, especially, peer-reviewed journals. Yes, some of us believe that microinvasive or endoscopic reconstructive mitral surgery will become a reality and will be performed widely. This may be the future; however, despite ungoverned enthusiasm at present, caution cannot be overemphasized. *Remember, our patients entrust confidence in us to be their advocates. We must not take this lightly as we proceed into the future.*

References

1. Baldwin JC: Minimally invasive port-access mitral valve surgery (Editorial; comment) J Thorac Cardiovasc Surg 115:563–564, 1998.
2. Lytle BW: Minimally invasive cardiac surgery (Editorial; comment) J Thorac Cardiovasc Surg 113:554–555, 1996.
3. Verrier ED: Minimally invasive port-access mitral valve surgery (Editorial). J Thorac Cardiovasc Surg 115:565–566, 1998.
4. Cosgrove DM, Sabik JF, Navia J: Minimally invasive valve operations. Ann Thorac Surg 65:1535–1538, 1998.
5. Gundry SR, Shattuck OH, Razzouk AJ, et al: Facile minimally invasive cardiac surgery via mini-sternotomy. Ann Thorac Surg 65:1100–1104, 1998.
6. Navia JL, Cosgrove DM: Minimally invasive mitral valve operations. Ann Thorac Surg 62:1542–1544, 1996.
7. Chitwood WR, Elbeery JR, Chapman WHH, et al: Video-assisted minimally invasive mitral valve surgery: The "micro-mitral" operation. J Thorac Cardiovasc Surg 113:413–414, 1997.
8. Falk V, Walther T, Diegeler R, et al: Echocardiographic monitoring of minimally invasive mitral valve surgery using an endoaortic clamp. J Heart Valve Dis 5:630–637, 1996.
9. Mohr FW, Falk V, Diegeler A, et al: Minimally invasive port-access mitral valve surgery. J Thorac Cardiovasc Surg 115:567–574, 1998.
10. Chitwood WR: Videoscopic minimally invasive mitral surgery: Trekking to a totally endoscopic operation. Heart Surg For 1:1–5, 1998.
11. Pompili MF, Yakub A, Siegel LC, et al: Port-acess mitral valve replacement: Initial clinical experience. Circulation 94 (suppl):I-533, 1996.
12. Grossi EA, Ribakove G, Schwartz DS, et al: Port-access approach for minimally invasive mitral valve surgery. *In* Cox JL, Sundt TM (eds): Operative Techniques in Cardiac and Thoracic Surgery: A Comparative Atlas, Vol 1. Philadelphia, WB Saunders, 1998, pp 32–46.
13. Arom KV, Emery RW: Minimally invasive mitral operations (Letter). Ann Thorac Surg 62:1542–1544, 1996.
14. Cohn LH, Adams DH, Couper GS, et al: Minimally invasive cardiac valve surgery improves patient satisfaction while reducing costs of cardiac valve replacement and repair. Ann Surg 226:421–426, 1997; discussion, 226:427–428, 1997.
15. Cohn LH: Parasternal approach for minimally invasive aortic valve surgery. *In* Cox JL, Sundt TM (eds): Operative Techniques in Cardiac and Thoracic Surgery: A Comparative Atlas, Vol 1. Philadelphia, WB Saunders, pp 54–61, 1998.

16. Cosgrove DM, Gillinov AM: Partial sternotomy for mitral valve operations. *In* Cox JL, Sundt TM (eds): Operative Techniques in Cardiac and Thoracic Surgery: A Comparative Atlas, Vol 1. Philadelphia, WB Saunders, pp 62–72, 1998.
17. Cosgrove DM: World-view Through 8 Centimeters. International Tele-symposium on Minimally Invasive Valve Surgery, Cleveland, OH, Cleveland Clinic Foundation September 27, 1997.
18. Colvin S, Galloway A. The New York University Experience with Port-Access Cardiac Surgery. Presented at the Heartport Satellite Meeting, Society for Thoracic Surgeons annual meeting, San Diego, January, 1997.
19. Smediera N: Presented at the ninth Cardiac and General Thoracic Minimally Invasive Valve Surgery Surgery Update, American College of Chest Physicians, Cancun, Mexico, December, 1997.
20. Aklog L, Adams DH, Couper GS, et al: Techniques and results of direct access minimally invasive mitral valve surgery: A paradigm for the future. J Thorac Cardiovasc Surg 116:705–715, 1998.
21. Colvin S: Symposium: Minimally invasive valve surgery. American Heart Association annual meeting, Orlando, FL, November, 1997.
22. Spencer FC, Galloway AC, Grossi EA, et al: Recent developments and evolving techniques for mitral valve reconstruction. Ann Thorac Surg 65:307–313, 1998.
23. Kaneko Y, Kohno T, Ohtsuka T, et al: Video-assisted observation in mitral valve surgery. J Thorac Cardiovasc Surg 111:279–280, 1996.
24. Carpentier A, Loulmet D, Carpentier A, et al: Chirurgie à coeur ouvert par vidéo-chirurgie et mini-thoracotomie—primier cas (valvuloplastie mitrale) opéré avec succès—(First open heart operation [mitral valvuloplasty] under videosurgery through a minithoracotomy.) C R Acad Sci III 319:219–223, 1996.
25. Chitwood WR, Elbeery JR, Moran JM: Minimally invasive mitral valve repair: Using a mini-thoracotomy and trans-thoracic aortic occlusion. Ann Thorac Surg 63:1477–1479, 1997.
26. Chitwood WR Jr, Wixon CL, Elbeery JR, et al: Video-assisted minimally invasive mitral valve surgery. J Thorac Cardiovasc Surg 14:773–780, 1997.
27. Chang CH, Lin PJ, Chu JJ, et al: Video-assisted cardiac surgery in closure of atrial septal defect. Ann Thorac Surg 62:697–701, 1996.
28. Tsai FC, Lin PJ, Chang CH, et al: Video-assisted cardiac surgery. Preliminary experience in reoperative mitral valve surgery. Chest 110:1603–1607, 1996.
29. Mohr F, Falk V: The evolution of minimally invasive mitral valve surgery—two year experience. Presented at the first annual meeting of the International Society for Minimally Invasive Cardiac Surgery, Minneapolis, MN, June 27, 1998.
30. Loulmet DF, Carpentier A, Cho PW, et al: Less invasive methods for mitral valve surgery. J Thorac Cardiovasc Surg 115:772–779, 1998.
31. Reichenspurner H, Bohm DH, Welz A, et al: Video-assisted mitral valve surgery using the Port-access technique and the 3-D Vista system—clinical experience with 35 patients. Presented at the first annual meeting of the International Society for Minimally Invasive Cardiac Surgery, Minneapolis, MN, June 27, 1998.
32. Flege JB Jr, Wolf RK: Venous drainage to the heart-lung machine via the internal jugular vein. Ann Thorac Surg 63:861, 1997.
33. Falk V, Walther T, Autschbach R, et al: Robot-assisted minimally invasive solo mitral valve operation. J Thorac Cardiovasc Surg 115:470–471, 1998.
34. Webb WR, Harrison LH Jr, Helmcke FR, et al: Carbon dioxide field flooding minimizes residual intracardiac air after open heart operations. Ann Thorac Surg 64:1489–1491, 1997.
35. Maisano F, Torracca L, Oppizzi M, et al: The-edge to-edge technique: A simplified method to correct mitral insufficiency. Eur J Cardiothorac Surg 13:240–246, 1998.

Chapter 73

Port Access Heart Valve Surgery

John S. Ikonomidis, James I. Fann, Thomas A. Burdon, and Mario F. Pompili

The field of mitral valve surgery has been marked by advances in biomaterials and innovative reparative techniques since the early 1960s,[1, 2, 5, 8, 10] but the conventional median sternotomy approach to surgical exposure of the mitral valve and the subvalvular apparatus has not changed significantly until recently. Primarily as a result of progress in video-assisted surgery and endovascular techniques since the 1980s, less invasive techniques to cardiac surgery have been proposed, and different techniques of mitral valve surgery through limited thoracotomy incisions are being evaluated in experimental and clinical settings.[3, 4, 7, 12, 13, 16–20, 22, 24]

In this chapter, we present indications for, and current status of, the port access technique of heart valve surgery. In its present form, the port access technique has been predominantly applied to mitral valve procedures; tricuspid valve surgery has been performed along with intracardiac repairs (e.g., atrial septal defects) in selected situations with minor modifications of the venous drainage cannulae. To date, although minimally invasive techniques have been employed in aortic valve surgery, the port access technique has not been routinely used, mainly because access to the ascending aorta in these less invasive procedures permits direct placement of an external cross-clamp. This chapter focuses on the port access technique of mitral valve repair or replacement.

Historical Background

The right thoracotomy approach has been used as an alternative to conventional median sternotomy to expose and access the mitral valve (Fig. 73–1).[11, 28] For this approach, peripheral cardiopulmonary bypass and hypothermic fibrillatory or cardioplegic arrest have been employed; use of video-assisted thoracoscopy has permitted smaller incisions for accessing the mitral valve.[3, 4–13] Chitwood and associates recently described their experience in 31 patients who underwent mitral valve procedures using a micromitral approach through a small 6-cm incision with the assistance of thoracoscopy.[3, 4] Mitral valve repair or replacement was performed with the support of peripheral cardiopulmonary bypass and fibrillatory arrest or cardioplegic arrest, using a transthoracically placed external aortic cross-clamp. The early mortality was 3.2%. Early follow-up suggested less perioperative pain and rapid recovery.

The port access system is a peripherally based endovascular system for cardiopulmonary bypass with cardioplegic arrest. Originally conceived by Peters in 1993, the endoaortic catheter has been modified and serves as the basis of the system.[16] The efficacy of the technique in achieving cardioplegic arrest and thereby permitting coronary revascularization and mitral valve procedures has been validated by investigators at Stanford University and New York University in the experimental and clinical setting.[17, 18, 21, 22] The feasibility of port access mitral valve procedures was demonstrated in 15 dogs by Pompili et al.[18] Through a small, rigid, oval port (3.5 cm × 1.7 cm) placed in the left fifth interspace, the mitral valve and subvalvular apparatus were assessed directly and with the assistance of a thoracoscope. The endoaortic clamp, placed in the femoral artery, was directed to the ascending aorta using fluoroscopic and transesophageal echocardiographic guidance. Peripheral cardiopulmonary bypass was instituted, and the endoaortic clamp balloon was inflated, achieving aortic occlusion. Antegrade and retrograde cardioplegia were instilled sequentially via the central lumen of the endoaortic clamp and via the percutaneously placed coronary sinus catheter, respectively. The mitral valve was exposed and replacement carried out. After closure of the left atriotomy, deairing maneuvers were performed and the animals weaned from cardiopulmonary bypass. The aortic cross-clamp time averaged 68 minutes and the cardiopulmonary bypass time 114 minutes.[18] Using the port-access approach to mitral valve replacement, Schwartz and associates demonstrated experimentally the recovery of left ventricular function at 30 and 60 minutes after cardiopulmonary bypass.[22] Preload recruitable stroke work returned to 96% and 85% of baseline at 30 and 60 minutes after conclusion of cardiopulmonary bypass. Transesophageal echocardiography demonstrated normal regional and global ventricular wall motion.[22] Thus, port access mitral valve replacement could be safely performed with good myocardial protection and recovery of left ventricular function.

Patient Selection

Mainly because of the requirement for peripheral cardiopulmonary bypass in using the port access system, patient selection criteria were established in an effort to recognize potential limitations of this technology. Additionally, because of the limited access to the left side of the heart through the smaller right thoracotomy incision, patients who had associated coronary artery disease were not considered candidates for port access mitral valve procedures. General exclusion criteria included significant associated cardiac pathology (e.g., coronary artery disease or other valvular disease) and severe peripheral vascular disease involving the iliofemoral artery or aorta (which would make femoral cannulation and endoaortic clamp insertion and deployment difficult or impossible).

Technical Considerations

Anesthesia and Monitoring

In all cases of port access surgery, the anesthesiologist plays a critical role and assumes increased responsibilities.

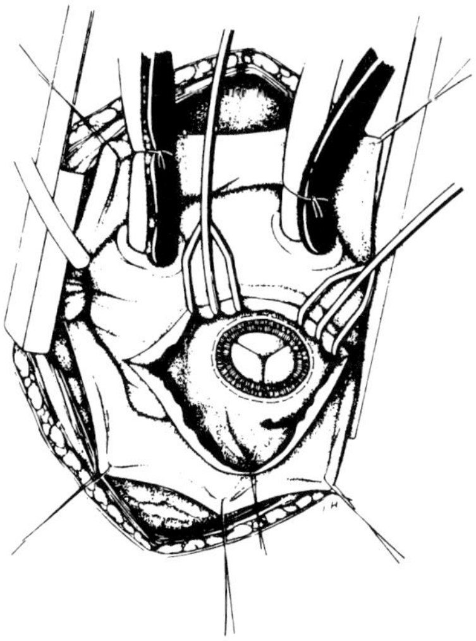

Figure 73–1. The right thoracotomy approach for mitral valve procedures. Bicaval cannulation is used along with femoral arterial cannulation for cardiopulmonary bypass. (Reprinted with permission from the Society of Thoracic Surgeons: Tribble CG, Killinger WA, Harman PK, et al: Anterolateral thoracotomy as an alternative to repeat median sternotomy for replacement of the mitral valve. Ann Thorac Surg 43:380–382, 1987.)

Following general anesthetic induction, a double-lumen endotracheal tube is placed to allow collapse of the right lung for left atriotomy exposure. Percutaneously placed via a jugular approach, an 8.5 French coronary sinus catheter is advanced into the coronary sinus under fluoroscopic or transesophageal echocardiographic guidance, or both. A second catheter, particularly important in mitral valve procedures, is a percutaneously placed 8.3 French pulmonary vent for assistance in venous drainage. The anesthesiologist, therefore, must have facility in operative transesophageal echocardiography for guiding catheter placement, assessing the ascending aorta for underlying pathology that could complicate endoaortic clamp passage, and monitoring endoaortic clamp positioning during the procedure.[6, 23] The position of the endoaortic clamp can also be indirectly monitored by continuous transduction of right and left radial artery pressures; the pressures in the radial artery lines should remain equal throughout the clamp time.[23] If there is a discrepancy in the radial artery pressures (e.g., the right radial pressure is less than the left radial pressure), this may indicate distal migration of the endoaortic clamp with occlusion of the innominate artery, mandating repositioning of the balloon portion of the catheter. Other monitoring strategies include surveillance of endoaortic balloon pressure and pulse-wave Doppler examination of the right carotid, right temporal, or right middle cerebral artery.[23]

Incision and Exposure

The patient is positioned supine with the right side slightly elevated. A limited right fourth interspace thoracotomy is made with or without resection of a short segment of the fourth rib. In our experience, a midportion of the fourth rib has been reflected inferiorly, leaving the intercostal vasculature intact. After completion of the procedure, the periosteum of the rib is approximated with the intercostal musculature of the third interspace, thereby closing the defect. A soft tissue retractor (6.5 to 9 cm in diameter) is placed in the interspace creating an oval port access (Fig. 73–2).[7] A 10-mm port is placed in the sixth interspace for introduction of a thoracoscope, if necessary. Under direct vision through the oval port, the pericardium is opened longitudinally anterior to the phrenic nerve, exposing the left atrium just anterior to the right superior pulmonary vein.

Establishment of Cardiopulmonary Bypass and Cardioplegic Arrest

As with port access coronary revascularization procedure, the left common femoral artery and vein are surgically exposed. Following systemic heparinization, venous drainage is accomplished using a thin-walled 28 French catheter inserted at the saphenofemoral junction and directed to the right atrial-superior vena caval junction.[26, 27] A 21 to 23 French arterial reinfusion catheter is inserted into the common femoral artery; this catheter contains a Y connector that allows arterial reinfusion from one side and insertion of the endoaortic clamp coaxially through the other side. The endoaortic clamp is a 10.5 French peripherally inserted triple-lumen catheter with an inflatable balloon at its distal end.[7, 15–27] The balloon is positioned over a guide wire in the ascending aorta using fluoroscopy and transesophageal echocardiography. The lumen used for balloon inflation is connected to a manometer for monitoring balloon pressure. Cardioplegic solution is delivered through a central lumen; this lumen also acts as an aortic root vent after cardioplegia delivery. A third smaller lumen serves as an aortic root pressure monitor. Cardiopulmonary bypass is instituted by using a standard circuit. Venous drainage can be kinetically assisted with a Biomedicus pump (Medtronic, Minneapolis, MN), maintain-

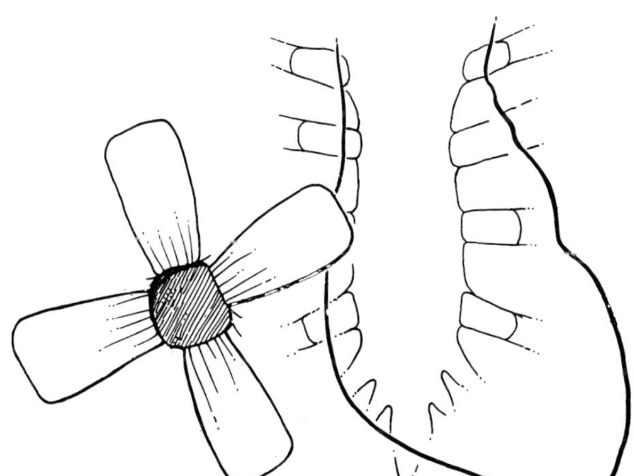

Figure 73–2. For port access mitral valve procedures, a limited right thoracotomy incision is made at the level of the fourth interspace. A soft-tissue retractor is placed and the right lung is deflated to permit access to the left atrium. (From Fann JI, Pompili MF, Burdon TA, et al: Minimally invasive mitral valve surgery. Semin Thorac Cardiovasc Surg 9:320–330, 1997, with permission.)

ing the siphon pressure between 40 and 90 mmHg.[26, 27] Systemic hypothermia (28 to 32°C) is generally employed. The endoaortic clamp is properly positioned with the aid of transesophageal echocardiography and contrast ascending aortography obtained under fluoroscopy. The aortic occlusion balloon is inflated using a mixture of saline and contrast dye (20 to 30%). A small amount of the dye is then infused into the aortic root to allow visualization of occlusion and proper position. Blood cardioplegia is administered in an antegrade fashion at flow rates of 250 to 300 ml/min, keeping the aortic pressure at 60 to 90 mmHg.[26, 27] After achieving antegrade cardioplegic arrest, retrograde cardioplegia can be delivered via the percutaneously placed coronary sinus catheter at a flow rate of 200 to 250 ml/min, keeping the coronary sinus pressure in the 30 to 50 mmHg range; the central lumen of the endoaortic clamp can be used as an aortic root vent.[24, 25]

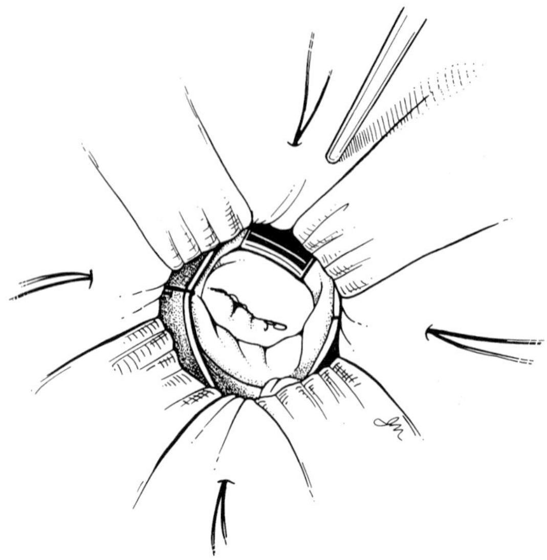

Figure 73–4. A left atrial retractor is placed through a separate stab incision, thereby directly exposing the mitral valve. (From Fann JI, Pompili MF, Burdon TA, et al: Minimally invasive mitral valve surgery. Semin Thorac Cardiovasc Surg 9:320–330, 1997, with permission.)

Mitral Valve Replacement or Repair

A standard left atriotomy is made, beginning at the level of the right superior pulmonary vein and extending inferiorly (Fig. 73–3).[7] The aortic root vent (or central lumen of the endoaortic clamp) is turned off during the mitral valve procedure to avoid entraining air into the aortic root. Retrograde cardioplegia is intermittently instilled during the valve procedure. A specially designed atrial retractor is placed through a small stab incision just medial to the limited thoracotomy incision. The mitral valve and subvalvular apparatus are visualized directly and with thoracoscopic assistance, if necessary (Fig. 73–4).[7] Standard valve repair or replacement techniques are carried out using long-shafted instruments to facilitate leaflet resection, suture placement, and knot tying (Fig. 73–5).[7] Occasionally, in smaller patients and those who have a shallow operative field, knot tying can be accomplished directly without using the knot-pushing device. Before completion of the atriotomy closure, initial dearing maneuvers include temporarily discontinuing pulmonary venting, inflating the lungs to displace residual air from the pulmonary veins, and increasing the patient's blood volume from the venous reservoir. The patient is placed in a Trendelenburg and left lateral decubitus position so that the left atriotomy site is the most nondependent region of the heart. The balloon of the endoaortic catheter is deflated, leaving the catheter in place for further deairing through the central lumen dur-

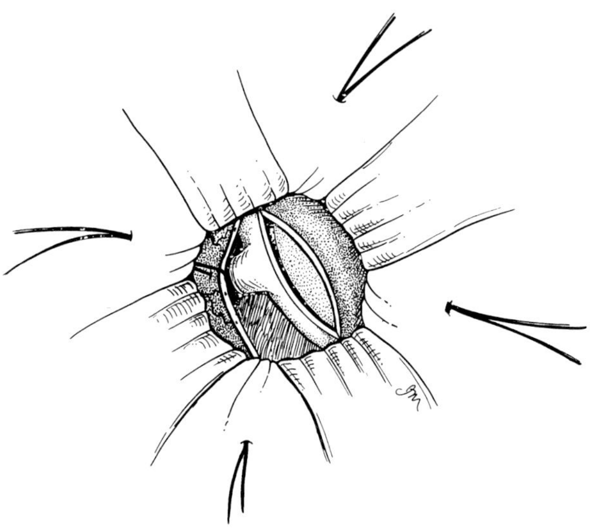

Figure 73–3. After a longitudinal pericardiotomy and placement of traction sutures, a left atriotomy is made beginning at the level of the right superior pulmonary vein and extending inferiorly. (From Fann JI, Pompili MF, Burdon TA, et al: Minimally invasive mitral valve surgery. Semin Thorac Cardiovasc Surg 9:320–330, 1997, with permission.)

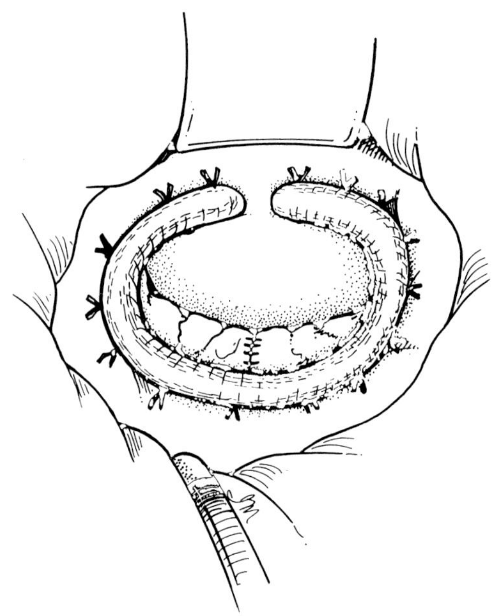

Figure 73–5. Using specially designed instruments, the mitral valve procedure is performed under direct vision (with thoracoscopic assistance, if necessary). (From Fann JI, Pompili MF, Burdon TA, et al: Minimally invasive mitral valve surgery. Semin Thorac Cardiovasc Surg 9:320–330, 1997, with permission.)

ing weaning from cardiopulmonary bypass. Additionally, with the heart decompressed, the aortic root can be accessed for direct placement of a pursestring suture followed by an aortic root vent to assist in further deairing. The endoaortic clamp is later removed. Temporary ventricular pacing wires are placed on the right ventricular wall. After weaning from cardiopulmonary bypass, the patient is decannulated and the anticoagulation reversed. A chest tube is placed into the right pleural cavity through the previous thoracoscope port.

Clinical Experience

The experience with port access mitral valve procedures has continued to increase since it was first performed in the clinical setting in 1995.[7, 9, 15, 19] In the initial clinical trial, 4 patients underwent port access mitral valve replacement for rheumatic valvular disease via a limited right anterior thoracotomy (mean incision length, 10 ± 3 cm).[19] There were no operative deaths. The average aortic cross-clamp time was 92 ± 18 minutes, and the mean cardiopulmonary bypass time was 138 ± 21 minutes. The mean operating time (from incision to skin closure) was 3 hours and 40 minutes. Intraoperative transesophageal echocardiography was used to assess prosthetic valve function; in 1 patient, a mild perivalvular leak was appreciated, and it was elected to follow this patient. One patient developed chest wall hemorrhage with resultant hypotension and required re-exploration; his course was complicated by a watershed cerebral infarct, presumably caused by hypotension and chronic respiratory failure that required tracheostomy. At 6 months follow-up, 3 patients had resumed full activity; the fourth patient continued to undergo rehabilitation. Following this initial experience, 10 patients underwent port access mitral valve procedures at Stanford University between May 1996 and January 1997.[7] The mean age of the patients (8 men and 2 women) was 54 ± 7 years; the average NYHA functional class was 2.7 ± 0.5. Nine patients had severe mitral regurgitation from myxomatous degeneration, and one had severe mitral regurgitation and moderate mitral stenosis from a rheumatic etiology. Two patients had markedly elevated pulmonary artery pressure (systolic > 70 mmHg). The left ventricular function of all but 2 patients was normal. Five patients underwent mitral valve replacement with a mechanical prosthesis because of extensive anterior and posterior leaflet pathology not deemed reparable. Five patients underwent mitral valve repair with quadrangular resection of the posterior leaflet and annuloplasty. There was no operative mortality. The mean incision length was 8.1 ± 2.5 cm. The aortic cross-clamp time averaged 99 ± 22 minutes, and the mean cardiopulmonary bypass time was 151 ± 52 minutes. The surgical time (i.e., skin to skin) averaged 4 hours and 21 minutes. All patients were extubated in less than 24 hours; the average stay in the intensive care unit was 1.7 ± 1.6 days. The total hospital stay averaged 4.3 ± 1.4 days. One patient who had a history of atrial arrhythmias underwent mitral valve replacement and developed third-degree atrioventricular block, requiring a prolonged stay in the intensive care unit and pacemaker placement; the same patient was found to have a perivalvular leak on follow-up, which required reoperation at 3 months. None of the patients required re-exploration for hemorrhage. One patient developed a groin seroma requiring drainage after discharge. All patients were well on follow-up. Thus, perioperative complications associated with port access mitral valve procedures in the early clinical experience were significant, but the complications cannot be considered unique to this technique and have also been reported with the conventional approach.

Mohr et al have reported their experience with 18 patients who underwent port access mitral valve repair for mitral regurgitation, stenosis, or both.[15] The length of the right minithoracotomy incision ranged from 3.8 to 6.5 cm. The mean duration of operation was 180 ± 33 minutes; the cardiopulmonary bypass times and the aortic cross-clamp times averaged 114 ± 21 minutes and 71 ± 16 minutes, respectively. The average time to extubation was 26 hours postoperatively. There was 1 early death due to a non-cardiac–related cause. One patient, who underwent quadrangular resection of the posterior leaflet, chordal replacement, and ring annuloplasty, was found to have persistent mitral regurgitation requiring mitral valve replacement. Two patients required postoperative exploration for hemorrhage, and 2 patients developed transient psychosis attributed to inadequate deairing of the heart. At a mean follow-up of 10 weeks, all patients were in NYHA functional class I or II. Echocardiography demonstrated adequacy of mitral valve repair in all patients, with only trivial mitral regurgitation in 5 patients.

Glower et al evaluated 39 patients who underwent mitral valve surgery using either the conventional median sternotomy approach (N = 20) or port access technique (N = 19).[9] Both groups were matched for age, sex, mitral pathology, ejection fraction, and comorbidity. Cardioplegic arrest times (119 ± 53 vs 99 ± 36 minutes) and cardiopulmonary bypass times (209 ± 67 vs 157 ± 36 minutes) were slightly longer for the port access technique. However, port access surgery permitted smaller incisions (8 ± 2 vs 26 ± 2 cm) and similar or shorter hospital stays (6 ± 4 vs 7 ± 3 days). By avoiding a median sternotomy, port access mitral valve surgery enabled a more rapid return to normal activity compared with the conventional approach (4 ± 2 vs 8 ± 2 weeks).

The early experience with port access mitral valve surgery has demonstrated advantages and disadvantages of this technique. A limited thoracotomy or access port requires no more operative time than a conventional sternotomy; however, the relatively deeper operative field for mitral valve procedures is associated with a distinct learning curve. This approach is somewhat facilitated by the specially designed shafted instruments. The average cross-clamp, cardiopulmonary bypass, and total operating room times are generally longer than with conventional techniques of mitral valve surgery; however, as the surgeon gains experience with the port access technique, the time required for the operation gradually decreases. Similarly, placement of the percutaneous pulmonary artery vent and retrograde cardioplegia catheters requires fluoroscopic guidance and technical expertise; again, the amount of time required decreases with increased experience. Proper positioning of the endoaortic clamp is important, because misplacement could result in left ventricular distention, unequal distribution of cardioplegia, or compromised perfusion of the arch vessels; therefore, close monitoring of the echocardiographic images and the radial artery lines is of utmost importance. A potential disadvantage is the inability to access the heart directly to ensure adequate deairing after the cardiotomy. Leaving the endoaortic catheter in place in the ascending aorta after deflation of the balloon and accessing the aortic root for direct placement of a venting catheter further ensure adequate deairing.

Summary

As a result of advances in video-assisted thoracoscopic surgery, techniques of minimally invasive mitral valve surgery using alternative incisions have been successfully performed at multiple centers. Less invasive methods promise less patient discomfort, less morbidity, and, possibly, lower overall cost, although current reports are predominantly anecdotal. The port access system is a catheter-based system that provides effective peripheral cardiopulmonary bypass, cardioplegic arrest, and ventricular decompression. This system enables the surgeon to perform various cardiac procedures, including mitral valve surgery, via smaller incisions in a still and bloodless field. The actual techniques employed in the replacement or repair are otherwise the same as those used in conventional procedures via a median sternotomy. As surgeons gain greater experience with port access mitral valve procedures, the operative times have decreased. Further clinical experience with long-term follow-up is necessary to fully evaluate the efficacy and patient benefit from the various techniques of minimally invasive mitral valve surgery.

References

1. Begos DG, Modlin EM: Laparoscopic cholecystectomy: From gimmick to gold standard. J Clin Gastroenterol 19:325–330, 1994.
2. Burke RP, Wernovsky G, van der Velde M, et al: Video-assisted thoracoscopic surgery for congenital heart disease. J Thorac Cardiovasc Surg 109:499–508, 1995.
3. Chitwood WR, Elbeery JR, Chapman WHH, et al: Video-assisted minimally invasive mitral valve surgery: The "micro-mitral" operation. J Thorac Cardiovasc Surg 113:413–414, 1997.
4. Chitwood WR, Wixon CL, Elbeery JR, et al: Video-assisted minimally invasive mitral valve surgery. J Thorac Cardiovasc Surg 114:773–782, 1997.
5. Deloche A, Jebara VA, Relland JY, et al: Valve repair with Carpentier techniques. The second decade. J Thorac Cardiovasc Surg 99:990–1002, 1990.
6. Falk V, Walther T, Diegeler A, et al: Echocardiographic monitoring of minimally invasive mitral valve surgery using an endoaortic clamp. J Heart Valve Dis 5:630–637, 1996.
7. Fann JI, Pompili MF, Burdon TA, et al: Minimally invasive mitral valve surgery. Semin Thorac Cardiovasc Surg 9:320–330, 1997.
8. Galloway AC, Colvin SB, Baumann FG, et al: Current concepts in mitral valve reconstruction for mitral insufficiency. Circulation 78(Suppl I): 97–105, 1988.
9. Glower DD, Landolfo K, Clements F, et al: Mitral valve operation via port-access versus median sternotomy. Abstract presented at the World Congress on Minimally Invasive Cardiac Surgery, Paris, May 1997.
10. Khan S, Chaux A, Matloff J, et al: The St. Jude Medical valve: Experience with 1000 cases. J Thorac Cardiovasc Surg 108: 1010–1020, 1994.
11. Kumar AS, Prasad S, Rai S, et al: Right thoracotomy revisited. Texas Heart J 20:40–41, 1993.
12. Landreneau RJ, Mack MJ, Hazelrigg SR, et al: Video-assisted thoracic surgery: Basic technical concepts and intercostal approach strategies. Ann Thorac Surg 54:800–807, 1992.
13. Lin PJ, Chang CH, Chu JJ, et al: Video-assisted mitral valve operations. Ann Thorac Surg 61:1781–1787, 1996.
14. Mack MJ, Aronoff RJ, Acuff TE, et al: Present role of thoracoscopy in the diagnosis and management of diseases of the chest. Ann Thorac Surg 54:401–409, 1992.
15. Mohr FW, Falk V, Diegeler A, et al: First results with video-assisted minimally invasive mitral valve repair using the port-access system. Abstract presented at the American Association for Thoracic Surgery, Washington, D.C., April 1997.
16. Peters WS: Minimally invasive cardiac surgery by cardioscopy. Aust J Thorac Cardiovasc Surg 2:152–154, 1993.
17. Peters WS, Siegel LC, Stevens JH, et al: Closed chest cardiopulmonary bypass and cardioplegia: Basis for less invasive cardiac surgery. Ann Thorac Surg 63:1748–1751, 1997.
18. Pompili MF, Stevens JH, Burdon TA, et al: Port-access mitral valve replacement in dogs. J Thorac Cardiovasc Surg 112: 1268–1274, 1964.
19. Pompili MF, Yakub A, Siegel LC, et al: Port-access mitral valve replacement: Initial clinical experience. Circulation 94(suppl I): I-533, 1996.
20. Reitz BA, Stevens JH, Burdon TA, et al: Port-access coronary artery bypass grafting: Lessons learned in a Phase I clinical trial (Abstract). Circulation 94:1294, 1996.
21. Schwartz DS, Ribakove GH, Grossi EA, et al: Minimally invasive cardiopulmonary bypass with cardioplegic arrest: A closed chest technique with equivalent myocardial protection. J Thorac Cardiovasc Surg 111:556–566, 1996.
22. Schwartz DS, Ribakove GH, Grossi EA, et al: Minimally invasive mitral valve replacement: Port-access technique, feasibility and myocardial function preservation. J Thorac Cardiovasc Surg 113:1022–1031, 1997.
23. Siegel LC, St. Goar FG, Stevens JH, et al: Monitoring considerations for port-access cardiac surgery. Circulation 96:562–568, 1997.
24. Stevens JH, Burdon TA, Peters WS, et al: Port-access coronary artery bypass grafting: A proposed surgical method. J Thorac Cardiovasc Surg 111:567–573, 1996.
25. Stevens JH, Burdon TA, Siegel LC, et al: Port-access coronary artery bypass with cardioplegic arrest: Acute and chronic canine studies. Ann Thorac Surg 62:435–441, 1996.
26. Toomasian JM, Peters WS, Siegel LC, et al: Extracorporeal circulation for port-access cardiac surgery. Perfusion 12:83–91, 1997.
27. Toomasian JM, Williams DL, Colvin SB, et al: Perfusion during coronary and mitral valve surgery utilizing minimally invasive port-access technology. J Extra-Corporeal Technol 29:66–72, 1997.
28. Tribble CG, Killinger WA, Harman PK, et al: Anterolateral thoracotomy as an alternative to repeat median sternotomy for replacement of the mitral valve. Ann Thorac Surg 43:380–382, 1987.

COMMENTARY

W. Randolph Chitwood, Jr.

In 1996, port access cardiac surgery was launched in the United States, largely by the efforts of this Stanford University group. This entirely new technologic concept began to bridge the innovation gap between traditional cardiac surgeons and intervention-based cardiology colleagues. This method alone gained more attention than any other new procedure in launching the new era of minimally invasive cardiac surgery. For the first time, cardiac surgeons considered widespread use of intravascular balloon catheters, inserted peripherally to occlude the aorta and administer cardioplegia.

In the last 2 years, well over 1000 coronary and valve operations have been done using port access methods. Despite multicenter adoption of these new devices, few large patient series have been reported to date. However, data are accruing that suggest the benefits of port access methods in performing minimally invasive coronary and mitral valve surgery. As with most new surgical techniques, surgeons have experienced an early learning curve with technique-related complications that include aortic dissections and endoclamp balloon dislodgement. Despite these concerns, experienced users have shown that these devices can facilitate even the most complex minimally invasive cardiac operations. Moreover, with increased institutional use, complications appear to decrease along with operative times.

In this chapter, Dr. Ikonomidis and associates at Stanford describe the experimental evolution of the port access method, as well as early clinical series. Moreover, detailed descriptions of the technique and indications for use are included. Also, patient exclusionary criteria are defined and include patients with severe iliofemoral arterial disease, diffuse aortic atherosclerosis, and significant cerebrovascular involvement. The potential of balloon dislodgement is mentioned; however, technique-induced retrograde aortic dissections are underemphasized. Caution regarding this dreaded complication is especially important for surgeons just beginning to adopt the technique. At the May 1997 meeting of the American Association for Thoracic Surgery, Mohr and associates presented the first 51 of their patients who had undergone port access mitral valve surgery at the University of Leipzig.[1] In this initial group, 2 retrograde aortic dissections occurred as did 6 balloon clamp dislodgements. Both complications resulted in severe neurologic injuries. The initial procedural mortality was 9.8%; however, by June of 1998 this had fallen to 4.0% for the overall series of 120 mitral patients. No aortic dissections occurred in the last 70 patients.[2] During the same period, Colvin and associates at New York University found the converse, experiencing a single retrograde dissection in over 200 mitral valve operations. Although their series mortality was 3.3% overall, the mortality was 1.1% for isolated mitral operations.[3] Those who have encountered retrograde dissections appear to have done so early in their experience, suggesting heightened caution at this time. As of January 1997, the Heartport International Registry showed that 412 patients worldwide had undergone a minimally invasive mitral operation using port access methods. The overall operative mortality was 3.2%, but it rose to 5.6% by 30 days. Of these patients, 57% underwent mitral repairs and 43% had prosthetic replacements. These data suggest that appropriate numbers of repairs are being done in most centers. By comparison, Cosgrove, Cohn, and our group have reported an operative mortality between 0% and 2.2% in over 350 minimally invasive mitral operations, each done using direct aortic clamping techniques. Moreover, Cosgrove and Cohn have reported significantly less operative cardiopulmonary perfusion and arrest times than noted when using either the port access method or our transthoracic clamp technique.[4–6] Thus, overall operative mortality, complication rates, operative times, and repair or replacement selection must be considered when selecting the best minimal access approach. Technique preference must not supersede clinical judgment.

Vanermin and Mohr have been able to reduce the minithoracotomy incision size to 4 cm for mitral surgery by using the port access method.[2] Other current thoracic and sternal minimally invasive cardiac incisions will be difficult to reduce to this size. Therefore, to achieve true micro-access, the port access method may provide a pathway for development of a truly endoscopic mitral operation. Moreover, to avoid the complications inherent in retrograde perfusion and aortic balloon occlusion, central aortic cannulation remains an important challenge. These and other technical solutions are being developed by several companies and may propel intra-aortic balloon occlusion even further. Although surgeons, cardiologists, and patients have become intrigued by the port access technique because it makes "intellectual sense," several factors must be stable before there will be greater acceptance by surgeons. Operative and perfusion or arrest times must decrease, and it is expected that they will fall. Also, operative mortality and complications must approximate or be less than both conventional and other current minimally invasive valve operations. Finally, surgeons practicing currently must be able to repair mitral valves with the same facility as they now do via the sternotomy.

Ikonomidis and the Stanford group are to be congratulated for their pioneering work and their comprehensive presentation in this chapter. The innovative spirit emanating from Stanford may be a major springboard for a Renaissance style of thinking in cardiac surgery. However, other surgeons must lend a hand to modify and improve these exciting new technologies for performing cardiac surgery. Careful data collection and critical reporting must remain effective monitors to determine our true successes—that is, *true benefits to our patients.*

References

1. Mohr FW, Falk V, Diegeler A, et al: Minimally invasive port-access mitral valve surgery. J Thorac Cardiovasc Surg 115:567–574, 1998.
2. Mohr F, Falk V: The evolution of minimally invasive mitral valve surgery—two year experience. Presented at the first annual meeting of the International Society for Minimally Invasive Cardiac Surgery, Minneapolis, MN, June 27, 1998.
3. Colvin S: Symposium: Minimally invasive valve surgery, American Heart Association Annual Meeting, Orlando, Florida, November 1997.

4. Cosgrove DM, Sabik JF, Navia J: Minimally invasive valve surgery. Ann Thorac Surg 1998:64 (in press).
5. Aklog L, Adams DH, Couper GS, et al: Techniques and results of minimally invasive mitral valve surgery in 100 patients: A paradigm for the future. J Thorac Cardiovasc Surg 1998 (in press).
6. Chitwood WR, Elbeery JR, Chapman WHH, et al: Video-assisted minimally invasive mitral valve surgery: The "micro-mitral" operation. J Thorac Cardiovasc Surg 113:413–414, 1997.

COMMENTARY

William S. Peters

Advances in surgical technique and technology in the late 1980s allowed the development of minimally invasive abdominal and thoracic surgical procedures to the point where some of these operations are currently considered routine and a first-line option. These procedures provide the definitive benefits of conventional operations while minimizing injury in accessing the body. In 1990, as an intern exposed to this rapid change, I asked myself, "What is, and how do we achieve, minimally invasive cardiac surgery?" In the previous year I had spent the elective period of my final year of medical training in the Cardiothoracic Surgical Unit at Greenlane Hospital, New Zealand, and taking what I had seen and learned, I understood that to achieve minimally invasive cardiac surgery, it was necessary to avoid or limit the chest incision and degree of rib retraction and dissection, and that the operating conditions that cardiopulmonary bypass and cardioplegia allow must be reproduced. I proposed a method of femorofemoral bypass and ascending aortic balloon catheter. The latter device was designed to effect aortic occlusion, antegrade cardioplegia infusion, and cardiac venting, thus mimicking the current standards of cardiac surgery, and providing a platform for recreating cardiac surgical procedures in a minimally invasive fashion. I focused on cardioscopy, right heart surgical procedures, and coronary artery bypass grafting. I proposed a double-balloon femoral venous cannula for bicaval drainage and right atrial isolation. Infusion of cold saline into the chambers of the heart allows the possibility of endoluminal, or cardioscopic, intervention in the aortic root, the aortic valve, the coronary arteries, and the right heart. This approach was obviously very complex and limited by the degree of intervention versus inspection. By using ports in the intercostal spaces, the right atrium could be entered, and tasks such as repair of an atrial septal defect were obvious. The idea for coronary artery bypass grafting evolved from this work, and I proposed a method of thoracoscopic internal mammary artery harvesting and using the endoluminal cardiopulmonary bypass system for constructing anastomoses on the arrested, bloodless heart via a small incision under the left breast.

After formulating these theoretical proposals, I set out to test several hypotheses; first, that the human ascending aorta could be occluded by a balloon catheter that would maintain its position against arterial perfusion pressure. This was achieved using an explanted human cadaveric heart and great vessels and a 30-ml 16 French Foley urinary catheter. The balloon was well positioned in the mid-ascending aorta, and there was no movement of the balloon up to 150 mmHg pressure in the distal aorta. Greatly encouraged, I successfully tested out thoracoscopic internal mammary artery (IMA) harvesting in a live anesthetized pig, and in a human cadaver I determined that access to the coronary arteries supplying the left ventricle was possible via a limited left anterior thoracotomy in the fourth intercostal space. This latter observation was made on the presumption that the heart was arrested and the balloon catheter vented, which allowed the heart to be manipulated, exposing the various coronary arteries for direct anastomosis. My original proposals and the results of these feasibility studies were published in *The Australasian Journal of Cardiac and Thoracic Surgery* in 1993.

John H. Stevens, a resident in Cardiothoracic Surgery at Stanford University Medical Center, California, proposed and tested a method of endoluminal aortic valve surgery, including valve replacement, using a very similar platform of femorofemoral bypass and an aortic balloon catheter. Stevens and associates extended its application to more practical applications, primarily in coronary artery bypass grafting and mitral valve replacement. Following my publication, I was contacted by Stevens and I joined the Stanford research and development effort in 1994. In preparing for initial clinical cases, we performed many acute and chronic canine studies evaluating techniques and devices. In the dog, the chest is deep anteroposteriorly, and this facilitated thoracoscopic IMA takedown and thoracomicroscopic IMA to left anterior descending coronary artery anastomosis. In human cadaver studies, the problems of a flatter chest were evident, and trials were conducted of the method of IMA dissection and the approach to the coronary arteries via a left anterior small thoracotomy. After attempting the first three clinical cases using the endoluminal cardiopulmonary bypass system and totally thoracoscopic left internal mammary artery (LIMA) to the left anterior descending coronary artery bypass graft—two of which converted to open procedures—a small anterior thoracotomy, with or without costal cartilage mobilization, was used. This method has proven to facilitate the time, accuracy, and number of anastomoses performed with minimal incisions. Mitral valve replacement was highly developed by Drs. Greg Ribakove (New York University) and Mario Pompili (Stanford). Because of the size and anatomy of the dog, the procedure and device development used an approach through the left atrial appendage. In human cadavers, both left and right hemithorax approaches were evaluated and found to be feasible. In practice, the right side is used because the exposure is uniformly better, but the approach is disadvantaged by the depth to the mitral annulus. The main concerns with this method are tying secure knots and deairing the heart. Developments, such as knot substitutes, ensure quicker and more secure prosthesis implantation. Risk of air embolism in minimally invasive valve procedures can be reduced—a high concentration of carbon dioxide is easily maintained within the closed chest cavity, and following deairing maneuvers, the carbon dioxide content of any gas that is retained in the cardiac chambers is quickly absorbed by the blood. We expanded the clinical platform to include bicaval venous drainage and right atrial isolation. Certainly, in preclinical studies, direct snaring or clamping of the cavae was preferable to balloon occlusion because it was simple, quick, and secure. The cavae were more compliant, and it was more difficult getting good balloon occlusion.

With the endovascular CPB platform, applying minimally invasive techniques to cardiovascular surgical problems is feasible. The bypass system makes it possible to duplicate the advantages of conventional open chest cardiac surgery by performing the same surgical correction via small chest wall ports. The Endoaortic Clamp has proven to be safe and effective in its 3 years of clinical use. The inflated Endoaortic Clamp balloon has a tendency to migrate if a significant pressure gradient exists across the balloon or if the balloon is inadequately filled. The minimum balloon volume occluding the ascending aorta can be calculated as the volume of a sphere using the radius of the ascending aorta as measured by transesophageal echocardiograpy. Avoiding a sternotomy may diminish the stress response to the operation and to cardiopulmonary bypass, reduce blood loss, eliminate the risk of delayed sternal healing and mediastinitis, shorten the rehabilitation period, and make redo surgery safer. A superior cosmetic result is achieved. Femoral arterial cannulation is associated with the risk of retrograde aortic dissection, embolism of atherosclerotic debris, limb ischemia, and lymph leak. The risks of femoral cannulation are offset to some extent by the avoidance of morbidity associated with sternotomy, aortic cannulation, and cross-clamping. The surgery is difficult and there is a significant learning curve. A dedicated team approach is very important to the success of this form of surgery. Dr. Mark Groh (Asheville) advocates the concept of "parallel tasking" to streamline the operative procedure. Patient selection based on history, examination, and appropriate investigation is very important.

I believe that the clinical results of port access cardiac surgery achieved to date in dedicated centers sets out a foundation for the further development of minimally invasive cardiac surgery and cardioscopy in a wide range of patients. As molecular surgery evolves, the endovascular cardiopulmonary bypass and cardioplegia system may also play a role in gene therapy targeted to the heart.

Section IX

Miscellaneous Cardiac Procedures

Chapter 74

Minimally Invasive Surgery for Congenital Heart Defects

Pyng Jing Lin, Jaw-Ji Chu, and Chau-Hsiung Chang

Surgical correction of simple congenital heart diseases, such as atrial septal defect (ASD) and ventricular septal defect (VSD), has been successful with minimal morbidity and mortality. However, the poor cosmetic effect and possible complications of median sternotomy are occasionally troublesome.[20]

Video-assisted laparoscopic surgical techniques have been applied in the milieu of abdominal or pelvic lesions since the late 1980s. These techniques have been introduced to treat intrathoracic lesions since the early 1990s. The aim of these surgeries is to lessen incisional pain, minimize incisional length, enhance functional recovery, and shorten hospital stay.[32]

Video-assisted thoracoscopic surgical treatment of congenital cardiovascular lesions was initiated in 1991 for treatment of patent ductus arteriosus.[21] It is now a standard procedure.[5–7, 14, 21–23, 37] However, it was not until 1995 that these minimally invasive surgical techniques were employed in treatment of congenital intracardiac lesions.[12, 42] Although there was some criticism of these procedures,[17, 36] minimally invasive surgery for correction of congenital heart lesions has been increasingly discussed in the literature.[13, 24]

In this review, we present the results we have achieved at Chang Gung Memorial Hospital, Taipei, Taiwan, with the use of minimally invasive surgical techniques in patients who have simple intracardiac congenital defects, ASD, or VSD.

Minimally Invasive Surgery for Atrial Septal Defect

After induction of general anesthesia, transesophageal echocardiography monitoring is set up and the diagnosis of ostium secundum is reconfirmed. The patient is placed in the left semi-decubitus position with exposure of the right groin. A right anterior submammary mini-thoracotomy (4 to 6 cm in length) (Fig. 74–1) is made through the fourth intercostal space.[12, 13] A small rib spreader is used for this incision to facilitate manipulation of the instruments. Cardiopulmonary bypass is established through cannulation of the right femoral artery and the right femoral vein[2–4, 19, 25, 26] or inferior vena cava via the right atrium. Systemic hypothermia (28.1 ± 2.9°C) is begun immediately after the start of cardiopulmonary bypass. The aorta is not cross-clamped. The heart is protected by continuous coronary perfusion while fibrillation is induced. Topical cooling is applied to facilitate fibrillation of the heart, enhance myocardial protection, and avoid deep hypothermia.

After the heart has been fibrillated, a 4-cm stab incision is made on the right atrium, which is then entered. The blood from the superior vena cava is cleared by a cardiotomy sucker, a cannula connected to the cardiopulmonary bypass system, or by clamping the superior vena cava for 10 to 15 minutes, being careful to avoid congestion or swelling of the head. For patients who have persistent left superior vena cava, a cardiotomy sucker placed in the coronary sinus can clear the operative field. An endoscope (Stryker Endoscopy, San Jose, CA) is inserted through a thoracostomy incision in some patients to assist the surgical repair of ASD. In most patients, the repair procedure can be performed under direct vision. The ASD is closed directly or by means of a knitted Dacron patch (Meadox Medicals, Inc., Oakland, NJ) or autologous pericardium. In patients who have ASD involving the sinus venosus, closure was performed successfully with the patch. During closure of the ASD, care is taken to fill the left atrium with blood. The air in the left atrium is carefully evacuated by rotating the operating table in all directions and expanding the lungs before completing closure of the ASD. After closure of the ASD, the right atriotomy is closed with a running suture. Before the heart starts beating again, there should be no obvious air bubble in the left atrium or left ventricle as noted by a transesophageal echocardiographic examination. Air in the left atrium, if any, can be vented through the right pulmonary vein, which is on the highest portion of the left atrium. The patient is then reversed to a head-down position. Cardioversion is easily achieved by placing two small cardioverter pads (CodeMaster, Hewlett-Packard Company, McMinnville, Oregon) on the surface of the heart.

Sinus rhythm is restored (this occurred in all of our patients). Cardiopulmonary bypass is terminated after the patient is rewarmed. Transesophageal echocardiographic examinations have shown complete closure of the ASD without any residual shunt, with the exception of 1 patient,

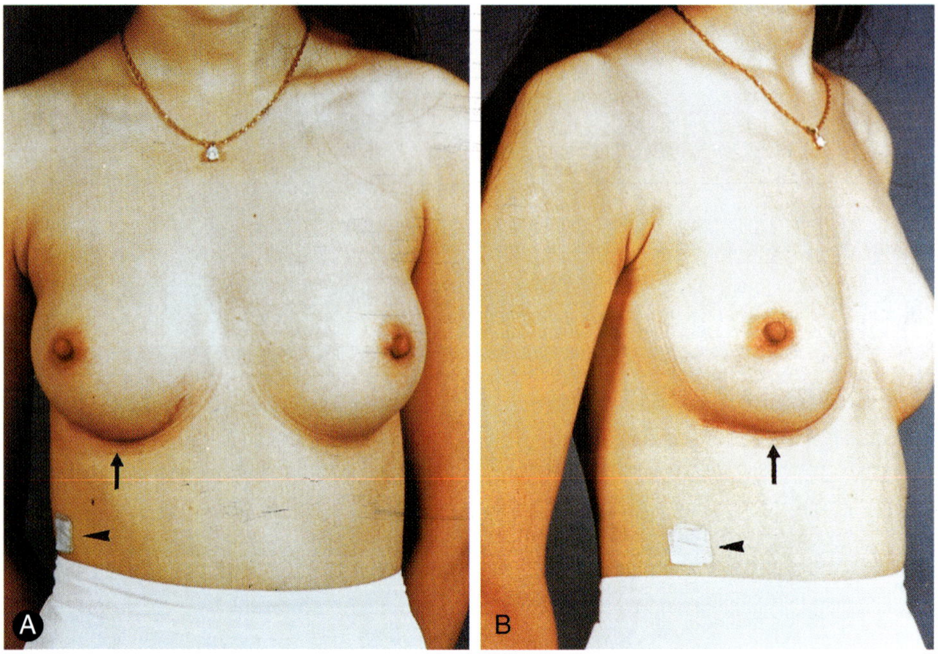

Figure 74–1. Photographs of a 22-year-old woman taken 1 month after minimally invasive surgical closure of atrial septal defect. Arrowhead indicates the thoracostomy created in the seventh intercostal space along the anterior axillary line for introduction of the endoscope and also for insertion of the pleural drain. The arrow indicates the submammary mini-thoracotomy incision.

whose shunt subsequently disappeared during the follow-up period. The thoracostomy incision used for insertion of the endoscope is then used for tubal drainage of the pericardial and pleural spaces. Hemostasis and closure of the incisions are easily achieved.

Comparison Between Minimally Invasive Surgery and Median Sternotomy in Patients With Atrial Septal Defect

Cardiopulmonary bypass time was significantly longer in patients who were treated with minimally invasive surgery than for those who underwent median sternotomy.[13] There was no difference between patients operated on via minimally invasive surgery and those who underwent median sternotomy in terms of operation time, transfusion of packed red blood cells, intensive care unit stay, and duration of chest tube insertion. However, length of incision, incidence of temporary pacemaker use, duration of endotracheal intubation, timing of first oral intake after operation, amount of drainage 24 hours postoperatively, total incidence of parenteral narcotic injection, and postoperative length of stay were significantly shorter and lower in patients who had minimally invasive surgery than in those who had median sternotomy. Resumption of normal activity, judged by return to school or work, was significantly faster in patients in the minimally invasive surgery group than in those in the median sternotomy group. These data indicate that minimally invasive surgery can lessen incisional pain, minimize incisional length, enhance functional recovery, and shorten hospital stay.

Minimally Invasive Surgery for Ventricular Septal Defect

After induction of general anesthesia, transesophageal echocardiographic monitoring is set up and the diagnosis of ventricular septal defect reconfirmed.[29] The patient is placed in a supine position with exposure of the left groin. Extracorporeal circulation is established through cannulation of the left femoral artery and the left femoral vein (Fig. 74–2*D*).[2–4, 19, 25, 26] Systemic hypothermia is begun immediately after the start of extracorporeal circulation. A left anterior parasternal mini-thoracotomy incision (see Fig. 74–2*A*) is made and the pleural space is entered through the division of the third (see Fig. 74–2*B*) or fourth costal cartilage in patients who have subarterial (Fig. 74–3*A*) or perimembranous ventricular septal defect. A 10-mm endoscope (Stryker Endoscopy, San Jose, CA) and other conventional surgical instruments are introduced through the thoracotomy incision. The left phrenic nerve is identified and the pericardium carefully incised longitudinally anterior to the phrenic nerve to expose the right ventricle (see Fig. 74–3*C*). The aorta is not cross-clamped. The heart is protected by continuous coronary perfusion with hypothermic fibrillatory arrest (rectal temperature 27.3 ± 3.0°C).

Topical cooling is applied to facilitate fibrillation of the heart. After the heart is fibrillated, a 1- to 2-cm incision is made on the right ventricular outflow tract, which is then entered. Care is taken to avoid injury to the major coronary artery branches. A cardiotomy suction tube is inserted into the right ventricle and the ventricular septal defect is identified with the assistance of the endoscope via projected images on the video monitor (see Fig. 74–3*A*). In patients who have mild aortic regurgitation, a suction catheter is inserted through a stab incision on the apex of the left ventricle. Conventional hand suturing for closure of the ventricular septal defect and ventriculotomy is performed smoothly through the thoracotomy incision with the guide of the endoscope.

The ventricular septal defect is identified and a small tube connected to the cardiotomy suction system is inserted into the left ventricle via the ventricular septal defect, which outlines the margin of the defect. The ventric-

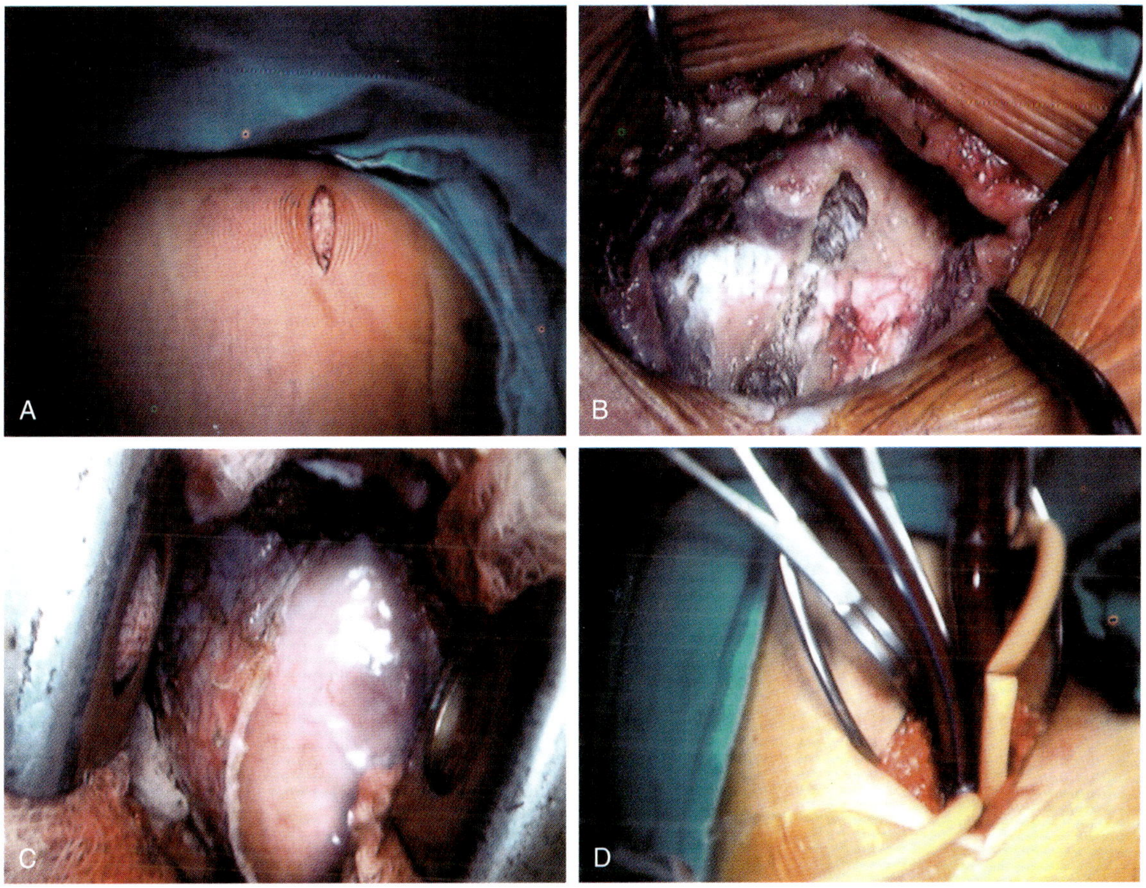

Figure 74–2. *A*, In a patient with ventricular septal defect, a 6-cm left parasternal incision was made. *B*, After division of the pectoralis major muscle, the third costal cartilage was divided. *C*, After longitudinal pericardiotomy, the right ventricular outflow tract was exposed. *D*, Cardiopulmonary bypass was established by cannulation of the femoral artery and the femoral vein.

ular septal defect is closed directly or by means of a patch (see Fig. 74–3*B*).

Before closure of the ventricular septal defect is completed, the air in the left ventricle is carefully evacuated by rotating the operating table in all directions and by inflating both lungs. A venting needle can be applied in the apex of the left ventricle to evacuate residual air, if any. There should be no obvious air bubble in the left atrium or left ventricle as recorded by transesophageal echocardiographic examination before the heart starts beating again. The patient is reversed to a head-down position. Cardioversion is easily performed by placing cardioverter pads on the surface of the heart. Sinus rhythm is resumed (this occurred in all of our patients). The right ventriculotomy is then closed directly with running suture or with a patch (see Fig. 74–3*C*).

Extracorporeal circulation is terminated after the patient is rewarmed. The femoral arteriotomy and venotomy are closed with 5-0 and 6-0 Prolene (Ethicon, Ltd., UK) interrupted sutures. Transesophageal echocardiographic examinations confirm complete closure of the ventricular septal defect without any residual shunt. The pericardium is closed with interrupted sutures. Dobutamine or sodium nitroprusside is not used. There is no AV block. However, a temporary pacemaker system is set up routinely. The pleural drainage tube is inserted. Hemostasis and closure of the incisions (see Fig. 74–3*D*) are easily achieved.

In our experience, duration of extracorporeal circulation is 40 ± 15 minutes. The operation time is 2.5 ± 0.5 hours. All our patients regained consciousness promptly after surgery. The endotracheal tube is removed on the operative night. Patients are transferred out of the intensive care unit on the first postoperative day. There has been no organ failure, and the postoperative course has been uneventful. The postoperative length of stay is 3 to 5 days (mean 4.5). There have been no wound, neurologic, or lower limb vascular complications. Follow-up transthoracic echocardiographic examination has not shown any residual shunt. All the patients are doing well.

Comment

Median sternotomy is the gold standard in the repair of congenital heart disease.[20] However, long incision length, postoperative pain, unsatisfactory cosmetic effect, and possible complications of sternotomy (e.g., mediastinitis, osteomyelitis) occasionally make repair of septal defects troublesome. In patients who have ASD, right anterior submammary mini-thoracotomy through the fourth intercostal space without excision of the ribs provides adequate

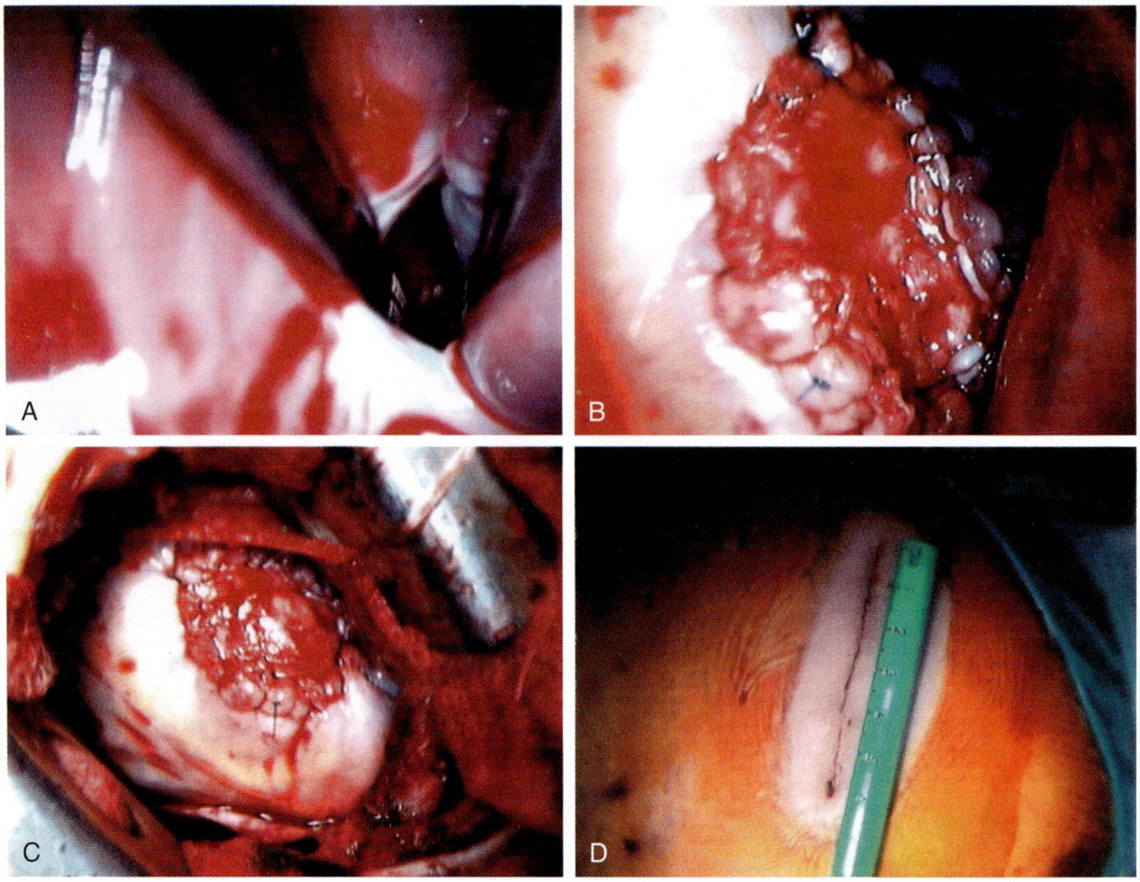

Figure 74–3. Minimally invasive surgical closure of subpulmonic ventricular septal defect. *A*, A subpulmonic ventricular septal defect was found. *B*, The ventricular septal defect was closed with a patch. *C*, The right ventricular outflow tract was closed with a patch. D, The left parasternal incision was closed.

exposure of the defect with excellent cosmetic healing (see Fig. 74–1). Left anterior parasternal mini-thoracotomy without resection of the costal cartilage of the third or fourth ribs can be performed for correction of ventricular septal defect. A small rib spreader, ports, trocars, or thoracoports can be used with these incisions to facilitate instrumentation. An endoscope can be inserted through the thoracotomy incision or through a separate thoracostomy incision for illumination or exploration of the lesions. The minimally invasive nature of this procedure reduces the incidence of postoperative mediastinitis and wound pain to a minimum.

Minimally invasive surgery for cardiac lesions can be performed on a beating heart[1, 5–9, 18, 24, 34, 35, 40, 41, 45, 48] with the use of a port access endovascular cardiopulmonary bypass system,[15, 38, 39, 43, 44] femorofemoral cardiopulmonary bypass with fibrillatory arrest (without aortic cross-clamping),[10, 12, 13, 27–29, 47] and cardiopulmonary bypass with aortic cross-clamping and cardioplegic arrest.[30, 31, 49, 50] In the correction of simple cardiac lesions with short cardiopulmonary bypass time, such as ASD or ventricular septal defect, femorofemoral cardiopulmonary bypass with fibrillatory arrest provides adequate myocardial protection and good tissue perfusion.[12, 13, 29] Topical cooling of the heart can be applied to facilitate fibrillation of the heart, enhance myocardial protection, and avoid deep hypothermia. Fibrillatory arrest can provide a quiet and steady operative field.

For pediatric patients who have ASD, the femoral vein may be too small to be cannulated. Cannulation with snaring of the inferior vena cava via the right atrium through the manipulation incision can be performed easily. The blood from the superior vena cava can be cleared by using the cardiotomy sucker, inserting the cannula connected to the cardiopulmonary bypass system, or temporarily clamping the superior vena cava . In our series, there was no organ failure postoperatively, and the patients regained consciousness promptly after the surgeries, indicating adequate tissue perfusion during cardiopulmonary bypass. The femoral artery and vein, although small in caliber in pediatric patients, can be easily repaired without stenosis. There were no vascular complications of the lower limbs in our patients.

Deairing is an important procedure in cardiac surgery, especially in minimally invasive surgery in which the aorta is not cross-clamped. Deairing can be accomplished by filling the left ventricle and then the left atrium with saline solution or blood; by expanding the lungs while rotating the operating table in all directions during air evacuation of the left ventricle and left atrium before complete closure of the atrial or ventricular septal defect; by inserting a venting needle into the right pulmonary vein (which is located on the superior portion of the left atrium) with the patient who has ASD in the left semi-decubitus position, or into the apex of the left ventricle of a patient who has ventricular septal defect, in order to evacuate the residual air, if any; by conducting a transesophageal echocardiographic examination to check for any residual air; and by keeping the patient in a head-down position before the heart resumes beating following the previously mentioned maneuvers.

Cardioversion can be easily performed by placing cardioverter pads on the surface of the heart through the mini-thoracotomy incision. Cardioversion can also be performed by taping an external cardioverter to the chest and the back of the patients before the start of the operation.

Direct or patch closure of the ASD can be successfully achieved through a right submammary incision under direct vision or under the guidance of the endoscope. In patients who have a sinus venosus type of ASD, patch closure is also feasible.

The choice of approach for VSD repair varies significantly among surgeons or centers performing this type of surgery. Repair of subarterial VSD can be accomplished through the pulmonary valve.[46] The right atrial approach is the route of choice for closure of other types of ventricular septal defect. A right atriotomy can reduce the prevalence of right bundle branch block but does not prevent late atrioventricular block.[16] Prevalence of ventricular arrhythmias increases with follow-up duration and age at evaluation, whether the surgical approach is through the right atrium or the ventricle.[16] This indicates that the right atrial approach cannot prevent the occurrence of ventricular arrhythmia. In our institute, subarterial or perimembranous septal defect is routinely closed through the transventricular route, which provides excellent exposure (see Fig. 74–3A).[11] We have not been able to document a significant adverse effect on mortality or morbidity resulting from the use of the ventricular approach, which is accomplished through an incision in the right ventricular outflow tract. The exposure of the VSD through the right ventricular outflow tract with the aid of video-assisted endoscope, has yielded excellent results in this series, and closure of the VSD can be easily accomplished by this approach.

We believe that minimally invasive thoracic surgeries can fulfill the promise of expediency, safety, minimal discomfort, diminished postoperative pain, quick functional recuperation, excellent cosmetic healing, shortened hospital stay, and, therefore, cost savings.[33] In our experience of minimally invasive surgery for ASD and VSD, there was no morbidity or mortality. All patients were satisfied with the cosmetic healing. These results indicate that minimally invasive surgery is a safe procedure with the expectation of benefit as previously mentioned. However, general and routine application of these procedures needs further long-term analysis of a larger series and comparison with results achieved by median sternotomy.

References

1. Acuff TE, Landreneau RJ, Griffith BP, et al: Minimally invasive coronary artery bypass grafting. Ann Thorac Surg 61: 135–137,1996.
2. Akins CW: Noncardioplegic myocardial preservation for coronary revascularization. J Thorac Cardiovasc Surg 88:174–181, 1984.
3. Akins CW, Carroll DL: Event-free survival following nonemergency myocardial revascularization during hypothermic fibrillatory arrest. Ann Thorac Surg 43:628–633, 1987.
4. Akins CW: 1987: Early and late results following emergency isolated myocardial revascularization during hypothermic fibrillatory arrest. Updated in 1994 by Cary W. Akins, MD. Ann Thorac Surg 1994;58:1205,1206.
5. Burke RP, Chang AC: Video-assisted thoracoscopic division of a vascular ring in an infant: A new operative technique. J Cardiac Surg 8:537–540, 1993.
6. Burke RP: Video-assisted thoracoscopic surgery for patent ductus arteriosus. Pediatrics 93:823–825,1994.
7. Burke RP, Wernovsky G, van der Velde M, et al: Video-assisted thoracoscopic surgery for congenital heart disease. J Thorac Cardiovasc Surg 109:499–507, 1995.
8. Calafiore AM, Angelini GD, Bergsland J, et al: Minimally invasive coronary artery bypass grafting. Ann Thorac Surg 62:1545–1548, 1996.
9. Calafiore AM, Teodori G, Di Giammarco G, et al: Minimally invasive coronary artery bypass grafting on a beating heart. Ann Thorac Surg 63(suppl 6):S72–S75, 1997.
10. Carpentier A, Loulmet D, Carpentier A, et al: First open heart operation (mitral valvuloplasty) under videosurgery through a minithoracotomy. C R Acad Sci Paris 319:219–223, 1996.
11. Chang CH, Lee MC, Hsieh MJ: Surgical treatment of supracristal type of ventricular septal defect. Scand J Thorac Cardiovasc Surg 22:221–225, 1988.
12. Chang CH, Lin PJ, Chu JJ, et al: Video-assisted cardiac surgery in closure of atrial septal defect. Ann Thorac Surg 62:697–701, 1996.
13. Chang CH, Lin PJ, Chu JJ, et al: Surgical closure of atrial septal defect. Minimally invasive cardiac surgery or median sternotomy? Surg Endosc 12:820–824, 1998.
14. Chu JJ, Chang CH, Lin PJ, et al: Video-assisted thoracoscopic surgery for interruption of patent ductus arteriosus in adult. Ann Thorac Surg 63:175–179, 1997.
15. Fann JI, Pompili MF, Stevens JH, et al: Port-access cardiac operations with cardioplegic arrest. Ann Thorac Surg 63(suppl 6):S35–S39, 1997.
16. Houyel L, Vaksmann G, Fournier A, et al: Ventricular arrhythmias after correction of ventricular septal defects. Importance of surgical approach. J Am Coll Cardiol 16:1224–1228, 1990.
17. Izzat MB, Yim AP: Minimally invasive direct atrial septal defect closure. Ann Thorac Surg 63:1831–1834, 1997.
18. King RC, Reece TB, Hurst JL, et al: Minimally invasive coronary artery bypass grafting decreases hospital stay and cost. Ann Surg 225:805–811, 1997.
19. Kirklin JW, Barratt-Boyes BG: Cardiopulmonary bypass established by peripheral cannulation. *In* Kirklin JW, Barratt-Boyes BG (eds): Cardiac Surgery, 2nd ed. New York, Churchill Livingstone, 1993, pp 110, 111.
20. Kirklin JW, Barratt-Boyes BG: Cardiac Surgery, 2nd ed. New York, Churchill Livingstone, 1993, pp 61–127.
21. Laborde F, Noirhomme P, Karam J, et al: A new video-assisted thoracoscopic surgical technique for interruption of patient ductus arteriosus in infants and children. J Thorac Cardiovasc Surg 105:278–280, 1993.
22. Laborde F, Folliguet T, Batisse A, et al: Video-assisted thoracoscopic surgical interruption: The technique of choice for patent ductus arteriosus. Routine experience in 230 pediatric cases. J Thorac Cardiovasc Surg 110:1681–1685, 1995.
23. Laborde F, Folliguet TA, Etienne PY, et al: Video-thoracoscopic surgical interruption of patent ductus arteriosus. Routine experience in 332 pediatric cases. Eur J Cardiothorac Surg 11:1052–1055, 1997.
24. Landreneau RJ, Mack MJ, Magovern JA, et al: "Keyhole" coronary artery bypass surgery. Ann Surg 224:453–462, 1996.
25. Lin PJ, Chang CH, Tan PPC, et al: Protection of the brain by ret-

rograde cerebral perfusion during circulatory arrest. J Thorac Cardiovasc Surg 108:969–974, 1994.
26. Lin PJ, Chang CH, Tan PPC, et al: Prolonged circulatory arrest in moderate hypothermia with retrograde cerebral perfusion: Is brain ischemic? Circulation 94(suppl II):169–172, 1996.
27. Lin PJ, Chang CH, Chu JJ, et al: Video-assisted mitral valve surgeries. Ann Thorac Surg 61:1781–1787, 1966.
28. Lin PJ, Chang CH, Chu JJ, et al: Video-assisted coronary artery bypass grafting during hypothermic fibrillatory arrest. Ann Thorac Surg 63:1113–1117, 1997.
29. Lin PJ, Chang CH, Chu JJ, et al: Minimally invasive cardiac surgical techniques in the closure of ventricular septal defect: An alternative approach. Ann Thorac Surg 65:165–169, 1998.
30. Lin PJ, Chang CH, Chu JJ, et al: Minimal access surgical techniques in coronary artery bypass grafting for triple vessels disease. Ann Thorac Surg 65:407–412, 1998.
31. Lin PJ, Chang CH, Chu JJ, et al: Minimally invasive coronary surgery in women. Chinese Med J (in press).
32. Liu HP, Chang CH, Lin PJ, et al: Video-assisted thoracic surgery—The Chang Gung experience. J Thorac Cardiovasc Surg 108:834–840, 1994.
33. Lumsden AB, Eaves FF III, Ofenloch JC, et al: Subcutaneous, video-assisted saphenous vein harvest: Report of the first 30 cases. Cardiovasc Surg 4:771–776, 1996.
34. Mack MJ, Acuff TE, Casimir-Ahn H, et al: Video-assisted coronary bypass grafting on the beating heart. Ann Thorac Surg 63(suppl 6):S100–S103, 1997.
35. Mack MJ, Brown DL, Sankaran A: Minimally invasive coronary bypass for protected left main coronary stenosis angioplasty. Ann Thorac Surg 64:545–546, 1997.
36. Mavroudis C: VATS ASD closure: A time not yet come. Ann Thorac Surg 62:638–639, 1996.
37. Rothenberg SS, Chang JH, Toews WH, et al: Thoracoscopic closure of patent ductus arteriosus: A less traumatic and more cost-effective technique. J Pediatr Surg 30:1057–1060, 1995.
38. Schwartz DS, Ribakove GH, Grossi EA, et al: Minimally invasive cardiopulmonary bypass with cardioplegic arrest: A closed chest technique with equivalent myocardial protection. J Thorac Cardiovasc Surg 111:556–566, 1996.
39. Schwartz DS, Ribakove GH, Grossi EA, et al: Single and multivessel port-access coronary artery bypass grafting with cardioplegic arrest: Technique and reproducibility. J Thorac Cardiovasc Surg 114:46–52, 1997.
40. Shennib H, Lee AG, Akin J: Safe and effective method of stabilization for coronary artery bypass grafting on the beating heart. Ann Thorac Surg 63:988–992, 1997.
41. Shennib H, Mack MJ, Lee AG: A survey on minimally invasive coronary artery bypass grafting. Ann Thorac Surg 64:110–115, 1997.
42. Shetty DP, Dixit MD, Gan MD, et al: Video-assisted closure of atrial septal defect [letter]. Ann Thorac Surg 62:940, 1996.
43. Stevens JH, Burdon TA, Peters WS, et al: Port-access coronary artery bypass grafting: A proposed surgical method. J Thorac Cardiovasc Surg 111:567–573, 1996.
44. Stevens JH, Burdon TA, Siegel LC, et al: Port-access coronary artery bypass with cardioplegic arrest: acute and chronic canine studies. Ann Thorac Surg 62:435–441, 1996.
45. Subramanian VA: Less invasive arterial CABG on a beating heart. Ann Thorac Surg 63(suppl 6):S68–S71, 1997.
46. Tharion J. Cartmill TB, Johnson DC, et al: Transpulmonary arterial repair of supracristal ventricular septal defects in infancy. J Thorac Cardiovasc Surg 80:948–950, 1980.
47. Tsai FC, Lin PJ, Chang CH, et al: Video-assisted cardiac surgery: Preliminary experience in reoperative mitral valve surgery. Chest 110:1603–1607, 1996.
48. Westaby S, Benetti FJ: Less invasive coronary surgery: Consensus from the Oxford meeting. Ann Thorac Surg 62:924–931, 1996.
49. Wu YC, Chang CH, Lin PJ, et al: Minimally invasive approach for coronary artery bypass surgery. Int J Cardiol 62(suppl 1):S111–S117, 1997.
50. Yeh CH, Chang CH, Lin PJ, et al: Totally minimally invasive cardiac surgery for coronary artery disease. Eur J Cardiothorac Surg 14(suppl 1):S43–S47, 1998.

COMMENTARY

Redmond P. Burke

Efforts to reduce the trauma of surgery for congenital heart disease have evolved rapidly in the past 5 years, progressing from thoracoscopic surgery for simple extracardiac lesions to intraoperative cardioscopy for facilitation of open-heart repairs. Endoscopic open-heart surgery, however, remains an elusive goal, and raises a central question—what is minimally invasive cardiac surgery? This definition forms the basis for critical evaluation of new approaches to congenital heart disease.

Surgery for congenital heart disease is traumatic on multiple levels beyond the incision. Tissue dissection, retraction, blood transfusion, cardiopulmonary bypass, prosthetic devices, long operative times, and ineffective repairs all contribute to this trauma. Truly minimally invasive cardiac surgery must address all of these elements. Unfortunately, an inordinate focus has been placed on the incision alone, and some surgeons have responded to this primarily cosmetic concern by reducing incision size and changing incision location. Paradoxically, these simple alterations in approach may actually increase surgical trauma, because they create more deviations from accepted practice than innovations in technique or instrumentation. No one has proven that a septal defect repair through a thoracotomy incision with endoscopic assistance is less invasive than the same repair performed through a median sternotomy, particularly when this approach requires cannulation of small femoral vessels in children, incisions near undeveloped breast tissue, division of costal cartilages, ventricular incisions, and deairing through the septal repair. A minimally invasive or endoscopic cardiac repair becomes a Pyrrhic victory for the surgeon if it is achieved at the cost of decreased visibility and dexterity, prolonged operating time, and compromised cardiac and neurologic protection. A beautiful surgical incision may hide an ugly cardiac repair.

The advent of endoscopic surgical imaging technology and endoscopic instrumentation has addressed some of these compromises—primarily, the loss of visualization produced by smaller incisions. However, significant technological advances must be made before we can achieve acceptable levels of dexterity, surgical precision, and neurologic and cardiac protection while operating in an endoscopic environment. Mistakes are being made because patients are being forced to fit currently available technology, instead of guiding emerging technology to fit the patient. New technology, such as virtual reality surgery, robotics, nanotechnology, three-dimensional imaging systems, imaging through blood, biocompatible prosthetic devices, and less inflammatory cardiopulmonary bypass, will allow us to reduce surgical trauma markedly in the coming years. The key to the future of less traumatic pediatric cardiac surgery will be the careful introduction and critical evaluation of these new technologies. The technology must be forced to fit the patient, while preserving the congenital heart surgeon's goal—a precise, accurate, rapid, gentle, and complete repair.

Chapter 75

Minimal Access Surgery for Patent Ductus Arteriosus

François Laborde and Thierry A. Folliguet

Patent ductus arteriosus (PDA) was first ligated surgically in 1939 by Gross and Hubbard.[1] Since then, the surgical technique, performed through a left thoracotomy, has evolved from an initially simple ligation to multiple transfixed ligatures, followed by titanium clipping, or suture and division. With improvements in anesthetic management and intensive perioperative care, this operation is able to be performed with no mortality, minimal morbidity, and decreased length of stay.[2]

The potential morbidity of thoracotomy in children, however, remains a problem, especially in neonates. Long-term post-thoracotomy pain is common,[3] and there is increased risk of postoperative pulmonary complications, such as atelectasis and pneumonia.[4] In addition, the incidence of thoracic scoliosis as a long-term complication in premature infants[5] is greater than 20 to 30%.

To circumvent these problems, we have developed a technique of PDA closure using video-assisted thoracoscopic surgery (VATS) in infants, children, and young adults. This approach leads to less discomfort and morbidity than that from classic surgical thoracotomy and provides an optimal rate of success.[6]

Pediatric VATS applications have been limited by a lack of equipment and techniques that are adaptable to small infants. However, the introduction of the small video camera has fostered the development of other surgical operations in children, such as vascular ring division, collateral interruption (arterial and venous), pericardial drainage, interruption of ductus, and diagnostic VATS (e.g., location of an aberrant coronary artery).[7, 8] We started performing VATS in the pediatric population in 1991 for closure of PDA, and, since then, we have performed 374 operations.

Indications

All children who are sent to our institution to undergo VATS manifest either isolated PDA or PDA associated with a more complex congenital lesion. We exclude from this population children who require early complex congenital repair using cardiopulmonary bypass, since ligation of their PDA is usually performed at the time of repair. Age itself does not represent a contraindication, because we have performed this technique in 8 premature infants. The only contraindications are diameter of the ductus larger than the size of the clip (9 mm) or calcification of the ductus. Both of these problems are encountered in older children or adults, who usually have a large but short ductus. In these patients, we recommend suture and division of the ductus via a thoracotomy. In children, the only contraindications are a previous thoracotomy with pleural adhesions or a right aortic arch requiring a contralateral approach.

In adults who have PDA, our decision to choose VATS is influenced by the size of the ductus, the amount of calcification, and the presence of pulmonary hypertension.

Patient Population

In our population of 374 patients, the mean weight was 9.1 kg (range, 1.2–55). Associated cardiac anomalies were atrial septal defect (ASD),[3] ventricular septal defect (VSD),[8] anomalous pulmonary venous return (APVR),[2] VSD and pulmonary artery stenosis,[1] and congenital aortic insufficiency.[1]

All procedures were performed by the same surgeon (François Laborde). The VATS procedure did not vary significantly from the standard procedure except for an increase in speed and efficiency (Table 75–1).

Data analysis was obtained prospectively for all patients. All complications were recorded, as well as hospital stay and procedure time.

To verify the intensity of the shunt, the size of the PDA, and the degree of pulmonary hypertension, including the presence of ductus calcification, all patients underwent transthoracic echocardiography performed at our institution by a physician. All other cardiac anomalies were recorded as well. A chest radiograph was also obtained, as well as routine preoperative blood work.

Procedure

General anesthesia is administered using pentothal at a dose of 5 to 10 mg/kg, vecuronium (Norcuron) at a dose of 0.1 mg/kg, fentanyl, or sufentanil at a dose of 0.5–1 mg/kg, and 1% to 2% enflurane (Ethrane). Intubation is performed with a straight endotracheal tube. A central line is placed via a jugular vein, and no arterial line is placed. Monitoring by electrocardiograph, oximeter, and capnograph is routine.

After general anesthesia is administered and intubation is complete, the patient is positioned on the right side as for a posterolateral thoracotomy (Fig. 75–1). The skin is prepared with two Betadine scrubs, a regular Vi-Drape dressing is placed, including a Steri-Drape. The surgeon and the scrub nurse are at the left side of the patient and the assistant is at the right side.

Two small incisions are made with a No. 11 blade in the left hemithorax. Each incision corresponds in size to the appropriate instruments for that position. The first incision is made just posterior to the left axillary line in the third in-

Table 75–1. Patient Population

Patients	Weight (kg)	Cardiac Anomalies	Prior Cardiac Surgery	Indomethacin Trials
N = 374	Mean 9.1 (1.2–55)	3 ASD 6 VSD 2 APVR 1 VSD PA stenosis 1 AI	3	1

ASD = atrial septal defect; VSD = ventricular septal defect; APVR = anomalous pulmonary venous return; VSD PA = ventricular septal defect and pulmonary artery stenosis; AI = aortic insufficiency.

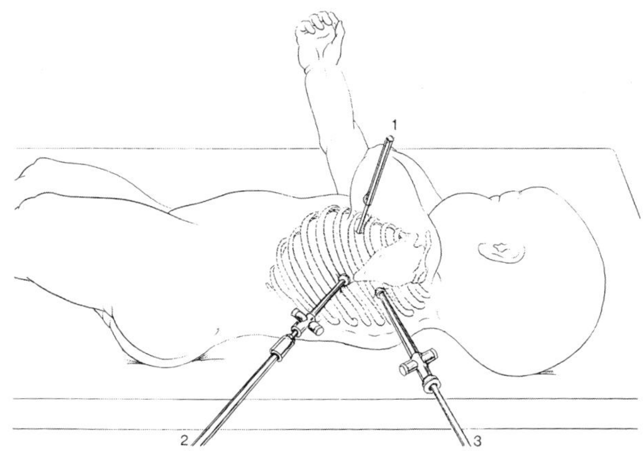

Figure 75–1. Illustration of ports and instruments for video thoracoscopic closure of patent ductus arteriosus (PDA), with placement of the patient on the operating table. 1: angled hooks retractor; 2: electrocautery hook; 3: camera. (From Folliguet T, Lagier A: Chirurgie cardiaque, un guide pour le praticien. Paris, Doin éditeur, 1997.)

tercostal space. The videoscope (4 mm) is introduced through this incision via a 5-mm trocar. A second incision is made in the third intercostal space at the midaxillary line. Two or three 60-degree right-angled hooks, 1 mm in diameter, are introduced directly through the incision, without any trocar, for lung retraction. A third incision is made in the fourth intercostal space, under the angle of the scapula, for the electrocautery hook, which is introduced via a 5-mm trocar (Figs. 75–2 and 75–3). Instruments are listed in Table 75–2.

The monitor is placed on the right side of the patient facing the surgeon. The cables also come from the right side and are clamped to the drape.

The upper lobe of the left lung is retracted inferomedially. The PDA is identified and the mediastinal pleura is opened with a cautery nerve hook. Electrocautery is placed on a low voltage and tested on the mediastinal pleura before dissection of the aorta is begun. The PDA is dissected clear of the surrounding tissue and the aorta is dissected from the PDA at the junction. The dissection on the aorta is continued on the aortic arch for a few centimeters to ensure adequate visualization of the different vascular structures. The pericardium is also dissected on the pulmonary side to protect the recurrent laryngeal nerve from traumatic injury (Fig. 75–4). The laryngeal nerve is usually seen and can, therefore, be preserved. It is essential to dissect the pleura on both sides of the PDA for

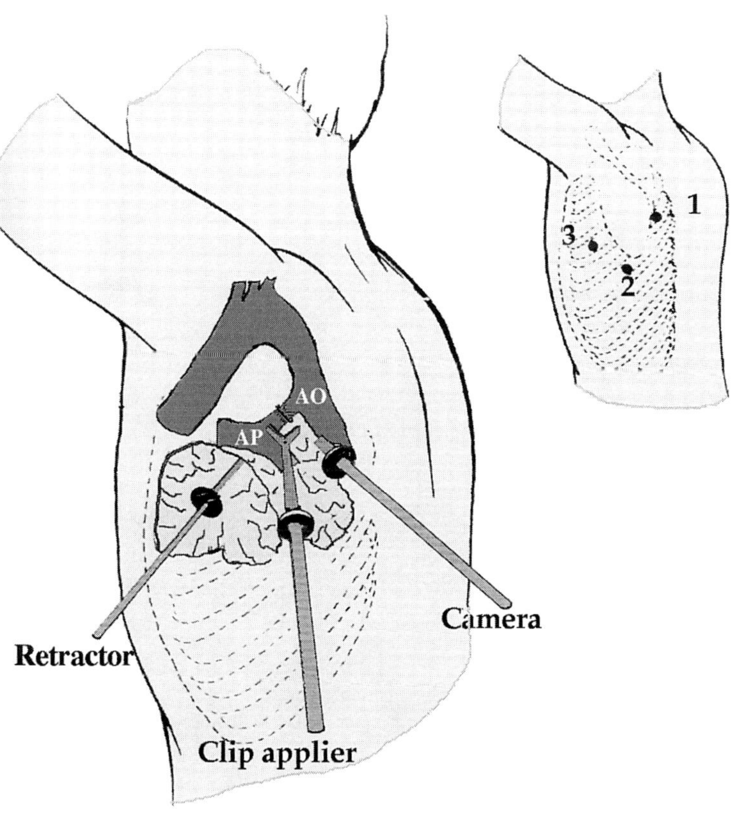

Figure 75–2. Position of the various thoracostomies and placement of the retractor clip applier and camera.

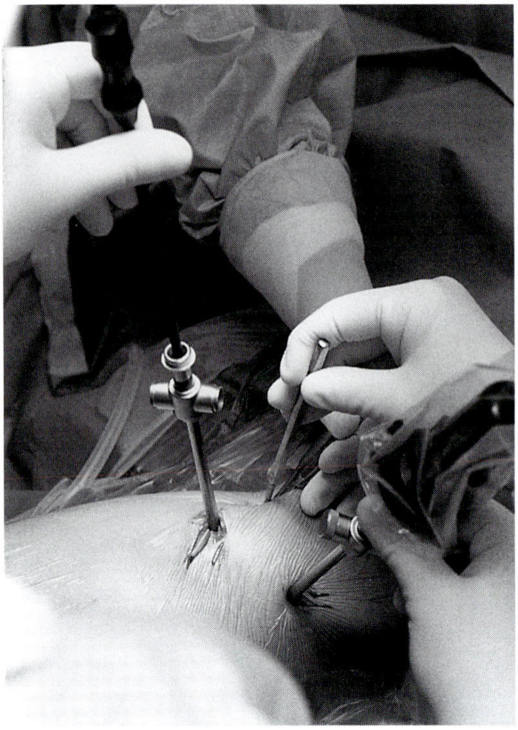

Figure 75–3. Placement of the camera, angled hook, and retractors.

proper placement of the clip. The ductus should be cleared of any adjacent fatty structures before placement of the clips. The clip applicator is introduced through the posterior thoracostomy after removal of the trocar. The first titanium clip (8 mm) is placed as distally as possible from the aortic junction on the pulmonary side (Fig. 75–5), and a second titanium clip is applied on the side proximal to the aorta (Figs. 75–6 and 75–7). After visual confirmation that both clips are adequately placed, the lung is inflated and a 2-mm diameter pleural suction catheter is placed through one of the thoracostomies before closure of the skin incision.

Postoperative Care

Transthoracic color-flow Doppler echocardiography is performed in the operating room or in the recovery room be-

Table 75–2. Instruments Used in Video-Assisted Thoracic Surgery (VATS)

Instruments	Diameter	Company
Camera		Storz
Monitor		Storz
Videoscope	4 mm	Storz
2 Trocars	5 mm	Wolf
3 Right-angle hooks		
Electrocautery hooks		Wolf
Suction device		
Clip applier	8 mm	Microfrance
Needle holder		

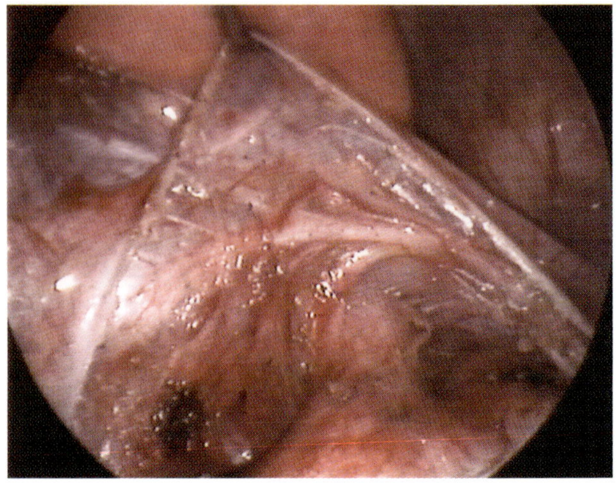

Figure 75–4. Recurrent laryngeal nerve.

fore extubation to assess the completeness of closure of the PDA. If a residual shunt is seen, the patient is immediately taken back to the operating room for reapplication of a new clip by a VATS procedure. Otherwise, if complete interruption is seen, extubation is performed and the patient is placed either in the intensive care unit or in a regular pediatric room, depending on age and previous symptoms of pulmonary hypertension. For most children who weigh less than 5 kg, extubation is performed in the intensive care unit (ICU) 4 to 6 hours after surgery. Length of ICU stay, depending on the condition and age of the patient, varies between 24 and 48 hours. The pleural suction catheter is usually removed the following day. A routine chest radiograph is obtained and a transthoracic echocardiogram is done before the patient is discharged. Postoperative pain protocol is started either in the ICU or on the floor and involves a combination of paracetamol (Prodafalgan) given intravenously or by mouth, combined with niflumic acid (Nifluril). Most patients can ambulate freely with minimal discomfort a few hours after surgery (Fig. 75–8).

After discharge, all patients are regularly followed by

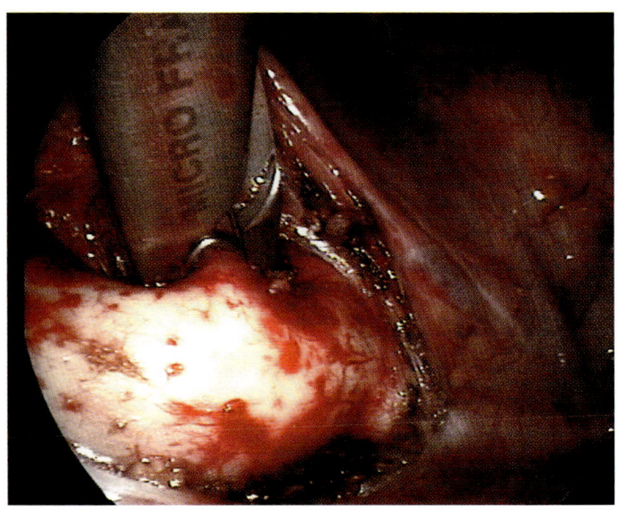

Figure 75–5. Placement of the first clip on the pulmonary side.

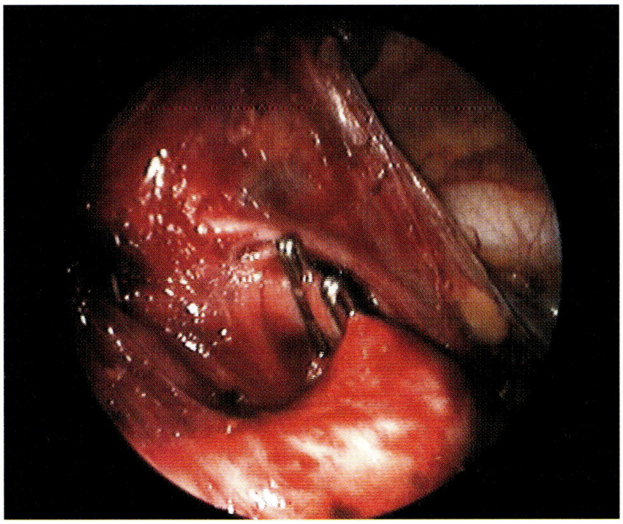

Figure 75–6. Placement of the second clip on the aortic side.

their personal pediatric cardiologists, who perform a complete physical and a transthoracic echocardiogram.

Results

Six patients had a persistent shunt following VATS. All these instances occurred early in our experience with this procedure (Table 75–3). Five patients had immediate interruption of the residual shunt (3 by VATS, 2 by thoracotomy). Subsequent echocardiography revealed persistent closure in these patients. A residual shunt with minimal flow was discovered in 1 asymptomatic patient following discharge. Recurrent laryngeal nerve dysfunction was noted immediately in 6 patients (1.6%) (5 transient, 1 persistent). Other complications included pneumothorax (2), chylothorax (1), which resolved spontaneously after 48 hours, reintubation secondary to laryngeal edema (1), and unexplained fevers persisting for 24 hours (2). There was no mortality or transfusion requirement. Mean operating time for the last 300 patients was 20 min-

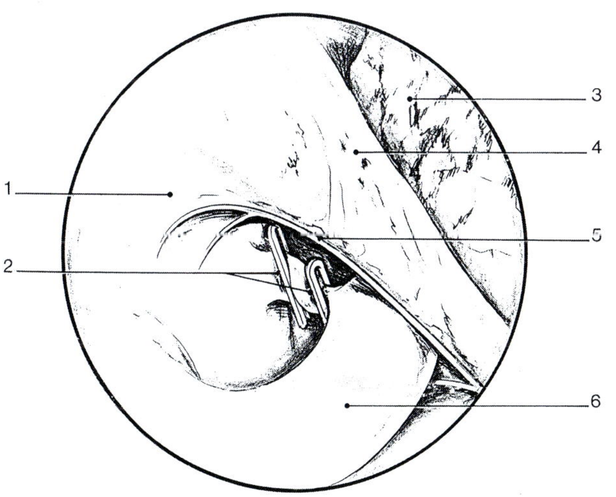

Figure 75–7. The PDA is dissected from surrounding tissue and the recurrent laryngeal nerve is visualized and resected. 1: mediastinal pleura; 2: clips applied on duct; 3: lung parenchyma; 4: pleura; 5: recurrent laryngeal nerve; 6: aorta. From Folliguet T, Lagier A: Chirurgie cardiaque, un guide pour le praticien. Paris, Doin éditeur, 1997.

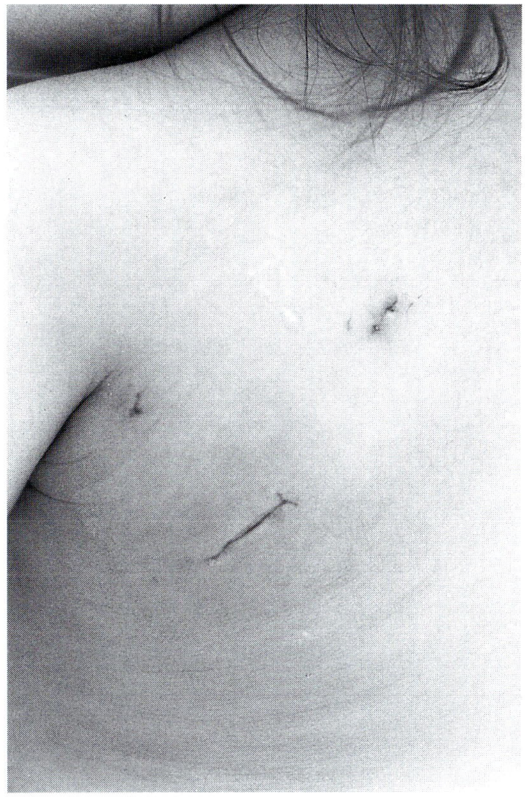

Figure 75–8. Result of the incisions 24 hours after closure.

Table 75–3. Results of Video-Assisted Thoracic Surgery (VATS)

Patients	N = 374
% Mortality	0
Reoperation for bleeding	0
Reoperation for inadequate ligation	5 (1.3%)
Conversion to thoracotomy	2 (0.5%)
Reoperation by VATS	3 (0.8%)
Persistent shunt	1 (0.26%)
Recurrent laryngeal dysfunction*	6 (1.6%)
Other complications	6 (1.6%)
	2 Pneumothorax†
	2 Unexplained fevers
	1 Reintubation for stridor
	1 Chylothorax‡
Total complications rate	18 (4.8%)
Extubation in operating room	237 (63.3%)
Length of stay (hr)	
Pts > 6 mo of age	48 ± 24
Pts < 6 mo of age	72 ± 24
Procedure time (min)	20 ± 15

* All resolved except one.
† Postoperative pneumothorax was prevented by the use of a small Silastic drain.
‡ Chylothorax resolved spontaneously after 48 hr.

utes ± 15 minutes and length of stay averaged 48 hours (patients > 6 months of age) and 72 hours (patients ≤ 6 months of age).

Discussion

In most older patients, division of the ductus is performed through a thoracotomy, whereas infants undergo closure with a clip. Excellent results of surgical closure of PDA in the neonatal ICU have been described.[9-13] The procedure consists of placement of one or two clips through a thoracotomy, generally via an extrapleural approach. The advantages of this procedure are low morbidity, lack of mortality, and reliable PDA closure. The application of metal clips near the aorta reduces the risk of recurrent laryngeal nerve injury and does not require complete mobilization of the ductus, reducing the risk of surgical bleeding.

Our technique of PDA closure by VATS[6] provides the same results without a thoracotomy (see Fig. 75–2). The persistent shunts that occurred after VATS in 6 patients early in our series were caused by incomplete dissection of the ductus, which nevertheless did permit correct placement of the clips over the ductus. No shunts occurred in our last 300 patients.

It is extremely important to dissect both sides of the ductus; this allows correct placement of the clips and prevents a residual shunt. Since we have been performing routine transthoracic echocardiography in the operating room or the recovery room, we have never had a child leave the operating room with a residual shunt. It is, therefore, essential to perform Doppler color flow echocardiography in the immediate postoperative phase, because residual ductal patency has been reported in patients without residual PDA auscultatory findings.[14]

The main complication of this procedure is transient paralysis of the left vocal cord (4.5%), the incidence of which is slightly higher than after an open surgical procedure.[2, 16] Risk factors are generally low weight, extensive dissection around the ductus, and the use of cautery to dissect the mediastinal pleura. To avoid this complication, it is important to use low-voltage electrocoagulation, minimal dissection around the ductus, and adequate retraction of the mediastinal pleura with visualization of the recurrent laryngeal nerve.

Transcatheter closure of the PDA using an umbrella as an occluding device has emerged as a primary therapy for a small PDA, because surgery can be avoided and, presumably, the cost is lower.[17–20] The disadvantage is persistent shunting, which occurs in 27% of patients at 6-week follow-up; this generally decreases 10 to 20% by 6-month follow-up.[21] Residual shunting correlates with the size of the ductus. Possible migration or embolization of the device may necessitate surgical removal.

Other complications associated with this procedure are hemolysis and bacterial endocarditis stemming from residual shunts. Moreover, this technique was, in the past, appropriate only for patients weighing more than 10 kg, because in smaller patients, the size of these vessels makes the use of the device difficult. We have applied clips over an endovascular device with a persistent shunt and have succeeded in obtaining ductus closure.

Refinements in catheter structure now allow this technique to be used in patients who weigh less than 10 kg. However, complications include device dislodgment, a 33% residual shunt at 6-month follow-up, and left pulmonary artery flow alteration in 9.9% of patients.[21]

New devices using coils have been used to occlude PDA, with a complete closure rate of approximately 75% on the day of the procedure, and this has also been performed in children weighing less than 10 kg.[22, 23]

One advantage of the transcatheter technique compared with thoracotomy closure is lower cost.[22, 23]

It is still too early to predict which technique will predominate in the future. Maybe size will determine the choice of procedure, with an endovascular approach and placement of coils for a small ductus and VATS for a large ductus.

The VATS technique can also be used in premature infants, as we and others have demonstrated with excellent results and no morbidity. It is possible to use this technique in the Pediatric ICU. The procedure can be performed quickly, with an average length of 15 to 20 minutes. No complications related to the procedure have been reported in this age group. Therefore, we believe that this technique can be safely applied to premature infants.

As mentioned previously, the only real contraindications for this procedure are diameter of the ductus greater than the size of the clip (9 mm) and calcification of the ductus, which occur in older children and adults.

Another approach described by Chu and associates is ligation of the ductus by video technique.[24] This technique allows treatment of a larger ductus, especially in adults. However, we are concerned with the fact that complete dissection around the ductus has to be made in order to achieve ligation. We believe there is a greater risk of injury and tearing of the ductus when this dissection is performed and when the knot is tied.

VATS for PDA can be performed with no mortality, no bleeding related to the procedure, and complete closure. Prospective efforts must be made to demonstrate reductions in cost, pulmonary injury, and hospital stay. We conclude that the technique described here is safe, that it can be performed with little morbidity, and can be learned easily. These findings are important for future cost-benefit considerations in the context of managed care.

References

1. Gross RE, Hubbard JP: Surgical ligation of a patent ductus arteriosus. Report of first successful case. JAMA 112:729–731, 1939.
2. Mavroudis C, Backer CL, Gevitz M: Forty-six years of patent ductus arteriosus division at Children's Memorial Hospital of Chicago. Standards for comparison. Ann Surg 220:402–410, 1994.
3. Dajczman E, Gordon A, Kreisman H, et al: Long-term post-thoracotomy pain. Chest 99:270–274, 1991.
4. Nomori H, Horio H, Fuyuno G, et al: Respiratory muscle strength after lung resection with special reference to age and procedures of thoracotomy. Eur J Cardiothorac Surg 10:352–358, 1996.
5. Shelton JE, Walburg JR, Schneider E: Functional scoliosis as a long term complication of surgical ligation for patent ductus arteriosus in premature infant. J Pediatr Surg 48A:855–857, 1986.
6. Laborde F, Folliguet T, Batisse A, et al: Video-assisted thoracoscopic surgical interruption: the technique of choice for patent

ductus arteriosus. Routine experience in 230 pediatric cases. J Thorac Cardiovasc Surg 110:1681–1685, 1995.

7. Burke RP, Wernovsky G, Van der Velde M, et al: Video-assisted thoracoscopic surgery for congenital heart disease. J Thorac Cardiovasc Surg 109:499–508, 1995.
8. Fôrster R: Thoracoscopic clipping of patent ductus arteriosus in premature infants. Ann Thorac Surg 56:1418–1420, 1993.
9. Taylor RL, Grover FL, Harman PK, et al: Operative closure of patent ductus arteriosus in premature infants in the neonatal intensive care unit. Am J Surg 152:704–708, 1986.
10. Palder SB, Schwartz MZ, Tyson KR, et al: Management of patent ductus arteriosus: A comparison of operative versus pharmacologic treatment. J Pediatr Surg 22:1171–1174, 1987.
11. Dasmahapatra BS, Pollock JC: Surgical closure of persistent ductus arteriosus in infants before 30 weeks gestation. J Cardiovasc Surg 27:675–678, 1986.
12. Eggert LD, Jung AJ, Mc Gough EC, et al: Surgical treatment of patent ductus arteriosus in preterm infants: Four-year experience with ligation in the newborn intensive care unit. Pediatr Cardiol 2:15–18, 1982.
13. Coster DD. Gorton MF, Grooters RK, et al: Surgical closure of the patent ductus arterious in the neonatal intensive care unit. Ann Thorac Surg 48:386–389, 1989.
14. Miles RH, DeLeon SY, Muraskas J, et al: Safety of patent ductus arteriosus closure in premature infants without tube thoracostomy. Ann Thorac Surg 59:668–670, 1995.
15. Sorensen KE, Kristensen BO, Hansen OK: Frequency of occurrence of residual ductal flow after surgical ligation by color-flow mapping. Am J Cardiol 67:653–654, 1991.
16. Fan LL, Campbell DN, Clarke DR, et al: Paralyzed left vocal cord associated with ligation of patent ductus arteriosus. J Thorac Cardiovasc Surg 98:611–613, 1989.
17. Porstmann W, Wierny L, Warnake H, et al: Catheter closure of patent ductus arteriosus; 62 cases treated without thoracostomy. Radiol Clin North Am 9:203–218, 1971.
18. Hosking MC, Benson LN, Musewe N, et al: Transcatheter occlusion of the persistently patent ductus arteriosus: Forty-month follow-up and prevalence of residual shunting. Circulation 84:2313–2317, 1991.
19. Khan AA, Yousef A, Mullins CE, et al: Experience with 205 procedures of transcatheter closure of ductus arteriosus in 182 patients, with special reference to residual shunts and long-term follow-up. J Thorac Cardiovasc Surg 104:1721–1727, 1992.
20. Gray DT, Fyler DC, Walker AM, et al: Clinical outcomes and costs of transcatheter as compared with surgical closure of patent ductus arteriosus. N Engl J Med 329:1517–1523, 1993.
21. Nykanen DG, Hayes AM, Benson LN, et al: Transcatheter patent ductus arteriosus occlusion: application in the small child. J Am Coll Cardiol 23:1666–1670, 1994.
22. Lloyd TR, Beekman RH III, Moore JW, et al: The PDA coil registry: 250 patient-years of followup. (Abstract). J Am Coll Cardiol 27:34A, 1996.
23. Shim D, Fedderly RT, Beekman RH III, et al: Followup of coil occlusion of patent ductus arteriosus. J Am Coll Cardiol 28:207–211, 1996.
24. Chu JJ, Chang H, Lin P J, et al: Video-assisted thoracoscopic operation for interruption for patent ductus arteriosus in adults. Ann Thorac Surg 63:175–179, 1997.

Chapter 76

Laser Revascularization of Ischemic Myocardium

Robert J. March

Coincident with the aggressive treatment of ischemic heart disease with advanced percutaneous and operative techniques, there is a growing number of patients with regional myocardial ischemia and unsuitable target vessels. Until recently, this group of patients was left incompletely revascularized, and further treatment consisted of maximal medical management. Patients with significant symptoms despite this approach are left with a poor quality of life and frequent hospitalizations for treatment of their refractory angina. Following several decades of research by many individuals targeting alternative methods of treating diffuse coronary artery disease, Mirhoseini and associates proposed using a carbon dioxide (CO_2) laser to create channels in ischemic myocardium as a means of improving the supply of oxygenated blood. A high-powered, gated CO_2 laser was introduced in 1990 so that this new procedure, transmyocardial laser revascularization (TMR), could be evaluated as a sole therapy, without the confounding benefit of coronary artery bypass (CAB). In August 1998, the Food and Drug Administration fully approved TMR with the CO_2 laser as primary treatment for patients with class III and IV chronic stable angina not treatable by conventional means. During the later phases of the CO_2 trials, investigations regarding the efficacy of other fiber-based systems began. The holmium: yttrium aluminum garnet (holmium:YAG) laser is now undergoing clinical trials via transthoracic and percutaneous approaches. The development of TMR and the methods used to deliver this novel therapy are reviewed in this chapter. Reference to data from ongoing trials, patient selection criteria, and procedural steps is also included. The 1-year results of the phase 3 randomized trial comparing TMR with the CO_2 laser to maximal medical management are emphasized, as this is the most mature study of its kind and has led the way for the evaluation of other similar devices.

Background and Clinical Trials

The anatomic design of the reptilian heart, the developing fetal human heart, and some hypoplastic left ventricles[1] reveal that myocardial perfusion is possible with a limited role for the epicardial coronary arteries. Reptiles successfully provide nutrients and oxygenated blood to the myocardium through channels that are directly connected to blood within the left ventricle. Wearn and colleagues' description of intramyocardial sinusoids,[2] which are in communication with the ventricular cavity, inspired the creation of alternative methods of revascularization that mimic the blood flow patterns seen in the reptilian heart. Early attempts to establish communications with this sinusoidal plexus included T-tube placement,[3] multiple needle punctures,[4–7] and implantation of the internal mammary artery.[8] These alternative methods of coronary revascularization, however, became overshadowed by the success of direct coronary artery grafting. One investigator continued to evaluate these alternative strategies in conjunction with coronary artery bypass grafting (CABG)[9, 10] to achieve complete revascularization. Because scarification[11] limited the efficacy and patency of needle-created channels as proposed by Sen, Mirhoseini and coworkers[12] systematically evaluated multiple laser types and found that the characteristics of the CO_2 laser led to the least amount of tissue destruction and to greater channel durability. Because of the infrared spectrum of this laser, it is rapidly absorbed by blood and water, thus allowing instantaneous tissue vaporization with minimal thermal conduction or acoustic damage. The latter injury is diminished because a driving catheter is not used and energy dissipation is largely from the endocardial and epicardial opening created by the channel. These characteristics of the CO_2 laser may provide a greater margin of safety when the procedure is performed on ventricles with lower ejection fractions. For impaired ventricles, there is a transient alteration in diastolic compliance and systolic performance secondary to the myocardial edema following lasing.[13–15] The author showed that there is no significant alteration in systolic or diastolic performance on long-term follow-up after TMR with the CO_2 laser.[16]

Initially, transmural channels were created with an 80-watt CO_2 laser on the cardioplegically arrested heart at the time of CABG.[9] Subsequently, Okada used a low-powered CO_2 laser on the fibrillating heart of a patient in whom a dense pericarditis prevented coronary bypass grafting.[17, 18] With the introduction of the Heart Laser,[19] a 1000-watt CO_2 laser (PLC Medical Systems, Inc.), in 1990, this new therapy could now be delivered in a gated fashion to the beating heart through a small left anterior thoracotomy. This allowed for the initiation of clinical investigations into the efficacy of this new therapy for the treatment of coronary artery disease without the overriding benefit of coronary grafting.

Phase 1 testing in 15 patients demonstrated that the Heart Laser was safe for human use. A nonrandomized, longitudinal United States (US) trial (phase 2) was then initiated and involved 201 patients at eight US sites. The group had an average anginal class of 3.8, and despite the presence of reversibly ischemic myocardium, they were not treatable with angioplasty, coronary bypass grafting, or further maximal medical management. Remarkably, 75% improved by at least two anginal classes at 1 year, and there was a significant reduction in the number of hospital admissions for angina in the year following TMR. Improved myocardial perfusion at 6 and 12 months postoperatively was demonstrated by a reduction in the number of reversible perfusion defects on thallium imaging.[20] This was not associated with an increase in the number of fixed defects. One institution used positron emission tomography (PET) imaging and demonstrated a significant improvement in the subendocardial-subepicardial perfusion ratio in its subset of patients.[21] Other investigators have shown improvements in perfusion[22] as well as stress tolerance[23] and a reduction in ischemic wall motion abnormalities[24] following TMR with the CO_2 laser. The operative mortality was 9%, with an 83% 1-year survival. An ejection fraction less than 40% and age older than 80 years were independent risk factors of late mortality.

As late follow-up for the phase 2 study, angina class was assessed in 70 patients after an average of 34 months (2380 total patient-months) following TMR.[25] With an average preoperative angina class of 3.8, there was considerable improvement to an average anginal class of 1.5 (P = .0001). This was not significantly different from their angina class of 1.4 at 12 months follow-up. Exercise treadmill testing using the Bruce protocol was improved by 28% between the time of enrollment and 24 months postoperatively. With a 3-year mortality of 78% in this group, long-term mortality was not significantly increased over that seen at 1 year of follow-up (83%). These findings support the concept that long-term angina relief and functional improvement can be provided for an otherwise untreatable group of patients.

To further evaluate the safety and efficacy of TMR and to compare this new therapy with continued maximal medical management, a prospective, centrally randomized, multicenter trial was initiated at 12 US sites.[26–28] From August 1995 to September 1996, 198 patients with symptomatic end-stage coronary artery disease were randomly assigned to undergo only TMR (97 patients) or to receive continued medical management (101 patients). As in phase 2, patients were required to have medically refractory angina (Canadian Cardiovascular Society [CCS] class III and IV) that was not amenable to coronary artery bypass grafting or percutaneous angioplasty. Radionuclide imaging confirmed the presence of reversibly ischemic myocardium and an ejection fraction of greater than 20%. Cross-over from the medical management group to the TMR group was allowed following the occurrence of an adverse clinical event, defined as a 48-hour admission requiring intravenous management of severe angina.

After randomization, there were no significant differences between the groups or among the participating institutions. Sixty-nine percent of the TMR group and 63% of the medical management group had class IV angina. More than half of both groups were considered at high risk according to the Cleveland Clinic CABG risk stratification model.[29] As shown in Figure 76–1, TMR was considerably more successful than medical management in reducing angina by at least two anginal classes at each follow-up. At 12 months, 72% of the TMR patients versus only 13% of the medical group experienced this improvement. These differences could not be explained on the basis of a change in cardioactive medications, as 83% of patients had no change or decrease in their medical regimen following successful TMR. Quality of life as measured by the SF-36 and Seattle Angina Questionnaire showed significant improvement for the TMR group compared with the medical group.

In terms of perfusion, thallium single photon emission computed tomography showed a significant difference at 12 months. There was a 20% improvement in myocardial perfusion for the TMR group and a 27% worsening in perfusion for the medical management group. Figure 76–2 shows that there were significantly fewer reversible perfusion defects for the TMR group than for the medical group at 3, 6 and 12 months follow-up. With respect to fixed defects, there was no significant difference between the two groups at any of the follow-up intervals.

Freedom from an unstable angina event at 12-month follow-up was significantly better for the TMR group (Fig. 76–3). As in phase 2, this resulted in a significant reduction in hospital admissions for those undergoing TMR. The hospitalization rate for unstable angina was 2% following TMR versus 69% after randomization to medical management. Additionally, the overall freedom from death, myocardial infarction, and class IV and unstable angina was 69% for those patients undergoing TMR compared with 15% for those continuing medical management ($P < .001$).

The 30-day operative mortality for TMR was 3%. There appeared to be a relationship between the perioperative mortality and the time interval from an episode of unstable angina (Fig. 76–4). A waiting period of 15 days after the last unstable angina episode is now recommended. As sug-

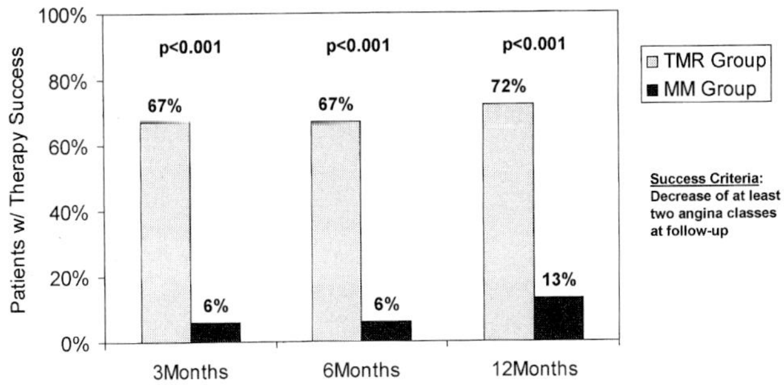

Figure 76–1. The percentage of therapy success (defined as a two-class improvement in angina) is shown for transmyocardial revascularization (TMR) versus medical management (MM) at 3, 6, and 12 months following study enrollment. (From March RJ: Transmyocardial laser revascularization with the CO_2 laser: One year results of a randomized, controlled trial. Semin Thorac Cardiovasc Surg 111:2–18, 1999.)

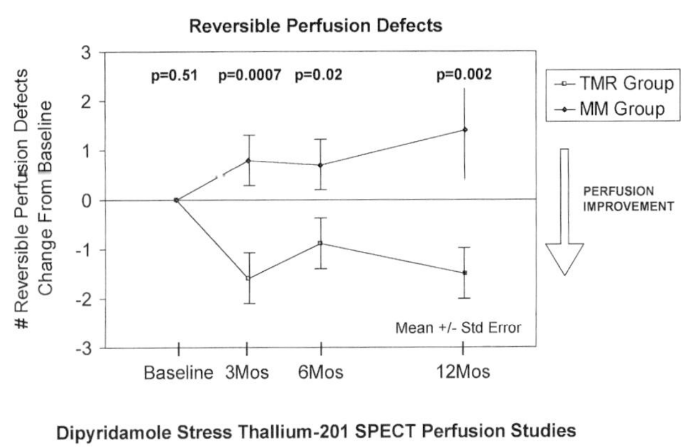

Figure 76–2. Left heart reversible perfusion defects. A reduction in reversible defects indicates improved perfusion following transmyocardial revascularization (TMR) versus worsening perfusion with medical management (MM) at 3, 6, and 12 months follow-up. (From March RJ: Transmyocardial laser revascularization with the CO_2 laser: One year results of a randomized, controlled trial. Semin Thorac Cardiovasc Surg 111:2–18, 1999.)

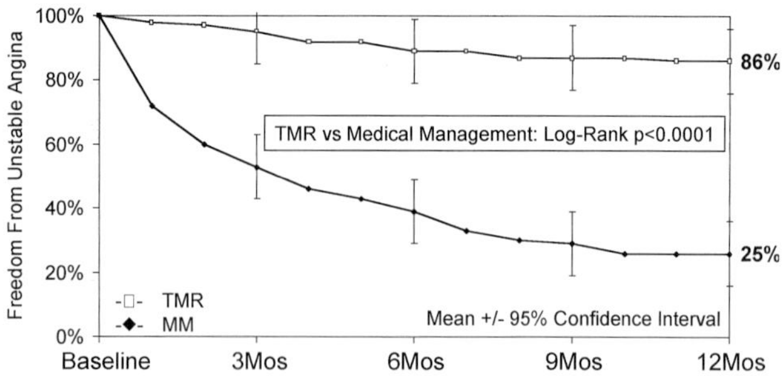

Figure 76–3. Kaplan-Meier estimator showing freedom from unstable angina during the first year of follow-up following transmyocardial revascularization (TMR) versus continued medical management (MM). (From March RJ: Transmyocardial laser revascularization with the CO_2 laser: One year results of a randomized, controlled trial. Semin Thorac Cardiovasc Surg 111: 2–18, 1999.)

gested by this author[30, 31] and others,[32] aggressive stabilization of the patient with intravenous nitrates, heparin, and an intra-aortic balloon pump (IABP) can lead to the safe performance of TMR, provided there is absence of ongoing myocardial injury. The Rush series of more than 90 patients included 15 with unstable angina and cross-overs from medical management who underwent TMR without operative mortality. The IABP usage rate was 60%.[30] Unstable angina must be differentiated from ongoing injury, because the latter is a definite contraindication for sole TMR. The ideal time for TMR is still during a period of clinical stability. Unstable angina was found to be the sole predictor of perioperative mortality on multivariate and univariate analysis. TMR did not negatively impact survival, as the 12-month survival for the TMR group was 85% and for those remaining in the medical group was 79% (not significant). Age and decreased ejection fraction predicted an increased late mortality for the TMR group, whereas the occurrence of acute myocardial infarction after enrollment negatively influenced the survival in both groups.

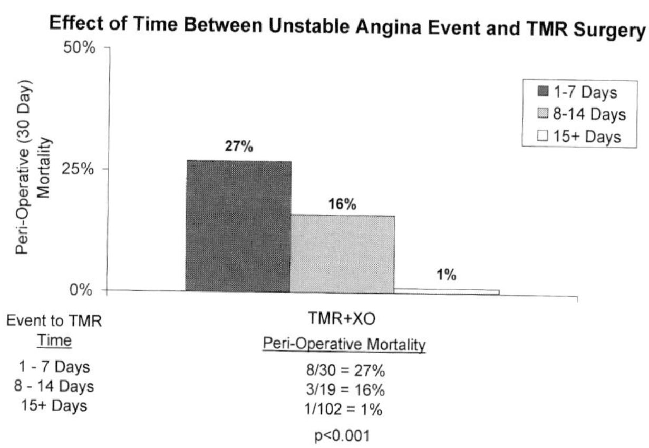

Figure 76–4. Perioperative mortality of transmyocardial revascularization (TMR) at increasing time intervals from an unstable angina episode, suggesting greater procedural safety when performed during a period of clinical stability. (From March RJ: Transmyocardial laser revascularization with the CO_2 laser: One year results of a randomized, controlled trial. Semin Thorac Cardiovasc Surg 111:2–18, 1999.)

In the cross-over group (cTMR), there was a significantly higher incidence of class IV and unstable angina after failure of medical management. According to the Cleveland Clinic CABG risk stratification model, 87% were considered to be at high operative risk. The desperate state of this group resulted in an operative mortality of 15%. As noted earlier, patient selection and preoperative stabilization may have reduced the risk of cTMR. After the first month following cTMR, the survival curve for these patients paralleled that of the initial TMR group and resulted in a 73% freedom from death at 12 months. Remarkably, follow-up at 12 months showed that 69% were in angina classes I and II.

Subsequent to the reporting of results with the CO_2 laser, trials began with another infrared laser, the holmium: YAG. The lower wattage allowed this system to be catheter based, and initial application was via a thoracotomy approach. Two versions became available: an electrocardiogram gated version (CardioGenesis Corp., Sunnyvale, CA) and a nongated system (Eclipse Surgical Technologies, Inc., Sunnyvale, CA). Recently, the results of a multicenter randomized comparison of TMR with the holmium laser (Eclipse) via a thoracotomy versus medical management in patients suffering class IV angina were reported.[33] The study was carried out from March 1996 to February 1997 and involved 160 patients with randomization between TMR (n = 74) and maximal medical management (n = 86). Although there were no differences between the two groups at 1-year follow-up in terms of myocardial perfusion benefit or mortality, there was a significant benefit to the TMR group in terms of angina class reduction, quality of life, and improved exercise tolerance. Other trials[34, 35] with the holmium:YAG support improved anginal class and exercise tolerance on early follow-up. No large series has reported a perfusion benefit.

Although TMR in its current form is minimally invasive, requiring a small left thoracotomy incision and minor manipulation of the beating heart, some groups have introduced thoracoscopic TMR.[36–38] On a limited basis, this approach has been shown to be feasible and safe, but its added benefit to an already minimal approach has been questioned.[39] Clinical investigations are now under way with at least two percutaneous holmium:YAG lasers to achieve percutaneous myocardial revascularization (PMR). These devices deliver 2 joules per pulse and after multiple activations lead to the creation of a partial-thickness endocardial channel approximately 5 to 6 mm in depth (Fig. 76–5). Treatment of the entire wall, as in TMR, is not possible without the risks of perforation. The results of a feasibility study with a gated holmium laser involving 30 patients at four institutions in Germany, Switzerland, and the United States were recently reported.[40] There was no procedure-related mortality, but one patient suffered pericardial tamponade. Other minor complications included bundle branch block in two patients, pericardial effusions in two, ventricular tachycardia in one patient, and nephropathy secondary to intravenous contrast in one patient. Further reports on this pilot study with 65 patients indicated an average anginal improvement of 1.2 classes at 3 months follow-up. Treadmill time increased more than 10% in 44% of the patients.[41] Early follow-up of 41 patients undergoing PMR with a nongated device indicated that 83% had improved by at least two angina classes.[42, 50] Of this group, one patient died after repeat PMR, and an-

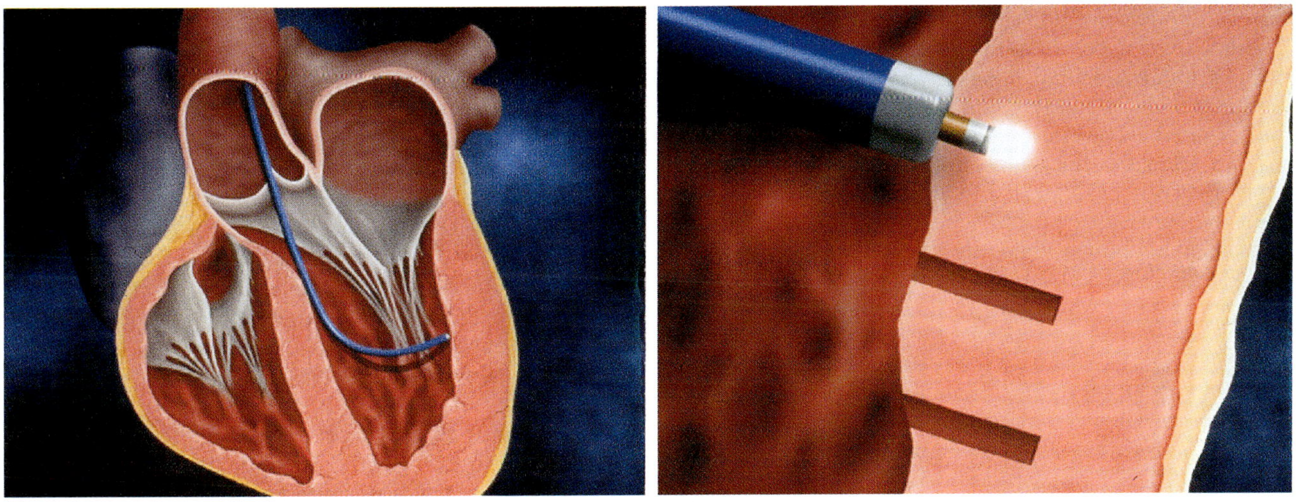

Figure 76–5. During percutaneous myocardial revascularization (PMR), the guiding catheter is positioned against the endocardium under fluoroscopic control. The fiber optic is advanced through the guiding catheter into endocardium as the device is activated. (Photo courtesy of Eclipse Surgical Technologies Inc., Sunnyvale, CA.)

other died after salvage CAB. Other complications included ventricular tachycardia, transient third-degree heart block, and one transient ischemic attack.

A randomized trial comparing PMR with medical management has been initiated at 12 centers in the United States and the United Kingdom. Six-month results were reported in March 1999. Inclusion criteria for the randomized trial include stable class III or IV angina (not amenable to percutaneous transluminal coronary angioplasty [PTCA] or CAB), documented ischemia, and an ejection fraction greater than 30%. Patients are excluded if there is a history of myocardial infarction in the preceding 3 months or an unstable angina admission within 14 days before study entry.

Patient Selection

A detailed clinical, anatomic, and functional analysis of the patient's coronary artery disease is necessary to determine the appropriateness of sole therapy with laser revascularization. The major determinants used to make this assessment are angina class, ejection fraction, and the presence of reversible ischemia. Patients considered for TMR are CCS angina class III or IV in the setting of maximal medical management. Review of the cardiac catheterization excludes the potential for coronary bypass grafting or PTCA. Conventional therapies, including maximal medical management, need to be optimized to ensure a clinically stable condition at the time of TMR or PMR. Biplane ventriculography offers the best estimate of the ejection fraction, which needs to be greater than 20% for TMR and greater than 30% for PMR. Echocardiography and multigated nuclear images are also used to measure ventricular function. However, the latter modality often overestimates the ejection fraction when compared with ventriculography. Finally, stress thallium imaging identifies regions of reversibly ischemic or hibernating myocardium. Fixed defects receive further analysis with PET to differentiate viable from scarred myocardium.

A stable pattern of angina suggests the absence of ongoing myocardial injury and is the best setting for TMR. Because the angina threshold increases gradually following TMR, acute myocardial ischemia will only be further aggravated by the operative procedure. Instead, aggressive measures such as intravenous nitrates, heparinization, and IABP insertion are instituted to stabilize the patient before TMR. Inability to stabilize the patient with these measures contraindicates sole TMR. If acute myocardial infarction has occurred, several weeks of recovery should be allowed before intervention. When sole TMR is used as a salvage measure in the setting of acute myocardial infarction, the results are uniformly poor. Instead, consideration should be given to conventional measures (PTCA or CABG) either alone or in combination with TMR. Close attention is paid to the pattern of angina in order to avoid intervention during ongoing or impending myocardial injury. At this time, TMR is not recommended as treatment for silent ischemia.

The operative risk of TMR is increased by left ventricular dysfunction unless specific measures are taken. Early in the experience with TMR, a low ejection fraction and greater than 2+ mitral insufficiency were associated with increased operative mortality.[44] To optimize ventricular function preoperatively and to minimize the effect of a decrease in ventricular compliance postoperatively, an IABP is placed when the left ventricular ejection fraction is less than 35%. The presence of mitral insufficiency greater than 2+ is thought to be a relative if not an absolute contraindication to TMR. Patients with mitral insufficiency up to 2+ are accepted if their ejection fraction is greater than 30%. Without mitral insufficiency, the patient would be considered a candidate for TMR with an ejection fraction as low as 20%. At lower ejection fractions, there is a greater need for more extensive areas of reversibly ischemic or hibernating myocardium. In other words, the presence of underperfused viable myocardium as an explanation for the reduced ejection fraction rather than scar tissue better supports the decision to proceed with TMR in the high-risk setting. Aside from its role in improving diastolic coronary perfusion, the IABP has had a great impact on lessening the myocardial workload, especially with the reduced ventricular compliance observed in the postoperative period. There is less aggravation of pre-existing mitral insufficiency by the early postoperative diastolic stiffness when the IABP is in place. Because revascularization is thought to take place gradually after TMR, a preference for mechanical support lessens the negative impact of the operative stress on myocardial oxygen consumption. For the same reason, inotropes are avoided if at all possible.

Stress thallium imaging, dobutamine echocardiography, and, if needed, positron emission tomography (PET) are used to determine the source of the patient's anginal symptoms. Because TMR treats the left ventricular free wall, a significant area of reversible ischemia must be identified in this region. Although PMR offers treatment limited to the endocardium, the left ventricular septum can be lased with this modality. As was shown in the early experience with TMR,[44] preserved perfusion to the anterior left ventricular wall was associated with fewer cardiac events following TMR. A patent left internal mammary graft to the left anterior descending coronary artery was most commonly found. The recommendation that one should not "lase in a desert," or rather myocardium, which is devoid of collateral vessels, is applicable to all forms of laser revascularization.

Contraindications to TMR include significant chronic obstructive lung disease, peripheral vascular occlusive disease preventing IABP insertion in the setting of low ejection fraction or unstable angina not responsive to intravenous nitrates and heparin, and fixed defects on thallium and PET imaging. Sole TMR and most likely PMR are not appropriate treatment for impending or ongoing myocardial injury. Protocols for the Eclipse holmium laser required the presence of CCS class IV angina. The PMR trials accepted patients with CCS class III and IV angina but specified a 3-month waiting period after myocardial infarction and a 14-day delay following an unstable angina event.

The ideal patient for TMR is one in whom a significant portion of myocardium has preserved epicardial blood flow either in the form of an undiseased native vessel or via a patent left internal mammary artery, ideally to the left anterior descending artery. Good underlying ventricular function without mitral insufficiency, as well as a stable clinical pattern of angina without recent infarction, offers the lowest risk for laser intervention.

Operative Procedure

Anesthetic considerations for TMR include avoidance of myocardial ischemia, management of one-lung or reduced double-lung ventilation, and control of perioperative pain. Continuous measurement of mixed venous oxygen saturation (oximetry Swan-Ganz catheter), ST segment analysis, and segmental wall motion changes observed with transesophageal echocardiography (TEE) give an early warning of myocardial ischemia. Additional benefits of continuous oximetry include detection of low cardiac output, hypoxemia, and anemia. Analysis with TEE identifies baseline and evolving segmental wall motion abnormalities and left ventricular filling. Diligent anesthetic support leads to rapid correction of these abnormalities and avoidance of spiraling ischemia in these end-stage patients. If standard measures fail to correct myocardial ischemia and low cardiac output, an IABP is inserted. Because the perfusion benefit from TMR is most likely delayed, inotropes are avoided to prevent a further increase in myocardial oxygen consumption. TEE is an important adjunct to TMR in order to determine the configuration of the mitral valve apparatus before and after lasing, to confirm endocardial penetration by the laser (Fig. 76–6), and to locate the papillary muscles and regions of myocardial thinning. One-lung ventilation is not imperative for the procedure, but collapse of the left lung provides optimal exposure, especially when left lung adhesions are encountered or when thoracoscopic TMR is performed. Hypoxemia is treated with continuous positive airway pressure applied to the collapsed lung. Reinflation of the left lung after creation of a pericardial cradle usually does not significantly compromise exposure. Finally, a thoracic epidural catheter is placed for perioperative pain management in all patients unless otherwise contraindicated by their coagulation status. This has been critical to on-table extubation, which reduces postoperative stress and greatly facilitates recognition of angina. Local anesthetics delivered into the epidural space perioperatively may have the added benefit of improved coronary blood flow and angina relief.[45] Intercostal nerve blocks with bupivacaine and epinephrine are used when thoracic epidural analgesia is ineffective or contraindicated.

For PMR, mild sedation is used as needed, and the catheters are introduced via the femoral arteries after infiltration with a local anesthetic. Biplane ventriculography and coronary angiography are carried out to define treat-

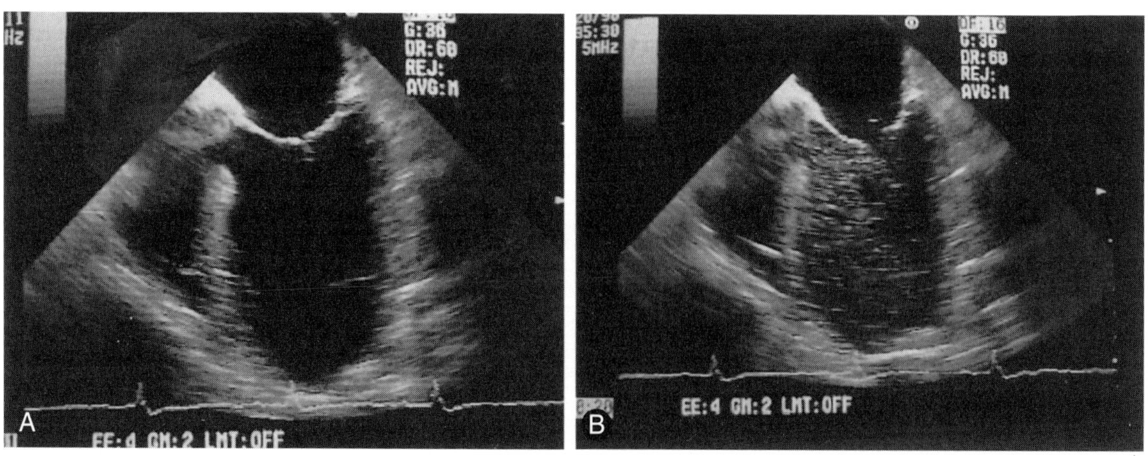

Figure 76–6. Long axis view of the left ventricle via transesophageal echocardiography showing the left ventricle before (A) and after (B) activation of the CO_2 laser. The intraventricular bubbles confirm endocardial penetration.

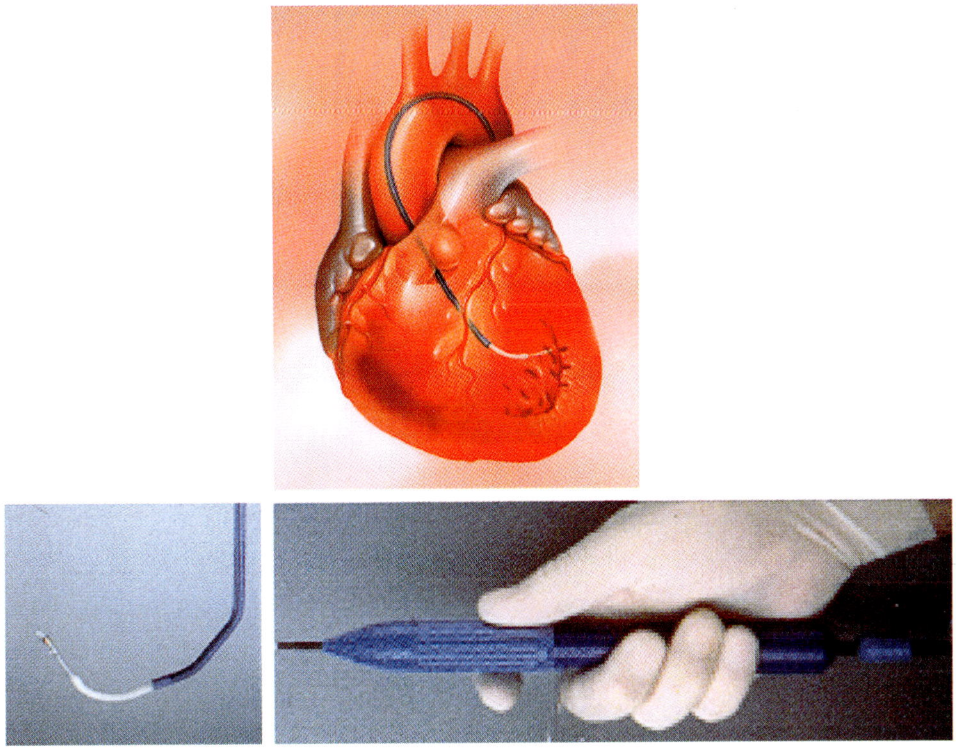

Figure 76–7. The steerability of the percutaneous myocardial revascularization (PMR) catheter is shown in a dual coaxial catheter system. At each channel site, four to six gated pulses are delivered to create a channel 5 to 6 mm deep. (Photo courtesy of CardioGenesis Corp., Sunnyvale, CA.)

ment areas. Generally both femoral arteries are used, with a 9 French sheath on one side and a smaller sheath on the other. After systemic anticoagulation, the 9 French guiding catheter is advanced into the left ventricle. With a coaxial catheter system, multiple positional adjustments can be made within the left ventricle (Fig. 76–7). The coronary anatomy of the intended treatment area is defined. The anterolateral region is best viewed in the left anterior oblique cranial angulation. The posterolateral and inferior areas of the left ventricle are visualized in the right anterior oblique caudal projections. The orthogonal view is useful for confirming endocardial fiber contact and fiber extension.[40] As in TMR, one channel is placed per cm^2 in the treatment area. Each channel is illustrated on tracing paper placed over the monitor screen. The ventricular outline and coronary vessels are included as a reference. Although most PMR systems use fluoroscopic guidance, one nonpenetrating holmium system uses electromechanical maps to reduce the need for fluoroscopy.[46] Two pulses of energy (2 joules/pulse) are delivered, as the catheter is advanced 1 to 2 mm. The total depth of catheter advancement is limited to 5 to 6 mm by nitinol petals near the distal end of the laser catheter. Most patients undergo treatment of one ischemic region, and the one channel per cm^2 spacing requirement determines the number of channels. Owing to the risk of tamponade, myocardium less than 8 mm thick is avoided. The advantages of this approach are that the septum can be treated and patients are generally discharged the day following the procedure.[67] Our institution has experience with the use of both TMR and PMR.

Surgical TMR is carried out by placing the patient in a 45-degree right lateral decubitus position, and the left arm is suspended at a right angle to the torso in an airplane arm holder to keep the latissimus dorsi muscle lateral to the incision. Because rotation of the table is required for optimal visualization, especially through a small incision, the ether screen is padded and used to support the left shoulder blade to prevent tension on the left arm (Fig. 76–8). The operative field encompasses the left chest and groin, as a left femoral arterial line is routinely used. This offers rapid access not only for percutaneous cardiopulmonary bypass support but also for IABP placement if low cardiac output or persistent myocardial ischemia occurs. Other adjuncts include external defibrillator patches over the right chest and left shoulder, temperature Foley catheter, lower extremity sequential compression devices, cell saver suction, and a carbon canister smoke evacuator.

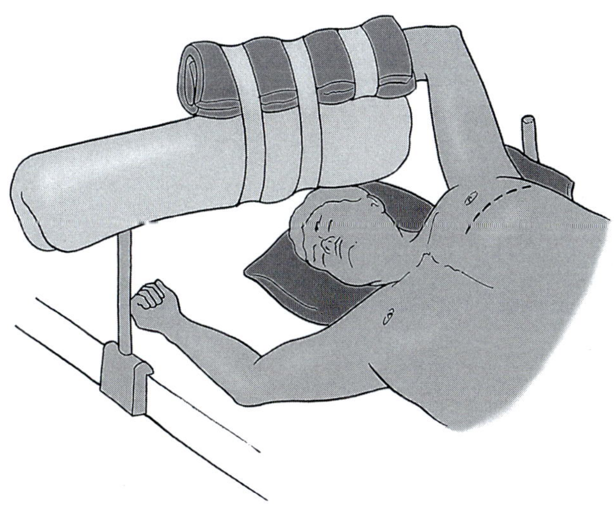

Figure 76–8. For transmyocardial revascularization (TMR), the patient is placed in a 45-degree right lateral decubitus position, and the left arm is suspended at a right angle to the torso in an airplane arm holder to keep the latissimus dorsi muscle lateral to the incision. The left scapula is supported to allow rotation of the table for optimal visualization through a small incision.

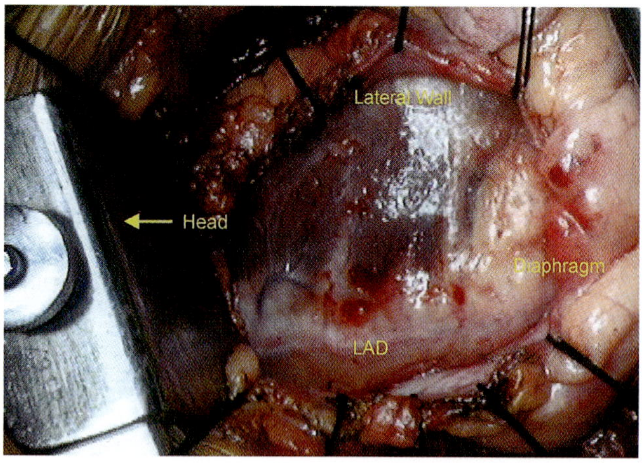

Figure 76–9. This operative photograph from the surgeon's perspective shows the left ventricular apex and diaphragm at the caudal portion of the incision. Lateral pericardial and caudal diaphragmatic retraction allows visualization of the entire left ventricular free wall. LAD = left anterior descending coronary artery.

The operative procedure involves a 6- to 10-cm left anterolateral thoracotomy incision centered over the point of maximal impulse or at the midclavicular line over the fifth intercostal space. The left chest is entered through the fifth intercostal space or the bed of the fifth rib. The latter is preferred in morbid obesity, a noncompliant chest wall, and significant cardiomegaly. The inferior border of the incision should ideally be at the level of the left ventricular apex and diaphragm (Fig. 76–9). This allows access to the inferoposterior left ventricular wall without tilting the ventricle cephalad and compromising hemodynamics. The left lung is decompressed and a vertical pericardiotomy performed anterior to the phrenic nerve. Pericardial stay sutures are placed, and gradual tension is applied as epicardial adhesions are divided. A sterile tongue blade provides countertraction to the epicardium as the base of the left ventricle is approached (Fig. 76–10). Manipulation of old vein grafts and dissection of the internal mammary artery pedicle are avoided. Exposure extends from the left anterior descending to the posterior descending coronary vessels. Because the length of the skin incision and pericardiotomy are limited, retraction of the lateral pericardium and diaphragm with a narrow Deaver or malleable retractor is essential to complete the dissection of the epicardial adhesions and to prevent dimpling of the epicardium by the head of the laser handpiece (Fig. 76–11). Epicardial pressure may bring the chordae closer to the endocardial surface and increase the likelihood of chordal severance during lasing (Fig. 76–12). Two small rib spreaders placed at right angles to each other provide the most stable exposure through the chest incision.

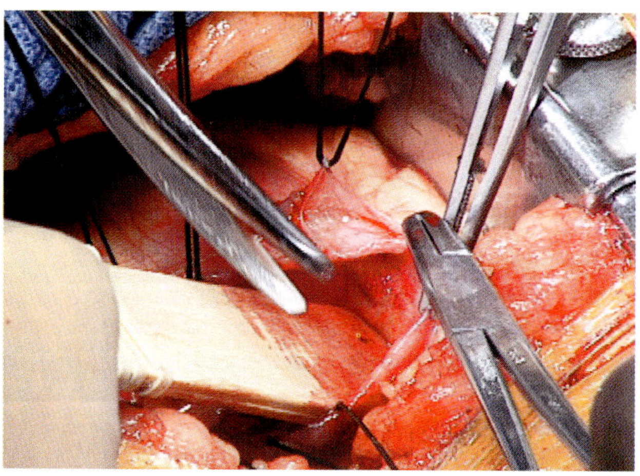

Figure 76–10. Multiple pericardial stay sutures and countertraction with a sterile tongue blade provide stable exposure for dissection of pericardial adhesions.

In the case of the CO_2 laser, the 6-foot articulating arm of the Heart Laser is dressed with a sterile sleeve and brought to the operative field, preferably over the right shoulder of the operating surgeon who is facing the patient (Fig. 76–13). In preparation for lasing, the anesthesiologist positions the TEE probe to provide a long axis view of the ventricular outflow tract to allow confirmation of endocardial penetration. Serum electrolytes (potassium and magnesium) and ventricular filling are optimized to reduce ventricular irritability and hemodynamic compromise, respectively. The basal regions of the left ventricle are generally treated first. The entire left ventricular free wall from the anterior to the posterior descending vessels is lased with channels placed at an arbitrary spacing of approximately one channel per cm^2 of epicardial surface. Areas of transmural scar are not treated. Five channels are placed at a time, and bleeding is controlled by direct pressure with a Ray-Tech sponge while the mirrored surface of the right-

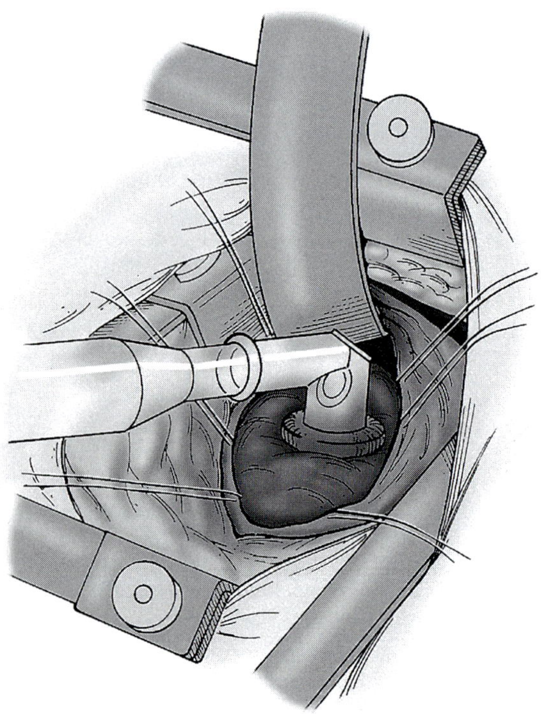

Figure 76–11. Lateral retraction with a narrow Deaver or malleable retractor provides additional exposure to prevent epicardial dimpling by the right-angle handpiece of the CO_2 laser. The right-angle configuration of the low-profile rib spreaders is also shown.

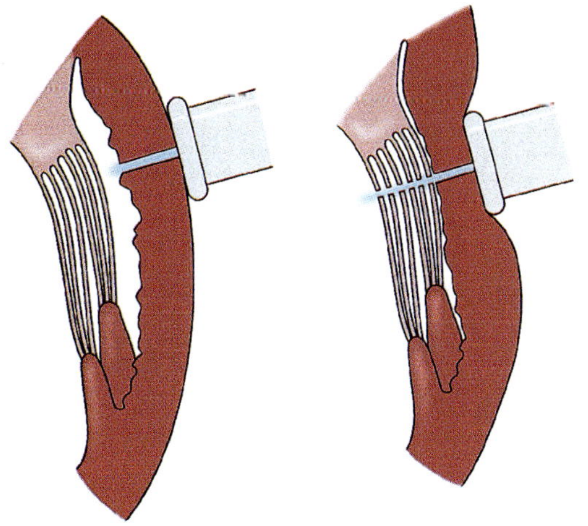

Figure 76–12. This cutaway view of the left ventricle shows the manner in which mitral valve chordae may be severed by the laser with epicardial dimpling and loss of the absorptive blood interface. Fortunately a rare complication, chordal severance has been described with the holmium:YAG and CO_2 lasers.

angle handpiece is cleaned. Headlight illumination, Deaver retraction of the pericardium and diaphragm, and epicardial stabilization with sterile tongue blades facilitate accurate channel placement away from epicardial vessels.

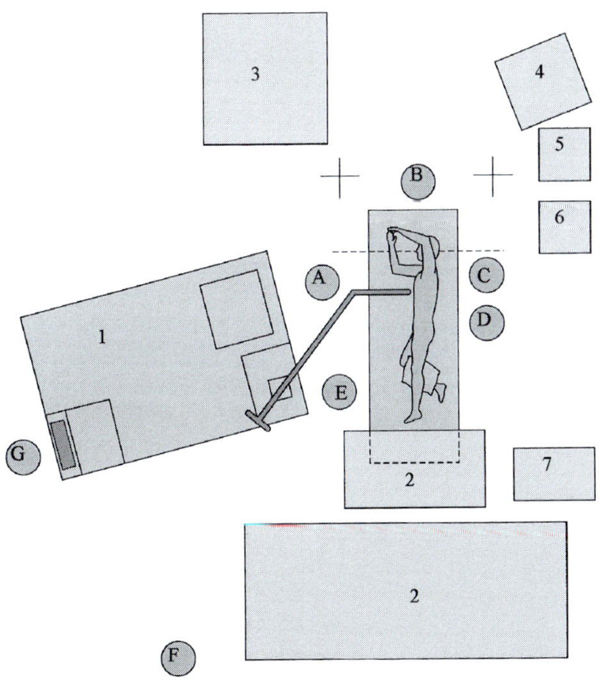

1. Heart Laser System
2. Surgical Table
3. Anesthesia Station
4. Transesophageal Echo
5. Defibrillator
6. Cell Saver
7. Smoke Evacuator

A. Surgeon
B. Anesthesiologist
C. First Assistant
D. Second Assistant
E. Scrub Nurse
F. Circulating Nurse
G. Laser Operator

Figure 76–13. The typical operating room setup for transmyocardial revascularization (TMR).

At the midventricular level, the region of the lateral obtuse marginal branch and an area approximately 1 cm lateral to the posterior septum identify the location of the anterolateral and posteromedial papillary muscles, respectively (Fig. 76–14). Pressure on the epicardium with the handpiece can also help identify the location of the papillary muscles as seen on the TEE image. Channel placement is generally avoided in these regions to reduce the risk of chordal disruption. Other factors that may increase the latter include inadequate left ventricular filling, epicardial dimpling with the head of the laser handpiece, an an excessively high energy setting at the time of activation. The anterior surface of the heart is treated with the straight handpiece (Fig. 76–15). An average of 30 channels are placed during the procedure. An excessive number of channels should be avoided, especially in hearts with a low baseline ejection fraction, as this may further decrease ventricular compliance. In general, we begin at 30 joules of energy. The pulse width is set automatically. The energy requirement varies directly with the amount of epicardial fat and the wall thickness (the base of the heart is thinner). The setting is lowered during combination procedures to reduce the amount of bleeding while on cardiopulmonary bypass. The intensity of intraventricular bubbles (acoustic effect) as seen on TEE is also used to gauge the level of energy required. Arrhythmias produced by activation of the laser have not occurred because device activation is gated to the R wave and only a single pulse is required to create the channel. Nevertheless, pediatric paddles and the external defibrillation system are available if needed.

After all regions have been treated, the pericardial sac is irrigated with warm saline, and each channel site is checked for bleeding. Epicardial sutures are rarely needed. If used, a superficial horizontal mattress of 6–0 prolene is placed. We have not found it necessary to use fibrin sealants, topical thrombin, or other agents to achieve hemostasis. Cell saver blood is then washed and returned to the patient. The pericardium is loosely approximated to allow for postoperative swelling, and a single chest tube is placed into the left chest gutter. In the presence of normothermia, adequate analgesia, and stable hemodynamics, the patient is extubated after return to the supine position.

Support for reduced cardiac output during the procedure is provided by insertion of an IABP via the left femoral arterial line. We have been able to anticipate the need for mechanical support based on clinical parameters and, except for one instance, have placed the IABP the day before the procedure.

In the case of TMR with the holmium laser, the operative exposure is similar.[47] A 20-watt holmium:YAG laser delivering 6 to 8 watts of power per pulse at a rate of 5 pulses per second is used. A flexible 1-mm fiber is used to create channels through the myocardium with three to eight activations of the device. Both available handpieces are malleable but differ in terms of electrocardiographic gating (Figs. 76–16 and 76–17). Channels are placed every square centimeter of the distal two thirds of the left ventricle. Pressure is applied to the epicardial surface every three to five channels to achieve hemostasis. Typically 30 to 50 channels are placed and arrhythmias are minimized if channels are placed slowly. Although a similar acoustic

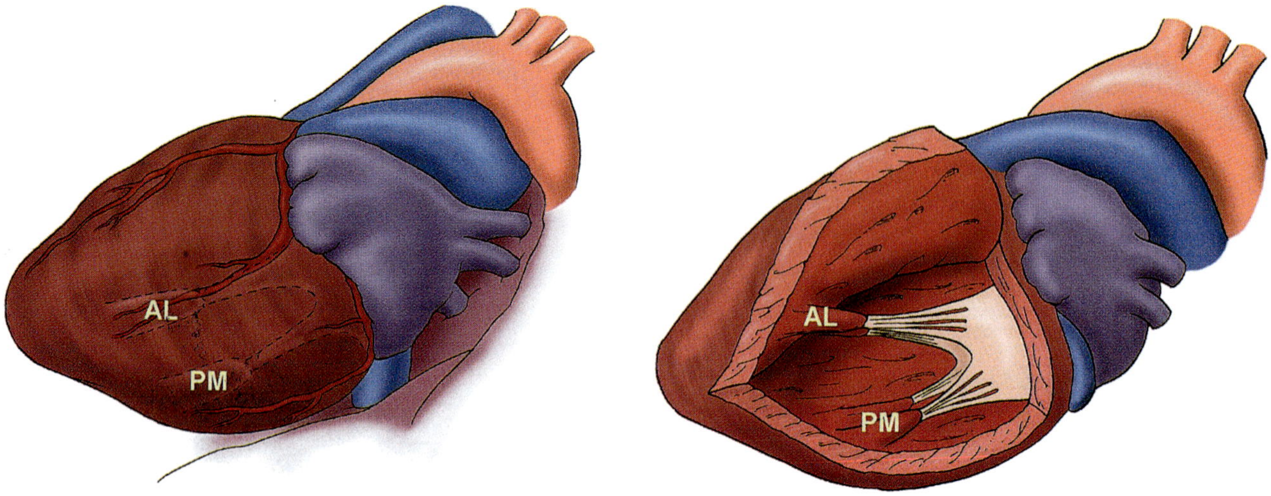

Figure 76–14. The locations of the anterolateral (AL) and posteromedial (PM) papillary muscle and chordal groups are shown as viewed from a left anterolateral thoracotomy.

effect is visualized within the ventricular cavity on TEE, tactile and auditory feedback to the experienced user of this device makes use of the TEE unnecessary.[47] As delineated earlier, TEE improves the safety of TMR through early detection of wall motion abnormalities and documentation of the functional mitral valve anatomy.

Postoperative Management

Intraoperative extubation is possible in the majority of patients. Postoperative care is similar to that of post-thoracotomy patients, with the exception that there is reduced ventricular compliance and a tendency toward myocardial ischemia in response to stress. A definite need for a higher left ventricular filling pressure is observed in the first 24 hours postoperatively. Diuretics are started on the first postoperative morning as mobilization of the third-space fluid begins. Mechanical support initiated prophylactically for a low preoperative ejection fraction is continued for 72 hours. If unstable angina was the indication, the IABP is removed earlier and continuous heparin is started 6 to 12 hours postoperatively. Such a patient would be converted to warfarin (Coumadin) for 3 months. Preoperative antianginals are restarted as dictated by tolerance of the pulse and blood pressure. These are continued at the same level for 3 months, at which point gradual weaning is initiated, depending on the clinical course and perfusion studies. Myocardial ischemia is aggressively treated with he-

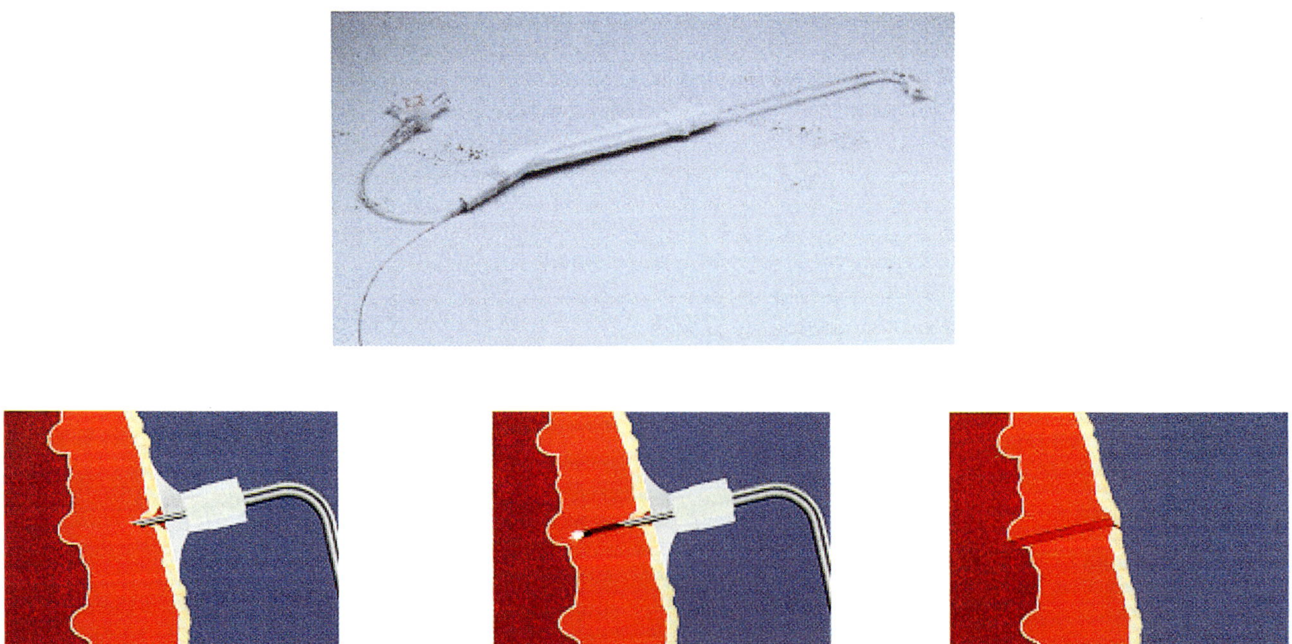

Figure 76–15. A straight handpiece is used for the anterior surface of the heart during gated activation of the CO_2 laser. A single pulse of 20 to 40 joules successfully penetrates the left ventricular wall. (Courtesy of Eclipse Surgical Technologies Inc., Sunnyvale, CA.)

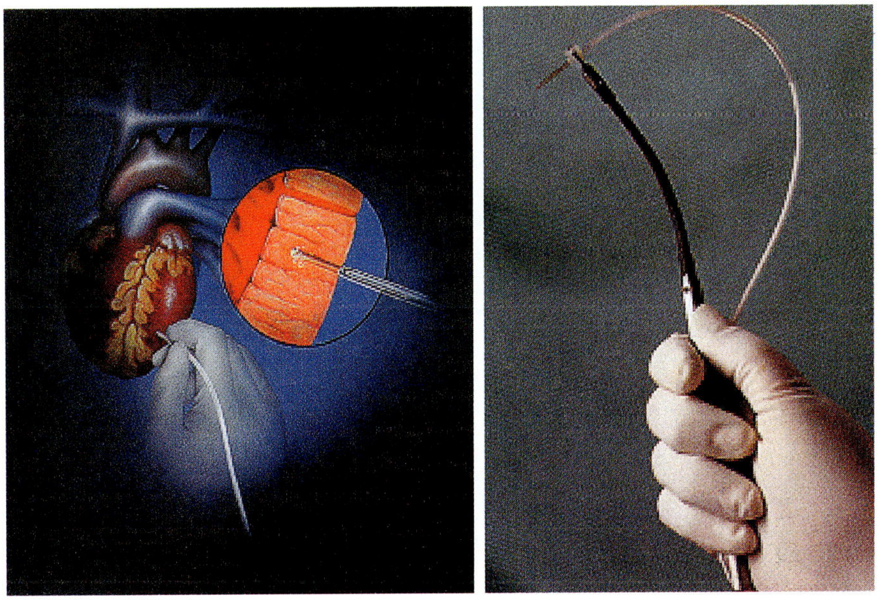

Figure 76–16. This malleable handpiece allows the fiber optic to be advanced from the epicardium to the endocardium during nongated activation of the holmium laser. A foot plate stabilizes the fiber. (Photo courtesy of Eclipse Surgical Technologies Inc., Sunnyvale, CA.)

parin, nitrates, and mechanical support. If intractable, salvage with percutaneous angioplasty is considered.

Low cardiac output may develop in the early postoperative period secondary to myocardial edema, recurrent ischemia, tamponade, or delayed chordal rupture. When the clinical circumstances are confounding, we move rapidly toward assessment with TEE. This can readily be compared to intraoperative images and appropriate therapy instituted. These patients are intolerant of any significant perioperative stress, so rapid identification of the etiology and institution of treatment are necessary. The amount of chest wall edema and air generally precludes adequate assessment with transthoracic echocardiography. The most common finding is inadequate ventricular filling followed by ischemia. If chordal rupture has occurred, the severity of the insufficiency and response to afterload reduction determine the necessity of repair. In general, this rare complication is poorly tolerated. The majority of patients are discharged 7 days after surgery without significant complications.

Discussion

The 12-month results of the randomized comparison of TMR with the CO_2 laser to maximal medical management confirm the superiority of TMR in significantly improving angina class, quality of life, and myocardial perfusion in patients with end-stage coronary artery disease. Coinciding with significant clinical improvement for the TMR group and lack of improvement for the medical management group was a 47% difference in perfusion in favor of those undergoing TMR. The perfusion benefit associated with CO_2 TMR has been corroborated by others.[20–22, 28] Sixty percent of patients initially randomized to medical management significantly worsened, and they were offered cross-over TMR. Significant clinical improvement was ob-

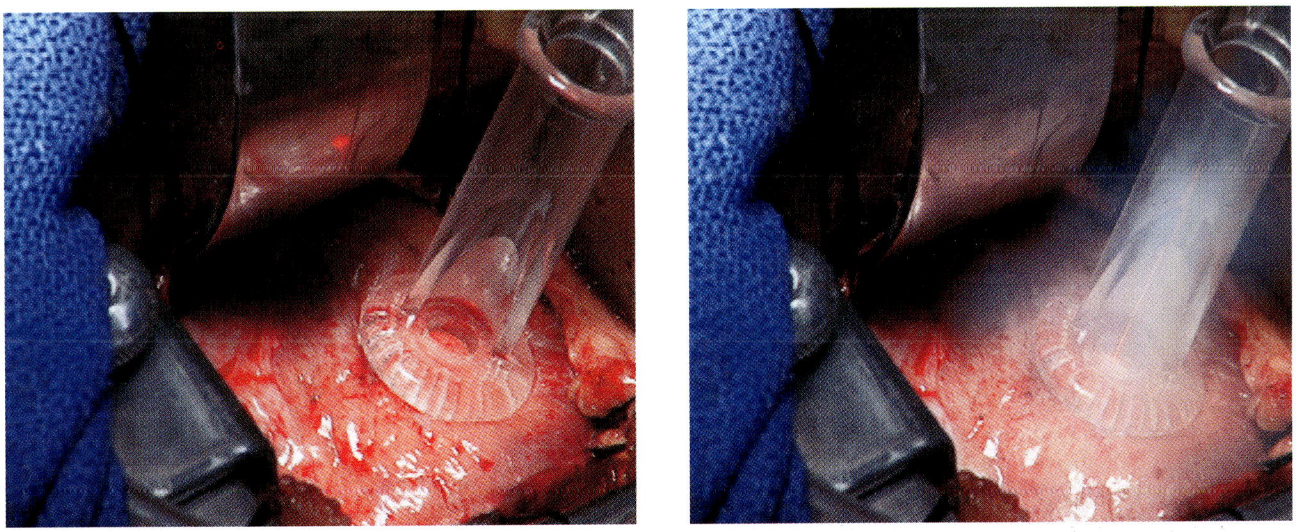

Figure 76–17. An intraoperative probe and reusable malleable handpiece facilitate transmural channel placement during gated activations of the holmium laser. (Photo courtesy of CardioGenesis Corp., Sunnyvale, CA.)

served after cTMR, but this was at the cost of a higher perioperative mortality. Proper patient selection, perioperative management, and a 15-day interval from the last unstable angina episode resulted in a 1% operative mortality. With over 400 patients treated during the various phases of the US trials with the CO_2 laser and over 4000 operations performed worldwide, significant lessons have been learned about the safe use of this new therapy. Intervention with TMR should be considered before clinical instability occurs.

With the success of the CO_2 trials, other catheter-based systems with lasers in the near infrared and ultraviolet[48] regions are under study. Favorable clinical response rates have been reported with TMR using a holmium:YAG laser in comparison to medical management.[33] There is some concern over the higher rate of ventricular arrhythmias and lack of perfusion benefit reported. Enrollment in a randomized study evaluating PMR with a holmium laser in contrast to medical management in terms of exercise tolerance and angina relief has been completed. Six-month follow-up was reported in March 1999.

The success of sole therapy with TMR for symptomatic end-stage coronary artery disease has prompted use of TMR in combination with coronary artery grafting in an attempt to offer complete revascularization. Trehan and colleagues used TMR to the circumflex region in conjunction with off-pump CAB to the left anterior descending and/or right coronary arteries in 56 patients.[49] Further evaluation with thallium imaging demonstrated an exponential improvement of perfusion indices in grafted areas, with a total gain of 33% and a linear improvement in lased areas with a total gain of 25% at 1-year follow-up. Others have reported the use of TMR in conjunction with CAB.[34, 51–53] The superiority of combination therapy has been suggested by a randomized study comparing combination therapy with a holmium laser versus CAB alone. Combination therapy was associated with significantly fewer cardiac events and a lower than predicted mortality rate than for patients undergoing CAB alone.[43, 57] Further evaluation is under way to determine the role of TMR in the treatment of cardiac allograft vasculopathy.[54–56] Trials are being initiated to evaluate the benefit of PMR as an adjunct to PTCA and stenting.

A better understanding of the mechanism by which TMR improves angina and myocardial perfusion should help identify the ideal patient for laser revascularization; the type of laser to be used; the route of therapy, either operative (transmural) or percutaneous (endocardial); and whether adjunctive procedures such as CAB or PTCA and stenting should also be performed.

Potential mechanisms include placebo effect, patent channels, stimulated angiogenesis, and denervation. With evidence that angina relief progressively improves after the procedure and persists up to 3 years, it is unlikely that a placebo effect contributes to the clinical benefit observed. Histologic studies in humans suggest that there is acute channel patency in specimens examined shortly after operation. When analysis was possible at greater intervals postoperatively, vascular spaces could be visualized within loose connective tissue representing the laser tract or channel remnant. Communication with and dilatation of adjacent vascular spaces can be identified in some specimens. Hearts from sole TMR patients examined up to 24 months after surgery show a greater density of scar within the channel remnants.[58] Whether durable endocardial connection persists is still debated.[59, 60]

The role of positive angiogenic regulators produced in response to laser-induced injury in ischemic myocardium is under investigation. In a canine model of coronary insufficiency, vascular endothelial growth factor (VEGF) injections distal to the arterial occlusion led to enhanced collateral blood flow.[61] Therapeutic angiogenesis has been successful in improving perfusion and function of ischemic swine myocardium following the injection of an adenovirus vector that transferred $VEGF_{121}$ cDNA to the myocardium.[62] It is known that tissue irradiation with a laser can produce heat-shock proteins and other substances that possess angiogenic properties.[63] In addition, it has been speculated that the initial channel thrombus observed histologically may contain growth factors and other mediators that stimulate angiogenesis in the surrounding myocardium.[13] Recently, the combination of gene therapy with CO_2 TMR was shown to significantly improve left ventricular performance in chronically ischemic porcine hearts compared with either therapy alone.[64] The angiogenic nature of TMR's effect is gaining greater support, and the combination of TMR with injectable growth factors may be important to further improving the efficacy of the procedure.

The holmium:YAG laser has recently been shown to destroy cardiac nerve fibers in the epicardium of canine hearts.[65] The possibility that denervation might contribute to the mechanism of clinical angina relief was suggested by the investigators. Loss of sympathetic innervation, however, would not explain the improvement in myocardial perfusion and segmental wall motion reported following TMR using the CO_2 laser.[20, 24, 26, 28] Lasers vary in the amount of tissue injury produced, with the holmium:YAG creating the greatest volume of damage[66] among the three lasers currently being investigated. Similar studies would have to be performed with each laser type to determine the contribution of denervation.

The future direction of TMR will depend on a thorough evaluation of the various lasers being proposed for clinical use. Thus far, follow-up has been most complete for patients undergoing TMR with the CO_2 laser. Further investigation is needed to determine the signature of a specific laser on ischemic myocardium. Determining the mechanism of action will help predict clinical improvement and indicate the safest method to achieve improved myocardial perfusion and angina relief in patients with advanced coronary artery disease. In the meantime, the procedural steps to safely carry out clinical TMR as sole therapy or as an adjunct have been reasonably well defined.

References

1. O'Connor W, Cash J, Cotrill C, et al: Ventriculocoronary connections in hypoplastic left hearts, an autopsy microscopy study. Circulation 665:1078–1086, 1982.
2. Wearn JT, Mettler SR, Klumpp TG, Zschiesche LJ: The nature of the vascular communications between the coronary arteries and the chambers of the heart. Am Heart J 9:143–164, 1933.

3. Massimo C, Boffi L: Myocardial revascularization by a new method of carrying blood directly from the left ventricle cavity into the coronary circulation. J Thorac Surg 34:257–264, 1957.
4. Sen PK, Udwadia TE, Kinare SG, Parulkar GB: Transmyocardial acupuncture, a new approach to myocardial revascularization. J Thorac Cardiovasc Surg 50:181–189, 1965.
5. White M, Hershey JE: Multiple transmyocardial puncture revascularization in refractory ventricular fibrillation due to myocardial ischemia. Ann Thorac Surg 6:557–563, 1968.
6. Sen PK. Daulatram J, Kinare SG, et al: Further studies in multiple transmyocardial acupuncture as a method of myocardial revascularization. Surgery 64:861–870, 1968.
7. Walter P, Hundeshagen H, Borst HG: Treatment of acute myocardial infarction by transmural blood supply from the left ventricular cavity. Eur Surg Res 3:130–138, 1971.
8. Vineberg A: Clinical and experimental studies in the treatment of coronary artery insufficiency by internal mammary artery implant. J Intern Coll Surg 22:503–518, 1954.
9. Mirhoseini M, Fisher JC, Cayton MM: Myocardial revascularization by laser: A clinical report. Lasers Surg Med 3:241–245, 1983.
10. Mirhoseini M, Shelgikar S, Cayton MM: New concepts in revascularization of the myocardium. Ann Thorac Surg 45:415–420, 1988.
11. Sen PK: Studies in myocardial revascularization. Indian J Med Res 57:415–433, 1969.
12. Mirhoseini M, Muckerheide M, Cayton MM: Transventricular revascularization by laser. Lasers Surg Med 2:187–198, 1982.
13. Fisher PE, Khomoto T, DeRosa CM, et al: Histologic analysis of transmyocardial channels: Comparison of CO_2 and holmium: YAG lasers. Ann Thorac Surg 64:466–472, 1997.
14. Fleischer KJ, Goldschmidt-Clermont PJ, Fonger JD, et al: One-month histologic response of transmyocardial laser channels with molecular intervention. Ann Thorac Surg 62:1051–1058, 1996.
15. Lutter G, Schwarzkopf J, Lutz C, et al: Histologic findings of transmyocardial laser channels after two hours. Ann Thorac Surg 65:1437–1439, 1998.
16. March RJ, Macioch JE, Donoghue J, et al: Transmyocardial laser revascularization preserves segmental left ventricular contractile reserve: A blinded echocardiographic evaluation (Abstract). American Heart Association 70th Scientific Sessions, November 1997.
17. Okada M, Ikuta H, Shimizu K, et al: Alternative method of myocardial revascularization by laser: Experimental and clinical study. Kobe J Med Sci 32:151–161, 1986.
18. Okada M: Transmyocardial laser revascularization: A long way to the first successful clinical application in the world. Ann Thorac Cardiovasc Surg 4:119–124, 1998.
19. Crew JR: Transmyocardial revascularization by CO_2 laser. Surg Tech Int 1:236–238, 1991.
20. Horvath KA, Cohn LH, Cooley DA, et al: Transmyocardial laser revascularization: Results of a multicenter trial with transmyocardial laser revascularization used as a sole therapy for end-stage coronary artery disease. J Thorac Cardiovasc Surg 113:645–654, 1997.
21. Cooley DA, Frazier OH, Kadipasaoglu KA, et al: Transmyocardial laser revascularization: Clinical experience with twelve month follow-up. J Thorac Cardiovasc Surg 111:791–799, 1996.
22. March RJ, Ali A, Bouzoukis M, et al: Effects of transmyocardial laser revascularization on myocardial perfusion. J Am Coll Cardiol 29(suppl A):121A, 1997.
23. Donoghue JA, Macioch JE, Neumann A, et al: Transmyocardial laser revascularization increases dobutamine-induced angina threshold in patients with refractory angina. J Am Coll Cardiol 226A, 1998.
24. Donovan CL, Landolfo KP, Lowe JE, et al: Improvement in inducible ischemia during dobutamine stress echocardiography after transmyocardial laser revascularization in patients with refractory angina pectoris. J Am Coll Cardiol 30:607–612, 1997.
25. Horvath KA, Cohn LH, Cooley DA, et al: Functional improvement, long term survival and angina relief after transmyocardial laser revascularization with a CO_2 laser. Circulation 98:I-217, 1998.
26. March RJ, Aranki S, Boyce SW, et al: Improved event free survival following transmyocardial laser revascularization versus medical management in patients with unreconstructable coronary artery disease. Presented at the 77th annual meeting of the American Association of Thoracic Surgery, Washington DC, May 1997.
27. PLC Medical Systems presentation to the FDA Advisory Panel, Circulatory System Devices, Gaithersburg, MD, April 24, 1998.
28. March RJ: Transmyocardial laser revascularization with the CO_2 laser: One year results of a randomized controlled trial. Semin Thorac Cardiovas Surg 11:12–19, 1999.
29. Higgins TL, Fawzy EG, Loop FD, et al: Stratification of morbidity and mortality outcome by preoperative risk factors in coronary artery bypass patients. JAMA 267:2344–2348, 1992.
30. March RJ: Transmyocardial laser revascularization: Current experience and future direction. J Clin Laser Med Surg 15: 301–307, 1997.
31. March RJ: Experience with transmyocardial laser revascularization. Asian Cardiovasc Thorac Ann 4:243–244, 1996.
32. Lutter G, Saurbier B, Nitzsche E, et al: Transmyocardial laser revascularization in patients with unstable angina and low ejection fraction. Eur J Cardiothorac Surg 13:21–26, 1998.
33. Allen KB, Fudge TL, Schoettle GP, et al: Prospective randomized multicenter trial of transmyocardial revascularization versus maximal medical management in patients with refractory class IV angina: 12-month results. Circulation 98 (suppl I):I-476, 1998.
34. Diegeler A, Schneider J, Lauer B, et al: Transmyocardial laser revascularization using the holmium:YAG laser for treatment of end-stage coronary artery disease. Eur J Cardiothorac Surg 13:392–397, 1998.
35. Milano A, Pratali S, Tartarini G, et al: Early results of transmyocardial revascularization with the holmium laser. Ann Thorac Surg 65:700–704, 1998.
36. Milano A, Pietrabissa A, Bortolotti U: Transmyocardial laser revascularization using a thoracoscopic approach. Am J Cardiol 79:538–539, 1997.
37. DeGuzman BJ, Lautz DB, Chen FY, et al: Thoracoscopic transmyocardial laser revascularization. Ann Thorac Surg 64:171–174, 1997.
38. Milano A, Pietrabissa A, Bortolotti U: Transmyocardial laser revascularization using a thoracoscopic approach. Am J Cardiol 79:538–539, 1997.
39. Vincent JG: Clinical experience with thoracoscopic TMR versus minimally invasive approach. Ann Thorac Surg 65:599–600, 1998.
40. Oesterle SN, Reifart NJ, Meier B, et al: Initial results of laser-based percutaneous myocardial revascularization for angina pectoris. Am J Cardiol 82:659–662, 1998.
41. Sanborn TA, Oesterle SN, Heuser RR, et al: Percutaneous myocardial revascularization with a holmium laser: A pilot multicenter feasibility trial.
42. Whitlow PL, Knopf D, O'Neill WW, et al: Percutaneous transmyocardial revascularization in patients with refractory angina. Circulation 98 (suppl I):I-87, 1998.
43. Oesterle S, Nguyen T, Allen KB: Percutaneous myocardial laser revascularization. J Interven Cardiol 11:S134–S136, 1998.
44. Frazier OH, Cooley DA, Kadipasaoglu KA, et al: Transmyocardial laser revascularization: Initial clinical results. Circulation 90:1–640, 1995.

45. Bloomberg S, Curaler I, Emanuelson H, et al: Thoracic epidural anesthesia in patients with unstable angina pectoris. Eur Heart J 10:437–444, 1989.
46. Kornowski R, Hong MK, Leon MB: Current perspectives on direct myocardial revascularization. Am J Cardiol 81:44E–48E, 1998.
47. Allen KB, Dowling RD, Heimansohn DA, et al: Transmyocardial revascularization utilizing a holmium:YAG laser. Eur J Cardiothorac Surg 14:S100–S104, 1998.
48. Mack CA, Magovern CJ, Hahn RT, et al: Channel patency and neovascularization after transmyocardial revascularization using an excimer laser: Results and comparisons to nonlased channels. Circulation 96(suppl 9):II65–II69, 1997.
49. Trehan N, Mishra M, Bapna R: Transmyocardial laser revascularization combined with coronary artery grafting without cardiopulmonary bypass. Eur J Cardiothorac Surg 12:276–284, 1997.
50. Knopf W, Londero H, Kaul U, et al: Feasibility study of percutaneous transluminal myocardial revascularization (PTMR) with a holmium laser and fiberoptic delivery system. J Am Coll Cardiol 131:235A, 1998.
51. Vincent JG, Bardos P, Kruse J, Maass D: End-stage coronary artery disease treated with the transmyocardial CO_2 laser revascularization: A chance for the inoperable patient. Eur J Cardiothorac Surg 11:888–894, 1997.
52. Krabatsch T, Tambeur L, Lieback E, et al: Transmyocardial laser revascularization in the treatment of end-stage coronary artery disease. Ann Thorac Cardiovasc Surg 4:64–71, 1998.
53. March RJ, Klontz B: Transmyocardial laser revascularization. *In* Cohen RJ, Mack MJ, Fonger JD, Landreneau RJ (eds): Minimally Invasive Cardiac Surgery. St Louis, Quality Medical Publishing, 1999, pp 329–336.
54. March RJ, Guynn T: Cardiac allograft vasculopathy: The potential role for transmyocardial laser revascularization. J Heart Lung Transplant 14:S242–S246, 1995.
55. Frazier OH, Kadipasaoglu KA, Radovancevic B, et al: Transmyocardial laser revascularization in allograft coronary artery disease. Ann Thorac Surg 65:1138–1141, 1998.
56. Malik FS, Mehra MR, Ventura HO, et al: Management of cardiac allograft vasculopathy by transmyocardial laser revascularization. Am J Cardiol 80:224–225, 1997.
57. Allen KB, Delrossi AJ, Realyvasquez F, et al: Transmyocardial revascularization combined with coronary artery bypass grafting versus coronary artery grafting alone: Results of a prospective randomized, multi-center trial. Circulation 98 (suppl I):I-217, 1998.
58. Rodriguez R: Personal communication.
59. Cooley DA, Frazier OH, Kadipasaoglu K, et al: Transmyocardial laser revascularization: Anatomic evidence of long term channel patency. Tex Heart Inst J 21:220–224, 1994.
60. Berkhoff D, Fisher PE, Apfelbaum M, et al: Histologic appearance of transmyocardial laser channels after 4 1/2 weeks. Ann Thorac Surg 61:1532–1535, 1996.
61. Banai S, Shou M, Jaktlish MT, et al: Enhancement of coronary collateral flow by intracoronary injection of vascular endothelial growth factor. J Am Coll Cardiol 19:936–22, 1992.
62. Mack CA, Patel SR, Schwarz EA, et al: Myocardial perfusion and function following adenovirus-mediated transfer of the $VEGF_{121}$ cDNA to ischemic porcine myocardium. Presented at the 77th annual meeting of the American Association of Thoracic Surgery, Washington, DC, May 1997.
63. Nakagawa K: Direct observation of laser generated free radicals from a myocardium target sac. Free Radic Biol Med 12:241–242, 1992.
64. Sayeed-Shah U, Mann MJ, Martin J, et al: Combined gene therapy with TMR improves hemodynamic performance in chronically ischemic porcine hearts. Circulation 98:I-217, 1998.
65. Kwong KF, Kanellopoulous GK, Nichols JC, et al: Transmyocardial laser treatment denervates canine myocardium. J Thorac Cardiovasc Surg 114:883–890, 1997.
66. Frazier OH, Kadipasaoglu KA, Cooley DA: Transmyocardial laser revascularization: Does it have a role in the treatment of ischemic heart disease? Tex Heart Inst J 25:24–29, 1998.
67. Snell RJ: Personal communication.

COMMENTARY

John E. Sanderson

In this excellent review, Dr. March has covered all aspects of transmyocardial laser revascularization. There seems little doubt now that the technique can produce symptomatic relief in patients with intractable angina. However, there is still an interesting debate about the mechanism involved. In particular, the controversy is still unresolved whether there is persistent channel patency after transmyocardial revascularization (TMR). If there is no channel patency, it is obvious that other mechanisms have to be considered, such as denervation or stimulation of angiogenesis. However, it would seem that "drilling" many holes into the myocardium is a rather obtuse way of denervating the heart or stimulating angiogenesis, and I am sure that there must be better ways to do this. The justification of TMR really hinges on the question of channel patency. Surprisingly, there are few human data available. One of the studies not mentioned by Dr. March is that by Gassler and associates.[1] In this study the authors had the opportunity to examine hearts in patients who had died without clinical evidence of persistent therapeutic effect at 3, 16, and 150 days after TMR. In the subjects who died on day 3, laser-induced channels were filled with abundant granulocytes, thrombosis, fibrous networks, and debris and were surrounded by severe myocardial necrosis. In addition, the epicardium and endocardium were obstructed by a fibrous network and microclots. In the patients who died on day 150, there was fibrous tissue mixed with a polymorphous, blood-filled capillary network and small veins that rarely had a continuous link to the left ventricular cavity. These patients were unresponsive to TMR, and the lack of channel patency may have been part of the reason. Alternatively, it could be that the mechanism of TMR is unrelated to channel patency, in which case this study is representative of what may be happening in most patients. All previous studies of laser-created channels were conducted using animal models with acutely induced myocardial ischemia. It would be surprising, however, if the tissue response to drilling holes in the myocardium were not similar to that which occurs in normal wound repair. In such cases there would be a mixture of granular tissue, lymphocytic response, generation of collagen, and fibrous scar tissue.

Dr. March believes that denervation is unlikely to contribute to clinical pain relief, as it would not explain the improvement in myocardial perfusion and segmental wall motion. This is not necessarily true. The coronary arteries are richly innervated by sympathetic nerve fibers and are involved in controlling coronary vasodilatation to match oxygen supply to demand.[2] With ischemia, α-adrenergic receptor stimulation may produce excess oxygen-free radicals and calcium overload and release endothelial factors that may potentiate ischemia.[3] Phentolamine (an α-blocker) given after thrombolysis has recently been shown to improve coronary blood flow and left ventricular function.[4] Thus removal of α-adrenergic stimulation by denervation may contribute significantly to improving coronary blood flow, myocardial function, and pain relief

TMR and percutaneous myocardial revascularization (PMR) have not been in use for very long, and there are few long-term mortality or randomized trial data. Allen and colleagues randomized 74 patients to TMR and 86 to maximal local management. At 1 year there was no difference in terms of myocardial perfusion benefit or mortality.[5] A recently published trial randomized 188 patients with refractory angina to TMR or medical management alone.[6] Although angina symptoms declined significantly, there was no significant or clinically important change in exercise time. Mortality at 1 year was not significantly higher in the TMR group than in the medical group. Laser revascularization must be considered a method of last resort.

References

1. Gassler N, Wintzer H-O, Stubbe H-M, et al: Transmyocardial laser revascularization: Histological features in human nonresponder myocardium circulation 95:371–375, 1997.
2. Heusch G: α-Adrenergic mechanisms in myocardial ischemia. Circulation 81:1–13, 1990.
3. Kern MJ: Appreciating α-adrenergic receptors and their role in ischemic left ventricular dysfunction. Circulation 99:468–471, 1999.
4. Gregorini L, Marco J, Kozakova M, et al: α-Adrenergic blockade improves recovery of myocardial perfusion and function after coronary stenting in patients with acute myocardial infarction. Circulation 99:482–490, 1999.
5. Allen KB, Fudge TL, Schoettle GP, et al: Prospective randomized multicenter trial of transmyocardial revascularization versus maximal medical management in patients with refractory class IV angina: 12-month results. (abstract) Circulation 98:I-476, 1998.
6. Schofield PM, Sharples LD, Caine N, et al: Transmyocardial laser revascularisation in patients with refractory angina: A randomised controlled trial. Lancet 353:519–524, 1999.

Chapter 77

Minimal Access Vein Harvesting for Coronary Artery Bypass

Leonardo Esteves Lima

Direct coronary surgery was first performed in the late 1950s, before cardiopulmonary bypass came into widespread use. In 1957, Bailey and associates were the first group to approach the problem of coronary occlusion directly.[1] The coronary anastomosis distal to the occlusion using the saphenous vein was experimentally considered by Murray and associates in 1954.[11] Sabiston performed the first right coronary artery bypass using the saphenous vein in 1962,[13] and Garrett and associates reported the first prolonged survival (7 years) of a patient operated on for a coronary bypass in 1973.[8] In 1968, Favaloro presented his work with routine saphenous vein graft coronary bypass.[7]

Coronary artery bypass grafting (CABG) is one of the most commonly performed surgical procedures in North America and Europe. Today, despite the availability of improved medical therapy and coronary angioplasty, surgical revascularization of the myocardium remains the treatment of choice for most advanced forms of coronary artery disease, and the saphenous vein is the most frequently used conduit.

Since we began using the autogenous greater saphenous vein as conduit for CABG, various open techniques have been used to harvest the saphenous vein. Traditional open techniques vary in incision length, ranging from a continuous incision from the groin to the ankle to multiple smaller interrupted incisions in the thigh and lower leg.

The complications of this procedure have not received great attention in the surgical literature,[3, 6, 16] but they are familiar to any active cardiovascular service where the leg is the primary site of vein harvest.[6] Both the long-leg incisions and interrupted incisions could lead to significant pain for the patient and potential postoperative wound complications, either major or minor. Major wound complications are rare[3]; however, impaired wound healing has been reported to be as high as 24%.[15, 16]

In all surgical fields, there has been a tendency toward minimizing access, shortening hospitalizations, and hastening recovery, as well as decreasing mortality, morbidity, and cost. Following this trend, the development of more effective and less expensive cardiovascular techniques is necessary.[5]

Minimally invasive vein harvesting (MIVH) aims to reduce complications and improve patient satisfaction. The first MIVH apparatus—the Vein Trap Atrium—was introduced in 1984. It was known as the "subcutaneous vein remover."[4, 12] This device never became popular. The disposable Vein Trap consists of a long, hard, hollow plastic cylindrical tube with two small scalpel blades imbedded in the circumferential edge at the leading end of the subcutaneous vein remover.

The Vein Trap technique, recommended for only thigh veins, involved making two small 3- to 4-cm incisions at the proximal and distal thigh. The device was rotated manually and then in a clockwise fashion while advancing the subcutaneous vein remover. This allowed the imbedded scalpel blades to sever tributaries simultaneously and to create a tunnel around the vein. This technique was blind, bloody, and traumatic, because no vein branches were ligated in situ. The leg wounds were packed tightly to prevent bleeding during the cardiopulmonary bypass. They were then closed and wrapped tightly with a compression Ace bandage.[4, 12]

Several other MIVH systems have since been introduced to the clinician and become commercially available: the Mini-Harvest System by Autosuture; the Endopath System by Ethicon Endo-Surgery, the Endosaph by General Surgical Innovations (GSI), and the Vasoview System by Origin.

This chapter details all these systems, which have been clinically evaluated in cardiac surgery by our group in La Pitié Hospital in Paris.

Review of Currently Available Minimally Invasive Vein Harvesting Systems

The Mini-Harvest System

Equipment. The Mini-Harvest System (Autosuture, a subsidiary of United States Surgical), consists of two right-angled retractors (one 6 cm long and the other 8 cm long) coupled to a light source (fiberoptic light). The retractor can be handled like a laryngoscope or fixed to a support, to provide self-retaining retraction (Fig. 77–1).

Technique. A 4-cm longitudinal incision is recommended at the mid-thigh on the medial border of the sartorius muscle, approximately 14 cm caudally from the groin crease. The mid-thigh incision avoids the groin area and so decreases potential wound infections from groin-related contaminants. The greater saphenous vein is then mobilized and branches ligated as with the standard open technique of vein harvesting. Using gentle blunt-finger dissection, the surgeon creates a subcutaneous tunnel just anterior to the saphenous vein both proximally and distally. The Mini-Harvest System is inserted into the distal tunnel, and tissues are retracted to provide lighted exposure of the tunnel. Working from within the tunnel, the surgeon can perform further dissection, clip ligation of the vein branches, and mobilization of the saphenous vein.

Vein mobilization is maximized by this second incision, approximately 4 cm long, made at the distal thigh, 8 cm proximal to the popliteal fossa. If needed, a third or fourth

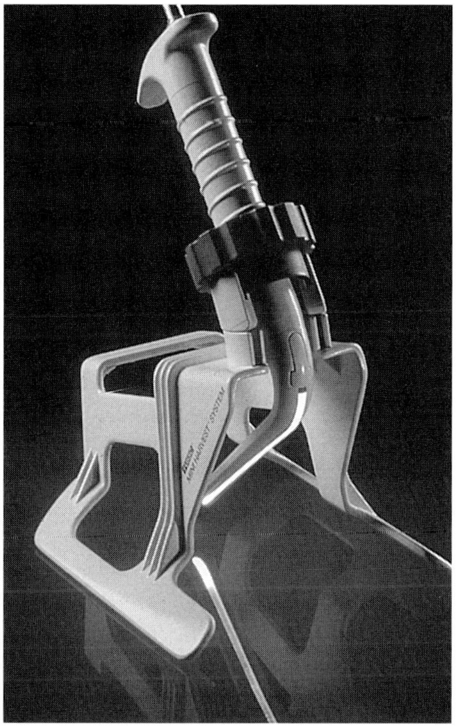

Figure 77–1. The Autosuture Mini-Harvest* System. (Autosuture, a subsidiary of United States Surgical, Norwalk, CT. Copyright © 1999 United States Surgical. All rights reserved. Reprinted with permission of United States Surgical.)

incision, approximately 4 cm (3 to 4 cm distal to the popliteal fossa), is made at the proximal and distal lower leg (6 to 7 cm proximal to the medial malleolus). Using similar open vein-harvesting techniques, the surgeon again mobilizes the saphenous vein and doubly ligates the vein branches. A tunnel is created both proximally and distally with blunt-finger dissection, making a connection with the tunnel that was made previously. The Mini-Harvest System is then inserted into the proximal and distal tunnels to complete vein dissection, mobilization, and branch ligation to the desired length, as previously described.

After ligating and cutting the distal end of the vein, the surgeon inserts the Mini-Harvest System into the proximal tunnel of the mid-thigh incision and performs further proximal mobilization of the vein to the saphenofemoral junction. The proximal saphenous vein stump may then be ligated and cut, and the vein removed by means of a pretied Autosuture Surgi-Tie device.

Standard open techniques and sutures are used for vein preparation and leg wound closure.[15]

Conclusion. The Mini-Harvest technique is similar to the interrupted incision used in the standard open technique, but it provides improved tunnel exposure and illumination.

The Endopath System

Equipment. This system (Ethicon Endo-Surgery, a subsidiary of Johnson & Johnson, Cincinnati, OH) consists of the Endopath Subcu-Dissector, the Endopath Subcu-Retractor (with a fiberoptic light attachment and 29.5-cm long retractor blade similar to a straight-blade laryngoscope), and the Endopath Vein Dissector. Unlike the Mini-Harvest System, the Endopath System requires the use of endoscopic equipment, including an endoscope (5 mm × 300 mm), endoscopic camera, video monitor, and endoscopic instruments. This vein-harvesting system allows the surgeon to use endoscopic instruments through a lighted retractor in an anterograde fashion. The Subcu-Retractor is held manually, allowing easier manipulation and retraction of tissues for optimal exposure (Fig. 77–2).

Technique. A 3- to 4-cm longitudinal incision is recommended. The incision should be made at the distal thigh, just proximal to the knee. Alternatively, the surgeon can start at the proximal thigh or at the distal lower leg, depending on personal preference. Once the saphenous vein is mobilized and the visible branches ligated, the surgeon using standard open vein-harvesting techniques, creates a subcutaneous tunnel just anterior to the greater saphenous vein, in the cephalad direction, using blunt-finger dissection initially. The Endopath Subcu Dissector is inserted into this proximal tunnel and under video monitor guidance advanced cephalad by manipulating it in a rocking motion for its full length while staying anterior to the vein.

When the tunnel is created, the Endopath Subcu Dissector is replaced by the Subcu-Retractor to keep the tissues retracted and the tunnel and vein exposed. Using the Endopath Vein Dissector and a 5-mm endoscopic clip applicator, the surgeon mobilizes the vein and doubly ligates and cuts the vein branches. Once the vein is mobilized, the Subcu-Dissector and Subcu Retractor are removed simultaneously under direct visualization to avoid inadvertent injury to the vein. The surgeon then reinserts the Subcu-Retractor to its full length while monitoring the transilluminated tip through the skin. A second smaller proximal thigh incision is made over the transilluminated area. Using both direct visualization—as with the standard open technique—and endoscopic visualization from inside the tunnel, the surgeon transects and ligates the vein and extracts it via the distal thigh wound. This procedure is repeated through a distal tunnel into the lower leg, approaching from the same distal thigh wound. A third incision is made at the lower leg to transect the distal end of the vein.[9]

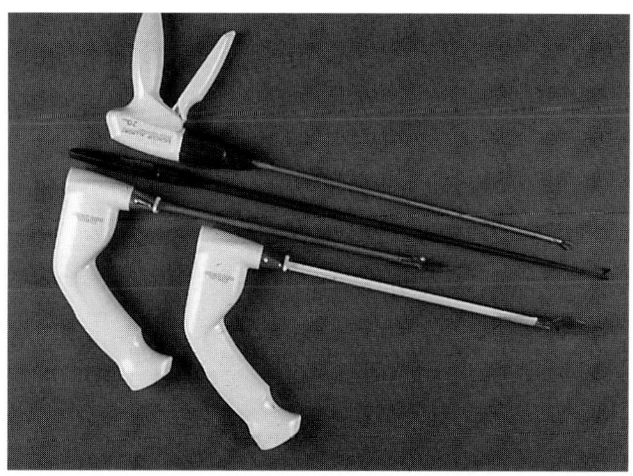

Figure 77–2. The Endopath System. (Courtesy of Ethicon Endo-Surgery, Paris.)

*Trademark of United States Surgical.

Conclusion. The Endopath technique uses an open-system endoscopic approach in which the operating tunnel is visualized through an open wound.

The Endosaph System

Equipment. The Endosaph System (General Surgical Innovations [GSI], Cupertino, CA) consists of a SAPHfinder surgical balloon dissector (with a fiberoptic light attachment, a 30-cm long malleable guide, a 120-cc attached balloon, and either a full tip or a 30-degree tip) (Fig. 77–3), and a Spacekeeper retractor (with a fiberoptic light attachment and a 30-cm long retractor blade similar to a straight-blade laryngoscope) and reusable hook and fork dissectors (Fig. 77–4).

Like the Endopath System, the Endosaph requires the use of endoscopic equipment, including a 30-degree endoscope (5 mm × 300 mm), an endoscopic camera, a video monitor, and endoscopic instruments. This vein-harvesting system allows the surgeon to use endoscopic instruments such as the Endopath System. The Spacekeeper retractor is held manually, allowing easier manipulation and retraction of tissues for optimal exposure (see Fig. 77–4).

Technique. A 3-cm incision is made just above the knee over the saphenous vein. The vein is mobilized and controlled with a vessel loop. A 30-degree endoscope (5-mm) is inserted into the SAPHfinder surgical balloon dissector. This provides an endoscopic view on the monitor to allow precise tracking of the saphenous vein and proper balloon positioning (see Fig. 77–3). The balloon is inserted subcutaneously along the anterior surface of the saphenous vein toward the groin. With the suction outlet closed, the balloon is inflated with saline solution to its recommended fill volume. Once the balloon is fully inflated, the dissection is complete. The balloon is emptied by opening the suction outlet. When the fluid has been completely evacuated, the SAPHfinder surgical balloon dissector is removed from the incision. The 30-degree endoscope (5 mm) is removed from the SAPHfinder surgical balloon dissector and inserted into the Spacekeeper retractor. The retractor is inserted into the dissected space (see Fig. 75–4). The appropriate Hook or Fork dissector instrument harvest the vein from its surrounding tissue bed. Tributaries are ligated with a clip applier. Endoscopic shears may then be used to divide the tributary. The dissection is continued until the desired length of the vessel has been completely harvested from its bed.

Additional incisions may be necessary to facilitate exposure. If access to more of the vein is required, a similar technique may be employed from the knee to the ankle. The Spacekeeper is then reinserted along its full length while monitoring the transilluminated tips through the skin. A second smaller proximal thigh incision is made over the transilluminated area.

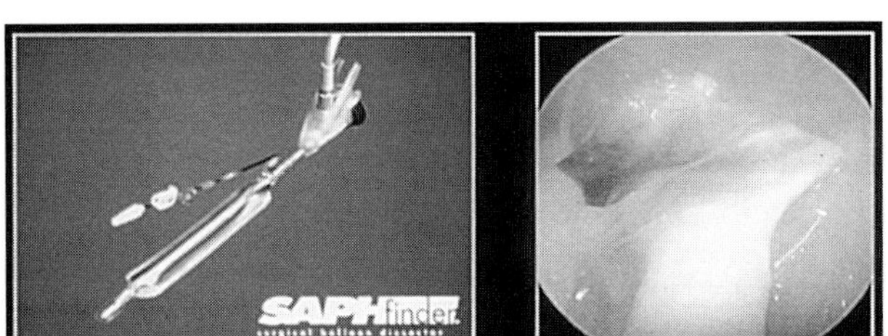

Figure 77–3. The Endosaph balloon dissector. (Courtesy of General Surgical Instruments, Cupertino, CA.)

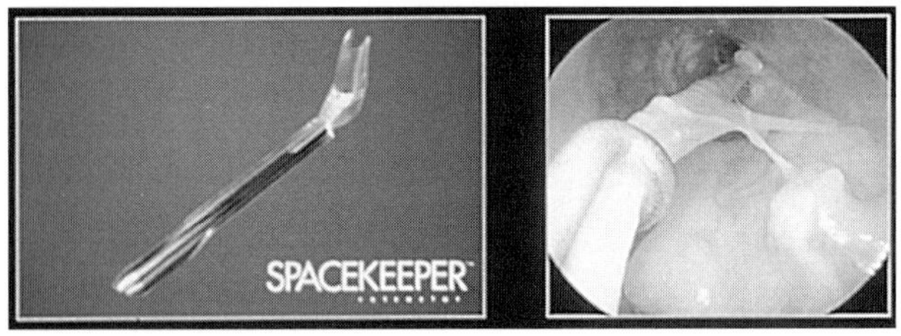

Figure 77–4. The Endosaph self-retaining distal retractor. (Courtesy of GSI.)

Using both direct visualization, as with the standard open technique, and endoscopic visualization from inside the tunnel, the surgeon transects and ligates the vein and extracts it via the distal thigh wound. Once the required length of vein has been harvested, the cavity is suction irrigated with saline solution and inspected under endoscopic visualization to ensure adequate hemostasis. The incisions are closed according to operator preference.

Conclusion. The Endosaph technique uses an open system endoscopic approach helped by a balloon to make the operating tunnel, which is visualized through an open wound.

The VASOVIEW System

Equipment. The VASOVIEW System (Origin, division of the Guidant Corporation, Indianapolis, IN), consists of two cannulas (balloon dissection and orbital dissector), one 10-mm Origin Blunt Tip Trocar (BTT) port, a 5-mm short trocar, and 5-mm bipolar scissors or forceps. The Balloon Dissection Cannula is a long (39 cm), hollow, transparent, hard plastic, cylindrical tube with a bullet-shaped tip and a 40-cc balloon near the tip. This device is used to create a subcutaneous tunnel. The second cannula, the orbital dissector, is 10 mm in diameter. It has an endoscopic ring dissector incorporated into the device that is used for vein skeletonization. The trocars are supplied to provide an airtight seal for maintaining insufflation of the tunnel during vein dissection (Fig. 77–5).

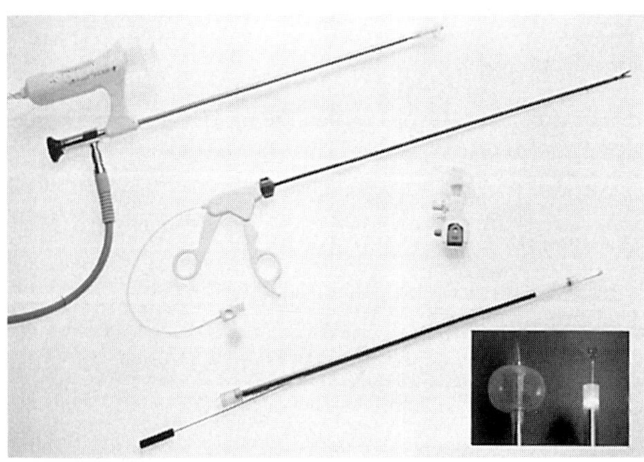

Figure 77–5. The VASOVIEW system.

Technique. A 2- to 2.5-cm horizontal incision is made at the distal thigh just proximal to the knee for harvesting the vein toward the groin. This smaller incision is important for maintaining an airtight seal around the BTT Port. The greater saphenous vein is then identified and dissected to the adventitial layer, with the side branches ligated and divided at the incision site. At this point, care must be taken to minimize mobilization and dissection of the vein through this small opening, because enlarging the opening could create a gross leak around the BTT port, with associated loss of insufflation in the tunnel. Using gentle blunt-finger dissection, the surgeon creates a subcutaneous tunnel. The VASOVIEW Balloon Dissection Cannula (VBDC) is advanced 4 to 5 cm, staying anterior to the vein. The BTT port is then inserted into the small tunnel and the BTT port balloon inflated with 20 to 30 ml of air to maintain an airtight seal. The tunnel is distended with carbon dioxide, with a flow rate of 3 L/min (low or medium flow) and a pressure of 10 to 12 mm Hg (Fig. 77–6). The VBDC is then advanced to its full length, staying anterior to the vein. The carbon dioxide helps visualization and aids dissection. If resistance is encountered at the site of a branch, the VBDC can be rotated and advanced further to avoid damaging the vein or its branches. When advancing the VBDC, the surgeon intermittently inflates the balloon with 40 ml of air while monitoring the progress of the transilluminated tip of the VASOVIEW system. Care must be taken to avoid advancing the VBDC while the balloon is inflated. Once the tunnel is created, the VBDC is removed slowly and intermittently inflated to further dilate the tunnel. Care should be taken not to dilate the tunnel near the wound.

The Orbital Dissector Cannula (VOC) with the ring dissector is advanced to the distal end of the tunnel and the dissection is begun working back towards the operator, using short axial strokes. The dissection ring is used to isolate and encircle the vein until the vein is completely skeletonized. The 5-mm short trocar is inserted 9 to 10 cm distal to the BTT port. The port placement may vary depending on the surgeon's judgment.

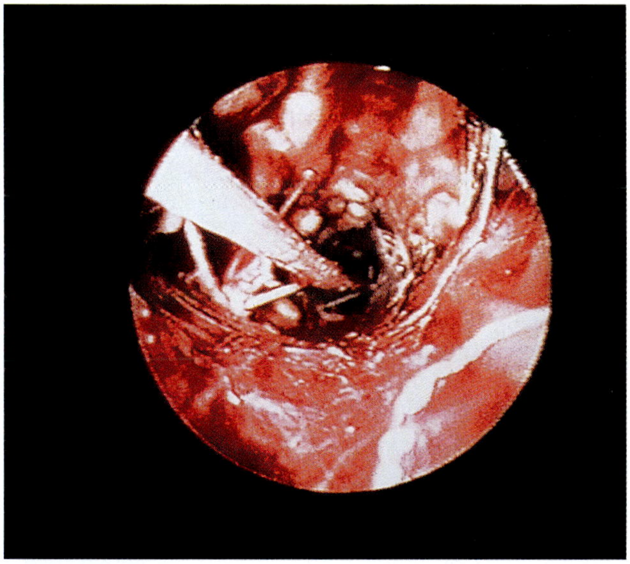

Figure 77–6. Saphenous vein dissection seen through a VASOVIEW system.

A 5-mm bipolar ligation instrument (either scissors or forceps) is guided through the short trocar. The instrument and the dissection ring are advanced to the first side branch. The dissection ring is used to isolate the tributary, enabling side-branch coagulation and division by the bipolar scissors. The process is repeated until the vein is completely detached.

When all tributaries have been ligated, the dissection ring is advanced along the length of the vein to ensure that all connective tissue has been dissected. Using a 30-ml syringe, the BTT is deflated and removed.

The ends of the saphenous vein are ligated using standard surgical techniques (e.g., sutures, clips) and the vein is removed through the incision at the knee.

If additional vein is needed, the VBDC is inserted in the opposite direction and the tunnel creation is repeated. The same procedure is followed for dissection, insufflation, skeletonization and side branch ligation.

Conclusion. The VASOVIEW system ensures a closed endoscopic approach, it requires ports and carbon dioxide to maintain adequate insufflation of the tunnel instead of a manually held retractor, facilitating manipulation exposure and dissection of tissues. Future developments of this technique are under way and hold the promise of further reducing the cost of use and operative times.

Personal Experience

We used all of the techniques described in this chapter. In our initial experience, 100 patients had greater saphenous vein (GSV) harvested by one of the minimally invasive techniques (MIT)—80% with the VASOVIEW system and 20% with other systems. These patients were compared prospectively with 100 patients who underwent the traditional open technique (OT).

There were 85 men and 15 women in the MIT group, and 89 men and 11 women in the OT group, with a mean age of 63.7 ± 9.5 years. There were 3 conversions to OT in the MIT group. Two of these resulted from a very superficial course of GSV, and 1 was as a result of bleeding. In the MIT group, 25% of the patients were obese and 11% had diabetes. In the OT group, 22% of the patients were obese and 9% had diabetes. Peripheral vascular disease was presented in 6% of the MIT group and 7% of the OT group. The harvest time averages 41 ± 10 minutes in the MIT group, and 42 ± 20 minutes in the OT group. The length of the harvest conduit averaged 37 ± 9 centimeters in the MIT group and 42 ± 5 centimeters in the OT group. The average length of the incision was 5 ± 4 cm in the MIT group and 38 ± 7 cm in the OT group.

The incidence of wound healing impairment was 0% in the MIT group and 11% in the OT group. There were only 9% of minor wound complications in the MIT group (2 hematomas and 7 instances of peripheral edema) and 60% in the OT group (50% peripheral edema, 5% hematoma, 4% drainage, and 6% wound edge separation). There were no major complications in the MIT group and 2 major complications in the OT group that required dressing and débridement.

The leg pain score was estimated by means of a Visual Analogue Scale, with a mean value of 1.3 ± 0.4 in the MIT group and 3 ± 2 in the OT group.

Discussion

Minimally invasive surgical techniques have now entered the arena of saphenous vein harvesting.[10] While MIVH techniques offer the potential advantages of reduced postoperative pain and fewer wound-healing complications, the quality of the conduit for coronary bypass is the highest priority, and, thus, new techniques of saphenous vein excision should be examined carefully. It is estimated that 694,000 CABG procedures were performed worldwide in 1998.[2] A majority of these will use both the internal mammary artery and the greater saphenous vein as conduits for complete revascularization of the myocardium. Current approaches to saphenous vein excision include a continuous incision from groin to ankle, which leaves a skin bridge at the knee region, and multiple small incisions along the entire length of the harvested vein. These techniques provide good exposure, but they cause considerable postoperative pain. The incidence of wound healing impairment after saphenous vein excision ranges from 1 to 43%, with the criteria being wound edge separation; cellulitis; drainage; or necrosis that requires dressing, antibiotics, or débridements.[3, 6, 15, 16]

Patients who have diabetes, peripheral vascular disease, immunosuppression, obesity, skin disorders, or poor connective tissues (e.g., resulting from aging), are at greater risk of potential leg wound complications.

Each of the techniques described here is distinctive. The Mini-Harvest System is essentially a standard open technique with improved visualization of the operative tunnel. The Endopath System and the Endosaph System are open-system endoscopic techniques. The VASOVIEW System can best be described as a truly endoscopic technique. With the Mini-Harvest System, the surgeon retracts tissues for tunnel exposure either manually with physical exertion or in a hands-free fashion, using a stand. The Endopath and Endosaph Systems use manual retraction, whereas the VASOVIEW System uses carbon dioxide insufflation to distend the operative tunnel. Operative equipment in addition to the included accessories is required for each system. The Mini-Harvest System requires the least amount of extra equipment, and the VASOVIEW System requires the most. All systems need a fiberoptic light source and standard open surgical instruments. With the Mini-Harvest System, the surgeon may also use the pretied Autosuture Surgi-Tie device for ligating the vein stump deep in the operative tunnel. The Endopath System requires an endoscope, a video camera and monitor, an endoscopic clip applicator, and endoscopic scissors. The VASOVIEW System requires the same equipment as the Endopath and Endosaph Systems, with the addition of gas insufflation.[9, 15]

All techniques maximize the benefits of fewer and smaller incisions. Assuming that an entire leg length of vein from groin to ankle needs to be harvested, the recommended number of incisions and incision lengths are four 4-cm incisions (longest) for the Mini-Harvest System, three 3- to 4-cm incisions for the Endopath and Endosaph systems, and three 2- to 2.5-cm incisions (shortest) for the VASOVIEW System. Longer than recommended incision lengths for the VASOVIEW System can potentially cause leakage of carbon dioxide gas around the BTT port and subsequent loss of tunnel distention and exposure. Smaller (2.5 to 3 cm) incisions with the Mini-Harvest System are achievable, but the smaller the incision, the more difficult the exposure. Skin incisions for the Endopath and Endosaph systems cannot be small, because the skin opening needs to be large enough for insertion of the Subcu-Retractor and the Spacekeeper Retractor. The length of the vein required often influences the number of incisions needed to harvest the vein. However, the distance of the skin bridge between each incision differs with each minimally invasive technique, and depends, in part, on the length of the particular system. Although the Mini-Harvest retractor blade is 6 cm long, using the technique of creating and connecting the operative tunnels, an approximately 12-cm tunnel and corresponding skin bridge can be made between each skin incision. The Endopath Subcu-Retractor and the Endosaph Spacekeeper are 30 cm long, providing a skin bridge along a distance of approximately 30 cm. The VASOVIEW System is 39 cm long, providing a corresponding skin bridge of approximately 40 cm (the longest distance of all the systems). Conceivably, the skin bridge distance can be nearly doubled for the latter three systems if a tunnel connection technique similar to the Mini-Harvest technique is used, but this would be technically challenging.

Visualization of the saphenous vein is direct with the Mini-Harvest System and indirect by video monitor with the other systems. Before the ring dissector is used for vein mobilization, the saphenous vein usually lies adherent to the floor of the operative tunnel with the Mini-Harvest, Endopath, and Endosaph systems. In contrast, the vein is usually found partially mobilized, hanging freely at the center of the tunnel in the VASOVIEW System, possibly secondary to the gas insufflation that mobilizes the vein along the dissected plane.

The learning curve is easiest with the Mini-Harvest System because the technique is essentially the standard open technique.[15] The Endopath and Endosaph systems have a mid-range level of difficulty in their learning curves because of their endoscopic and video monitor visualization. The VASOVIEW System has the steepest learning curve, primarily because of the need to work completely endoscopically. Early attempts at minimally invasive vein harvesting may take as long as 2 hours, regardless which system is used. However, minimally invasive vein-harvesting times are competitive with standard open techniques once the system is mastered. Two operators may be needed in the initially learning phase in the Endopath and Endosaph systems. In contrast, the surgeon can operate independently from the beginning with the VASOVIEW System.

The VASOVIEW System uses bipolar scissors or forceps to cut and coagulate tributaries. This facilitates dissection and saves time. The other systems use traditional endoscopic clip appliers and scissors.

At the present time, some studies comparing MIVH systems with traditional techniques suggest a better result with fewer wound complications with these systems, as shown by our experience.

Clearly, the complications associated with the conventional approach for harvesting the saphenous vein present considerable cost implications. Besides the patient benefits from a dramatically smaller incision, clinical studies of hospital costs associated with the conventional procedure have demonstrated a cumulative cost of 47.44 United States dollars (USD) for 64 patients, or 688 USD per patient.[14]

Even though there is an added cost for each vein-harvesting system, ranging from 120 USD to approximately 500 USD, this may be offset by the benefits of minimally invasive techniques.

Conclusion

Based on our initial clinical experience and that of other authors, it seems that these less invasive approaches are not only clinically effective but may reduce patient pain and postoperative wound complications. These techniques offer many advantages over the standard methods. Certainly MIVH requires a learning curve; however, the benefits of these techniques typically outweigh the pitfalls, once operator skills are mastered.

As fewer minimally invasive products enter this highly competitive market, randomized trials will be necessary to compare these new approaches with standard open vein-harvesting techniques. These trials will require lengthy follow-up.

References

1. Bailey C, May A, Lemon W: Survival after coronary endarterectomy in men. JAMA:167, 1957.
2. American Health Consultants: Cardiovascular Device Update, 1997.
3. De Laria GA, Hunter JA, Golden MD, et al: Leg wound complications associated with coronary revascularization. J Thorac Cardiovasc Surg 81:403–407, 1981.
4. Dorsey JS: Harvesting the greater saphenous vein with a subcutaneous vein remover. Can J Surg 28:13, 14, 1985.
5. Esteves Lima L, Nataf P, Gandjbakhch I, et al: Thoracoscopic IMA dissection and direct suture (La Pitié Technique). *In* Emery RW: Techniques for Minimally Invasive Direct Coronary Artery Bypass Surgery, 1st ed: Philadelphia, Hanley & Belfus, 1997, pp 55–62.
7. Favaloro RG: Saphenous vein autograft replacement of severe segmental coronary artery occlusion. Ann Thorac Surg 10:97–111, 1970.
8. Garrett HE, Dennid EW, DeBakey ME: Aorto-coronary bypass with saphenous vein graft: Seven year follow-up. JAMA 223:792–794, 1973.
9. Lee J: Minimally invasive vein harvesting. Surg Phys Assist Nov/Dec: 25–32, 1996.
10. Lumsden AB, Eaves FF, Ofenloch JC, et al: Subcutaneous video-assisted saphenous vein harvest: Report of the first 30 cases. Cardiovasc Surg 4:771–776, 1996.
11. Murray G, Porcheron R, Hilario J, et al: Anastomosis of a systemic artery to the coronary. Can Med Assoc J 1:594–597, 1954.
12. Rashid A, Fabri B, Meade JB: Subcutaneous technique for saphenous vein harvest. Ann Thorac Surg 37:169, 170, 1984.
13. Sabiston DC: The coronary circulation. Johns Hopkins J 134:314, 1974.
14. Schwartz ME, Harrington EB, Schanzer H: Wound complications after in situ bypass. J Vasc Surg 7:802–807, 1988.
15. Tevaearai HT, Mueller XM, Von Segesser LK: Minimally invasive harvest of the saphenous vein for coronary artery bypass grafting. Ann Thorac Surg 63:S119–S121, 1997.
16. Utley JR, Thomasen BS, Wallace KS: Preoperative correlates of impaired wound healing after saphenous vein excision. J Thorac Cardiovasc Surg 98:147–149, 1989.

COMMENTARY

Thierry A. Folliguet

Coronary artery bypass grafting is now one of the most extensively performed cardiac operations. This surgery requires various conduits, with the saphenous vein remaining a conduit of choice. Although greater saphenous vein harvesting is performed mostly through an extended medial lower incision, other techniques with multiple incisions have been described, including a technique using endoscopic harvesting. We have used essentially two systems for minimal access vein harvesting (MIVH) in approximately 70 patients: the Endopath system (Ethicon Endo-Surgery), and the VASOVIEW system manufactured by Origin. Our results are somewhat similar to those of the Pitié group, as the patients in the MIVH group experienced almost no pain, and can ambulate without any leg discomfort. We feel that both systems are adequate and provide excellent results. The VASOVIEW has the advantage of allowing one person to perform the entire procedure, with excellent visibility; however, the learning curve and therefore the time required at the beginning is greater than when using the Endopath system. This latter system is therefore more convenient when starting MIVH, and requires less material. It is also possible to use conventional scissors and clips applier, allowing a more "classical vein dissection." One problem is the cost of these devices which remains somewhat high, including the camera and light source. However, we feel that MIVH should now be a routine procedure in order to provide increased patient comfort.

COMMENTARY

Clinton T. Lloyd and Gianni D. Angelini

This is a well-written review on the background and clinical evaluation of a number of minimally invasive techniques currently available for the harvesting of the greater saphenous vein. The advantages and disadvantages of the various techniques have been carefully evaluated and presented. This is certainly a novel approach that will come into practice among most units in the near future, as in our own.

A number of points should be addressed with regard to the implementation of this technique routinely. The cost is certainly the main issue restraining most units from adopting its use. Although this can potentially be offset by the gain in expenditure on reduced hospital stay and infection control, cost becomes of theoretical importance when these problems are managed outside of the unit's budget, for example in district hospitals or by general practitioners. One means by which this initial expenditure may be reduced is to develop a reusable system. We have been using Storz equipment (Karl Storz Endoscopy, Dundee, UK), a reusable sterilized system, with success, although some instruments such as the clip applicator are still disposable.

A second concern is the learning curve invariably associated with new techniques. In the United Kingdom, it is mostly the role of junior surgeons, who rotate through the various specialties, to harvest the vein. Dedicated vein harvesters are few but will become more commonplace, and certainly this group of surgeons will need to become familiar with these newer techniques. Reduction in harvest time has been shown over a one-year (100-case) period from 75 minutes to 35 minutes,[1] which is clinically acceptable.

The role of these instrumental techniques on vein function has yet to be fully evaluated. Vessel injury has been shown in our department to induce smooth muscle cell proliferation and neointimal formation.[2] Although the storage solution affects the endothelial function following the harvest,[3] mechanical trauma may provide the nidus for injury site. Endothelial integrity following minimal harvesting techniques has been evaluated recently in the animal model.[4] Both functional (vasoactive substance release) and morphological (lack of endothelial cell retraction or intimal fissuring) integrity seem to be preserved and compare favorably with open harvesting techniques, but whether this will translate to the clinical setting is yet to be established.

References

1. Davis Z, Jacobs K, Zhang M, et al: Endoscopic vein harvest for coronary artery bypass grafting: Technique and outcomes. J Thorac Cardiovasc Surg 116:228–235, 1998.
2. Angelini G, Soyombo A, Newby A: Smooth muscle cell proliferation in response to injury in an organ culture of human saphenous vein. Eur J Vasc Surg 5:5–12, 1991.
3. Zerkowski H-R, Knocks M, Konerding M, et al: Endothelial damage of the venous graft in CABG. Influence of solutions used for storage and rinsing on endothelial function. Eur J Cardiothoracic Surg 7:376–382, 1993.
4. Cable D, Dearani J, Pfeifer E, et al: Minimally invasive saphenous vein harvesting: Endothelial integrity and early clinical results. Ann Thorac Surg 66:139–143, 1998.

Chapter 78

Minimally Invasive Surgery for Pericardial Diseases

Hui-Ping Liu

Pericardial disease has been a topic of interest for centuries. Surgical indications for pericardial diseases include two large categories of patients—those who have some type of effusive pericarditis (with or without tamponade) unresponsive to medical therapy, and those who have chronic constrictive pericarditis. Pericardial effusions can result from either acute or chronic processes, primary or secondary, which involve the pericardium and these disease processes can be primary or secondary to other diseases (e.g., cancer). Frequently, pericardial effusion can be diagnosed by means of clinical evaluation and echo-guided aspiration. The selection of appropriate therapy is related to the nature of the underlying disease state. Modes of therapy have included surgical drainage, pericardiocentesis, chemotherapy, and installation of sclerosing agents into the pericardium. General indications for surgical drainage have included life-threatening tamponade, when there is a reasonable expectation that the patient will survive the underlying disease process; failure to control by medical therapy; presence of a constrictive component; and need for histologic documentation of etiology. The technique of thoracoscopic pericardiectomy provides some potential advantages over the standard subxiphoid approach. The thoracoscopic technique allows biopsy over a much broader area of the pericardium. An additional advantage of this approach is the ability of the surgeon to biopsy, manage, or both, pleural and pulmonary lesions simultaneously. This chapter describes our experience with the thoracoscopic management of pericardial diseases.

Preoperative Evaluation

Patient Selection. Patients considered for thoracoscopic management of pericardial disease must be able to tolerate general anesthesia and single-lung ventilation. Those who are likely to have a dense, obliterated pleural space, such as patients who have a history of previous thoracotomy, empyema, or tuberculosis, should be evaluated cautiously. Specific attention should be given also to pulmonary and cardiac function, including the possibility of an underlying constrictive component or pericardial disease. Cardiac tamponade physiology and the amount of pericardial effusion are usually evaluated using two-dimensional echocardiography. Patients who would be hemodynamically compromised by anesthetic induction, or those who have marginal cardiopulmonary reserve, are poor candidates for thoracoscopic pericardial surgery.

Anesthesia. Whenever possible, the procedure should be conducted under single-lung ventilation to expose the pericardium. However, one-lung ventilation may be difficult on some occasions. When only pericardial drainage is required, the procedure may be conducted temporarily disconnecting the endotracheal tube, which causes intermittent apnea in the patient. If this is impossible, one should perform subxiphoid drainage.

Positioning and Setup. The patient is positioned in a 45-degree off-center position, and a roll is placed under the side to be approached. This position permits an immediate subxiphoid approach should hemodynamic measurements reveal instability during thoracoscopic maneuvers. The pericardiectomy may be performed from either pleural cavity. The presence of an associated pleural or lung abnormality requiring diagnostic or therapeutic intervention may dictate the preferred side. A very large pericardial effusion may take up a significant portion of the left pleural space, limiting room to manipulate on that side. The right chest cavity normally provides greater space, better exposure, and more space for thoracoscopic manipulation.[3]

Surgical Technique

The first incision is generally placed in the sixth intercostal space along the midaxillary line. The pleural cavity is entered by blunt dissection. The space is then palpated digitally to determine whether adhesions are present. If the lung is free of the pleural wall, an 11-mm trocar is inserted into the chest cavity, through which a 10-mm, zero-degree telescope is passed. The chest cavity is explored carefully. Two additional intercostal incisions are made along the anterior axillary line at approximately the fourth and seventh intercostal spaces. Adjustments may be necessary depending on the patient's anatomy. The pericardium and entire chest cavity (including the diaphragm, the mediastinum and the lung parenchyma) are carefully examined. The phrenic nerve is identified and kept in view throughout the procedure. A stab incision is made by the electrocautery on the surface of the distended pericardium (Fig. 78–1). A conventional sharp Kelly clamp is then used to carefully penetrate the stabbed hole, allowing pericardial fluid to drain into the pleural space (Fig. 78–2). The hole is then dilated, grasped with forceps (Fig. 78–3), with use of electrocautery, a patch of pericardium is resected to create an adequate pericardiopleural window with an average size of 4 × 3 cm (Fig. 78–4). The fluid is sent for cytologic evaluation and the specimen is sent for pathologic analysis or microbiologic analysis when indicated. Concomitant lung or pleural abnormalities are visually and digitally inspected. Thoracoscopic biopsies are performed on any abnormal tissue identified. If a bilateral pericardiectomy is indicated, the left and right pericardium is resected se-

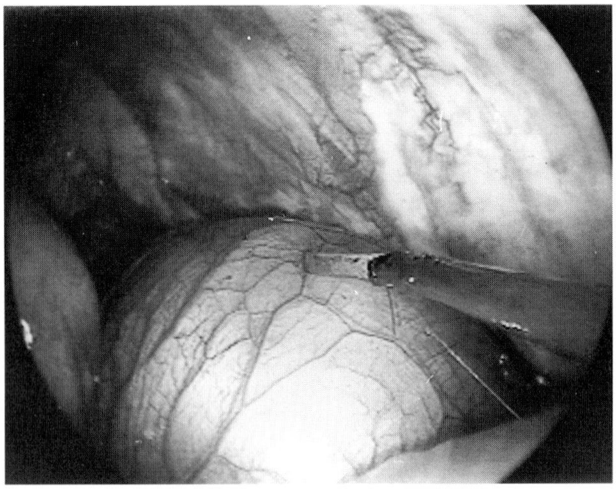

Figure 78–1. Stab incision created on the surface of the distended pericardium using electrocautery.

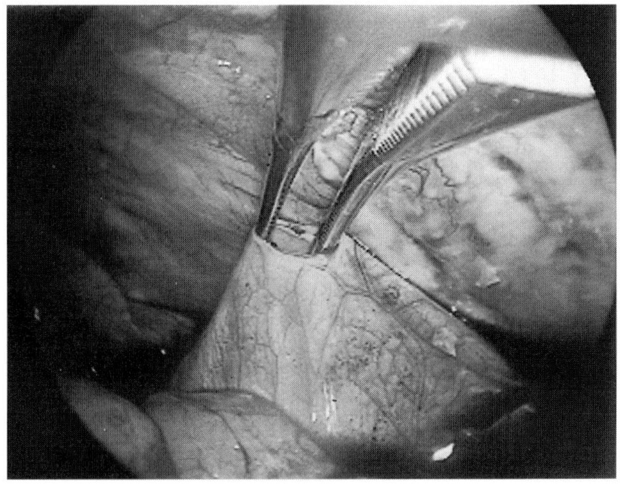

Figure 78–3. The pericardium hole was dilated using a Kelly clamp.

quentially to a maximal extent as in an open procedure. After completing the procedure, a 32 French chest tube is placed in the pleura through the inferior incision, which has already been made.

Personal Experience

Sixty-eight patients who were sonographically documented to have underlying massive pericardial effusion were submitted to diagnostic or therapeutic (or both) thoracoscopic pericardial drainage and examination of lung or pleura as part of their operation. There were 42 men and 26 women, with a median age of 58 years. The indications for the thoracoscopic approach are listed in Table 78–1. Thoracoscopic intervention was based on the need for relieving pericardial effusion in all patients and, concomitantly, establishing a diagnosis in patients who had abnormal lung and pleural disorders. In 14 patients, the subxiphoid approach was not used for fear of the adhesions from previous procedures. These included 8 patients who had recurrent effusion, 4 patients who had a previous heart procedure, and 2 patients who received a previous substernal route reconstruction following esophagectomy. The causes of pericardial effusion are summarized as follows: lung cancer, 14; metastatic (unknown primary), 9; esophageal cancer, 2; uremia, 6; postcardiac procedure (blood clot), 4; tuberculosis, 11; and chronic inflammation, 22. There were 29 patients who received thoracoscopic pericardial decompression followed by thoracoscopic evaluation of lung or pleural abnormalities identified on the chest roentgenogram. Seventeen new patients were found to have a lung malignancy. Pleural and diaphragmatic metastatic deposits of unknown primary (poorly differentiated adenocarcinoma) were confirmed in 7 patients. There were 5 patients who did not have thoracoscopic evidence of malignancies, although they were clinically suspected to have pleural or lung tumor. Two patients with mixed effusive and constrictive pericarditis (tuberculous) received bilateral sequential thoracoscopic maximal pericardiectomy. Blood clot was evacuated thoracoscopically in the patients

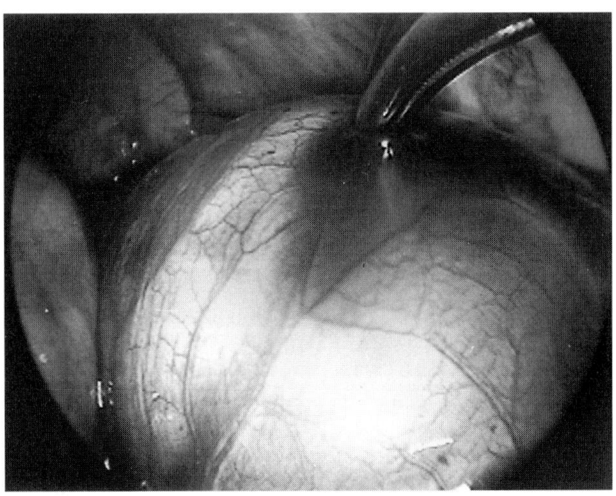

Figure 78–2. Kelly clamp used to penetrate the stabbed hole to allow pericardial fluid to drain into pleural space.

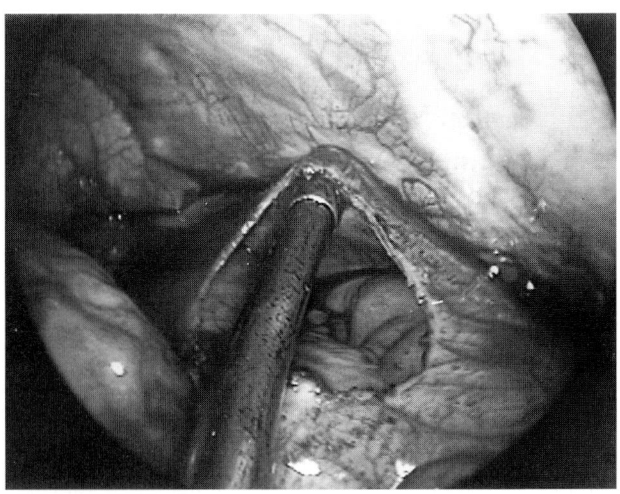

Figure 78–4. Pericardiopleural window with average size 4 × 3 cm.

Table 78–1. Indications for Thoracoscopic Pericardial Drainage

Massive pericardial effusion	23
Concomitant with pleural effusion	19
Concomitant with lung or pleural mass	10
Recurrent/loculated pericardial effusion*	8
After heart procedure (CABG and subxiphoid pacemaker implantation)*	4
After substernal esophagogastrostomy (esoph. ca.)*	2
Constrictive pericarditis (early phase)	2

*Thoracoscopy performed to avoid subxiphoid scarring from previous procedures.
CABG = coronary artery bypass grafting; esoph. ca. = esophageal cancer.

who had delayed tamponade after a heart procedure. Forty-six patients had thoracoscopic pericardial drainage performed through the right side of the chest and 22 through the left side of the chest. In the series, 5 patients received subxiphoid decompression first because of low arterial blood pressure after the induction. Subsequent thoracoscopic examination and lung biopsies were performed when the patient became hemodynamically stable. All patients tolerated the procedure well. There were no intraoperative or postoperative complications related to the procedures. Twenty-four patiens who had proven malignancies were referred to medical oncologists for further therapy. No recurrence of pericardial effusion was noted over a mean follow-up period of 12.5 months. Two patients who received bilateral thoracoscopic maximal pericardiectomy showed no residual constriction by echocardiogram at 16 months and 27 months, respectively, after the procedure.

Discussion

Surgical intervention for the diagnosis and treatment of pericardial disease has been evolving during this century.[1–3] The appropriate treatment of persistent and recurrent pericardial effusion depends on the underlying disease and clinical symptoms. Various surgical approaches have been used to treat effusive pericardial disease.[4–16] Standard approaches for pericardial drainage include a subxiphoid approach and a left or right anterior thoracotomy with creation of a pericardial window. Recently, video-assisted thoracic surgery (VATS) in the management of pericardial diseases has been used increasingly.[5, 7, 16] Yim and Ho[16] have suggested a theoretical advantage in using a video-assisted subxiphoid approach, so that more of the pericardium can be excised. Their approach provides a minimally invasive alternative for creation of a pericardial window or pericardiectomy, which can be especially useful for patients who are at high risk for thoracotomy or for patients who have dense pleural adhesions. In addition to being therapeutic for pericardial effusion, thoracoscopy can prove very useful for diagnosis, es pecially in patients who have concomitant lung or pleural pathology. In such circumstances, the thoracoscopic approach can provide an accurate diagnosis when pleural biopsy and fluid etiology have failed to do so. Echo-guided needle biopsy is of value, in our experience, only for large, peripherally located tumors but is of little or no use for tumors confined to the diaphragm or the visceral or mediastinal pleura. Basically, the goals of thoracoscopy in the management of pleural or pericardial effusion are searching for the cause and giving appropriate treatment to initiate promptly. Undoubtedly, thoracoscopy has been established as a valuable adjunct in the management of such disorders. It allows excellent visualization of both pleural and pericardial surfaces. A larger window of the pericardium can be excised through the thoracoscopic approach than through the subxiphoid route, which may lead to a lower incidence of recurrence.[11, 12] It also produces less pulmonary morbidity than anterolateral thoracotomy.

Pleuropulmonary abnormalities were present preoperatively in 29 of our 68 patients (42.7%). As previously mentioned, 17 patients had concomitant lung malignancy, and pleural or diaphragmatic metastatic deposits were confirmed in 7 patients. The other 5 abnormal lung lesions were sampled and proved to be caused by chronic inflammation. All of these diagnoses would not have been made if only a subxiphoid approach had been used. For patients who had delayed tamponade after their heart operation, the subxiphoid approach was avoided and retained blood was easily drained by thoracoscopic techniques. Recurrent loculated pericardial effusions were frequently located posteriorly, and these could not be readily drained without open thoracotomy, whereas such an effusion could be drained easily by VATS. Additionally, bilateral thoracoscopic pericardiectomy can be performed in patients who have an early state of mixed effusive and constrictive pericarditis, and thus late constriction can be avoided. The subxiphoid route usually does not permit an adequate resection.

Thoracoscopy is a new technique, not a new operation. Use of this technique should not compromise the primary diagnostic and therapeutic goals set forth for the patient. Surgeons who lose sight of their priorities may do harm to their patients. This is particularly true in patients who require emergent pericardial decompression. In patients with unstable hemodynamic measurements, the surgeon should perform the drainage immediately instead of wasting time to prepare for a thoracoscopic approach. Clearly, a subxiphoid route is the simplest and fastest approach for pericardial decompression. We strongly recommend the subxiphoid approach for relieving the pericardial effusion if the patient demonstrates hemodynamic instability and has no concomitant lung or pleural abnormalities. In some patients who have a known malignancy at a nearly terminal stage, the simple subxiphoid procedure should always be used to relieve the effusion. Thoracoscopy is not indicated in such patients, who have a short life expectancy and little hope of effective treatment for their malignancy.

In conclusion, thoracoscopy provides excellent visualization of the pericardium. Thoracoscopic management of effusive pericardial disease is an effective and promising alternative for treating the disease. The ability to investigate pleuropulmonary disorders simultaneously can be of great benefit to patients who present with both abnormalities. The goals in these patients are to relieve the effusion, make a definite diagnosis, and create an adequate pleuropericardial window with the lowest possible morbidity. We believe the thoracoscopic approach is the most favorable and attractive alternative fulfilling the aforementioned requirements. However, despite the availability of the thoracoscopic technique, one should not forget the use of the simple subxiphoid approach under certain circumstances, as described in this chapter. Thoracoscopy should be used in carefully selected patients who have the proper indications to benefit greatly from this procedure.

References

1. Gregory JR, McMutrey MJ, Mountain CF: A surgical approach to the treatment of pericardial effusion in cancer patients. Am J Clin Oncol 8:319, 1985.
2. Hankins JR, Satterfield JR, Aisner J, et al: Pericardial window for malignant pericardial effusion. Ann Thorac Surg 30:465, 1980.
3. Hazelrigg SR, Mack MJ, Landreneau RJ, et al: Thoracoscopic pericardiectomy for effusive pericardial disease. Ann Thorac Surg 56:792–795, 1993.
4. Kopecky SL, Callahan JA, Tajik AJ: Percutaneous pericardial catheter drainage: Report of 42 consecutive cases. Am J Cardiol 58:633–635, 1986.
5. Krasna MJ, Mack MJ: Pericardiectomy. *In* Atlas of thoracoscopic surgery. St. Louis, Quality Medical Publishing, Inc. 1994, pp 129–137.
6. Little AG, Kremser PC, Wade JL, et al: Operation for diagnosis and treatment of pericardial effusions. Surgery 96:738–744, 1984.
7. Mack MJ, Landreneau RJ, Hazelrigg SR, et al: Videothoracoscopic management of benign and malignant pericardial effusions. Chest 103:390–395, 1993.
8. Miller JI: Pericardiectomy. *In* Hurst JW (ed): Update Three: The Heart. New York, McGraw-Hill, 1980, pp 147–159.
9. Miller JI: Pericardiectomy: Current indications, concepts, and results in a university center. Ann Thorac Surg 1:40–45, 1982.
10. Naunheim KS, Kesler KA, Fiore AC, et al: Pericardial drainage: Subxiphoid vs transthoracic approach. Eur J Cardiothorac Surg 5:99–104, 1991.
11. Piehler JM, Pluth JR, Schaff HV, et al: Surgical management of effusive pericardial disease. J Thorac Cardiovasc Surg 90:506–516, 1985.
12. Santos GH, Frater RWM: The subxiphoid approach in the treatment of pericardial effusion. Ann Thorac Surg 23:467–470, 1977.
13. Spodick DH: Medical history of the pericardium. Am J Cardiol 26:447, 1970.
14. Spodick DH. The normal and diseased pericardium, current concepts of pericardial physiology, diagnosis and treatment. J Am Coll Cardiol 1:240–251, 1983.
15. Sugimoto JT, Little AG, Ferguson MK, et al: Pericardial window: Mechanisms of efficacy. Ann Thorac Surg 50:442–445, 1990.
16. Yim APC, Ho JKS: Video-assisted subxiphoid pericardiectomy. J Laparoendosc Surg 5:193–198, 1995.

COMMENTARY

Stephen R. Hazelrigg

Dr. Liu makes a clear presentation of the role of video-assisted thoracic surgery (VATS) in pericardial disease. We would emphasize that the presumed advantage of VATS over the subxiphoid route is the ability to resect more of the pericardium and thus decrease the risk of recurrence or later constriction. It has no advantage over the subxiphoid route in malignant cases with short expected survival times in whom the simplest method of drainage should be used (catheter or subxiphoid).

As described, the fibrinous pericardium may be resected but requires an advanced technical skill level. True constriction still is probably best managed by open techniques.

Section X

Future Technologies

Chapter 79

Robotic Surgery

Volkmar Falk

The surgeon in his room (at a cardiac center in Touston 2050) has everything automatically delivered to him. His orders are executed by a computerized dispatcher of instruments. Should additional help be necessary, a robot is available.

A. Carpentier, *J Thorac Cardiovasc Surg 1983;86:323*

For many years, the concept of total endoscopic cardiac surgery has been on the verge of introduction. Despite numerous efforts and the introduction of various techniques for both minimally invasive coronary artery bypass graft and valve procedures,[1–3] as well as the development of closed chest bypass systems[4] and stabilizers, totally endoscopic procedures could not be established because of technical limitations. Cardiac surgeons were faced with the same problems that have challenged those in other specialties working in an endoscopic environment; they are handicapped by the limited intracorporeal mobility of endoscopic instruments.[5] The use of rigid, long instruments through a fixed incision point leads to impaired tissue manipulation (fulcrum effect); force feedback is lost because of the friction of instruments inside the ports. To perform a complete motion, 6 degrees of freedom are required. The human hand allows 20 degrees of freedom, whereas the human palm has 7 degrees of freedom, summing up the possible motions in the shoulder, elbow, and wrist. In contrast, currently available endoscopic instruments have only 4 degrees of freedom (up-down, left-right, in-out, rotation plus an additional degree of freedom for grip), leading to a great reduction of manual dexterity. The loss of full control of the tip of the endoscopic instrument results in a limitation of possible motions necessary to perform a surgical manipulation. Some motions may even become impossible, rendering easy tasks like knot tying difficult, thereby requiring a lot of training and skill. More complex surgical maneuvers like suturing a coronary anastomosis may not be performed successfully given the high-quality standard and the time constraints inherent in cardiac surgery. In addition, standard endoscopic instruments do not perform favorably from an ergonomic point of view because the surgeon cannot rest the arms and wrists. The limited range of motion inside the body has to be compensated, in part, by large and unnatural movements externally, leading to fatigue and loss of concentration.

Videoscopic imaging plays a major role in endoscopic surgery. The use of videoscopic images, however, not only diminishes the field of view but also decreases resolution and reduces depth perception. Although higher in resolution, two-dimensional images render positioning of instruments inside the body more difficult because of the lack of stereoscopic depth. High magnification and working with long instruments also amplifies the surgeon's tremor. Hand-held videoscopic guidance not only promotes communication misunderstandings but also causes the surgeon to become distracted by constantly moving targets.

In an effort to overcome these limitations and to enhance dexterity and facilitate endoscopic surgery, computer-enhanced surgical robots have been developed.[6] Along with the use of robotic devices, the concept of telepresence surgery with the surgeon working at a remote distance from the patient has evolved.

Basic Mechanics

Robots are designed to perform high-precision tasks repetitively or to work in an environment that is not suitable for humans. Whatever purpose a robot is designed for, it should adhere to the three laws of robotics originally published by Isaac Asimov:

1. A robot may not injure a human being or, through interaction, allow a human being to come to harm.
2. A robot must obey the orders received from humans except when such orders conflict with the first law.
3. A robot must protect its own existence provided such protection does not conflict with the first or second law.

These laws are of special importance for robotic devices used to operate on the human body.[7] The basic construction principle of currently used robots is that of arm manipulators with a serial architecture of joints and links. The last element in this series is the surgical instrument that is also called the end-effector. Joint motion is provided by mechanical actuators that are electrically or hydraulically driven. Two categories of robots are used clinically. In so-called off-line systems, the device is preprogrammed for a specific task, which is then performed autonomously. An example of this type of robot is the so called Robodoc, a surgical manipulator used in orthopedics to preshape the femur for total hip replacement.[8] The complexity of cardiac surgery requires a different type of robot. The robotic devices currently under investigation for use in cardiac surgery are supervised on-line systems. The operator is in steady control of the system via a human-machine interface. The concept of these robots is to combine human skills, such as judgment and perception, by computer-enhanced technology with the precise mechanics of a robot for performance of delicate surgical tasks.[9]

Voice-Activated Robotic Arm

The automated endoscope system for optimal positioning (AESOP, Computer Motion, Goleta, CA) is mainly used to guide a videoscope or retractor. The arm can be attached to standard operating tables and is controlled via the surgeon's voice. The arm has six articulating joints, four of which are powered and two of which are passive. Microprocessors continuously assess the actual position of each joint. Excessive external forces (manual displacement, contact with tissue) that are applied to the system lead to a mismatch between the calculated and actual position, which puts the system on hold automatically. To prevent any injury from the arm's being too close to the body, one can set a lower limit that the system will not exceed under any circumstances. The motion itself can be continuous or incremental, depending on what is needed to enhance exposure. The arm is able to store information and to return to various positions on request. The videoscope or a retractor is coupled to the robotic arm via adjustable magnetic couplers that can be resterilized. Motion control of the robot is performed via voice activation (Fig. 79–1). Automatic recognition of human speech is realized by a speaker-dependent model that is trained to the idiosyncrasies of an individual's voice. In principle, words are converted into frames that are then matched by the computer with stored phone models. The match scores for phones are calculated and, by statistical analysis, compared with match scores for words.[10] The best word match is then chosen. Since this model is speaker-dependent, acquisition of training data is necessary. Before the robotic arm is used, a voice card is recorded that stores the individual phones. During surgery, the surgeon addresses the robot via a microphone and directs its movements by simple one- or two-word commands. The system provides a stable and tremor-free picture and obviates the need for an assistant to hold the camera. The voice control mode allows continuous surgery to proceed without interruption for videoscope repositioning. Lens cleanings are necessary less often because of the absence of inadvertent camera contact with tissue.[11] The system has been used successfully for internal thoracic artery (ITA) harvesting as well as for minimally invasive mitral valve surgery, enabling solo operation technique.[12]

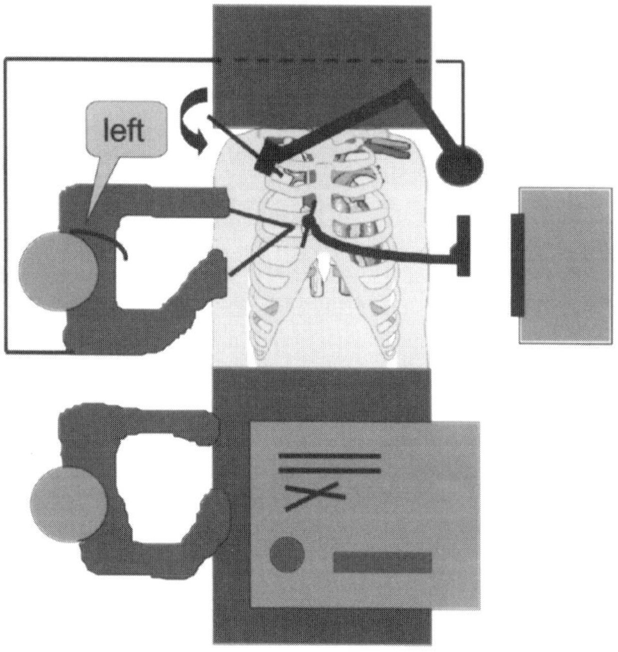

Figure 79–1. Principle of mitral valve solo operation using a voice-controlled robotic arm for videoscopic guidance. The robotic arm directs the videoscope according to simple one- or two-word commands.

Remote Computer-Enhanced Surgery

Remote computer-enhanced surgery is based on the concept of telepresence surgery. The surgeon no longer manipulates the tissue directly but acts via a human-machine interface using surgical manipulators. The surgeon is seated in an ergonomically favorable position at a console (Fig. 79–2). A two- or three-dimensional thoracoscopic image is displayed on a video screen. At the console, the surgeon manipulates two instrument handles that trigger highly sensitive motion sensors for each component of a given movement (shoulder, elbow, wrist, hand movement). These data are then processed by a computer and transferred to surgical manipulators that perform the same motion inside the chest. In order to enhance precision, motion scaling is used. A motion scale of 5 : 1 moves the tool 1 cm inside the chest for every 5 cm of motion at the master control. In addition, unintended movements caused by tremor can be filtered by the computer. Human tremor occurs with a frequency of 6 to 10 Hz. By applying a 6-Hz motion filter, tremor is reduced at the surgical manipulators. It is possible at any time to temporarily break the slave tools from following the masters, enabling repositioning of the master within its workspace while the position of the instruments remains unchanged. This allows the surgeon to work in the most favorable ergonomic position at all times, while simultaneously providing optimal hand-eye alignment. Some force feedback is provided so that tissue contact (inside body forces, i.e., bony resistance) as well as external forces (collision of slaves) are reflected at the master. However, small forces exerted with soft tissue manipulation are not felt at the console.

Two systems are currently under investigation for use in cardiac surgery. The Zeus-System (Computer Motion) consists of three independent arms that can be freely mounted to the operating table and that interact through a microprocessor. The camera arm is voice-controlled, whereas the instrument-holding arms are triggered by operating the master manipulator handles from the console where a two- or three-dimensional videoscopic image is displayed. The instruments have 4 degrees of freedom. In a plastic model of coronary anastomoses, the system proved to be effective, creating patent anastomoses at an

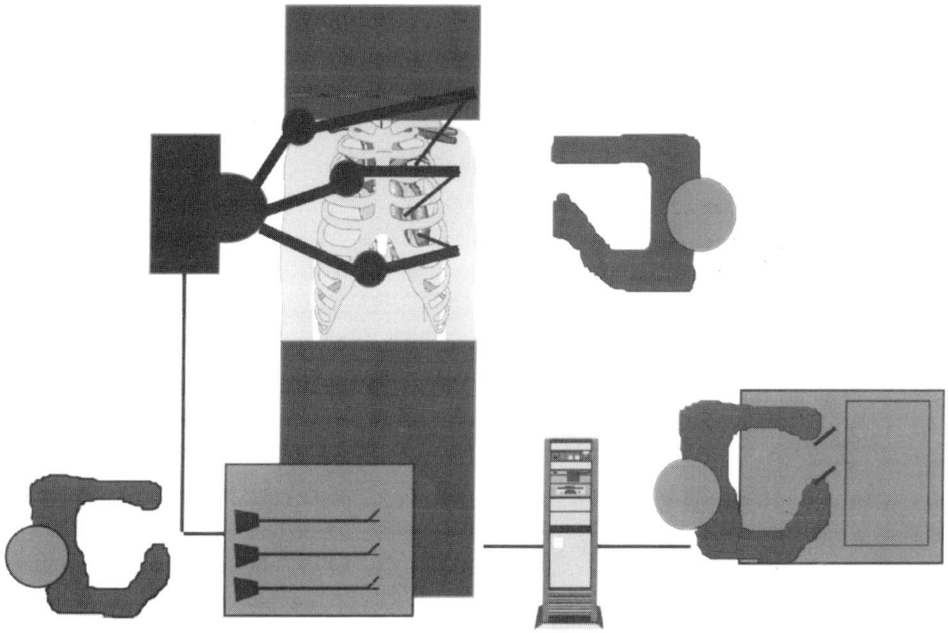

Figure 79–2. Set-up for computer-enhanced coronary artery bypass surgery. The surgeon is seated at a console and acts by master manipulator handles. Through a computer interface, hand movements are reproduced precisely in the operative field. Motion scaling and tremor filtering allow for micromovements.

average time of 46 ± 12 minutes.[13] Acute and chronic animal studies are currently being performed.

The Intuitive System (Intuitive Surgical, Mountain View, CA) consists of a cart with a column that supports three robotic arms. The surgical manipulators have 3 degrees of freedom (pitch, yaw, and insertion) and provide motion coupling to the end-effector, an exchangeable instrument. The central arm holds a 10-mm-diameter high-resolution three-dimensional videoscope (two three-CCD cameras) and can be operated from the console by switching control of the right master manipulator handle from control of the right instrument arm to the central arm. The two instrument-holding arms are placed left and right to the videoscope. The instruments add another 4 degrees of freedom by means of an endowrist that allows the tip of the instrument to be articulated in all directions (remote center kinematics). The endowrist technology provides a total of 7 degrees of freedom (six degrees of freedom plus gripper) inside the chest (Fig. 79–3). Thus, no special surgical technique is required to operate the system because all movements are readily transferred to the tip of the instruments. Grip strength is programmable and differs for the various end-effectors (grasper, fine needle holder, and so on), with lesser grip strength for instruments intended to handle delicate tissue. Using the endowrist, it is possible to suture even along a line perpendicular to the shaft, which is virtually impossible using rigid endoscopic instruments. Not only does the system provide full control of the tip of the instrument, allowing any intended motion, but it also provides ambidexterity. Motion scaling and tremor filtering add to the precision of the system (Fig. 79–4).

Technique of Computer-Enhanced Coronary Artery Bypass Graft Surgery

Using the Intuitive System, the robotic arms are placed to the right side of the patient. After positioning the patient in a 30-degree right lateral decubitus position with the left arm flexed and suspended overhead and after deflating the left lung, three ports are created to enter the left thorax in the third, fourth and sixth intercostal spaces. Carbon dioxide is used to insufflate (ITP <10 mm Hg) in order to enhance visualization of the ITA and to increase the space between the pericardium and the chest wall. A 30-degree angled scope is used. The ITA is harvested using low energy electrocautery. Alternatively, a subxiphoidal approach may be chosen. After preparation of the pedicle, femorofemoral bypass is established and an endoaortic clamp (Heartport, Redwood City, CA) is advanced into the ascending aorta under transesophageal echocardio-

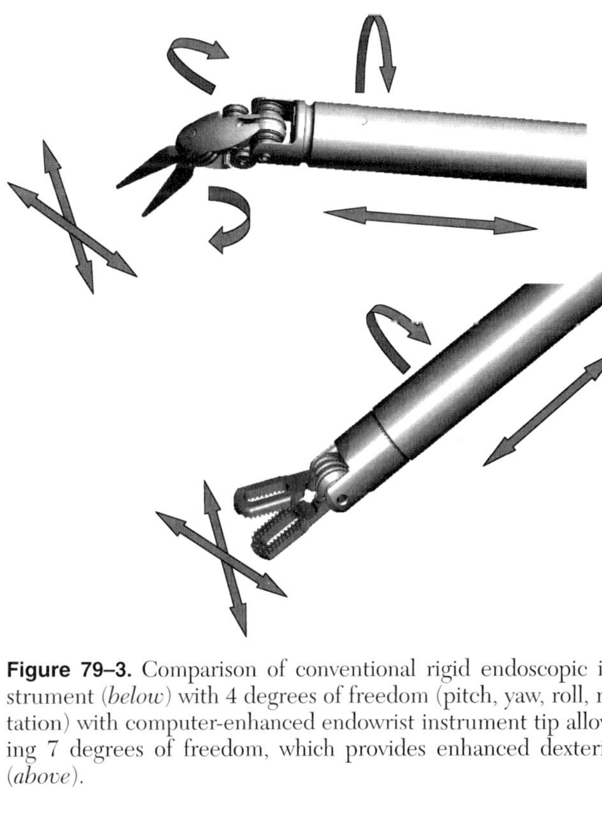

Figure 79–3. Comparison of conventional rigid endoscopic instrument (*below*) with 4 degrees of freedom (pitch, yaw, roll, rotation) with computer-enhanced endowrist instrument tip allowing 7 degrees of freedom, which provides enhanced dexterity (*above*).

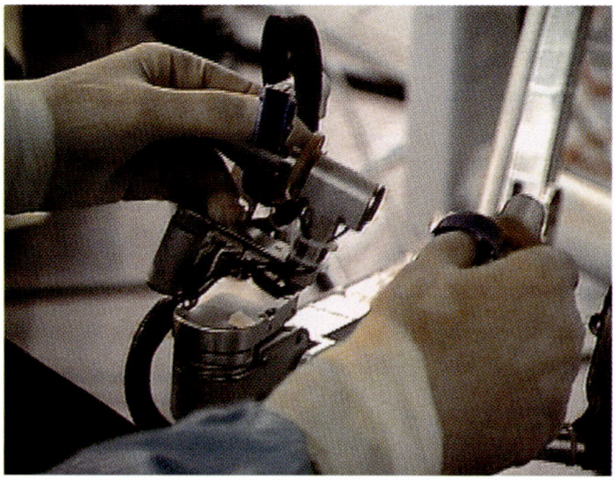

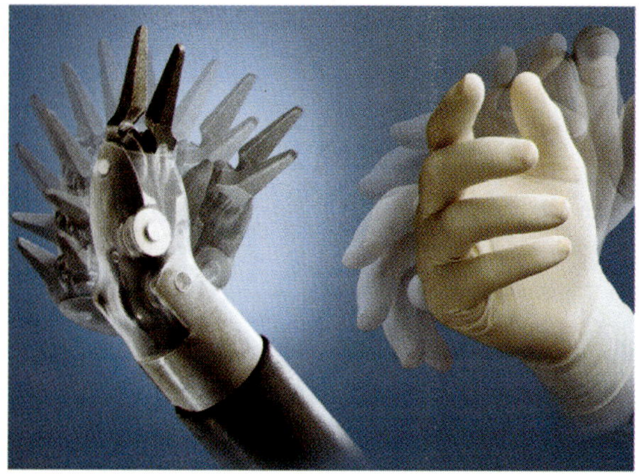

Figure 79–4. *A*, Master manipulator handles (*left*) and *B*, effectors (*right*) move simultaneously (online system).

graphic guidance. A high-resolution 0-degree three-dimensional videoscope is used. The pericardium is opened and the target artery is identified. The endoclamp is then inflated and the heart arrested using antegrade crystalloid cardioplegia. The arteriotomy is performed remotely using a blade and extending it with scissors. The coronary anastomosis is performed with short double-armed 7–0 Prolene sutures using the parachute technique. After completion of the anastomosis, the robotic arms are removed from the table. Endoscopic thermal coronary angiography and transit-time flow measurements may be performed to document graft patency.[14] The system has been used successfully in cadavers and animal studies (Fig. 79–5).[15] Initial clinical trials have demonstrated the feasibility of robot-assisted remote coronary artery bypass grafting.

Computer-Enhanced Mitral Valve Surgery

For computer-enhanced mitral valve surgery, a minithoracotomy is performed in the fourth intercostal space, and a small retractor housing a left atrial venting line is placed. A left atrial retractor is inserted parasternally in the right sixth intercostal space and is mounted to a passive manipulator arm. After femorofemoral cardiopulmonary bypass is initiated and the heart is arrested using the port access technique with endoaortic clamping, the left atrium is opened.[3] Two ports are created at the second and fifth intercostal spaces for entry of the instruments. The robot is placed on the left side of the operating table and the instruments are inserted. Mitral valve repair, including ring implantation, is performed remotely from the console.

Patient Selection

Despite using the most advanced technology one can still do the wrong operation.

H. Troidl, *Langenbecks Arch 1996;Suppl II:727–741*

The described techniques for computer-enhanced robotic surgery are currently based on the use of femorofemoral cardiopulmonary bypass. Therefore, all patients with pe-

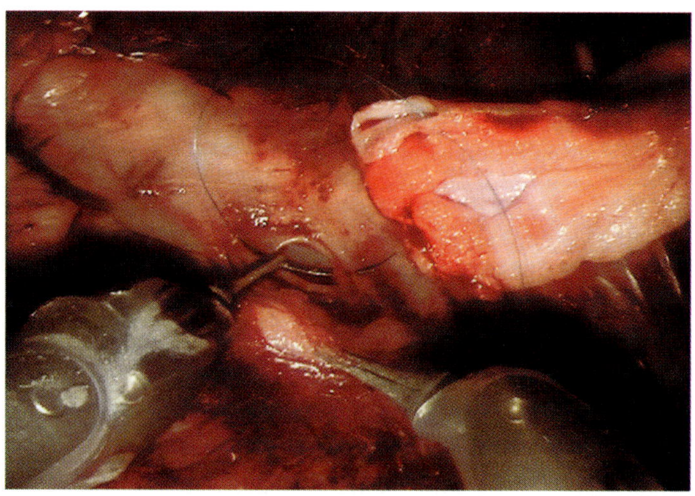

Figure 79–5. Coronary anastomosis (sheep) performed remotely using the Intuitive System with endowrist technology.

ripheral artery disease or an atheromatous aorta must be excluded. So far, no beating heart procedures have been performed, and coronary artery bypass surgery has been performed only for single-vessel disease. However, with further refinements of the technology and different access routes, multivessel revascularizations seem possible. For mitral valve surgery, the contraindications for femoral cannulation again have to be considered. Patients who have severe calcified mitral valve lesions or a heavily calcified mitral valve ring should be excluded, because the currently available instruments may not be strong enough to manipulate stenotic valves. Reoperations may be performed, but in the presence of severe pleural adhesions, the potential of injury from introducing trocars and working with endoscopic instruments has to be taken into account. Creation of a pneumothorax by insufflating carbon dioxide can lead to hemodynamic impairment. Patients who have poor cardiac function should, therefore, be excluded from an endoscopic approach requiring high intrathoracic pressures to gain exposure.

One has to acknowledge that some patients may be frightened by the idea of having a robot operating on them while the surgeon is located at a remote distance from the operating table. It is, therefore, necessary to explain to the patient that at any time the surgeon can take over without delay. The patient should also understand that the robot does not operate autonomously but is under the surgeon's constant control and only translates the outside hand movements into precise micromovements inside the chest.

Pitfalls and Limitations

Defining the optimal port location is sometimes difficult because the anatomy of the chest and heart varies. Since 10-mm ports are created (as opposed to small stab incisions with conventional endoscopic ITA-harvesting techniques[1, 16]) for the robotic arms, multiple repositioning maneuvers may cause some trauma. Because of size, the robotic arms may collide in extreme positions, leading to sudden and inadvertent movements of the end-effectors. Set-up time needs to be shortened, but this can be expected with faster software routines. With available systems, camera movements are isolated, leaving instruments in their location. Larger movements, therefore, require multiple adjustments in order not to lose sight of the instruments. Software changes will solve this problem. The loss of tactile feedback impairs the manipulation of both tissue and suturing material. Thin sutures (such as 8–0 Prolene) used for coronary anastomoses may break because there is little control of the exerted force acting on the suture. Customized suture material is necessary to perform coronary anastomoses. A double-armed suture 7 cm long seems to be ideal. Longer sutures are difficult to handle. Considering suture material, threads with less or no memory but increased strength are desirable. The implementation of force scaling (i.e., different force modes for various tasks) could also improve the handling of microscopic structures. In contrast, excessive tissue (i.e., epicardial fat) is sometimes not easy to excise and displace, because the small instrument tips are built to deal with delicate tissue. Hemostasis is also a concern, because the available clip appliers allow only single clip placement. Electrocautery may be used, but the smoke that results impairs visualization. If suction is applied, intrathoracic pressure will drop because of the loss of carbon dioxide, and exposure will be impaired. The use of telepresence surgery systems with 4 degrees of freedom has been shown to be associated with longer operating times for gastrotomy closures and arteriotomy closures.[16–18] An increase in the number of degrees of freedom (dexterity enhancement) may therefore be required to achieve operating times comparable with those of conventional surgery.

Further Developments

A variety of developments will help improve the current systems. Automated instrument tracking and image-guided triangulation using position markers at the tip of the instrument may improve orientation. Improvement of the human-machine interface is necessary. A haptic interface providing tactile and force feedback from force sensors at the tips of the instruments will possibly improve the manipulation of tissue and thin sutures. According to Madhani and associates, however, forces beyond 0.4 N cannot be felt. Displacement of soft tissue of 6 mm will create forces of only 0.2 to 0.6 N and, therefore, can hardly be felt, whereas a 1-mm displacement can already be seen. It is debatable whether force reflection is indeed required.[6]

Versatile, flexible multitask effectors could eliminate the need for instrument changes that currently require an assistant. The integration of a Harmonic scalpel for harvesting the ITA could overcome some problems associated with electrocautery (smoke, heat, bleeding of side branches). Endoscopic stabilizers could enable robot-assisted beating heart procedures. Besides mechanical stabilizers, techniques for virtual immobilization of the heart are being investigated. In this approach, the complex forward motion of the contracting heart is recognized and analyzed by computer. The position of the instruments relative to the heart is held fixed by moving the instruments in the same direction as the heart. The surgeon at the console will not be aware of the system moving but will be presented the image of a virtually arrested heart. Tissue manipulation can therefore be performed with the comfort of having a nonmoving target while the system corrects any motion performed at the console according to the actual position of the heart. New anastomotic devices (stapling or suturing devices) may work as add-on technology to the robotic systems. They will decrease the time necessary for performing an anastomosis and will enable work on the beating heart. Alternative implanting techniques for valves may also be considered for use with the robotic system.

New technologies will require a different form of teaching. Therefore, a structured teaching process must be developed. In minimally invasive cardiac surgery, as in other minimally invasive procedures, modern teaching modalities of the digital classroom with three-dimensional interactive multimedia applications will replace the concept of the one-to-one apprenticeship training that has been in use unchanged in surgical specialties for a century.[20, 21] Similar to simulation programs in aviation, computer-based training in a virtual environment with visual and force feedback surgical trainers, which allow real-time

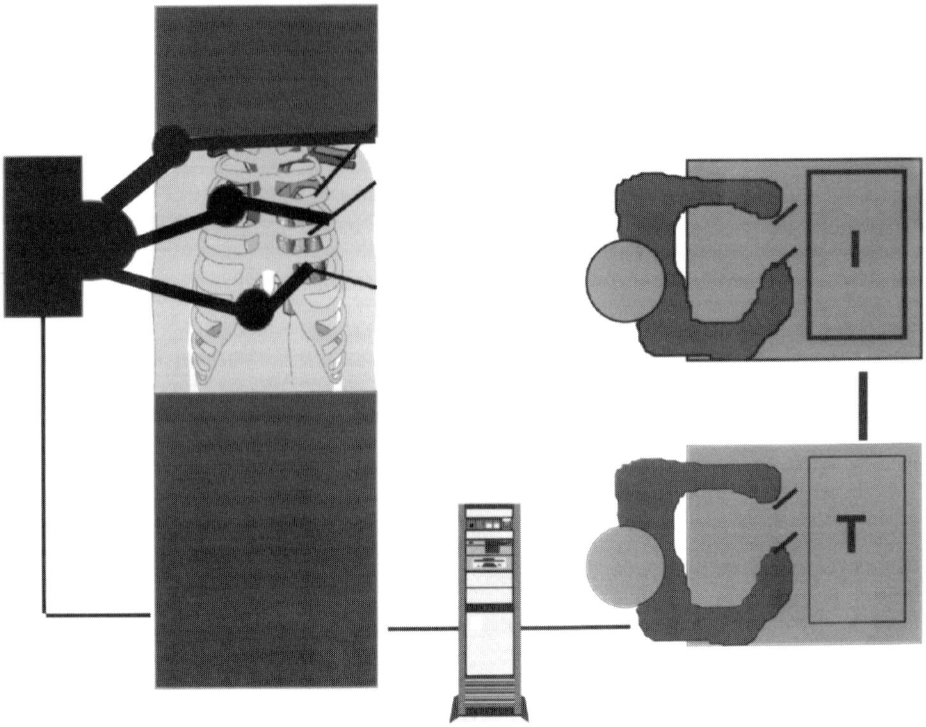

Figure 79–6. The future of surgical training by telementoring. By coupling two consoles, the instructor (I) can demonstrate to or correct a surgical manipulation of the trainee (T).

simulation of dextrous endoscopic instruments, will ultimately change the tradition of surgical education.[22] For the first time, it is possible to introduce telementoring into cardiac surgery. By coupling two consoles, it will be possible for a senior instructor to control a primary surgeon. The instructor will have exactly the same detailed view of the operating field and will be able to demonstrate or correct a surgical manipulation from his or her console (Fig. 79–6). The use of telepresence surgery may also enable specialists to operate or assist an operation in a remote location if telecommunication capabilities will allow online data transfer.[18, 23] Microrobots that are small enough to work inside blood vessels and navigate independently are currently being developed. However, energy storage and the difficulties in constructing powerful microactuators limit the use of these devices.

References

1. Mack M, Acuff T, Yong P, et al: Minimally invasive thoracoscopically assisted coronary artery bypass surgery. Eur J Cardiothorac Surg 12:20–24, 1997.
2. Nataf P, Lima L, Regan M, et al: Thoracoscopic internal mammary artery harvesting: Technical considerations. Ann Thorac Surg 63:S104–106, 1997.
3. Mohr FW, Falk V, Diegeler A, et al: Minimally invasive port-access mitral valve surgery. J Thorac Cardiovasc Surg 115: 567–576, 1998.
4. Stevens JH, Burdon TA, Peters WS, et al: Port-access coronary artery bypass grafting: A proposed surgical method. J Thorac Cardiovasc Surg 111:567–573, 1996.
5. Scott-Connor CE, Berci G: Unsolved problems in endoscopic surgery. Surg Endosc 7:281–282, 1993.
6. Madhani AJ, Niemeyer G, Salisbury JK: The black falcon: A teleoperated surgical instrument for minimally invasive surgery. Proceedings of the IEEE/RSJ International Conference on Intelligent Robots and Systems, 1998, (in press).
7. Cain P, Kazanides P, Zuhars J, et al: Safety considerations in a surgical robot. Biomed Sci Instrum 29:291–294, 1993.
8. Paul HA, Barger WL, Mittelstadt B, et al: Development of a surgical robot for cementless hip arthroplasty. Clin Orthop 285: 57–66, 1992.
9. Cadeddu JA, Stoianovici D, Kavoussi LR: Robotics in urologic surgery. Urology 49:501–507, 1997.
10. Sackier JM, Wooters C, Jacobs L, et al: Voice activation of a surgical robot. Am J Surg 174:406–409, 1997.
11. Kavoussi LP, Moore RG, Adams JB, Partin AW: Comparison of robotic versus human laparoscopic camera control. J Urol 154: 2134–2136, 1994.
12. Falk V, Walther T, Autschbach R, et al: Robot assisted minimally invasive solo mitral valve operation. J Thorac Cardiovasc Surg 115:470–471, 1998.
13. Garcia-Ruiz A, Smedira NG, Loop FD, et al: Robotic surgical instruments for dexterity enhancement in thoracoscopic coronary artery bypass graft. J Laparoendosc Adv Surg Tech 7: 277–283, 1997.
14. Falk V, Diegeler A, Walther T, et al: Intraoperative patency control of arterial grafts in minimally invasive coronary artery bypass graft surgery using endoscopic thermal coronary angiography. J Thorac Cardiovasc 114:507–509, 1997.
15. Falk V, Gummert J, Moll F, et al: Remote computer enhanced coronary anastomosis. Eur J Cardiothorac Surg (in press).
16. Ohtsuka T, Wolf RK, Hiratzka LF, et al: Thoracoscopic internal mammary harvest for MIDCABG using the harmonic scalpel. Ann Thorac Surg 63(suppl):S107–S109, 1997.
17. Bowersox JC, Shaw A, Jensen J, et al: Vascular applications of telepresence surgery: Initial feasability studies in swine. J Vasc Surg 23:281–287, 1996.
18. Bowersox JC, Cordts PR, LaPorta AJ: Use of an intuitive telemanipulator system for remote trauma surgery: An experimental study. J Am Coll Surg 186:615–621, 1998.
19. Tendick F, Mori T, Way LW: Future of laparoscopic surgery. *In* Way LW, Bhoyrul S, Mori T (eds): Fundamentals of Laparoscopic Surgery, New York, Churchill Livingstone, pp 235–252.
20. Satava RM: Advanced simulation technologies for surgical education. Am Col Surg 81:77–81, 1996.

21. Geis WP, Kim HC, McAfee PC, et al: Synergistic benefits of combined technologies in complex minimally invasive surgical procedures. Clinical experience and educational processes. Surg Endosc 10:1025–8, 1996.
22. Kuehnapfel UG, Neisius B: CAD based graphical computer simulation in endoscopic surgery. Endosc Surg Allied Technol 1:181–183, 1993.
23. Schurr MO, Breitwieser H, Melzer A, et al: Experimental telemanipulation in endoscopic surgery. Surg Laparosc Endosc 6: 167–175, 1996.

COMMENTARY

W. Randolph Chitwood, Jr.

In this unique chapter on robotic surgery, Dr. Falk has provided us a look into the future of telemicroaccess heart surgery. He and his colleague, Professor Friedrich Mohr, have been true innovators in applying robotic techniques to cardiac surgery. They have a large experience in using the AESOP 3000 voice-activated robot for camera control during videoscopic mitral valve surgery. This chapter represents a primer for cardiac surgeons interested in these devices. Falk defines the mechanical advantages of fully articulated robotic devices, which provide 7 degrees of freedom, or the same as the human wrist. He projects the important notion that this is not surgery performed by an electronically minded, mechanical device at some long distance; rather, it represents a true intracardiac telepresence. Thus, the surgeon is doing all the manipulation, not the robot. The robot merely filters motion artifact, scales motion, enhances accuracy, and allows the surgeon to operate within a cardiac chamber by placing the activated portion of the tiny instrument precisely at the desired site. Dexterity is enhanced without losing complete control. Falk carefully details the basic mechanics of these electronic devices in a way that most surgeons can understand so they can appreciate the potential utility. He transcends the engineering jargon and writes in terms that we can appreciate from experiences in clinical practice.

During robotic cardiac surgery using these devices, the electromechanical instrument remains the central effector. However, videoscopic secondary vision is equally important. Falk emphasizes the importance of three-dimensional visualization during robotic cardiac surgery. Additionally, tracking the instrument tips during excursion around the surgical field is necessary. All three must be coordinated, and Falk conveys the interdependence of these components. He describes current techniques for voice-activated tracking of instruments during both manual and robotic manipulation. Currently, we routinely use the voice-activated robot (AESOP 3000) for camera control in videoscopic mitral surgery. This truly facilitates these operations—it works!.

Finally, the chapter describes the techniques used in Leipzig to perform coronary surgery and mitral repairs with the Intuitive robotic system. I had the pleasure of being present in Leipzig in early June 1998 during the initial mitral valve repair and coronary grafting trials. Thus, having seen this truly interactive surgical robot used clinically (Intuitive System), and from my experience experimentally, I must emphasize the magnitude of future applicability of these devices. During the week I was there, the group performed eight operations using this device without patient complications. One week earlier, Carpentier had performed the first successful mitral repair with the system in Paris. Based on these clinical successes, others should appreciate the potential future of robotics in cardiac surgery. Despite this early enthusiasm, Falk emphasizes the pitfalls in using this new technology. In the concluding section, he gives the reader a glimpse of future innovations in this area but warns surgeons that new training methods will be needed to reap the benefits and minimize deficiencies inherent in a learning curve. In summary, Dr. Falk has hurled us past the concept that surgical robots are cold, thoughtless, humanoid figures to thoughts of a reliable, enabling technology that can facilitate future cardiac surgeons in their quest for less traumatic operations. Clearly, our patients will benefit most if we are cautious. Although mechanical size, cavitary access, and visualization still remain important issues before these methods can be established, we should follow this work enthusiastically. The next century promises to be really exciting!

Chapter 80

Facilitated Approaches to Vascular End-to-Side Anastomoses

Robin H. Heijmen, Paul F. Gründeman, and Cornelius Borst

Recent progress in off-pump, beating heart coronary artery bypass grafting (>10,000 procedures in 1997) and initiatives toward progressively reduced surgical access warrant an intensified search for facilitated approaches to vascular end-to-side anastomoses.

Coronary artery bypass grafting without cardiopulmonary bypass requires temporary occlusion of the coronary artery. Interruption of coronary flow, however, may result in regional myocardial ischemia and its sequelae.

A large variety of innovative anastomotic techniques have been explored to reduce or eliminate occlusive anastomosis time. Coronary shunting techniques, including the use of distal perfusion cannulas, intraluminal coronary shunts, and a temporary luminal arteriotomy seal, enable persistent coronary perfusion while suturing. An alternative approach to the prevention of myocardial ischemia is accelerated tissue bonding, including the use of tissue adhesives, laser tissue welding, and mechanical anastomotic stapling devices. In one center, a truly nonocclusive end-to-side anastomosis technique is being applied clinically in cerebral artery bypass grafting.

It is anticipated that in combination with the thoracoscopic application of local coronary stabilization and robotic surgery, a greatly facilitated coronary anastomosis technique will enable closed chest, off-pump coronary bypass grafting in the near future.

The Need for a Facilitated Coronary Anastomosis Technique

Since the early 1990s, coronary artery bypass grafting (CABG) on the beating heart has gained interest[1, 2] and is rapidly evolving as coronary motion can now be restrained adequately with mechanical stabilization devices.[3–5] It is estimated that in 1997 more than 10,000 CABG procedures were performed on the beating heart. Off-pump, beating heart CABG, however, requires temporary interruption of coronary blood flow to obtain a bloodless surgical field for optimal visualization of the distal anastomosis site. To date, the coronary artery anastomosis is sutured under direct vision through a median sternotomy (full access) or mini-thoracotomy (limited access). However, performing a coronary anastomosis on a beating heart, particularly via limited access, is technically demanding. Video-assisted, closed-chest CABG may further complicate the procedure and prolong anastomosis time and, hence, the ischemic period.

The potential risk of regional myocardial ischemic injury caused by prolonged coronary occlusion may be reduced by (1) ischemic preconditioning[6, 7] or pharmacologic and mechanical cardioprotective techniques[8] or by (2) (intraluminal) coronary shunting[9–11] to enable persistent coronary perfusion while suturing. An alternative approach to the prevention of myocardial ischemia is accelerated tissue bonding[12] to replace the tedious, often time-consuming process of manual suturing.

This chapter discusses facilitated approaches to vascular end-to-side anastomoses to reduce or eliminate occlusive anastomosis time. Coronary shunting techniques, including the use of distal perfusion cannulas, intraluminal coronary shunts, and a novel temporary luminal arteriotomy seal are reviewed, as are accelerated tissue bonding techniques, including tissue adhesives, laser tissue welding, and mechanical anastomotic stapling devices. In addition, a true nonocclusive, end-to-side anastomosis technique is described.

First, various hemostatic techniques in use for interruption of coronary flow are presented. Next, the potential limitations of coronary occlusion, regional myocardial ischemia, and retrograde coronary flow are briefly reviewed to delineate the rationale for the intensified search for facilitated alternative anastomosis techniques.

Interruption of Coronary Flow

Hemostatic Techniques

In the majority of patients, the anastomosis is performed while the recipient coronary artery is temporarily occluded proximally and distally by means of silicone or polypropylene suture loops,[13, 14] with buttressed either a pledget or a small piece of silicone tubing. Snaring of the coronary artery, without applying traction to improve stabilization, does not cause endothelial dysfunction at the proximal and distal snare sites.[15] Passage of a needle twice around the coronary artery, however, carries the risk of accidentally puncturing perforating or septal branches. Subsequent bleeding at the site of passage of the suture may impair visibility of the arteriotomy.

Various other techniques have been described to prevent blood from flooding the anastomotic area after arteriotomy, including graduated probes,[16] Fogarty biliary catheters,[17] catheter stents,[18] intravascular (balloon) occluders, occlusive balloons applied extravascularly,[19] and coronary clamps.[19, 20] In our institution, recipient coronary artery flow is temporarily interrupted by means of two separately applied microvascular Acland clamps proximally and distally to the anastomosis site, in both experimental[21] and clinical[22] settings. The microvascular Acland clamps[23] are used routinely in plastic surgical practice and are considered atraumatic.[21] In a recent study by Perrault and associates,[19] however, coronary artery clamping with a vascular bulldog clamp, even with a perivascular cushion, resulted in marked endothelial cell injury and loss, and hence endothelial dysfunction.

Regional Myocardial Ischemia

Interruption of existing residual or collateral coronary flow results in regional myocardial ischemia, which may prompt rate, rhythm, or conduction disturbances; deterioration of pump function; and acute myocardial infarction. In the majority of patients, however, the short ischemia period during construction of the graft is remarkably well tolerated without a rise in cardiac troponin levels, indicative of myocardial cell death.[24, 25] This may be attributed to a well-developed collateral coronary circulation in patients who have high-grade proximal stenosis or occlusion.

It is inferred that the severity of preocclusion stenosis and the site of coronary occlusion play a crucial role in the magnitude and consequence of myocardial ischemia induced by interruption of coronary flow.[26] It is conceivable that expanding the indication for coronary bypass surgery without cardiopulmonary bypass to patients who have three-vessel disease, lesser grade proximal stenosis, and unstable angina will enlarge the group of patients at risk for coronary flow interruption because of the cumulative effect of short ischemia periods and the absence of adequate collateral coronary flow. In addition, less invasive or true thoracoscopic approaches are likely to prolong the anastomosis time and, hence, the ischemic period. It is hard to predict, however, which patient will fail to tolerate the period of coronary flow interruption.

To reduce susceptibility to ischemic injury, the myocardium can be preconditioned by 5 minutes of stop-flow ischemia, that is, ischemic preconditioning.[6, 7] Tolerance to ischemia may also be enhanced by mechanical unloading or pharmacologic agents.[8]

Retrograde Coronary Flow

Collateral flow via perforating branches that happen to be located in the isolated coronary segment often produces retrograde flow that wells up in the arteriotomy and obscures its edges. Suboptimal visualization of the coronary anastomosis site carries the risk of imperfect anastomotic suturing. Saline solution irrigation through a syringe or gas jet insufflation,[27] although recently associated with endothelial cell injury and loss,[19] can be effective for optimizing visualization of the anastomotic area. It is inferred, however, that retrograde flow occurs at the expense of distal myocardial perfusion by collateral circulation,[28] which may result in hemodynamic deterioration.

Coronary Shunting

In a few cases, coronary blood flow interruption during CABG on the beating heart is not tolerated, and regional myocardial ischemia leads to serious ventricular arrhythmias or hemodynamic deterioration, or both, necessitating conversion to a conventional procedure with cardiopulmonary bypass[4, 28] or insertion of a coronary shunt.[29, 30]

Distal Perfusion Cannula

The use of coronary shunt to provide continuous distal coronary perfusion while suturing was originally described by Trapp and associate in 1975.[9] A perfusion cannula placed in the ascending aorta and the coronary arteriotomy maintained distal perfusion while the surgeon sutured around the catheter. Just before finishing the anastomosis, the catheter was removed and the suture line completed. Occasionally, reports have been published demonstrating the use of coronary shunts to repair operatively severed aortocoronary bypass grafts.[31, 32] Coulson and associates[33] delineated the advantages of a coronary perfusion cannula during CABG on the beating heart and advocated its use to facilitate training of the operative procedure.[34]

Intraluminal Coronary Shunt

In 1977, Franzone and associates[10] described an alternative intraluminal coronary shunt technique, which consisted of a series of silicone tubings of various calibers with beveled edges. Application of this shunt during CABG on the beating heart was associated with a reduced incidence of persistent myocardial ischemia and intraoperative myocardial infarction postoperatively.[10] Rivetti and associate[35] reported their results using a comparable intraluminal shunt during CABG without cardiopulmonary bypass.

None of these coronary shunting techniques has ever been widely used. This may be attributed to their inability to provide a bloodless arteriotomy without snaring the recipient artery proximally and distally, their obstruction to residual blood flow because their inner diameter is often flow-limiting, or their cumbersome and possibly traumatic retrieval through the small residual opening on completion of the anastomosis. In addition, isolating a segment of the recipient coronary artery by inserting an intraluminal tubular shunt (Fig. 80–1) blocks antegrade residual or retrograde collateral flow in many of the (perforating) side branches, which may result in regional myocardial ischemia and its sequelae.[35]

Temporary Luminal Arteriotomy Seal

To enable anastomotic suturing in a bloodless surgical field in combination with persistent distal perfusion and without blocking the entrance to side branches, a temporary luminal arteriotomy seal (TLAS) has been described (Figs. 80–2 and 80–3).[11, 36] Figure 80–3 schematically summarizes the application of the TLAS.

The success of the TLAS may be attributed to the following:

1. Intra-arterial, transmural pressure
2. Elastic properties of the polyurethane material, because its radius of curvature is larger than the radius of the recipient artery

After initial assessment of the TLAS in a porcine carotid artery bypass graft model,[11] in which the seal enabled bloodless anastomosis suturing without obstructing recipient artery blood flow with minimal damage to the arterial wall, the feasibility was explored of applying a TLAS for end-to-side coronary anastomosis suturing on the beating heart in the pig.[36] After only a short learning period, in-

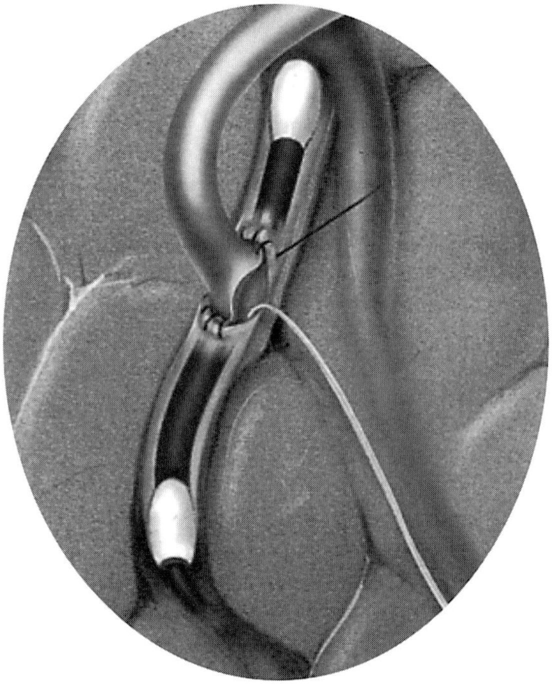

Figure 80–1. Schematic representation of a commercially available intraluminal coronary shunt. Immediately after arteriotomy, a properly sized shunt is introduced proximally and distally into the coronary artery, after which coronary blood flow is restored. An encircling retention suture at the midpoint of the shunt is used for withdrawal after completion of the anastomosis.

sertion and retrieval of the seal required about 20 and 10 seconds, respectively. Coronary artery occlusion time was limited to about 80 seconds. As a consequence, none of the animals experienced serious rate, rhythm, or conduction disturbances during the anastomotic procedure. Because of its low profile and the relative expansion of the artery at arteriotomy, a minimal decrease in the cross-sectional area of the recipient artery lumen was achieved, and consequently no obstruction to coronary blood flow was observed.[36] The study in the porcine coronary artery supported the previous findings in the carotid artery concerning arterial wall damage and subsequent healing.[11] Because of its design, the seal contacts only about half the circumference of the recipient artery and, consequently, endothelial damage was found to be localized and limited to the area covered by the seal. Re-endothelialization, therefore, may be accelerated by spread of endothelial cells from the side of the artery opposite the arteriotomy, rather than from minute side branches (vasa vasorum) and the proximal and distal, nonoccluded segments. This was supported by the preliminary finding of endothelial-like cells already observed at the suture line 7 days postoperatively.[36] Furthermore, the flimsy seal caused no medial necrosis and at 28 days, all anastomoses remained patent, with minimal intimal hyperplasia.

The experimental evaluation of the TLAS was extended in postmortem atherosclerotic human coronary arteries perfused at various pressures.[85] At all anastomosis sites, the seal provided a bloodless operative field. Irregular luminal wall surface and low transmural pressure did not frustrate sealing.

To date, the seal has been used in experimental settings only. The TLAS, however, holds promise for clinical application and may expand the indications for CABG on the beating heart and facilitate the development of true port hold, closed chest, off-pump coronary surgery.

In addition to coronary anastomosis suturing, a modified seal might be employed during proximal anastomosis suturing. This would obviate the need for the side clamp on the ascending aorta and would further reduce the risk of adverse cerebral effects by particulate emboli.[37]

Accelerated Tissue Bonding

Tissue Adhesives

The use of adhesive substances for vascular anastomoses has been studied by many investigators. Generally, two groups of adhesives can be distinguished: fibrin glue and the cyanoacrylate glues.

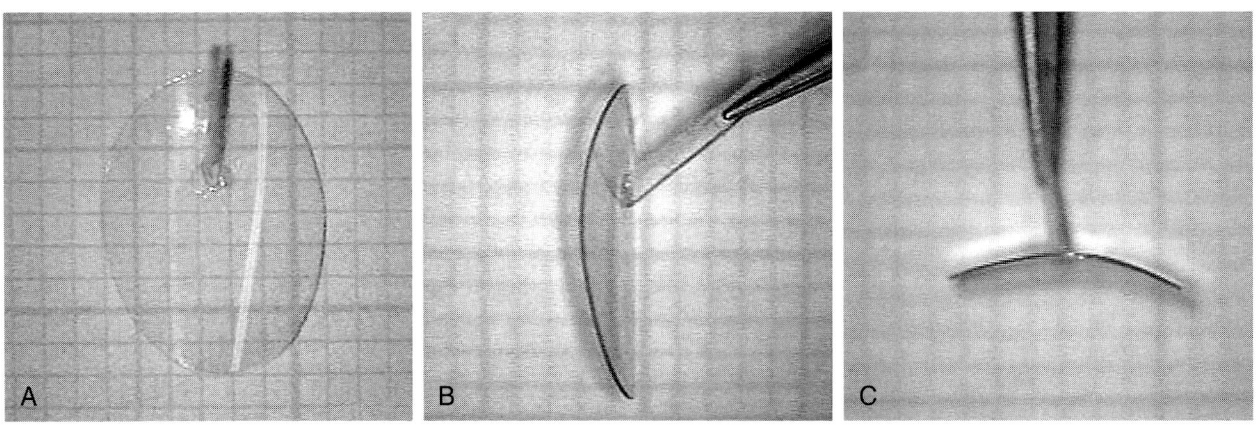

Figure 80–2. Top (*A*), lateral (*B*), and frontal (*C*) view of the temporary luminal arteriotomy seal. The 200-μm-thick seal is made from a polyurethane balloon skin material. The seal's oval and convex shape conforms to the elliptic arteriotomy that results from a linear incision in the pressurized coronary artery. The dorsal fin is used for insertion, positioning and retrieval of the seal. (Reprinted with permission from the Society of Thoracic Surgeons. From Heijmen RH, Borst C, van Dalen R, et al: Temporary luminal arteriotomy seal: II. Coronary artery bypass grafting on the beating heart. Ann Thorac Surg 66:471–476, 1998.)

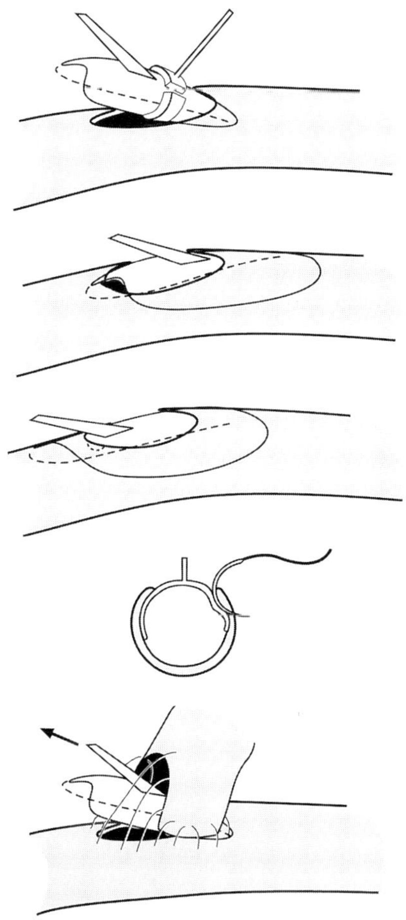

Figure 80–3. Schematic representation of the temporary luminal arteriotomy seal (TLAS) and its application. After interruption of recipient artery blood flow and arteriotomy, the TLAS, which is prefolded in a small cannula segment, is inserted into the artery (*A*), where it unfolds owing to the flexibility of the material (*B*). After positioning the seal correctly inside the artery, usually after about 80-cm second interruption, blood flow is restored (*C*). During suturing, the flimsy seal gives way when a needle is inserted between the seal and the arterial wall, without producing a leak (*D*). After finishing the suturing, coronary blood flow is briefly interrupted again, the TLAS is grasped, sliding it toward the heel of the anastomosis and withdrawing it in the axial direction from the artery past the suture (*E*), which subsequently is tightened to complete the anastomosis. (Reprinted with permission from the Society of Thoracic Surgeons. Modified from Heijmen RH, Borst C, van Dalen R, et al: Temporary luminal arteriotomy seal: II. Coronary artery bypass grafting on the beating heart. Ann Thorac Surg 66:471–476, 1998.)

The fibrin glue consolidates by aggregation of fibrin monomers when its two components (i.e. fibrinogen and thrombin) are merged.[38] Its homology with the latter part of the clotting cascade clearly reflects the risk of thromboembolic complications when fibrin glue accidentally reaches the intravascular compartment. Because of its increased thrombogenicity[39] and insufficient tensile strength to support sutureless anastomoses,[40] there has been a general reluctance to use fibrin glue for vascular anastomoses. Negatively charged fibrin glue has been proposed to prevent intraluminal thrombus formation.[41]

As an alternative to fibrin glue, cyanoacrylate adhesives have been studied in experimental vascular surgery. Although successful sutureless arterial anastomoses have been reported,[42, 43] the main limitation of cyanoacrylate glue is its potential histotoxicity, which may be attributed to the adhesive's heat of polymerization, as well as toxic degradation products.[44] The application of cyanoacrylate adhesive to the outer surface of the anastomotic line caused severe adventitial and medial necrosis,[44] resulting in a thinned vascular wall and, ultimately, aneurysm formation.[45–47] In addition, cyanoacrylate hardens completely, and, as a result, the anastomotic line lacks elasticity.[48]

A novel photopolymerizable glue, polyethylene glycol 400 diacrylate, was introduced, which effectively sealed vessel puncture sites and anastomotic junctions.[49] The glue was found to be nontoxic to living tissue[50] and nonthrombogenic in a vascular thrombosis model,[49] but unfortunately was not effective enough to support a sutureless anastomosis.[49]

Laser Tissue Welding

Since the advent of laser tissue welding for vascular anastomosis by Jain[51] in 1980, there has been a progressive effort to refine the laser-assisted vascular anastomosis technique and to use this modality in clinical practice. In contrast to the sutureless anastomosis originally described by Jain, most surgeons advocate a hybrid technique, in which three to four stay sutures are used to coapt the vessel edges, after which the laser beam is applied to the gap between two adjacent sutures while traction is applied to them.[52–55] The time required for laser-assisted anastomosis has been substantially less than that required for conventional techniques, with at least equivalent patency rates.[52–55] However, the reported incidence of pseudoaneurysm formation and anastomotic disruption has limited its clinical application.[55, 56] It is inferred that inadvertent overapplication of laser energy, resulting in full-thickness vessel wall degeneration, is responsible for aneurysm formation, because the anastomotic tensile and bursting strength was found to be sufficient to withstand higher than arterial blood pressure at different time intervals.[53, 57] Infrared tissue surface temperature feedback of the laser output has been described to keep tissue surface temperature from exceeding a predetermined value.[58, 59] The feasibility of using laser tissue welding in experimental CABG has already been demonstrated.[60, 61] However, further surgical refinements and study of the optimal laser parameters needed to produce a reliable weld are required before clinical application.

Mechanical Anastomotic Stapling Devices

A number of mechanical anastomotic stapling devices have been proposed in an effort to reduce occlusive anastomosis time.[12] In the late 1940s, the Russian engineer Gudov constructed a circular stapler apparatus that enabled end-to-end vascular anastomosis by mechanical means.[62] Both vessel ends were threaded through and everted across two bushings that were each held by a clamp, opposed, and,[62] subsequently stapled. The successful clinical application of the Russian stapler in peripheral vascular and coronary surgery was reported by Androsov[63] and Kolesov,[62] respectively. Since then, individual modifications of this stapler have been described by Vogelfanger and Beattie,[64] Mallina and associates,[65] and Inokuchi.[66] However, the requirement of a relatively long segment of nondiseased vessel on either side for adequate eversion, the suitability for end-to-end anastomoses only, and the technical complexity and cumbersome handling of these staplers, have limited their clinical application.

In the late 1960s, simplified mechanical stapling devices for end-to-side anastomosis entered the field of vascular surgery.[12, 67–70] Aside from individual modifications, the primary principle was based on the insertion and subsequent stapling of the everted distal end of the graft in the recipient vessel. Despite the authors' claims to simplicity and the efficacy of the accelerated anastomotic procedure, the use of semiautomated mechanical stapling devices has generally waned in the present era. This may in part be ascribed to improvements in magnification, suture material, and instrumentation, which have made direct anastomotic suturing the technique of choice in microvascular surgery.

In the early 1990s, the concept of a sutureless, mechanically constructed anastomosis was revised by Kirsch and associates,[71] who introduced a new method of microvascular reconstruction based on the principle of flanged, intimal approximation by interrupted application of arcuate-legged, nonpenetrating clips. After extensive experimental testing,[71–73] in which the clips proved biologically and technically at least equivalent[72] if not superior[74] to the penetrating microsuture, successful clipped anastomoses were performed in both the peripheral[72, 74] and coronary circulation.[75] Symmetric eversion of the vessel edges by means of a special forceps, however, as well as proper application of the clips requires training.

To facilitate symmetric eversion of the vessel edges and to enable circumferential clip application by a single maneuver for rapid end-to-side anastomosis, a novel One-Shot anastomotic stapler prototype has been developed (Figs. 80–4 and 80–5), based on earlier designs of semiautomated mechanical anastomotic devices. Preliminary results suggest that this stapler prototype shows promise as a facilitated end-to-side anastomotic device.[86]

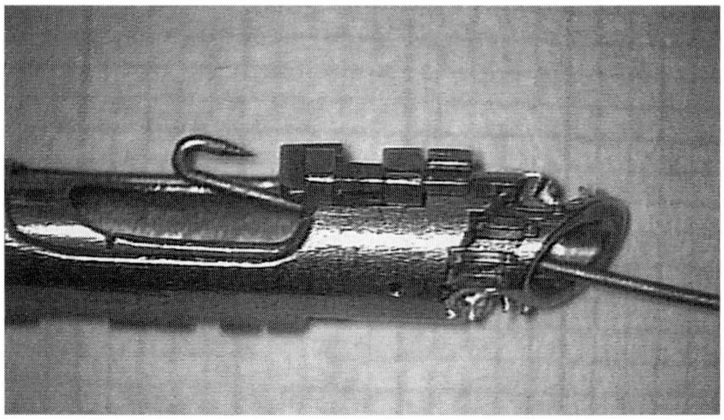

Figure 80–4. Close-up of the tip of the One-Shot anastomotic stapler prototype (U.S. Surgical Corporation, Norwalk, CT). The device consists of a clip cartridge, which is loaded circumferentially with 12 equally spaced clips, attached to a firing handle that serves for simultaneous, circumferential clip closure. The graft is pulled through the clip cartridge by the hook, everted across the anvil, and subsequently hooked on the lower jaws of the clips. The everted distal end of the graft is inserted in the arteriotomy, after which the firing handles are squeezed, closing the clips across the everted edges of the graft and recipient vessel. Resqueezing the firing handle allows the clip cartridge to split and enables removal of the graft from within it. (From Heijmen RH, Hinchliffe P, Borst C, et al: A novel one-shot anastomotic stapler prototype for coronary bypass grafting on the beating heart: Feasibility in the pig. J Thorac Cardiovasc Surg 117: 117–125, 1999, with permission.)

Nonocclusive End-to-Side Anastomosis Technique

All the innovative techniques described previously, including intraluminal coronary shunting, tissue adhesives, laser welding, and mechanical anastomotic stapling devices, have reduced but not eliminated occlusive anastomosis time.

In neurosurgery, Tulleken and associates[76–80] revisited the concept of a nonocclusive laser-assisted anastomosis technique originally described by Yahr and associates[81] and developed an alternative end-to-side anastomosis technique that does not require interruption of flow in the recipient (cerebral) artery. After the everted graft has been connected with the exterior of the recipient artery, a laser punch catheter removes the partitioning wall of the latter (Fig. 80–6). This elegant approach has been applied successfully to CABG on the beating heart in the pig.[3] Tulleken's technique, however, requires apposition of the intima of the graft to the thrombogenic adventitia of the recipient artery, leaving an adventitial rim inside the lumen.[78] This is in contrast to current surgical practice, which dictates apposition of both intimas. In both experimental and clinical studies,[76–80] Tulleken and associates have reported patency rates up to 90%. Qualitative assessment by scanning electron microscopy of the adventitial rim in the rabbit showed no early thrombus formation and

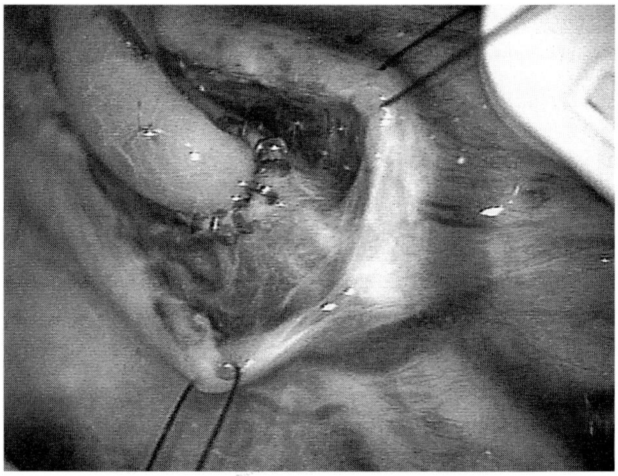

Figure 80–5. Stapled left internal mammary artery to left anterior descending coronary artery anastomosis on the beating heart in the pig, after restoration of graft blood flow. The left anterior descending coronary artery was immobilized with the Octopus Tissue Stabilizer (Medtronic, Inc., Minneapolis, MN) (*upper right corner*). To improve visualization, two sutures were passed through the epicardium on either side of the left anterior descending coronary artery. (From Heijmen RH, Hinchliffe P, Borst C, et al: A novel one-shot anastomotic stapler prototype for coronary bypass grafting on the beating heart: Feasibility in the pig. J Thorac Cardiovasc Surg 117:117–125, 1999, with permission.)

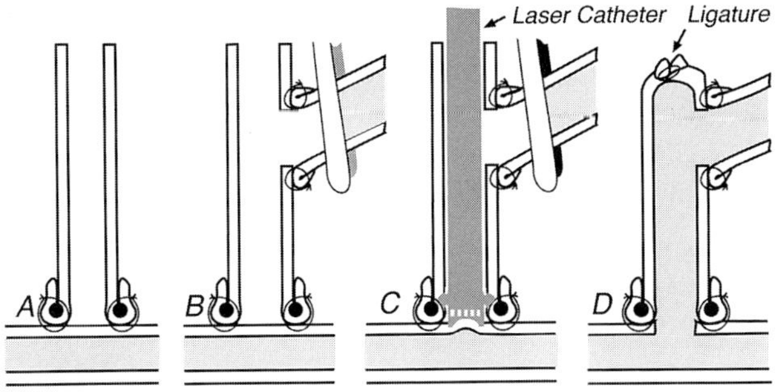

Figure 80–6. Schematic representation of a nonocclusive end-to-side anastomosis technique developed by Tulleken and colleagues.[3, 7–80] An everted short segment of the graft is connected to the exterior of the recipient artery (*A*). Next, the graft is sutured end-to-side to the short segment close to its open end (*B*). A laser punch catheter is introduced into the segment and removes the partitioning wall of the recipient artery by laser ablation (*C*). The open end of the short segment of the graft is closed, and graft blood flow is restored (*D*). (Reprinted with permission from the American College of Cardiology. From Borst C, Jansen EWL, Tulleken CAF, et al: Coronary artery bypass grafting without cardiopulmonary bypass and without interruption of native coronary flow using a novel anastomosis site restraining device ["Octopus"]. J Am Coll Cardiol 27:1356–1364, 1996.)

complete re-endothelialization at 6 weeks.[76–78] On the beating porcine heart, however, the laser punch catheter failed to remove the punched-out coronary arterial wall disk properly in 25% of cases.[3] This increased the incidence of primary anastomotic closure.

In atherosclerotic human coronary arteries, a mechanical device may eventually be required to perform the arteriotomy effectively and at low cost. In a porcine carotid artery bypass graft model, in which the arteriotomy was made by a mechanical punch rather than by a laser punch catheter, intima-adventitia apposition was associated with serious initial thrombotic phenomena, although in all animals, after 4 weeks it yielded a patent anastomosis with a small intimal hyperplasia response that was comparable with conventional intima-intima apposition.[82]

Conclusion

Various facilitated approaches to vascular end-to-side anastomoses have been described to reduce or ultimately eliminate occlusive anastomosis time. These innovative procedures generally include

1. Coronary shunting techniques, which enable manual suturing without time constraint due to persistent distal perfusion
2. Accelerated tissue-bonding techniques, which rely mostly on alternative tissue bonding during interruption of coronary flow

To date, the laser-assisted anastomotic procedure developed by Tulleken and associates[3, 76–80] is the only truly nonocclusive, end-to-side anastomosis technique available.

Robotic devices have been developed to enhance precision and surgical dexterity,[83] facilitating true endoscopic coronary anastomosis suturing.[84] It is anticipated that in combination with the thoracoscopic application of local coronary stabilization and robotic surgery, a greatly facilitated coronary anastomosis technique will enable closed chest off-pump coronary bypass grafting in the near future.

References

1. Borst C (ed): Towards Minimally Invasive Coronary Artery Bypass Grafting. Ann Thorac Surg 63(Suppl):S1–142, 1997.
2. Borst C, Jansen EWL, Gründeman PF: Less invasive coronary artery bypass grafting: Without cardiopulmonary bypass and via reduced surgical access (Editorial). Heart 77:302–303, 1997.
3. Borst C, Jansen EWL, Tulleken CAF, et al: Coronary artery bypass grafting without cardiopulmonary bypass and without interruption of native coronary flow using a novel anastomosis site restraining device ("Octopus"). J Am Coll Cardiol 27:1356–1364, 1996.
4. Shennib H, Lee AGL, Akin J: Safe and effective method of stabilization for coronary artery bypass grafting on the beating heart. Ann Thorac Surg 63:988–992, 1997.
5. Borst C, Santamore WP, Smedira NG, Bredée JJ: Minimally invasive coronary artery bypass grafting: On the beating heart and via limited access. Ann Thorac Surg 63:S1–5, 1997.
6. Murry CE, Jennings RB, Reimer KA: Preconditioning with ischemia: A delay of lethal cell injury in ischemic myocardium. Circulation 74:1124–1136, 1986.
7. Alkhulaifa AM, Yellon DM, Pugsley WB: Preconditioning the human heart during aortocoronary bypass surgery. Eur J Cardiothorac Surg 8:270–276, 1994.
8. Flameng WJ: Role of myocardial protection for coronary artery bypass grafting on the beating heart. Ann Thorac Surg 63:S18–22, 1997.
9. Trapp WG, Bisarya R: Placement of coronary artery bypass graft without pump oxygenator. Ann Thorac Surg 19:1–9, 1975.
10. Franzone AJ, Wallsh E, Stertzer SH, et al: Reduced incidence of intraoperative myocardial infarction during coronary bypass surgery with use of intracoronary shunt technique. Am J Cardiol 39:1017–1020, 1977.
11. Heijmen RH, Borst C, van Dalen R, et al. Temporary luminal arteriotomy seal for bypass grafting. Ann Thorac Surg 65:1093–1099, 1998.
12. Werker PMN, Kon M: Review of facilitated approaches to vascular anastomosis surgery. Ann Thorac Surg 63:S122–127, 1997.
13. Buffolo E, Andrade JCS, Branco JNR, et al: Coronary artery bypass grafting without cardiopulmonary bypass. Ann Thorac Surg 61:63–66, 1996.
14. Benetti FJ, Mariani MA, Sani G, et al: Video-assisted minimally invasive coronary operations without cardiopulmonary bypass: A multicenter study. J Thorac Cardiovasc Surg 112:1478–1484, 1996.
15. Perrault LP, Menasché P, Bidouard J-P, et al: Snaring of the target vessel in less invasive bypass operations does not cause endothelial dysfunction. Ann Thorac Surg 63:751–755, 1997.
16. Parsonnet V, Gilbert L, Gielchinsky I: Graduated probes for coronary bypass surgery. J Thorac Cardiovasc Surg 68:424–427, 1974.
17. Grow JB Sr, Brantigan CO: Use of a Fogarty biliary catheter to create a bloodless field for saphenous vein–coronary artery anastomosis. J Thorac Cardiovasc Surg 69:105–106, 1975.
18. Ludington LG, Kafrouni G, Peterson MH, et al: Technique for using soft, flexible catheter stents in aortocoronary vein bypass operations. Ann Thorac Surg 21:328–332, 1976.
19. Perrault LP, Menasché P, Wassef M, et al: Endothelial effects of hemostatic devices for continuous cardioplegia or minimally invasive operations. Ann Thorac Surg 62:1158–1163, 1996.

20. Abhay SW, Kole SD: Clamp for coronary artery operations. Ann Thorac Surg 65:1475–1476, 1998.
21. Jansen EWL, Gründeman PF, Mansvelt Beck HJ, et al: Experimental off-pump grafting of a circumflex branch via sternotomy using a suction device. Ann Thorac Surg 63:S93–96, 1997.
22. Jansen EWL, Gründeman PF, Borst C, et al: Less invasive off-pump CABG using a suction device for immobilization: The "octopus" method. Eur J Cardiothorac Surg 12:406–412, 1997.
23. Acland RD: Microvascular anastomosis: A device for holding stay sutures and a new vascular clamp. Surgery 75:185–187, 1974.
24. Birdi I, Caputo M, Hutter JA, et al: Troponin I release during minimally invasive coronary artery surgery. J Thorac Cardiovasc Surg 114:509–510, 1997.
25. Hadjinikalaou LK, Cohen AS, Aitkenhead H, et al: Troponin-T in minimally invasive coronary operations (Correspondence). Ann Thorac Surg 63:1511–1512, 1997.
26. Airaksinen KEJ, Ikäheimo MJ, Huikuri HV: Stenosis severity and the occurrence of ventricular ectopic activity during acute coronary occlusion during balloon angioplasty. Am J Cardiol 76:346–349, 1995.
27. Teoh KHT, Panos AL, Harmantas AA, et al: Optimal visualization of coronary artery anastomoses by gas jet. Ann Thorac Surg 52:564, 1991.
28. Jansen EWL: Towards minimally invasive coronary artery bypass grafting. PhD Thesis, Utrecht, the Netherlands, Utrecht University, 1998.
29. Levinson MM, Fooks GS: Coronary grafting using a temporary intraluminal shunt instead of heart-lung bypass. Ann Thorac Surg 60:1800–1801, 1995.
30. Borges MF, Spohn PK, Coulson AS: Arrhythmia/ischemia management during minimally invasive cardiac operations. Ann Thorac Surg 64:843–844, 1997.
31. Robison RJ, Brown JW, Deschner WP, King RD: Intraluminal shunting of operatively severed aortocoronary saphenous vein grafts. Ann Thorac Surg 42:475–476, 1986.
32. Carrel T, Pasic M, Turina M: Use of an intraluminal shunt to repair a coronary bypass graft injury during resternotomy. J Thorac Cardiovasc Surg 109:178–179, 1995.
33. Coulson A, Bakhshay S, Quarnstrom J, Spohn P: Temporary coronary artery perfusion catheter during minimally invasive coronary surgery. Chest 113:514–520, 1998.
34. Coulson A: Minimally invasive coronary artery surgery (Letter). J Thorac Cardiovasc Surg 115:486–487, 1998.
35. Rivetti LA, Gandra SMA: Initial experience using an intraluminal shunt during revascularization of the beating heart. Ann Thorac Surg 63:1742–1747, 1997.
36. Heijmen RH, Borst C, van Dalen R, et al: Temporary luminal arteriotomy seal: II. Coronary artery bypass grafting on the beating heart. Ann Thorac Surg 66:471–476, 1998.
37. Roach GW, Kanchuger M, Mangano CM, et al: Adverse cerebral outcomes after coronary bypass surgery. N Engl J Med 335:1857–1863, 1996.
38. Matras H: Fibrin seal: The state of the art. J Oral Maxillofac Surg 43:605–611, 1985.
39. Bschorer R, Frerich B, Wolburg H, et al: Fibrin sealing and histometrical changes in conventionally sutured microvascular anastomoses. J Craniomaxillofac Surg 21:192–198, 1993.
40. Flahiff C, Feldman D, Saltz R, Huang S: Mechanical properties of fibrin adhesives for blood vessel anastomosis. J Biomater Res 26:481–491, 1992.
41. Dowbak GM, Rohrich RJ, Robinson JB Jr, Peden E: Effectiveness of a new non-thrombogenic bio-adhesive in microvascular anastomoses. J Reconstr Microsurg 10:383–386, 1994.
42. Weissberg D, Schwartz P, Goetz R: Nonsuture end-to-side anastomosis of small blood vessels. Surg Gynecol Obstet 123:341–346, 1966.
43. Takenaka H, Esato K, Ohara M, Zempo N: Sutureless anastomosis of blood vessels using cyanoacrylate adhesives. Surg Today 22:46–54, 1992.
44. Vinters HV, Galil KA, Lundie MJ, Kaufmann JCE: The histotoxicity of cyanoacrylate. A selective review. Neuroradiology 27:279–291, 1985.
45. Weissberg D, Goetz RH: Necrosis of arterial wall following application of methyl 2-cyanoacrylate. Surg Gynecol Obstet 119:1248–1252, 1964.
46. Woodward SC, Herrman JB, Cameron JL, et al: Histotoxicity of cyanoacrylate tissue adhesive in the rat. Ann Surg 162: 113–122, 1965.
47. Green AR, Milling MAP, Green ART: Butylcyanoacrylate adhesive in microvascular surgery: An experimental pilot study. J Reconstr Microsurg 2:103–105, 1986.
48. Middleton WG, Matthews W, Chiasson DA: Histoacryl glue in microvascular surgery. J Otolaryngol 20:363–366, 1991.
49. Dumanian GA, Dascombe W, Hong C, et al: A new photopolymerizable blood vessel glue that seals human vessel anastomoses without augmenting thrombogenicity. Plast Reconstr Surg 95:901–907, 1995.
50. Pathak CP, Sawhney AS, Hubbel JA: Rapid photopolymerization of immunoprotective gels in contact with cells and tissue. J Am Chem Soc 114:8311–8315, 1992.
51. Jain KK: Sutureless microvascular anastomosis using a neodymium-YAG laser. J Microsurg 1:436–439, 1980.
52. Neblett CR, Morris JR, Thomsen S: Laser-assisted microsurgical anastomosis. Neurosurgery 19:914–934, 1986.
53. Nakata S, Campbell CD, Pick R, Repogle RL: End-to-side and end-to-end vascular anastomoses with a carbon dioxide laser. J Thorac Cardiovasc Surg 98:57–62, 1989.
54. Ruiz-Razura A, Lan M, Cohen BE: The laser-assisted end-to-side microvascular anastomosis. Plast Reconstr Surg 83:511–517, 1989.
55. McCarthy WJ, LoCicero J, Hartz RS, Yao JST: Patency of laser-assisted anastomoses in small vessels: One year follow-up. Surgery 102:319–326, 1987.
56. Quigley MR, Bailes JE, Kwaam HC, et al: Aneurysm formation after low power carbon dioxide laser-assisted vascular anastomosis. Neurosurgery 18:292–299, 1986.
57. Flemming AFS, Bown SG, Colles MJ, Brough MD: Comparison of laser-assisted and conventionally sutured microvascular anastomoses by bursting pressure: a reanalysis and further studies. Microsurgery 11:25–33, 1990.
58. Springer TA, Welch AJ: Temperature control during laser vessel welding. Appl Optics 32:517–525, 1993.
59. Cilesiz I, Thompsen S, Welch AJ: Controlled temperature tissue fusion: Argon laser welding of rat intestine in vivo. Part 1. Lasers Surg Med 21:269–277, 1997.
60. Nakata S, Campbell CD, Repogle RL: Experimental aortocoronary artery bypass grafting using a Co_2 laser on the dog: Acute experiment. Ann Thorac Surg 48:628–631, 1989.
61. Basu S, Marini CP, Coons MS, et al: Internal mammary coronary artery anastomosis by Co_2 laser: An acute experimental study. J Cardiac Surg 6:286–293, 1991.
62. Olearchyk AS, Vasilii I Kolesov: A pioneer of coronary revascularization by internal mammary-coronary artery grafting. J Thorac Cardiovasc Surg 96:13–18, 1988.
63. Androsov PI: New method of surgical treatment of blood vessel lesions. Arch Surg 73:902–910, 1956.
64. Vogelfanger IJ, Beattie WG: A concept of automation in vascular surgery: A preliminary report on a mechanical instrument for arterial anastomosis. Can J Surg 1:262–265, 1958.
65. Mallina RF, Miller RR, Cooper P, Christie SG: Surgical stapling. Sci Am 207:802–810, 1962.
66. Inokuchi K: A new type of blood vessel suturing apparatus. Arch Surg 77:954–957, 1958.
67. Inokuchi K: Stapling device for end-to-side anastomosis of blood vessel. Arch Surg 82:337–341, 1961.

68. Kahn DR, Mallina RF, Wilson WS, Sloan H: Use of the American and Russian vascular staplers for coronary artery anastomoses in calves. J Thorac Cardiovasc Surg 50:699–706, 1965.
69. Lee S, Wong L, Orloff MJ, Nahum AM: A review of vascular anastomosis with mechanical aids and nonsuture techniques. Head Neck Surg 3:58–65, 1980.
70. Ragnarsson R, Berggren A, Östrup LT, Gilbert RW: Arterial end-to-side anastomosis with the UNILINK system. Ann Plast Surg 22:405–415, 1989.
71. Kirsch WM, Zhu YH, Hardesty RA, Chapolini R: A new method for microvascular anastomosis. Am Surg 58:722–727, 1992.
72. Boeckx WD, Darius O, van den Hof B, van Holder C: Scanning electron microscopic analysis of the stapled microvascular anastomosis in the rabbit. Ann Thorac Surg 63:S128–134, 1997.
73. Leppäniemi A, Wherry D, Pikoulis E, et al: Arterial and venous repair with vascular clips: Comparison with suture closure. J Vasc Surg 26:24–28, 1997.
74. Schild AF: Use of a vascular staple device for creation of AV fistulas and bridge grafts for hemodialysis. *In* Henry ML, Ferguson RM (eds): Vascular Access for Hemodialysis—V. Chicago, Precept Press, 1997, pp 95–102.
75. Nataf P, Kirsch W, Hill AC, et al: Nonpenetrating clips for coronary anastomosis. Ann Thorac Surg 63:S135–137, 1997.
76. Tulleken CAF, van Dieren A, Verdaasdonk RM, Berendsen W: End-to-side anastomosis of small vessels using an ND:YAG laser with a hemispherical contact probe. J Neurosurg 76:546–549, 1992.
77. Tulleken CAF, Verdaasdonk RM, Berendsen W, Mali WPTM: Use of the excimer laser in high-flow bypass surgery of the brain. J Neurosurg 78:477–480, 1993.
78. Tulleken CAF, Verdaasdonk RM: First clinical experience with Excimer assisted high flow bypass surgery of the brain. Acta Neurochir (Wien) 134:66–70, 1995.
79. Tulleken CAF, Verdaasdonk RM, Mansvelt Beck RJ, Mali WPTM: The modified excimer laser-assisted high-flow bypass operation. Surg Neurol 46:424–429, 1996.
80. Tulleken CAF, Verdaasdonk RM, Mansvelt Beck HJ: Non-occlusive Excimer laser-assisted end-to-side anastomosis. Ann Thorac Surg 63:S138–142, 1997.
81. Yahr WZ, Strully KJ, Hurwitt ES: Non-occlusive small arterial anastomosis with a neodymium laser. Surg Forum 15:224–226, 1964.
82. Heijmen RH, Gründeman PF, Borst C: Intima-adventitia apposition in end-to-side arterial anastomosis. An experimental study in the pig. Ann Thorac Surg 65:705–711, 1998.
83. Buckingham RA, Buckingham RO: Robots in operating theatres. BMJ 311:1479–1482, 1995.
84. Garcia-Ruiz A, Smedira NG, Loop FD, et al: Robotic surgical instruments for dexterity enhancement in thoracoscopic coronary artery bypass graft. J Laparoendosc Adv Surg Tech A 7:277–283, 1997.
85. Heijmen RH, Borst C, Mouës CM, et al: Temporary luminal arteriotomy seal: III. Postmortem atherosclerotic human coronary artery. Am Thorac Surg 67:120–123, 1999.
86. Heijmen RH, Hinchliffe P, Borst C, et al: A novel one-shot anastomotic stapler prototype for coronary bypass grafting on the beating heart: Feasibility in the pig. J Thorac Cardiovasc Surg 117:117–125, 1999.

Chapter 81

Therapeutic Angiogenesis

James F. Symes

Present day therapy for ischemia resulting from coronary artery disease relies on reducing myocardial oxygen demand, preventing further disease progression, or using percutaneous angioplasty or coronary artery bypass to restore blood flow. Before the advent of direct coronary revascularization, surgeons atttempted to enhance myocardial perfusion by stimulating blood vessel growth with indirect methods such as transplantation of highly vascular tissue (omental or muscle flaps), epicardial poudrage, or manipulation of the coronary venous system.[7, 70] Recent advances in our understanding of the stimuli and control mechanisms involved in the development of new blood vessels, particularly collateral formation resulting from coronary artery obstructive disease, have renewed interest in the concept of promoting neovascularization as an alternative means of treating myocardial ischemia. In 1993, Hockel[26] proposed the term *therapeutic angiogenesis* to describe interventions aimed at inducing local growth of blood vessels in areas of hypovascularity. Since then, this term has been used primarily to refer to the pharmacologic induction of collateral artery growth using angiogenic growth factors.

This chapter briefly reviews the rapidly expanding field of angiogenesis research that forms the basis for preliminary clinical trials currently being undertaken. It begins with a review of our understanding of the molecular basis of angiogenesis and collateral formation, then reviews the preclinical studies on which the current clinical trials are based, and focuses on some of the many issues that are being addressed in the field of therapeutic angiogenesis, with particular reference to the treatment of coronary artery disease.

Blood Vessel Growth and Development

Angiogenesis and Vasculogenesis

Vasculogenesis and angiogenesis are the processes responsible for the embryologic development of circulatory system.[16] Vasculogenesis refers to the in situ formation of blood vessels from progenitor endothelial cells or angioblasts.[47] Angiogenesis involves extension of the primitive vasculature, that is, new capillaries sprout from a pre-existing network, which by definition implicates differentiated endothelial cells as the responsible cellular element. Full development of the circulatory system involves recurrent remodeling as some vessels regress and others branch or are invested with a multilayer architecture characteristic of medium to large arteries and veins. This extensive endothelial cell proliferative activity constitutes the basis for angiogenesis during embryologic development and contrasts markedly with the endothelial cell quiescence observed in adults in whom the interval for endothelial cell turnover is estimated to be in excess of 1000 days.[15]

In established blood vessels in mature organisms, the quiescent, nonproliferative state remains the norm until proliferative activity is provoked by pathologic stimuli, for example, wound inflammation, ischemia, or tumor growth. Indeed much of our basic understanding of the biologic mechanisms involved in angiogenesis derives from the work of Folkman[13] in relation to mechanisms of inhibiting tumor growth and metastasis. D'Amore and Thompson[10] subsequently described the classic paradigm for angiogenesis, which is disruption of the basement membrane and surrounding matrix; migration, adhesion, and proliferation of endothelial cells; and the formation of new three-dimensional capillary tubules (Fig. 81–1). Because pathologic entities such as solid tumor growth and diabetic retinopathy are dependent on angiogenesis, studies aimed at improving perfusion to ischemic tissues by means of stimulation of new vessel development (i.e., therapeutic angiogenesis) must keep in focus the avoidance of excessive or widespread neovascularization in other organs or tissues.

Angiogenic Cytokines

Over the past 15 years, a series of polypeptide growth factors has been purified, sequenced, and demonstrated to be responsible for both natural and pathologic angiogenesis. These angiogenic cytokines all share the ability to act as mitogens for endothelial cells (Table 81–1).

Endothelial Cell Mitogens. One of the more potent endothelial mitogens is vascular endothelial growth factor (VEGF), also known as vascular permeability factor.[11] Recent observations suggest that VEGF is actually a family of growth factors that interact with different receptors to induce endothelial mitogenesis.[71] The recently described VEGF B is particularly highly expressed in cardiac tissues.[40] The critical importance of VEGF in initial vascular development is emphasized by the fact that removal of the VEGF gene is lethal early in embryogenesis in animals heterozygous for this mutation.[12] Four homodimeric species of VEGF have been identified, each monomer having 121, 165, 189, or 206 amino acids, respectively, with different secretion patterns for each.[66] Despite the variations in secretion and binding patterns, no differences with regard to anatomic or physiologic evidence of angiogenesis could be demonstrated between the 121, 165, or 189 isoforms in studies carried out in our laboratory in a rabbit ischemic hind limb model.[62] These data, combined with those of Houck and colleagues[25] regarding the proteolytically clipped VEGF species that result from the action of plasmin on the 165 and 189 isoforms, suggest that perhaps the key role of plasminogen activation in angiogenesis involves cleaving the longer VEGF form to release a soluble VEGF 121–like species as the final common mediator of angiogenesis in vivo.[42]

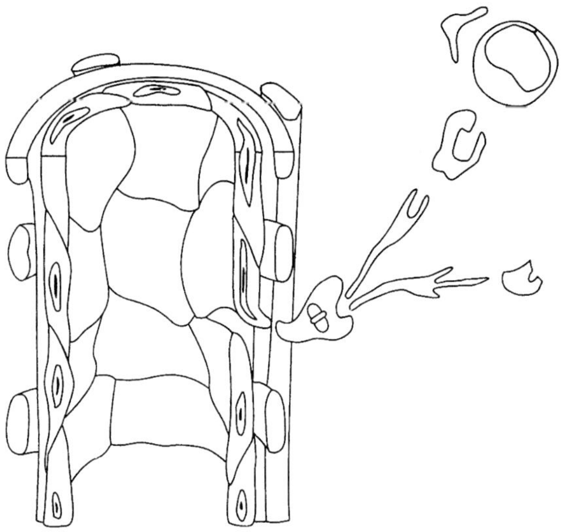

Figure 81–1. Paradigm for angiogenesis. Activated endothelial cells separate from their basement membrane, migrate, proliferate, and remodel to form a new lumen, thus generating new blood vessels or sprouts from the parent vessel. (From D'Amore PA, Thompson RW: Mechanisms of angiogenesis. Ann Rev Physiol 49:453–464, 1997, with permission.)

Other widely studied growth factors include those in the fibroblast growth factor family especially FGF-1 (αFGF) and FGF-2 (βFGF.)[14] Like VEGF, FGFs bind heparin-like components of the extracellular matrix on the surface of endothelial and smooth muscle cells, thereby facilitating attachment of these growth factors to their high-affinity receptors.[71] In addition to their roles in the specific aspects of initial development, VEGF, the FGFs and their receptors are expressed by endothelial cells in capillaries that sprout in response to pathologic conditions. Angiogenic cytoknes such as VEGF and the FGFs, which are capable of stimulating angiogenesis in vitro, are commonly referred to as direct cytokines.[59] Indirect cytokines are growth factors such as platelet-derived growth factor, which are involved in the angiogenic process in vivo but act through an intermediary. PDGF treatment of human vascular smooth muscle cells, for example, induces VEGF and βFGF mRNA expression.

Synergism of Angiogenic Cytokines

In addition to the various actions of the direct and indirect cytokines in the angiogenic process, studies from several groups have disclosed evidence for a synergistic effect of certain growth factors in vitro. Pepper and associates demonstrated, for example, that when VEGF and βFGF were added simultaneously to cultures of microvascular endothelial cells grown on the surface of three-dimensional collagen gels, their ability to stimulate the formation of capillary-like tubules exceeded the additive effect of either growth factor used separately.[41] Similarly, results of in vivo studies in our laboratory (Fig. 81–2) demonstrated that both the extent of collateral formation and the luminal diameter of the stem artery were significantly greater in the VEGF plus βFGF group than the additive effect of either VEGF or βFGF administered separately.[1] The fundamental basis for the synergistic effect most likely is a function of the differing and independent receptor systems responsible for signaling the mitogenic effects of each cytokine on endothelial cells. In addition, the ability of βFGF to stimulate other cell types such as smooth muscle cells may be important in this setting.

Site-Specific Effects of Angiogenic Cytokines

Effective therapeutic angiogenesis as a treatment modality for ischemic syndromes will depend on avoidance of indis-

Table 81–1. Endothelial Growth Factors and Their Receptors

Growth Factors	Endothelial Cell Receptors	Tissue Distribution
FGF-1 (acidic) heart	FGFR-1,2,3,4	Brain, bone matrix, kidney, EC, retina, heart, others
FGF-2 (basic)	FGFR-1,2	Brain, retina, pituitary, kidney, placenta, testes, monocytes, corpus luteum, heart, many others
FGF-4	FGFR-1,2	Embryonic tissue
FGF-5	Unknown	Neonatal brain, central nervous system
VEGF-A	VEGFR-1 (flt 1)(fms) VEGFR-2 kdr/flk	Pituitary cells, monocytes (macrophages), smooth muscle, heart, lung, skeletal muscle, prostate
VEGF-B	Unknown	Heart, skeletal muscle, pancreas, prostate, many others
VEGF-C	flt 4(VEGFR-3)/VEGFR-2	Heart, placenta, ovary, small intestine, others
HGF (scatter factor)	cmet	Lung, liver, skin, blood, many others
PDGF-BB	PDGFRβ	Platelets, malignant cells, macrophages, EC, fibroblasts, VSMC, glial cells, astrocytes, myoblasts, kidney cells

Modified from Ware JA, Simons MC: Angiogenesis in ischemic heart disease. Nat Med 3:158–164, 1997, with permission.
EC = endothelial cells; VSMC = vascular smooth muscle cells.

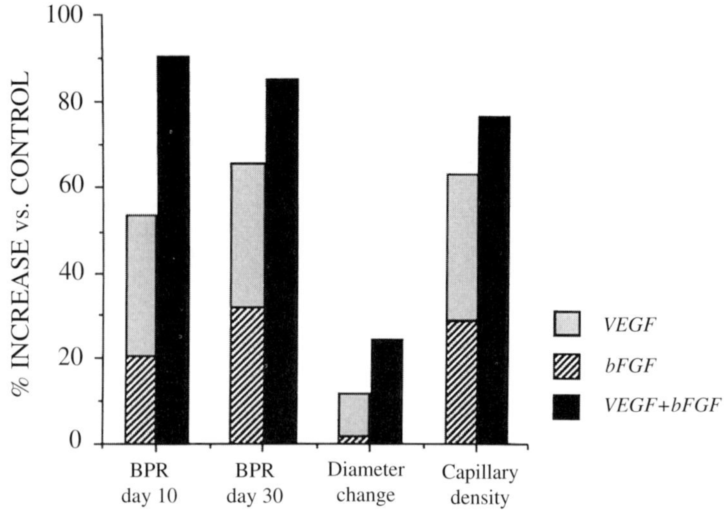

Figure 81–2. Synergistic effect of VEGF plus βFGF. Percent increase in blood pressure ratio (BPR) on day 10 and day 30; in angiographic luminal diameter of stem artery and in capillary density contrasting the additive result of VEGF and βFGF administered alone (left, composite bar) vs. VEGF and βFGF administered together (right, black bar). In each instance, the combined administration group exceeds the additive effects of VEGF and βFGF alone. (From Bauters C, Asahara J, Zheng LP: Synergistic effect of vascular endothelial growth factor and basis fibroblast growth factor on angiogenesis in vivo. Circulation 92(Suppl II):II-365–II371, 1995, with permission.)

criminate, widespread promotion of neovascularization. In this context, there is, in fact, important evidence that angiogenesis occurring in response to stimuli, such as tissue ischemia, may be site-specific. Studies in a variety of animal models using αFGF,[46] βFGF,[2] VEGF,[6, 60] and scatter factor[72] have shown that systemic administration of angiogenic cytokines selectively produces neovascularization in the ischemic limb. Clinically, patients with peripheral vascular disease have been shown to have detectable levels of circulating bFGF, yet evidence of angiogenesis in these patients appears limited to the ischemic lower extremity.[50] We have documented circulating levels of VEGF after intramuscular injection of the gene encoding for VEGF, again with evidence of angiogenesis occurring only in the ischemic limb being treated.[3]

Accumulating data strongly suggest that, at least in the case of VEGF, regional ischemia is the principal factor responsible for localization of angiogenesis. Experiments performed on endothelial cells in vitro suggest that the basis for this localized activity is upregulation of the VEGF receptor in response to hypoxia.[28] In a study of Brogi and associates,[9] for example, an increase in mRNA levels of the VEGF-specific tyrosine kinase receptor KDR on human umbilical vein endothelial cells was observed when these human umbilical vein endothelial cells (HUVECs) were treated 3 hours with conditioned medium from hypoxic myoblasts (Fig. 81–3). This increased binding was shown to be due to a marked increase in the number of KDR receptors available.

Interaction with Nitric Oxide

Data from a number of recent studies strongly support the importance of the endothelial-derived relaxing factor nitric oxide (NO) in the angiogenic process. Studies by Brock and associates[8] and Ku and associates[33] have demonstrated that VEGF receptor binding is associated with increased endothelial cell production of NO. Ku, for example, observed dose-dependent relaxation of isolated canine coronary arteries induced by VEGF, which could be abolished by pretreatment with N^G-monomethyl-L-arginine (L-NMMA), an NO synthase inhibitor. Selke and associates[57] studied the microvascular responses to VEGF and βFGF in isolated porcine coronary vessels and demonstrated an enhanced relaxation response to both cytokines in the collateral dependent ischemic region, which differed from that seen in the normally perfused region of the heart. This was associated with an increased expression of both VEGF receptors (flt-1, flk-1) as well as βFGF receptor 1 in this collateral perfused region. Measurements performed in our own laboratory have confirmed that application of VEGF to freshly excised arterial segments with intact endothelium will result in a dose-dependent increase in the production or release of NO, or both.[69] Murohara and associates[39] demonstrated that dietary supplementation with the NO precursor L-arginine enhanced angiogenesis in the ischemic rabbit hind limb and that angiogenesis was significantly impaired in a murine model of hind limb ischemia when the gene encoding for endothe-

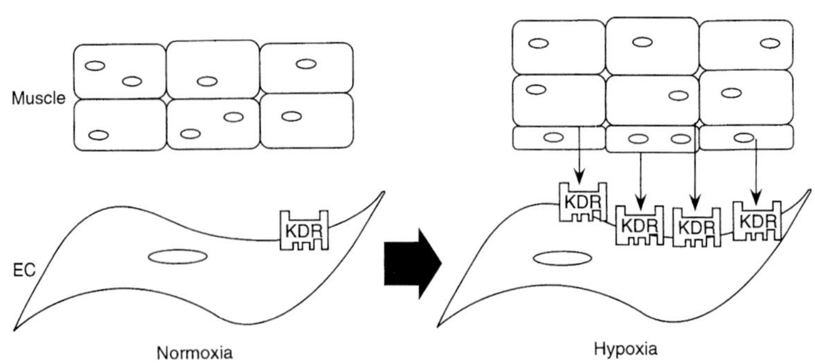

Figure 81–3. Factors secreted by hypoxic myocytes upregulate VEGF receptor expression on endothelial cells within the hypoxic milieu. This localized receptor expression may help explain the site-specific effects of VEGF in regions of tissue ischemia. (From Comprehensive Cardiovascular Medicine, Chapter 115. Isner JM: Angiogenesis. p 2987, with permission.)

lial nitric oxide synthase (eNOS) was missing. Further, this impaired angiogenesis in eNOS knockout mice was not improved by administration of VEGF, suggesting that eNOS acts downstream from VEGF. Finally, studies from our laboratory and others have documented endothelium-dependent hypotension in response to systemic administration of VEGF and to some degree βFGF.[23] This hypotensive effect may have negative implications for the administration of angiogenic growth factors in patients with myocardial ischemia. Nonetheless, the ability of VEGF, for example, to improve endothelium-dependent vasomotor function of collateral vessels as demonstrated by Bauters and associates,[5] suggests an additional potential benefit of carefully regulated administration of this angiogenic cytokine (Fig. 81–4).

Myocardial Ischemia, Collateral Formation, and Angiogenesis

Collateral circulation in the heart develops as a compensatory mechanism to supply oxygenated blood to myocardium jeopardized by coronary occlusive lesions. Indeed, when coronary collaterals are well developed, even severe proximal left main disease can be compensated and clinical outcomes are clearly better.[52] Why the collateral circulation is adequate is some circumstances but inadequate in others has been the subject of considerable investigation over the past decade. As a result, our understanding of the development of collateral circulation has been greatly enhanced.

Collateral development in response to myocardial ischemia may occur as a result of recruitment and enlargement of pre-existing epicardial vessels (so-called arteriogenesis) or as a result of true angiogenesis with budding of capillaries from pre-existing vascular structures leading to new microvessels.[54] Both processes appear to be important and probably occur by different mechanisms. Despite extensive research, the interrelationship of the two processes is as yet not clearly understood.

Hypoxia-induced augmentation of expression of endothelial mitogens, such as VEGF and the FGF family, as well as their specific receptors (flk-1 and flt-1 in the case of VEGF and FGF receptor 1 in the case of FGF), has been demonstrated in response to myocardial ischemia.[21] In addition, the inflammatory reaction resulting from myocardial necrosis, including the presence of macrophages and neutrophils, is sufficient to produce angiogenesis in the ischemic or infarcted myocardium.[36] Upregulation of specific receptors is critical to the process of angiogenesis as demonstrated by the fact that infusion of growth factors into normal hearts does not result in angiogenesis.[54] The observation that specific binding sites for VEGF, for example, exist in the normal heart in the presence of the ligand without significant vascular proliferation suggests the existence of natural inhibitors that must be interfered with in order for angiogenesis to occur in response to ischemic stimuli.[43]

In addition to its function as an endothelial cell mitogen, VEGF increases vascular permeability in response to ischemia and infarction, leading to the presence of inflammatory cells in the ischemic tissue. This function appears to be equally important to VEGF's sentinel contribution to the angiogenic process.[71]

Extensive studies by Schaper[54] and others have demonstrated that an important contributor to collateral development is in situ enlargement of pre-existing arterial connections into true collateral arteries. These vessels enlarge and develop in areas remote from the ischemic stimulus, perhaps by other mechanisms such as increased shear stress and pressure gradients. Indeed Schaper has demonstrated that these mechanical forces increase the secretion of monocyte chemotactic protein 1 in cultured human endothelial cells, leading to increased monocyte adhesion.[31] These monocytes are potentially capable of producing large amounts of growth factors and thus stimulating collateral development even in the absence of a direct ischemic stimulus.

Taken together, these studies clearly document the critical role played by angiogenic growth factors, particularly VEGF and βFGF, in the process of coronary collateral development. This opens the door to the possibility of therapeutic augmentation of collateral development and perfusion of ischemic myocardium by enhanced delivery of these angiogenic cytokines.

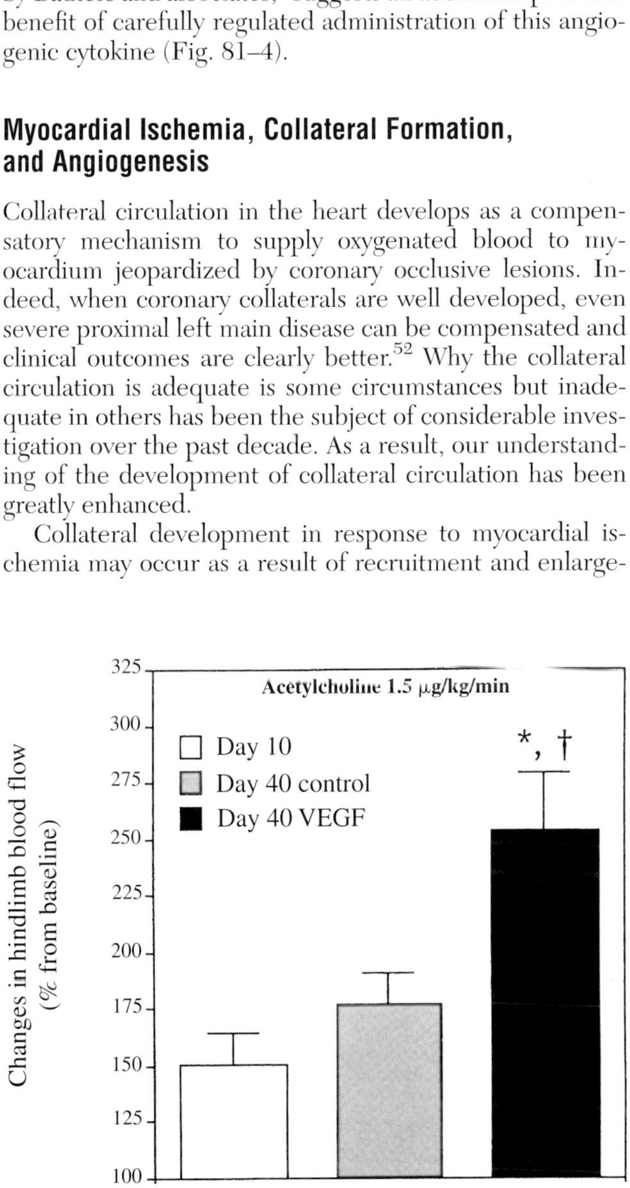

Figure 81–4. Blood flow response to infusion of acetylcholine (l^{-1}-min^{-1}) in the ischemic limb day 10 and on day 40 (30 days after saline or VEGF infusion). Animals receiving VEGF demonstrate a significant ($P < .01$ vs. day 10, $P < .05$ vs. day 40 controls) increase in endothelium-dependent vasomotor response. (From Bauters C, Asahara T, Zheng LP: Recovery of disturbed endothelium-dependent flow in the collateral-perfused rabbit ischemic hind limb after administration of vascular endothelial growth factor. Circulation 91:2802–2809, 1995, with permission.)

Preclinical Studies of Therapeutic Angiogenesis

The goal of therapeutic angiogenesis as outlined by Höckel and associates,[26] is controlled stimulation of new blood vessel formation to reduce the unfavorable tissue effects caused by ischemia. The feasibility of obtaining this goal has been greatly advanced by the recent availability of recombinant formulations of human growth factor proteins capable of stimulating endothelial cell proliferation and capillary formation.

Studies in the Ischemic Limb

To test the potential efficacy of this strategy of stimulating collateral formation by the administration of angiogenic cytokines, it was necessary to establish an appropriate animal model. Such a model was developed by Pu and associates[45] in the hind limb of New Zealand white rabbits, and, as a result, much of our current understanding of the angiogenic process has been derived from testing it in this setting. The angiographic demonstration by Pu of increased collateral formation accompanied by a significant improvement in calf blood pressure ratio in this model after intramuscular administration of endothelial cell growth factor (FGF-1) was probably the first documentation of angiogenesis in vivo.[44] Shortly thereafter, Baffour and associates,[2] using a similar model of rabbit hind limb ischemia, showed a significant improvement in tissue perfusion after daily intramuscular injections of βFGF. Subsequent studies in this model by Takeshita and associates,[60, 64] using VEGF administered by intramuscular injection[60] as well as by a single intra-arterial injection into the iliac artery perfusing the ischemic limb,[64] demonstrated angiographic as well as histologic evidence of new vessel growth and enlargement seen 10 to 30 days after growth factor administration (Fig. 81–5). This anatomic evidence of increased vascularity was further augmented by studies by Bauters and associates[4] using a Doppler flow probe advanced into the internal iliac artery to record flow velocity. A single intra-arterial bolus of VEGF resulted in significant improvement in blood flow to the ischemic limb 30 days later, compared with control animals receiving saline only. Takeshita and associates[61] used bromodioxide uridine labeling to show that maximal endothelial cell proliferation occurred 5 days after administration of a single intra-arterial bolus of VEGF and was confined to the so-called midzone collaterals.

An additional potentially important effect of VEGF is its ability to improve disturbed endothelium-dependent flow in collateral vessels as demonstrated by the study of Bauters and associates.[5] In vivo flow measurements in the ischemic limb showed that a 500-μg bolus of VEGF greatly improved the collateral vessels' response to the endothelium-dependent vasodilator acetylcholine compared with saline-treated controls (see Fig. 81–4). Finally, this animal model was used to study the impact of hyperlipidemia on collateral vessel development. Van Belle and associates[68] induced ischemia in the hindlimb of both Watanabe hyperlipidemic rabbits and normal rabbits and demonstrated that the hyperlipidemic rabbits had a significantly impaired ability to form spontaneous collaterals compared with normal rabbits, but that this could be significantly improved by administration of VEGF.

These studies confirmed the hypothesis that exogenous administration of angiogenic cytokines could produce both anatomic and physiologic evidence of significantly augmented collateral development in the settings of severe chronic limb ischemia.

Studies of Myocardial Ischemia

Yanagisawa-Miwa and associates[75] are generally credited with the first demonstration that administration of βFGF to a model of acute myocardial infarction could result in significant histologic evidence of angiogenesis as well as a significant improvement in myocardial function and reduction of infarct size. Because of the acuteness of this model, however, alternative mechanisms for the beneficial effects of βFGF, such as improved endothelium-independent vasomotor function or perhaps increased myocyte viability and resistance to injury, likely explained the results.

The demonstration that administration of growth factors could improve chronic myocardial ischemia has been made by a number of investigators using a porcine model of myocardial ischemia created by application of an ameroid constrictor to the left circumflex coronary artery. Using this model, calcium alginate microcapsules containing βFGF have been used to deliver the growth factor continuously over several weeks, resulting in a reduction in infarct size and better myocardial perfusion and contractility in the ischemic zone.[19] Similar beneficial results were obtained by daily injection of βFGF into an indwelling catheter in the left atrium in dogs.[34]

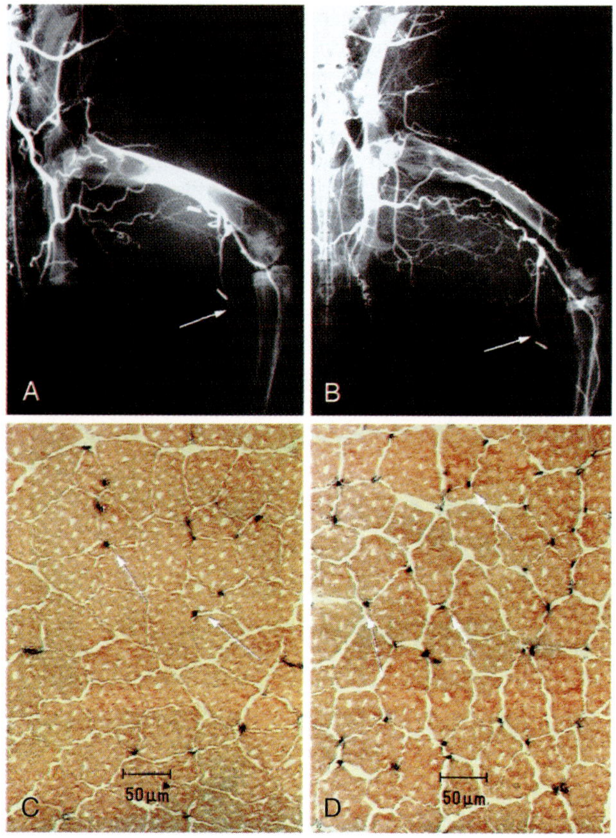

Figure 81–5. Angiograms of control (*A*) and VEGF-treated rabbits (*B*) at day 30, comparing collateral artery development in the medial thigh region. Distal arterial reconstitution of these 4-second films barely apparent in the control group was readily seen in the VEGF-treated group (*arrows*). Alkaline phosphatase staining of ischemic limb muscle harvested at day 40 is seen in the control group (*C*) and VEGF-treated group (*D*). Dark blue dots indicate capillaries counterstained with eosin. (From Takeshita S, Pu L-Q, Stein LA: Intramuscular administration of vascular endothelial growth factor induces dose-dependent collateral artery augmentation in a rabbit model of chronic limb ischemia. Circulation 90:II-228–II234, 1994, with permission.)

Injection of a single bolus (500 μg) of VEGF directly into the left coronary ostium of pigs 4 weeks after application of the ameroid constrictor to the left circumflex artery also resulted in evidence of improved myocardial perfusion and function based on microsphere flow studies and two-dimensional echocardiography.[20] However, this mode of administration of VEGF resulted in significant NO-mediated hypotension, whereas long-term perivascular administration of VEGF produced similar improvements in myocardial perfusion without the hypotensive effect.[18] As indicated that the abnormal vasomotor responses seen in the presence of ischemia can be ameliorated by the administration of both bFGF and VEGF. Thus, when taken together, the results of these preclinical studies suggest that exogenous administration of angiogenic proteins, particularly βFGF and VEGF, can significantly improve myocardial perfusion secondary to coronary artery occlusive disease.

Therapeutic Angiogenesis by Gene Transfer

Somatic gene therapy is the introduction and expression of recombinant genes in somatic cells for the purpose of treating a disease. Although this concept dates back only to 1989, it is already being tested in numerous clinical trials involving patients with a variety of disease processes, including cardiovascular disease. The studies alluded to earlier supply abundant data supporting the potential utility of recombinant protein therapy for stimulating angiogenesis both in the myocardium and in the treatment of lower extremity vascular insufficiency. The considerable expense associated with production of recombinant protein formulations for clinical use, combined with the demonstrated need to deliver the protein over a period of several days or weeks, has led a number of investigators to consider transferring the gene encoding that protein into the tissues directly.[28] The successful transfer of DNA into a host cell involves a number of complex steps, including isolation of the segment of DNA encoding a specific protein and attachment to a suitable initiation sequence to permit replication and expression known as a vector. Once produced, the vector must then be introduced into the cell either by ex vivo, indirect transfer or by in vivo direct transfer. Because in vivo transfer is technically easier and can be accomplished in a single procedure, it tends to be more clinically relevant to most gene therapy strategies for cardiovascular disease.[51]

Studies carried out in a number of laboratories over the past few years have demonstrated that efficient transfection of the myocardium can be accomplished by direct intramuscular administration of the DNA, as originally described by Wolff and colleagues.[73] More efficient transfection has been demonstrated with the use of replication-deficient adenoviral vectors by direct intramyocardial injection and also by intracoronary infusion of the DNA.[35] Adenovirus-mediated gene transfer does not result in stable incorporation of the transgene into the host gene, so the expression is by definition transient. However, treatment of myocardial ischemia may be achieved effectively and safely with relatively brief transgene expression. Indeed, Giordano and associates[17] demonstrated significant improvement in myocardial blood flow and contractile function after intracoronary injection of a recombinant adenovirus expressing human fibroblast growth factor 5 in a porcine model of chronic myocardial ischemia. Mack and associates[37] used the same animal model to demonstrate enhanced myocardial perfusion and function after direct intramyocardial injection of an adenoviral vector expressing $VEGF_{121}$ (Fig. 81–6).

Concern with regard to the potential for inflammatory or immunologic reactions, or both, stimulated by the use of adenoviral vectors led us to focus on the use of naked plasmid DNA. $VEGF_{165}$, because of its ability to be secreted from intact cells, lends itself well to gene therapy strategies using naked DNA, in which the transfection efficiency may be somewhat lower. This concept was confirmed in studies by Takeshita and associates[63] using intra-arterial administration of $VEGF_{165}$ applied to a balloon catheter, as well as by Tsurumi and associates[67] who administered the VEGF DNA directly into the muscle of the ischemic limb. Both studies demonstrated enhanced collateral development, improved perfusion, and increased capillary density in the rabbit ischemic hind limb model, similar to that seen with the administration of the recombinant VEGF protein. Studies in our laboratory using the porcine model of myocardial ischemia have demonstrated that direct intramyocardial injection of $VEGF_{165}$ DNA can enhance collateral development in the ischemic circumflex territory (Fig. 81–7).[65] These preclinical studies have prepared the groundwork for phase I clinical trials using both

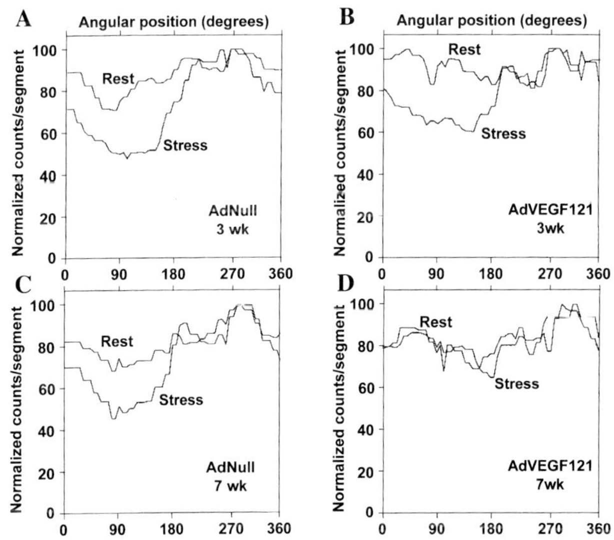

Figure 81–6. Quantitative assessment of regional stress induced myocardial ischemia with sestamibi SPECT imaging. Extent and severity of myocardial ischemia was determined from the difference between the rest and stress curves. *A*, Control treated animal at 3 weeks. *B*, Same animal at 7 weeks. *C*, $AD_{GV}VEGF_{121}$–treated animal at 3 weeks. *D*, The same animal at 7 weeks. There is a marked decrease in both the area and maximal severity of ischemia at 7 weeks in the $AD_{GV}VEGF_{121}$–treated animal compared with the control. (Modified from Mack et al: Biologic bypass with the use of adenovirus-mediated gene transfer of the complementary deoxyribonucleic acid for vascular endothelial growth factor 121 improves myocardial perfusion and function in the ischemic porcine heart. J Thorac Cardiovasc Surg 115:168–177, 1998, with permission.)

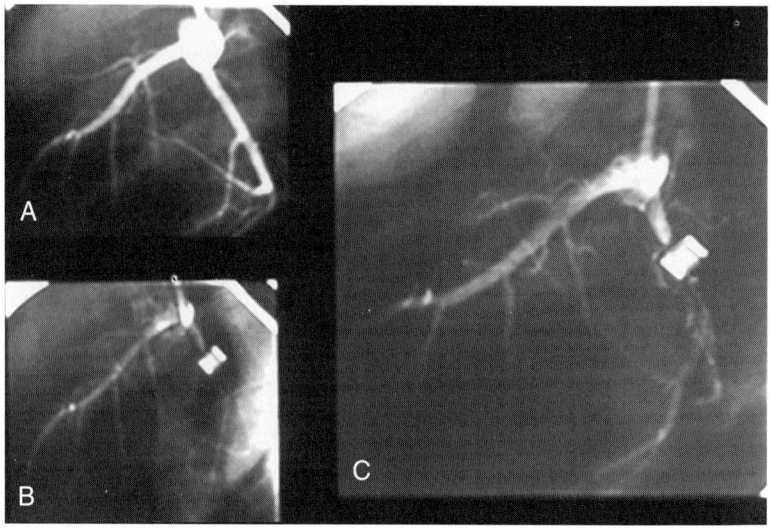

Figure 81–7. Serial angiograms at baseline (*A*), 3 weeks after placement of ameroid constrictor (*B*), and 4 weeks after intramyocardial administration of phVEGF$_{165}$ (*C*) showing improved filling of the distal circumflex system in a porcine model of chronic myocardial ischemia.

intramuscular and intracoronary gene therapy strategies in the treatment of myocardial and peripheral arterial ischemia.

Clinical Trials of Therapeutic Angiogenesis

Critical Limb Ischemia

Despite the profound impact of direct revascularization procedures, an increasing number of patients with coronary artery disease and peripheral vascular disease are deemed "inoperable" because of diffuse obliteration of target vessels or absence of useable conduits, or both. In the case of peripheral vascular disease, there is no effective medical treatment for critical limb ischemia and such patients are at high risk for amputation and limb loss. It is perhaps not surprising that the first Food and Drug Administration approved protocol for therapeutic angiogenesis involved treatment of patients with advanced critical limb ischemia by gene transfer with vascular endothelial growth factor.[30] In this study, which began at our center in 1994, patients with otherwise untreatable advanced limb ischemia initially received phVEGF$_{165}$ via a hydrogel-coated angioplasty balloon catheter that was advanced into the arterial system of the affected ischemic limb. In that dose-escalating trial, angiographic evidence of collateral development, as well as the formation of spider angiomas in the foot a week after gene transfer, was seen in the first patient to receive 2000 μg of VEGF DNA.[29] Subsequently, the use of intramuscular gene transfer of phVEGF$_{165}$, employed initially as a means of treating patients whose vascular disease was too extensive to permit an intra-arterial approach, was shown by Baumgartner and colleagues[3] to result in circulating levels of VEGF detectable by enzyme-linked immunosorbent assay as well as reproducible hemodynamic and angiographic improvement (Fig. 81–8). Furthermore, a subgroup of patients presenting with advanced thromboangiitis obliterans (Buerger's disease), who had necrotic lesions of their toes despite multiple attempts at other forms of therapy, showed improvement in perfusion after two 2000-μg doses of intramuscular VEGF 4 weeks apart.[27] Indeed limb salvage was achieved in two patients who had already been advised elsewhere to undergo below-the-knee (BK) amputation (Fig. 81–9). To date, some 25 patients have been treated with this protocol, with minimal evidence of adverse effects aside from transient peripheral edema, perhaps related to the increased vascular permeability, which is a known effect of VEGF. These preliminary results support the concept that gene therapy with naked

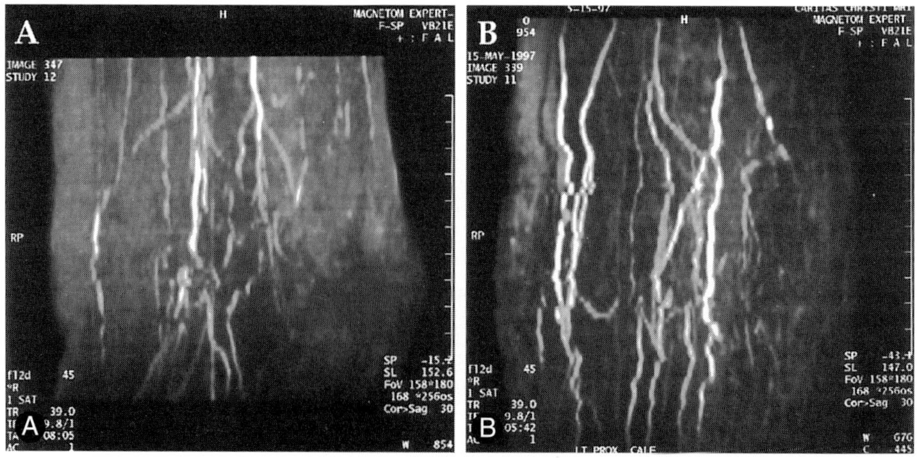

Figure 81–8. Representative magnetic resonance angiogram in a patient with critical limb ischemia performed without contrast injection before (*A*) and 8 weeks after (*B*) intramuscular VEGF gene therapy. Signal enhancement and increased vessel visibility both consistent with improved flow are seen in the angiogram obtained after gene therapy.

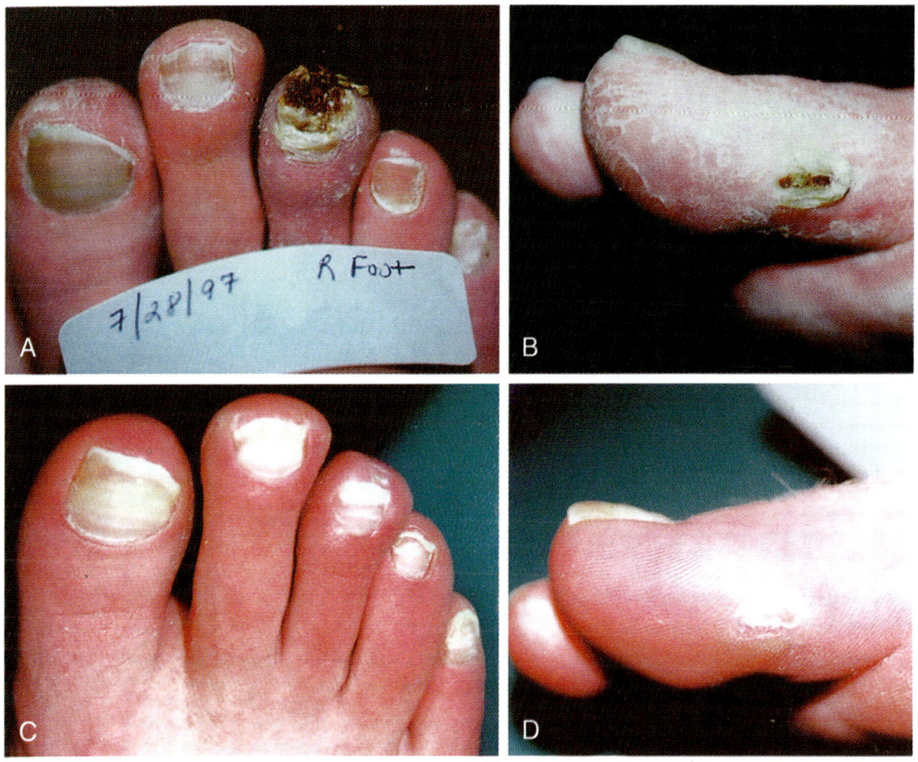

Figure 81–9. Photographs of the toes of a patient with Buerger's disease taken before (*A, C*) and 3 months after (*B, D*) administration of intramuscular VEGF gene therapy. The necrotic lesion on the third toe, as well as that on the medial aspect of the great toe, have healed completely.

DNA may be capable of producing meaningful biologic outcomes without adverse consequences, possibly because of the relatively low level of VEGF secreted over a prolonged period (approximately 1 to 2 weeks). The promotion of angiogenesis seems to be site-specific and to occur primarily in the ischemic region, as would have been predicted by the preclinical studies indicating that upregulation of the principal high-affinity kdr receptor for VEGF occurred exclusively in the presence of hypoxia. The somewhat more dramatic improvement seen in patients with Buerger's disease, who tend by definition to be relatively young and free of diffuse atherosclerosis, may be a function not only of age but also the absence of hypercholesterolemia and diabetes, three factors that have been shown to impair collateral vessel development.[48, 49, 68] In the peripheral vascular field, two additional trials are currently under way using βFGF protein, primarily in patients with claudication, but no results have yet been published in the literature.

Myocardial Ischemia

Schumacher and associates[55] were among the first to report on the use of angiogenic growth factors to treat myocardial ischemia in patients. In their study, FGF-1 was administered by direct intramyocardial injection after completion of coronary bypass surgery, which included an internal mammary artery graft to the left anterior descending coronary artery in 20 patients with three-vessel coronary disease. Twelve weeks later, they documented angiographic evidence of a dense capillary network in the region of the internal mammary artery graft using digital angiography. Later, Selke and colleagues[56] reported preliminary results on a feasibility study in which βFGF protein incorporated into heparin alginate beads was implanted on the epicardial surface in a region of an ungraftable coronary artery at the time of coronary bypass surgery.[56] This preliminary study demonstrated some evidence of increased perfusion in the already vascularized territory on exercise sestamibi scans performed 3 months after surgery. In a phase I clinical trial using a single injection of VEGF protein into the coronary circulation in patients with demonstrable reversible ischemia who were not candidates for direct revascularization, 7 of 15 patients were shown to have improved perfusion on 60-day follow-up perfusion scans.[22] On the basis of this preliminary trial, a phase II study is now under way.

At least three phase I trials are currently in progress using gene transfer techniques for the treatment of myocardial ischemia. Rosengart and associates are injecting an adenoviral vector containing the 121 isoform of VEGF into the myocardium in patients undergoing coronary bypass surgery who have a territory that is unable to be revascularized. Hammond's group plans a randomized study in which exertional angina and good ventricular function will be investigated. Finally, our group has recently embarked on a phase I clinical trial using naked (nonviral) $VEGF_{165}$ DNA. This material (essentially the same construct used in patients with critical limb ischemia) is injected directly into the myocardium in patients who have medically intractable angina and who are not candidates for coronary revascularization because of advanced diffuse disease or an absence of conduits, or both. The DNA is administered through a mini–anterior thoracotomy incision without any other concomitant revascularization procedure. It is hoped that this will allow us to document more definitively the safety of gene therapy for myocardial angiogenesis, as well as its efficacy, since the results will not be complicated by any other revascularization procedure. In the first eight patients to complete the study (unpublished data), significant relief of angina as well as some evidence of improved myocardial perfusion on sestamibi scans has been documented (Fig. 81–10).

Transmyocardial Laser Revascularization

Another approach to the treatment of medically intractable angina in patients who are unsuitable for direct revascularization is transmyocardial laser revascularization (TMR). The first reported use of a CO_2 laser to create epicardial transmyocardial laser channels by Mirhoseini and colleagues[38] in 1983 stimulated a number of clinical trials recently culminating in the Food and Drug Administration approval of the CO_2 laser device for TMR.[24] Despite evidence of improvement in angina in many of these patients, combined with studies showing increased myocardial perfusion, the precise mechanism by which TMR works remain a mystery. Histologic studies have suggested that the majority of laser channels become occluded early, and evidence of blood flow from the ventricular cavity to the myocardium has not been forthcoming.[32] The demonstration of increased angiogenesis in regions of myocardium treated by TMR, combined with the fact that the increased perfusion is usually seen days to weeks after the procedure, suggests that an important mechanism may be stimulation of angiogenesis.[74] Indeed, one study combining TMR with administration of angiogenic growth factors suggested that this approach appears to provide superior improvement in myocardial perfusion compared with TMR alone.[53] Further investigation of this interesting observation will be needed to determine whether TMR, with its increased risk, actually enhances the angiogenic effect of growth factor administration alone.

Controversies and Future Perspectives

Despite the numerous advances in the field of therapeutic angiogenesis that have been described in the preceding sections of this chapter, a great deal of research remains to be done to determine the extent to which this therapeutic modality may be applicable to the treatment of coronary artery disease. Ongoing basic research will help to elucidate further the mechanisms involved in the process of collateral development. This, will, in turn, resolve the controversy over the extent to which pre-existing collaterals and new vessel formation each contribute separately to collateral growth, how they are interrelated, and the sequence of events that occurs in response to the ischemic stimulus. In addition, it will provide data to determine which growth factors administered alone or in combination are most effective in enhancing collateral growth and improving myocardial perfusion. As research moves into the treatment of patients who have coronary artery disease, the focus will be on resolving such issues as whether the best approach is administration of the recombinant protein or its gene. Protein therapy will require refinements in the mode of administration and its duration, whereas the need for adjunctive viral vectors or other mechanisms to enhance transfection efficiency will need to be resolved if gene therapy is to be the primary approach. The best mode of delivery needs to be determined and the question of whether administration of angiogenic growth factors can be effective as the sole therapy in patients with advanced coronary disease or will be used primarily as an adjunct to other revascularization techniques needs to be answered. At present, therapeutic angiogenesis is focused primarily on stimulating microvascular proliferation and thus would seem unlikely to be able to overcome the effects of high-grade proximal occlusive disease. Conversely,

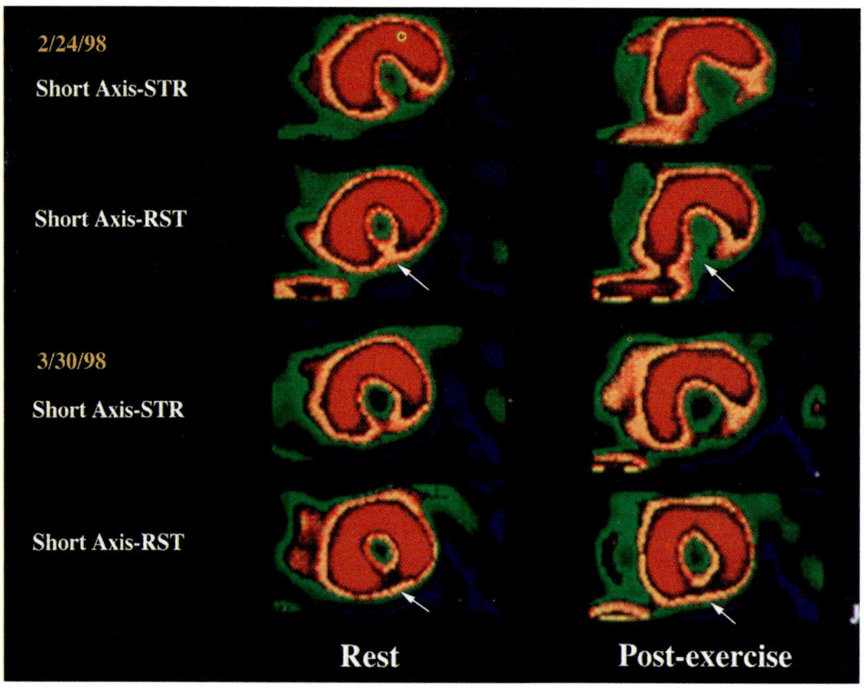

Figure 81–10. Representative short-axis views of sestamibi scans in a patient before (2/24/98) and one month after (3/30/98) direct intramyocardial administration of $VEGF_{165}$ DNA via a left anterior thoracotomy. The resting image of 2/24/98 shows a significant area of inferolateral ischemia which increased after exercise (*arrows*). By comparison, on 3/30/98 the ischemic area is smaller and does not change with exercise.

if it were possible to revascularize a large area of ischemic myocardium resulting from multivessel disease by means of an off-pump single internal mammary artery bypass procedure combined with intramyocardial administration of an angiogenic cytokine, one might have a durable, minimally invasive approach to complete coronary revascularization. Thus, although patients who are not candidates for any form of direct revascularization may eventually benefit from catheter-based, percutaneous administration of angiogenic growth factors, it would appear likely that cardiac surgeons will continue to have a major role in the treatment of coronary artery disease in the era of angiogenic therapy.

References

1. Asahara T, Bauters C, Zheng LP, et al: Synergistic effect of vascular endothelial growth factor and basic fibroblast growth factor on angiogenesis in vivo. Circulation 92:II-365–II-371, 1995.
2. Baffour R, Berman J, Garb JL, et al: Enhanced angiogenesis and growths of collaterals by in vivo administration of recombinant basic fibroblast growth factor in a rabbit model of acute lower limb ischemia: Dose-response effect of basic fibroblast growth factor. J Vasc Surg 16:181–191, 1992.
3. Baumgartner I, Pieczek A, Manor O, et al: Constitutive expression of phVEGF$_{165}$ following intramuscular gene transfer promotes collateral vessel development in patients with critical limb ischemia. Circulation 97:1114–1123, 1998.
4. Bauters C, Asahara T, Zheng LP, et al: Physiologic assessment of augmented vascularity induced by VEGF in ischemic rabbit hindlimb. Am J Physiol 267:H1263–H1271, 1994.
5. Bauters C, Asahara T, Zheng LP, et al: Recovery of disturbed endothelium-dependent flow in the collateral-perfused rabbit ischemic hind limb after administration of vascular endothelial growth factor. Circulation 91:2802–2809, 1995.
6. Bauters C, Asahara T, Zheng LP, et al: Site-specific therapeutic angiogenesis following systemic administration of vascular endothelial growth factor. J Vasc Surg 21:314–325, 1995.
7. Beck CS: The development of a new blood supply to the heart by operation. Ann Surg 102:801–813, 1935.
8. Brock TA, Dvorak HF, Senger DR: Tumor-secreted vascular permeability factor increases cytosolic Ca^{2+} and von Willebrand factor release in human endothelial cells. Am J Pathol 138:213–221, 1991.
9. Brogi E, Schatteman G, Wu T, et al: Hypoxia-induced paracrine regulation of VEGF receptor expression. J Clin Invest 97:469–476, 1996.
10. D'Amore PA, Thompson RW: Mechanisms of angiogenesis. Annu Rev Physiol 49:453–464, 1987.
11. Dvorak HF, Brown LF, Detmar M, et al: Vascular permeability factor/vascular endothelial growth factor, microvascular hyperpermeability, and angiogenesis. Am J Pathol 146:1029–1039, 1995.
12. Ferrara N, Carver-Moore K, Chen H, et al: Heterozygous embryonic lethality induced by targeted inactivation of the VEGF gene. Nature 380:439–442, 1996.
13. Folkman J: Tumor angiogenesis. *In* Becker FF (ed): Cancer Biology, New York, Plenum Press, 1975, pp 355–388.
14. Folkman J, Klagsbrun M: Angiogenic factors. Science 235: 442–447, 1987.
15. Folkman J, Shing Y: Angiogenesis. J Biol Chem 267: 10931–10934, 1992.
16. Gilbert SF: Developmental Biology, 4th ed. Sunderland, MA, Sinauer Associates, 1997, p 342.
17. Giordano FJ, Ping P, McKirnan D, et al: Intracoronary gene transfer of fibroblast growth factor-5 increases blood flow and contractile function in an ischemic region of the heart. Nat Med 2:534–539, 1996.
18. Harada K, Friedman M, Lopez JJ, et al: Vascular endothelial growth factor in chronic myocardial ischemia. Am J Physiol 270:H1791–H1802, 1996.
19. Harada K, Grossman W, Friedman M, et al: Basic fibroblasts growth factor improves myocardial function in chronically ischemic porcine hearts. J Clin Invest 94:623–630, 1994.
20. Hariawala M, Horowitz JR, Esakof D, et al: VEGF improves myocardial blood flow but produces EDRF-mediated hypotension in porcine hearts. J Surg Res 63:77–82, 1996.
21. Hashimoto E, Ogita T, Nakaoka T, et al: Rapid induction of vascular endothelial growth factor expression by transient ischemia in rat heart. Am J Physiol 267:H1948–H1954, 1994.
22. Henry TD, Rocha-Sing K, Isner JM, et al: Results of intracoronary recombinant human vascular endothelial growth factor (rhVEGF) administration trial. J Am Coll Cardiol 31:65A, 1998.
23. Horowitz JR, Rivard A, van der Zee R, et al: Vascular endothelial growth factor/vascular permeability factor produces nitric oxide–dependent hypotension. Arterioscler Thromb Vasc Biol 17:2793–2800, 1997.
24. Horvath KA, Cohn LH, Cooley DA, et al: Transmyocardial laser revascularization: Results of a multicenter trial with transmyocardial laser revascularization used as the sole therapy for end-stage coronary artery disease. J Thorac Cardiovasc Surg 113:645–654, 1997.
25. Houck KA, Leung DW, Rowland AM, et al: Dual regulation of vascular endothelial growth factor bioavailability by genetic and proteolytic mechanisms. J Biol Chem 267:26031–26037, 1992.
26. Höckel M, Schlenger K, Doctrow S, et al: Therapeutic angiogenesis. Arch Surg 128:423–429, 1993.
27. Isner JM, Baumgartner I, Rauh G, et al: Treatment of thromboangiitis obliterans (Buerger's disease) by intramuscular gene transfer of vascular endothelial growth factor: Preliminary clinical results. J Vasc Surg 28:964–975, 1998.
28. Isner JM: Angiogenesis: *In* Topol EJ (ed): Textbook of Cardiovascular Medicine. Philadelphia: Lippincott-Raven, 1998, pp 2491–2518.
29. Isner JM, Pieczek A, Schainfeld R, et al: Clinical evidence of angiogenesis following arterial gene transfer of phVEGF$_{165}$. Lancet 348:370–374, 1996.
30. Isner JM, Walsh K, Symes JF, et al: Arterial gene therapy for therapeutic angiogenesis in patients with peripheral artery disease. Circulation 91:2687–2692, 1995.
31. Ito WD, Anas M, Winkler B, et al: Monocytochemotactic protein-I increased collateral and peripheral conductome after femoral artery occlusion. Circ Res 80:829–837, 1997.
32. Kohmoto T, Fisher PE, Gu A, et al: Does blood flow through Holmum:Yag transmyocardial laser channels? Ann Thorac Surg 61:861–868, 1996.
33. Ku DD, Zaleski JK, Liu S, et al: Vascular endothelial growth factor induces EDRF-dependent relaxation in coronary arteries. Am J Physiol 265:H586–H592, 1993.
34. Lazarous DF, Schemowitz M, Shou M, et al: Effects of chronic systemic administration of basic fibroblast growth factor on collateral development in the canine heart. Circulation 91:145–153, 1995.
35. Leiden JM, Barr E: In Vivo Gene Transfer into the Heart: Gene Therapeutics. Methods and Applications of Direct Gene Transfer. Boston, Birkhauer, 1994.
36. Li J, Brown LF, Hibberd MG, et al: VEGF, *flk*-1, and *flt*-1 expression in a rat myocardial infarction model of angiogenesis. Am J Physiol 270:H1803–H1811, 1996.
37. Mack CA, Patel SR, Schwaz EA, et al: Biologic bypass with the use of adenovirus-mediated gene transfer of the complemen-

tary deoxyribonucleic acid for vascular endothelial growth factor 121 improves myocardial perfusion and function in the ischemic porcine heart. J Thorac Cardiovasc Surg 115:168–177, 1998.
38. Mirhoseini M, Fisher JC, Cayton MM: Myocardial revascularization by laser. Lasers Surg Med 3:241–245, 1983.
39. Murohara T, Asahara T, Silver M, et al: Nitric oxide synthase modulates angiogenesis in response to tissue ischemia. J Clin Invest 101:2567–2578, 1998.
40. Olofsson B, Pajusola K, Kaipainen A, et al: Vascular endothelial growth factor B, a novel growth factor for endothelial cells. Proc Natl Acad Sci USA 93:2576–2581, 1996.
41. Pepper MS, Ferrara N, Orci L, et al: Potent synergism between vascular endothelial growth factor and basic fibroblast growth factor in the induction of angiogenesis in vitro. Biochem Biophys Res Commun 189:824–831, 1992.
42. Pepper MS, Montesano R: Proteolytic balance and capillary morphogenesis. Cell Differ Dev 32:319–328, 1990.
43. Peters KG, de Vries C, Williams LT: Vascular endothelial growth factor receptor expression during embryogenesis and tissue repair suggests a role in endothelial differentiation and blood vessel growth. Proc Natl Acad Sci USA 90:8915–8919, 1993.
44. Pu L, Lachapelle K, Graham A, et al: Angiogenic stimulation: A new approach for severe chronic limb ischemia. Surg Forum 42:365–367, 1991.
45. Pu LQ, Jackson S, Lachapelle KJ, et al: A persistent hind limb ischemia model in the rabbit. J Invest Surg 7:49–60, 1994.
46. Pu LQ, Sniderman AD, Brassard R, et al: Enhanced revascularization of the ischemic limb by means of angiogenic therapy. Circulation 88:208–215, 1993.
47. Risau W: Differentiation of endothelium. FASEB J 9:926–933, 1995.
48. Rivard A, Silver M, Fabre J-E, et al: Diabetes impairs angiogenesis in limb ischemia. Circulation 96:I-95, 1997.
49. Rivard A, Fabre J-E, Silver M, et al: Age-dependent impairment of angiogenesis (Abstract). Circulation 96:I-18, 1997.
50. Rohovsky S, Kearney M, Pieczek A, et al: Elevated levels of basic fibroblast growth factor in patients with limb ischemia. Am Heart J 132:1015–1019, 1996.
51. Rowland RT, Cleveland JC, Meng X, et al: Potential gene therapy strategies in the treatment of cardiovascular disease. Ann Thorac Surg 60:721–728, 1995.
52. Sasayama S, Fujita M: Recent insights into coronary collateral circulation. Circulation 85:1197–1204, 1992.
53. Sayeed-Shah U, Mann M, Martin J, et al: Complete reversal of ischemic wall motion abnormalities by combined use of gene therapy with transomy cardial laser revascularization (Abstract). 78th Meeting of the American Association for Thoracic Surgery, May 3–6, 1998 Boston, 1998.
54. Schaper W: Molecular mechanisms of coronary collateral growth. Circ Res 79:911–919, 1996.
55. Schumacher B, Pecher P, von Specht BU, et al: Induction of neoangiogenesis in ischemic myocardium by human growth factors: First clinical results of a new treatment of coronary heart disease. Circulation 97:645–650, 1998.
56. Selke FW, Laham RJ, Edelman ER, et al: Therapeutic angiogenesis with basic fibroblast growth factor: Technique and early results. Ann Thorac Surg 65:1540–1544, 1998.
57. Selke FW, Wang SY, Stamler A, et al: Enhanced microvascular relaxations to VEGF and βFGF in chronically ischemic porcine myocardium. Am J Physiol 271:H713–H720, 1996.
58. Selke FW, Wang SY, Friedman M, et al: Basic FGF enhances endothelium-dependent relaxation of the collateral-perfused coronary microcirculation. Am J Physiol 267:H1303–H1311, 1994.
59. Symes JF, Sniderman AD: Angiogenesis: Potential therapy for ischemic disease. Curr Opin Lipidiol 5:305–312, 1994.
60. Takeshita S, Pu L-Q, Zheng L, et al: Vascular endothelial growth factor induces dose-dependent revascularization in a rabbit model of persistent limb ischemia. Circulation 90:II-228–II-234, 1994.
61. Takeshita S, Rossow ST, Kearney M, et al: Time course of increased cellular proliferation in collateral arteries following administration of vascular endothelial growth factor in a rabbit model of lower limb vascular insufficiency. Am J Pathol 147:1649–1660, 1995.
62. Takeshita S, Tsurumi Y, Couffinhal T, et al: Gene transfer of naked DNA encoding for three isoforms of vascular endothelial growth factor stimulates collateral development in vivo. Lab Invest 75:487–502, 1996.
63. Takeshita S, Weir L, Chen D, et al: Therapeutic angiogenesis following arterial gene transfer of vascular endothelial growth factor in a rabbit model of hindlimb ischemia. Biochem Biophys Res Commun 227:628–635, 1996.
64. Takeshita S, Zheng LP, Asahara T, et al: Therapeutic angiogenesis: A single intra-arterial bolus of vascular endothelial growth factor augments collateral vessel formation in a rabbit ischemic hind limb (Abstract). Circulation 88:I-370, 1993.
65. Tio RA, Lebherz C, Scheuermann T, et al: Evidence of collateral development following intramyocardial gene therapy with vascular endothelial growth factor. Surg Forum XLIX:220–221, 1998.
66. Tischer E, Mitchell R, Hartmann T, et al: The human gene for vascular endothelial growth factor: Multiple protein forms are encoded through alternative exon splicing. J Biol Chem 266:11947–11954, 1991.
67. Tsurumi Y, Takeshita S, Chen D, et al: Direct intramuscular gene transfer of naked DNA encoding vascular endothelial growth factor augments collateral development and tissue perfusion. Circulation 94:3281–3290, 1996.
68. Van Belle E, Rivard A, Chen D, et al: Hypercholesterolemia attenuates angiogenesis but does not preclude augmentation by angiogenic cytokines. Circulation 96:2667–2674, 1997.
69. van der Zee R, Murohara T, Luo Z, et al: Vascular endothelial growth factor (VEGF)/vascular permeability factor (VPF) augments nitric oxide release from quiescent rabbit and human vascular endothelium. Circulation 95:1030–1037, 1997.
70. Vineberg AM: Development of an anastomosis between the coronary vessels and a transplanted animal mammary artery. Can Med Assn J 55:117–119, 1946.
71. Ware JA, Simons M: Angiogenesis in ischemic heart disease. Nat Med 3:158–164, 1997.
72. Witzenbichler B, Van Belle E, Chang L, et al: Scatter factor (SF) induces vascular endothelial growth factor (VEGF) expression in vascular smooth muscle cells (VSMC) and acts synergistic to VEGF on endothelial cell (EC) migration in vitro (Abstract). Circulation 94:I-593–I-594, 1996.
73. Wolff JA, Malone RW, Williams P, et al: Direct gene transfer into mouse muscle in vivo. Science 247:1465–1468, 1990.
74. Yamumoto N, Kohmoto T, Gu A, et al: Angiogenesis is enhanced in ischemic canine myocardium by transmyocardial laser revascularization. J Am Coll Cardiol 31:1426–1433, 1998.
75. Yanagisawa-Miwa A, Uchida Y, Nakamura F, et al: Salvage of infarcted myocardium by angiogenic action of basic fibroblast growth factor. Science 257:1401–1403, 1992.

Chapter 82

Future of Minimally Invasive Cardiac Surgery

Michael J. Mack

For many years, coronary artery bypass surgery was performed essentially the same way; now, things have changed. The performance of heart surgery using cardiopulmonary bypass, ischemic cardioplegic arrest, myocardial preservation, oxygenation and pump technology, and instrumentation has improved so that more than 600,000 coronary artery bypass graft operations and a total of 800,000 cardiac operations are performed annually worldwide with generally good results by most cardiac surgeons in virtually every corner of the world.[1] However, despite upgrades (e.g., membrane oxygenators, myocardial preservation, arterial conduits), after the great breakthrough of coronary artery bypass surgery in the late 1960s, there have been no major strategic changes.[2] However, there has been a major paradigm shift in the way coronary artery bypass grafting is approached.[3] "Less is more" is the theme of the new millennium. Whether on a beating heart or an arrested heart, through limited access or full access approach, as stand-alone therapy or in conjunction with other methods of myocardial revascularization, innovative concepts and techniques are being introduced in the cardiac surgical arena. Whether this is merely a sidelight in the history of coronary revascularization or a true strategic infliction point in cardiac surgery remains to be seen. Its true value will be defined only by well-performed studies documenting clear outcome advantages over conventional techniques.[4] Until now, most claims of superiority of minimally invasive cardiac surgery have rested on anecdotal reports, registries, and uncontrolled studies.[5–7] In order to predict the future, we have to first look at what the present tells us about the recent past, that is, the first 3 years of minimally invasive coronary surgery.

Current Status of Minimally Invasive Coronary Surgery

Minimally Invasive Direct Coronary Artery Bypass (MIDCAB)

In 1998 an estimated 600,000 coronary bypass operations were performed, of which an estimated 40,000 (7%) were beating-heart procedures, and another 4000 were performed by a port access approach.[1] Concerns regarding beating-heart surgery exist, especially concerning the technical ability to perform an accurate anastomosis on a beating heart.[4] Using angiographic patency as the benchmark, numerous series now exist attesting to the graft patency of the MIDCAB procedure (Table 82–1).[8] This can be compared with existing published series of left internal mammary artery to left anterior descending artery grafts by conventional techniques (Table 82–2). It should be emphasized that all series were performed with stabilization by experienced surgeons after a learning curve, and similar results generally cannot be expected from a less experienced center. More recent results from Cremer, Kayser, and Boonstra and their colleagues all support MIDCAB patency rates of 95 to 97%.[9–11]

Recently, there appears to be a shift to high-risk patients (old, with poor left ventricular function) using targeted revascularization, either alone or in conjunction with catheter-based procedures.

Off-Pump Coronary Artery Bypass (OPCAB)

The application of the MIDCAB procedure in which coronary revascularization is performed on a beating heart through a limited access incision seems to have reached a plateau. The reasons for this include more clear determination of appropriate indications, limited application to single-vessel disease, and the increasing use of new stents for the management of proximal left anterior descending coronary artery disease. Currently, the real growth area in minimally invasive coronary artery surgery appears to be in OPCAB procedures.[12–14] There are a number of reasons for this. First, because the procedures are performed through a median sternotomy, although performed on a beating heart, the procedures are easier for surgeons to learn. Second, it significantly broadens the application of minimally invasive surgery by allowing multivessel coronary artery disease to be approached, as opposed to the narrow niche of the MIDCAB procedure. Third, innovative techniques and technologies have facilitated the OPCAB procedure; therefore, it is being more widely applied. One example is posterior pericardial stay sutures placed for presentation of the posterior surface of the heart, as described by Professor Lima from Recife, Brazil. In this technique, sutures are placed in the pericardium just anterior to the left superior and inferior pulmonary veins, and by traction on these sutures, the apex of the heart is displaced out of the chest cavity (Fig. 82–1). Surprisingly, the hemodynamic compromise caused by this aggressive distraction of the heart is not severe in most cases, allowing off-pump techniques to be used even when the posterior circulation is in need of revascularization (Fig. 82–2). In addition, significant improvement in the newest generation of stabilizers allows a broader application of beating-heart surgery. With the aid of additional devices such as micropumps for assisting the right side of the heart, as addressed later, the majority of coronary artery disease will be able to be treated successfully with beating-heart techniques. Many believe that within the next decade, conventional cardiopulmonary bypass will prove unnecessary for most coronary revascularization.

Table 82–1. Published Series of Left Internal Mammary Artery Graft Patency in Minimally Invasive Coronary Artery Bypass

Author	Year	No. Studied / No. Operated	% Angio/OP	Interval of Postoperative Study	Graft Patency (%)	Exclusions/Notes
Schaff	1996	15/16	94	Intraoperative	100	3 revised
Calafiore	1996	231/434	62	1–26 d	93	Additional 4% had stenosis >50%
Subramanian	1997	169/189	89	24–36 hr	92	Stenosis = occlusion
Gill	1997	29/29	100	4–6 hr	97.5	Additional 19% had stenosis >50%
Mack	1998	100/103	97	38 intraoperative; 62 48–96 hr	99	Additional 8% had stenosis >50%
Cremer	1998	220/296	74		98.2	Additional 4.8% had stenosis ≥50%
Kayser	1998	201/299	68		97.2	Additional 5.3% had stenosis ≥50%

% Angio/OP = percentage of patients operated upon who had intraoperative or postoperative coronary angiography.

Port Access Coronary Artery Bypass

There has been some broader application of port access coronary bypass grafting to multivessel coronary artery disease. Refinements in the Heartport platform, including direct thoracic cannulation (see later), have allowed multivessel disease to be revascularized through a limited access incision.[15] Although port access technology has been used mainly for mitral valve procedures, port access techniques are being applied more frequently to multivessel coronary artery disease. The definitive demonstration of benefit has not yet occurred, and published series are still relatively small and limited.

Minimally Invasive Valve Procedures

Numerous series now exist of successful application of minimal access techniques for valve surgery.[16–18] A number of published series of mitral valve repair and replacement showed acceptable mortality, comparable valve repair rates to open procedures, and safety of the procedure.[19] However, no randomized study of open versus minimal access valve procedures that demonstrates benefit exists. Numerous series of aortic valve replacement performed through minimal access incisions—either a limited right anterior thoracotomy or partial median sternotomy incision—have been published. Although many surgeons believe that there is subjective benefit, including quicker recovery and less morbidity in terms of pain and respiratory adverse effects, no definitive objective demonstration of benefit exists.

New Technology

Significant enabling technology has been introduced for the expansion of minimally invasive cardiac surgical techniques, both for beating-heart surgery and for limited access surgery.

Stabilizers

Commercial manufacturers (at least six) have introduced stabilization devices for beating-heart surgery. Some of the original stabilization devices have undergone incremental improvements, and the second and third generations of these devices have now been introduced. The Octopus 2 (Medtronic Inc., Minneapolis, MN) is a suction stabilization system that has been made more user-friendly and allows not only stabilization but also presentation of various surfaces of the heart (Fig. 82–3). When it is used in conjunction with pericardial traction sutures, most target areas of the heart in the majority of patients can now be accessed by beating-heart techniques. Cardio Thoracic Systems (Cupertino, CA) has recently introduced the newest upgrade for stabilization devices specific to off-pump coronary bypass procedures (Fig. 82–4). It allows greater versatility for stabilization of the posterior surfaces of the heart and for placement of pericardial stay sutures. Development in this area of user-friendly stabilization is rapid, and it is anticipated that even the instruments mentioned here will soon be on the way to becoming obsolete.

Table 82–2. Results of Early Angiography (≤1 Month) After Conventional Coronary Artery Bypass

Author	Year	No. Studied / No. Operated	% Studied	Interval	Graft Patency (%)	Exclusions/Notes
Barner	1976	139/307	45	20 d	95	Nonsurvivors
Geha	1979	175/208	82	2 wk	99	6 nonsurvivors (3%)
Tyras	1980	527/765	69	1 mo	95	Nonsurvivors (1.4%)
Grondin	1984	37/40	92	1 mo	97	2 nonsurvivors, 1 patient declined
Ivert	1988	91/99	92	2 wk	94	2 nonsurvivors
Gill	1997	25/25	100	4–6 hr	96	
Berger (IMAGE)	1997	645/768	84	10.8 d	98.8	Additional 7.8% had graft stenosis >50%

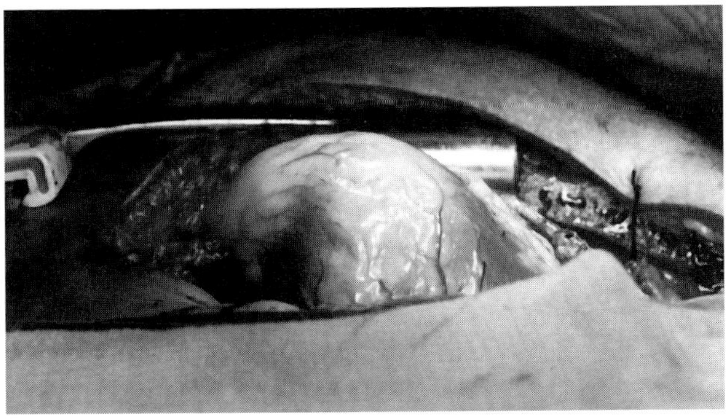

Figure 82–1. Pericardial traction sutures posterior on the left side allow distraction of the apex of the heart out of the pericardial cavity and access to the posterior wall.

Circulatory Support

Port access surgery has relied on peripheral access via the femoral artery for circulatory support and for placement of the endoaortic balloon occluder. Reports of aortic dissection and inability to place the platform when significant peripheral vascular disease exists have limited application of the port access technique.[20] More recently, the EndoDirect system has allowed central aortic cannulation with a trocar-type aortic cannula that allows placement through a 12-mm port into the ascending aorta. The cannula is introduced into the right side of the aorta at the base of the innominate artery for mitral valve procedures and into the left side of the aorta on the underside of the arch through the first intercostal space for coronary artery bypass grafting. The benefits of this system are avoidance of peripheral cannulation and minimization of the concerns of retrograde aortic dissection. Potential migration of the endoaortic balloon is minimized by placement directly through the cannula into the ascending aorta.

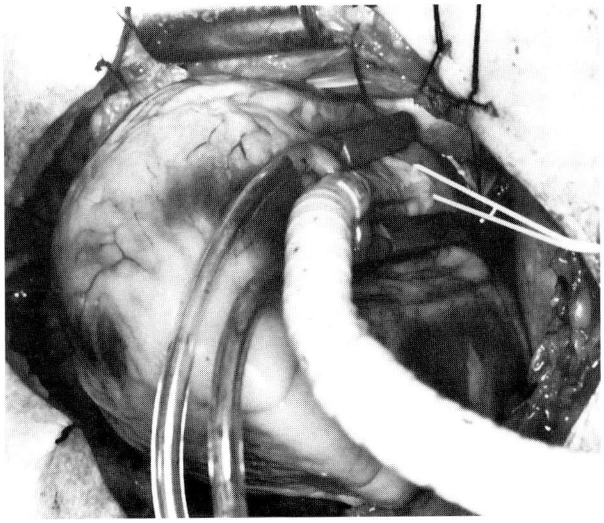

Figure 82–3. Octopus 2 Stabilizer (Courtesy of Medtronic Inc., Minneapolis, MN).

Ventricular Assist Devices

Significant interest has been generated in many centers regarding circulatory assistance for off-pump beating-heart surgery. Micropump systems have been developed that allow univentricular or biventricular assist support without oxygenation (Fig. 82–5). The principle behind these support systems is that by eliminating the oxygenator from cardiopulmonary bypass, the major component inducing the systemic inflammation response is eliminated. Although significant interest exists in support of the left side of the heart, more intriguing is the interest in support of the right side of the heart. It appears that in beating-heart surgery the impairment of systemic circulatory hemodynamics is due to obstruction of flow to the *right* rather than to the *left* side of the heart. Distortions in the right ventricle and pulmonary outflow tract during manipulations for accessing the inferior and posterior circulation seem to be

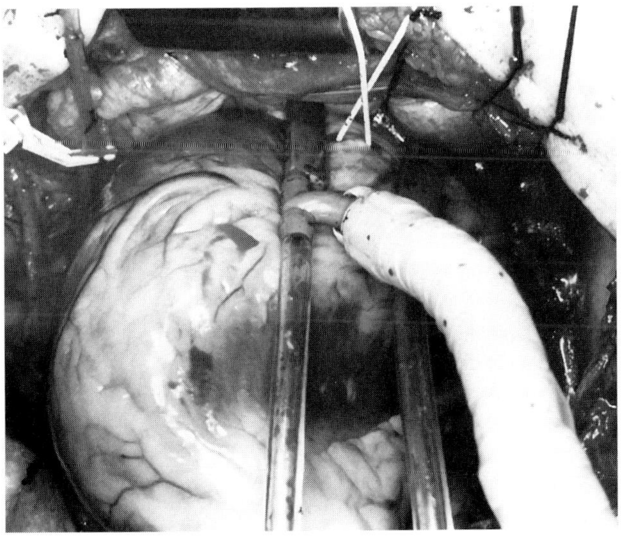

Figure 82–2. Stabilization and presentation of the circumflex coronary system.

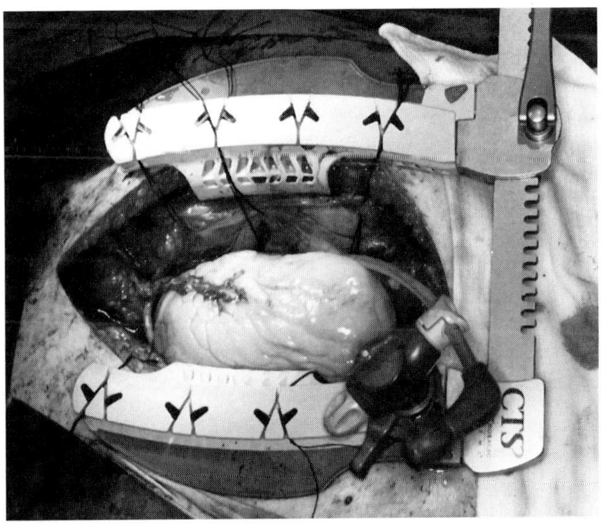

Figure 82–4. Ultima Refractor and Stabilizer (Courtesy of Cardio-Thoracic Systems, Inc., Cupertino, CA).

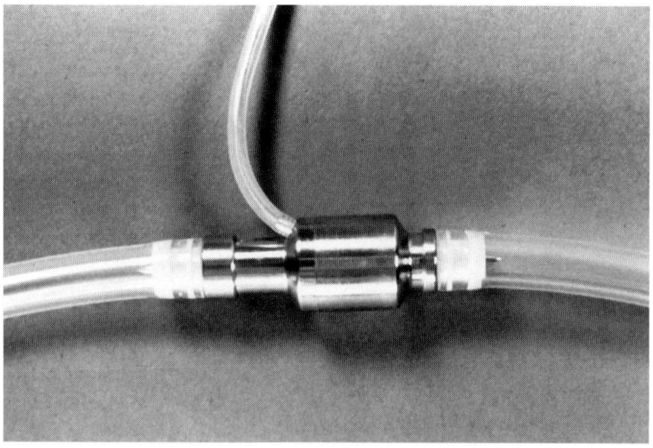

Figure 82–5. Jarvik Axial Flow Micropump.

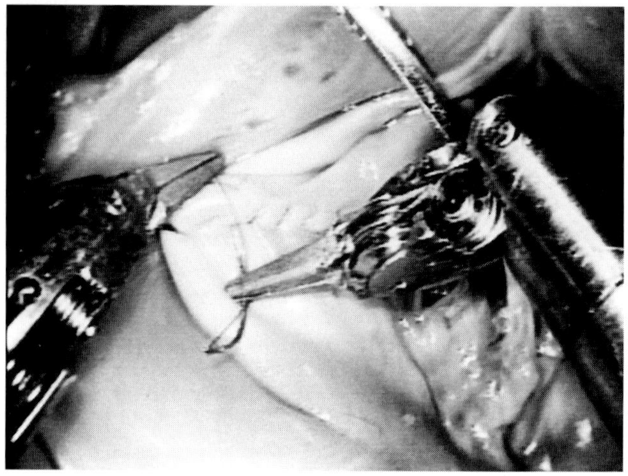

Figure 82–6. "Endowrists" articulating robotic endoscopic instrumentation. (Courtesy of Intuitive Surgical, Inc., Mountain View, CA).

the cause of hemodynamic instability associated with off-pump surgery. The institution of support of the right side of the heart by a micropump offers the potential benefit of circulatory support for off-pump procedures yet minimization of the adverse systemic inflammatory effects associated with conventional circulatory support. In addition, the avoidance of cannulation of the arterial circulation further minimizes potentially adverse effects (dissection, embolization) of conventional cardiopulmonary bypass.

Robotics

Recently there has been intense interest in the field of robotics for coronary artery bypass surgery (see Chapter 79). The principle behind robotics in surgery is the introduction of computer assistance for the enhanced precision necessary for endoscopic surgery. Whereas limited access procedures render suturing for performance of a vascular anastomosis prohibitively difficult because of the length of instrumentation, the fulcrum effect of the chest wall, and the requirement for video assistance, robotics can facilitate endoscopic suturing.[21]

Robotics offers the benefits of scaled motion, tremor filtration, and remote telemanipulation. Essentially, robotics inserts a microchip between the surgeon's hands and the tips of the instruments. This allows more precision when endoscopic suturing is performed. Scaled motion allows the surgeon to scale up or scale down the instrument motion relative to the hand motion. For example, in a 4:1 scale, for every 4 cm the surgeon's hands move, the tip of the instrument moves 1 cm. In a similar manner, any tremor of the surgeon's hands—not a factor in conventional surgery, but magnified with video endoscopic surgery—is totally filtered out. Although the original idea behind the introduction of robotics in surgery was remote telemanipulation, it appears that the practicality of this application is nonexistent at the present time.

Two commercially available robotics systems exist for coronary bypass surgery. The Intuitive System (Intuitive Surgical, Mountain View, CA) offers the unique aspect of articulated instrumentation (endowrists) within the thoracic cavity. These "wrists" offer greater versatility in 7 degrees of freedom, which allows significant user-friendliness and a decreased learning curve (Fig. 82–6). Numerous coronary bypass procedures, mitral valve procedures, and repair of simple intracardiac defects (n = 30) have been performed with robotic assistance at Hôpital Broussais in Paris, France, Leipzig, Germany, and Aalst, Belgium, using the Intuitive System.[22]

Another commercially available system, Zeus (Computer Motion, Goleta, CA), offers other advantages and disadvantages. Although articulation (wrists) is not available in this system, the instruments are smaller, the setup required for the system is less, and the bulkiness is somewhat decreased compared with the Intuitive System (Fig. 82–7). Clinical trials using the Zeus system for endoscopic bypass surgery have been introduced in Munich, Germany, and Hershey, Pennsylvania.[23] Although it is too early to tell whether there will be a significant "value added" component to robotics systems in enabling endoscopic coronary bypass procedures, such systems offer intriguing technological applications to bypass surgery.

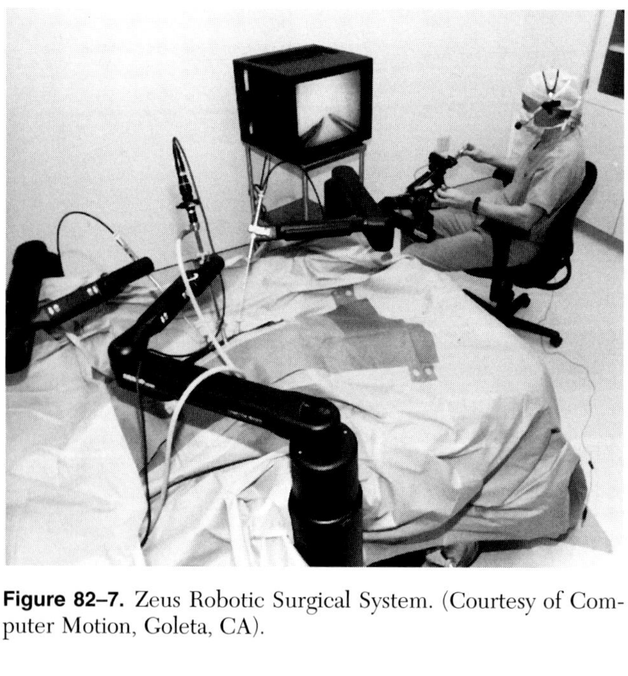

Figure 82–7. Zeus Robotic Surgical System. (Courtesy of Computer Motion, Goleta, CA).

Numerous other devices and products to facilitate anastomosis have been introduced. These include an enhanced mechanical anastomotic device, the one-shot device introduced for a nonsutured anastomosis, and vascular glues and sealants.[24]

Visualization

In the quest for endoscopic coronary bypass surgery, visualization is paramount. The ability to perform precise microvascular procedures using two-dimensional visualization is problematic. The introduction of three-dimensional visualization is a significant enhancement of technology that may ultimately lead to totally endoscopic procedures. Currently, two three-dimensional video systems exist. One is incorporated in the Intuitive Surgical robotics system, and the other is manufactured by Vista (Fig. 82–8). Although the degree of resolution with these three-dimensional systems does not yet approach that of two-dimensional systems, it is hoped that with digital enhancement and more user-friendly systems, the degree of resolution will compare favorably with two-dimensional systems and offer a facilitated means for endoscopic coronary bypass surgery.

Other Devices

Although there is no consensus on the definition of minimally invasive cardiac surgery, numerous ingenious methods have been developed that minimize the adverse effects of conventional bypass surgery. Some of the more devastating complications of conventional cardiac surgery are the neurologic sequelae associated with aortic cannulation, aortic manipulation, and cardiopulmonary bypass. The source of a significant number of these adverse neurologic consequences are atherosclerotic emboli from the ascending aorta.[25] An aortic filter (Embol-X) has been introduced with aortic cannulation to serve as a filter, or a trap, to catch atherosclerotic debris from the aorta during cardiopulmonary bypass (Fig. 82–9*B*). Although it has been demonstrated that this filtering system actually catches atherosclerotic debris and although it has been introduced into early clinical human trials, a definitive demonstration of benefit and decrease of neurologic consequences has yet to occur.

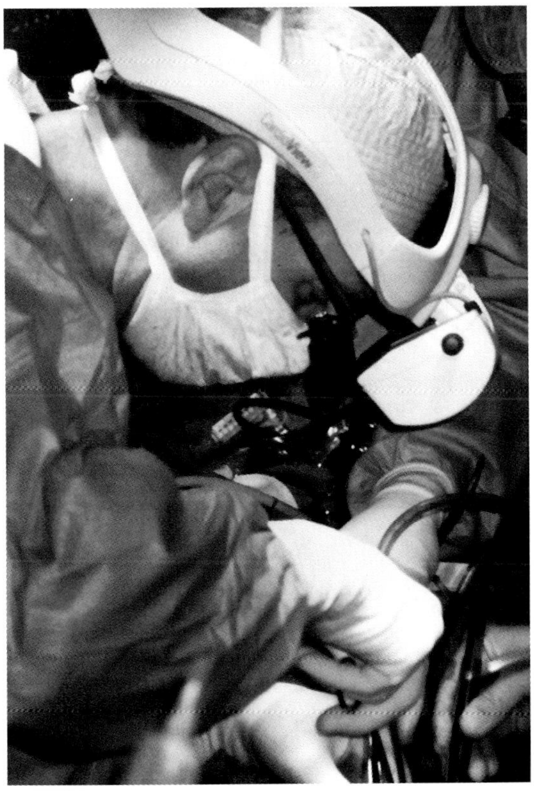

Figure 82–8. 3-D Head Mounted Display. (Courtesy of Vista.)

Alternative Methods of Coronary Revascularization

Various alternative methods of myocardial revascularization have been developed and implemented. Many of these techniques are adaptable to minimally invasive techniques.

Transmyocardial Laser Revascularization (TMR)

TMR has recently been approved for myocardial revascularization (see Chapter 76). The technique involves drilling multiple holes in an area of ischemic myocardium that cannot be revascularized by conventional surgical or catheter-based techniques, and it appears to improve clinical status and possibly improve local ischemia (Fig. 82–10).[26–28] Although numerous mechanisms for improvement have been hypothesized, including sympathetic denervation, placebo effect, and the opening of new blood channels, none of these explains the clinical benefit that appears to occur with this technique. Probably the most viable mechanism of benefit is angiogenesis induced by the myocardial injury caused by the laser channel.[29] A recent study of TMR in combination with gene therapy induced greater degrees of angiogenesis than either did alone.[30] Although these procedures are usually performed through a limited access thoracotomy or by an open approach in conjunction with conventional bypass surgery, the technique is easily adapted to the minimally invasive approach and has been performed on a limited basis totally thoracoscopically.

Gene Therapy

Numerous genes or gene products have been identified that induce angiogenesis in ischemic muscle and myocardium.[31–33] Currently, the two most common factors used are vascular endothelial growth factor (VEGF) and β-fibroblast growth factor (βFGF). Both have been demonstrated to induce angiogenesis in ischemic muscle. Although the ability to induce angiogenesis has been demonstrated by gene therapy, the mechanism of delivery, whether to introduce it directly into the muscle or by transcoronary means, and whether to use it as stand-alone or adjunctive therapy have yet to be determined. If clinical benefit is clearly demonstrated by this technique, minimally invasive approaches have been developed that are capable of easily delivering gene therapy into the myocardium (see Chapter 81).

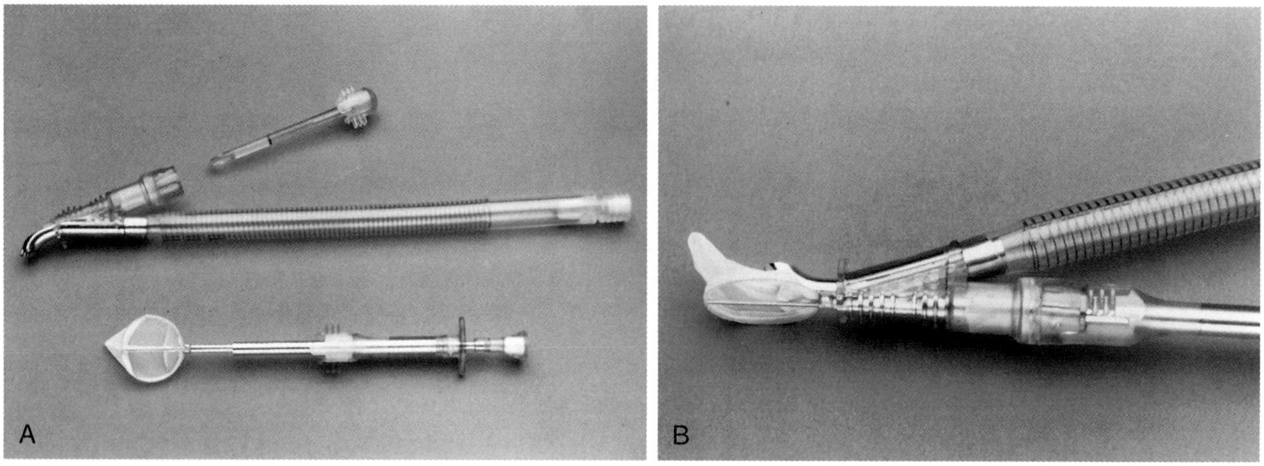

Figure 82–9. *A*, *B*, Intra-aortic filter and cannula system to protect the cerebral circulation (Embol-X).

Direct Myocardial Revascularization

Some interest has been shown in a concept of direct myocardial revascularization in which new channels are opened between the left ventricle, coronary sinus, or coronary veins directly into a coronary artery (Fig. 82–11).[34] Although this concept is at an early stage of development, it is hoped that this alternative therapy will offer a new modality for revascularization in patients who are not candidates for more conventional therapy.

Hybrid Procedures

The concept of combining minimally invasive cardiac surgical procedures with catheter-based procedures and achieving a synergistic therapeutic effect is an intriguing one (see Chapter 58). The logic behind this approach is that a left internal mammary artery is placed at the left anterior descending artery, and a catheter-based procedure is used to access other vessels of the circulation (right coronary and/or circumflex arteries) that are amenable to catheter-based therapy. Published series exist,[35] but the experience is small. The ultimate role of hybrid procedures in coronary revascularization, although yet to be determined, will probably be quite limited. Problems include the logistics and expense associated with the performance of two procedures and the lack of a common room in which both procedures can be performed at the same time, as well as selection of appropriate patients for the procedures. This will continue to be an area of interest that may or may not be a viable alternative for coronary revascularization integrating minimally invasive cardiac surgery into patient care.

In the field of coronary revascularization, the trend in surgical revascularization is toward greater simplicity, whereas catheter-based procedures are becoming more complex (Fig. 82–12). Although there is intense interest in eliminating cardiopulmonary bypass and using minimal access incisions in cardiac surgery, interventional cardiology is adding stents and brachytherapy to catheter-based procedures.[36, 37] Because both areas are evolving rapidly, it is difficult to say which therapy is appropriate for which pa-

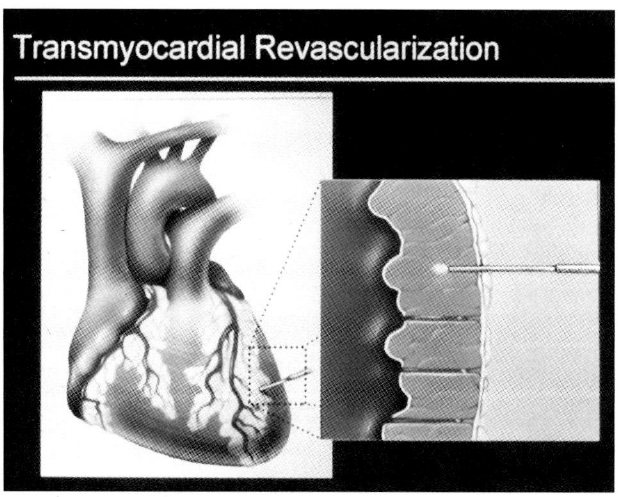

Figure 82–10. Diagram illustrating the technique of transmyocardial laser revascularization (TMR).

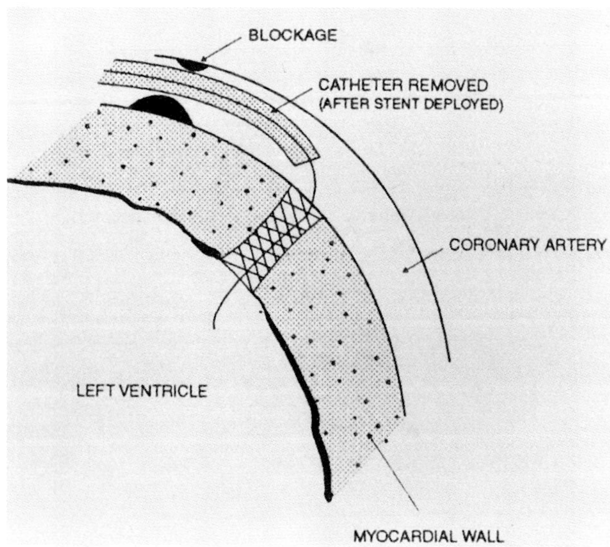

Figure 82–11. Concept of direct myocardial revascularization by construction of a left ventricle coronary shunt.

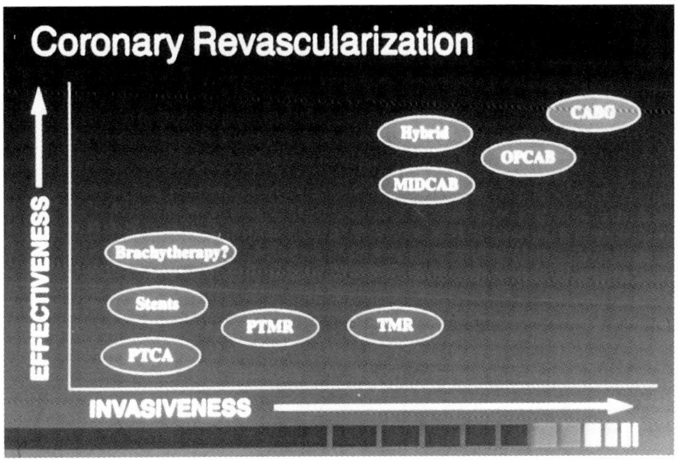

Figure 82–12. As cardiology becomes more invasive to increase effectiveness, cardiac surgery is attempting to become less invasive without sacrificing effectiveness.

tient. Although catheter-based procedures have traditionally been the least invasive form of coronary revascularization, their lack of long-term effectiveness has been their shortcoming. Attempts at improving the effectiveness of catheter-based therapy naturally lead to the more invasive nature of the procedures.

In a similar manner, coronary bypass surgery by conventional techniques has had maximal long-term effectiveness but maximal invasiveness as well. Minimally invasive surgery attempts to decrease the invasiveness of surgical revascularization yet maintain a long-term effectiveness; therefore, the balance between invasiveness and effectiveness more closely approaches that of catheter-based procedures. There are two published series that compare catheter-based procedures and minimally invasive cardiac surgical procedures for types B2 and C lesions of the left anterior descending artery. Both series demonstrate that the mortality and morbidity of the two procedures are essentially the same; however, the need for target vessel revascularization at 6 months and 1 year significantly increases with catheter-based procedures.[11, 38] I anticipate that as both fields progress and as the approach to coronary revascularization becomes more integrated, determining populations for each of these therapies will become more clearly defined.

This is an exciting time in the history of cardiac surgery. The field of minimally invasive cardiac surgery has served as a stimulus for rejuvenating the innovative techniques of cardiac surgery and redefining the field of coronary revascularization. The possibilities are limited only by imagination and ingenuity. Over the past few years, there has been a significant paradigm shift in thought processes. However, a balance needs to be struck between innovation and rigidity, with too much of either being destructive. If the appropriate balance between acceptance of proven standards and open-mindedness to change is attained, the evolutionary process of developing better methods of treating our patients will be the product of our endeavors.[39]

References

1. American Heart Association: 1998 Heart and Stroke Statistical Update.
2. Baudet E: Cardiac surgery in the 21st century: The future is now? Eur J Cardiothorac Surg 14:545–553, 1998.
3. Loop FD: Coronary artery surgery: The end of the beginning. Eur J Cardiothorac Surg 14:554–571, 1998.
4. Bonchek LI, Ullyot DJ: Minimally invasive coronary bypass: A dissenting opinion. Circulation 98:495–497, 1998.
5. Subramanian VA, Sani G, Benetti FJ, Calafiore AM: Minimally invasive coronary bypass surgery: A multi-center report of preliminary clinical experience. Circulation 92(suppl I):I–645, 1995.
6. Calafiore AM, Gallina S, Iaco A, et al: Minimally invasive mammary artery Doppler flow velocity evaluation in minimally invasive coronary operations. Ann Thorac Surg 66:1236–1241, 1998.
7. Gulielmos V, Knaut M, Wagner FM, Schuler S: Minimally invasive surgical technique for the treatment of multivessel coronary artery disease. Ann Thorac Surg 65:1331–1334, 1998.
8. Mack MJ, Osborne JA, Shennib H: Arterial graft patency in coronary artery bypass grafting: What do we really know? Ann Thorac Surg 66:1055–1059, 1998.
9. Cremer J, Mugge A, Wittwer T, et al: Early angiographic results after revascularization by minimally invasive direct coronary artery bypass (MIDCAB). Presented at the 12th annual meeting of the European Association for Cardio-Thoracic Surgery, 1998.
10. Kayser S, Diegeler A, Matin M, et al: Angiographic control after minimally invasive coronary bypass surgery. Presented at the 12th annual meeting of the European Association for Cardio-Thoracic Surgery, 1998.
11. Boonstra PW, van Boven AJ, Grandjean JG, et al: PTCA with stenting compared to off-pump coronary surgery with a left internal mammary artery in patients with single vessel disease of the left anterior descending artery: 6 months angiographic follow-up results of a prospective clinical trial. Circulation 98(suppl):1119, 1998.
12. Spooner TH, Dyrud PE, Monson BK, et al: Coronary artery bypass on the beating heart with the Octopus: A North American experience. Ann Thorac Surg 66:1032–1035, 1998.
13. Massetti M, Babatasi G, Lotti A, et al: Less invasive cardiac operations through a median sternotomy: 100 consecutive cases. Ann Thorac Surg 66:1050–1054, 1998.
14. Puskas JD, Wright CE, Ronson RS, et al: Off-pump multivessel coronary bypass via sternotomy is safe and effective. Ann Thorac Surg 66:1068–1072, 1998.
15. Reichenspurner H, Boehm DH, Welz A, et al: Minimally invasive coronary artery bypass grafting: Port-access approach versus off-pump techniques. Ann Thorac Surg 66:1036–1040, 1998.
16. Cohn LH, Adams DH, Couper GS, et al: Minimally invasive cardiac valve surgery improves patient satisfaction while reducing costs of cardiac valve replacement and repair. Ann Thorac Surg 226:421–428, 1997.
17. Cohn LH, Adams DH, Couper GS, et al: Minimally invasive aortic valve replacement. Semin Thorac Cardiovasc Surg 9:331–336, 1997.

18. Cosgrove DM III, Sabik JF, Navie J: Minimally invasive valve operations. Ann Thorac Surg 65:1535–1539, 1998.
19. Chitwood WR, Elbeery JR, Chapman WHH, et al: Video-assisted minimally invasive mitral valve surgery: The "micromitral" operation. J Thorac Cardiovasc Surg 113:413–414, 1997.
20. Cooley DA: Minimally invasive valve surgery versus the conventional approach. Ann Thorac Surg 66:1101–1105, 1998.
21. Stephenson ER Jr, Sankholkar S, Ducko CT, Damiano RJ Jr: Successful endoscopic coronary artery bypass grafting: An acute large animal trial. J Thorac Cardiovasc Surg 116: 131–138, 1998.
22. Intuitive Surgical Systems: Personal communication.
23. Reichenspurner H, Damiano R, Mack M, et al: Experimental and first clinical use of the voice-controlled and computer-assisted surgical system Zeus™ for endoscopic coronary artery bypass grafting. J Thorac Cardiovasc Surg (in press).
24. Nataf P, Hinchliffe P, Manzo S, et al: Facilitated vascular anastomoses: The one-shot device. Ann Thorac Surg 66:1041–1044, 1998.
25. Taylor KM: Brain damage during cardiopulmonary bypass. Ann Thorac Surg 65:S20–S26, 1998.
26. Mirhoseini M, Fisher JC, Cayton MM: Myocardial revascularization by laser. Lasers Surg Med 3:241–245, 1983.
27. Horvath KA, Cohn LH, Cooley DA, et al: Transmyocardial laser revascularization: Results of a multicenter trial with transmyocardial laser revascularization used as the sole therapy for end-stage coronary artery disease. J Thorac Cardiovasc Surg 113:645–654, 1997.
28. Kohmoto T, Fisher PE, Gu A, et al: Does blood flow through holmium:YAG transmyocardial laser channels? Ann Thorac Surg 61:861–868, 1996.
29. Yamumoto N, Kohmoto T, Gu A, et al: Angiogenesis is enhanced in ischemic canine myocardium by transmyocardial laser revascularization. J Am Coll Cardiol 31:1426–1433, 1998.
30. Sayeed-Shah U, Mann M, Martin J, et al: Complete reversal of ischemic wall motion abnormalities by combined use of gene therapy with transmyocardial laser revascularization (Abstract). Presented at 78th meeting of the American Association for Thoracic Surgery, Boston, May 3–6, 1998.
31. Olofsson B, Pajusola K, Kaipainen A, et al: Vascular endothelial growth factor B, a novel growth factor for endothelial cells. Proc Natl Acad Sci USA 93:2576–2581, 1996.
32. Selke FW, Laham RJ, Edelman ER, et al: Therapeutic angiogenesis with basic fibroblast growth factor: Technique and early results. Ann Thorac Surg 65:1540–1544, 1998.
33. Schumacher B, Pecher P, von Specht BU, et al: Induction of neoangiogenesis in ischemic myocardium by human growth factors: First clinical results of a new treatment of coronary heart disease. Circulation 97:645–650, 1998.
34. Oesterle SN: Beyond stents: Third-generation coronary devices. Ann Thorac Surg 66:1045–1049, 1998.
35. Riess FC, Schofer J, Kremer P, et al: Beating heart operations including hybrid revascularization: Initial experiences. Ann Thorac Surg 66:1076–1081, 1998.
36. Teirstein PS, Massullo V, Jani S, et al: Catheter-based radiotherapy to inhibit restenosis after coronary stenting. N Engl J Med 336:1697–1703, 1997.
37. Serruys PW, Levendag PC: Intracoronary brachytherapy: The death knell of restenosis or just another episode of a never-ending story? Circulation 96:709–712, 1997.
38. Schuler GC, Diegeler A, Spyrantis NA, et al: Minimal invasive bypass surgery versus PTCA + stent in high grade proximal lesions of the LAD: A prospective randomized trial. Circulation 98 (suppl):1121, 1998.
39. Mack M, Damiano R, Matheny R, et al: Inertia of success—a response to minimally invasive coronary bypass, a dissenting opinion. Circulation 99:1404–1406, 1999.

Chapter 83

Future Technologies for Surgical Applications*

Richard M. Satava and Shaun B. Jones

The modern era of surgery began at the end of the 19th century when medicine encountered the Industrial Age with its wealth of revolutionary technologies, such as anesthesia, asepsis, microscopy, and new materials. As this century closes, the Information Age is diffusing into medicine, and a revolution of even greater magnitude is occurring. To understand the change, it is necessary to look outside of medicine to society as a whole and find the underlying principles to apply within our discipline. Futurists have been hawking the coming era; however, it took a pragmatist like Nicholas Negroponte of the Massachusetts Institute of Technology Media Laboratory in his book, *Being Digital,* to focus our attention on the critical element.[1]

Negroponte introduced the concept of "bits instead of atoms" to describe how we can represent the real world and the objects in it by a computer or information representation—which will be referred to in this chapter as "information equivalents." The example he uses to illustrate his concept is that of the facsimile machine. For more than 4000 years, messages have been transmitted from one person to another by sending the actual atoms, such as clay tablets, papyrus, or paper. With the facsimile machine, the same messages can be sent virtually in an instant (and at greatly reduced cost) by sending the bits (data) over telephone lines rather than the atoms (letters). In our profession, the object of attention is the patient, or, more specifically, the human body.

Fortunately, in 1994, the information equivalent of the human body became available from the National Library of Medicine as "The Visible Human."[2] At the same time, robotic and computer-assisted surgical technologies were beginning to emerge, trying to convert our hand motions and sense of touch into information by using sensors, effectors, and a computer. It was also at that time that a National Science Foundation workshop on virtual reality (VR) informally asked the question: How much of what a physician does can be represented by information? Figure 83–1 illustrates a number of these analogies. During laparoscopic surgery, the surgeon does not look at the patient's organs but at a video monitor with an image of the organs (information equivalent of the organs).

When surgery is finished and the patient is in the recovery room, the surgeon looks at the vital signs monitor for the heart rate and blood pressure (equivalent of taking the pulse and touching). The medical record is evolving into an electronic file, and nearly all of our imaging has changed from film (atoms) to digital images (bits). Surgical education is using computer-aided instruction, compact disk-read only memory (CD-ROM), and VR to supplement cadaver and animal models. With the new research in robotics, even our hand motions are being changed to electronic signals and sent from one place to another. The future of medicine is no longer blood and guts but bits and bytes.

The relevance is that Information Age technologies are based upon this metaphor, using technologies such as diagnostic imaging for visualization; sensors for vital signs and physiologic parameters; microelectronic machine systems (MEMS) for new instruments; computers and telecommunications for database and record keeping; and artificial intelligence for decision support, quality assurance, and outcomes analysis. These are the engines of empowerment, not only for the physician but for the patient as well. Although the vast field of surgical applications of biotechnology and genetic engineering is not addressed here, it is pertinent to point out that desoxyribonucleic acid (DNA) is, in its very essence, information—a fancy set of bits and bytes represented by the base pairs instead of zeros and ones. It is this commonality of information that enables us to tie together a whole new concept of how surgery could evolve into an entire medical ecosystem. Discoveries in microsensors permit new imaging devices, which enable new forms of image-based surgery. It is an upward spiral: One discovery providing a giant step forward toward the next technology and elevating the whole system logarithmically. This offers an explanation as to why we are all so overwhelmed by the rapidity of our changing profession.

Nonetheless, today's surgeons-to-be are not uncomfortable with the rapidly changing technologies. They "surf the net," get instant news from CNN, watch MTV, and conquer video games with ease. They are the "Nintendo" surgeons, who were born, raised, educated, and now trained with Information Age tools. They absorb information by osmosis, displaying all the intuitive ability they exercise to master native language. Their ability to cope with, and even demand, new technologies confirms that this is a major direction of the future. One of their fundamental tools is the ability to understand the world in the form of three-dimensional (3-D) visualization (once again, replacing atoms with bits). There is a speculative scenario that can be used as a framework to illuminate the integrating power of this concept. It is referred to as the "doorway to the future" and it extrapolates 20, 50, or perhaps 100 years into the future.

Imagine this future scenario. As a patient visits her surgeon for a consult, she passes through the office door and, just as we are scanned today by airport security, she is scanned by multiple imaging modalities (perhaps computed tomography [CT], magnetic resonance imaging [MRI], or ultrasound). As she places her hand on a pad on the desk, both physiologic vital signs and biochemical parameters are acquired instantly and noninvasively by

*The opinions or assertions contained herein are the private views of the authors and are not to be construed as official, or as reflecting the views of the Department of the Army, the Department of the Navy, the Advanced Research Projects Agency, or the Department of Defense.

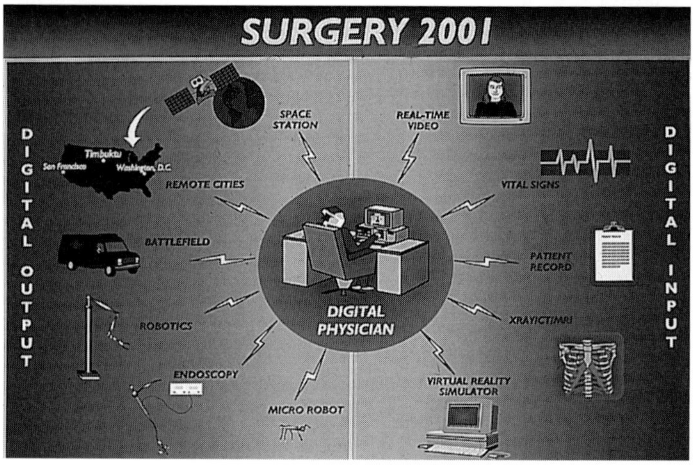

Figure 83–1. Graphic representation of information equivalents.

means of hyperspectral analysis, as is done today by noninvasive acquisition of oxygen saturation or pulse by pulse oximeters. The data are all collected and then displayed as a 3-D image of the patient (looking like the Visible Human), not only with correct anatomic structure but also with all the biochemical and other data added to the correct organ systems. If she complains of right chest pain, the surgeon can rotate the image, tap or click on the lung or aorta, and have the relevant data displayed, such as oxygen saturation, blood pressure, or heart rate. If an abnormality is seen, such as a pulmonary nodule, a virtual bronchoscopy can be done on the image by "flying through" the bronchus, providing the same view as an actual bronchoscopy. If a lesion is found, the image can be used for patient education, illustrating exactly what the specific problem is. Should this require a complicated procedure, the image can be used for preoperative surgical planning or imported into a surgical simulator to practice a resection on the patient's virtual anatomy to achieve the optimal procedure.

At the time of surgery, the image can be imported onto the video monitor during the thoracoscopic procedure, and through data fusion the two images can be displayed simultaneously as an intraoperative navigation tool (see later discussion on stereotactic navigation). At the postoperative follow-up visit, the patient is scanned again by comparison of data sets compiled pre- and postoperatively and by digital subtraction techniques; the difference between the two data sets is automatic outcomes analysis. The record is a data set, so it can be stored on a credit card (the US military is using a prototype called the personal information card [PIC]) or kept on a Web server to be distributed worldwide over the Internet for consultation. Thus, by considering the medical record as a 3-D image of the patient, the entire spectrum of patient care can be integrated and continuously updated.

The purpose of the preceding scenario is to provide a rationale for the importance of understanding how information can empower us, and to get a glimpse through the looking glass at the way in which the next generation of surgeons will view the world. To bring the scenario out of the speculative and rhetorical realm and into the real world, the technologies that support the views expressed in this chapter will be held up to the scrutiny of science. Only when these new discoveries have been properly evaluated by rigorous testing and clinical trials can they take their place in the framework of the future. It is our postulate that these technologies are based upon proven scientific principles, but they have to respond successfully to significant challenges in development, clinical trials, and commercialization before they can become the standard of practice for surgical applications. Three areas represent an arbitrary division of surgical applications for the new technologies: Diagnostics, therapeutics, and surgical education.

Diagnostics

In the area of diagnostics, noninvasive microsensors for physiologic and biochemical data and portable 3-D imaging systems will obtain information for the surgeon. A wearable system for soldiers (developed by Sarcos, Inc., Salt Lake City, UT) called the Personnel Status Monitor (PSM)[3] was field-tested in 1996 (Fig. 83–2). This system consists of a geolocation position satellite (GPS) locator, telecommunications, and a suite of vital signs (e.g., pulse rate, temperature, respiration); the medic has a hand-held

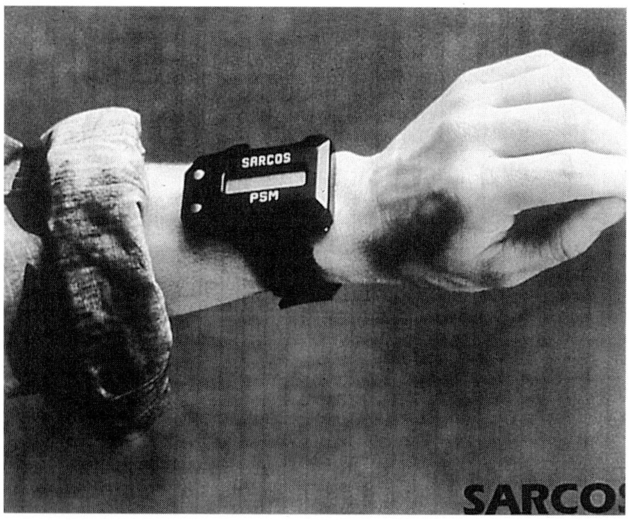

Figure 83–2. Personnel Status Monitor. (Courtesy of Stephen Jacobsen, Sarcos, Inc, Salt Lake City, UT.)

receiving unit. When a soldier is wounded, the medic is instantly alerted, and the unit displays the casualty's location and vital signs, so the medic can find and triage the wounded immediately. To complement this, a "Smart Tee Shirt" (Fig. 83–3) is being developed by Naval Research and Development at San Diego, California.[4] Sensors are woven into the fabric (fiberoptic and pizoelectric materials) or embroidered onto strategic locations (electrocardiograph [ECG] leads) and their signals are read by the PSM system for remote transmission. Although the initial application is for the battlefield, it is clear that such a technology, when produced as a consumer product, can be used equally well for health and fitness, intensive care patients, in the operating theater, or for nursing home invalids. These monitoring devices emphasize the trend toward point-of-service health care.

A number of new 3-D imaging modalities are being developed, most with the intent of miniaturizing. Small, portable CT and MRI scanners will make these imaging modalities affordable and available. Significant progress is occurring in the ultrasound field. Taking sophisticated digital signal-processing algorithms from the satellite-image community, Sandia National Labs in Albuquerque, New Mexico, is refining the clarity of ultrasound to approach that of CT or MRI scans (Fig. 83–4). In addition, full 3-D representations can be made from serial slices.[4] In September 1996, the US military used a Battelle-Pacific Northwest Labs prototype portable 3-D ultrasound system in Bosnia (Fig. 83–5). With this unit, full 3-D ultrasound images were acquired in field hospitals (MASH) and sent back to a radiologist at Walter Reed Army Medical Center or Madigan Army Medical Center for interpretation and immediate report to the field hospital.[5] There were no radiologists in Bosnia, but the combat surgeons had access to this information. In 1998, the same system was used to transmit a 3-D image of a shoulder injury from Mount Everest Base Camp Telemedicine Clinic (17,700 ft elevation) to radiologists and surgeons at Yale University School of Medicine.

There are also new miniaturization discoveries that will allow the next generation of 3-D ultrasound to be handheld, such that physicians of the future will have both a stethoscope to hear inside the body and an ultrasound image to see inside the body. Ten years ago, Professor Hans Troidl of Cologne, Germany, stated in his presidential address to the European Association of Endoscopic Surgeons that ". . . ultrasound will be the visual stethoscope of the future." Progress is such that this is no longer a technology issue, but rather one of practicality and cost.

In addition to the new ultrasound modalities, there is emerging virtual endoscopy that uses standard, high-resolution CT and MRI scanning techniques. The virtual endoscopy is created by taking a standard helical CT scan and processing the cross-sections on the computer into full 3-D models of specific organs, such as the heart, lungs, or bronchus. Using the sophisticated terrain-tracking techniques of a military pilot, the operator can "fly through" the organ, which gives the same view as if an actual endoscopic procedure were taking place. There are numerous

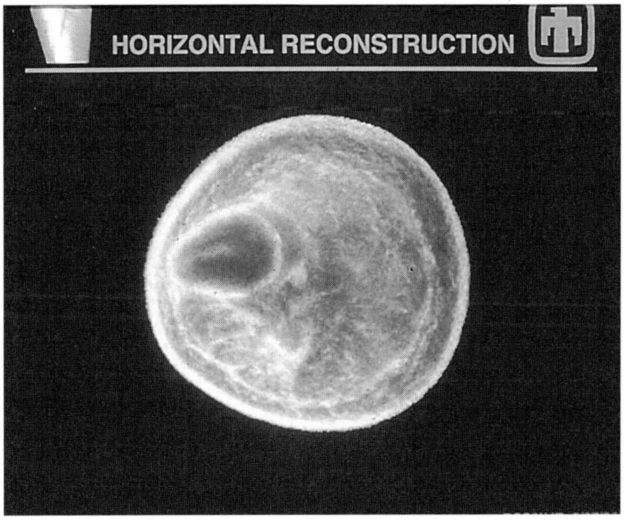

Figure 83–4. Cross-section of a three-dimensional (3-D) ultrasound image. (Courtesy of Alan Morimoto, Sandia National Labs, Albuquerque, NM.)

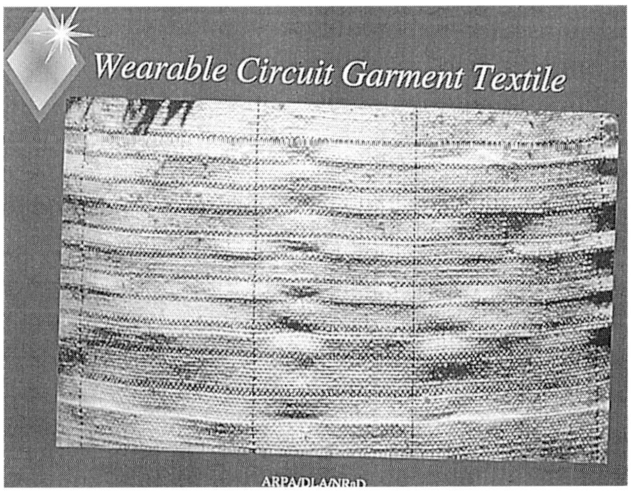

Figure 83–3. "Smart Tee Shirt" showing woven fiberoptic sensors. (Courtesy of Eric Lind, Naval Research and Development, San Diego, CA.)

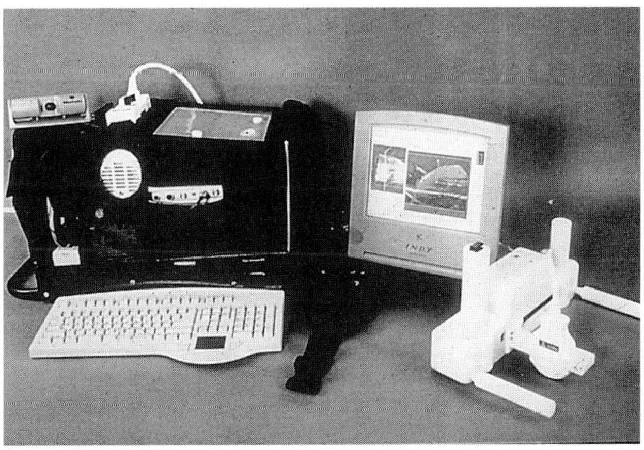

Figure 83–5. 3-D portable tele-ultrasound system. (Courtesy of Pacific Northwest National Laboratory, Richland, WA.)

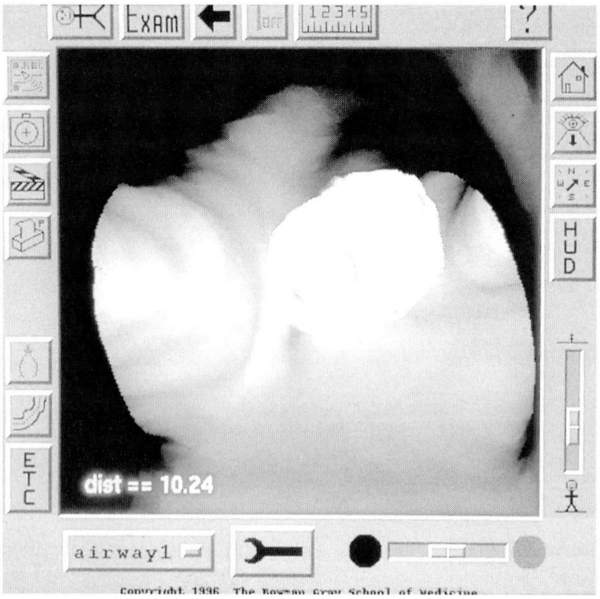

Figure 83–6. Virtual bronchoscopy showing the trachea and carina (Courtesy of Dr. David Vining, Bowman Gray Medical Center, Winston-Salem, NC.)

investigators in this field, including Sandy Napel of Stanford University, Richard Robb of Mayo Clinic, Ron Kikinis of Brigham and Women's Hospital, and Bill Lorensen of General Electric Medical Research Center. An example of virtual bronchoscopy (Fig. 83–6), provided by David Vining of Bowman-Gray Medical Center, gives a view of the trachea at the carina, and Figure 83–7 shows the same view, except that the trachea is transparent to allow visualization of the subcarinal node.[6]

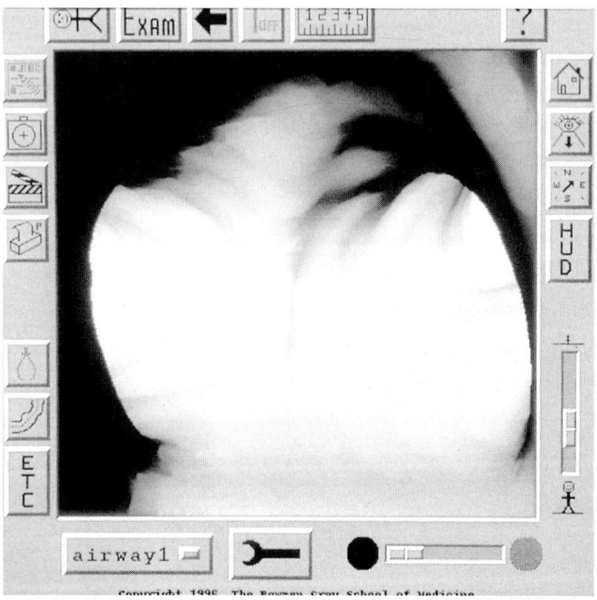

Figure 83–7. Virtual bronchoscopy showing the trachea and carina with a transparency of the wall to reveal subcarinal lymph node. (Courtesy of Dr. David Vining, Bowman Gray Medical Center, Winston-Salem, NC.)

The advantages of virtual endoscopy are not only having the opportunity to view the anatomy from many different perspectives and viewpoints, but also getting the same view without having to subject the patient to the minimal risks of bronchoscopy. Admittedly we are not able to perform biopsies or therapeutic procedures on virtual images. However, a great majority (perhaps as many as 80%) of bronchoscopic examinations are performed for screening purposes and result in a negative or normal examination. Therefore, being able to perform virtual screening procedures would dramatically reduce costs and make those procedures that are performed more cost-effective (because they will be done for known or highly suspicious lesions). Today, the images from helical CT scans have a resolution of 0.03 mm, and preliminary laboratory work has shown more than 95% accuracy for known lesions 3 mm or larger in size.[7]

Therapeutics

Along with the well-known benefits, laparoscopic surgery has imposed some significant difficulties for surgeons because of the loss of 3-D vision, dexterity, and the sense of touch. A number of systems have been devised to regain those lost qualities, using various computer-assisted, image-guided, and robotic systems. After Robodoc for hip replacement, the Green-SRI International telepresence surgery system (Figs. 83–8, 83–9)

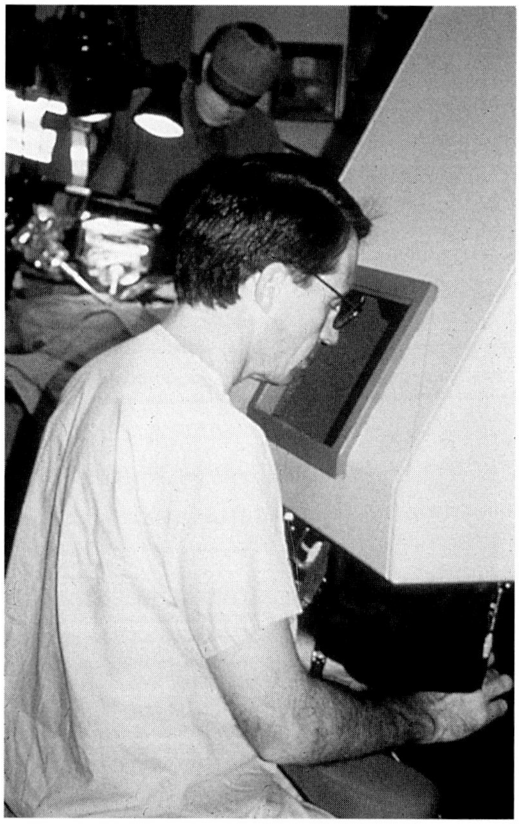

Figure 83–8. Surgeon workstation, telepresence surgery. (Courtesy of SRI International, Menlo Park, CA.)

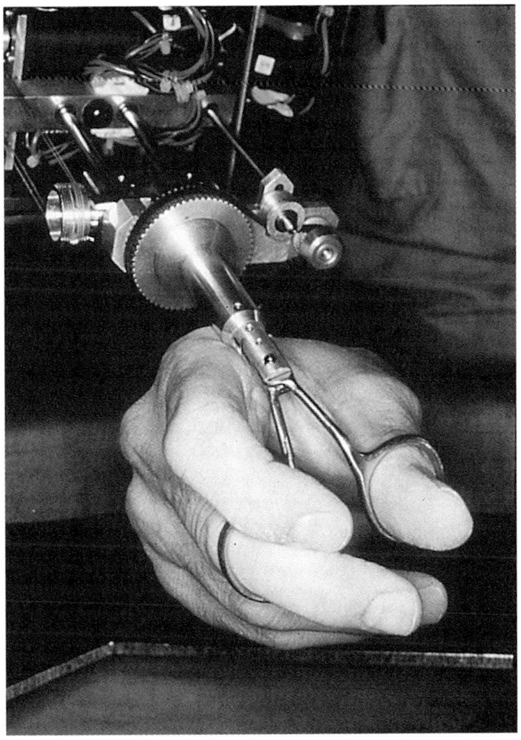

Figure 83–9. Surgical handle input device, telepresence surgery. (Courtesy of SRI International, Menlo Park, CA.)

was developed.[8] This system, like all current teleoperation systems, has been devised to increase the dexterity of the surgeon. However, it is mediated through a computer, so it automatically has the capabilities of a remote surgical system as well (Fig. 83–10). This system is currently being commercialized (by Intuitive Surgical Inc.), and human-use studies are being conducted in Belgium.

Some other systems, such as the Zeus system[9] (Computer Motion Inc.) (Fig. 83–11), the Paradex system[10] (Microdexterity Systems) (Fig. 83–12), and Ian Hunter's system at Massachusetts Institute of Technology,[11] are adding sophisticated motion tracking, tremor filtration, and scalability for dexterity enhancement. Other researchers in the laboratory, including Professor Blake Hannaford of the University of Washington,[12] are experimenting with tactile sensation added to the instruments. One of the target applications will be minimally invasive surgery upon the beating heart. The goal is to produce a system with the same or greater dexterity than the human hand via a minimally invasive approach that rules out cardiopulmonary bypass. Today, a significant part of the cost, operative time, and complications of coronary artery surgery is strictly related to placing the patient on cardiopulmonary bypass. The motion-tracking, dexterity-enhancing capabilities of these systems under development all aim to eliminate the need for cardiopulmonary bypass and thus gain the advantages previously noted.

Interestingly enough, all these systems work through a computer interface and, therefore, they inherently

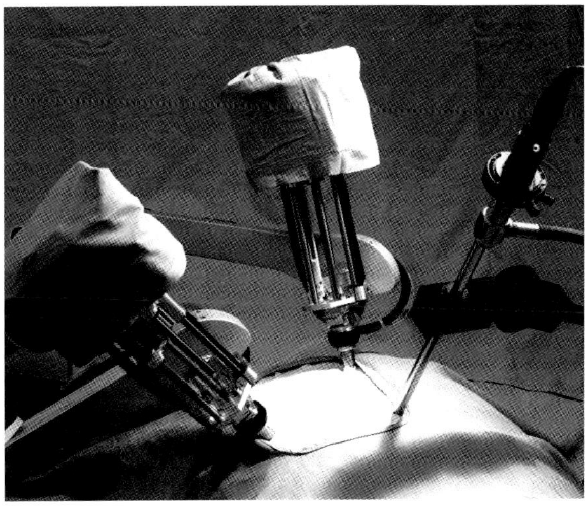

Figure 83–10. Remote manipulators, telepresence surgery. (Courtesy of SRI International, Menlo Park, CA.)

constitute a remote telepresence surgical workstation. Although the cost benefit analysis of implementing the cardiac application appears viable, there are questions of the need for remote surgery. Thus, early acceptance of these newly emerging technologies may well be seen first in the cardiovascular surgery arena, only later migrating to other areas of surgery. We must be mindful that other robotic systems have been used for neurology (stereotactic neurosurgery), urology (prostate surgery), orthopedics (hip and knee surgery), and ophthalmology (eye surgery), but they have gained less than universal acceptance. The prolonged period of clinical trials and US Food and Drug Administration (FDA) approval is currently under way and will continue until these systems will be able to merge into the mainstream of clinical surgery. The value to the average surgeon will be the chance to enhance his or her skills beyond current human limits, and the benefit to the patient will be ready access to a high quality of surgical care.

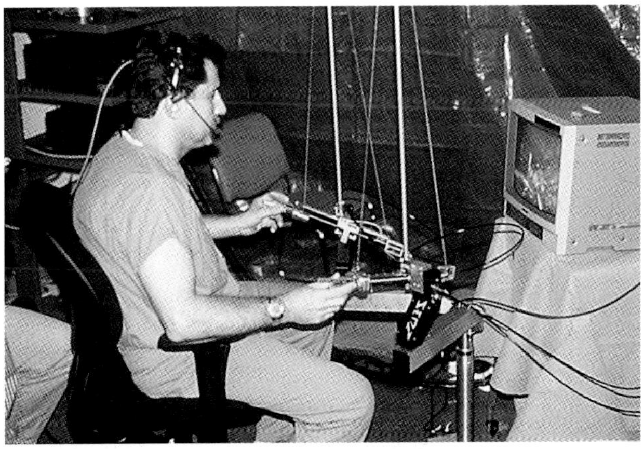

Figure 83–11. Zeus telepresence surgery system. (Courtesy of Yulun Wang, Computer Motion Inc., Goleta, CA.)

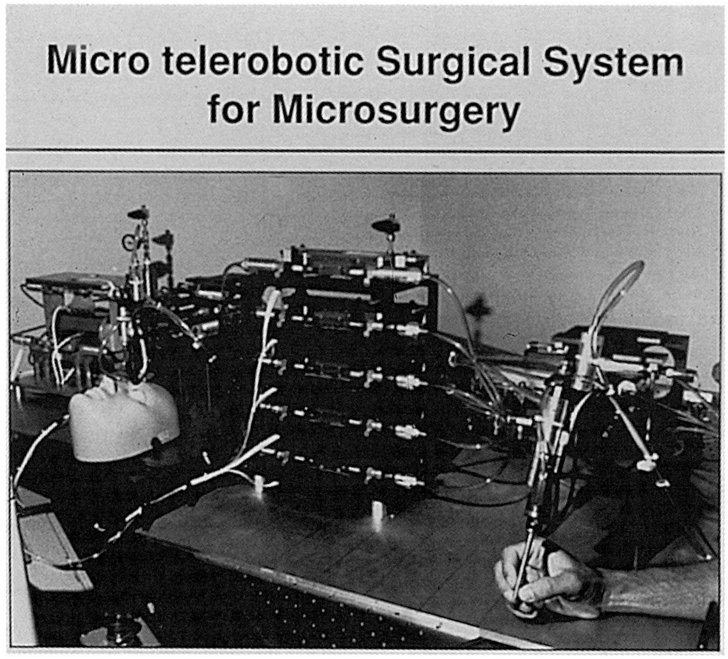

Figure 83–12. Paradex microdexterity system. (Courtesy of Steven Charles, Microdexterity Inc, Memphis, TN.)

Surgical Education

One of the advantages of telesurgical systems is that the surgeon looks into a video image rather than directly at the patient. By replacing the real-time video image with a computer model of the patient or the disease, the system automatically becomes a virtual reality surgical simulator.[13] This can be applied to an enormous number of fields, in medicine (endoscopy, radiology, angioplasty), nursing (intravenous needle placement), and surgery (many different procedures). Simulations can occur in models at many different levels, from simple graphic objects that represent various organs or tissues to highly complex environments that portray multiple systems. Basic simulators can provide instruction, such as demonstrating an intravenous needle, whereas more complex models can actually perform procedures such as angioplasty, or complete operations, such as laparoscopic cholecystectomy. However, the more complicated the environment simulated, the less realistic the images. Even with current high-performance computers, there is not enough computational power to display all the aspects needed to achieve simulation. These requirements include visual fidelity to the appearance and properties of tissues, the dynamic changes to tissues, the contact detection between surgical instruments and tissues, and the drawing of objects in real time in high-resolution full color at least 40 times per second.

Thus, all simulations are the result of tradeoffs of the above components. Will the simulator have cartoon-like organs that behave like real organs in real time, or will they be photorealistic but not have any properties (e.g., bleeding when cut, changing shape when poked), and will they be displayed on the monitor in a jerking motion at only a few frames per second? Until we have much greater computer power, we must match the educational need with the technological capability. Simulators such as the Limb Trauma Simulator (MusculoGraphics) (Fig. 83–13) or the Anastomosis Simulator[15] (Boston Dynamics Incorporated[14]) provide a training opportunity but they also serve as skills performance assessment tools. As the instrument handles of the simulator are manipulated to perform the surgical simulation, the system can also track such things as hand motions, applied pressures, and accuracy and precision of needle placement. These data can be compiled into a full analysis of individual skills for objective feedback that will enhance training, or they may even be used for credentialing.

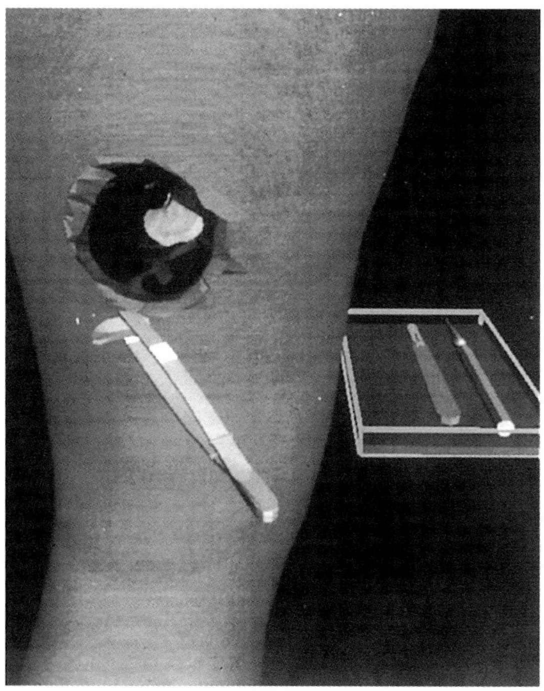

Figure 83–13. Gunshot wound of the thigh on the Leg Trauma Simulator. (Courtesy of Scott Delp, MusculoGraphics, Inc., Chicago, IL.)

Early implementations are ongoing in the areas discussed previously. They are also used to complement the current Advanced Trauma and Life Saving (ATLS) course. The key elements in all these simulators are their contributions to educational content, curriculum, and assessment rather than their technical capabilities. To improve surgical training, efforts must be focused as much upon nontechnical areas as on the simulators' capabilities.

Current Status

All the technologies discussed in this chapter are laboratory prototypes. They must be validated in clinical trials and reduced to commercial product. Moreover, FDA approval must be obtained. This is a stringent process, and some of the technologies will fail to meet the standards of clinical efficacy, cost effectiveness, and practicality. There are, however, some overall trends that will probably persist. Miniaturization of diagnostic biosensor systems will continue, with sensors embedded, so they will be wireless, nonencumbering, noninvasive, ubiquitous, and transparent to the patient. Portable or hand-held imaging devices will also be ubiquitous and embedded. Therapeutic systems will soon prove their efficacy in enhancing dexterity in surgical procedures; however, there are significant technical barriers that must be overcome for this technology to prove clinically relevant in remote surgery. Even when the technical problems are solved, the question of practical needs must be considered.

It is attractive to postulate that providing surgical expertise in remote areas through telepresence surgery will greatly improve access to health care, but the slow acceptance of telemedicine has shown that barriers in the areas of reimbursement and licensure as well as legal, social, and behavioral issues, can frequently impede, if not prevent, the implementation of what appears a priori to be a great benefit. Surgical education will begin to follow the 40-year proven record of flight simulators. As medical simulators improve in quality and are reduced in cost, their value in training, skill assessment, and, ultimately, credentialing will be apparent just as flight simulators have become the mainstays of the aviation industry on the basis of their incredible safety record. The challenge of employing virtual reality for medical simulation of the human body is in an order of magnitude far more complex than that of flight simulators, but the obstacles to success are, nonetheless, able to be surmounted.

Conclusion

What has been presented is a survey of developing medical devices and technologies that will radically alter the direction of medicine and surgery, shaping a milieu in which the information equivalent of the human body will play a central role. Many of the devices will acquire information (through sensors or imagers) to build the virtual representation. Powerful informatics tools will process information that will be relayed through therapeutic devices to produce results, such as an enhanced surgical procedure, virtual endoscopy, or an entirely new way to display information. The same images will become the centerpiece for future education.

As a word of caution, however, we must not be so enamored by the technology that we ignore the reason for these advances—the patient. There is a sacred trust embodied in the Hippocratic oath that must be the final measure of any of these concepts or devices. Every surgeon has accepted personal stewardship for the safety and interest of his or her patients, and to that end we must not rush to embrace or reject technical advances; rather, we must carefully and prudently evaluate which of these advances will yield the greatest benefit to patients.

References

1. Negroponte N: Being Digital. New York, Alfred A. Knopf, Inc., 1995, pp 11–20.
2. Spitzer V, Ackerman MJ, Scherzinger AL, et al: The visible male: A technical report. J Am Med Information Assn 3: 118–130, 1996.
3. Satava RM: Virtual reality and telepresence for military medicine. Comput Biol Med 25:229–236, 1995.
4. Lind EJ, Jayaraman S, Park S, et al: A sensate liner for biomedical monitoring applications. *In* Westwood JD, Hoffman HM, Stredney D, et al (Eds). Medicine Meets Virtual Reality. Art, Science, Technology: Healthcare Revolution. Amsterdam, IOS Press, 1998, pp 258–264.
5. Macedonia CR, Littlefield RJ, Cleman J, et al: Ultrasound telepresence: A preliminary report. J Ultrasound Med. In press, 1998.
6. Vining DN, Padhani AR, Wood S, et al: Virtual bronchoscopy: A new perspective for viewing the transbronchial tree. Radiology 189:438, 1993.
7. Napel, S: Personal communication.
8. Hill JW, Holst PA, Jesen JF, et al: Telepresence interface with applications to microsurgery and surgical simulation. *In* Westwood JD, Hoffman HM, Stredney D, et al. (Eds). Medicine Meets Virtual Reality. Art, Science, Technology: Healthcare Revolution. Amsterdam: IOS Press, 1998. pp 96–102.
9. Garcia-Ruiz A, Smedira NG, Loop FD, et al: Robotic surgical instruments for dexterity enhancement in thoracoscopic coronary artery bypass graft. Laparoendoscopic Adv Surg Tech 7:5, 1997.
10. Charles S, Das H, Ohm T, et al: Dexterity-enhanced telerobotic microsurgery. Proceedings of the Eighth International Conference on Advanced Robotics, Piscataway, NJ: IEEE Service Center, 1997, pp 5–10.
11. Hunter IW, Doukoglou TD, Lafontaine SR, et al: A teleoperated microsurgical robot and associated virtual environment for eye surgery. Presence 1:265–280, 1993.
12. Hannaford B, Trujillo J, Sinanan M, et al: Computerized endoscopic surgical grasper. *In* Westwood JD, Hoffman HM, Stredney D, et al. (Eds). Medicine Meets Virtual Reality. Art, Science, Technology: Healthcare Revolution. Amsterdam: IOS Press, 1998, pp 265–271.
13. Hill JW, Holst PA, Jesen JF, et al: Telepresence interface with applications to microsurgery and surgical simulation. *In* Westwood JD, Hoffman HM, Stredney D, Weghorst SJ (Eds): Medicine Meets Virtual Reality. Art, Science, Technology: Healthcare Revolution. Amsterdam, IOS Press, 1998, pp 96–102.
14. Playter R, Raibert M: A virtual surgery simulator using advanced haptic feedback. Min Invas Ther Allied Technol 6: 117–121, 1997.
15. Delp SL, Loan P, Cagatay B, Rosen J: Surgical simulation: An emerging technology for training in emergency medicine. Presence 6:147–159, 1997.

COMMENTARY

Ralph Damiano

The chapter by Drs. Satava and Jones provides an engaging summary of future technologies that will revolutionize surgery over the next decade. The technology of the Information Age, which has transformed our society and its industrial infrastructure, will have a similar impact on medicine. The same forces that have created the high technology business giants of Intel and Microsoft will likewise transform our medical practice. These new technologies will empower surgeons in ways not yet imaginable, allowing us not only to perform the operations we presently do more safely and with less morbidity, but also to open up a whole new range of therapeutics that has before now been considered impossible.

As the authors aptly state, "the future of medicine is no longer blood and guts but bits and bytes." Already much of our information has become digital in nature—radiography and other imaging modalities, medical records, textbooks, journals, professional communications, and the wealth of medical information available on the Internet. The information equivalent of the human body is now available as "The Visible Human." In the operating room, we have become dependent on electronic video images to display our operative fields and monitor our patients' vital signs and other physiologic data. In the next decade, computers and robots will be introduced into the operating room and will even transform our actual manual operative techniques. This should not only enhance surgical dexterity, but also allow us to perform very complicated operations in a minimally invasive manner.

Our entire operating room may soon be controlled by computers, empowering the surgeon to have all the equipment in the operating room (e.g., monitors, lights, table, electrocautery, suction devices, cameras, video monitors) under his or her direct control and eventually to provide direct access on video monitors to imaging studies, the medical record, and the Internet. The same technology will have a dramatic impact on surgical education, allowing us to train our residents on virtual reality simulators, enhancing not only the educational process but also patient safety.

As one of the most sophisticated and expensive specialties, cardiothoracic surgery will be one of the first areas to see the impact of these new technologies. The high cost of cardiothoracic surgery will make the use of advanced computer and robotic technology easy to justify, particularly if it can be employed to develop minimally invasive approaches that will decrease length of postoperative stay and morbidity. Robotically assisted endoscopic coronary bypass grafting is already a reality in the animal laboratory. The day is not far off when we will be able to perform endoscopic cardiothoracic surgery. If this can significantly improve results and the quality of care without escalating costs, this technology will certainly be embraced by our community.

While we are undoubtedly on the cusp of an exciting new era in surgery, we must remember, as Drs. Satava and Jones so aptly conclude, "we must not be so enamored by the technology that we ignore the reason for these advances—the patient." As we enter the Medical Information Age, it is our professional responsibility to our patients to evaluate each advance carefully and rationally and judge it not by its technologic ingenuity but by its medical benefit. We must also possess the courage and strength to be able to reinvent ourselves and our specialty continually in what will certainly be a time of rapid evolution of new technology and techniques. We are all in for an exciting ride that will profoundly change the world of surgery over the next decade.

INDEX

Note: Page numbers in *italics* refer to illustrations; page numbers followed by t refer to tables.

C

D

E

N

O

S

ISBN 0-7216-7723-1